KT-436-856

NURSING RESEARCH
Generating and Assessing Evidence for Nursing Practice

Eleventh Edition

Denise F. Polit, PhD, FAAN
President
Humanalysis, Inc.
Saratoga Springs, New York, and
Adjunct Professor
Griffith University School of Nursing
Brisbane, Australia
(www.denisepolit.com)

Cheryl Tatano Beck, DNSc, CNM, FAAN
Distinguished Professor
School of Nursing
University of Connecticut
Storrs, Connecticut

. Wolters Kluwer

Philadelphia · Baltimore · New York · London
Buenos Aires · Hong Kong · Sydney · Tokyo

Not authorised for sale in United States, Canada, Australia, New Zealand, Puerto Rico, and U.S. Virgin Islands.

Vice President and Publisher: Julie K. Stegman
Director of Nursing Content Publishing: Renee Gagliardi
Acquisitions Editor: Mark Foss
Director of Product Development: Jennifer K. Forestieri
Senior Development Editor: Meredith L. Brittain
Editorial Coordinator: David Murphy
Marketing Manager: Brittany Clements
Editorial Assistant: Molly Kennedy
Design Coordinator: Stephen Druding
Art Director, Illustration: Jennifer Clements
Production Project Manager: Barton Dudlick
Manufacturing Coordinator: Karin Duffield
Prepress Vendor: TNQ Technologies

Eleventh Edition

Copyright © 2021 Wolters Kluwer.

Copyright © 2017 Wolters Kluwer. Copyright © 2012 Wolters Kluwer Health | Lippincott Williams & Wilkins. Copyright © 2008, 2004, 1999 by Lippincott Williams & Wilkins. Copyright © 1995, 1991, 1987, 1983, 1978 by J. B. Lippincott Company.

All rights reserved. This book is protected by copyright. No part of this book may be reproduced or transmitted in any form or by any means, including as photocopies or scanned-in or other electronic copies, or utilized by any information storage and retrieval system without written permission from the copyright owner, except for brief quotations embodied in critical articles and reviews. Materials appearing in this book prepared by individuals as part of their official duties as US government employees are not covered by the abovementioned copyright. To request permission, please contact Wolters Kluwer at Two Commerce Square, 2001 Market Street, Philadelphia, PA 19103, via email at permissions@lww.com, or via our website at shop.lww.com (products and services).

9 8 7 6 5 4 3 2 1

Printed in China

Library of Congress Cataloging-in-Publication Data

ISBN-13: 978-1-975110-64-2

Cataloging in Publication data available on request from publisher.

This work is provided "as is," and the publisher disclaims any and all warranties, express or implied, including any warranties as to accuracy, comprehensiveness, or currency of the content of this work.

This work is no substitute for individual patient assessment based upon healthcare professionals' examination of each patient and consideration of, among other things, age, weight, gender, current or prior medical conditions, medication history, laboratory data, and other factors unique to the patient. The publisher does not provide medical advice or guidance, and this work is merely a reference tool. Healthcare professionals, and not the publisher, are solely responsible for the use of this work including all medical judgments and for any resulting diagnosis and treatments.

Given continuous, rapid advances in medical science and health information, independent professional verification of medical diagnoses, indications, appropriate pharmaceutical selections and dosages, and treatment options should be made, and healthcare professionals should consult a variety of sources. When prescribing medication, healthcare professionals are advised to consult the product information sheet (the manufacturer's package insert) accompanying each drug to verify, among other things, conditions of use, warnings, and side effects and identify any changes in dosage schedule or contraindications, particularly if the medication to be administered is new, infrequently used, or has a narrow therapeutic range. To the maximum extent permitted under applicable law, no responsibility is assumed by the publisher for any injury and/or damage to persons or property, as a matter of products liability, negligence law or otherwise, or from any reference to or use by any person of this work.

shop.lww.com

RRS1911

TO

The memory of Denise's husband:

Alan A. Janosy, 1943-2019

Acknowledgments

This 11th edition, like the previous 10 editions, depended on the contributions of dozens of people. Many faculty and students who used the text have made invaluable suggestions for its improvement, and to all of you we are very grateful. In addition to all those who assisted us during the past 40 years with the earlier editions, the following individuals deserve special mention.

We would like to acknowledge the comments of reviewers of the previous edition of this book, anonymous to us initially, whose feedback influenced our revisions. Faculty at Griffith University in Australia made useful suggestions and inspired the inclusion of some new content. Valori Banfi, reference librarian at the University of Connecticut, provided ongoing assistance. Dr. Carrie Morgan Eaton at the University of Connecticut provided regular feedback. Dr. Deborah Dillon McDonald and Dr. Xiaomei Cong were extraordinarily generous in giving us access to NINR grant application material for the *Resource Manual*.

We also extend our thanks to those who helped to turn the manuscript into a finished product. The staff at Wolters Kluwer has been of great assistance to us over the years. We are indebted to Mark Foss, Meredith Brittain, David Murphy, Brittany Clements, Barton Dudlick, and all the others behind the scenes for their fine contributions.

Finally, we thank our family and friends. Our husbands Alan and Chuck have become accustomed to our demanding schedules, but we recognize that their support involves a lot of patience and many sacrifices.

Reviewers

Kelley M. Anderson, PhD, FNP, CHFN-K
Associate Professor
Department of Professional Nursing Practice
Georgetown University
Washington, District of Columbia

Debra Bacharz, PhD, MSN, RN
Professor of Nursing, Leach College of Nursing
University of St. Francis
Joliet, Illinois

Kimberly Balko, PhD, RN
Assistant Professor
Department of Nursing
SUNY Empire State College
Saratoga Springs, New York

Susan A. Bonis, PhD, RN
Assistant Clinical Professor
College of Nursing
University of Wisconsin—Milwaukee
Milwaukee, Wisconsin

Barbara Brewer, PhD, RN, MALS, MBA
Associate Professor
College of Nursing
The University of Arizona
Tucson, Arizona

Kathleen A. Fagan, PhD, RN, APN
Associate Professor
Graduate Nursing
School of Nursing
Felician University
Lodi, New Jersey

Tracia Forman, PhD, RN-BC, CNE
Assistant Professor
Department of Nursing
University of Texas Rio Grande Valley
Brownsville, Texas

LaDawna R. Goering, DNP, APN, ANP-BC
Assistant Professor
Department of Nursing
Northern Illinois University
DeKalb, Illinois

Rebecca W. Grizzle, PhD, RN, MSN, NP-C
Clinical Assistant Professor
College of Nursing
Sacred Heart University
Fairfield, Connecticut

Ashlyn Johnson, DNP, FNP-BC
Assistant Professor of Nursing
MSN Program (FNP & PMHNP Tracks)
Mount Marty College
Yankton, South Dakota

Kara Misto, PhD, RN
Assistant Professor
School of Nursing
Rhode Island College
Providence, Rhode Island

Stephen J. Stapleton, PhD, MS, RN, CEN, FAEN
Associate Professor
Mennonite College of Nursing
Illinois State University
Normal, Illinois

Debbie Stayer, PhD, RN-BC, CCRN-K
Assistant Professor
Department of Nursing
Bloomsburg University
Bloomsburg, Pennsylvania

Kathleen Thompson, PhD, RN, CNE
Clinical Professor
Department of Nursing
University of Tennessee, Knoxville
Knoxville, Tennessee

Ann Tritak, EdD, RN
Associate Dean
Department of Graduate Nursing
Felician University
Lodi, New Jersey

Shelly Wells, PhD, MBA, MS, APRN-CNS
Division Chair and Professor
Division of Nursing
Northwestern Oklahoma State University
Alva, Oklahoma

Kelli D. Whittington, PhD, RN, CNE
Chair, Division of Nursing
McKendree University
Lebanon, Illinois

Preface

Research methodology is a dynamic enterprise. Even after writing 10 editions of this book, we have continued to draw new material and inspiration from ground-breaking advances in research methods and in nurse researchers' use of those methods. It is thrilling to share many of those developments in this new edition. We expect that many of the new methodologic and technological enhancements will be translated into powerful evidence for nursing practice. Four years ago, we considered the 10th edition as a watershed edition of a classic textbook, having added two new chapters. We are persuaded, however, that this 11th edition is even better than the previous one. We have retained many features that made this book a classic textbook and resource, including its focus on research as a support for evidence-based nursing, but have introduced important innovations that we hope will help to shape the future of nursing research.

NEW TO THIS EDITION

New Chapters

We are excited to have added two new chapters to this edition. The first new chapter (Chapter 12) focuses on quality improvement and improvement science. Quality improvement (QI) has not historically been considered "research" because knowledge from QI has been deemed too localized to be of broad interest. Yet, QI initiatives undertaken by interprofessional teams often yield important lessons for healthcare professionals in diverse settings. In the new chapter, we discuss methods and frameworks that can be used to develop and assess improvement projects.

We are particularly enthusiastic about our second new chapter, which concerns the applicability, generalizability, and relevance of research evidence (Chapter 31). There is growing awareness that approaches being used to support evidence-based practice (EBP) have limitations in terms of their *applicability* to individual patients or subgroups of patients. EBP efforts prioritize rigorous evidence from tightly controlled studies with select populations that often exclude many patients typically seen in real-world settings. Moreover, evidence for EBP usually represents *average effects* for these atypical populations. Our new chapter describes a range of cutting-edge strategies for generating *practice-based evidence* that is patient-centered. We discuss such approaches as comparative effectiveness research, pragmatic clinical trials, adaptive interventions, SMART designs, subgroup (moderator) analyses, and multivariable risk-stratified analyses for better understanding the diversity of treatment effects. This chapter is consistent with the emerging interest in *precision healthcare*.

Extensively Revised Chapters

We have made major revisions to two chapters in this book. We have revamped Chapter 2, the chapter on evidence-based practice, to better guide efficient evidence searches (e.g., via the 6S hierarchy of preappraised evidence) and for ranking evidence on traditional level-of-evidence (LOE) scales. We have also extensively revised another chapter that has relevance for EBP: the chapter on systematic reviews (Chapter 30). The types of reviews being undertaken, and the methods used to conduct them, have expanded considerably in recent years. We describe in some detail the GRADE system for assessing the degree of *confidence* a review team has in the estimated effects of an intervention on key outcomes. We also describe differences in two broad approaches to qualitative syntheses, distinguishing interpretive approaches (metasyntheses) from aggregative approaches using meta-aggregation.

New and Added Content

Throughout the book, we have included material on methodologic innovations that have arisen in nursing, medicine, and the social sciences during the past 4 to 5 years. The many additions and changes are too numerous to describe here. One deserves special mention, however: we have revised the chapter on qualitative data analysis (Chapter 25) to provide greater support for the actual tasks of coding and categorizing data.

The inclusion of two new chapters and the expansion of others made it challenging to keep the textbook to a manageable length. Our solution was to include some content in supplements that are available online. Every chapter has an online supplement (and some chapters in this edition have two supplements), which gave us the opportunity to add a considerable amount of new material. For example, one new supplement is devoted to the conduct of plausibility analyses as a tool for strengthening internal validity in nonrandomized intervention studies. Other supplements include a description of various randomization methods such as urn randomization, an overview of item response theory, and a description of statistical process control.

Here is a complete list of the supplements for the 33 chapters of the textbook:

1. The History of Nursing Research
2. A. Evaluating Clinical Practice Guidelines— AGREE II
   B. Evidence-Based Practice in an Organizational Context
3. Deductive and Inductive Reasoning
4. Complex Relationships and Hypotheses
5. A. Finding Evidence for a Clinical Query
   B. Literature Review Summary Tables
6. Prominent Conceptual Models of Nursing Used by Nurse Researchers, and a Guide to Middle-Range Theories
7. Historical Background on Unethical Research Conduct
8. Research Control
9. Randomization Strategies
10. A. Selected Experimental and Quasi-Experimental Designs: Diagrams, Uses, and Drawbacks/Validity Threats
    B. Plausibility Assessments and Other Strategies When Randomization is Not Possible
11. Other Specific Types of Research
12. Statistical Process Control
13. Sample Recruitment and Retention
14. Other Types of Structured Self-Reports
15. Cross-Cultural Validity and the Adaptation/ Translation of Measures
16. Overview of Item Response Theory
17. SPSS Analysis of Descriptive Statistics
18. SPSS Analysis of Inferential Statistics
19. SPSS Analysis and Multivariate Statistics
20. Some Preliminary Steps in Quantitative Analysis Using SPSS
21. Clinical Significance Assessment with the Jacobson–Truax Approach
22. Historical Nursing Research and Other Types of Qualitative Inquiry
23. Models of Generalizability in Qualitative Research
24. Additional Types of Unstructured Self-Reports
25. Transcribing Qualitative Data
26. Whittemore and Colleagues' Framework of Quality Criteria in Qualitative Research
27. Transforming Quantitative and Qualitative Data
28. Complex Intervention Development: Additional Resources
29. Examples of Various Pilot and Feasibility Objectives
30. A. Publication Bias in Systematic Reviews
    B. Supplementary Resources for Qualitative Evidence Synthesis
31. The RE-AIM Framework

32. A. Tips for Publishing Reports on Pilot Intervention Studies
    B. Impact Factor and Publication Information for Selected Nursing Journals
33. Proposals for Pilot Intervention Studies

Another feature of this edition concerns readers' access to references we cited. To the extent possible, the studies we have chosen as examples of research methods are published as open-access articles. These studies are identified in the reference list at the end of each chapter, and a link to the articles is included in the accompanying *Resource Manual for Nursing Research,* 11th Edition (available for separate purchase) in the online Toolkit (for more information, see the section "A Comprehensive Package for Teaching and Learning" later in this preface.) In addition, one Wolters Kluwer article per chapter that is available on the book's companion website is also identified in each chapter's reference list.

We hope that our many revisions will help users of this book to maximize their learning experience.

ORGANIZATION OF THE TEXT

The content of this edition is organized into six main parts.

- **Part 1—Foundations of Nursing Research and Evidence-Based Practice** introduces fundamental concepts in nursing research. Chapter 1 briefly summarizes the history and future of nursing research, discusses the philosophical underpinnings of qualitative research versus quantitative research, and describes major purposes of nursing research. Chapter 2, extensively revised, offers guidance on using research to support evidence-based practice. Chapter 3 introduces readers to key research terms and presents an overview of steps in the research process for both qualitative and quantitative studies.
- **Part 2—Conceptualizing and Planning a Study to Generate Evidence for Nursing** further sets the stage for learning about the research process by discussing issues relating to a study's conceptualization: the formulation of research questions and hypotheses (Chapter 4), the review of relevant research (Chapter 5), the development of theoretical and conceptual contexts (Chapter 6), and the fostering of ethically acceptable approaches in doing research (Chapter 7). Chapter 8 provides an overview of important issues that researchers must attend to during the planning of any study.
- **Part 3—Designing and Conducting Quantitative Studies to Generate Evidence for Nursing** presents material on undertaking quantitative nursing studies. Chapter 9 describes fundamental principles of quantitative research design, and Chapter 10 focuses on methods to enhance the rigor of a quantitative study, including mechanisms of research control. Chapter 11 examines research with different and distinct purposes, such as noninferiority trials, realist evaluations, surveys, and outcomes research. Chapter 12, a new chapter in this edition, is devoted to methods used in quality improvement and improvement science. Chapter 13 presents strategies for sampling study participants in quantitative research. Chapter 14 describes structured data collection methods that yield quantitative information. Chapter 15 discusses the concept of measurement and then focuses on methods of assessing the quality of formal measuring instruments. In this edition, we describe methods to assess the properties of point-in-time measurements (reliability and validity) and longitudinal measurements—i.e., change scores (reliability of change scores and responsiveness). Chapter 16 presents material on how to develop high-quality self-report instruments. Chapters 17, 18, and 19 present an overview of univariate, bivariate, and multivariate statistical analyses, respectively. Chapter 20 describes the development of an overall analytic strategy for quantitative studies, including material on handling missing data. Chapter 21, a chapter that was added in the 10th edition, discusses the issue of interpreting results and making inferences about clinical significance.
- **Part 4—Designing and Conducting Qualitative Studies to Generate Evidence for Nursing** presents material on undertaking qualitative nursing

studies. Chapter 22 is devoted to research designs and approaches for qualitative studies, including information on critical theory, feminist, and participatory action research. Chapter 23 discusses strategies for sampling study participants in qualitative inquiries. Chapter 24 describes methods of gathering unstructured self-report and observational data for qualitative studies. Chapter 25 discusses methods of analyzing qualitative data, with specific information on grounded theory, phenomenologic, and ethnographic analyses. Greater guidance on coding qualitative data has been added to this edition. Chapter 26 elaborates on methods qualitative researchers can use to enhance (and assess) integrity and trustworthiness throughout their inquiries.

- **Part 5—Designing and Conducting Mixed Methods Studies to Generate Evidence for Nursing** presents material on mixed methods nursing studies. Chapter 27 discusses a broad range of issues, including asking mixed methods questions, designing a study to address the questions, sampling participants in mixed methods research, and analyzing and integrating qualitative and quantitative data. Chapter 28 presents information about using mixed methods approaches in the development of complex nursing interventions. In Chapter 29, a chapter that was new in the 10th edition, we provide suggestions for designing and conducting pilot studies and using data from the pilots to make decisions about "next steps."

- **Part 6—Building an Evidence Base for Nursing Practice** provides additional information on linking research and clinical practice. Chapter 30 offers an overview of methods of conducting systematic reviews that support EBP. In this greatly expanded chapter in this edition, we provide guidance on conducting meta-analyses (and an evaluation of confidence in the evidence using the GRADE system), meta-syntheses, qualitative evidence syntheses using meta-aggregation, and mixed studies reviews. Chapter 31, a new chapter in this edition, offers cutting-edge advice on strategies to enhance the *applicability* of practice-based evidence

to clinical decisions for individuals and sub-groups. Chapter 32 discusses the dissemination of evidence—how to prepare a research report (including theses and dissertations) and how to publish research findings. The concluding chapter (Chapter 33) offers suggestions and guidelines on developing research proposals and obtaining financial support; it includes information about applying for NIH grants and interpreting scores from NIH's scoring system.

KEY FEATURES

This textbook was designed to be helpful to those who are learning how to do research, as well as to those who are learning to appraise research reports critically and to use research findings in practice. Many of the features successfully used in previous editions have been retained in this 11th edition. Among the basic principles that helped to shape this and earlier editions of this book are (1) an unswerving conviction that the development of research skills is critical to the nursing profession, (2) a fundamental belief that research is intellectually and professionally rewarding, and (3) a steadfast opinion that learning about research methods does not need to be intimidating nor dull. Consistent with these principles, we have tried to present the fundamentals of research methods in a way that both facilitates understanding and arouses curiosity and interest. Key features of our approach include the following:

- **Research examples.** Each chapter concludes with one or two actual research examples designed to highlight methodologic features described in the chapter and to sharpen the reader's critical thinking skills. In addition, many research examples are used throughout the book to illustrate key points and to stimulate ideas for a study. Many examples used in this edition are published as open-access articles that can be used for further learning and classroom discussion.

- **Specific practical tips on doing research.** The textbook is filled with practical suggestions on how to translate the abstract notions of research methods into realistic strategies for conducting research. Every chapter includes several tips for applying the chapter's lessons to real-life situations. These tips are an acknowledgment that there is often a gap between what gets taught in research methods textbooks and what a researcher needs to know to conduct a study.

- **Critical appraisal guidelines.** Almost all chapters include guidelines for conducting a critical appraisal of various aspects of a research report.
- **A comprehensive index.** We have crafted an exceptionally thorough index. We know that our book is used as a reference book as well as a textbook, and we recognize how crucial it is to access needed information efficiently.
- **Aids to student learning.** This book includes several additional features designed to enhance and reinforce learning, including the following: succinct, bulleted summaries at the end of each chapter; tables and figures that provide examples and graphic materials in support of the text discussion; and a detailed glossary.
- **Clear, user-friendly style.** Our writing style is designed to be easily digestible and nonintimidating. Concepts are introduced carefully and systematically, difficult ideas are presented clearly, and readers are assumed to have no prior exposure to technical terms.

A COMPREHENSIVE PACKAGE FOR TEACHING AND LEARNING

To further facilitate teaching and learning, a carefully designed ancillary package has been developed to assist faculty and students.

Resources for Instructors

Tools to assist you with teaching your course are available upon adoption of this text at http://thepoint.lww.com/Polit11e.

- An **e-Book** gives you access to the book's full text and images online.

- The **Test Generator** lets you put together exclusive new tests from a bank containing more than 790 questions to help you in assessing your students' understanding of the material.
- **PowerPoint Presentations** summarizing key points in each chapter provide an easy way for you to integrate the textbook with your students' classroom experience, either via slide shows or handouts. Multiple-choice and true/false questions are integrated into the presentations to promote class participation and allow you to use i-clicker technology.
- An **Image Bank** of all the images in the book allows you to use these illustrations in your PowerPoint slides or as you see fit in your course.
- Other helpful resources include **Answers to Application Exercises** (the exercises are found in the student resources) and **Strategies for Effective Teaching.**

Contact your sales representative for more details and ordering information.

Resources for Students

An exciting set of free resources is available to help students review material and become even more familiar with vital concepts. Students can access all these resources at http://thepoint.lww.com/Polit11e using the codes printed in the front of their textbooks.

- **Chapter supplements** include material to enhance the content of each chapter (the full list of these supplements is included earlier in this preface).
- **Application Exercises** test methodologic skills with short-answer and essay questions related to research studies.
- **Journal Articles** offer access to current research available in Wolters Kluwer journals.
- A **Spanish–English Audio Glossary** provides helpful terms and phrases for communicating with patients who speak Spanish.
- A description of **Nursing Professional Roles and Responsibilities** provides information about these functions.

Resource Manual for Nursing Research, 11th Edition

Available for separate purchase, **Resource Manual for Nursing Research, 11th Edition** augments the textbook in important ways. The manual itself provides students with exercises that correspond to each text chapter, with opportunities to carefully glean information from and critically appraise actual studies. The appendices include 13 research journal articles in their entirety, plus portions of two successful grant applications for studies funded by the National Institute of Nursing Research. The 13 reports cover a range of nursing inquiries, including qualitative, quantitative, and mixed methods studies, an instrument development study, an evidence-based practice project, a quality improvement project, and two systematic reviews. Full critiques of two of the reports are also included and can serve as models for a comprehensive critical appraisal.

- **The online Toolkit to the *Resource Manual*** is a "must have" innovation that will save considerable time for both students and seasoned researchers. Included on the manual's companion webpage, the Toolkit offers dozens of research resources in Word documents that can be downloaded and used or adapted in research projects. The resources reflect best-practice research material, most of which has been pretested and refined in our own research. The Toolkit originated with our realization that in our technologically advanced environment, it is possible to not only *illustrate* methodologic tools as graphics in the textbook but also to make them directly available for use and adaptation. Thus, we have included dozens of documents in Word format that can readily be used in research projects, without requiring researchers to "reinvent the wheel" or tediously retype material from the textbook. Examples include informed consent forms, a demographic questionnaire, content validity forms, templates for statistical tables, and a coding sheet for a meta-analysis—to name only a few. The Toolkit also lists relevant and useful websites for each chapter, which can be "clicked" on directly without having to retype the URL and risk a typographical error. Links to open-access articles cited in the textbook, as well as other open-access articles relevant to each chapter, are included in the Toolkit.

A COMPREHENSIVE, DIGITAL, INTEGRATED COURSE SOLUTION: *LIPPINCOTT® COURSEPOINT*

The same trusted solution, innovation and unmatched support that you have come to expect from *Lippincott CoursePoint* is now enhanced with more engaging learning tools and deeper analytics to help prepare students for practice. This powerfully integrated, digital learning solution combines learning tools, case studies, real-time data, and the most trusted nursing education content on the market to make curriculum-wide learning more efficient and to meet students where they are at in their learning. And now, it is easier than ever for instructors and students to use, giving them everything they need for course and curriculum success!

Lippincott CoursePoint includes:

- Engaging course content provides a variety of learning tools to engage students of all learning styles.
- A more personalized learning approach gives students the content and tools they need at the moment they need it, giving them data for more focused remediation and helping to boost their confidence and competence.
- Powerful tools, including varying levels of case studies, interactive learning activities, and adaptive learning powered by PrepU, help students learn the critical thinking and clinical judgment skills to help them become practice-ready nurses.

- Unparalleled reporting provides in-depth dashboards with several data points to track student progress and help identify strengths and weaknesses.
- Unmatched support includes training coaches, product trainers, and nursing education consultants to help educators and students implement CoursePoint with ease.

It is our hope that the content, style, and organization of *Nursing Research,* 11th Edition continue to meet the needs of a broad spectrum of nursing students and nurse researchers. We also hope that the book will help to foster enthusiasm for the kinds of discoveries that research can produce and for the knowledge that will help support an evidence-based nursing practice.

DENISE F. POLIT, PhD, FAAN

CHERYL TATANO BECK, DNSC, CNM, FAAN

Table of Contents

Part 1

FOUNDATIONS OF NURSING RESEARCH AND EVIDENCE-BASED PRACTICE

Introduction to Nursing Research in an Evidence-Based Practice Environment

NURSING RESEARCH IN PERSPECTIVE

In all parts of the world, nursing has experienced a profound culture change. Nurses are increasingly expected to understand and conduct research, and to base their professional practice, in part, on research evidence—that is, to adopt an **evidence-based practice (EBP)**. EBP involves using the best evidence (as well as clinical judgment and patient preferences and circumstances) in making patient care decisions, and "best evidence" typically comes from research conducted by nurses and other healthcare professionals.

What is Nursing Research?

Research is systematic inquiry that relies on disciplined methods to answer questions or solve problems. Nurses are increasingly engaged in disciplined studies that benefit nursing and its clients. **Nursing research** is systematic inquiry designed to generate evidence about issues of importance to the nursing profession, including nursing practice, education, administration, and informatics. In this book, we emphasize **clinical nursing research** aimed at guiding nursing practice and improving the health and quality of life of nurses' clients.

Nursing research has experienced remarkable growth in the past few decades, providing nurses with a growing evidence base from which to practice. Yet many questions persist, and mechanisms for incorporating research innovations into nursing practice still are in development.

Examples of Nursing Research Questions:
- How effective is a web-based intervention in improving parent-adolescent communication about sexuality and sexual health? (Varas-Díaz et al., 2019)
- What are the experiences of college students who are newly diagnosed with type 1 diabetes mellitus? (Saylor et al., 2019)

The Importance of Research in Nursing

Findings from rigorous research provide evidence for informing nurses' decisions. Nurses have come to accept the desirability of incorporating research evidence into their actions, if the evidence shows that the actions are clinically appropriate and result in positive patient outcomes.

In some countries, research plays an important role in nursing credentialing and status. For example, the American Nurses Credentialing Center—an arm of the American Nurses Association and a prestigious credentialing organization in the United States—developed a Magnet Recognition Program to acknowledge healthcare organizations that provide high-quality nursing care. The 2019 Magnet application manual incorporates revisions that strengthen evidence-based requirements (Graystone, 2017). Indeed, applicants must now submit at least three nursing studies, indicating that Magnet hospitals must not only be involved in EBP but also in the creation of new practice knowledge. The good news is that there is growing evidence that the focus on research and EBP may have important payoffs. For example, Barnes and coresearchers (2016) found that Magnet hospitals had lower rates of central line–associated bloodstream infection than non-Magnet hospitals, even when differences in other hospital characteristics were taken into account. And McCaughey et al. (2019) found that patients treated at a Magnet hospital were more satisfied with their care than patients in non-Magnet hospitals.

Changes to nursing practice now occur regularly because of EBP efforts. Practice changes often are local initiatives that are not publicized, but broader clinical changes are also occurring based on accumulating research evidence about beneficial practice innovations.

Example of Evidence-Based Practice:

"Kangaroo care" (the holding of diaper-clad infants skin-to-skin by parents) is now routinely practiced in neonatal intensive care units (NICUs), but before 2000, only a minority of NICUs offered kangaroo care options. Expanded adoption of this practice reflects mounting evidence that early skin-to-skin contact has benefits without negative side effects (e.g., Johnston et al., 2017; Moore et al., 2016). Some of that evidence came from rigorous studies conducted by nurse researchers (e.g., Bastani et al., 2017; Billner-Garcia et al., 2018; Cho et al., 2016).

The Consumer–Producer Continuum in Nursing Research

Most nurses are likely to engage in research activities along a continuum of participation. At one end are *consumers of nursing research*, who read research reports or research summaries to keep up-to-date on findings that might affect their practice. EBP depends on well-informed research consumers.

At the other end of the continuum are *producers of nursing research*: nurses who conduct research. At one time, most nurse researchers were academics who taught in nursing schools, but research is increasingly being conducted by clinical nurses who seek solutions to recurring problems in patient care.

Between these end points on the continuum lie a variety of research activities that are undertaken by nurses. Even if you never personally carry out a study, you may (1) contribute to an idea for a clinical study; (2) gather information for a study; (3) advise clients about participating in research; (4) seek answers to a clinical problem by searching for and appraising research evidence; or (5) discuss the implications of a study in a **journal club** in your practice setting, which involves meetings (in groups or online) to discuss research articles. Understanding research can improve the depth and breadth of every nurse's professional practice.

TIP The Cochrane Collaboration, an important organization for EBP, offers an online journal club resource with podcasts, slides, and discussion questions (http://www.cochranejournalclub.com). Journal clubs can help to create an environment of lifelong learning and can foster a commitment to EBP (Gardner et al., 2016). Links to some articles about journal clubs are provided in the Toolkit in the accompanying *Resource Manual*.

Nursing Research in Historical Perspective

Table 1.1 summarizes some of the key events in the historical evolution of nursing research. An expanded summary of the history of nursing research appears in the Supplement to this chapter on thePoint. 🅢

Most people would agree that research in nursing began with Florence Nightingale in the 1850s. Her most well-known research contribution involved an analysis of factors affecting soldier mortality and morbidity during the Crimean War. Based on skillful analyses, she was successful in effecting changes in nursing care—and, more generally, in public health. After Nightingale's work, research was absent from the nursing literature until the early 1900s, but most early studies concerned nurses' education rather than patient care.

TABLE 1.1 • Historical Landmarks in Nursing Research

YEAR	EVENT
1859	Nightingale's *Notes on Nursing* is published.
1900	*American Journal of Nursing* begins publication.
1923	Columbia University establishes first doctoral program for nurses.
	Goldmark Report with recommendations for nursing education is published.
1936	Sigma Theta Tau awards first nursing research grant in the United States.
1948	Brown publishes report on inadequacies of nursing education.
1952	The journal *Nursing Research* begins publication.
1955	Inception of the American Nurses' Foundation to sponsor nursing research.
1957	Establishment of nursing research center at Walter Reed Army Institute of Research.
1963	*International Journal of Nursing Studies* begins publication.
1965	American Nurses' Association (ANA) sponsors nursing research conferences.
1969	*Canadian Journal of Nursing Research* begins publication.
1972	ANA establishes a Commission on Research and Council of Nurse Researchers.
1976	Stetler and Marram publish guidelines on assessing research for use in practice.
	Journal of Advanced Nursing begins publication.
1982	Conduct and Utilization of Research in Nursing (CURN) project publishes report.
1983	*Annual Review of Nursing* Research begins publication.
1985	ANA Cabinet on Nursing Research establishes research priorities.
1986	National Center for Nursing Research (NCNR) is established within U.S. National Institutes of Health.
1988	Conference on Research Priorities is convened by NCNR.
1989	The U.S. Agency for Health Care Policy and Research (AHCPR) is established.
1993	NCNR becomes a full institute, the National Institute of Nursing Research (NINR).
	The Cochrane Collaboration is established.
	Magnet Recognition Program makes first awards.
1995	Joanna Briggs Institute, an EBP collaborative, is established in Australia.
1997	Canadian Health Services Research Foundation is established with federal funding.
1998	The European Academy of Nursing Science (EANS) is launched.
1999	AHCPR is renamed Agency for Healthcare Research and Quality (AHRQ).
2000	NINR's annual funding exceeds $100 million.
	The Canadian Institute of Health Research is launched.
	Council for the Advancement of Nursing Science (CANS) is established.
2005	The Quality & Safety Education for Nurses (QSEN) initiative is inaugurated.
2006	NINR issues strategic plan for 2006-2010.
2010	The Institute of Medicine publishes a report, *The Future of Nursing,* that includes research priorities and recommendations for lifelong learning.
2011	NINR celebrates 25th anniversary and issues a new strategic plan.
2016	NINR issues *The NINR Strategic Plan: Advancing Science, Improving Lives.*
2019	NINR budget exceeds $145 million.

In the 1950s, research by nurses began to accelerate. For example, the American Nurses' Foundation, which is devoted to the promotion of nursing research, was founded. The surge in the number of studies conducted in the 1950s created the need for a new journal; *Nursing Research* came into being in 1952. As shown in Table 1.1, dissemination opportunities in professional journals grew steadily thereafter.

In the 1960s, nursing leaders expressed concern about the shortage of research on practice issues. Professional nursing organizations, such as the Western Interstate Council for Higher Education in Nursing, established research priorities, and practice-oriented research on various clinical topics began to emerge in the literature.

During the 1970s, improvements in client care became a more visible research priority, and guidance on assessing research for application in practice settings emerged. Also, nursing research expanded internationally. For example, the Workgroup of European Nurse Researchers was established in 1978 to develop greater communication and opportunities for partnerships among 25 European National Nurses Associations.

In the United States, the National Center for Nursing Research (NCNR) at the National Institutes of Health (NIH) was established in 1986. Several forces outside of nursing also helped to shape the nursing research landscape in the 1980s. A group from the McMaster Medical School in Canada designed a clinical learning strategy that was called evidence-based medicine (EBM). EBM, which promulgated the view that research findings were superior to the opinions of authorities as a basis for clinical decisions, constituted a profound shift for medical education and practice, and has had a major effect on all healthcare professions.

Nursing research was strengthened and given more visibility when NCNR was promoted to full institute status within the NIH. In 1993, the **National Institute of Nursing Research (NINR)** was established, helping to put nursing research more into the mainstream of health research. Funding opportunities for nursing research expanded in other countries as well.

Current and Future Directions for Nursing Research

Nursing research continues to develop at a rapid pace and will undoubtedly flourish throughout the 21st century. Broadly speaking, the priority for future nursing research will be the promotion of excellence in nursing science. Toward this end, nurse researchers and practicing nurses will be sharpening their research skills and using those skills to address emerging issues of importance to the profession and its clientele. Among the trends we foresee for the early 21st century are the following:

- *Continued focus on EBP.* Encouragement for nurses to engage in evidence-based patient care and lifelong learning is sure to continue. In turn, improvements will be needed both in the quality of studies and in nurses' skills in locating, understanding, critically appraising, and using relevant study results. Relatedly, there is an emerging interest in **translational research**, which involves research on how findings from studies can best be translated into practice.

- *Accelerating emphasis on research synthesis.* Research syntheses that integrate research evidence across studies are the cornerstone of EBP. Of particular importance is a type of synthesis called **systematic reviews**, which rigorously integrate research information on a research question. Clinical practice guidelines typically rely on such systematic reviews. We offer some guidance on how to create, as well as how to appraise, research syntheses in this book.

- *Expanded local research and quality improvement efforts in healthcare settings.* Projects designed to solve local problems are increasing. This trend will be reinforced as more hospitals apply for (and are recertified for) Magnet status in the United States and in other countries. Mechanisms need to be developed to ensure that evidence from these projects becomes available to others facing similar problems.

- *Strengthening of* **interprofessional collaboration**. Collaboration of nurses with researchers in related fields has expanded in the 21st century as researchers address fundamental healthcare problems. In turn, such collaborative efforts could lead to nurse researchers playing a more prominent role in national and international healthcare policies. One major recommendation in the Institute of Medicine's influential 2010 report *The Future of Nursing* was that nurses should be full partners with physicians and other healthcare professionals in redesigning health care.

- *Increased emphasis on patient-centeredness.* **Patient centeredness** has become a central concern in health care, as well as in research. In the United States, the Patient-Centered Outcomes Research Institute (PCORI) funds research focused on assisting patients and their caregivers to make well-informed healthcare decisions. Efforts are increasing to ensure that research is relevant to patients and that patients play a role in setting research priorities. **Comparative effectiveness research**, which involves direct comparisons of alternative treatments, has emerged as an important tool for patient-centered research.

- *Relatedly, greater interest in the* **applicability** *of research.* More attention is being paid to figuring out how study results can be applied to individual patients or groups of patients. A limitation of the current EBP model is that standard strategies offer evidence on *average effects* of healthcare interventions under ideal circumstances. Ideas are emerging about how best to enhance the applicability of research in real-world settings.

- *Growing interest in defining and ascertaining* **clinical significance**. Research findings increasingly must meet the test of being clinically significant, and patients have taken center-stage in efforts to define clinical significance.

- *Growing interest in* **precision health care** *and* **symptom science**. NINR has embraced research in these areas (Cashion & Grady, 2015). Symptom science involves research to study the underlying behavioral and molecular mechanisms of symptoms, irrespective of the health disorder. The Precision Healthcare Initiative is helping to advance nursing *omic* research (e.g., genomic, microbiomic).

What are nurse researchers likely to be studying in the future? Although there is rich diversity in research interests—as we illustrate throughout this book in our research examples—research priorities have been articulated by several nursing organizations, including NINR, Sigma Theta Tau International, and other nursing organizations throughout the world. For example, the primary areas of interest articulated in the 2016 NINR strategic plan were Symptom Science: Promoting Personalized Health Strategies; Wellness: Promoting Health and Preventing Disease; Self-Management: Improving Quality of Life for Individuals with Chronic Illness; and End-of-Life and Palliative Care: The Science of Compassion. Two cross-cutting areas of emphasis were promoting innovation and developing innovative strategies for research careers (NINR, 2016). And in 2017, the Science Committee of the Council for the Advancement of Nursing Science (CANS) in the United States identified four priorities: precision science, big data and data analytics, determinants of health, and global health (Eckardt, 2017).

SOURCES OF EVIDENCE FOR NURSING PRACTICE

Nurses make clinical decisions based on knowledge from many sources, including coursework, textbooks, and their own clinical experience. Because evidence is constantly evolving, learning about best practice nursing will persist throughout your career.

Some of what you have learned is based on systematic research, but some is not. What *are* the sources of evidence for nursing practice? Until recently, knowledge primarily was handed down from one generation to the next based on experience, trial and error, tradition, and expert opinion. A brief discussion of some alternative sources of evidence shows how research-based information is different.

Tradition and Authority

Decisions are sometimes based on custom or tradition. Certain "truths" are accepted as given, and such "knowledge" is so much a part of a common heritage that few seek validation. Some nursing interventions are based on custom and "unit culture" rather than on sound evidence. Indeed, one analysis suggested that some "sacred cows" (ineffective traditional habits) persisted even in a healthcare center recognized as a leader in EBP (Hanrahan et al., 2015).

Another common source of information is an authority, a person with specialized expertise. Reliance on authorities (such as faculty or textbook authors) is unavoidable but imperfect: authorities are not infallible, particularly if their expertise is based primarily on personal experience or out-of-date materials.

Clinical Experience and Trial and Error

Clinical experience is a functional source of knowledge and plays an important role in EBP. Yet personal clinical experience has some limitations as a knowledge source because each nurse's experience is too narrow to be generally useful. Moreover, the same objective event is often perceived differently by different nurses.

Trial and error involves trying alternatives successively until a solution to a problem is found. Trial and error may offer a practical means of securing knowledge, but the method tends to be haphazard and solutions may be idiosyncratic.

Logical Reasoning

Solutions to some problems are developed by logical reasoning, which combines experience, the intellect, and formal systems of thought. **Inductive reasoning** involves developing generalizations from specific observations. For example, a nurse may observe the anxious behavior of (specific) hospitalized children and conclude that (in general) children's separation from their parents is stressful. **Deductive reasoning** involves developing specific predictions from general principles. For example, if we assume that separation anxiety occurs in hospitalized children (in general), then we might predict that (specific) children in a hospital whose parents do not room-in will manifest symptoms of stress. Both types of reasoning are useful for understanding phenomena, and both play a role in research. Logical reasoning by itself, however, is limited because the validity of reasoning depends on the accuracy of the initial premises.

Assembled Information

In making clinical decisions, healthcare professionals rely on information that has been assembled for a various purposes. For example, local, national, and international *benchmarking data* provide information on such issues as infection rates or the rates of various procedures (e.g., cesarean births) and can facilitate evaluations of clinical practices. *Cost data*—information on the costs associated with certain procedures, policies, or practices—are sometimes used as a factor in clinical decision-making. *Quality improvement and risk data*, such as medication error reports, can be used to assess the need for practice changes. Such sources are useful, but they do not provide a mechanism for making clinical decisions or guiding improvements.

Disciplined Research

Research conducted in a disciplined framework is the best method of acquiring knowledge. Nursing research combines logical reasoning with other features to create evidence that, although fallible, tends to be especially reliable. Carefully synthesized findings from rigorous research are especially valuable. The current emphasis on EBP requires nurses to base their clinical practice to the greatest extent possible on research-based findings rather than on tradition, authority, intuition, or personal experience—although nursing will always remain a rich blend of art and science.

PARADIGMS AND METHODS FOR NURSING RESEARCH

A **paradigm** is a world view, a general perspective on the complexities of the world. Paradigms for human inquiry are often characterized in terms of the ways in which they respond to basic philosophical questions, such as, "What is the nature of reality?" and "What is the relationship between the inquirer and those being studied?"

Disciplined inquiry in nursing has been conducted mainly within two broad paradigms, *positivism* and *constructivism*. This section describes these two paradigms and outlines the research methods associated with them. In later chapters, we describe the *transformative paradigm* that underpins *critical theory research* (Chapter 22) and a *pragmatism paradigm* that underlies *mixed methods research* (Chapter 27).

The Positivist Paradigm

The paradigm that dominated healthcare research for decades is called **positivism** (or *logical positivism*). Positivism is rooted in 19th century thought, guided by such philosophers as Newton and Locke. Positivism reflects a broader cultural phenomenon (*modernism*) that emphasizes the rational and the scientific.

A fundamental assumption of positivists is that there is a reality *out there* that can be studied and known. (An **assumption** is a basic principle that is believed to be true without proof.) Adherents of positivism assume that nature is basically ordered and regular and that reality exists independent of human observation (Table 1.2). The related assumption of **determinism** refers to the positivists' belief that phenomena are not haphazard but rather have antecedent causes. If a person has a cerebrovascular accident, a positivist assumes that there must be a reason that can be potentially identified. Within this paradigm, much research activity is aimed at understanding the underlying causes of phenomena.

Positivists value objectivity and attempt to hold personal beliefs and biases in check. The positivists' scientific approach involves using orderly procedures with tight controls of the research situation to test hunches about the phenomena being studied.

Strict positivist thinking has been challenged, and few researchers adhere to the tenets of pure positivism. In the **postpositivist paradigm**, there is a belief in reality and a desire to understand it, but postpositivists recognize the impossibility of total objectivity. They do, however, see objectivity as a goal and strive to be as neutral as possible. Postpositivists also recognize the obstacles to knowing reality with certainty and therefore seek *probabilistic* evidence—i.e., learning what the true state of a phenomenon *probably* is. This modified positivist position remains a dominant force in healthcare research. For the sake of simplicity, we refer to it as positivism.

The Constructivist Paradigm

The **constructivist paradigm** (also called the *naturalistic paradigm*) began as a countermovement to positivism with writers such as Weber and Kant. Just as positivism reflects the cultural phenomenon of modernism that burgeoned after the industrial revolution, naturalism is an outgrowth of the cultural transformation called *postmodernism*. Postmodern thinking emphasizes the value of *deconstruction*, taking apart old ideas and structures, and *reconstruction*, putting ideas and structures together in new ways. The constructivist paradigm represents a major alternative system for conducting disciplined research in nursing. Table 1.2 compares the major assumptions of the positivist and constructivist paradigms.

For the naturalistic inquirer, reality is not a fixed entity but rather is a construction of the people participating in the research; reality exists within a context, and many constructions are possible. Naturalists thus take the position of relativism: if there are multiple interpretations of reality that exist in people's minds, then there is no process by which the ultimate truth or falsity of the constructions can be determined.

The constructivist paradigm assumes that knowledge is maximized when the distance between the researcher and those under study is minimized. The voices and interpretations of study participants are crucial to understanding the phenomenon of interest. Findings in a constructivist inquiry are the product of the interaction between the inquirer and the participants.

Paradigms and Methods: Quantitative and Qualitative Research

Research methods are the techniques researchers use to structure a study and to gather and analyze information relevant to the research question. The two alternative paradigms correspond

TABLE 1.2 • Major Assumptions of the Positivist and Constructivist Paradigms

PHILOSOPHICAL QUESTION	POSITIVIST PARADIGM ASSUMPTION	CONSTRUCTIVIST PARADIGM ASSUMPTION
What is the nature of reality?	Reality exists; there is a real world driven by real natural causes	Reality is multiple and subjective, mentally constructed by individuals
In what way is the researcher related to those being researched?	The researcher is independent from those being researched; findings are not influenced by the researcher	The researcher interacts with those being researched; findings are the creation of the interactive process
What is the role of values in the inquiry?	Values and biases are to be held in check; objectivity is sought	Subjectivity and values are inevitable and desirable
What are the best methods for obtaining evidence?	Deductive processes → hypothesis testing	Inductive processes → hypothesis generation
	Emphasis on discrete, specific concepts	Emphasis on entirety of a phenomenon, holistic
	Focus on the objective and quantifiable	Focus on the subjective and nonquantifiable
	Outsider knowledge—researcher is external, separate	Insider knowledge—researcher is part of the process
	Fixed, prespecified design	Flexible, emergent design
	Controls over context	Context-bound
	Large, representative samples	Small, information-rich samples
	Measured (quantitative) information	Narrative (unstructured) information
	Statistical analysis	Qualitative analysis
	Seeks generalizations	Seeks in-depth understanding

to different approaches to developing evidence. A key methodologic distinction is between **quantitative research**, which is most closely allied with positivism, and **qualitative research**, which is associated with constructivist inquiry—although positivists sometimes undertake qualitative studies and constructivist researchers sometimes collect quantitative information. This section provides an overview of the methods associated with the two paradigms.

The Scientific Method and Quantitative Research

The traditional **scientific method** refers to a set of orderly, disciplined procedures used to acquire information. Quantitative researchers use deductive reasoning to generate predictions that are tested in the real world. They typically move in a systematic fashion from the definition of a problem and the selection of concepts on which to focus, to the solution of the problem. By **systematic**, we mean that the investigator progresses logically through a series of steps, according to a prespecified plan of action.

Quantitative researchers use various control strategies. **Control** involves imposing conditions on the research situation so that biases are minimized and validity is maximized. Control mechanisms are discussed at length later in this book.

Quantitative researchers gather **empirical evidence**—evidence that is rooted in objective reality and gathered through the senses (e.g., through sight or hearing). Observations of the presence or absence of skin inflammation, patients' agitation, or infant birth weight are all examples of empirical observations. Reliance on empirical evidence means that findings are grounded in reality rather than in researchers' personal beliefs.

Evidence for a study in the positivist paradigm is gathered according to an established plan, using structured methods to collect needed information. Usually the information gathered is **quantitative**—that is, numeric information that is obtained through a formal *measurement* and is analyzed statistically.

A traditional scientific study strives to go beyond the specifics of a research situation. For example, quantitative researchers are typically not as focused on understanding why a *particular* person has a stroke as in understanding what factors influence its occurrence in people generally. The degree to which research findings can be generalized to individuals other than those who participated in a study is called **generalizability**.

The scientific method has enjoyed considerable stature as a method of inquiry and has been used productively by nurse researchers studying a wide range of nursing problems. This approach cannot, however, solve all nursing problems. One important limitation—common to both quantitative and qualitative research—is that research cannot be used to answer moral or ethical questions. Many intriguing questions about humans fall into this area—questions such as whether euthanasia should be practiced or abortion should be legal.

The traditional research approach also must address measurement challenges. To study a phenomenon, quantitative researchers try to measure it using numeric values that express quantity. For example, if the phenomenon of interest is patient stress, researchers would want to assess if patients' stress is high or low. Physiologic phenomena like blood pressure can be measured with great accuracy and precision, but measuring psychological phenomena (e.g., stress, resilience, depression) is challenging.

Another issue is that nursing research focuses on humans, who are inherently complex and diverse. Quantitative studies typically concentrate on relatively few concepts (e.g., weight gain, fatigue, pain). Complexities tend to be controlled and, if possible, eliminated, rather than studied directly, and this narrowness of focus can sometimes obscure insights. Quantitative research within the positivist paradigm has been accused of an inflexibility of vision that fails to capture the full breadth of human experience.

Constructivist Methods and Qualitative Research

Researchers in constructivist traditions emphasize the inherent complexity of humans, their ability to shape and create their own experiences, and the idea that truth is a composite of realities. Constructivist studies are thus focused on understanding the human experience as it is lived, usually through the collection and analysis of **qualitative** materials that are narrative and subjective.

Researchers who criticize the scientific method believe that it is overly *reductionist*—that is, it reduces human experience to the few concepts under investigation, and those concepts are defined in advance by the researcher rather than emerging from the perspective of those under study. Constructivist researchers tend to emphasize the dynamic and holistic aspects of human life and attempt to capture those aspects in their entirety.

Flexible, evolving procedures are used to capitalize on findings that emerge during the study. Constructivist inquiry often takes place in the **field** (i.e., in naturalistic settings), sometimes over an extended time period. In constructivist research, the collection of information and its analysis typically progress concurrently; as researchers sift through information, insights are gained, new questions emerge, and further evidence is sought to amplify or confirm the insights. Through an inductive process, researchers integrate information to develop a theory or description that helps illuminate the phenomenon of interest.

Constructivist studies yield rich, in-depth information that can elucidate varied dimensions of a complicated phenomenon. Findings from qualitative research are typically grounded in the real-life experiences of people with first-hard knowledge of a phenomenon. Nevertheless, the approach has several limitations. Human beings are used directly as the instrument through which information is gathered, and humans are extremely intelligent and sensitive—but fallible—tools. The subjectivity that enriches the analytic insights of skillful researchers can yield trivial and obvious "findings" among less competent ones.

Another potential limitation involves the subjectivity of constructivist inquiry, which sometimes raises concerns about the idiosyncratic nature of the conclusions. Would two constructivist researchers studying the same phenomenon in similar settings arrive at similar conclusions? The situation is further complicated by the fact that most constructivist studies involve a small group of participants. Thus, the generalizability of findings from constructivist inquiries is sometimes a potential concern.

Multiple Paradigms and Nursing Research

Paradigms should be viewed as lenses that help to sharpen our focus on phenomena, not as blinders that limit intellectual curiosity. Nursing knowledge would be thin if there were not a rich array of methods available within the two paradigms—methods that are often complementary in their strengths and limitations. We believe that intellectual pluralism is advantageous.

We have emphasized differences between the two paradigms and associated methods so that distinctions would be easy to understand. Subsequent chapters of this book elaborate further on differences in terminology, methods, and research products. It is equally important to note, however, that the two main paradigms have many features in common, only some of which are mentioned here:

- *Ultimate goals.* The aim of disciplined research, regardless of paradigm, is to answer questions and solve problems. Both quantitative and qualitative researchers seek to capture the truth about an aspect of the world in which they are interested, and both groups can make meaningful contributions to evidence for nursing practice.
- *External evidence.* Although the word *empiricism* has come to be associated with the classic scientific method, researchers in both traditions gather and analyze evidence empirically, that is, through their senses.
- *Reliance on human cooperation.* Human cooperation is essential in both qualitative and quantitative research. To understand people's circumstances and experiences, researchers must persuade them to participate in the investigation *and* to speak and act candidly.
- *Ethical constraints.* Research with human beings is guided by ethical principles that sometimes are at odds with research goals. Ethical dilemmas sometimes confront researchers, regardless of paradigm or method.
- *Fallibility of disciplined research.* Virtually all studies have limitations. Every research question can be addressed in many ways, and inevitably there are tradeoffs. The fallibility of any single study makes it important to understand and critically appraise researchers' methodologic decisions when evaluating evidence quality.

Thus, despite philosophic and methodologic differences, researchers using traditional scientific or constructivist methods face many similar challenges. The selection of an appropriate method depends on researchers' personal philosophy and on the research question. If a researcher asks, "What are the effects of cryotherapy on nausea and oral mucositis in patients undergoing chemotherapy?" the researcher needs to study effects by carefully measuring patient outcomes. On the other hand, if a researcher asks, "What is the process by which parents learn to cope with the death of a child?" the researcher would be hard pressed to quantify such a process. Personal world views of researchers help to shape their questions.

In reading about the alternative paradigms for nursing research, you likely were more attracted to one of the two paradigms. It is important, however, to learn about both approaches to disciplined inquiry and to recognize their respective strengths and limitations. In this textbook, we describe methods associated with both qualitative and quantitative research to assist you in becoming *methodologically bilingual*. This is especially important because large numbers of nurse researchers are now undertaking **mixed methods research** that involves the collection and analysis of both qualitative and quantitative data (Chapters 27-29).

THE PURPOSES OF NURSING RESEARCH

The general purpose of nursing research is to answer questions and solve problems of relevance to nursing. Specific purposes can be classified in various ways. For example, a distinction sometimes is made between basic and applied research. **Basic research** is undertaken to discover general principles of human behavior and biophysiologic processes. Some basic research (*bench research*) is performed in laboratory settings and focuses on the molecular and cellular mechanisms that underlie disease. **Applied research** is aimed at examining how basic principles can be used to solve practice problems. Nurse researchers undertake both types of research.

Another way to classify research purposes concerns the extent to which studies provide explanatory information. Specific study goals can range along a descriptive/explanatory continuum, but a fundamental distinction is between studies whose primary intent is to *describe* phenomena and those that are **cause-probing**—that is, designed to illuminate the underlying causes of phenomena. The descriptive/explanatory continuum includes studies whose purposes are identification, description, exploration, prediction/control, and explanation of health-related phenomena. For each purpose, various types of question are addressed—some more amenable to qualitative than to quantitative inquiry,

and vice versa. Table 1.3 gives examples of questions asked for these purposes.

In both nursing and medicine, several books have been written to facilitate evidence-based practice, and these books categorize studies in terms of the types of information needed by clinicians (Guyatt et al., 2015; Melnyk & Fineout-Overholt, 2015). These writers focus on several types of clinical purposes: Therapy/intervention; Diagnosis/assessment; Prognosis; Etiology (causation)/prevention of harm; Description; and Meaning/process.

Therapy/Intervention

Therapy/intervention questions are addressed by healthcare researchers who want to learn about the effects of specific actions, products, or processes. Typically, researchers addressing this type of question are evaluating whether a new treatment or a practice change has beneficial effects.

The name "Therapy" for this category originates from promoters of EBP in medicine who focused on studies of the effects of "therapeutic" medical interventions, such as new drugs or surgical procedures. However, this category should be thought of more broadly to include research on the effects of alternative ways of doing things, usually with the intent of testing strategies for making improvements. *Therapy questions are foundational for evidence-based decision-making.* Evidence for changes to nursing practice, nursing education, and nursing administration comes from studies that have specifically tested the effects of intervening in a particular way. Table 1.4 provides some examples of studies in which nurse researchers addressed diverse Therapy/intervention questions. If such questions are answered in a rigorous fashion, the evidence might suggest a practice change or the implementation of an institutional innovation.

Studies in this category range from evaluations of highly specific treatments (e.g., comparing two types of cooling blankets for febrile patients) to assessments of complex multisession interventions designed to change behaviors (e.g., nurse-led health promotion programs). **Intervention research** is essential for evidence-based practice, and nurses are increasingly engaging in this type of

TABLE 1.3 • Research Purposes and Questions on the Description/Explanation Continuum

PURPOSE	TYPES OF QUESTIONS: QUANTITATIVE RESEARCH	TYPES OF QUESTIONS: QUALITATIVE RESEARCH
Identification		What is this phenomenon? What is its name?
Description	How prevalent is the phenomenon? How often does the phenomenon occur? How intense is the phenomenon?	What are the dimensions or characteristics of the phenomenon? What is important about the phenomenon?
Exploration	What factors are related to the phenomenon? What are the antecedents of the phenomenon?	What is the full nature of the phenomenon? What is really going on here? How is the phenomenon experienced? What is the process by which the phenomenon evolves?
Explanation	What is the underlying cause of the phenomenon? Does the theory explain the phenomenon?	How does the phenomenon work? What does the phenomenon mean? How did the phenomenon occur?
Prediction	If phenomenon X occurs, will phenomenon Y follow? What will happen if we modify a phenomenon or introduce an intervention?	–
Control	Can the occurrence of the phenomenon be prevented or controlled?	–

research. Research addressing Therapy questions is inherently cause-probing: the researcher wants to know if a certain intervention will *cause* improved outcomes.

Diagnosis/Assessment

A burgeoning number of nursing studies concern the rigorous development and evaluation of formal instruments to screen, diagnose, and assess patients and to measure important clinical outcomes—that is, they address **Diagnosis/assessment questions**. High-quality instruments with documented accuracy are essential for both clinical practice and research. Typically, the question being addressed is: Does this new instrument yield reliable and valid

information about an outcome, situation, or condition of importance to nursing? Studies addressing Diagnosis questions are not cause-probing.

Example of a Study Aimed at Diagnosis/ Assessment
Kang and colleagues (2018) developed and evaluated the Automated Medical Error Assessment System, which was incorporated into an electronic health record system.

Prognosis

Researchers who ask **Prognosis questions** strive to understand the outcomes that are associated with a disease or a health problem (i.e., its consequences),

TABLE 1.4 • Examples of Therapy/Intervention Questions

THERAPY/INTERVENTION QUESTION	AREA OF FOCUS
Does an education intervention improve teenagers' knowledge and behaviors relating to contraception? (Pivatti et al., 2019)	Nursing practice
Do muscle relaxation or nature sounds reduce fatigue in patients with heart failure? (Seifi et al., 2018)	Nursing practice
Does a nurse-led phone follow-up education program reduce cardiovascular risk among patients with cardiovascular disease? (Zhou et al., 2018)	Nursing practice
Does a simulation-based palliative care communication skill workshop improve self-perception of skills in expressing empathy and discussing spiritual issues among healthcare workers and students? (Brown et al., 2018)	Interprofessional education
Does simulation improve the ability of first year nursing students to learn vital signs? (Eyikara & Baykara, 2018)	Nursing education
Does a bundle of interventions to support nurses' engagement in evidence-based practice (EBP) increase their knowledge, attitudes, and use of library resources? (Carter et al., 2018)	Nursing administration

to estimate the probability they will occur, and to predict the types of people for whom the outcomes are most likely. Such studies facilitate the development of long-term care plans for patients and can suggest the need for appropriate interventions. For example, Prognosis studies provide valuable information for guiding patients to make lifestyle choices or to be vigilant for key symptoms. Prognosis questions are typically cause-probing; the researcher wants to know if, for example, a certain disease or behavior causes subsequent adverse outcomes.

Example of a Study Aimed at Prognosis
Galazzi and colleagues (2018) studied the long-term quality of life outcomes of patients with severe respiratory failure who had undergone extracorporeal membrane oxygenation.

Etiology (Causation)/Prevention of Harm

Nurses encounter patients who face potentially harmful exposures as a result of environmental agents or because of personal behaviors or characteristics. Providing information to patients about such

harms and how best to avoid them depends on the availability of accurate evidence about factors that contribute to health risks. For example, there would be no smoking cessation programs if research had not provided strong evidence that smoking cigarettes causes or contributes to a wide range of health problems. Thus, identifying factors that affect or cause illness, mortality, or morbidity is an important purpose of many nursing studies. **Etiology questions** are inherently cause-probing—the purpose is to understand factors that cause health problems.

Example of a Study Aimed at Identifying and Preventing Harm
Philpott and Corcoran (2018) did a study to identify factors that put men at risk of paternal postnatal depression in Ireland. The risk factors examined included a prior history of depression, economic circumstances, marital status, and availability of paternity leave.

Description

Description questions are not in a category typically identified in EBP-related classification schemes, but so many nursing studies have a descriptive purpose that we include it here. Examples of phenomena that nurse researchers have described include patients' pain, physical function, confusion, and levels of depression. Quantitative description focuses on the prevalence, size, intensity, and measurable attributes of phenomena. Qualitative researchers, by contrast, describe the dimensions or the evolution of phenomena.

> **Example of a Quantitative Study Aimed at Description**
> Schoenfisch and colleagues (2019) did a study to describe hospital nursing staff's use of lift or transfer devices. They found that only 40% of the nurses used equipment for at least half of lifts/transfers.

> **Example of a Qualitative Study Aimed at Description**
> Dose and Rhudy (2018) undertook a study to describe what was important to patients newly diagnosed with advanced cancer and receiving dignity therapy during cancer treatment.

Meaning/Process

Designing effective interventions, motivating people to comply with treatments and health promotion activities, and providing sensitive advice to patients are among the many healthcare activities that can benefit from understanding clients' perspectives. Research that provides evidence about what health and illness mean to clients, what barriers to positive health practices they face, and what processes they experience in a transition through a healthcare crisis are important to evidence-based nursing practice. Studies that address **Meaning/process questions** are seldom focused on identifying the underlying causes of phenomena but might offer important clues.

> **Example of a Study Aimed at Understanding Meaning/Process**
> Qin and coresearchers (2019) studied the process by which women experienced a cognitive–behavioral transition after undergoing pregnancy termination for fetal anomaly.

Study Purposes and Evidence-Based Practice

Studies that address Therapy/intervention questions provide the most direct evidence for EBP. If we want to know, for example, whether wedge-shaped foam cushions are more effective in preventing heel pressure ulcers than standard foam pillows, we would need to look for rigorous studies that have addressed this Therapy question. However, other questions also play a role in improving the quality of nursing care, albeit in different ways.

Table 1.5 presents examples of different types of questions relating to cigarette smoking, using the study purpose categories we just described. The findings from studies relating to only one of these questions is directly *actionable*—the Therapy question. If there is strong evidence that nurse-led smoking cessation programs are effective in reducing smoking among young adults, we might consider initiating such a program in our own community.

If the other questions in Table 1.5 were answered in rigorous studies, the evidence could also play a role in guiding efforts to improve nursing practice—but not as directly. Answers to some of these questions might help to target those most in need of an intervention. For example, based on studies addressing the Diagnosis question, we could launch a prevention effort aimed at teenagers with high scores on the evidence-based Smoking Susceptibility Index, or results from an Etiology study might lead us to offer a smoking-cessation initiative in low-income neighborhoods. Evidence from the Prognosis question might prompt us to develop a strong program of emotional support for patients with lung cancer. We might be motivated to implement an intervention for high school students if we knew that rates of smoking were high (the Description question). And, if we knew that a high percentage of smokers in our community had been unsuccessful in efforts to quit, we might design an intervention with that information in mind. The stories from long-term smokers who failed to quit despite efforts to do so (the Meaning question) could lead us to involve them in the design of an intervention for hardened smokers.

TABLE 1.5 • Different Categories of Questions Related to Cigarette Smoking

TYPE OF QUESTION	EXAMPLE OF A RELATED RESEARCH QUESTION ON CIGARETTE SMOKING
Therapy/ intervention	Does a nurse-led smoking cessation program for young adults reduce smoking?
Diagnosis/ assessment	Is our Smoking Susceptibility Index a valid and reliable measure of propensity to initiate smoking in teenagers?
Prognosis	Is a diagnosis of smoking-related lung cancer associated with increased risk of suicidal ideation?
Etiology (causation)/ prevention of harm	Does being poor increase the risk that a person will smoke cigarettes?
Description	What percentage of high school students smoke 1+ packs of cigarettes/ week, and what percentage of smokers have tried to quit?
Meaning/process	What is it like for long-term smokers to attempt and fail at quitting?

Nurse researchers are making strides in addressing all types of questions about important health problems—but evidence regarding what "works" to address problems comes from studies focused on Therapy questions. Evidence about the scope of a problem, factors affecting the problem, the consequences of the problem, and the meaning of the problem can, however, play a crucial role in efforts to design better interventions, to aim our resources at those in greatest need, and to provide appropriate guidance to clients in everyday practice.

ASSISTANCE FOR USERS OF NURSING RESEARCH

This book is designed primarily to help you develop skills for conducting research, but in an environment that stresses EBP, it is extremely important to hone your skills in reading, evaluating, and using nursing studies. We provide specific guidance to consumers in most chapters by including guidelines for critically appraising aspects of a study covered in the chapter. The questions in Box 1.1 are designed to assist you in using the information in this chapter in an overall preliminary assessment of a research report.

TIP The *Resource Manual* (RM) for this book offers rich opportunities to practice your critical appraisal skills. The RM's Toolkit on the**Point** includes Box 1.1 as a Word document, which will allow you to adapt these questions, if desired, and to input answers to them directly in a Word document without having to retype the questions.

RESEARCH EXAMPLES

Each chapter of this book presents brief descriptions of studies conducted by nurse researchers, focusing on aspects emphasized in the chapter. Read the full journal articles to learn more about the methods and results of these studies.

Research Example of a Quantitative Study

Study: Promoting heart health among rural African Americans (Abbott et al., 2018)

Study purpose: The purpose of the study, which addressed a Therapy question, was to evaluate a culturally relevant health promotion intervention designed to reduce cardiovascular disease risk in rural African American adults—the "With Every Heartbeat is Life" program.

BOX 1.1 Questions for a Preliminary Overview of a Research Report

1. How relevant is the research question in this study to the actual practice of nursing? Does the study focus on a topic that is a priority area for nursing research?
2. Was the research quantitative or qualitative?
3. What was the underlying purpose (or purposes) of the study—identification, description, exploration, explanation, or prediction and control? Does the purpose correspond to an EBP focus such as Therapy/intervention, Diagnosis/assessment, Prognosis, Etiology (causation)/prevention of harm, Description, or Meaning/process?
4. Is this study fundamentally cause-probing?
5. What might be some clinical implications of this research? To what type of people and settings is the research most relevant? If the findings are valid, how might I use the results of this study in my clinical work?

Study methods: Twelve rural churches in two counties of northern Florida were assigned, at random, to either receive the intervention (six churches) or not receive it (the other six churches). Pastors and community members from the churches then recruited people to participate in the study. A total of 115 adults were in the intervention group, and 114 were in the group not receiving the intervention (the control group). Those in the intervention group received the weekly, 90-minute cardiovascular health promotion intervention for 6 weeks, whereas those in the control group did not receive any health promotion education. Everyone who participated in the study completed questionnaires before the start of the study and 6 weeks later at the end of the study. The questionnaires were used to gather information about participants' attitudes, intentions, and self-efficacy to increase the consumption of produce, reduce dietary saturated fat intake, and increase exercise.

Key findings: Those in the intervention group had significantly greater improvements than those in the control group on most of the outcomes. For example, participants who received the program had significantly greater intentions to increase produce consumption and reduce dietary fat intake. Self-efficacy for healthy choices also increased significantly more among participants in the intervention group.

Conclusions: Abbott and colleagues concluded that nurse-led interventions in community settings can potentially reduce cardiovascular disease risk.

Research Example of a Qualitative Study

Study: "I can never be too comfortable"—Race, gender, and emotion at the hospital bedside (Cottingham et al., 2018)

Study purpose: The purpose of this descriptive study was to explore how gender and race intersect to shape the emotion practice of nurses as they experience, manage, and reflect on their emotions in the workplace.

Study methods: As part of a larger study of nurses and emotional labor, audio diaries were elicited from a sample of 48 nurses who were diverse with respect to gender (both women and men) and race (white, black, and Asian). Study participants were given a digital voice recorder and were instructed to make a recording after six consecutive shifts. They were asked to reflect on how they felt during and after their last shift, to describe things that influenced their emotions, and to explain how they responded to their own emotions. Participants were not asked to specifically reflect on experiences related to race. Each recording was transcribed for analysis.

Key findings: Analysis of the audio diary data revealed "a disproportionate emotional labor that emerges among women nurses of color in the white institutional space of American health care" (p. 145). Women of color were found to experience an emotional "double shift" in negotiating interactions between patients, coworkers, and supervisors. These women were found to have experiences that added to job-related stress and that resulted in depleted emotional resources that negatively influenced patient care.

Conclusions: The researchers expressed the hope that their study would help to make more visible the toll of the intersection of race and gender on emotional labor in nursing.

SUMMARY POINTS

- **Nursing research** is systematic inquiry undertaken to develop evidence on problems of importance to nurses. Nurses are adopting an **evidence-based practice (EBP)** that incorporates research findings into their clinical decisions.
- Nurses can participate in a range of research-related activities that span a continuum from being *consumers of research* (those who read and evaluate studies) to being *producers of research* (those who design and undertake studies). Engagement with research often occurs in practice settings through participation in a **journal club**.
- Nursing research began with Florence Nightingale but developed slowly until its rapid acceleration in the 1950s. Since the 1980s, the focus has been on **clinical nursing research**—that is, on problems relating to clinical practice.
- The **National Institute of Nursing Research (NINR)**, established at the U.S. National Institutes of Health in 1993, affirms the stature of nursing research in the United States.
- Contemporary issues in nursing research include the growth of EBP, expansion of local research and quality improvement efforts, research synthesis through **systematic reviews**, **interprofessional** studies, **patient-centeredness** in both clinical care and in research, interest in the **applicability** of research to individual patients or groups, interest in precision health care and symptom science, and efforts to measure the **clinical significance** of research results.
- Disciplined research stands in contrast to other knowledge sources for nursing practice, such as tradition, authority, personal experience, trial and error, and logical reasoning.

- Nursing research is conducted mainly within one of two broad **paradigms**—world views with underlying **assumptions** about reality: the positivist and the constructivist paradigms.
- In the **positivist paradigm**, it is assumed that there is an objective reality and that natural phenomena are orderly. The assumption of **determinism** is the belief that phenomena result from prior causes and are not haphazard.
- In the **constructivist** (*naturalistic*) **paradigm**, it is assumed that reality is not fixed, but it is a construction of human minds; "truth" is a composite of multiple constructions of reality.
- The positivist paradigm is associated with **quantitative research**—the collection and analysis of numeric information. Quantitative research is typically conducted within the traditional **scientific method**, which is a systematic, controlled process. Quantitative researchers gather and analyze **empirical evidence** (evidence collected through the human senses) and strive for **generalizability** of their findings.
- Researchers within the constructivist paradigm emphasize understanding the human experience as it is lived through the collection and analysis of subjective, narrative materials using flexible procedures that evolve in the **field**; this paradigm is associated with **qualitative research**.
- **Basic research** is designed to extend the knowledge base for the sake of knowledge itself. **Applied research** focuses on discovering solutions to immediate problems.
- A fundamental distinction, especially relevant in quantitative research, is between studies whose primary intent is to *describe* phenomena and those that are **cause-probing**—i.e., designed to illuminate underlying causes of phenomena. Specific research purposes on the description/explanation continuum include identification, description, exploration, prediction/control, and explanation.
- Nursing studies can be classified in terms of several EBP-related aims: **Therapy/intervention**; **Diagnosis/assessment**; **Prognosis**; **Etiology** (causation)/prevention of **harm**; **Description**; and **Meaning/process**. Rigorous answers to Therapy questions are foundational for EBP.

STUDY ACTIVITIES

Study activities are available to instructors on thePoint.

REFERENCES CITED IN CHAPTER 1

**Abbott, L., Williams, C., Slate, E., & Gropper, S. (2018). Promoting heart health among rural African Americans. *Journal of Cardiovascular Nursing, 33*, E8–E14.

*Barnes, H., Reardon, J., & McHugh, M. (2016). Magnet® hospital recognition linked to lower central line-associated bloodstream infection rates. *Research in Nursing & Health, 39*, 96–104.

Bastani, F., Rajai, N., Farsi, Z., & Als, H. (2017). The effects of kangaroo care on the sleep-wake states of preterm infants. *Journal of Nursing Research, 25*, 231–239.

Billner-Garcia, R., Spilkerm, A., & Goyak, D. (2018). Skin to skin contact: newborn temperature stability in the operating room. *MCN: American Journal of Maternal-Child Nursing, 43*, 158–163.

Brown, C., Back, A., Ford, D., Kross, E., Downey, L., Shannon, S., ... Engelberg, R. (2018). Self-assessment scores improve after simulation-based palliative care communication skill workshop. *American Journal of Hospice & Palliative Care, 35*, 45–51.

Carter, E., Rivera, R., Gallagher, K., & Cato, K. (2018). Targeted interventions to advance a culture of inquiry at a large, multicampus hospital among nurses. *Journal of Nursing Administration, 48*, 18–24.

*Cashion, A. K., & Grady, P. (2015). The National Institutes of Health/National Institutes of Nursing Research intramural research program and the development of the NIH Symptom Science Model. *Nursing Outlook, 63*, 484–487.

Cho, E., Kim, S., Kwon, M., Cho, H., Kim, E., Jun, E., & Lee, S. (2016). The effects of kangaroo care in the neonatal intensive care unit on the physiological functions of preterm infants, maternal-infant attachment, and maternal stress. *Journal of Pediatric Nursing, 31*, 430–438.

Cottingham, M., Johnson, A., & Erickson, R. (2018). "I can never be too comfortable": race, gender, and emotion at the hospital bedside. *Qualitative Health Research, 28*, 145–158.

Dose, A., & Rhudy, L. (2018). Perspectives of newly diagnosed advanced cancer patients receiving dignity therapy during cancer treatment. *Supportive Care in Cancer, 26*, 187–195.

Eckardt, P., Culley, J., Corwin, E., Richmond, T., Dougherty, C., Pickler, R., ... DeVon, H. (2017). National nursing science priorities: creating a shared vision. *Nursing Outlook, 65*, 726–736.

Eyikara, E., & Baykara, Z. (2018). Effect of simulation on the ability of first year nursing students to learn vital signs. *Nurse Education Today, 60*, 101–106.

Galazzi, A., Brambilla, A., Grasselli, G., Pesenti, A., Fumagali, R., & Lucchini, A. (2018). Quality of life of adult survivors after extra corporeal membrane axygenation (ECMO). *Dimensions of Critical Care Nursing, 37*, 12–17.

Gardner, K., Kanaskie, M., Knehans, A., Salisbury, S., Doheny, K., & Schirm, V. (2016). Implementing and sustaining evidence based practice through a nursing journal club. *Applied Nursing Research, 31*, 139–145.

Graystone, R. (2017). The 2014 Magnet® Application Manual: nursing excellence standards evolving with practice. *Journal of Nursing Administration, 47*, 527–528.

Guyatt, G., Rennie, D., Meade, M., & Cook, D. (2015). *Users' guide to the medical literature: essentials of evidence-based clinical practice* (3rd ed.). New York: McGraw Hill.

Hanrahan, K., Wagner, M., Matthews, G., Stewart, S., Dawson, C., Greiner, J., ... Williamson, A. (2015). Sacred cows gone to pasture: a systematic evaluation and integration of evidence-based practice. *Worldviews on Evidence-Based Nursing, 12*, 3–11.

*Institute of Medicine. (2010). *The future of nursing: leading change, advancing health*. Washington, DC: The National Academies Press.

Johnston, C., Campbell-Yeo, M., Disher, T., Benoit, B., Fernandes, A., Streiner, D., ... Zee, R. (2017). Skin-to-skin care for procedural pain in neonates. *Cochrane Database of Systematic Reviews*, CD0008435.

Kang, M., Jin, Y., Jin, T., & Lee, S. (2018). Automated medication error risk assessment system (Auto-MERAS). *Journal of Nursing Care Quality, 33*, 86–93.

McCaughey, D., McGhan, G., Rathert, C., Williams, J., & Hearld, K. (2019). Magnetic work environments: patient experience outcomes in Magnet versus non-Magnet hospitals. *Health Care Management Review* (in press).

Melnyk, B. M., & Fineout-Overholt, E. (2015). *Evidence-based practice in nursing and healthcare: a guide to best practice* (3rd ed.). Philadelphia: Lippincott Williams & Wilkins.

Moore, E. R., Bergman, N., Anderson, G., & Medley, N. (2016). Early skin-to-skin contact for mothers and their health newborn infants. *Cochrane Database of Systematic Reviews*, CD0003519.

*National Institute of Nursing Research. (2016). *The NINR strategic plan: advancing science, improving lives*. Bethesda, MD: NINR.

Philpott, L., & Corcoran, P. (2018). Paternal postnatal depression in Ireland: prevalence and associated factors. *Midwifery, 56*, 121–127.

Pivatti, A., Osis, M., & deMorales Lopes, M. (2019). The use of educational strategies for promotion of knowledge, attitudes and contraceptive practice among teenagers: a randomized clinical trial. *Nurse Education Today, 72*, 18–26.

Qin, C., Chen, W., Deng, Y., Li, Y., Mi, C., Sun, L., & Tang, S. (2019). Cognition, emotion, and behaviour in women undergoing pregnancy termination for foetal anomaly: a grounded theory analysis. *Midwifery, 68*, 84–90.

Saylor, J., Hanna, K., & Calamaro, C. (2019). Experiences of students who are newly diagnosed with type 1 diabetes mellitus. *Journal of Pediatric Nursing, 44*, 74–80.

Schoenfisch, A., Kucera, K., Lipscomb, H., McIlvaine, J., Becherer, L., James, T., & Avent, S. (2019). Use of assisteive devices to lift/transfer, and reposition hospital patients. *Nursing Research, 68,* 3–12.

Seifi, L., Najafi Ghezeljeh, T., & Haghani, H. (2018). Comparison of the effects of Benson muscle relaxation and nature sounds on the fatigue of patients with heart failure. *Holistic Nursing Practice, 32,* 27–34.

Varas-Díaz, N., Betancourt-Díaz, E., Lozano, A., Huang, L., DiNapoli, L., Hanlon, A., & Villaruel, A. (2019). Testing the efficacy of a web-based parent-adolescent sexual communication intervention among Puerto Ricans. *Family & Community Health, 42,* 30–43.

Zhou, Y., Liao, J., Feng, F., Ji, M., Zhao, C., & Wang, X. (2018). Effects of a nurse-led phone follow-up education program based on the self-efficacy among patients with cardiovascular disease. *Journal of Cardiovascular Nursing, 33,* E15–E23.

*A link to this open-access article is provided in the Toolkit for Chapter 1 in the Resource Manual. ✖

**This journal article is available on thePoint *for this chapter.*

Evidence-Based Nursing: Translating Research Evidence into Practice

Evidence-based practice (EBP) has been a major force in the health professions for the past few decades. In nursing, many organizations and initiatives have promoted EBP. For example, EBP has been named as one of the six core competencies in the Quality and Safety Education for Nurses (QSEN) initiative (Cronenwett, 2012).

This book will help you to develop skills to generate, and to evaluate, research evidence for nursing practice. Before we delve into the "how-tos" of research, we discuss key aspects of EBP to clarify the key role that research plays in EBP.

BACKGROUND OF EVIDENCE-BASED NURSING PRACTICE

This section provides a context for understanding evidence-based nursing practice and closely related concepts.

Definition of Evidence-Based Practice

Dozens of definitions of evidence-based practice have been proposed. Here is the one offered by Melnyk and Fineout-Overholt (2019) in their textbook on EBP: "A paradigm and lifelong problem-solving approach to clinical decision making that involves the conscientious use of the best available evidence (including a systematic search for and critical appraisal of the most relevant evidence to answer a clinical question) with one's own clinical expertise and patient values and preferences to improve outcomes for individuals, communities, and systems" (p. 753). This definition, like many others, declares that EBP is a *decision-making* (or *problem-solving*) *process*. Most definitions also include the idea that EBP is built on a "three-legged stool," each "leg" of which is essential to the process: *best evidence, clinical expertise*, and *patient preferences and values*. Figure 2.1 depicts these concepts.

> **TIP** Scott and McSherry (2009), in their review of evidence-based nursing concepts, identified 13 overlapping but distinct definitions of evidence-based nursing and EBP—and many more definitions have emerged. A few alternative definitions of EBP are presented in a table in the Toolkit of the accompanying *Resource Manual*.

Best Evidence
A basic feature of EBP as a clinical problem-solving strategy is that it de-emphasizes decisions based on tradition or expert opinions. The emphasis is on identifying and evaluating the best available research evidence as a tool for solving problems.

FIGURE 2.1 Evidence-based practice components.

> **TIP** The consequences of *not* using research evidence can be devastating. For example, from 1956 through the 1980s, Dr. Benjamin Spock—who was considered an expert on the care of infants—published a top-selling book, *Baby and Child Care*. Spock advised putting babies on their stomachs to sleep. In their systematic review, Gilbert and colleagues (2005) wrote, "Advice to put infants to sleep on the front for nearly half a century was contrary to evidence from 1970 that this was likely to be harmful" (p. 874). They estimated that if medical advice had been guided by research evidence, over 60,000 infant deaths might have been prevented.

There continues to be debate about what qualifies as "*best*" evidence. Numerous organizations and authors have created *evidence hierarchies* that rank evidence sources according to the degree to which they provide unbiased evidence to guide clinical decisions. We discuss evidence hierarchies in more detail later in this chapter. Evidence, however, whether "best" or not, is never by itself a sufficient basis for clinical decision-making.

Patient Values and Preferences
Patient-centered care has been defined by the Institute of Medicine (2001) as "providing care that is respectful of and responsive to individual patient preferences, needs and values, and ensuring that patient values *guide* all clinical decisions." Patient-centered care is an important feature of EBP.

"Patient preferences" encompass several concepts, including patient preferences for type of treatment; preferences for being involved in decision-making; patients' social or cultural values; preferences about involving family members in healthcare decisions; patients' priorities regarding quality of life issues; and their spiritual or religious values. Decisions also require understanding patients' circumstances, such as the resources at their disposal. Nurses thus need the skills to elicit and understand patient preferences—and to communicate information about "best evidence" to patients.

Clinical Expertise and Experiential Evidence
Decision-making in clinical practice ultimately relies on clinicians' expertise, which is an amalgam of academic knowledge gained during training and continuing education, experiences with patient care, and interdisciplinary sharing of new knowledge. David Sackett, the pioneer of evidence-based medicine, strongly advocated for the importance of clinical expertise in making decisions because even very strong research evidence may not be appropriate or applicable for individual patients.

Newhouse (2007) also stressed the importance of *experiential evidence*, which is internal evidence from local monitoring or evidence-gathering efforts, such as quality improvement projects. Clinical expertise and experiential evidence, combined with patient preferences, guide how "best evidence" can be used to make healthcare decisions.

Evidence-Based Practice and Related Concepts

During the 1980s, concern about research utilization began to emerge. **Research utilization (RU)** is the use of findings from a study in a practical application. In RU, the emphasis is on translating new knowledge into real-world applications. EBP is a broader concept than RU because it integrates research findings with other factors, as just noted. Also, whereas RU begins with the research itself

(How can I put this new knowledge to use in my clinical setting?), the start-point in EBP typically is a clinical question (What does the evidence suggest is the best approach to solving this clinical problem?).

During the 1980s and 1990s, RU projects were undertaken by numerous hospitals and nursing organizations. These projects were institutional attempts to implement changes in nursing practice based on research findings. During the 1990s, however, the call for research utilization was superseded by the push for EBP.

The EBP movement originated in the fields of medicine and epidemiology during the 1990s. British epidemiologist Archie Cochrane criticized healthcare practitioners for failing to incorporate research evidence into their decision-making. His work led to the establishment of the **Cochrane Collaboration**, an international partnership with centers established in 43 countries. The Collaboration prepares and disseminates reviews of research evidence and has a goal of making Cochrane "the home of evidence" relating to healthcare decision-making.

> **TIP** The Cochrane Collaboration publishes a series called *Making a Difference*, which presents stories of how evidence from Cochrane reviews has made impacts on real-world decision-making and patient outcomes. For example, one article in this series focused on the benefits of continuity of midwife care (http://www.cochrane.org/news/cochrane-making-difference-midwifery).

Also during the 1990s, a group from McMaster Medical School in Canada (led by Dr. David Sackett) developed a clinical learning strategy, which they called *evidence-based medicine*. The evidence-based medicine movement has shifted to a broader conception of using best evidence by all healthcare practitioners (not just physicians) in a multidisciplinary team. EBP is considered a major shift for healthcare education and practice. In the EBP environment, a skillful clinician can no longer rely on a repository of memorized information but rather must be a lifelong learner who is adept in accessing, evaluating, and using new evidence.

> **TIP** A debate has emerged concerning whether the term "evidence-based practice" should be replaced with "*evidence-informed practice*" (EIP). Those who advocate for EIP have argued that the word "based" suggests a stance in which patient preferences are not sufficiently considered in clinical decisions (e.g., Glasziou, 2005). Yet, as noted by Melnyk and Newhouse (2014), all current models of EBP incorporate clinicians' expertise and patients' preferences. They argued that "Changing terms now…will only create confusion at a critical time where progress is being made in accelerating EBP" (p. 348). We concur and use the term EBP throughout this book.

Knowledge translation (KT) is a related term that is often associated with efforts to enhance systematic change in clinical practice. The term was coined by the Canadian Institutes of Health Research (CIHR), which defined KT as "the exchange, synthesis, and ethically-sound application of knowledge—within a complex system of interactions among researchers and users—to accelerate the capture of the benefits of research for Canadians through improved health, more effective services and products, and a strengthened health care system" (CIHR, 2004). The World Health Organization (WHO) (2005) adapted the CIHR's definition and defined KT as "the synthesis, exchange, and application of knowledge by relevant stakeholders to accelerate the benefits of global and local innovation in strengthening health systems and improving people's health." Institutional projects aimed at KT often use methods and models that are similar to organizational EBP projects.

Translational research has emerged as a discipline devoted to developing methods to promote knowledge translation and the use of evidence. Translational science involves the study of interventions, implementation processes, and contextual factors that affect the uptake of new evidence in healthcare practice (Titler, 2014). In nursing, the need for translational research was an important impetus for the development of the Doctor of Nursing Practice degree. We discuss translational research in Chapter 11.

EBP can be undertaken by individual nurses working with patients or as a project taken on by a team within a healthcare organization. Organizational EBP projects share certain features with **quality improvement (QI)** efforts. We describe methodologic strategies for quality improvement in Chapter 12.

> **TIP** EBP is widely endorsed in nursing, but its adoption often faces many challenges. Some of the obstacles include nurses' lack of research appraisal skills; their misperceptions about EBP; heavy patient loads and lack of time; nurses' and administrators' resistance to change; and lack of autonomy about practice decisions. Factors that facilitate EBP include strong organizational support; the availability of EBP mentors and resources; collaboration among healthcare professionals; and participation in journal clubs (Gardner et al., 2016; Newhouse & Spring, 2010).

RESOURCES FOR EVIDENCE-BASED PRACTICE IN NURSING

Although EBP can present challenges to nurses, resources to support EBP are increasingly available. We offer some guidance and urge you to explore other ideas with your colleagues, mentors, and health information experts.

Preprocessed and Preappraised Evidence

Searching for best evidence requires skill, especially because of the accelerating pace of evidence production. Thousands of studies of relevance to nurses are published each month in professional journals. These **primary studies** are not preappraised for quality or clinical utility.

Fortunately, finding evidence useful for practice is often facilitated by the availability of evidence sources that are preprocessed (synthesized) and sometimes preappraised. DiCenso and colleagues (2009) have created a "6S" hierarchy of evidence sources, which is intended as a guide to evidence retrieval. The 6S hierarchy, typically shown as a pyramid, places five types of preprocessed evidence at the top, and individual studies at the bottom. The hierarchy is intended to help you see how to proceed with an evidence search. A clinician seeking evidence would start at the top of the hierarchy and work downward if appropriate evidence was lacking at a given level. Table 2.1 shows the **6S hierarchy** and provides examples at each level. In this section, we describe each evidence source, starting at the bottom of the hierarchy because higher levels build on the ones that precede them.

> **TIP** The 6S hierarchy does not imply a gradient of evidence in terms of *quality*, but rather in terms of ease in retrieving relevant evidence to address a clinical question. At all levels, the evidence should be assessed for quality and relevance.

Level 6 in the 6S Hierarchy: Single Studies

Reports describing a single original study are at the base of the 6S hierarchy because single studies are not ready for immediate use in making EBP decisions. At a minimum, individual primary studies need to be critically appraised for their rigor and their relevance to clinical problems. Clinicians searching for best evidence for a clinical query would start with a single study *only* if evidence from higher levels was unavailable or was judged to be flawed. We describe the major source of research reports (journal articles) in Chapter 3 and provide guidance in searching for studies in Chapter 5.

Level 5 in the 6S Hierarchy: Synopses of Single Studies

A synopsis of a study provides a brief overview of the research, often with sufficient detail to understand the evidence. As noted by DiCenso et al. (2009), a synopsis offers three advantages over the original report: (1) the brevity of the synopsis makes it more readily accessible to practitioners; (2) the study was likely chosen for abstraction because an expert believed the study was important; and (3) the synopsis is sometimes accompanied by commentary about the clinical utility of the evidence (i.e., preappraised). Several evidence-based journals include synopses of original studies, including *Evidence-Based Nursing, Evidence-Based*

TABLE 2.1 • The "6S" Hierarchy of Evidence Sources[a]

EVIDENCE SOURCE	DESCRIPTION/EXAMPLES	EXAMPLES OF RESOURCES
1. Systems ↓	• Computerized decision support systems	• In some electronic health records systems
2. Summaries ↓	• Evidence-based clinical practice guidelines • Online EBP summary resources	• U.S. National Guidelines Clearinghouse • Registered Nurses Association of Ontario Best Practices • EBSCO Nursing Reference Center; JBI COnNECT+; UpToDate
3. Synopses of syntheses ↓	• Synopses published in evidence-based abstraction journals or compiled by organizations	• *Evidence-Based Nursing* • DARE Database of Reviews of Evidence • The Centre for Reviews and Dissemination (CRD)
4. Syntheses ↓	• Systematic reviews • Rapid reviews	• Joanna Briggs Institute Database • Cochrane Database • AHRQ Evidence Reports • *BMC Systematic Reviews*
5. Synopses of studies ↓	• Brief summaries of single studies, often with commentary on clinical applicability	• *Evidence-Based Nursing* • *ACP Journal Club*
6. Single original studies	• Not preprocessed, primary studies published in journals	• PubMed (MEDLINE) • CINAHL

[a]The "6S" hierarchy depicting the efficiency of evidence retrieval for different sources was proposed by DiCenso et al., 2009.
AHRQ, Agency for Healthcare Research and Quality; EBP, evidence-based practice.

Midwifery, ACP Journal Club, and *The Online Journal of Knowledge Synthesis for Nursing*.

Level 4 in the 6S Hierarchy: Syntheses

Evidence-based practice relies on meticulous integration and synthesis of research evidence on a topic. The importance of such syntheses has given rise to many different types of research review (Grant & Booth, 2009), but the best known and most widely respected type of synthesis is the systematic review. A systematic review is not just a literature review, such as ones we describe in Chapter 5. A systematic review is in itself a methodical, scholarly inquiry that follows many of the same steps as those for primary studies and that yields a summary of current best evidence at the time the review was written. Chapter 30 offers guidance on conducting and critically appraising systematic reviews and describes a few other types of synthesis, such as *scoping reviews, realist reviews*, and *umbrella reviews*.

Systematic reviewers sometimes integrate findings from quantitative studies using statistical methods, in what is called a **meta-analysis**. Meta-analysts treat the findings from a study as one piece of information. The findings from multiple studies on the same topic are combined and analyzed statistically. Instead of individual people being the **unit**

of analysis (the basic entity of a statistical analysis) as in most primary studies, meta-analysts use findings from individual studies as the unit of analysis. Meta-analysis is an objective method of integrating a body of findings and of observing patterns that might otherwise have gone undetected.

Example of a Meta-Analysis

Zhang and colleagues (2018) conducted a meta-analysis of the effectiveness of psychological interventions for patients with osteoarthritis. Their analysis included findings from 12 randomized controlled trials. They found that psychological interventions could reduce pain and fatigue and improve self-efficacy, but the researchers concluded that better confirmatory evidence is needed.

Systematic reviews of qualitative studies often take the form of metasyntheses, which are rich resources for EBP (Beck, 2009). A **metasynthesis**, which involves integrating qualitative research findings on a topic, is less about reducing information and more about amplifying and interpreting it. For certain qualitative questions, an approach to systematic synthesis called **meta-aggregation** may be appropriate, as we describe in Chapter 30. Strategies have also been developed for **systematic mixed studies review** (also called *mixed research syntheses*), which are efforts to integrate and synthesize both quantitative and qualitative evidence on a topic (Heyvaert et al., 2017; Sandelowski et al., 2013).

Example of a Mixed Studies Review

Beck and Woynar (2017) conducted a mixed studies review on posttraumatic stress in mothers while their preterm infants are in the neonatal intensive care unit. They synthesized a total of 37 studies: 25 were quantitative and 12 were qualitative.

Many systematic reviews are published in professional research journals that can be accessed using standard literature search procedures; others are available in dedicated databases. A major example is the Cochrane Database of Systematic Reviews, which contains thousands of systematic reviews. Most Cochrane reviews involve meta-analyses, and most of them relate to healthcare interventions—but the Cochrane Collaboration

now also includes qualitative evidence syntheses. Cochrane reviews are done with great rigor and have the advantage of being checked and updated regularly.

In recent years, a type of synthesis called a **rapid review** (or *rapid evidence assessment*) has emerged (Khangura et al., 2012). These streamlined reviews are less rigorous than systematic reviews but are typically completed in a period of weeks, rather than months or years. Rapid reviews are described in Chapter 30.

TIP Many resources are available for finding systematic reviews. For example, the Joanna Briggs Institute in Australia (http://joannabriggs.org/) and the Centre for Reviews and Dissemination at the University of York in England (http://www.york.ac.uk/inst/crd/index.htm) produce useful systematic reviews. We provide links to many of these resources (as well as to other EBP-related websites) in the Toolkit of the accompanying *Resource Manual*.

Level 3 in the 6S Hierarchy: Synopses of Syntheses

Synopses of systematic reviews make rigorously integrated evidence even more handy for practitioners seeking answers to clinical queries. Many abstract journals mentioned in connection with Level 5 synopses of studies (e.g., *Evidence-Based Nursing, Evidence-Based Midwifery*) also include synopses of selected systematic reviews. The Cochrane Collaboration is working toward making their reviews more accessible by creating plain-language summaries of systematic review findings. A link to such a summary is included in the Toolkit of the accompanying *Resource Manual* ✪.

Level 2 in the 6S Hierarchy: Summaries

For some clinical questions, best evidence may be conveniently available in "Summaries," which include online EBP summary resources and clinical practice guidelines.

Dozens of evidence-based point-of-care resources for healthcare professionals have become available. These web-based resources are designed to provide rapidly accessible evidence-based information (and, sometimes, guidance) that is periodically updated. Campbell and colleagues (2015) undertook a quantitative evaluation of the content, breadth, quality, and rigor of 20 online point-of-care summary resources. Their assessment led them to conclude that the top five were UpToDate, Nursing Reference Center, Mosby's Nursing Consult, BMJ Best Practice, and the Joanna Briggs Institute's COnNECT+. Kwag and colleagues (2016), who focused on evidence summaries for physicians, also came to the conclusion that UpToDate and BMJ Best Practice were two of the best and most reliable resources out of the 23 they evaluated.

Evidence-based **clinical practice guidelines**, like systematic reviews, represent efforts to distill a large body of evidence into a manageable form, but guidelines differ from reviews in a number of respects. First, clinical practice guidelines, which are usually based on systematic reviews, give specific recommendations for evidence-based decision-making. Second, guidelines attempt to address all issues relevant to a clinical decision, including balancing benefits and risks. Third, systematic reviews are evidence-driven—that is, they are undertaken when a body of evidence has been produced and needs to be synthesized. Guidelines, by contrast, are "necessity-driven" (Straus et al., 2011, p. 125), meaning that guidelines are developed to guide clinical practice—even when available evidence is limited or of unexceptional quality. Fourth, systematic reviews are done by researchers, but guideline development typically involves the consensus of a group of researchers, experts, and clinicians. For this reason, guidelines based on the same evidence may result in different recommendations. Differences across guidelines sometimes reflect genuine contextual factors—for example, guidelines appropriate in the United States may be unsuitable in India.

It can be challenging to find clinical practice guidelines because there is no single guideline repository. One approach is to search for guidelines in comprehensive guideline databases. For example, in the United States, nursing and other healthcare guidelines are maintained by the National Guideline Clearinghouse (www.guideline.gov),

and similar databases are available in other countries. An important nursing guideline resource comes from the Registered Nurses Association of Ontario (RNAO) (www.rnao.org/bestpractices).

In addition to looking for guidelines in national clearinghouses and in the websites of professional organizations, you can search bibliographic databases such as MEDLINE or EMBASE. Search terms such as the following can be used: *practice guideline, clinical practice guideline, best practice guideline, evidence-based guideline*, and *consensus statement*. Be aware, though, that a standard search for guidelines in bibliographic databases will yield many references—but often a frustrating mixture of citations to not only the actual guidelines, but also to commentaries, anecdotes, implementation studies, and so on.

Example of a Nursing Clinical Practice Guideline

In 2017, the Registered Nurses Association of Ontario (RNAO) published the second edition of a best practice guideline called *"Adult asthma care: Promoting control of asthma."* The guideline is intended for use "by nurses and other members of the interprofessional healthcare team to enhance the quality of their practice pertaining to the assessment and management of adult asthma."

There are many topics for which practice guidelines have not yet been developed, but the opposite problem is also true: the dramatic increase in the number of guidelines means that there are sometimes multiple guidelines on the same topic. Worse yet, because of variation in the rigor of guideline development and in interpretations of the evidence, different guidelines sometimes offer different and even conflicting recommendations. Thus, those who wish to adopt clinical practice guidelines to address a clinical problem are urged to critically appraise them to identify ones that are based on the strongest and most up-to-date evidence, have been meticulously developed, are user-friendly, and are appropriate for local use.

Several guideline appraisal instruments are available, but the one that has gained the broadest support is the Appraisal of Guidelines Research and Evaluation (AGREE) Instrument, now in its second version (Brouwers et al., 2010). This tool has been translated into many languages and has been endorsed by the World Health Organization. Further information about the AGREE II instrument is provided in Supplement A to Chapter 2 on thePoint. 🅢 A shorter and simpler tool for evaluating guideline quality is called the iCAHE Guideline Quality Checklist (Grimmer et al., 2014). A "mini-checklist" (MIChe) for assessing guideline quality for daily practice use has also been proposed (Siebenhofer et al., 2016).

> **TIP** The U.S. Agency for Healthcare Research and Quality (AHRQ) offers "guideline syntheses" that provide systematic comparisons of agreement and disagreement among selected guidelines on the same topic (https://www.guidelines.gov/syntheses/index).

One final issue is that guidelines change more slowly than original research or syntheses. If a high-quality guideline is not recent, it is advisable to determine whether more up-to-date evidence would alter (or strengthen) the guideline's recommendations. It has been recommended that, to avoid obsolescence, guidelines should be reassessed every 3 years.

> **TIP** In addition to clinical guidelines, evidence-based **care bundles** are being developed. The concept of care bundles, developed by the Institute for Healthcare Initiatives (www.ihi.org), refers to a set of interventions to treat or prevent a specific cluster of symptoms. There is evidence that a bundle of strategies produces better outcomes than a single intervention.

Level 1 in the 6S Hierarchy: Systems

In a perfect world, evidence-based clinical information systems would link rigorous, up-to-date evidence (e.g., from summaries or syntheses) about a problem with information about a *particular* patient from the patient's electronic health record. Clinicians would then, with best evidence in hand, incorporate their own expertise and patient preferences in arriving at a course of action. Although few current systems match this ideal, some computerized decision support systems have been developed for particular problems, including decisional

support tools available on laptops and smartphones. We can expect progress on such systems in the years ahead.

> **Example of a Clinical Decision Support Systems**
> Gengo e Silva and colleagues (2018) described an electronic decision support system in a Brazilian hospital that links nursing diagnoses, outcomes, and interventions performed by nurses caring for medical and surgical patients.

Evidence Hierarchies and Level of Evidence Scales

The EBP movement has led to a proliferation of different **evidence hierarchies,** which are intended to show a ranking of evidence sources in terms of their risk of bias. (These are distinct from the 6S hierarchy discussed in the previous section, which rank evidence sources in terms of the ease and efficiency of finding answers to clinical questions.) Evidence hierarchies are often presented as pyramids, with the highest ranking sources—those presumed to have the least bias for making inferences about the effects of an intervention—at the top.

The hierarchies form **level of evidence (LOE) scales** that rank order types of evidence. Level I evidence usually is considered the best (least biased) type of evidence, and almost all leveling schemes put systematic reviews at the top level. Some LOE scales have only three levels, while others have 10 or more levels.

Figure 2.2 shows our eight-level evidence hierarchy for Therapy/intervention questions. This hierarchy ranks sources of evidence with respect to the *readiness* of an intervention to be put to use in practice. In our scheme, the Level I evidence source is a systematic review of a type of study called a *randomized controlled trial* (RCT), which is the "gold standard" type of study for Therapy questions. An individual RCT is a Level II evidence source in our hierarchy. Going down the "rungs" of the evidence hierarchy for Therapy questions results in evidence with a higher risk of bias in answering questions about "what works." For example, Level III evidence comes from a type of study called quasi-experiments (The terms in Figure 2.2 are explained

FIGURE 2.2 Polit–Beck evidence hierarchy/levels of evidence scale for therapy questions.

later in the book). Of course, there continue to be clinical practice questions for which there is relatively little research evidence. In such situations, nursing practice must rely on other sources, including internal evidence from pathophysiologic data, local projects, and expert opinion (Level VIII). As Straus and colleagues (2011) have noted, one benefit of the EBP movement is that a new research agenda can emerge when clinical questions arise for which there is no satisfactory evidence.

TIP Several alternative LOE scales that you may want to consider using are presented in the Toolkit in the accompanying *Resource Manual*.

Hierarchies and Level of Evidence Scales: Some Caveats

Although evidence hierarchies are intended as an EBP resource, considerable confusion exists regarding LOE scales. The fact that there are dozens from which to choose exacerbates this confusion.

One important issue that is seldom acknowledged is that different types of questions require different hierarchies. An evidence hierarchy for Prognosis questions, for example, is different from

the hierarchy for Therapy questions. The concept of evidence hierarchies arose in medicine, with the goal of informing decisions about medical interventions—thus early evidence hierarchies explicitly ranked evidence for Therapy/intervention questions. Few of the currently published hierarchies make this point clear, the major exceptions being the LOE hierarchies created by the Oxford Centre for Evidence-Based Medicine (http://www.cebm.net/ocebm-levels-of-evidence/) and the Joanna Briggs Institute (http://joannabriggs.org/jbi-approach.html). We also provide LOE scales in this book for different types of questions (see Chapter 9). As we noted in Chapter 1, evidence for non-Therapy questions can play a role in EBP, but such evidence does not directly support practice changes.

TIP As an example, if we wanted to know whether drinking alcohol during pregnancy puts the women at higher risk of a miscarriage (an Etiology question), we would not find "best evidence" from a systematic review of RCTs. Pregnant women would never be assigned at random to a "drinking" versus nondrinking condition to assess whether miscarriage rates are higher in the drinking group.

A second issue is that LOE scales have been used for different purposes. Some writers suggest that LOE scales are similar to the 6S hierarchy—the highest level offers the best starting place in a search for evidence. Others, however, use evidence hierarchies to "level" or grade evidence sources, implying that higher levels provide better quality evidence. As pointed out by Levin (2014), an evidence hierarchy "is not meant to provide a quality rating for evidence retrieved in the search for an answer" (p. 6). The Oxford Centre for Evidence-Based Medicine concurs: the levels in their scheme are "NOT intended to provide you with a definitive judgment about the quality of evidence. There will inevitably be cases where 'lower level' evidence…will provide stronger evidence than a 'higher level' study" (Howick et al., 2011, p. 2). A critical appraisal of each study or evidence source, regardless of level, is needed to make a final determination of the *quality of evidence*.

Related to this second issue is the fact that some LOE scales conflate risk of bias levels with terms implying quality. For example, in Melnyk and Fineout-Overholt's (2019) evidence hierarchy (Box 1.3), Level II is defined as *well-designed RCTs*.

Another word of caution: evidence hierarchies are seldom sufficiently detailed to include the full range of possible evidence sources. Users of LOE scales often must "read between the lines" and use some judgment. For example, in our hierarchy, if a systematic review included both RCTs *and* nonrandomized trials, we would still consider this Level I evidence. However, if a systematic review included several nonrandomized trials but no RCTs, we might consider this to be evidence somewhere between Levels I and II. As another example, in the Melnyk and Fineout-Overholt (2019) hierarchy, there is no level specified for RCTs that are not especially "well-designed."

As noted by Levin (2014), those who wish to use an LOE scale must choose one that matches their needs from the many that exist, keeping in mind that "leveling" a study based on the chosen scale is not a substitute for a critical appraisal of the evidence.

TIP Evidence hierarchies and LOE scales are rather firmly entrenched in the EBP literature, but they are not without controversy. Concern was expressed initially by critics who felt that qualitative evidence was being undervalued. For example, for Therapy questions, qualitative studies are typically near the bottom of the hierarchy. Another criticism of these ranking systems is that they focus exclusively on the risk of certain types of bias, but not on biases that might undermine the applicability of evidence in real-world settings (e.g., Goodman, 2014). We discuss this important concern about EBP in Chapter 31.

Systems for a Body of Evidence

It is important to note that LOE scales are typically used to "level" an individual piece of evidence, such as a single study. Other systems exist, however, for grading an entire body of evidence with regard to the *strength of evidence*. By far the most widely used system is the Grading of Recommendations Assessment, Development, and Evaluation (GRADE) system (Guyatt et al., 2008). The GRADE system involves two components—grading the quality of an overall body of evidence and ranking the strength of recommendations based on that evidence. GRADE is used with increasing frequency in systematic reviews and in the development of clinical practice guidelines. We discuss GRADE at some length in Chapter 30.

Models for Evidence-Based Practice

Models of EBP are important resources for designing and implementing EBP projects in practice settings. Some models focus on the use of research from the perspective of individual clinicians (e.g., the Stetler Model), but most focus on institutional EBP efforts (e.g., the Iowa Model). Another way to categorize existing models is to distinguish process-oriented models (e.g., the Iowa Model) and models that are explicitly mentor models, such as the ARCC-E (Advanced Research and Clinical Practice Through Close Collaboration in Education) model.

The many worthy EBP models are too numerous to list comprehensively, but a few are shown in Box 2.1. Melnyk and Fineout-Overholt (2019)

BOX 2.1 Selected Models for Evidence-Based Practice

- ACE Star Model of Knowledge Transformation (Stevens, 2012)
- Advancing Research and Clinical Practice Through Close Collaboration in Education (ARCC-E) Model (Melnyk & Fineout-Overholt, 2019)
- Diffusion of Innovations Model (Rogers, 1995)
- Iowa Model of Evidence-Based Practice to Promote Quality Care (Buckwalter et al., 2017; Titler et al., 2001)
- Johns Hopkins Nursing EBP Model (Dearholt & Deng, 2012)
- Promoting Action on Research Implementation in Health Services (PARiHS) Model (Harvey & Kitson, 2016; Rycroft-Malone et al., 2013),
- Stetler Model of Research Utilization (Stetler, 2010)

provide a good synthesis of several EBP models, and Schaffer and colleagues (2013) identify features to consider in selecting a model to plan an EBP project. Although each model offers different perspectives on how to translate research findings into practice, several of the steps and procedures are similar across the models. Figure 2.3 shows a diagram of one prominent EBP model, the revised **Iowa Model** of EBP (Buckwalter et al., 2017).

Example of Using an Evidence-Based Practice Model

Saqe-Rockoff and colleagues (2018) used the Iowa Model in their EBP project designed to improve thermoregulation for trauma patients in the emergency department.

INDIVIDUAL AND ORGANIZATIONAL EVIDENCE-BASED PRACTICE

Individual nurses make many decisions and convey important healthcare information and advice to patients, and so they have ample opportunity to put research into practice. Here are three clinical scenarios that provide examples of such opportunities:

- Clinical Scenario 1. You work in an allergy clinic and notice how difficult it is for many children to undergo allergy scratch tests. You wonder if an interactive distraction intervention would help reduce children's anxiety when they are being tested.

- Clinical Scenario 2. You work in a rehabilitation hospital, and one of your elderly patients, who had total hip replacement, tells you she is planning a long airplane trip to visit her daughter after rehabilitation treatments are completed. You know that a long plane ride will increase her risk of deep vein thrombosis and wonder if compression stockings are an effective in-flight treatment for her. You decide to look for the best evidence to answer this question.

- Clinical Scenario 3. You are caring for a hospitalized cardiac patient who tells you that he has sleep apnea. He confides in you that he is reluctant to undergo continuous positive airway pressure (CPAP) treatment because he worries it will hinder intimacy with his wife. You wonder if there is any evidence about what it is like to experience CPAP treatment so that you can better address your patient's concerns.

In these and thousands of other clinical situations, research evidence can be put to good use to improve the quality of nursing care. Thus, individual nurses need to have the skills to personally search for, appraise, and apply evidence in their practice.

For some clinical scenarios that trigger an EBP effort, individual nurses have sufficient autonomy to implement research-informed actions on their own (e.g., answering patients' questions about experiences with CPAP). In other situations, however, decisions are best made among a team of nurses (or with an interprofessional team) working together to solve a common clinical problem. Institutional EBP efforts typically result in a formal policy or protocol affecting the practice of many nurses and other staff.

The Iowa Model Revised: Evidence-Based Practice to Promote Excellence in Health Care

Identify Triggering Issues / Opportunities
- Clinical or patient identified issue
- Organization, state, or national initiative
- Data / new evidence
- Accrediting agency requirements / regulations
- Philosophy of care

State the Question or Purpose

Is this topic a priority?
- No → **Consider another Issue / opportunity**
- Yes ↓

Form a Team

Assemble, Appraise and Synthesize Body of Evidence
- Conduct systematic search
- Weigh quality, quantity, consistency, and risk

← **Reassemble**

Is there sufficient evidence?
- No → **Conduct research**
- Yes ↓

Design and Pilot the Practice Change
- Engage patients and verify preferences
- Consider resources, constraints, and approval
- Develop localized protocol
- Create an evaluation plan
- Collect baseline data
- Develop an implementation plan
- Prepare clinicians and materials
- Promote adoption
- Collect and report post-pilot data

← **Redesign**

Is change appropriate for adoption in practice?
- No → **Consider alternatives**
- Yes ↓

Integrate and Sustain the Practice Change
- Identify and engage key personnel
- Hardwire change into system
- Monitor key indicators through quality improvement
- Reinfuse as needed

Disseminate Results

◆ = a decision point

DO NOT REPRODUCE WITHOUT PERMISSION

©University of Iowa Hospitals and Clinics, Revised June 2015
To request permission to use or reproduce, go to
https://uihc.org/evidence-based-practice/

FIGURE 2.3 Revised Iowa Model of Evidence-Based Practice to Promote Quality Care Iowa Model Collaborative. (2017). Iowa model of evidence-based practice: revisions and validation. *Worldviews on Evidence-Based Nursing*, 14(3), 175-182. doi:10.1111/wvn.12223. Used/reprinted with permission from the University of Iowa Hospitals and Clinics, copyright 2015. For permission to use or reproduce, please contact the University of Iowa Hospitals and Clinics at 319-384-9098.

Many of the steps in institutional EBP projects are the same as those we describe in the next section, but additional issues are of relevance at the organizational level. For example, as shown in the Iowa Model (Figure 2.3), some of the activities include assessing whether the question is an organizational priority, forming a team, and conducting a formal evaluation. We offer further information about organizational EBP efforts in Supplement B for Chapter 2 on thePoint 🅢.

MAJOR STEPS IN EVIDENCE-BASED PRACTICE

In this section, we provide an overview of how research evidence can be put to use in clinical settings. In describing the basic steps in the EBP process, we use a mnemonic device (the 5As) that we have adapted from several sources (e.g., Guyatt et al., 2015; EBP blogs by nurse educator Cathy Thompson [https://nursingeducationexpert.com]).

- Step 1: **Ask**—Ask a well-worded clinical question that can be answered with research evidence;
- Step 2: **Acquire**—Search for and retrieve the best evidence to answer the clinical question;
- Step 3: **Appraise**—Critically appraise the evidence for validity and applicability to the problem and situation;
- Step 4: **Apply**—After integrating the evidence with clinical expertise, patient preferences, and local context, apply it to clinical practice; and
- Step 5: **Assess**—Evaluate the outcome of the practice change.

The EBP process cannot be undertaken in a vacuum, however. A precondition for the entire undertaking is to have an openness to change and a desire to provide the best possible care, based on evidence showing benefits to patient outcomes. Melnyk and Fineout-Overholt (2019) call this Step 0: Cultivating a spirit of inquiry. Johnson and Fineout-Overholt (2005) noted that "getting from zero to one" involves having nurses be reflective about their clinical practice. An additional step after Step 5 might be to disseminate information about the EBP project.

Step 1: Ask a Well-worded Clinical Question

A crucial first step in EBP involves converting information needs into well-worded clinical questions that can be answered with research evidence. You might wonder, though, where do the questions come from? Some EBP models distinguish two types of "triggers" for an EBP undertaking: (1) *problem-focused triggers*—a clinical practice problem in need of solution, or (2) *knowledge-focused triggers*—readings in the research literature. Problem-focused triggers may arise in the normal course of clinical practice and include both patient-identified and clinician-identified issues. The Iowa Model (Figure 2.3) includes examples of both types of trigger in the top box.

EBP experts distinguish between background and foreground questions. *Background questions* are foundational questions about a clinical issue, for example: What is cancer cachexia (progressive body wasting), and what is its pathophysiology? Answers to such background questions are typically found in textbooks. *Foreground questions,* by contrast, are those that can be answered based on current research evidence on diagnosing, assessing, or treating patients, or on understanding the meaning or prognosis of their health problems. For example, we may wonder, is a fish oil–enhanced nutritional supplement effective in stabilizing weight in patients with advanced cancer? The answer to such a Therapy question may provide direction on how to address the needs of patients with cachexia. In other words, foreground questions seek the specific information needed to make clinical decisions.

Most guidance for EBP uses the acronyms PIO and PICO to help practitioners develop well-worded questions. In the PICO form, the clinical question is worded to identify four components:

1. P: the *Population* or *patients* (What are key characteristics of the patients or people?)
2. I: the *Intervention*, *influence*, or *exposure* (What is the intervention or therapy of interest? Or what is a potentially harmful or beneficial influence?)
3. C: an explicit *Comparison* to the "I" component (With what is the intervention or influence being compared?)
4. O: the *Outcome* (What is the outcome or consequence in which we are interested?)

Applying this scheme to our question about cachexia, our *population* (P) is cancer patients with cachexia; the *intervention* (I) is fish oil–enhanced nutritional supplements; and the *outcome* (O) is weight stabilization. In this question, the *comparison* is not formally stated, but the implied "C" is the *absence* of fish oil–enhanced supplements—the question is in a PIO format. However, when there is an explicit comparison of interest, the full PICO question is required. For example, we might be interested in learning whether fish oil–enhanced supplements (I) are better than melatonin (C) in stabilizing weight (O) in patients with cancer (P).

For questions that can best be answered with qualitative information (e.g., about the meaning of an experience or health problem), two components are most relevant:

1. the *population* (What are the characteristics of the patients or clients?) and
2. the *situation* (What conditions, experiences, or circumstances are we interested in understanding?)

For example, suppose our question was "What is it like to suffer from cachexia?" In this case, the question calls for rich qualitative information; the *population* is patients with advanced cancer, and the *situation* is the experience of cachexia.

In addition to the basic PICO components, other components may be used in an evidence search. For example, some EBP experts suggest adding a "T" component (PICOT) to designate a time frame. For example, take the following question: Among caregivers of people with dementia (P), what is the effect of participation in a caregiver intervention (I), compared with not participating in the intervention (C) on quality of life (O) 6 months after enrollment (T)? Other experts, however, consider the time frame as part of the outcome: e.g., quality of life 6 months after enrollment (O). Still others prefer to search for the PICO elements without filtering out evidence from studies that used a different period of follow-up, such as 4 months after enrollment.

TIP The Cochrane Collaboration has launched a PICO project—a *Strategy to 2020* initiative—to annotate its systematic reviews with PICO component identification to facilitate retrieval efforts.

Table 2.2 offers question templates for asking well-framed clinical foreground questions for specific types of questions. The right-hand column includes questions with an explicit comparison (PICO questions), while the middle column does not (PIO). The questions are categorized in a manner similar to that discussed in Chapter 1 (EBP purposes), as featured in Table 1.3. Note that although there are some differences in components across question types, there is always a P component.

TIP The Toolkit for Chapter 2 in the accompanying *Resource Manual* includes Table 2.2 in a Word file that can be adapted for your use, so that the template questions can be readily "filled in." .

Step 2: Acquire Research Evidence

By asking clinical questions in a well-worded form, you should be able to more effectively search the research literature for the information you need. Using the templates in Table 2.2, the information inserted into the blanks constitutes *keywords* for undertaking an electronic search.

Earlier in this chapter, we described resources to facilitate an efficient search for evidence. As shown in the 6S hierarchy (Table 2.1), there is a range of preappraised evidence sources that can help you acquire evidence regarding your question. Starting with preappraised evidence might lead you to a quick answer—and potentially to a better answer than would be possible if you had to start at the bottom rung with individual studies. Researchers who prepare systematic reviews and synopses usually have excellent research skills and use established standards to evaluate the evidence. Thus, when preprocessed evidence is available to answer a clinical question, you may not need to look any farther, unless the review is not recent or is of poor quality. When high-quality preprocessed evidence cannot be located or is old, you will need to look for best evidence in primary studies, using strategies we describe in Chapter 5.

TABLE 2.2 • Question Templates for Selected Clinical Foreground Questions: PIO and PICO

TYPE OF QUESTION	PIO QUESTION TEMPLATE (QUESTIONS WITHOUT AN EXPLICIT COMPARISON)	PICO QUESTION TEMPLATE (QUESTIONS WITH AN EXPLICIT COMPARISON)
Therapy/ treatment/ intervention	In _____ (**Population**), what is the effect of _____ (**Intervention**) on _____ (**Outcome**)?	In _____ (**Population**), what is the effect of _____ (**Intervention**), in comparison to _____ (**Comparative/alternative** intervention), on _____ (**Outcome**)?
Diagnosis/ assessment	For _____ (**Population**), does _____ (**Identifying tool/** procedure) yield accurate and appropriate diagnostic/assessment information about _____ (**Outcome**)?	For _____ (**Population**), does _____ (**Identifying tool/** procedure) yield more accurate or more appropriate diagnostic/ assessment information than _____ (**Comparative tool/** procedure) about _____ (**Outcome**)?
Prognosis	In _____ (**Population**), does _____ (**Influence/exposure to** disease or condition) increase the risk of _____ (**Outcome**)?	In _____ (**Population**), does _____ (**Influence/exposure to** disease or condition), relative to _____ (**Comparative disease/** condition OR absence of the disease/ condition) increase the risk of _____ (**Outcome**)?
Etiology/ harm	In _____ (**Population**), does _____ (**Influence/exposure/** characteristic) increase the risk of _____ (**Outcome**)?	In _____ (**Population**), does _____ (**Influence/exposure/** characteristic) compared to _____ (**Comparative influence/** exposure OR lack of influence or exposure) increase the risk of _____ (**Outcome**)?
Description (prevalence/ incidence)	In _____ (**Population**), how prevalent is _____ (**Outcome**)?	*Explicit comparisons are not typical, except to compare different populations*
Meaning or process	What is it like for _____ (**Population**) to experience (condition, illness, circumstance)? OR What is the process by which _____ (**Population**) cope with, adapt to, or live with (condition, illness, circumstance)?	*Explicit comparisons are not typical in these types of questions*

TIP In Chapter 5, we describe the free internet resource, PubMed, which offers a special
tool for those seeking evidence for clinical decisions. Guidance on conducting a clinical query
search is provided in the online Supplement A
to Chapter 5. **$** Another important database,
CINAHL, allows users to restrict a search with an
"EBP" limiter.

Step 3: Appraise the Evidence

The evidence acquired in Step 2 of the EBP process
should be appraised before taking clinical action.
Critical appraisal for EBP may involve several types
of assessments. Various criteria have been proposed
for EBP appraisals, including the following:

1. *Quality:* To what extent is the evidence valid—
   that is, how serious is the risk of bias?
2. *Magnitude:* How large is the effect of the intervention or influence (I) on the outcome (O) in
   the population of interest (P)? Are the effects
   clinically significant?
3. *Quantity:* How much evidence is there? How many
   studies have been conducted, and did those studies
   involve a large number of study participants?
4. *Consistency:* How consistent are the findings
   across various studies?
5. *Applicability:* To what extent is the evidence relevant to my clinical situation and patients?

Evidence Quality

The first appraisal issue is the extent to which the
findings in a research report are valid. That is, were
the study methods sufficiently rigorous that the evidence has a low risk of bias? Melnyk and Fineout-
Overholt (2019) propose the following formula:
Level of evidence (e.g., Figure 2.2) + quality of
evidence = strength of evidence. Thus, in coming
to a conclusion about the quality of the evidence, it
is insufficient to simply "level" the evidence using
an LOE scale—it must also be appraised. We offer
guidance on appraising the quality of evidence from
primary studies throughout this book, and Chapter
5 includes an appraisal worksheet.

   If there are several primary studies and no existing systematic review, you would need to draw

conclusions about the body of evidence taken as a
whole. The previously mentioned GRADE system
(Guyatt et al., 2008) is being used increasingly to
summarize evidence quality for a body of evidence
in systematic reviews (Chapter 30).

Magnitude of Effects

The appraisal criterion relating to magnitude considers how powerful the effects of an intervention
or influence are. Estimating the magnitude of the
effect for quantitative findings is especially important when an intervention is costly or when there
are potentially negative side effects. If, for example, there is good evidence that an intervention is
only marginally effective in improving a health
problem, it is important to consider other factors
(e.g., evidence regarding its effects on quality of
life). There are various ways to quantify the magnitude of effects, such as an *effect size index* that we
describe later in this book.

   The magnitude of effects also has a bearing on
clinical significance. We discuss how to assess the
clinical significance of study findings in Chapter 21.

Quantity and Consistency of Evidence

A rigorously conducted primary study of a randomized controlled trial offers especially strong
evidence about the effect of an intervention on an
outcome of interest. But *multiple* RCTs are better
than a single study. Moreover, large-scale studies
(such as multisite studies) with a large number of
study participants are especially desirable.

   If there are multiple studies that address your
clinical query, however, the strength of the evidence
is likely to be diminished if there are inconsistent results across studies. In the GRADE system,
inconsistency of results leads to a lower quality-of-
evidence grade. When the results of different studies do not corroborate each other, it is likely that
further research will have an impact on confidence
about an intervention's effect.

Applicability

It is also important to appraise the evidence in
terms of its relevance for the clinical situation at
hand—that is, for *your* patient in a specific clinical
setting. Best practice evidence can most readily be

applied to an individual patient in your care if he or she is similar to people in the study or studies under review. Would your patient have qualified for participation in the study—or is there some factor such as age, illness severity, or comorbidity that would have excluded him or her? Practitioners must reach conclusions about the applicability of research evidence, but researchers also bear some responsibility for enhancing the applicability of their work. As we discuss in Chapter 31, concerns about the fact that "best evidence" is usually about "average" patients from restricted populations has made the issue of applicability increasingly salient.

> **TIP** An appraisal of evidence for use in your practice may involve additional factors. In particular, costs are likely to be an important consideration. Some interventions are expensive, and so the amount of resources needed to put best evidence into practice would need to be factored into any decision. Of course, the cost of *not* taking action is also important.

Actions Based on Evidence Appraisals

Appraisals of the evidence may lead you to different courses of action. You may reach this point and conclude that the evidence is not sufficiently sound, or that the likely effect is too small, or that the cost of applying the evidence is too high. The evidence may suggest that "usual care" is the best strategy—or it may lead you to pose an alternative clinical query. You may also consider the possibility of undertaking your own study to add to the body of evidence relating to your original clinical question. If, however, the initial appraisal of evidence suggests a promising clinical action, then you can proceed to the next step.

Step 4: Apply the Evidence

As the definition for EBP implies, research evidence needs to be integrated with your own clinical expertise and knowledge of your clinical setting. You may be aware of factors that would make implementation of the evidence, no matter how sound or promising, inadvisable. Patient preferences and values are also important. A discussion with the patient may reveal negative attitudes toward a potentially beneficial course of action, contraindications (e.g., comorbidities), or possible impediments (e.g., lack of health insurance).

Armed with rigorous evidence, your own clinical know-how, and information about your patient's circumstances, you can use the resulting information to make an evidence-based decision or provide research-informed advice. Although the steps in the process, as just described, may seem complicated, in reality the process can be efficient—*if* there is an adequate evidence base and especially if it has been skillfully preprocessed. EBP is most challenging when findings from research are contradictory, inconclusive, or "thin"—that is to say, when better quality evidence is needed.

One final issue is the importance of integrating evidence from qualitative research, which can provide rich insights about how patients experience a problem, or about barriers to complying with a treatment. A new intervention with strong potential benefits may fail to achieve desired outcomes if it is not implemented with sensitivity and understanding of the patients' perspectives. As Morse (2005) so aptly noted, evidence from an RCT may tell you whether a pill is effective, but qualitative research can help you understand why patients may not swallow the pill.

Step 5: Assess the Outcomes of the Practice Change

One last step in many EBP efforts concerns evaluating the outcomes of the practice change. Did you achieve the desired outcomes? Were patients satisfied with the results?

Straus and colleagues (2011) remind us that part of the ongoing evaluation involves how well you are performing EBP. They offer self-evaluation questions that relate to the EBP steps, such as asking answerable questions (Am I asking any clinical questions at all? Am I asking well-formulated question?) and acquiring external evidence (Do I know the best sources of current evidence? Am I becoming more efficient in my searching?).

TIP Every nurse can play a role in using research evidence. Here are some strategies:

- *Read widely and critically.* Professionally accountable nurses keep abreast of important research developments relating to their specialty by reading professional journals.
- *Attend professional conferences.* Conference attendees have opportunities to meet researchers and to explore practice implications of new research.
- *Insist on evidence that a procedure is effective.* Every time nurses or nursing students are told about a standard nursing procedure, they have a right to ask: Why? Nurses need to develop expectations that the clinical decisions they make are based on sound, evidence-based rationales.
- *Become involved in a journal club.* Many organizations that employ nurses sponsor journal clubs that review studies with potential relevance to practice.
- *Pursue and participate in EBP projects.* Several studies have found that nurses who are involved in research activities (e.g., an EBP project or data collection activities) develop more positive attitudes toward research and better research skills.

RESEARCH EXAMPLE

Thousands of EBP projects are underway in practice settings. Many that have been described in the nursing literature offer information about planning and implementing such an endeavor. One is described here, and another full article is included in the *Resource Manual.*

Study: Implementation of the MEDFRAT to promote quality care and decrease falls in community hospital emergency rooms (McCarty et al., 2018).

Purpose: An interprofessional team undertook an evidence-based practice implementation project at a large healthcare delivery system with 12 emergency departments (EDs). The focus of the project was to decrease falls in community hospital EDs.

Framework: The project used the Iowa Model as its guiding framework. The EBP team identified a problem-focused trigger—the inconsistent use of fall-risk assessments and variation in falls in the EDs.

Approach: The project team assembled relevant literature to identify an appropriate assessment tool for use in emergency departments. The team selected the Memorial Emergency Department Fall-Risk Assessment Tool (MEDFRAT) because it was simple to use (only six questions) and had been validated for use in EDs (i.e., it had evidence-based utility). The tool creates two risk-stratification levels, and each has suggested fall-risk prevention interventions. For example, possible interventions included hourly rounding, bed in low position, bedside alarms, and locating patients into view of the nurses' station. Information systems staff built the MEDFRAT into the electronic medical record. The team then created and implemented a 1-hour education session about falls for nurses in the EDs. The EDs in the project were visited over a 4-month period, with 60 nurses attending the sessions. The participating nurses offered feedback and further suggestions. Several nurses mentioned the lack of bedside alarms, and so portable alarms were ordered. Another suggestion concerned the use of different colored grip socks to identify patients at high risk of a fall. Overall, the nurses' reactions to MEDFRAT were unanimously positive.

Evaluation: The MEDFRAT has been implemented in all 12 EDs in the system. Baseline levels of falls in the ED over a 4-year period ranged from 0 (in EDs with under 10 beds) to 76 in the ED with the most beds. Data regarding the effectiveness of the intervention were not available when the report was written, but short-term outcomes and longer-term outcomes (decrease in ED falls) are being monitored.

Conclusions: The authors of the report concluded that the Iowa Model was a useful framework. They were optimistic about the outcomes and about using the Iowa Model to implement other evidence-based nursing interventions in their setting.

SUMMARY POINTS

- **Evidence-based practice (EBP)** is the conscientious integration of current best evidence and other factors in making clinical decisions. The three main components of EBP are (1) best research evidence; (2) your own clinical experience and knowledge; and (3) patient preferences, values, and circumstances.

- Two underpinnings of the EBP movement are the **Cochrane Collaboration** (which is based on the work of British epidemiologist Archie Cochrane) and the clinical learning strategy called *evidence-based medicine* developed at the McMaster Medical School.

- **Research utilization (RU)** and EBP are overlapping concepts that concern efforts to use research as a basis for clinical decisions, but RU *starts* with a research-based innovation that gets evaluated for possible use in practice.

- **Knowledge translation (KT)** is a term used primarily about system-wide efforts to enhance systematic change in clinical practice or policies. **Translational research** is a discipline devoted to developing methods to promote knowledge translation and the use of evidence.

- Resources to support EBP are growing at a phenomenal pace. Preprocessed (synthesized) and preappraised evidence is especially useful and efficient in addressing clinical queries. The **6S hierarchy** of preappraised evidence offers a guide for efficient evidence searches. This hierarchy includes (6) systems at the pinnacle; (5) summaries; (4) synopses of syntheses; (3) syntheses; (2) synopses of single studies; and (1) individual primary studies, which are not preappraised, at the base.

- Systematic reviews (Syntheses) have been considered the cornerstone of EBP. **Systematic reviews** are rigorous integrations of research evidence from multiple studies on a topic. Systematic reviews can involve either narrative approaches to integration (including **metasynthesis** and **meta-aggregation** of qualitative studies) or quantitative methods (**meta-analysis**) that integrate findings statistically by using individual studies as the **unit of analysis**. The emergence of **rapid reviews** reflects the need for less rigorous, but more timely, syntheses of evidence.

- Evidence-based **clinical practice guidelines** are a major example of preappraised evidence

in the "Summaries" category of the 6S hierarchy. These guidelines combine a synthesis and appraisal of research evidence from a systematic review with specific recommendations for clinical decision-making. Clinical practice guidelines should be carefully and systematically appraised, for example, using the Appraisal of Guidelines Research and Evaluation (*AGREE II*) instrument.

- The EBP movement has given rise to a proliferation of **evidence hierarchies** that provide a preliminary guidepost for finding "best" evidence—evidence with the lowest risk of bias. Evidence hierarchies reflect **level of evidence (LOE) scales** that rank order types of evidence source. Most published LOE scales are appropriate only for Therapy/intervention questions. In LOEs for Therapy questions, systematic reviews of *randomized controlled trials* (RCTs) are considered Level I sources. However, at every level, the quality of the evidence must be appraised: Strength of evidence = level + quality.

- Many models of EBP have been developed, including models that provide a framework for individual clinicians (e.g., the **Stetler model**) and others for organizations or teams of clinicians (e.g., the **Iowa Model** of Evidence-Based Practice to Promote Quality Care).

- Although organizational projects include additional steps, the most basic steps in EBP for both individuals and team are as follows (the 5As): *Ask* a well-worded clinical question; *Acquire* the best evidence to answer the question; *Appraise* and synthesize the evidence; *Apply* the evidence, after integrating it with patient preferences and clinical expertise; and *Assess* the effects of the practice change.

- A widely used scheme for asking well-worded clinical questions involves four primary components, an acronym for which is **PICO**: Population or patients (P), Intervention or influence (I), Comparison (C), and Outcome (O).

- An appraisal of the evidence involves such considerations as the quality of the evidence, in terms of the risk of bias; the magnitude of the effects and their clinical importance;

the quantity of evidence; the consistency of evidence across studies; and the applicability of the evidence to particular settings and patients.

STUDY ACTIVITIES

Study activities are available to instructors on thePoint.

REFERENCES CITED IN CHAPTER 2

Beck C. (2009). Metasynthesis: a goldmine for evidence-based practice. *AORN Journal*, 90, 701–702.

Beck C. T., & Woynar J. (2017). Posttraumatic stress in mothers while their preterm infants are in the newborn intensive care unit: a mixed research synthesis. *Advances in Nursing Science*, 40, 337–355.

*Brouwers M., Kho M., Browman G., Burgers J., Cluzeau F., Feder G., … Zitzelsberger L. for the AGREE Next Steps Consortium. (2010). AGREE II: advancing guideline development, reporting and evaluation in health care. *Canadian Medical Association Journal*, 182, E839–E842.

Buckwalter K., Cullen L., Hanrahan K., Kleiber C., McCarthy A., Rakel B., … Tucker S. (2017). Iowa model of evidence-based practice: revisions and validation. *Worldviews on Evidence-Based Nursing*, 14, 175–182.

Campbell J. M., Umapathysivam K., Xue Y., & Lockwood C. (2015). Evidence-based practice point-of-care resources: a quantitative evaluation of quality, rigor, and content. *Worldviews on Evidence-Based Nursing*, 12, 313–327.

CIHR (2004). *Knowledge translation strategy 2004–2009: innovation in action*. Ottawa, ON: Canadian Institutes of Health Research.

Cronenwett L. R. (2012). A national initiative: quality and safety education for nurses (QSEN). In Sherwood G., & Barnsteiner J. (Eds.), *Quality and safety in nursing: a competency approach to improving outcomes*. Ames, IA: John Wiley & Sons.

Dearholt D., & Dang D,. (Eds.). (2012). *Johns Hopkins nursing evidence-based practice: model and guidelines*. Indianapolis, IN: Sigma Theta Tau International.

DiCenso A., Bayley L., & Haynes B. (2009). Accessing pre-appraised evidence: fine-tuning the 5S model into a 6S model. *Evidence-based Nursing*, 12, 99–101.

Gardner K., Kanaskie M., Knehans A., Salisbury S., Doheny K., & Schirm V. (2016). Implementing and syustaining evidence based practice through a nursing journal club. *Applied Nursing Research*, 31, 139–145.

Gengo e Silva R., Dos Santos Diogo R., da Cruz D., Ortiz D., Ortiz D., Peres H., & Moorhead S. (2018). Linkages of nursing diagnoses, outcomes, and interventions performed by nurses caring for medical and surgical patients using a decision support system. *International Journal of Nursing Knowledge*, 29, 269–275.

*Gilbert R., Salanti G., Harden M., & See S. (2005). Infant sleeping position and the sudden infant death syndrome: systematic review of observational studies and historical review of recommendations from 1940 to 2002. *International Journal of Epidemiology*, 34, 874–887.

Glasziou P. (2005). Evidence-based medicine: does it make a difference? Make it evidence informed with a little wisdom. *British Medical Journal*, 330(7482), 92.

*Goodman C. S. (2014). *HTA 101: introduction to health technology assessment*. Washington, DC: National Information Center on Health Services Research and Health Care Technology.

*Grant M., & Booth A. (2009). A typology of reviews: an analysis of 14 review types and associated methodologies. *Health Information and Libraries Journal*, 26, 91–108.

*Grimmer K., Dizon J., Milanese S., King E., Beaton K., Thorpe O., … Kumar S. (2014). Efficient clinical evaluation of guideline quality: development and testing of a new tool. *BMC Medical Research Methodology*, 14, 63.

*Guyatt G., Oxman A., Vist G., Kunz R., Falck-Ytter Y., Alonso-Coello P., … GRADE Working Group (2008). GRADE: an emerging consensus on rating quality of evidence and strength of recommendations. *BMJ*, 336, 924–926.

Guyatt G., Rennie D., Meade M., & Cook D. (2015). *Users' guide to the medical literature: essentials of evidence-based clinical practice* (3rd ed.). New York: McGraw Hill.

*Harvey G., & Kitson A. (2016). PARIHS revisited: from heuristic to integrated framework for the successful implementation of knowledge into practice. *Implementation Science*, 11, 33.

Heyvaert M., Hannes K., & Onghena P. (2017). *Using mixed methods research synthesis for literature reviews*. Los Angeles: Sage Publications.

*Howick J., Chalmers I., Glasziou P., Greenhalgh T., Heneghan C., Liberati A., … Thornton H. (2011).*The 2011 Oxford CEBM levels of evidence: introductory document*. Oxford: Centre for Evidence-Based Medicine.

*Institute of Medicine. (2001). *Crossing the quality chasm: a new health care system for the 21st century*. Washington, DC: National Academic Press.

Johnston L., & Fineout-Overholt E. (2005). Teaching EBP: "Getting from zero to one." moving from recognizing and admitting uncertainties to asking searchable, answerable questions. *Worldviews on Evidence-Based Nursing*, 2, 98–102.

*Khangura S., Konnyu K., Cushman R., Grimshaw J., & Moher D. (2012). Evidence summaries: the evolution of a rapid review approach. *Systematic Reviews*, 1, 10.

*Kwag K. H., Gonzalez-Lorenzo M., Banzi R., Bonovos S., & Moja L. (2016). Providing doctors with high-quality informatation: an updated evaluation of web-based point-of-care information summaries. *Journal of Medical Internet Research*, 18, e15.

Levin R. F. (2014). Levels, grades, and strength of evidence: "What's it all about, Alfie?". *Research and Theory for Nursing Practice*, 28, 5–8.

*McCarty C., Woehrle T., Waring S., Taran A., & Kitch L. (2018). Implementation of the MEDFRAT to promote quality care and decrease falls in community hospital emergency rooms. *Journal of Emergency Nursing*, 44, 280–284.

Melnyk B.M., & Fineout-Overholt E. (2019). *Evidence-based practice in nursing and health care* (4th ed.). Philadelphia: Lippincott Williams & Wilkins.

Melnyk B. M., & Newhouse R. (2014). Evidence-based practice versus evidence-informed practice: a debate that could stall forward momentum in improving health care quality, safety, patient outcomes, and costs. *Worldviews on Evidence-Based Nursing*, 11, 347–349.

Morse J. M. (2005). Beyond the clinical trial: expanding criteria for evidence. *Qualitative Health Research*, 15, 3–4.

Newhouse R. P. (2007). Diffusing confusion among evidence-based practice, quality improvement, and research. *Journal of Nursing Administration*, 37, 432–435.

*Newhouse R. P., & Spring B. (2010). Interdisciplinary evidence-based practice: moving from silos to synergy. *Nursing Outlook*, 58, 309–317.

Registered Nurses' Association of Ontario (2017). *Adult asthma care: promoting control of asthma* (2nd ed.). Retrieved from http://rnao.ca/bpg/guidelines/adult-asthma-care.

Rogers E. M. (1995). *Diffusion of innovations* (4th ed.). New York: Free Press.

*Rycroft-Malone J., Seers K., Chandler J., Hawkes C., Crichton N., Allen C., … Strunin L. (2013). The role of evidence, context, and facilitation in an implementation trial: implications for the development of the PARIHS framework. *Implementation Science*, 8, 28.

**Saqe-Rockoff A., Schubert F., Ciardiello A., & Douglas E. (2018). Improving thermoregulation for trauma patients in the emergency department: an evidence-based project. *Journal of Trauma Nursing*, 25, 14–20.

Sandelowski M., Voils C. I., Crandell J. L., & Leeman J. (2013). Synthesizing qualitative and quantitative research findings. In Beck C. T. (Ed.). *Routledge international handbook of qualitative nursing research* (pp. 347–356). New York: Routledge.

Schaffer M. A., Sandau K., & Diedrick L. (2013). Evidence-based practice models for organizational change: overview and practical applications. *Journal of Advanced Nursing*, 69, 1197–1209.

Scott K., & McSherry R. (2009). Evidence-based nursing: clarifying the concepts for nurses in practice. *Journal of Clinical Nursing*, 18, 1085–1095.

*Siebenhofer A., Semlitsch T., Herbom T., Siering U., Kopp I., & Hartig J. (2016). Validation and reliability of a guideline appraisal mini-chicklist for daily practice use. *BMC Medical Research Methodology*, 16, 39.

Stetler C. B. (2010). Stetler model. In Rycroft-Malone J. & Bucknall T. (Eds.), *Models and frameworks for implementing evidence-based practice: linking evidence to action* (pp. 51–77). Malden, MA: Wiley-Blackwell.

Stevens K. R. (2012). *Star model of EBP: knowledge transformation. Academic center for evidence-based practice.* San Antonio, TX: The University of Texas Health Science Center at San Antonio.

Straus S. E., Glasziou P., Richardson W., & Haynes R. (2011). *Evidence-based medicine: how to practice and teach it* (4th ed.). Toronto: Churchill Livingstone.

Titler M. (2014). Overview of evidence-based practice and translation science. *Nursing Clinics of North America*, 49, 269–274.

Titler M. G., Kleiber C., Steelman V., Rakel B., Budreau G., Everett L., … Goode C. (2001). The Iowa model of evidence-based practice to promote quality care. *Critical Care Nursing Clinics of North America*, 13, 497–509.

*World Health Organization (2005). *Bridging the "Know-Do" gap: meeting on knowledge translation in global health.* Retrieved June 20, 2019, from https://www.measureevaluation.org/resources/training/capacity-building-resources/high-impact-research-training-curricula/bridging-the-know-do-gap.pdf.

Zhang L., Fu T., Zhang Q., Yin R., Zhu L., He Y., … Shen B. (2018). Effects of psychological interventions for patients with osteoarthritis: a systematic review and meta-analysis. *Psychology, Health, and Medicine*, 23, 1–17.

A link to this open-access article is provided in the Toolkit for Chapter 2 in the Resource Manual. ✳

This journal article is available on thePoint for this chapter.

3

Key Concepts and Steps in Qualitative and Quantitative Research

This chapter covers a lot of ground—but, for many of you, it is familiar ground. If you have taken an earlier research course, this chapter will be a review of key terms and steps in the research process. If you have no previous exposure to research methods, this chapter offers basic grounding in research terminology.

Research, like any discipline, has its own *jargon*. Some terms are used by both qualitative and quantitative researchers, but others are used mainly by one or the other group. Also, some nursing research jargon has its roots in the social sciences, but sometimes different terms for the same concepts are used in medical research; we cover both.

FUNDAMENTAL RESEARCH TERMS AND CONCEPTS

When researchers address a problem—regardless of the underlying paradigm—they undertake a **study** (or an **investigation**). Studies involve people cooperating with each other in different roles.

The Faces and Places of Research

Studies with humans involve two groups: those doing research and those providing the information. In a quantitative study, the people being studied are called **subjects** or **study participants** (Table 3.1). In a qualitative study, those under study are called study participants or **informants**. Collectively, study participants comprise the **sample**.

The person who conducts a study is the **researcher** or **investigator**. Studies are often done by a team; the person directing the study is the **principal investigator (PI)**. Increasingly, nurse researchers are working as a part of interdisciplinary research teams. In large-scale projects, dozens of individuals may be involved in planning and conducting the study.

Research can be undertaken in a variety of *settings*—the specific places where information is gathered. Some studies take place in *naturalistic settings* in the field, such as in people's homes, but some studies are done in laboratory or clinical settings. Qualitative researchers are especially likely to engage in **fieldwork** in natural settings because they are interested in the contexts of people's experiences. The *site* is the overall location for the research—it could be an entire community (e.g., a Haitian neighborhood in Miami) or an institution (e.g., a hospital in Toronto). Researchers sometimes undertake **multisite studies** because the use of multiple sites offers a larger or more diverse sample of participants.

The Building Blocks of Research

Phenomena, Concepts, and Constructs

Research involves abstractions. For example, *pain*, *fatigue*, and *obesity* are abstractions of human characteristics. These abstractions are called **concepts** or, in qualitative studies, **phenomena**.

TABLE 3.1 • Key Terms in Quantitative and Qualitative Research

CONCEPT	QUANTITATIVE TERM	QUALITATIVE TERM
Person contributing information	Subject Study participant –	– Study participant Informant, key informant
Person undertaking the study	Researcher Investigator	Researcher Investigator
That which is being investigated	– Concepts Constructs Variables	Phenomena Concepts – –
System of organizing concepts	Theory, theoretical framework Conceptual framework, conceptual model	Theory Conceptual framework, sensitizing framework
Information gathered	Data (numerical values)	Data (narrative descriptions)
Connections between concepts	Relationships (cause-and-effect, associative)	Patterns of association
Logical reasoning processes	Deductive reasoning	Inductive reasoning

Researchers also use the term **construct**, which refers to an abstraction inferred from situations or behaviors—but often one that is deliberately invented or constructed. For example, *self-care* in Orem's model of health maintenance is a construct. The terms *construct* and *concept* are sometimes used interchangeably, but by convention, a construct typically refers to a more complex abstraction than a concept.

Theories and Conceptual Models

A **theory** is a systematic explanation of some aspect of reality. Theories, which knit concepts together into a coherent system, play a role in both qualitative and quantitative research.

Quantitative researchers may start with a theory or *conceptual model* (distinctions are discussed in Chapter 6). Based on theory, researchers predict how phenomena will behave in the real world *if the theory is true*. Researchers use *deductive reasoning* to go from a theory to specific predictions, which are tested through research; study results are used to support, reject, or modify the theory.

In qualitative research, theories may be used in various ways. Sometimes conceptual or **sensitizing frameworks**, derived from qualitative research traditions we describe later in this chapter, offer an orienting world view. In such studies, the framework helps to guide the inquiry and to interpret the findings. In other qualitative studies, theory is the *product* of the research: the investigators use information from participants *inductively* to develop a theory rooted in the participants' experiences.

 Deductive and inductive logical reasoning processes are described more fully in the Supplement to this chapter on the book's website, the Point.

Variables

In quantitative studies, concepts often are called **variables**. A variable, as the name implies, is something that varies. Weight, fatigue, and stress are variables—each varies from one person to another. In fact, most aspects of humans are variables. If everyone weighed 150 pounds, weight would not be a variable but rather would be a *constant*. It is precisely because people and conditions *do* vary that most research is conducted. Quantitative researchers seek to understand how or why things vary and to learn if differences in one variable are related to differences in another. For example, lung cancer research focuses on the variable of lung cancer, which is a variable because not everyone has this disease. Researchers have studied factors that might be linked to lung cancer, such as cigarette smoking. Smoking is also a variable because not everyone smokes. A variable, then, is any quality of a person, group, or situation that takes on different values.

When an attribute is highly varied in the group under study, the group is **heterogeneous** with respect to that variable. If the amount of variability is limited, the group is **homogeneous**. For example, for the variable height, a sample of 2-year-old children would be more homogeneous than a sample of 21-year-olds.

Characteristics of Variables. Variables may be inherent characteristics of people, such as their age or blood type. Sometimes, however, researchers *create* a variable. For example, if a researcher tests the effectiveness of patient-controlled analgesia as opposed to intramuscular analgesia in relieving pain after surgery, some patients would be given patient-controlled analgesia and others would receive intramuscular analgesia. In the context of the study, method of pain management is a variable because different patients get different analgesic methods.

Some variables take on a wide range of values that can be represented on a continuum. For example, a person's age is a *continuous variable* that can, in theory, assume an infinite number of values between two points. For example, between 1 and 2 pounds for the variable *weight*, the number of values is limitless (e.g., 1.05, 1.3333, and so on). Other variables take on only a few values. *Discrete variables* convey quantitative information (e.g., number of children), but *categorical variables* involve placing people into categories (e.g., gender, blood type). Categorical variables with only two categories (e.g., alive/dead) are *dichotomous variables.*

Dependent and Independent Variables. Many studies seek to unravel and understand causes of phenomena. Does a nursing intervention *cause* improvements in patient outcomes? Does smoking *cause* lung cancer? The presumed cause is the **independent variable**, and the presumed effect is the **dependent variable** (or the **outcome variable**). The dependent variable corresponds to the "O" (outcome) of the PICO scheme discussed in Chapter 2. The independent variable corresponds to the "I" (the intervention, influence, or exposure), *plus* the "C" (the comparison). In doing an evidence search, you might want to learn about the effects of an intervention or influence (I), compared with *any* alternative, on an outcome (O). In a study, however, researchers must always specify the comparator (the "C") that they will investigate.

Variation in the dependent variable is presumed to *depend on* variation in the independent variable. For example, researchers study the extent to which lung cancer (the dependent variable) depends on smoking (the independent variable). Or, investigators might study the extent to which patients' pain (the dependent variable) depends on certain nursing actions (the independent variable). The dependent variable is the outcome that researchers want to understand, explain, or predict.

The terms *independent variable* and *dependent variable* are also used to indicate *direction of influence* rather than a causal link. For example, suppose a researcher studied the role of gender in the mental health (O) of spousal caregivers of patients with dementia (P) and found lower depression for wives than for husbands (I and C). We could not conclude that depression was *caused* by gender. Yet the direction of influence clearly runs from gender to depression: patients' level of depression does not influence their gender. Even without a cause-and-effect connection, it is appropriate to consider depression as the outcome variable and gender as an independent variable.

Most outcomes have multiple causes or influences. If we were studying factors that influence obesity, as measured by people's body mass index (the dependent variable), we might consider height, physical activity, and diet as independent variables in this Etiology question. Two or more *dependent* variables also may be of interest. For example, a researcher may compare the effects of alternative nursing interventions for children with cystic fibrosis (a Therapy question). Several dependent variables could be used to assess treatment effectiveness, such as length of hospital stay, number of recurrent respiratory infections, and so on. It is common to design studies with multiple independent and dependent variables.

Variables are not *inherently* dependent or independent. A dependent variable in one study could be an independent variable in another. For example, a study might examine the effect of an exercise intervention versus no intervention (the independent variable) on osteoporosis (the dependent variable) to answer a Therapy question. Another study might investigate the effect of osteoporosis versus no osteoporosis (the independent variable) on bone fracture incidence (the dependent variable) to address a Prognosis question. In short, whether a variable is independent or dependent is a function of the role that it plays in a particular study.

Example of Independent and Dependent Variables

Research question (Etiology/Harm question): Is dietary vitamin C deficiency associated with cardiac event–free survival in adults with heart failure? (Wu et al., 2019)

   Independent variable: Dietary vitamin C deficiency (vs. no deficiency).

   Dependent variable: Cardiac event–free survival versus a cardiac event.

Conceptual and Operational Definitions

Concepts are abstractions of observable phenomena, and researchers' world views shape how those concepts are defined. A **conceptual definition** presents the abstract or theoretical meaning of concepts under study. Even seemingly straightforward terms need to be conceptually defined. The classic example is the concept of *caring*. Morse et al. (1990) examined how researchers and theorists defined *caring* and identified five classes of conceptual definition: as a human trait; a moral imperative; an affect; an interpersonal relationship; and a therapeutic intervention. More recently Andersson et al. (2015) found that nurses offered multiple interpretations of caring. Researchers undertaking studies of caring need to clarify which conceptual definition they have adopted.

In qualitative studies, conceptual definitions of key phenomena may be a major end product, reflecting an intent to have the meaning of concepts defined by those being studied. In quantitative studies, however, researchers must define concepts at the outset because they must decide how the variables will be observed and measured. An **operational definition** specifies what the researchers must do to measure the concept and collect needed information.

Variables differ in the ease with which they can be operationalized. The variable weight, for example, is easy to define and measure. We might operationally define weight as the amount that an object weighs, to the nearest half pound. This definition designates that weight will be measured using one system (pounds) rather than another (grams). We could also specify that weight will be measured using a digital scale with participants fully undressed after 10 hours of fasting. This operational definition clarifies what we mean by the variable *weight*.

Few variables are operationalized as easily as weight. Most variables can be measured in different ways, and researchers must choose the one that best captures the variables as they conceptualize them. Take, for example, *anxiety*, which can be defined in terms of both physiologic and psychological functioning. For researchers choosing to emphasize physiologic aspects, the operational definition might involve a measurement of salivary cortisol. If researchers conceptualize anxiety as a psychological state, the operational definition might be people's scores on a patient-reported test such as the State Anxiety Scale. Readers of research articles may not agree with how variables were conceptualized and measured, but definitional precision is important for communicating exactly what concepts mean within the study.

TIP Operationalizing a concept is often a two-part process that involves deciding (1) how to accurately measure the variable and (2) how to represent it in an analysis. For example, a person's age might be obtained by asking them to report their birthdate but operationalized in an analysis in relation to a threshold (e.g., younger than 65 years vs. 65 years or older).

Example of Conceptual and Operational Definitions

Rafferty et al. (2017) developed a measure called the Culture of Care Barometer (CoCB) to measure the culture of care in healthcare organizations. They defined "culture of care" conceptually as the shared beliefs, norms, and routines through which the environment of a healthcare organization can be interpreted and understood. This construct was operationalized in the CoCB through a series of 30 questions to staff. Two examples are, "I have the resources I need to do a good job" and "I feel supported to develop my potential."

Data

Research **data** (singular, datum) are the pieces of information obtained in a study. In quantitative studies, researchers define their variables and then collect relevant data from study participants. Quantitative researchers collect primarily **quantitative data**—data in numeric form. For example, suppose *depression* was a key variable in a quantitative study. We

might ask participants, "Thinking about the past week, how depressed would you say you have been on a scale from 0 to 10, where 0 means 'not at all' and 10 means 'the most possible'?" Box 3.1 presents quantitative data for three fictitious people. Subjects provided a number along a 0 to 10 continuum representing their degree of depression—*9* for subject 1 (a high level of depression), *0* for subject 2 (no depression), and *4* for subject 3 (mild depression). The numeric values for all participants, collectively, would comprise the data on depression in this study.

In qualitative studies, researchers collect **qualitative data**, that is, narrative descriptions. Narrative information can be obtained by having conversations with participants, by making detailed notes about how people behave, or by obtaining narrative records, such as diaries. Suppose we were studying depression qualitatively. Box 3.2 presents qualitative data for three people responding conversationally to the question, "Tell me about how you've been feeling lately—have you felt sad or depressed

BOX 3.1   Example of Quantitative Data

Question: Thinking about the past week, how depressed would you say you have been on a scale from 0 to 10, where 0 means "not at all" and 10 means "the most possible"?

Data: 9 (Subject 1)
0 (Subject 2)
4 (Subject 3)

BOX 3.2   Example of Qualitative Data

Question: Tell me about how you've been feeling lately—have you felt sad or depressed at all, or have you generally been in good spirits?

Data: "Well, actually, I've been pretty depressed lately, to tell you the truth. I wake up each morning and I can't seem to think of anything to look forward to. I mope around the house all day, kind of in despair. I just can't seem to shake the blues, and I've begun to think I need to go see a shrink." (Participant 1)

"I can't remember ever feeling better in my life. I just got promoted to a new job that makes me feel like I can really get ahead in my company. And I've just gotten engaged to a really great guy who is very special." (Participant 2)

"I've had a few ups and downs the past week, but basically things are on a pretty even keel. I don't have too many complaints." (Participant 3)

at all, or have you generally been in good spirits?" The data consist of rich narrative descriptions of participant's emotional state.

Relationships

Researchers are rarely interested in isolated concepts, except in descriptive studies. For example, a researcher might describe the percentage of patients receiving intravenous (IV) therapy who experience IV infiltration. In this example, the variable is IV infiltration versus no infiltration. Usually, however, researchers study phenomena in relation to other phenomena—that is, they focus on relationships. A **relationship** is a bond or a connection between phenomena. For example, researchers repeatedly have found a *relationship* between cigarette smoking and lung cancer. Both qualitative and quantitative studies examine relationships, but in different ways.

In quantitative studies, researchers examine the relationship between the independent and dependent variables. Researchers ask whether variation in the dependent variable (the outcome) is systematically related to variation in the independent variable. Relationships are usually expressed in quantitative terms, such as *more than*, *less than*, and so on. For example, let us consider a person's weight as our dependent variable. What variables are related to (associated with) body weight? Some possibilities are height, caloric intake, and exercise. For each independent variable, we can make a prediction about its relationship to the outcome variable:

Height: Taller people will weigh more than shorter people.
Caloric intake: People with higher caloric intake will be heavier than those with lower caloric intake.
Exercise: The lower the amount of exercise, the greater the person's weight.

Each statement expresses a predicted relationship between weight (the dependent variable) and a measurable independent variable. Terms like *more than* and *heavier than* imply that as we observe a change in one variable, we are likely to observe a change in weight. If Alex is taller than Tom, we would predict (in the absence of other information) that Alex is heavier than Tom.

Quantitative studies can address one or more of the following questions about relationships:

- Does a relationship between variables *exist*? (e.g., Is cigarette smoking related to lung cancer?)
- What is the *direction* of the relationship between variables? (e.g., Are people who smoke *more* likely or *less* likely to develop lung cancer than those who do not?)
- How *strong* is the relationship between the variables? (e.g., How great is the risk that smokers will develop lung cancer?)
- What is the *nature* of the relationship between variables? (e.g., Does smoking *cause* lung cancer? Does some other factor *cause* both smoking and lung cancer?)

Variables can be related in different ways. One type of relationship is a **cause-and-effect** (or **causal**) **relationship**. Within the positivist paradigm, natural phenomena have antecedent causes that are presumably discoverable. In our example about a person's weight, we might speculate that there is a causal relationship between caloric intake and weight: we might predict that consuming more calories causes weight gain. Many quantitative studies are *cause-probing*—they seek to illuminate the causes of phenomena.

Example of a Study of Causal Relationships

Lee et al. (2019a) evaluated the effect of California's safe patient handling legislation on musculoskeletal injury prevention among nurses.

Not all relationships between variables can be interpreted as causal ones. There is a relationship, for example, between a person's pulmonary artery and tympanic temperatures: people with high readings on one tend to have high readings on the other. We cannot say, however, that pulmonary artery temperature *caused* tympanic temperature, nor vice versa. This type of relationship is a **functional** (or **associative**) **relationship** rather than a causal one.

Example of a Study of Associative Relationships
Fox et al. (2018) studied the relationship between various risk factors (including age and sex) and severe respiratory depression (SRD) among adults with acute prescription opioid overdose. Age was associated with higher risk of SRD.

Qualitative researchers are not concerned with quantifying relationships nor in testing causal relationships. Qualitative researchers seek patterns of association as a way to illuminate the underlying meaning and dimensionality of phenomena. Patterns of interconnected themes and processes are identified as a means of understanding the whole.

Example of a Qualitative Study of Patterns
MacArtney et al. (2017) explored what steps patients with cancer in three countries (Denmark, England, and Sweden) took to arrive at their original cancer diagnosis. In-depth interviews with 155 men and women revealed two distinct patterns: (1) those who left their primary care consultation with a plan about what should happen next and (2) those who were unclear about next steps. The second pattern extended over many weeks of uncertainty. Patients from Sweden were more likely to follow the first pattern.

MAJOR CLASSES OF QUANTITATIVE AND QUALITATIVE RESEARCH

Researchers usually work within a paradigm that is consistent with their world view and that gives rise to questions that excite their curiosity. The maturity of the focal concept also may lead to one or the other paradigm: when little is known about a phenomenon, a qualitative approach may be more fruitful than a quantitative one. In this section, we briefly describe broad categories of quantitative and qualitative research.

Quantitative Research: Experimental and Nonexperimental Studies

A basic distinction in quantitative studies is between experimental and nonexperimental research. In **experimental research**, researchers actively introduce an intervention or treatment—most often, to address Therapy questions. In **nonexperimental research**, researchers are bystanders—they collect data without intervening (most often, to address Etiology, Prognosis, or Description questions). For example, if a researcher gave bran flakes to one group of people and prune juice to another to evaluate which method facilitated elimination more effectively, the study would be experimental because the researcher intervened in the normal course of things. If, on the other hand, a researcher compared elimination patterns of two groups whose regular eating patterns differed, the study would be nonexperimental because there is no intervention. In medical research, an experimental study usually is called a **clinical trial** and a nonexperimental inquiry is called an **observational study**. A *randomized controlled trial* or RCT is a particular type of clinical trial.

> **TIP** On the evidence hierarchy shown in Figure 2.1, the two levels directly below systematic reviews (RCTs and quasi-experiments) involve interventions.

Experimental studies are explicitly cause-probing—they test whether an intervention *causes* changes in the dependent variable. Sometimes nonexperimental studies also explore causal relationships, but the resulting evidence is usually less conclusive. Experimental studies offer the possibility of greater control over confounding influences than nonexperimental studies, and so causal inferences are more plausible.

Example of Experimental Research
Mitchell et al. (2018) are testing the effectiveness of an online therapy program (ReaDySpeech) for people with dysarthria following a stroke.

In this example of a study addressing a Therapy question, the researchers intervened by giving some stroke patients the special intervention but not giving it to others. In other words, the researcher *controlled* the independent variable, which in this case was receipt versus nonreceipt of the ReaDySpeech intervention.

Example of Nonexperimental Research
Chung and Sohn (2018) studied the relationship between nurse staffing levels on in-hospital mortality (after taking into account such factors as patient comorbidities) among stroke inpatients from 615 hospitals in Korea. Better staffing was associated with lower rates of mortality.

In this nonexperimental study to address an Etiology/Harm question, the researchers did not intervene in any way—they did not have control over nurse staffing. They were interested in a similar population as in the previous example (stroke patients), but their intent was to examine existing relationships rather than to test a potential solution to a problem.

Qualitative Research: Disciplinary Traditions

The majority of qualitative nursing studies can best be described as **qualitative descriptive research**. Many qualitative studies, however, are rooted in research traditions that originated in anthropology, sociology, and psychology. Three such traditions that are prominent in qualitative nursing research are briefly described here. Chapter 22 provides a fuller discussion of these traditions and the methods associated with them.

Grounded theory research, with roots in sociology, seeks to describe and understand the key social psychological processes that occur in social settings. Most grounded theory studies focus on a developing social experience—the social and psychological processes that characterize an event or episode. A major component of grounded theory is the discovery of not only the basic social psychological problem but also a *core variable* that is central in explaining what is going on in that social scene. Grounded theory researchers strive to generate explanations of phenomena that are grounded in reality. Grounded theory was developed in the 1960s by two sociologists, Glaser and Strauss (1967).

Example of a Grounded Theory Study
Hsieh et al. (2018) conducted a grounded theory study in Taiwan to explore ischemic stroke patients' decision-making process regarding the use of Western medicine and complementary and alternative medicine (CAM).

Phenomenology is concerned with the lived experiences of humans. Phenomenology is an approach to thinking about what life experiences of people are like and what they mean. The phenomenologic researcher asks the questions: What is the *essence* of this phenomenon as experienced by these people? Or, what is the meaning of the phenomenon to those who experience it?

Example of a Phenomenologic Study
Lee et al. (2019b) conducted in-depth interviews to explore the social adjustment experiences of adolescents with Tourette syndrome.

Ethnography, the primary research tradition in anthropology, provides a framework for studying the patterns, lifeways, and experiences of a defined cultural group in a holistic manner. Ethnographers typically engage in extensive fieldwork, often participating in the life of the culture under study. Ethnographic research can be concerned with broadly defined cultures (e.g., Syrian refugee communities), but sometimes focuses on more narrowly defined cultures (e.g., the culture of an intensive care unit). Ethnographers strive to learn from members of a cultural group, to understand their world view, and to describe their customs and norms.

Example of an Ethnographic Study
Ahlstedt et al. (2019) conducted an ethnographic study of Swedish nurses to explore nurses' workday events to better understand what influences nurses' decision to keep working.

MAJOR STEPS IN A QUANTITATIVE STUDY

In quantitative studies, researchers move from the beginning of a study (posing a question) to the end point (obtaining an answer) in a reasonably linear sequence of steps that is broadly similar across studies. In some studies, the steps overlap; in others, some steps are unnecessary. Still, a general flow of activities is typical in a quantitative study (see Figure 3.1). This section describes that flow, and the next section explains how qualitative studies differ.

Phase 1: The Conceptual Phase

Early steps in a quantitative study typically have a strong conceptual element. Activities include reading, conceptualizing, theorizing, and reviewing ideas with colleagues or advisers. During this phase, researchers call on such skills as creativity, deductive reasoning, and a firm grounding in previous research on a topic of interest.

Step 1: Formulating and Delimiting the Problem

Quantitative researchers begin by identifying an interesting, significant research problem and

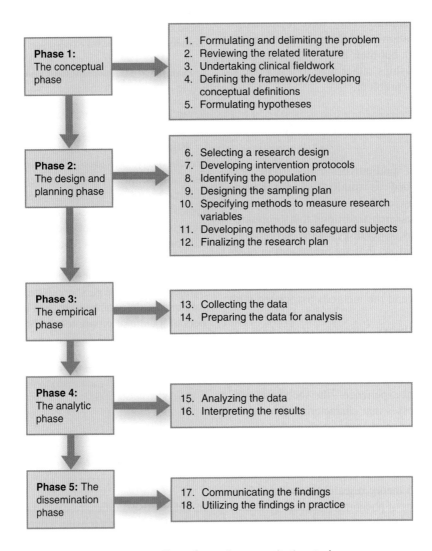

Phase 1:
The conceptual phase

1. Formulating and delimiting the problem
2. Reviewing the related literature
3. Undertaking clinical fieldwork
4. Defining the framework/developing conceptual definitions
5. Formulating hypotheses

Phase 2:
The design and planning phase

6. Selecting a research design
7. Developing intervention protocols
8. Identifying the population
9. Designing the sampling plan
10. Specifying methods to measure research variables
11. Developing methods to safeguard subjects
12. Finalizing the research plan

Phase 3:
The empirical phase

13. Collecting the data
14. Preparing the data for analysis

Phase 4:
The analytic phase

15. Analyzing the data
16. Interpreting the results

Phase 5: The dissemination phase

17. Communicating the findings
18. Utilizing the findings in practice

FIGURE 3.1 Flow of steps in a quantitative study.

formulating **research questions**. Good research requires starting with good questions. In developing research questions, nurse researchers must attend to substantive issues (What kind of new evidence is needed?); theoretical issues (Is there a conceptual context for understanding this problem?); clinical issues (How could evidence from this study be used in clinical practice?); methodologic issues (How can this question best be studied to yield high-quality evidence?); and ethical issues (Can this question be rigorously addressed in an ethical manner?)

> **TIP** A critical ingredient in developing good research questions is personal interest. Begin with topics that fascinate you or about which you have a passionate interest.

Step 2: Reviewing the Related Literature

Quantitative research is conducted in a context of previous knowledge. Quantitative researchers typically strive to understand what is already known about a topic by undertaking a literature review. A thorough **literature review** provides a foundation on which to base new evidence and usually is conducted before data are collected. For clinical problems, it may also be necessary to learn the "status quo" of current procedures and to review existing practice guidelines.

Step 3: Undertaking Clinical Fieldwork

Unless the research problem originated in a clinical setting, researchers embarking on a clinical nursing study benefit from spending time in relevant clinical settings, discussing the problem with clinicians and administrators, and observing current practices. Clinical fieldwork can provide perspectives on recent clinical trends, diagnostic procedures, and relevant healthcare delivery models; it can also help researchers better understand clients and the settings in which care is provided. Such fieldwork can also be valuable in gaining access to an appropriate site or in developing research strategies. For example, in the course of clinical fieldwork, researchers might discover the need for research staff who are bilingual.

Step 4: Defining the Framework and Developing Conceptual Definitions

Theory transcends the specifics of a particular time, place, and group and characterizes regularities in the relationships among variables. When quantitative research is performed within the context of a theoretical framework, the findings often have broader significance and utility. Even when the research question is not embedded in a theory, researchers should have a conceptual rationale and a clear vision of the concepts under study.

Step 5: Formulating Hypotheses

Hypotheses state researcher's predictions about relationships between study variables. The research question identifies the study concepts and asks how the concepts might be related; a hypothesis is the predicted answer. For example, the research question might be: Is preeclamptic toxemia related to stress during pregnancy? This might be translated into the following hypothesis: Women with high levels of stress during pregnancy will be more likely than women with lower stress to experience preeclamptic toxemia. Most quantitative studies involve testing hypotheses through statistical analysis.

Phase 2: The Design and Planning Phase

In the second major phase of a quantitative study, researchers decide on the methods they will use to address the research question. Researchers make many methodologic decisions, which have important implications for the integrity and generalizability of the resulting evidence.

Step 6: Selecting a Research Design

The **research design** is the overall plan for obtaining answers to the research questions. In designing the study, researchers select a specific design from the many experimental and nonexperimental research designs that are available. Research designs specify how often data will be collected, what types of comparisons will be made, and where the study will take place. Researchers also identify strategies to minimize biases and to maximize the *applicability* of their research to real-life settings. The research design is the architectural backbone of the study.

Step 7: Developing Protocols for the Intervention

In experimental research, researchers create an intervention (the independent variable) and need to articulate its features. For example, if we were interested in testing the effect of biofeedback on hypertension, the independent variable would be exposure to biofeedback compared with either an alternative treatment (e.g., relaxation) or no treatment. An **intervention protocol** for the study must be developed, specifying exactly what the biofeedback treatment would entail (e.g., what type of feedback, who would administer it, how frequently and over how long a period the treatment would last, and so on) *and* what the alternative condition would be. The goal of such protocols is to ensure that all people in each group are treated in the same way. (In nonexperimental research, this step is not necessary.)

Step 8: Identifying the Population

Quantitative researchers need to clarify the group to whom study results can be generalized—that is, they must identify the population to be studied. A **population** is *all* the individuals or objects with common, defining characteristics (the "P" component in PICO questions). For example, the population of interest might be all patients undergoing chemotherapy in Atlanta.

Step 9: Designing the Sampling Plan

Researchers collect data from a sample, which is a subset of the population. Using samples is more feasible than collecting data from an entire population, but the risk is that the sample might not reflect the population's traits. In a quantitative study, a sample's adequacy is assessed by its size and **representativeness**. The quality of the sample depends on how typical, or representative, the sample is of the population. The **sampling plan** specifies how the sample will be selected and recruited and how many subjects there will be.

Step 10: Specifying Methods to Measure Research Variables

Quantitative researchers must identify methods to measure their research variables. The primary methods of data collection are *self-reports* (e.g.,

interviews), *observations* (e.g., observing the sleep-wake state of infants), and *biophysiologic measurements (biomarkers)*. Self-reports from patients are the largest class of data collection methods in nursing research. The task of selecting measures of research variables and developing a **data collection plan** is complex and challenging.

Step 11: Developing Methods to Safeguard Human/Animal Rights

Most nursing research involves humans, and so procedures need to be developed to ensure that the study adheres to ethical principles. A formal review by an ethics committee is usually required.

Step 12: Reviewing and Finalizing the Research Plan

Before collecting their data, researchers often take steps to ensure that plans will work smoothly. For example, they may evaluate the *readability* of written materials to assess if participants with low reading skills can comprehend them, or they may *pretest* their measuring instruments to see if they work well. Normally, researchers also have their research plan critiqued by peers, consultants, or other reviewers before implementing it. Researchers seeking financial support submit a **proposal** to a funding source, and reviewers usually suggest improvements.

TIP For major studies, researchers often undertake a small-scale pilot study to test their research plans. Strategies for designing effective pilot studies are described in Chapter 29.

Phase 3: The Empirical Phase

The empirical phase of quantitative studies involves collecting data and preparing the data for analysis. Often, the empirical phase is the most time-consuming part of the investigation. Data collection typically requires months of work.

Step 13: Collecting the Data

The actual collection of data in quantitative studies often proceeds according to a preestablished plan. A *data collection protocol* typically spells out procedures for training data collection staff; for actually collecting data (e.g., the location and timing of gathering the data); and for recording information. Technological advances have expanded possibilities for automating data collection.

Step 14: Preparing the Data for Analysis

Data collected in a quantitative study must be prepared for analysis. One preliminary step is *coding*, which involves translating verbal data into numeric form (e.g., coding gender as "1" for females, "2" for males, and "3" for other). Another step may involve transferring the data from written documents onto computer files for analysis.

Phase 4: The Analytic Phase

Quantitative data must be subjected to analysis and interpretation, which occur in the fourth major phase of a project.

Step 15: Analyzing the Data

Quantitative researchers analyze their data through **statistical analyses**, which include simple procedures (e.g., computing an average) as well as ones that are complex. Some analytic methods are computationally formidable, but the underlying logic of statistical tests is fairly easy to grasp. Computers have eliminated the need to get bogged down with mathematic operations.

Step 16: Interpreting the Results

Interpretation involves making sense of study results and examining their implications. Researchers attempt to explain the findings in light of prior evidence, theory, and their own clinical experience—and in light of the adequacy of the methods they used in the study. Interpretation also involves drawing conclusions about the *clinical significance* of the results, envisioning how the new evidence can be used in nursing practice, and suggesting what further research is needed.

Phase 5: The Dissemination Phase

In the analytic phase, the researcher comes full circle: questions posed at the outset are answered. Researchers' responsibilities are not completed, however, until study results are disseminated.

Step 17: Communicating the Findings

A study cannot contribute evidence to nursing practice if the results are not shared. Another—and often final—task of a study is the preparation of a **research report** that summarizes the study. Research reports can take various forms: dissertations, journal articles, conference presentations, and so on. Journal articles—reports appearing in professional journals such as *Nursing Research*—usually are the most useful because they are available to a broad, international audience. We discuss journal articles later in this chapter.

Step 18: Utilizing the Findings in Practice

Ideally, the concluding step of a high-quality study is to plan for the use of the evidence in practice settings. Although nurse researchers may not themselves be able to implement a plan for using research findings, they can contribute to the process by making recommendations for utilizing the evidence, by ensuring that adequate information has been provided for a systematic review, and by pursuing opportunities to disseminate the findings to clinicians.

ACTIVITIES IN A QUALITATIVE STUDY

Quantitative research involves a fairly linear progression of tasks—researchers plan the steps to be taken to maximize study integrity and then follow those steps as faithfully as possible. In qualitative studies, by contrast, the progression is closer to a circle than to a straight line—qualitative researchers continually examine and interpret data and make decisions about how to proceed based on what has already been discovered (Figure 3.2).

Because qualitative researchers have a flexible approach, we cannot show the flow of activities precisely—the flow varies from one study to another, and researchers themselves do not know exactly how the study will unfold. We provide a sense of how qualitative studies are conducted, however, by describing major activities and indicating when they might be performed.

FIGURE 3.2 Flow of activities in a qualitative study.

Conceptualizing and Planning a Qualitative Study

Identifying the Research Problem

Qualitative researchers usually begin with a broad topic area, focusing on an aspect of a topic that is poorly understood and about which little is known. Qualitative researchers often proceed with a fairly broad initial question, which may be narrowed and clarified on the basis of self-reflection and discussion with others. The specific focus and questions are usually delineated more clearly once the study is underway.

Doing a Literature Review

Qualitative researchers do not all agree about the value of doing an upfront literature review. Some believe that researchers should not consult the literature before collecting data because prior studies could influence conceptualization of the focal phenomenon. In this view, the phenomena should

be explicated based on participants' viewpoints rather than on prior knowledge. Those sharing this opinion often do a literature review at the end of the study. Other researchers conduct a brief preliminary review to get a general grounding. Still others believe that a full early literature review is appropriate. In any case, qualitative researchers typically find a small body of relevant previous work because of the types of question they ask.

Selecting and Gaining Entrée Into Research Sites

Before going into the field, qualitative researchers must identify an appropriate site. For example, if the topic is the health beliefs of the urban poor, an inner-city neighborhood with low-income residents must be identified. Researchers may need to engage in anticipatory fieldwork to identify a suitable and information-rich environment for the study. In some cases, researchers have ready access to the study site, but in others, they need to **gain entrée**. A site may be well suited to the needs of the research, but if researchers cannot "get in," the study cannot proceed. Gaining entrée typically involves negotiations with **gatekeepers** who have the authority to permit entry into their world.

> **TIP** The process of gaining entrée is usually associated with doing fieldwork in qualitative studies, but quantitative researchers often need to gain entrée into sites for collecting data as well.

Developing an Overall Approach in Qualitative Studies

Quantitative researchers do not collect data until they have finalized their research design. Qualitative researchers, by contrast, use an **emergent design** that materializes during the course of data collection. Certain design features may be guided by the qualitative research tradition within which the researcher is working, but few qualitative studies follow rigidly structured designs that prohibit changes while in the field. Although qualitative researchers do not always know in advance exactly how the study will progress, they nevertheless must have some sense of how much time is available for fieldwork and must also arrange for and test needed equipment, such as laptop computers or cameras.

Addressing Ethical Issues

Qualitative researchers, like quantitative researchers, must also develop plans for addressing ethical issues—and, indeed, there are special concerns in qualitative studies because of the more intimate nature of the relationship that typically develops between researchers and study participants. Chapter 7 describes these concerns.

Conducting a Qualitative Study

In qualitative studies, the tasks of sampling, data collection, data analysis, and interpretation typically take place iteratively. Qualitative researchers begin by talking with or observing a few people who have first-hand experience with the phenomenon under study. The discussions and observations are loosely structured, allowing for the expression of a full range of beliefs, feelings, and behaviors. Analysis and interpretation are ongoing, concurrent activities that guide choices about the kinds of people to sample next and the types of questions to ask or observations to make.

The process of data analysis involves clustering together related types of narrative information into a coherent scheme. As analysis and interpretation progress, researchers begin to identify **themes** and categories (or stages in a process), which are used to build a rich description or theory of the phenomenon. The kinds of data obtained and the people selected as participants tend to become increasingly purposeful as the conceptualization is developed and refined. Concept development shapes the sampling process—as a conceptualization or theory emerges, the researcher seeks participants who can confirm and enrich the theoretical understandings, as well as participants who can potentially challenge them and lead to further theoretical development.

Quantitative researchers decide upfront how many people to include in a study, but qualitative researchers' sampling decisions are guided by the data. Qualitative researchers use the principle of **data saturation**, which occurs when themes and categories in the data become repetitive and redundant, such that no new information can be gleaned by further data collection.

Quantitative researchers seek to collect high-quality data by measuring their variables with methods that have been found to be reliable and valid. Qualitative researchers, by contrast, are the main data collection instrument and must take steps to demonstrate the *trustworthiness* of the data. The central feature of these efforts is to confirm that the findings accurately reflect the experiences and viewpoints of participants rather than the researcher's perceptions. One confirmatory activity, for example, involves going back to participants and sharing interpretations with them so that they can evaluate whether the researcher's thematic analysis is consistent with their experiences.

Disseminating Qualitative Findings

Qualitative nurse researchers also share their findings with others at conferences and in journal articles. Regardless of researchers' positions about *when* a literature review should be conducted, a summary of prior research is usually offered in qualitative reports as a means of providing context for the study.

Quantitative reports almost never contain **raw data**—that is, data in the form they were collected, which are numeric values. Qualitative reports, by contrast, are usually filled with rich verbatim passages directly from participants. The excerpts are used in an evidentiary fashion to support or illustrate researchers' interpretations and thematic construction.

> **Example of Raw Data in a Qualitative Report**
> Nijboer and Van der Cingel (2019) did an in-depth study of the perceptions of novice nurses in the Netherlands on compassion. The nurses identified four themes, one of which was compassion as part of the nurses' professional identity. Here is an illustrative quote: "I am convinced that I have to be a nurse. Being compassionate and being a nurse is a part of who I am" (p. 87).

Like quantitative researchers, qualitative nurse researchers want their findings used by others. Qualitative findings sometimes are the basis for formulating hypotheses that are tested by quantitative researchers, for developing measuring instruments for both research and clinical purposes, and for designing effective nursing interventions. Qualitative studies help to shape nurses' perceptions of a problem or situation, their conceptualizations of potential solutions, and their understanding of patients' concerns and experiences.

RESEARCH JOURNAL ARTICLES

Research **journal articles**, which summarize the background, design, and results of a study, are the primary method of disseminating research evidence. This section reviews the content and style of research journal articles to ensure that you will be equipped to delve into the research literature. A more detailed discussion of the structure of journal articles is presented in Chapter 32, which provides guidance on writing research reports.

Content of Journal Articles

Many quantitative and qualitative journal articles follow a conventional organization called the **IMRAD format**. This format involves organizing material into four main sections—Introduction, Methods, Results, and Discussion. The text of the report is usually preceded by an abstract and followed by cited references.

The Abstract

The **abstract** is a brief description of the study placed at the beginning of the article. The abstract answers, in about 250 words, the following: What were the research questions? What methods did the researcher use to address the questions? What did the researcher find? And, what are the implications? Readers review abstracts to assess whether the entire report is of interest. Some journals have moved from traditional abstracts—single paragraphs summarizing the study's main features—to longer, structured abstracts with specific headings. For example, in the journal *Nursing Research*, abstracts are organized under the following headings: Background, Objectives, Method, Results, and Conclusions.

The Introduction

The introduction communicates the research problem and its context. The introduction, which often is not be specifically labeled "Introduction," follows immediately after the abstract. This section typically describes the following: (1) the central phenomena, concepts, or variables under study; (2) the population of interest; (3) the current state of evidence, based on a brief literature review; (4) the theoretical framework; (5) the study purpose, research questions, or hypotheses to be tested; and (6) the study's significance. Thus, the introduction sets the stage for a description of what the researcher did and what was learned. The introduction corresponds roughly to the conceptual phase of a study.

The Method Section

The method section describes the methods used to answer the research questions. This section lays out methodologic decisions made in the design and planning phase and may offer rationales for those decisions. In a quantitative study, the method section usually describes the following: (1) the research design; (2) the sampling plan for selecting participants from the population of interest; (3) methods of data collection and specific instruments used; (4) study procedures (including ethical safeguards); and (5) analytic procedures and methods.

Qualitative researchers discuss many of the same issues, but with different emphases. For example, a qualitative study often provides more information about the research setting and the study context, and less information on sampling. Also, because formal instruments are not used to collect qualitative data, there is less discussion about data collection methods. Reports of qualitative studies may also include descriptions of the researchers' efforts to enhance the trustworthiness of the study.

The Results Section

The results section presents the **findings** from the data analyses. The text summarizes key findings, and (in quantitative reports) tables provide greater detail. Virtually all results sections contain a description of the participants (e.g., their average age, percentage male/female).

In quantitative studies, the results section provides information about the **statistical tests** used to test hypotheses and to evaluate the believability of the findings. For example, if the percentage of smokers who smoke two packs or more daily is computed to be 40%, how *probable* is it that the percentage is accurate? If the researcher finds that the average number of cigarettes smoked weekly is lower for those in an intervention group than for those not getting the intervention, how *probable* is it that the intervention effect is *real*? Statistical tests help to answer such questions. Researchers typically report the following:

- *The names of statistical tests used.* Different tests are appropriate for different situations but are based on common principles. You do not have to know the names of all statistical tests—there are dozens of them—to comprehend the findings.
- *The value of the calculated statistic.* Computers are used to calculate a numeric value for the statistical test used. The value allows researchers to draw conclusions about the results. The *actual* numeric value of the statistic, however, is not inherently meaningful and need not concern you.
- *The statistical significance.* A critical piece of information is whether the value of the statistic was significant (not to be confused with important or clinically relevant). When researchers say that results are **statistically significant**, it means the findings are probably reliable and replicable with a new sample. Research reports indicate the **level of significance**, which is an index of how probable it is that the findings are reliable. For example, if a report says that a finding was significant at the .05 level, this means that only 5 times out of 100 ($5 \div 100 = .05$) would the result be spurious. In other words, 95 times out of 100, similar results would be obtained with a new sample. Readers can have a high degree of confidence—but not total assurance—that the result is reliable.

Example From the Results Section of a Quantitative Study

Caldwell et al. (2018) tested a tailored smoking cessation intervention for parents of young children, to reduce children's exposure to tobacco smoke. A total of 453 parents, recruited from 14 elementary schools, were assigned, at random, to either receive the intervention or to serve as a nonintervention control group. Saliva cotinine was measured at the start of the study and then at the end of the intervention 2 years later. In the intervention group, average cotinine levels dropped from 239.9 to 99.3, whereas in the control group average cotinine levels increased from 221.1 to 239.0, $F = 5.72$, $p = .004$.

In this study addressing a Therapy question, Caldwell et al. found improvement over time (from an initial measurement to a second measurement after the intervention was completed), in the intervention parents' levels of salivary cotinine—but not among parents in the control group. This finding is very reliable: less than four times in 1,000

($p < .004$) would a group difference as great as that observed have occurred as a fluke. To understand this finding, you do not have to understand what an F statistic is, nor do you need to worry about the actual value of the statistic, 5.72.

Results sections of qualitative reports often have several subsections, the headings of which correspond to the themes, processes, or categories identified in the data. Excerpts from the raw data are presented to support and provide a rich description of the thematic analysis. The results section of qualitative studies may also present the researcher's emerging theory about the phenomenon under study.

The Discussion Section

In the discussion section, researchers draw conclusions about what the results mean, and how the evidence can be used in practice. The discussion in both qualitative and quantitative reports may include the following elements: (1) the degree to which results are consistent with previous research; (2) an interpretation of the results and their clinical significance; (3) implications for clinical practice and for future and research; and (4) study limitations and ramifications for the integrity of the results. Researchers are in the best position to point out sample deficiencies, design problems, weaknesses in data collection, and so forth. A discussion section that presents these limitations demonstrates to readers that the author was aware of these limitations and probably took them into account in interpreting the findings.

The Style of Research Journal Articles

Research reports tell a story. However, the style in which many research journal articles are written—especially reports of quantitative studies—makes it difficult for many readers to figure out the story or become intrigued by it. To unaccustomed audiences, research reports may seem stuffy, pedantic, and overwhelming. Four factors contribute to this impression:

- *Compactness.* Journal space is limited, so authors compress a lot of information into a short space. Interesting, personalized aspects of the study are not reported. Even in qualitative studies, only a handful of supporting quotes can be included.
- *Jargon.* The authors of research reports use terms that may seem esoteric.
- *Objectivity.* Quantitative researchers tell their stories objectively, in a way that may make them sound impersonal. For example, most quantitative reports are written in the passive voice (i.e., personal pronouns are avoided), which tends to make a report less lively than use of the active voice. Qualitative reports, by contrast, are more personal and written in a more conversational style.
- *Statistical information.* Quantitative reports summarize the results of statistical analyses. Numbers and statistical symbols can intimidate readers who do not have statistical training.

In this textbook we try to assist you in dealing with these issues and strive to encourage you to tell *your* research stories in a manner that makes them accessible to practicing nurses.

Tips on Reading Research Reports

As you progress through this book, you will acquire skills for evaluating research reports critically. Some preliminary hints on digesting research reports follow.

- Grow accustomed to the style of research articles by reading them frequently, even though you may not yet understand all the technical points.
- Read from an article that has been downloaded and printed so that you can highlight portions and write marginal notes (or use software that allows you to do this in pdf files).
- Read articles slowly. Skim the article first to get major points and then read it more carefully a second time.
- On the second reading of a journal article, train yourself to be an *active* reader. Reading actively means that you constantly monitor yourself to assess your understanding of what you are reading. If you have problems, go back and reread difficult

BOX 3.3 Additional Questions for a Preliminary Review of a Research Report

1. What is the study all about? What are the main phenomena, concepts, or constructs under investigation?
2. If the study is quantitative, what are the independent and dependent variables? What are the PICO elements—and for what type of question (Therapy, Prognosis, etc.)?
3. Do the researchers examine relationships or patterns of association among variables or concepts? Does the report imply the possibility of a causal relationship?
4. Are key concepts clearly defined, both conceptually and operationally?
5. What type of study does it appear to be, in terms of types described in this chapter: Quantitative—experimental? nonexperimental? Qualitative—descriptive? grounded theory? phenomenologic? ethnographic?
6. Does the report provide any information to suggest how long the study took to complete?
7. Does the format of the report conform to the traditional IMRAD format? If not, in what ways does it differ?

passages or make notes so that you can ask some-one for clarification. In most cases, that "someone" will be your research instructor, but also consider contacting researchers themselves via email.

- Some people find it helpful to use a structured reading method when reading research reports. One such method is called the SQ3R Reading Technique, which involves five steps: *Survey, Question, Read, Recite, and Review.* We provide basic guidance about this method in Chapter 3 of the Toolkit in the accompanying *Resource Manual.* ✪
- Keep this textbook with you as a reference while you are reading articles so that you can look up unfamiliar terms in the glossary or index.
- Try not to get "turned off" by statistical infor-mation. Try to grasp the gist of the story without letting numbers frustrate you.
- Until you become accustomed to research journal articles, you may want to "translate" them by expanding compact paragraphs into looser constructions, by translating jargon into familiar terms, by recasting the report into an active voice, and by summarizing find-ings with words rather than numbers (Chapter 3 in the accompanying *Resource Manual* has an example of such a translation).

GENERAL QUESTIONS IN REVIEWING A RESEARCH STUDY

Most chapters of this book contain guidelines to help you evaluate different aspects of a research report critically, focusing primarily on the research-ers' methodologic decisions. Box 3.3 ✪ presents some further suggestions for performing a prelimi-nary overview of a research report, drawing on con-cepts explained in this chapter. These guidelines supplement those presented in Box 1.1, Chapter 1.

RESEARCH EXAMPLES

In this section, we illustrate the progression of activities and discuss the time schedule of two studies (one quantitative and the other qualitative) conducted by the second author of this book.

Project Schedule for a Quantitative Study

Study: Postpartum depressive symptomatology: Results from a two-stage U.S. national survey (Beck et al., 2011).

Study purpose: Beck and colleagues undertook a study to estimate the prevalence of mothers experiencing elevated postpartum depressive symptom levels in the United States and to explore factors that contributed to variability in symptom levels.

Study methods: This study required a little less than 3 years to complete. Key activities and methodologic decisions included the following:

Phase 1. Conceptual Phase: 1 Month. Beck had been a member of the Listening to Mothers II National Advisory Council. Data for their national survey (the Childbirth Connection: Listening to Mothers II U.S. National Survey) had already been collected when Beck was approached to analyze the variables in the survey relating to postpartum depressive (PPD) symptoms. The first phase took only 1 month because data collection was already completed, and Beck, a world expert on PPD, just needed to update a review of the literature.

Phase 2. Design and Planning Phase: 3 Months. The design phase entailed identifying which of the hundreds of variables on the national survey the researchers would focus on in their analysis. Also, their research questions were formalized and approval from a human subjects committee was obtained during this phase.

Phase 3. Empirical Phase: 0 Months. In this study, the data from nearly 1,000 postpartum women had already been collected.

Phase 4. Analytic Phase: 12 months. Statistical analyses were performed to (1) estimate the percentage of new mothers experiencing elevated postpartum depressive symptom levels and (2) identify which demographic, antepartum, intrapartum, and postpartum variables were significantly related to these elevated symptom levels.

Phase 5. Dissemination Phase: 18 Months. The researchers prepared and submitted their report to the *Journal of Midwifery & Women's Health* for possible publication. It was accepted within 5 months and was "in press" (awaiting publication) another 4 months before being published. The article received the *Journal of Midwifery & Women's Health* 2012 Best Research Article Award.

Project Schedule for a Qualitative Study

Study: Posttraumatic growth after birth trauma: "I was broken, now I am unbreakable" (Beck & Watson, 2016)

Study Purpose: The purpose of this study was to describe the meaning of mothers' experiences of posttraumatic growth after experiencing a traumatic childbirth.

Study Methods: This study required a little less than 4 years to complete. Key activities and methodologic decisions included the following:

Phase 1. Conceptual phase: 4 months. Beck and Watson had conducted a number of qualitative studies on traumatic childbirth and the negative consequences for mothers (e.g., the impact of the traumatic birth on their breastfeeding experiences and subsequent childbirth). This was their first study on posttraumatic growth, so they needed time to review relevant studies and to read about the theory of posttraumatic growth.

Phase 2. Design and planning phase: 3 months. Beck and Watson chose a phenomenologic design for this study. They had conducted several phenomenologic studies so designing this new study did not require a lengthy time period. Once their proposal was finalized, it was submitted to the university's committee on ethics for approval.

Phase 3. Empirical/analytic phrases: 2 years. A recruitment notice was placed on the website of Trauma and Birth Stress, a charitable trust located in New Zealand. Fifteen mothers sent narratives about their posttraumatic growth after a previous traumatic birth to Beck via the Internet. It took 18 months to recruit the sample. Analysis of the mothers' stories took an additional 6 months. Four themes emerged from the data analysis: (1) opening oneself up to a new present, (2) achieving a new level of relationship nakedness, (3) fortifying spiritual-mindedness, and (4) forging new paths.

Phase 4. Dissemination phase: 1 year, 1 month. It took approximately 4 months to prepare the manuscript reporting this study. It was submitted to the *MCN: The American Journal of Maternal Child Nursing* on December 1, 2015. This journal had an unusually rapid response, and 1 month later on January 4, 2016, Beck and Watson received a "revise-and-resubmit" decision from the journal. Only minor revisions were needed, and so on January 11, 2016, the authors submitted their revised manuscript. One week later, on January 19, 2016, Beck and Watson received notification that their manuscript had been accepted for publication, and the article was published in the September/October issue of 2016.

SUMMARY POINTS

- The people who provide information to the **researchers** (*investigators*) in a study are called **subjects** or **study participants** (in quantitative research) or study participants or **informants** in qualitative research; collectively the participants comprise the **sample**.
- The *site* is the overall location for the research; researchers sometimes engage in **multisite studies**. *Settings* are the types of places where data collection occurs. Settings can range from totally naturalistic environments to formal research locations.
- Researchers investigate **concepts** (or **constructs**) and **phenomena**, which are abstractions or mental representations inferred from behavior or characteristics.
- Concepts are the building blocks of **theories**, which are systematic explanations of some aspect of the real world.
- In quantitative studies, concepts are called variables. A **variable** is an attribute that takes on different values (i.e., that varies from one person to another). Groups that vary with respect to an attribute are **heterogeneous**; groups with limited variability are **homogeneous**.
- The **dependent** (or **outcome**) **variable** is the behavior or characteristic the researcher is interested in explaining, predicting, or affecting (the "O" in the PICO scheme). The **independent variable** is the presumed cause of, antecedent to, or influence on the dependent variable. The independent variable corresponds to the "I" and the "C" components in the PICO scheme.
- A **conceptual definition** describes the abstract or theoretical meaning of a concept being studied. An **operational definition** specifies how the variable will be measured.
- **Data**—information collected during a study—may take the form of narrative information (**qualitative data**) or numeric values (**quantitative data**).
- A **relationship** is a bond or connection between two variables. Quantitative researchers examine the relationship between the independent variable and dependent variable.

- When the independent variable is a cause of the dependent variable, the relationship is a **cause-and-effect** (or **causal**) **relationship**. In an **associative** (*functional*) **relationship**, variables are related, but in a noncausal way.
- A key distinction in quantitative studies is between **experimental research**, in which researchers introduce an intervention, and **nonexperimental** (or **observational**) **research**, in which researchers observe existing phenomena without intervening.
- Qualitative research sometimes is rooted in research traditions that originate in other disciplines. Three such traditions are grounded theory, phenomenology, and ethnography.
- **Grounded theory** seeks to describe and understand key social psychological processes that occur in social settings.
- **Phenomenology** focuses on the lived experiences of humans and is an approach to learning what the life experiences of people are like and what they mean.
- **Ethnography** provides a framework for studying the meanings, patterns, and lifeways of a culture in a holistic fashion.
- Quantitative researchers usually progress in a fairly linear fashion from asking research questions to answering them. The main phases in a quantitative study are the conceptual, planning, empirical, analytic, and dissemination phases.
- The *conceptual phase* involves (1) defining the problem to be studied; (2) doing a **literature review;** (3) engaging in **clinical fieldwork** for clinical studies; (4) developing a framework and conceptual definitions; and (5) formulating **hypotheses** to be tested.
- The *planning phase* entails (6) selecting a **research design**; (7) developing **intervention protocols** if the study is experimental; (8) specifying the **population**; (9) developing a **sampling plan**; (10) specifying methods to measure research variables; (11) developing strategies to safeguard the rights of participants; and (12) finalizing the research plan (e.g., *pretesting* instruments).
- The *empirical phase* involves (13) collecting data and (14) preparing data for analysis.

- The *analytic phase* involves (15) analyzing data through **statistical analysis** and (16) interpreting the results.
- The *dissemination phase* entails (17) communicating the findings in a **research report** and (18) promoting the use of the study evidence in nursing practice.
- The flow of activities in a qualitative study is more flexible and less linear. Qualitative studies typically involve an **emergent design** that evolves during data collection.
- Qualitative researchers begin with a broad question regarding a phenomenon, often focusing on a little-studied aspect. In the early phase of a qualitative study, researchers select a site and seek to **gain entrée** into it, which typically involves enlisting the cooperation of **gatekeepers**.
- Once in the field, qualitative researchers select informants, collect data, and then analyze and interpret them in an iterative fashion. Knowledge gained during data collection helps to shape the design of the study and the selection of participants.
- Early analysis in qualitative research leads to refinements in sampling and data collection, until **data saturation** (redundancy of information) is achieved.
- Both qualitative and quantitative researchers disseminate their findings, often in **journal articles** that concisely communicate what the researchers did and what they found.
- Journal articles typically consist of an **abstract** (a brief synopsis) and four major sections in an **IMRAD format**: an **I**ntroduction (explanation of the study problem and its context); **M**ethod section (the strategies used to address the problem); **R**esults section (study findings); **a**nd **D**iscussion (interpretation of the findings).
- Research reports can be difficult to read because they are dense and contain a lot of jargon. Quantitative research reports may be intimidating at first because, compared with qualitative reports, they are more impersonal and include statistical information.
- **Statistical tests** are procedures for testing research hypotheses and evaluating the believability of the findings. Findings that are **statistically significant** are ones that have a high probability of being "real."

STUDY ACTIVITIES

Study activities are available to instructors on thePoint.

REFERENCES CITED IN CHAPTER 3

Ahlstedt, C., Eriksson-Lindvall, C., Holmström, I., & Muntlin-Athlin, A. (2019). What makes registered nurses remain in work? An ethnographic study. *International Journal of Nursing Studies, 89*, 32–38.

*Andersson, E., Willman, A., Sjöström-Strand, A., & Borglin, G. (2015). Registered nurses' descriptions of caring: A phenomenographic interview study. *BMC Nursing, 14*, 16.

Beck, C. T., Gable, R. K., Sakala, C., & Declercq, E. R. (2011). Postpartum depressive symptomatology: Results from a two-stage U.S. national survey. *Journal of Midwifery & Women's Health, 56*, 427–435.

Beck, C. T., & Watson, S. (2016). Postraumatic growth after birth trauma: "I was broken, now I am unbreakable". *MCN: The American Journal of Maternal Child Nursing, 41*, 264–271.

Caldwell, A., Tingen, M., Nguyen, J., Andrews, J., Heath, J., Waller, J., & Treiber, F. (2018). Parental smoking cessation: Impacting children's tobacco exposure in the home. *Pediatrics, 141*, S96–S106.

Chung, W., & Sohn, M. (2018). The impact of nurse staffing on in-hospital mortality of stroke patients in Korea. *Journal of Cardiovascular Disease, 22*, 47–54.

Fox, L., Hoffman, R., Vlahov, D., & Manini, A. (2018). Risk factors for severe respiratory depression from prescription opioid overdose. *Addiction, 113*, 59–66.

Glaser, B. G., & Strauss, A. L. (1967). *The discovery of grounded theory: Strategies for qualitative research.* Chicago: Aldine.

Hsieh, C., Wang, S., Chuang, Y., & Chen, H. (2018). Ischemic stroke patients' decision-making process in their use of Western medicine and alternative and complementary medicine. *Holistic Nursing Practice, 32*, 17–26.

Lee, S., Lee, J., & Harrison, R. (2019a). Impact of California's safe patient handling legislation on mulculoskeletal injury prevention among nurses. *American Journal of Industrial Medicine, 62*, 50–58.

Lee, M., Wang, H., Chen, C., & Lee, M. (2019b). Social adjustment experiences of adolescents with Tourette syndrome. *Journal of Clinical Nursing, 28*, 279–288.

*MacArtney, J., Malmstrom, M., Overgaard Nielsen, T., Evans, J., Bernhardson, B., Hajdarevic, S., … Ziebland, S. (2017). Patients initial steps to cancer diagnosis in Denmark, England and Sweden: What can a qualitative, cross-country comparison of narrative interviews tell us about potentially modifiable factors? *BMJ Open, 7*(11), e018210.

*Mitchell, C., Bowen, A., Tyson, S., & Conroy, P. (2018). A feasibility randomized controlled trial of ReaDySpeech for people with dysarthria after stroke. *Clinical Rehabilitation, 32,* 1037–1046.

Morse, J. M., Solberg, S. M., Neander, W. L., Bottorff, J. L., & Johnson, J. L. (1990). Concepts of caring and caring as a concept. *Advances in Nursing Science, 13,* 1–14.

Nijboer, A., & Van der Cingel, M. (2019). Compassion: Use it or lose it?: A study into the perceptions of novice nurses on compassion: A qualitative approach. *Nurse Education Today, 72,* 84–89.

*Rafferty, A. M., Philippou, J., Fitzpatrick, J., Pike, G., & Ball, J. (2017). Development and testing of the "culture of care barometer" (CoCB) in healthcare organisations. *BMJ Open, 7,* e016677.

**Wu, J., Song, E., Moser, D., & Lennie, T. (2019). Dietary vitamin C deficiency is associated with health-related quality of life and cardiac event-free survival in adults with heart failure. *Journal of Cardiovascular Nursing, 34,* 29–35.

*A link to this open-access article is provided in the Toolkit for Chapter 3 in the **Resource Manual**.

**This journal article is available on thePoint for this chapter.

Part 2

CONCEPTUALIZING AND PLANNING A STUDY TO GENERATE EVIDENCE FOR NURSING

4

Research Problems, Research Questions, and Hypotheses

OVERVIEW OF RESEARCH PROBLEMS

Studies begin, much like evidence-based practice (EBP) efforts, with a problem that needs to be solved or a question that needs to be answered. This chapter discusses the development of research problems. We begin by clarifying some relevant terms.

Basic Terminology

At a general level, a researcher selects a *topic* or a *phenomenon* on which to focus. Examples of research topics are claustrophobia during MRI tests, pain management for sickle cell disease, and nutrition during pregnancy. Within broad topic areas are many potential research problems. In this section, we illustrate various terms using the topic *side effects of chemotherapy.*

A **research problem** is an enigmatic or troubling condition. Researchers identify a research problem within a broad topic of interest. The purpose of research is to "solve" the problem—or to contribute to its solution—by generating relevant, high-quality evidence. Researchers articulate the problem in a **problem statement** that also presents a rationale for the study.

Many reports include a **statement of purpose** (or purpose statement), which summarizes the goal of the study. **Research questions** are the specific queries researchers want to answer in addressing the problem. Research questions guide the types of data to collect in a study. Researchers who make predictions about answers to research questions pose **hypotheses** that are tested in the study.

These terms are not always consistently defined in research methods textbooks, and differences among them are often subtle. Table 4.1 illustrates the terms as we define them.

Research Problems and Paradigms

Some research problems are better suited to qualitative versus quantitative methods. Quantitative studies usually focus on concepts that are fairly well developed, about which there is existing evidence, and for which reliable methods of measurement have been (or can be) developed. For example, a quantitative study might be undertaken to explore whether older people with chronic illness who continue working are less (or more) depressed than those who retire. There are relatively good measures of depression that would yield quantitative information about the level of depression in a sample of employed and retired seniors who are chronically ill.

Qualitative studies are often undertaken because a researcher wants to develop a rich and context-bound understanding of a poorly understood phenomenon. Researchers often initiate a qualitative study to heighten awareness

TABLE 4.1 • Example of Terms Relating to Research Problems

TERM	EXAMPLE
Topic/focus	Side effects of chemotherapy
Research problem (simple problem statement)	Nausea and vomiting are common side effects among patients on chemotherapy, and interventions to date have been only moderately successful in reducing these effects. One issue concerns the efficacy of alternative means of administering antiemetic therapies.
Statement of purpose	The purpose of the study is to test an intervention to reduce chemotherapy-induced side effects—specifically, to compare the effectiveness of patient-controlled and nurse-administered antiemetic therapy for controlling nausea and vomiting in patients on chemotherapy.
Research questions	What is the relative effectiveness of patient-controlled antiemetic therapy versus nurse-controlled antiemetic therapy with regard to (1) medication consumption and (2) control of nausea and vomiting in patients on chemotherapy?
Hypotheses	Patients receiving antiemetic therapy by a patient-controlled pump will (1) be less nauseous, (2) vomit less, and (3) consume less medication than patients receiving the therapy by nurse administration.

and create a dialogue about a phenomenon. Qualitative methods would not be well suited to comparing levels of depression among employed and retired seniors, but they would be ideal for exploring, for example, the meaning or experience of depression among chronically ill retirees. Thus, the nature of the research question is linked to paradigms and to research traditions within paradigms.

Sources of Research Problems

Where do ideas for research problems come from? At a basic level, research topics originate with researchers' interests. Because research is a time-consuming enterprise, curiosity about and interest in a topic are essential. Research reports rarely indicate the source of researchers' inspiration, but a variety of explicit sources can fuel their interest, including the following:

- *Clinical experience.* Nurses' everyday clinical experience is a rich source of ideas for research inquiries. Immediate problems that need a solution—analogous to problem-focused triggers discussed in Chapter 2—may generate

enthusiasm and have high potential for clinical relevance.
- *Patients' involvement.* Increasingly, researchers are turning to patients and other key stakeholders for input in identifying important issues for research. *Patient-centered outcomes research (PCOR)* has become increasingly prominent.
- *Quality improvement efforts.* Important clinical questions sometimes emerge in the context of findings from quality improvement studies. Personal involvement on a quality improvement team can sometimes lead to ideas for a study. In Chapter 12, we discuss a process called *root cause analysis* that can suggest a research focus.
- *Nursing literature.* Ideas for studies sometimes come from reading the nursing literature. Research articles may suggest problems indirectly by stimulating the reader's curiosity and directly by pointing out needed research.
- *Social issues.* Topics are sometimes suggested by global social or political issues of relevance to the healthcare community. For example, the feminist movement raised questions about such topics as gender equity in health care. Public

awareness about health disparities has led to research on healthcare access and culturally sensitive interventions.

- *Ideas from external sources.* External sources and direct suggestions can sometimes provide the impetus for a research idea. For example, ideas for studies may emerge from brainstorming with other nurses.

Additionally, researchers who have developed a program of research on a topic area may get inspiration for "next steps" from their own findings or from a discussion of those findings with others.

Example of a Problem Source in a Program of Research

Beck, one of this book's authors, conducted a study with two collaborators (Beck et al., 2015) on secondary traumatic stress among certified nurse midwives (CNMs). Beck has developed a strong research program on postpartum depression and traumatic births. She and Gable had previously conducted a study with labor and delivery nurses and their experiences of secondary traumatic stress caring for women during traumatic births. When Beck presented the findings of this study at conferences, certified CNMs in the audience often said "You should research us too. We also have secondary traumatic stress."

TIP Personal experiences in clinical settings are a provocative source of research ideas and questions. Here are some hints:

- Watch for a recurring problem and see if you can discern a pattern in situations that lead to the problem.
  Example: Why do so many patients complain of being tired after being transferred from a coronary care unit to a progressive care unit?
- Think about aspects of your work that are frustrating or do not result in the intended outcome—then try to identify factors contributing to the problem that could be changed.
  Example: Why is suppertime so frustrating in a nursing home?
- Critically examine your own clinical decisions. Are they based on tradition, or are they based on systematic evidence that supports their efficacy?
  Example: What would happen if you used the return of flatus to assess the return of GI motility after abdominal surgery, rather than listening to bowel sounds?

DEVELOPING AND REFINING RESEARCH PROBLEMS

Procedures for developing a research problem are difficult to describe. The process is rarely a smooth and orderly one; there are likely to be false starts, inspirations, and setbacks. The few suggestions offered here are not intended to imply that there are techniques for making this first step easy but rather to encourage you to persevere in the absence of instant success.

Selecting a Topic

Developing a research problem is a creative process—and it is a process that is sometimes best done in teams. The teams can include other nurses, mentors, interdisciplinary partners, patients, or other community members.

In the early stages of initiating research ideas, try not to be too self-critical. It is better to relax and jot down topics of interest as they come to mind. It does not matter if the ideas are abstract or concrete, broad or specific, technical or colloquial—the important point is to put ideas on paper.

After this first step, ideas can be sorted in terms of interest, knowledge about the topics, and the perceived feasibility of turning the ideas into a study. When the most fruitful topic area has been selected, the list should not be discarded; it may be necessary to return to it.

TIP The process of selecting and refining a research problem usually takes longer than you might think. The process involves starting with some preliminary ideas; having discussions with colleagues, advisers, or stakeholders; perusing the research literature; looking at what is happening in clinical settings; and a lot of reflection.

Narrowing the Topic

Once you have identified a topic of interest, you can begin to ask some broad questions that can lead you to a researchable problem. Examples of question stems that might help to focus an inquiry include the following:

- What is going on with ...?
- What is the process by which ...?

- What is the meaning of ...?
- What would happen if ...?
- What influences or causes ...?
- What are the consequences of...?
- What factors contribute to ...?

Early criticism of ideas can be counterproductive. Try not to jump to the conclusion that an idea sounds trivial or uninspired without giving it more careful consideration or exploring it with others. Another potential danger is that new researchers sometimes develop problems that are too broad in scope. The transformation of a general topic into a workable problem often is accomplished in uneven steps. Each step should result in progress toward the goals of narrowing the scope of the problem and sharpening the concepts.

As researchers move from general topics to more specific ideas, several possible research problems may emerge. Consider the following example. Suppose you were working on a medical unit and were puzzled by that fact that some patients always complained about having to wait for pain medication when certain nurses were assigned to them. The general problem is discrepancy in patient complaints regarding pain medications. You might ask: What accounts for the discrepancy? How can I improve the situation? These are not research questions, but they may lead you to ask such questions as the following: How do the two groups of nurses differ? or What characteristics do the complaining patients share? At this point, you may observe that the cultural and ethnic background of the patients and nurses could be relevant. This may lead you to search the literature for studies about culture and ethnicity in relation to nursing care, or it may prompt you to discuss your observations with others. These efforts may result in several research questions, such as the following:

- What is the nature of patient complaints among patients of different cultural backgrounds?
- Is the cultural background of nurses related to the frequency with which they dispense pain medication?
- Does the number of patient complaints increase when patients are of dissimilar cultural backgrounds as opposed to when they are of the same cultural background as nurses?

- Do nurses' dispensing behaviors change as a function of the similarity between their own cultural background and that of patients?

These questions stem from the same problem, yet each would be studied differently. Some suggest a qualitative approach and others suggest a quantitative one. A quantitative researcher might be curious about cultural or ethnic differences in nurses' dispensing behaviors. Both ethnicity and nurses' dispensing behaviors are variables that can be operationalized. A qualitative researcher would likely be more interested in understanding the *essence* of patients' complaints, their *experience* of frustration, or the *process* by which the problem got resolved.

Researchers choose a problem to study based on several factors, including its inherent interest and its compatibility with a paradigm of preference. In addition, tentative problems vary in their feasibility and worth. A critical evaluation of ideas is appropriate at this point.

Evaluating Research Problems

Although there are no rules for selecting a research problem, four important considerations to keep in mind are the problem's significance, researchability, feasibility, and interest to you.

Significance of the Problem

A crucial factor in selecting a problem is its significance to nursing. Evidence from the study should have potential to contribute meaningfully to nursing; the new study should be the right "next step" in building an evidence base. The right next step could be an original study, but it could also be a *replication* to answer previously asked questions with greater rigor or with a different population.

TIP In evaluating the significance of an idea, ask the following kinds of questions: Is the problem important to nursing and its clients? Will patient care benefit from the evidence? Will the findings challenge (or lend support to) existing practices? If the answer to all these questions is "no," then the problem probably should be abandoned.

Researchability of the Problem

Not all problems are amenable to research inquiry. Questions of a moral or ethical nature, although provocative, cannot be researched. For example, should assisted suicide be legalized? There are no *right* or *wrong* answers to this question, only points of view. Of course, related questions could be researched, such as: Do patients living with high levels of pain hold more favorable attitudes toward assisted suicide than those with less pain? What moral dilemmas are perceived by nurses who might be involved in assisted suicide? The findings from studies addressing such questions would have no bearing on whether assisted suicide should be legalized, but they could be useful in developing a better understanding of key issues.

Feasibility of the Problem

A third consideration concerns feasibility, which encompasses several issues. Not all of the following factors are universally relevant, but they should be kept in mind in making a decision.

Time. Most studies have deadlines or completion goals, so the problem must be one that can be studied in the allotted time. It is prudent to be conservative in estimating time for the various tasks because research activities typically require more time than anticipated.

Researcher experience. Ideally, the problem should relate to a topic about which you have some prior knowledge or experience. Also, beginning researchers should avoid problems that might require the development of a new measuring instrument or that demand complex analyses.

Availability of study participants. In any study involving humans, researchers need to consider whether people with the desired characteristics will be available and willing to cooperate. Researchers may need to put considerable effort into recruiting participants or may need to offer a monetary incentive.

Cooperation of others. It may be necessary to gain entrée into an appropriate community or setting and to develop the trust of gatekeepers. In institutional settings (e.g., hospitals), access to clients, personnel, or records requires authorization.

Ethical considerations. A research problem may be unfeasible if the study would pose unfair or unethical demands on participants. The ethical issues discussed in Chapter 7 should be reviewed when considering a study's feasibility.

Facilities and equipment. All studies have resource requirements, although needs are sometimes modest. It is prudent to consider what facilities and equipment will be needed and whether they will be available.

Money. Monetary needs for studies vary widely, ranging from $100 or less for small student projects to hundreds of thousands of dollars for large-scale research. If you are on a limited budget, you should think carefully about projected expenses before selecting a problem. Major categories of research-related expenditures include:

- Personnel costs—payments to research assistants (e.g., for interviewing, coding, data entry, transcribing, statistical consulting)
- Participant costs—payments to participants as an incentive for their cooperation or to offset their expenses (e.g., parking, babysitting costs)
- Supplies—paper, memory sticks, postage, and so forth
- Printing and duplication—costs for reproducing forms, questionnaires, and so on
- Equipment—computers and software, audio- or video-recorders, calculators, and the like
- Laboratory fees for the analysis of biophysiologic data
- Transportation costs (e.g., travel to participants' homes)

TIP If your study involves testing a new procedure or intervention, you should also consider the feasibility of ultimately implementing it in real-world settings, should it prove effective. If the innovation requires a lot of resources, there may be little interest in adopting it, even if it results in improvements.

Researcher Interest

Even if a tentative problem is researchable, significant, and feasible, there is one more criterion: your own interest in the problem. Genuine curiosity about a research problem is an important prerequisite to a successful study. A lot of time and energy are expended in a study; there is little sense devoting these resources to a project about which you are not enthusiastic.

> **TIP** New researchers often seek suggestions about a topic area, and such assistance may be helpful in getting started. Nevertheless, it is unwise to be talked into a topic in which you have limited interest. If you do not find a problem appealing at the beginning of a study, you are likely to regret your choice later.

COMMUNICATING RESEARCH PROBLEMS AND QUESTIONS

Every study needs a problem statement—an articulation of what is problematic and is the impetus for the research. Most research reports also present a statement of purpose, research questions, or hypotheses.

Many people do not understand problem statements and may have trouble identifying them in a research article—not to mention developing one. A problem statement often begins with the very first sentence after the abstract. Specific research questions, purposes, or hypotheses appear later in the introduction. Typically, however, researchers *begin* their inquiry by identifying their research question and *then* develop an argument in their problem statement to present the rationale for the new research. This section follows that sequence by describing statements of purpose and research questions, followed by a discussion of problem statements.

Statements of Purpose

Many researchers articulate their research goals in a statement of purpose, worded declaratively. It is usually easy to identify a purpose statement because the word *purpose* is explicitly stated "The purpose of this study was..."—although sometimes the words *aim*, *goal*, or *objective* are used instead, as in "The goal of this study was...."

In a quantitative study, a statement of purpose identifies the key study variables and their possible interrelationships, as well as the population of interest (i.e., the PICO elements).

> **Example of a Statement of Purpose From a Quantitative Study**
> "Aim: This study examined the effects of a music intervention on anxiety, depression, and psychosomatic symptoms of oncology nurses" (Ploukou & Panagopoulou, 2018, p. 77).

In this purpose statement for a Therapy question, the population (P) is oncology nurses. The aim is to assess whether a music intervention (I) compared with no music intervention (C)—which together comprise the independent variable—has an effect on the nurses' anxiety, depression, and psychosomatic symptoms, which are the dependent variables (the Os).

In qualitative studies, the statement of purpose indicates the key concept or phenomenon, and the people under study.

> **Example of a Statement of Purpose From a Qualitative Study**
> The aims of this study were "to explore the experiences of adherence to endocrine therapy in women with breast cancer and their perceptions of the challenges they face in adhering to their medication" (Iacorossi et al., 2018, p. E57).

This statement indicates that the central phenomenon in this study was the experiences of medication adherence and related challenges among women with breast cancer (P).

The statement of purpose communicates more than just the nature of the problem. Researchers' selection of verbs in a purpose statement suggests how they sought to solve the problem, or the state of knowledge on the topic. A study whose purpose is to *explore* or *describe* a phenomenon is likely an investigation of a little-researched topic, sometimes involving a qualitative approach. A purpose statement for a qualitative study may also use verbs such as *understand*, *discover*, or *develop*. Statements of purpose in qualitative studies may "encode" the tradition of inquiry, not only through the researcher's choice of verbs but also through the use of "buzz words" associated with those traditions, as follows:

- *Grounded theory:* Processes; social structures; social interactions
- *Phenomenologic studies:* Experience; lived experience; meaning; essence
- *Ethnographic studies:* Culture; roles; lifeways; cultural behavior

Quantitative researchers also suggest the nature of the inquiry through their selection of verbs. A statement indicating that the study's purpose is to *test* or *evaluate* something (e.g., an intervention) suggests an experimental design. A study whose purpose is to *examine* or *explore* the relationship between two variables likely involves a nonexperimental design. Sometimes the verb is ambiguous: a purpose statement indicating that an intent to *compare* could be referring to a comparison of alternative treatments (using an experimental approach) or a comparison of preexisting groups (using a nonexperimental approach). In any event, verbs such as *test*, *evaluate*, and *compare* suggest an existing knowledge base and quantifiable variables.

The verbs in a purpose statement should connote objectivity. A statement of purpose indicating that the study goal was to *prove*, *demonstrate*, or *show* something suggests a bias. The word *determine* should usually be avoided as well because research methods almost never provide definitive answers to research questions.

> **TIP** Unfortunately, some reports fail to state the study purpose clearly, leaving readers to infer the purpose from such sources as the title of the report. In other reports, the purpose may be difficult to find. Researchers often state their purpose toward the end of the report's introduction.

Research Questions

Research questions are sometimes direct rewordings of purpose statements, phrased interrogatively rather than declaratively, as in the following example:

- *Purpose:* The purpose of this study was to assess the relationship between the functional dependence level of renal transplant recipients and their rate of recovery.

- *Question:* What is the relationship between the functional dependence level (I and C: higher versus lower levels) of renal transplant recipients (P) and their rate of recovery (O)?

Questions have the advantage of simplicity and directness—they invite an answer and help to focus attention on the kinds of data needed to provide that answer. Some research reports thus omit a statement of purpose and state only research questions. Other researchers use a set of research questions to clarify or lend greater specificity to a global purpose statement.

Research Questions in Quantitative Studies

In Chapter 2, we discussed the framing of clinical foreground questions to guide an EBP inquiry. Many of the EBP question templates in Table 2.1 could yield questions to guide a study as well, but *researchers* tend to conceptualize their questions in terms of their *variables*. Take, for example, the Therapy question in Table 2.1, which states, "In (Population), what is the effect of (Intervention) on (Outcome)?" A researcher would likely think of the question in these terms: "In (population), what is the effect of (independent variable) on (dependent variable)?" Thus, in quantitative studies research questions identify the population (P) under study, the key study variables (I, C, and O components), and possible relationships among the variables. The variables are all quantifiable concepts.

Most research questions concern relationships, so many quantitative research questions could be articulated using a general template: "In (population), what is the relationship between (independent variable or IV) and (dependent variable or DV)?" Variations include the following:

- *Therapy/intervention:* In (population), what is the effect of (IV: intervention versus an alternative) on (DV)?
- *Prognosis:* In (population), does (IV: presence of disease or illness versus its absence) affect or increase the risk of (DV: adverse consequences)?
- *Etiology/harm:* In (population), does (IV: exposure versus nonexposure) cause or increase the risk of (DV: disease, health problem)?

Clinical foreground questions for an EBP-focused search and a question for a study sometimes differ. As shown in Table 2.1, sometimes clinicians ask PICO questions about explicit comparisons (e.g., they want to compare intervention A with intervention B) and sometimes they do not (e.g., they want to learn the effects of intervention A, compared with those of any other intervention or to the absence of an intervention, PIO questions). In a research question, there must *always* be a designated comparison because the independent variable must be operationally defined; this definition would articulate the specific "I" and "C" being studied.

TIP Research questions are sometimes more complex than clinical foreground questions for EBP. They may include, in addition to the independent and dependent variable, elements called moderator variables or mediating variables. A **moderator variable** is a variable that influences the strength or direction of a a relationship between two variables (e.g., a person's age might moderate the effect of exercise on physical function). A **mediating variable** is one that acts like a "go-between" in a link between two variables (e.g., a smoking cessation intervention may affect smoking behavior through the intervention's effect on motivation to quit). The Supplement for this chapter on this book's website describes the role of moderating and mediating variables in complex research questions. 🅢

Some research questions are primarily descriptive. As examples, here are some descriptive questions that could be addressed in a study on nurses' use of humor:

- What is the frequency with which nurses use humor as a complementary therapy with hospitalized patients with cancer?
- What are the reactions of hospitalized cancer patients to nurses' use of humor?
- What are the characteristics of nurses who use humor as a complementary therapy with hospitalized patients with cancer?
- Is my *Use of Humor Scale* a reliable and valid measure of nurses' use of humor with patients in clinical settings?

Answers to such questions might, if addressed in a methodologically sound study, be useful in developing interventions for reducing stress in patients with cancer.

Example of a Research Question From a Quantitative Study
Lechner and colleagues (2018) studied skin condition and skin care in German care facilities. Here is one research question: *What is the prevalence of dry skin in nursing home residents and hospital patients and is the prevalence higher in nursing homes or hospitals?*

TIP The Toolkit section of Chapter 4 of the accompanying *Resource Manual* includes question templates in a Word document that can be "filled in" to generate many types of research questions for both qualitative and quantitative studies.

Research Questions in Qualitative Studies

Research questions for qualitative studies state the phenomenon of interest and the group or population of interest. Researchers in the various qualitative traditions vary in their conceptualization of what types of questions are important. Grounded theory researchers are likely to ask *process* questions, phenomenologists tend to ask *meaning* questions, and ethnographers generally ask *descriptive* questions about cultures. Special terms associated with the various traditions, noted previously, are likely to be incorporated into the research questions.

Example of a Research Question From a Phenomenologic Study
What is the lived experience of children with spina bifida in the West Bank, Palestine (Nahal et al., 2019)?

Not all qualitative studies are rooted in a specific research tradition. Many researchers use qualitative methods to describe or explore phenomena without focusing on cultures, meaning, or social processes.

Example of a Research Question From a Descriptive Qualitative Study
In their descriptive qualitative study, Dial and Holmes (2018) asked, "What are the successful self-care hygienic strategies that patients of size use to care for themselves at home?"

In qualitative studies, research questions may evolve over the course of the study. Researchers begin with a *focus* that defines the broad boundaries of the study, but the boundaries are not cast in stone.

The boundaries "can be altered and, in the typical naturalistic inquiry, will be" (Lincoln & Guba, 1985, p. 228). The naturalist begins with a research question that provides a general starting point but does not prohibit discovery. The emergent nature of qualitative inquiry means that research questions can be modified as new data make it relevant to do so.

Problem Statements

Problem statements express the dilemma or troubling situation that needs investigation and that provide a rationale for a new inquiry. A good problem statement is a well-structured formulation of what is problematic, what "needs fixing," or what is poorly understood. Problem statements, especially for quantitative studies, often have most of the following six components:

1. *Problem identification:* What is wrong with the current situation?
2. *Background:* What is the context of the problem that readers need to understand?
3. *Scope of the problem:* How big a problem is it? How many people are affected?
4. *Consequences of the problem:* What are the costs of *not* fixing the problem?
5. *Knowledge gaps:* What information about the problem is lacking?
6. *Proposed solution:* How would the proposed study contribute to the solution of the problem?

These components, taken together, form the **argument** for the study—researchers try to

persuade readers that the rationale for undertaking the study is sound.

> **TIP** The Toolkit section of Chapter 4 of the accompanying *Resource Manual* includes these six questions in a Word document that can be "filled in" and reorganized as needed, as an aid to developing a problem statement.

Suppose our topic was humor as a complementary therapy for reducing stress in hospitalized patients with cancer. Our research question is, "What is the effect of nurses' use of humor on stress and natural killer cell activity in hospitalized patients with cancer?" Box 4.1 presents a rough draft of a problem statement for such a study. This problem statement is a reasonable first draft. The draft has several, but not all, of the six components.

Box 4.2 illustrates how the problem statement could be strengthened by adding information about scope (component 3), long-term consequences (component 4), and possible solutions (component 6). This second draft builds a more compelling argument for new research: millions of people are affected by cancer, and the disease has adverse consequences not only for those diagnosed and their families but also for society. The revised problem statement also suggests a basis for the new study by describing a solution on which the new study might build.

As this example suggests, the problem statement is usually interwoven with supportive evidence from the research literature. In many research articles, it

BOX 4.1 Draft Problem Statement on Humor and Stress

A diagnosis of cancer is associated with high levels of stress. Sizable numbers of patients who receive a cancer diagnosis describe feelings of uncertainty, fear, anger, and loss of control. Interpersonal relationships, psychological functioning, and role performance have all been found to suffer following cancer diagnosis and treatment.

A variety of alternative/complementary therapies have been developed in an effort to decrease the harmful effects of stress on psychological and physiological functioning, and resources devoted to these therapies (money and staff) have increased in recent years. However, many of these therapies have not been carefully evaluated to determine their efficacy, safety, or cost-effectiveness. For example, the use of humor has been recommended as a therapeutic device to improve quality of life, decrease stress, and perhaps improve immune functioning, but the evidence to support this claim is limited.

BOX 4.2 Some Possible Improvements to Problem Statement on Humor and Stress

Each year, more than 1 million people are diagnosed with cancer, which remains one of the top causes of death among both men and women (reference citations). Numerous studies have documented that a diagnosis of cancer is associated with high levels of stress. Sizable numbers of patients who receive a cancer diagnosis describe feelings of uncertainty, fear, anger, and loss of control (citations). Interpersonal relationships, psychological functioning, and role performance have all been found to suffer following cancer diagnosis and treatment (citations). These stressful outcomes can, in turn, adversely affect health, long-term prognosis, and medical costs among cancer survivors (citations).

A variety of alternative/complementary therapies have been developed in an effort to decrease the harmful effects of stress on psychological and physiological functioning, and resources devoted to these therapies (money and staff) have increased in recent years (citations). However, many of these therapies have not been carefully evaluated to determine their efficacy, safety, or cost-effectiveness. For example, the use of humor has been recommended as a therapeutic device to improve quality of life, decrease stress, and perhaps improve immune functioning (citations), but the evidence to support this claim is limited. Preliminary findings from a recent small-scale endocrinology study with a healthy sample exposed to a humorous intervention (citation) holds promise for further inquiry with immuno-compromised populations.

is difficult to disentangle the problem statement from the literature review, unless there is a subsection specifically labeled "Literature Review."

Problem statements for a qualitative study similarly express the nature of the problem, its context, its scope, and information needed to address it, as in the following abridged example:

Example of a Problem Statement From a Qualitative Study

"Rheumatoid arthritis (RA) and psoriatic arthritis (PsA) are inflammatory diseases characterised by chronic arthritis that can result in considerable disease burden. Disease activity and symptoms of RA and PsA can contribute to reduced physical, emotional or psychosocial health and well-being…A physically active lifestyle is associated with reduced risk of several diseases…However, only a minority of people with RA participate in health-promoting physical activities… In addition, people with RA report high levels of pain-catastrophising exhibited as high levels of self-rated pain associated with increased fear-avoidance behaviour towards physical activity…This study was conducted to gain better insight into fear-avoidance beliefs in relation to physical activity among people experiencing moderate-to-severe rheumatic pain." (Lööf & Johansson, 2019, p. 322).

Qualitative studies embedded in a particular research tradition usually incorporate terms in their problem statements that foreshadow the tradition. For example, the problem statement in a grounded theory study might refer to the need to generate a theory relating to social processes. A problem statement for a phenomenologic study might note the need to gain insight into people's experiences or the meanings they attribute to those experiences. And an ethnographer might indicate the need to understand how cultural forces affect people's health behaviors.

RESEARCH HYPOTHESES

A hypothesis is a prediction, almost always a prediction about the relationship between variables.[1] In qualitative studies, researchers do not have an a priori hypothesis, in part because there is too little known to justify a prediction and in part because qualitative researchers want the inquiry to be guided by participants' viewpoints rather than by their own hunches. Thus, our discussion here focuses on hypotheses in quantitative research.

---

[1]Although this does not occur with great frequency, it is possible to make a hypothesis about a specific value. For example, we might hypothesize that the rate of medication compliance in a specific population is 60%. Chapter 18 has an example.

Function of Hypotheses in Quantitative Research

Research questions, as we have seen, are usually queries about relationships between variables. Hypotheses are predicted answers to these queries. For instance, the research question might ask: Does sexual abuse in childhood affect the development of irritable bowel syndrome in women? The researcher might predict the following: Women (P) who were sexually abused in childhood (I) have a higher incidence of irritable bowel syndrome (O) than women who were not (C).

Hypotheses sometimes follow from a theory. Scientists reason from theories to hypotheses and test those hypotheses in the real world. Take, as an example, the theory of reinforcement, which maintains that behavior that is positively reinforced (rewarded) tends to be learned or repeated. Predictions based on this theory could be tested. For example, we could test the following hypothesis: Pediatric patients (P) who are given a reward (e.g., a toy) (I) when they undergo nursing procedures tend to be more cooperative during those procedures (O) than nonrewarded peers (C). This hypothesis can be put to a test, and the theory gains credibility if it is supported with real data.

Even in the absence of a theory, well-conceived hypotheses offer direction and suggest explanations. For example, suppose we hypothesized that cue-based feedings compared with traditional methods of feeding for preterm infants will shorten the time to full oral feedings and discharge from the NICU. We could justify our speculation based on earlier studies or clinical observations, or both. *The development of predictions forces researchers to think logically and to tie together earlier research findings.*

Now let us suppose the preceding hypothesis is not confirmed: we find that time to full oral feedings and discharge is similar for preterm infants on cue-based feedings and traditional methods of feeding. *The failure of data to support a prediction forces researchers to analyze theory or previous research critically, to consider study limitations, and to explore alternative explanations for the findings.* The use of hypotheses tends to induce critical thinking and encourages careful interpretation of the evidence.

To illustrate further the utility of hypotheses, suppose we conducted the study guided only by the research question, Is there a relationship between feeding method in preterm infants and the length of time to full oral feedings and NICU discharge? The investigator without a hypothesis is apparently prepared to accept any results. The problem is that it is almost always possible to explain something superficially after the fact, no matter what the findings are. Hypotheses reduce the risk that spurious results will be misconstrued.

> **TIP** Consider whether it might be appropriate to develop hypotheses that predict different effects of the independent variable on the outcome for different subgroups of people—that is, to consider the effects of *moderator* variables. For example, would you predict the effects of an intervention to be different for males and females? Testing such hypotheses might facilitate greater applicability of the evidence to specific types of patient (Chapter 31).

Characteristics of Testable Hypotheses

Testable hypotheses state the expected relationship between the independent variable (the presumed cause or antecedent) and the dependent variable (the presumed effect or outcome) within a population.

> **Example of a Research Hypothesis**
> Palesh and colleagues (2018) hypothesized that, among women with advanced breast cancer, a greater degree of physical activity is associated with longer survival.

In this example, the population is women with advanced breast cancer, the independent variable is amount of physical activity, and the dependent variable is length of time before death. The hypothesis predicts that these two variables are related within the population—greater physical activity is predicted to be associated with longer survival.

Hypotheses that do not make a relational statement are difficult to test. Take the following example: *Pregnant women who receive prenatal instruction about postpartum experiences are not likely to experience postpartum depression.* This statement expresses no anticipated relationship—there is only one variable (postpartum depression), and a relationship requires at least two variables.

The problem is that without a prediction about an anticipated relationship, the hypothesis is difficult to test using standard statistical procedures. In our example, how would we know whether the hypothesis was supported—what standard could be used to decide whether to accept or reject it? To illustrate this concretely, suppose we asked a group of mothers who had been given instruction on postpartum experiences the following question 1 month after delivery: On the whole, how depressed have you been since you gave birth? Would you say (1) extremely depressed, (2) moderately depressed, (3) a little depressed, or (4) not at all depressed?

Based on responses to this question, how could we compare the actual outcome with the predicted outcome? Would *all* the women have to say they were "not at all depressed?" Would the prediction be supported if 51% of the women said they were "not at all depressed" or "a little depressed?" It is difficult to test the accuracy of the prediction.

A test is simple, however, if we modify the prediction as follows: Pregnant women who receive prenatal instruction are less likely to experience postpartum depression than those with no prenatal instruction. Here, the outcome variable (O) is the women's depression, and the independent variable is receipt (I) versus nonreceipt (C) of prenatal instruction. The relational aspect of the prediction is embodied in the phrase *less than*. If a hypothesis lacks a phrase such as *more than*, *less than*, *greater than*, *different from*, *related to*, *associated with*, or something similar, it is probably not amenable to statistical testing. To test this revised hypothesis, we could ask two groups of women with different prenatal instruction experiences to respond to the question on depression and then compare the average responses of the two groups. The absolute degree of depression of either group would not be at issue.

Hypotheses should be based on justifiable rationales. Hypotheses often follow from previous research findings or are deduced from a theory. When a new area is being investigated, the researcher may have to turn to logical reasoning or clinical experience to justify predictions.

The Derivation of Hypotheses

Many students ask, How do I go about developing hypotheses? Two basic processes—induction and deduction—are the intellectual machinery involved in deriving hypotheses (The Supplement to Chapter 3 **S** on the Point thePoint book's website described induction and deduction).

An **inductive hypothesis** is inferred from observations. Researchers observe certain patterns among phenomena and then make predictions based on the observations. An important source for inductive hypotheses is clinical experiences. For example, a nurse might notice that presurgical patients who ask a lot of questions about pain have a more difficult time than other patients in learning postoperative procedures. The nurse could formulate a hypothesis, such as: Patients who are stressed by fear of pain have more difficulty in deep breathing and coughing after surgery than patients who are not stressed. Qualitative studies are an important source of inspiration for inductive hypotheses.

> **Example of Deriving an Inductive Hypothesis**
> LoGiudice and Beck (2016) conducted a phenomenological study of the experience of childbearing from eight survivors of sexual abuse. One of the themes from this study was "Overprotection: Keeping my child safe." A hypothesis that can be derived from this qualitative finding might be as follows: Women who are survivors of sexual abuse will be more overprotective of their children than mothers who have not experienced sexual abuse.

Inductive hypotheses begin with specific observations and move toward generalizations. **Deductive hypotheses** have theories or prior knowledge as a starting point, as in our earlier example about reinforcement theory. Researchers deduce that if the theory is true, then certain outcomes can be expected. If hypotheses are supported, then the theory is strengthened. The advancement of nursing knowledge depends on both inductive and deductive hypotheses. Researchers need to be organizers of concepts (think inductively), logicians (think deductively), and critics and skeptics of resulting formulations, constantly demanding evidence.

Wording of Hypotheses

A good hypothesis is worded clearly and concisely and in the present tense. Researchers make predictions about relationships that exist in the population and not just about a relationship that will be revealed in a particular sample. There are various types of hypotheses.

Directional Versus Nondirectional Hypotheses

Hypotheses can be stated in a number of ways, as in the following example:

1. Older patients are more likely to fall than younger patients.
2. There is a relationship between the age of a patient and the risk of falling.
3. The older the patient, the greater the risk that he or she will fall.
4. Older patients differ from younger ones with respect to their risk of falling.
5. Younger patients tend to be less at risk of a fall than older patients.

In each example, the hypothesis indicates the population (patients), the independent variable (patients' age), the dependent variable (a fall), and the anticipated relationship between them.

Hypotheses can be either directional or nondirectional. A **directional hypothesis** is one that specifies not only the existence but the expected direction of the relationship between variables. In our example, hypotheses 1, 3, and 5 are directional because there is an explicit prediction that older patients are more likely to fall than younger ones. A **nondirectional hypothesis** does not state the direction of the relationship, as illustrated by versions 2 and 4. These hypotheses predict that a patient's age and risk of falling are related, but they do not stipulate whether the researcher thinks that *older* patients or *younger* ones are at greater risk.

Hypotheses derived from theory are almost always directional because theories provide a rationale for expecting variables to be related in a certain way. Existing studies also offer a basis for directional hypotheses. When there is no theory or related research, when findings of prior studies are contradictory, or when researchers' own experience leads to ambivalence, nondirectional hypotheses may be appropriate. Some people argue, in fact, that nondirectional hypotheses are preferable because they connote impartiality. Directional hypotheses, it is said, imply that researchers are intellectually committed to certain outcomes, and such a commitment might lead to bias. Yet, researchers typically *do* have hunches about outcomes, whether they state them explicitly or not. We prefer directional hypotheses when there is a reasonable basis for them because they clarify the study's framework and demonstrate that researchers have thought critically about the study variables.

> **TIP** Hypotheses can be either *simple hypotheses* (ones with one independent variable and one dependent variable) or *complex hypotheses* (ones with three or more variables—for example, with multiple independent or dependent variables). Information about complex hypotheses is available in the Supplement for this chapter on thePoint. $\boldsymbol{S}$

Research Versus Null Hypotheses

Hypotheses can be described as either research hypotheses or null hypotheses. **Research hypotheses** (also called *scientific* hypotheses) are statements of expected relationships between variables. All hypotheses presented thus far are research hypotheses that state actual predictions.

Statistical inference uses a logic that may be confusing. This logic requires that hypotheses be expressed as an expected *absence* of a relationship. **Null hypotheses** (or *statistical hypotheses*) state that there is no relationship between the independent and dependent variables. The null form of the hypothesis used in our example might be: "Patients' age is unrelated to their risk of falling" or "Older patients are just as likely as younger patients to fall." The null hypothesis might be compared with the assumption of innocence of an accused criminal in many justice systems: the variables are assumed to be "innocent" of any relationship until they can be shown "guilty" through appropriate statistical procedures. The null hypothesis represents the formal statement of this assumption of "innocence."

Researchers typically state research rather than null hypotheses. Indeed, you should avoid stating hypotheses in null form in a proposal or a report because this gives an amateurish impression. In statistical testing, underlying null hypotheses are assumed without being stated. If the researcher's *actual* research hypothesis is that no relationship among variables exists, complex procedures are needed to test it.

Hypothesis Testing and Proof

Hypotheses are formally tested through statistical analysis. Researchers use statistics to test whether their hypotheses have a high probability of being correct (i.e., have a $p < .05$). Statistical analysis does not offer proof; it only supports inferences that a hypothesis is *probably* correct (or not). Hypotheses are never *proved* or *disproved*; rather, they are *supported* or *rejected*. Findings are always tentative. Hypotheses come to be increasingly supported with evidence from multiple studies.

Let us look at why this is so. Suppose we hypothesized that height and weight are related. We predict that, on average, tall people weigh more than short people. We then obtain height and weight measurements from a sample and analyze the data. Now suppose we happened by chance to get a sample that consisted of short, heavy people, and tall, thin people. Our results might indicate that there is no relationship between height and weight. But we would not be justified in concluding that this study *proved* or *demonstrated* that height and weight are unrelated.

This example illustrates the difficulty of using observations from a sample to draw definitive conclusions about a population. Issues such as the accuracy of the measures, the effects of uncontrolled variables, and idiosyncrasies of the study sample prevent researchers from concluding that hypotheses are proved.

> **TIP** If a researcher uses any statistical tests (as is true in most quantitative studies), it means that there were underlying hypotheses—regardless of whether the researcher explicitly stated them—because statistical tests are designed to test hypotheses. In planning a quantitative study of your own, do not hesitate to state hypotheses.

CRITICAL APPRAISAL OF RESEARCH PROBLEMS, RESEARCH QUESTIONS, AND HYPOTHESES

In appraising research articles, you need to evaluate whether researchers have adequately communicated their problem. The problem statement, purpose, research questions, and hypotheses set the stage for a description of what the researchers did and what they learned. You should not have to dig deeply to decipher the research problem or the questions.

A critical appraisal of the research problem is multidimensional. Substantively, you need to consider whether the problem has significance for nursing. Studies that build in a meaningful way on existing knowledge are well-poised to contribute to evidence-based nursing practice. Researchers who develop a systematic **program of research**, designing new studies based on their own earlier findings, are especially likely to make important contributions (Conn, 2004). For example, Cheryl Beck's series of studies relating to postpartum depression and traumatic births have influenced women's health care worldwide. Also, research problems stemming from established research priorities (Chapter 1) have a high likelihood of yielding important new evidence for nurses because they reflect expert opinion about areas of needed research.

Another dimension in appraising the research problem is methodologic—in particular, whether the research problem is compatible with the chosen research paradigm and its associated methods. You should also evaluate whether the statement of purpose or research questions have been properly worded and lend themselves to empirical inquiry.

In a quantitative study, if the research article does not contain explicit hypotheses, you need to consider whether their absence is justified. If there are hypotheses, you should evaluate whether they are logically connected to the problem and are consistent with existing evidence or relevant theory. The wording of hypotheses should also be assessed. To be testable, the hypothesis should contain a prediction about the relationship between two or more measurable variables. Specific

BOX 4.3 Guidelines for Critically Appraising Research Problems, Research Questions, and Hypotheses

1. What is the research problem? Is the problem statement easy to locate and is it clearly stated? Does the problem statement build a cogent and persuasive argument for the new study?
2. Does the problem have significance for nursing? How might the research contribute to nursing practice, administration, education, or policy?
3. Is there a good fit between the research problem and the paradigm in which the research was conducted? Is there a good fit between the problem and the qualitative research tradition (if applicable)?
4. Does the report formally present a statement of purpose, research question, and/or hypotheses? Is this information communicated clearly and concisely, and is it placed in a logical and useful location?
5. Are purpose statements or questions worded appropriately? For example, are key concepts/variables identified and is the population of interest specified? Are verbs used appropriately to suggest the nature of the inquiry and/or the research tradition?
6. If there are no formal hypotheses, is their absence justified? Are statistical tests used in analyzing the data despite the absence of stated hypotheses?
7. Do hypotheses (if any) flow from a theory or previous research? Is there a justifiable basis for the predictions?
8. Are hypotheses (if any) properly worded—do they state a predicted relationship between two or more variables? Are they directional or nondirectional, and is there a rationale for how they were stated? Are they presented as research or as null hypotheses?

guidelines for critically appraising research problems, research questions, and hypotheses are presented in Box 4.3. ❖

RESEARCH EXAMPLES

This section describes how the research problem and research questions were communicated in two nursing studies, one quantitative and one qualitative.

Research Example of a Quantitative Study

Study: Effectiveness of a patient-centred, empowerment-based intervention programme among patients with poorly controlled type 2 diabetes (Cheng et al., 2018).

Problem statement (Excerpt; citations omitted to streamline presentation): "Despite extensive advances and collective prioritization of evidence-based diabetes management, poor glycaemic control still remains common in many countries… Adherence to diabetes self-management regimen continues to be the most significant determinant to attain glycaemic target. Patients with poorly controlled type 2 diabetes find enormous difficulty

synthesizing self-management recommendations in the dynamic and complex daily context. There is a great call to support and empower them to take a proactive self-management role in the disease trajectory. A flourishing body of studies have illustrated that patient-centred, empowerment-based approach could boost patients' engagement in and commitment to diabetes self-management." (p. 44).

Statement of purpose: The aim of this study was "to evaluate the effectiveness of a patient-centred, empowerment-based programme on glycaemic control and self-management behaviours among patients with poorly controlled type 2 diabetes." (p.43).

Research question: Although not formally stated by the researchers, we can state their Therapy question as follows: Among patients with poorly controlled type 2 diabetes (P), does participation in a patient-centered self-management program (I), compared with non-participation (C), lead to improvements in HbA1c levels and self-management behaviors (O)?

Hypotheses: The researchers hypothesized that compared with study participants who do not receive the intervention, patients who receive the intervention program will have (1) significantly optimized glycaemic control and (2) better self-management behaviors.

Study methods: The study was conducted in two tertiary hospitals in China. A total of 242 eligible patients were recruited and were allocated, at random, to either receive or not receive the intervention. Those in the intervention group received a 6-week self-management program; the control group received general health education and post discharge follow-up. The key outcomes were HbA1c levels and scores on a measure of self-management behaviors.

Key findings: HbA1c values declined in both groups, and group differences at follow-up were not statistically significant. However, patients in the intervention group exhibited significant improvements in diet management and blood glucose self-monitoring both in the short term (8-week follow-up) and longer term (20-week follow-up).

Research Example of a Qualitative Study

Study: Patients' perceptions and experiences of living with a surgical wound healing by secondary intention (McCaughan et al., 2018).

Problem statement (Excerpt; citations omitted to streamline presentation): Most surgeries in the United Kingdom "result in a wound that heals by primary intention; that is to say, the incision is closed by fixing the edges together with sutures (stitches), staples, adhesive glue, or clips. However, some wounds may be left open to heal…Healing occurs through the growth of new tissue from the base of the wound upwards, a process described as 'healing by secondary intention.' …Management of open surgical wounds requires intensive treatment that may involve prolonged periods of hospitalisation for patients and/or further surgical intervention…While there is an expansive literature relating to patients' experiences of chronic wounds, such as leg ulcers, evidence concerning the impact on patients of experiencing an open surgical wound is lacking." (p. 30).

Statement of purpose: The objective of this study was "to explore patients' views and experiences of living with a surgical wound healing by secondary intention" (p. 29).

Research questions: The patients' experiences were explored by asking such questions as "How has this wound impacted on your daily life?" and "What effect has the wound had on your relationship with your immediate family or friends?"

Method: 20 patients from two locations in the north of England who had a surgical wound healing by secondary intention participated in the study. The researchers made efforts to recruit patients of different gender, age, wound duration, and type of surgery. The study was designed in collaboration with three patient advisers. Study participants were interviewed in-depth, with interviews continuing until data saturation occurred.

Key findings: The patients reported that alarm, shock, and disbelief were their initial reactions to their surgical wound healing. Wound-associated factors had a profound negative impact on their daily life, physical and psychosocial functioning, and well-being. Feelings of powerlessness and frustration were common, and many expressed dissatisfaction with the perceived lack of continuity of care in relation to wound management.

SUMMARY POINTS

- A **research problem** is a perplexing or enigmatic situation that a researcher wants to address through disciplined inquiry. Researchers usually identify a broad *topic*, narrow the problem scope, and identify questions consistent with a paradigm of choice.
- Common sources of ideas for nursing research problems are clinical experience, patient queries, relevant literature, quality improvement initiatives, social issues, and external suggestions.
- Key criteria in selecting a research problem are that the problem should be clinically important; researchable; feasible; and of personal interest.
- Feasibility involves the issues of time, researcher skills, cooperation of participants and other people, availability of facilities and equipment, adequacy of resources, and ethical considerations.
- Researchers communicate their goals as problem statements, statements of purpose, research questions, or hypotheses.
- **Problem statements,** which articulate the nature, context, and significance of a problem, include several components organized to form an **argument** for a new study: problem identification; the background, scope, and consequences

of the problem; knowledge gaps; and possible solutions to the problem.

- A **statement of purpose,** which summarizes the overall study goal, identifies key concepts or variables and the population. Purpose statements often communicate, through the use of verbs and other key terms, the underlying research tradition of qualitative studies, or whether study is experimental or nonexperimental in quantitative ones.
- A **research question** is the specific query researchers want to answer in addressing the research problem. In quantitative studies, research questions usually focus on relationships between variables.
- In quantitative studies, a **hypothesis** is a statement of predicted relationships between two or more variables. Complex hypotheses may involve a **moderator variable** (a variable that alters the strength or direction of a relationship between two variables) or a **mediating variable** that acts as a "go-between" in the link between two variables.
- **Directional hypotheses** predict the direction of a relationship; **nondirectional hypotheses** predict the existence of relationships, not their direction.
- **Research hypotheses** predict the existence of relationships; **null hypotheses**, which express the absence of a relationship, are the hypotheses subjected to statistical testing.
- Hypotheses are never proved or disproved in an ultimate sense—they are accepted or rejected, supported or not supported by the research data.

STUDY ACTIVITIES

Study activities are available to instructors on thePoint.

REFERENCES CITED IN CHAPTER 4

Beck, C. T., LoGiudice, J., & Gable, R. K. (2015). A mixed methods study of secondary traumatic stress in certified nurse-midwives: shaken belief in the birth process. *Journal of Midwifery & Women's Health, 60,* 16–23.

Cheng, L., Sit, J., Choi, K., Chair, S., Li, X., Wu, Y., ... Tao, M. (2018). Effectiveness of a patient-centred, empowerment-based intervention programme among patients with poorly controlled type 2 diabetes. *International Journal of Nursing Studies, 79,* 43–51.

Conn, V. (2004). Building a research trajectory. *Western Journal of Nursing Research, 26,* 592–594.

Dial, M., & Holmes, J. (2018). "I do the best I can;" Personal care preferences of patients of size. *Applied Nursing Research, 39,* 259–264.

Iacorossi, L., Gambalunga, F., Fabi, A., Giannarelli, D., Marchetti, A., Piredda, M., & DeMarinis, M. (2018). Adherence to oral administration of endocrine treatment in patients with breast cancer. *Cancer Nursing, 41,* E57–E63.

*Lechner, A., Lahmann, N., Lichterfeld-Kottner, A., Müller-Werdan, U., Blume-Peytavi, U., & Kottner, J. (2018). Dry skin and the use of leave-on products in nursing care: a prevalence study in nursing homes and hospitals. *Nursing Open, 6,* 189–196.

Lincoln, Y. S., & Guba, E. G. (1985). *Naturalistic inquiry.* Newbury Park, CA: Sage.

LoGiudice, J. A., & Beck, C. T. (2016). The lived experience of childbearing from survivors of sexual abuse: "it was the best of times, it was the worst of times". *Journal of Midwifery & Women's Health, 61,* 474–481.

Lööf, H., & Johansson, U. (2019). "A body in transformation"—an empirical phenomenological study about fear-avoidance beliefs toward physical activity among persons experiencing moderate to severe rheumatic pain. *Journal of Clinical Nursing, 28,* 321–329.

McCaughan, D., Sheard, L., Cullum, N., Dunville, J., & Chetter, I. (2018). Patients' perceptions and experiences of living with a surgical would healing by secondary intention. *International Journal of Nursing Studies, 77,* 29–38.

Nahal, M., Axelsson, A., Iman, A., & Wigert, H. (2019). Palestinian children's narratives about living with spina bifida: stigma, vulnerability, and social exclusion. *Child: Care, Health, and Development, 45,* 54–62.

**Palesh, O., Kamen, C., Sharp, S., Golden, A., Neri, E., Spiegel, D., & Koopman, C. (2018). Physical activity and survival in women with advanced breast cancer. *Cancer Nursing, 41,* E31–E38.

Ploukou, S., & Panagopoulou, E. (2018). Playing music improves well-being of oncology nurses. *Applied Nursing Research, 39,* 77–80.

A link to this open-access article is provided in the Toolkit for Chapter 4 in the **Resource Manual**. ✪

**This journal article is available on* thePoint *for this chapter.*

5

Literature Reviews: Finding and Critically Appraising Evidence

A research **literature review** is a written synthesis and appraisal of evidence on a research problem. Researchers typically undertake a literature review as an early step in conducting a study. This chapter describes activities associated with literature reviews, including locating and critically appraising studies.

SOME LITERATURE REVIEW BASICS

Before discussing the steps involved in doing a research-based literature review, we briefly discuss some general issues.

Purposes of Research Literature Reviews

Healthcare professionals are undertaking many different types of research synthesis, several of which are specifically intended to support evidence-based practice. Grant and Booth (2009) identified 14 different types of synthesis—and even more review types are now appearing in the literature. We described one type of synthesis (systematic reviews) in Chapter 2, and several others will be discussed in Chapter 30. In this chapter, we focus primarily on narrative literature reviews that researchers prepare during the conduct of a new study.

TIP A *narrative literature review* is one in which the findings from the studies under review are integrated using the judgments of the reviewers, rather than through statistical integration—as in a meta-analysis. Until meta-analytic techniques were developed, all reviews were narrative reviews.

Once a research problem and research questions have been identified, a thorough literature review is essential. Literature reviews provide researchers with information to guide a high-quality study, such as information about the following:

- The scope and complexity of the identified research problem (for the argument);
- What other researchers have found in relation to the research question;
- The quality and quantity of existing evidence;
- The contexts and locales in which research has been conducted;
- The characteristics of the people who have served as study participants;
- Theoretical underpinnings of completed studies;
- Methodologic strategies that have been used to address the question; and
- Gaps in the existing evidence base—the type of new evidence that is needed.

This list suggests that a good literature review requires thorough familiarity with available evidence. As Garrard (2017) has advised, you must strive to *own* the literature on a topic to be confident of preparing a high-quality review.

The term "reviewing the literature" is often used to refer to the *process* of identifying, locating, and reading relevant sources of research evidence—that is, conducting a literature review. However, researchers will ultimately need to summarize what they have learned in written form. The length of the product depends on its purpose. Written narrative literature reviews may take the following forms:

- *A review embedded in a research report.* Literature reviews in the introduction to a research report provide readers with an overview of existing evidence and contribute to the argument for new research. These reviews are usually only two to three double-spaced pages, and so only key studies can be cited. The emphasis is on summarizing and critiquing an overall body of evidence and demonstrating the need for a new study.
- *A review in a research proposal.* A literature review in a proposal (often, to request financial support) provides context and illuminates the rationale for new research. The length of such reviews is specified in proposal guidelines; sometimes it is just a few pages. When this is the case, the review must reflect expertise on the topic in a succinct fashion.
- *A review in a thesis or dissertation.* Dissertations in the traditional format (see Chapter 32) often include a thorough, critical literature review. An entire chapter may be devoted to the review, and such chapters are often 20 to 30 pages long. These reviews typically include an evaluation of the overall body of literature as well as critiques of key individual studies. They may also describe relevant theoretical foundations for the study.

In all three cases, the review is not simply a knowledge synthesis: the review provides a context for readers of the report or proposal and offers a justification for a new inquiry. Such reviews also can demonstrate the researcher's competence and thoroughness.

Additionally, nurses sometimes prepare free-standing narrative reviews that are not necessarily done in connection with a planned new study. A written review may be undertaken as a course requirement in graduate school or for publication in a journal. As an example, Gleason et al. (2018) published a literature review on the prevalence of atrial fibrillation symptoms and the relationship between such symptoms and patients' sex, race, and psychological distress. Such free-standing reviews are usually 15 to 25 pages long.

Literature Reviews in Qualitative Research

Quantitative researchers almost always do an upfront literature review, but qualitative researchers have varying opinions about reviewing the literature before doing a new study. Some of the differences reflect viewpoints associated with qualitative research traditions.

Grounded theory researchers often collect and analyze their data before reviewing the literature. Researchers turn to the literature once the grounded theory is sufficiently developed, seeking to relate the theory to prior findings. Glaser (1978) warned that, "It's hard enough to generate one's own ideas without the 'rich' detailment provided by literature in the same field" (p. 31). Thus, grounded theory researchers may defer doing a literature review, but then later consider how previous research fits with or extends the emerging theory.

Phenomenologists often undertake a search for relevant materials at the outset of a study, looking in particular for experiential descriptions of the phenomenon being studied (Munhall, 2012). The purpose is to expand the researcher's understanding of the phenomenon from multiple perspectives, and this may include an examination of artistic sources in which the phenomenon is described (e.g., in novels or poetry).

Even though "ethnography starts with a conscious attitude of almost complete ignorance" (Spradley, 1979, p. 4), literature relating to the chosen cultural problem is often reviewed before data collection. A second, more thorough literature review is often done during data analysis and interpretation so that findings can be compared with previous findings.

Regardless of tradition, if funding is sought for a qualitative project, an upfront literature review is usually necessary. Proposal reviewers need to understand the context for a proposed study when deciding whether it should be funded.

Sources for a Research Review

Written **source materials** vary in their quality and content. In performing a literature review, you will have to decide what to read and what to include in a written review. You may begin your search with broad reference sources on a topic (e.g., textbooks), but ultimately you will mostly be retrieving information from articles published in professional journals.

Findings from prior completed studies are the most important type of information for a research review. You should rely mostly on **primary source** research reports, which are descriptions of studies written by the researchers who conducted them.

> **TIP** Study *protocols* are an additional type of primary source—they are descriptions of the design and methods for studies that are underway but have not yet been completed. These protocols, which are available in *registries* and sometimes in journals, allow researchers to understand what new evidence will *become* available and hence can help you avoid unwanted duplication.

Secondary sources are descriptions of studies prepared by someone other than the original researcher. Literature reviews, for example, are secondary sources. If reviews are recent, they are very useful because they provide an overview of the topic and a valuable bibliography. Secondary sources are not substitutes for primary sources because they typically fail to provide much detail about studies and may not be completely objective.

In addition to research reports, your search may yield nonresearch references, such as case reports, anecdotes, editorials, or clinical descriptions. Nonresearch materials may broaden understanding of a problem, demonstrate a need for research, or describe aspects of clinical practice. These writings may help in formulating research ideas, but they usually have limited utility in written research reviews because they do not address the central question: What is the current state of *evidence* on this research problem?

Primary and Secondary Questions for a Review

For free-standing literature reviews, reviewers may summarize evidence about a single focused question, such as: *Do virtual reality goggles (I) reduce pain (O) in patients undergoing wound care procedures (P)?* For those who are undertaking a literature review as part of a new study, the *primary question* for the literature review is the same as the research question for the new study. The researcher wants to know: What is the current state of knowledge on the question that I will be addressing in *my* study?

If you are doing a review for a new study, you inevitably will need to search for current evidence on several *secondary questions* because you need to develop an argument for the new study. An example will clarify this point.

Suppose that we were conducting a study to address the following question: *Among nurses working in hospitals (P), what characteristics of the nurses or their practice settings (I) are associated with their management of children's pain (O)?* Such a question might arise in the context of a perceived problem, such as a concern that nurses' treatment of children's pain is not always optimal. A simplified statement of the problem might be as follows:

Many children are hospitalized annually and many hospitalized children experience high levels of pain. Although effective analgesic and nonpharmacologic methods of controlling children's pain exist, and although there are reliable methods of assessing children's pain, previous studies have found that nurses do not always manage children's pain effectively.

This rudimentary problem statement suggests a number of *secondary questions* for which up-to-date evidence needs to be found. Examples of such secondary questions include the following:

- How many children are hospitalized each year?
- What levels of pain do hospitalized children typically experience?

- How can pain in hospitalized children be reliably assessed?
- How knowledgeable are nurses about pain assessment and pain management strategies for children?

Thus, a literature review tends to be a multi-pronged task when it is done in preparation for a new study. It is important to identify all questions for which information from the research literature needs to be retrieved.

Major Steps and Strategies in a Narrative Literature Review

Conducting a literature review is a little like doing a full study, in the sense that reviewers start with a question, formulate and implement a plan for gathering information, and then analyze and interpret the information. The "findings" are then summarized in a written product.

Figure 5.1 outlines key steps in the literature review process. As the figure shows, there are several potential feedback loops, with opportunities to retrace earlier steps in search of more information. This chapter discusses each step, but some steps are elaborated in Chapter 30 in our discussion of systematic reviews.

Conducting a high-quality literature review is more than a mechanical exercise—it is an art and a science. Several qualities characterize a high-quality review. First, the review must be comprehensive, thorough, and up-to-date. To "own" the literature

(Garrard, 2017), you must be determined to become an expert on your topic, which means that you need to be diligent in hunting down leads for possible sources of evidence.

> **TIP** Locating all relevant information on a research question is like being a detective. The literature retrieval tools we discuss in this chapter are essential aids, but there inevitably needs to be some digging for the clues to evidence on a topic. Be prepared for sleuthing.

Second, a high-quality review is systematic. Decision rules should be clear, and criteria for including or excluding a study need to be explicit. This is because a third characteristic of a good review is that it is reproducible, which means that another diligent reviewer would be able to apply the same decision rules and criteria and come to similar conclusions about the evidence.

Another desirable attribute of a literature review is the absence of bias. This is more easily achieved when systematic rules for evaluating information are followed or when a team of researchers participates in the review—as is almost always the case in systematic reviews. Finally, reviewers should strive for a review that is insightful and that is more than "the sum of its parts." Reviewers can contribute to knowledge through an astute synthesis of the evidence.

Doing a literature review is somewhat similar to doing a qualitative study: you will need a flexible

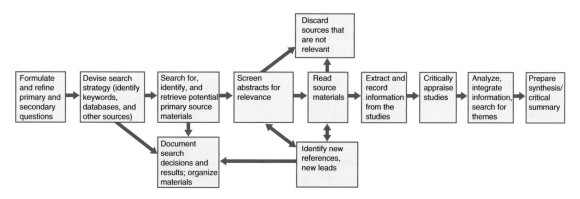

FIGURE 5.1 Flow of tasks in a literature review.

and creative approach to "data collection." Leads for relevant studies should be pursued until "saturation" is achieved—i.e., until your search strategies yield redundant information about studies to include. Finally, the analysis of your "data" will typically involve the identification of important themes in the literature.

Organization in Literature Reviews

The importance of being well-organized in conducting a literature review cannot be overemphasized. As discussed in "Documentation in Literature Retrieval" later in this chapter, we encourage you to document all your decisions and products, and documentation needs to be maintained in an organized framework.

You may prefer to use traditional methods of searching, retrieving, and storing information. For example, you may retrieve a journal article, print or photocopy it, and write notes in the margin. If you do this, you will still need to develop a cataloging system that enables you to find a particular article (e.g., alphabetical filing by last name of the first author).

Increasingly, journal articles are retrieved as portable document files (pdf) and read online using Adobe software, which permits you to highlight text passages and enter marginal comments. If this is your approach, you should create a folder on your computer or in the cloud to store these articles, naming each file in a manner that will allow you to easily locate it. For example, here is how we named the file storing the previously mentioned Gleason et al. (2018) literature review: Gleason2018JCNAtrialFibSymptoms. pdf. This file name indicates the last name of the first author, year of publication, an abbreviation for the journal (JCN = *Journal of Cardiovascular Nursing*), and a brief phrase about the topic. This system would result in a document folder with articles listed alphabetically by the first authors' last names.

You may opt to use reference management software that will help you to stay organized—as well as help you retrieve articles, maintain a reference library and notes, insert citations into papers, and create a bibliography when you write up your review. Popular reference management software that can be used with either Windows for PCs or Macs includes EndNote (free for the Basic version), Mendelay (also free), and RefWorks. Many other reference management software packages are available (for example, see https://en.wikipedia.org/wiki/Comparison_of_reference_management_software).

It is wise to think ahead about the various components of your literature review effort and to have a plan for how to organize them—most likely this will involve the creation of various file folders that will be stored on your computer or in the cloud. For example, if you are not using reference management software, you should create a master folder (e.g., labeled "Pain_Management_Children"), with multiple subfolders. For example, one subfolder could store the source documents (e.g., the pdf journal article files), another could store documentation of your search strategy and results, and another subfolder could save drafts of your actual literature review.

Another organizational tool—one that is essential for a systematic review—is a flow chart that documents your progress in identifying, retrieving, screening, and selecting source materials. Figure 5.2 presents an example of such a flow chart with fictitious numbers (n =) shown in each box. This figure shows that the reviewer started with 400 possible source documents, of which only 15 were used in the final literature review.

LOCATING RELEVANT LITERATURE FOR A RESEARCH REVIEW

As shown in Figure 5.1, an early step in a literature review is devising a strategy to locate relevant studies. The ability to locate research documents on a topic is an important skill that requires adaptability. Sophisticated new search strategies and tools are being introduced regularly. We urge you to consult with librarians, colleagues, or faculty for suggestions. Reference librarians in health libraries are especially valuable and often serve on teams conducting systematic reviews.

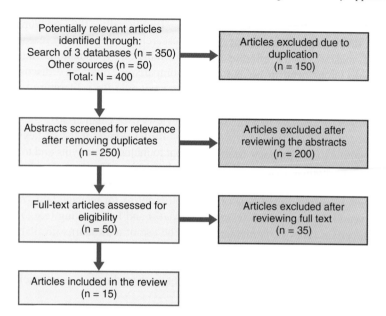

FIGURE 5.2 Example of a flow chart documenting literature search progress.

Formulating a Search Strategy

There are many ways to search for research evidence. Searching is inevitably an iterative process that evolves as new "leads" are discovered based on information you have already retrieved.

Search Strategy Options

Cooper (2017) has identified several search strategies, one of which we describe in some detail in this chapter: searching for references in **bibliographic databases**. Database searches, which can be done efficiently from computers and tablets, are likely to yield the largest number of research references—indeed, sometimes the yield can be overwhelming. Databases are searched primarily for key variables (e.g., pain management) but can also be searched for the names of researchers who have played a key role in a field.

Another approach, called the *ancestry approach* (also called *snowballing, footnote chasing,* or *pearl growing*), involves using references cited in recent relevant studies to track down earlier research on the same topic (the "ancestors"). This is an ongoing process that can be used to not only identify earlier

relevant studies, but also to discover new search terms for subsequent electronic searches.

A third method, the *descendancy approach,* is to find a pivotal early study and to search forward in citation indexes to find more recent studies ("descendants") that cited the key study. Other strategies exist for tracking down what is called the *grey literature*, which refers to studies with more limited distribution, such as conference papers, unpublished reports, and so on. We describe these strategies in Chapter 30 on systematic reviews. If your intent is to "own" the literature, then you will likely want to adopt many of these strategies.

TIP You may be tempted to begin a literature search through an Internet search engine, such as Google, Yahoo, or Bing. Such a search is likely to yield a lot of "hits" on your topic but is unlikely to give you full bibliographic information on relevant *research*. However, such searches can provide useful leads for *search terms*. Also, an Internet search may be the appropriate route for finding answers to secondary questions, such as: How many children are hospitalized annually? This information is more likely to be found in government reports, which are available online, than in research articles.

Eligibility Criteria Specifications

Search plans also involve decisions about the criteria that would make a study eligible for your review. These decisions need to be explicit to guide your search of bibliographic databases. Search limits are most often managed in databases through the use of *filters* (or *limiters* in some bibliographic software).

If you are not multilingual, you may need to constrain your search to studies written in your own language. You may want to limit your search to studies conducted within a certain time frame (e.g., within the past 15 years). You may also want to exclude studies with certain types of participants. For instance, in our example of a literature search about nurses' management of children's pain, we might want to exclude studies in which the children were neonates.

Constraining your search might help you to avoid irrelevant material but be cautious about putting too many restrictions on your search, especially initially. You can always make decisions to exclude studies at a later point.

> **TIP** Be sure not to limit your search to articles exclusively in the nursing literature (e.g., in the nursing subset of records in the database called PubMed). Researchers in many disciplines engage in research relevant to nursing. Also, many nurse researchers publish in nonnursing journals, increasingly as members of interprofessional teams. Moreover, in some databases (e.g., PubMed), some journals with many articles contributed by nurse researchers are not coded as being in the nursing subset (e.g., *Qualitative Health Research*, *Birth*), whereas some journals that are in the nursing subset have articles mostly *not* written by nurse authors (e.g., *Journal of Wound Care*).

Identifying Keywords

Reviewers seeking articles for their reviews begin with a set of search terms, often called **keywords**. Thus, an important early task is to identify and make a written list of the keywords that will be used to search bibliographic databases. The keyword list will be augmented as your search proceeds.

Traditionally, the keywords are your main research variables. Many researchers use the PICO formulation (population, intervention/influence, comparison, outcome) discussed in Chapter 2 as keywords for a literature search, although this may not always be the best strategy for systematic reviews (See Chapter 30).

In developing a list of keywords, it is important to include synonyms and to think broadly about related terms. For example, if we were searching for articles on *teenage smoking*, you should consider other terms for teenage (e.g., *adolescent, children, youth*) and for smoking (e.g., *tobacco, cigarettes*). The use of a thesaurus (available in word processing software) for identifying synonyms is recommended—but take note of keywords specified by researchers themselves in articles you locate.

Searching Bibliographic Databases

Reviewers typically begin by searching bibliographic databases that can be accessed by computer. The databases contain entries for millions of journal articles, and the articles are coded by professional indexers to facilitate retrieval. For example, articles may be coded for language used (e.g., English), subject matter (e.g., pain), journal subset (e.g., nursing), and so on. Some databases can be accessed free of charge (e.g., PubMed, Google Scholar), whereas others are sold commercially—but they are often available through hospital or university libraries. Most database programs are user-friendly, offering menu-driven systems with on-screen support so that retrieval can proceed with minimal instruction.

Getting Started With a Bibliographic Database

Before searching an electronic database, you should become familiar with the features of the software used to access the database. The software gives you options for limiting your search, combining the results of two searches, saving your search, and sending you notifications of new citations relevant to your search. Most programs have tutorials that can improve the efficiency and effectiveness of your search.

In most databases, there are two major strategies for searching. One method is to search for standardized **subject headings** (subject codes) that are assigned by indexers (usually professionals with Master's degrees or higher in relevant disciplines). The subject headings differ from one database to another. It is useful to learn about the relevant subject codes because they offer a path to retrieving articles that use different words to describe the same concept. Another major advantage is that indexers code the articles based on a reading of the entire article (not just the abstract), and they code for *meaning* and not just words. Subject codes for databases can be located in the database's thesaurus or reference tools.

An alternative strategy is to enter your own keywords into a search field. Such a search is an important supplement to searching using the database's controlled vocabulary because indexers are not infallible. However, such keyword searches are limited to searching for words in the article's title or abstract (*not in the full text*), and so if concepts are not mentioned in the title or abstract, the article will not be retrieved.

Most bibliographic software has automatic term mapping capabilities. *Mapping* is a feature that facilitates a search using your own keywords. The software translates ("maps") the keywords you enter into the most plausible subject codes. Nevertheless, it is important to undertake both a keyword search and a subject code search because they yield overlapping but nonidentical results.

General Database Search Features

Some features of an electronic search are similar across databases. One feature is the use of **Boolean operators** to expand or delimit a search. Three widely used Boolean operators are AND, OR, and NOT (in all caps for some databases). The operator AND delimits a search. If we searched for *pain* AND *child,* the software would retrieve only records that have both terms. The operator *OR* expands the search: *pain* OR *child* could be used in a search to retrieve records with either term. Finally, *NOT* narrows a search: *pain* NOT *child* would retrieve all records with pain that did not include the term child. Note that when using multiple Boolean operators, they are processed from left to right. For example, the search phrase *teenage* AND *smoking* OR *cigarettes* would retrieve (1) records that include both teenage and smoking and (2) *all* records with cigarettes, whether or not the article is about teenage smokers. Parentheses can be used to reorder the terms: *teenage* AND (*smoking* OR *cigarettes*). Boolean operators also can be used to combine searches for keyword terms and the last names of prominent researchers in a field, for example, *teenage* AND (*smoking* OR *cigarettes*) AND Kulbok (a researcher).

> **TIP** Be extremely careful using the "NOT" operator because you run the risk of inadvertently removing relevant articles. For example, if you were searching for studies of female teenage smokers and used "NOT male" in the search field, the software would remove any article that included both male and female participants.

Truncation symbols are another useful tool for searching databases. These symbols vary from one database to another, but their function is to expand the search. A **truncation symbol** (often an asterisk, *) expands a search term to include all forms of a root word. For example, a search for *child** would instruct the computer to search for any word that begins with "child" such as children, childhood, or childrearing. For each database, it is important to learn what these special symbols are and how they work. For example, many databases require at least three letters at the beginning of a search term before a truncation symbol can be used. (e.g., ca* would not be allowed).

Some databases (but not PubMed) allow for a **wildcard symbol**—often a question mark—that can be inserted into the middle of a search term to allow for alternative spellings. For example, in databases that allow wildcards, a search for *behavio?r* would retrieve records with either *behavior* or *behaviour.*

Although truncation and wildcard symbols can sometimes be useful, they have one major drawback: in most databases, the use of special symbols turns off a software's mapping feature.

For example, a search for *child** would retrieve records in which any form of "child" appeared in text fields, but it would not map any of these concepts onto the database's subject heading codes. It may be preferable to use a Boolean operator to list all terms of interest (e.g., *child* OR *children*), which would look for either term in a text word search of the title and abstract *and* would map onto the appropriate subject code.

Another issue concerns phrase searching in which you want words to be kept together (e.g., *blood pressure*). Some bibliometric software would treat this as *blood AND pressure* and would search for records with both terms somewhere in text fields, even if they are not contiguous. Quotation marks sometimes can be used to ensure that the words are searched in combination, as in "blood pressure." PubMed recommends, however, that you do not use quotation marks until you have first tried a search without them. PubMed automatically searches for phrases during its mapping process—i.e., in searching for relevant subject heading codes.

Key Electronic Databases for Nurse Researchers

Two bibliographic databases that are especially useful for nurse researchers are the **C**umulative **I**ndex to **N**ursing and **A**llied **H**ealth **L**iterature (CINAHL) and **Med**ical Literature On-**Line** (MEDLINE, accessed through PubMed), which we discuss in the next sections. We also briefly discuss Google Scholar. Other potentially useful bibliographic databases/search engines for nurses include the following:

- **B**ritish **N**ursing **I**ndex (BNI)
- Cochrane Central Register of Controlled Trials (CENTRAL)
- Cochrane Database of Systematic Reviews
- **D**atabase **of P**romoting **H**ealth **E**ffectiveness **R**eviews (DoPHER)
- **E**xcerpta **M**edica data**base** (EMBASE)
- **H**ealth **a**nd **P**sychosocial **I**nstruments database (HaPI)
- **Psy**chology **Info**rmation (PsycINFO)

In addition, the ISI Web of Knowledge and Scopus are two *citation indexes* for retrieving articles that cite a source article.

Note that a search strategy that works well in one database does not always produce good results in another. Thus, it is important to explore strategies in each database and to understand how each database is structured—for example, what subject codes are used, how they are organized in a hierarchy, and what special features are available.

> **TIP** In the following sections, we provide specific information about using CINAHL and MEDLINE via PubMed. Note, however, that databases and the software through which they are accessed change periodically, and so our instructions may not be up-to-date.

Cumulative Index to Nursing and Allied Health Literature

CINAHL is an important bibliographic database: it covers references to virtually all English-language nursing and allied health journals, and includes books, dissertations, and selected conference proceedings in nursing and allied health fields. There are several versions of the CINAHL database (e.g., CINAHL Plus, CINAHL Complete), each with somewhat different features relating to full text availability and journal coverage.

The CINAHL database indexes material from more than 5,000 journals dating from 1981 and contains more than 6 million records. In addition to providing bibliographic information for references (i.e., author, title, journal, year of publication, volume, and page numbers), CINAHL provides abstracts of most citations. Links to the actual article are sometimes provided. We illustrate features of CINAHL but note that some features may be different at your institution.

At the outset, you might begin with a "basic search" by simply entering keywords or phrases relevant to your primary question. As you begin to enter your term into the search box, autocomplete suggestions will display, and you can click on the one that is the best match. In the basic search screen, you can limit your search in a number of ways, for example, limiting the records retrieved to those with certain features (e.g., only ones with abstracts; only research articles); to a specific range of publication dates (e.g., only those from 2010 to the present); or to those in specific languages (e.g., English). The search screen allows you to expand your search by clicking an option labeled "Apply related words."

As an example, suppose we were interested in recent research on nurses' pain management for children. If we did a keyword search for *pain management*, we would get about 18,000 records. Searching for *pain management AND child AND nurse* would bring the number down to about 400 (we did not truncate child* because this would retrieve records for some irrelevant terms associated with pain, such as *childhood*). We could pare the number down to about 160 by limiting the search to research articles with abstracts published since 2000.

The full records for the 160 references would then be displayed on the monitor in a Search Results list. There is a "sort" option at the top of the list that allows you to sort the references based on several criteria, such as publication date, author's last name, and relevance. From the Results list, we could place promising references into a folder for later scrutiny by clicking on a file icon in the upper right corner of each entry. We could then save the folder, print it, or export it to reference manager software such as EndNote.

An example of an abridged CINAHL record entry for a study identified through the search on the management of children's pain is presented in Figure 5.3. The record begins with the article title, the authors' names and affiliation, and source. The source indicates the following:

- Name of the journal (*Pain Management Nursing*)
- Year and month of publication (Feb 2015)
- Volume (16)
- Issue (1)
- Page numbers (40-50)

The record also shows the major and minor CINAHL subject headings that were coded by the indexers. Any of these headings could have been used to retrieve this reference. Note that the subject headings include substantive codes, such as *Postoperative Pain*, and methodologic codes (e.g., *Correlational Studies*), person characteristic codes (e.g., *Child*), and a location code (*Singapore*). Next, the abstract for the study is shown. Based on the abstract, we might be able to decide whether this reference was pertinent. Each entry shows an accession number that is the unique identifier for each record in the CINAHL database, as well as other identifying numbers.

An important feature of CINAHL helps you to find other relevant references once a good one has been found. In Figure 5.3 you can see that the record offers many embedded links on which you can click. For example, you could click on any of the authors' names to see if they published other related articles. There is also a sidebar link in each record called *Times Cited in this Database* (if there has been a citation), with which you could retrieve records for articles that had cited this paper (for a descendancy search). Another link is labeled *Find Similar Results* that suggests other relevant references.

In CINAHL, you can also explore the structure of the database's thesaurus to get additional leads for searching. The tool bar at the top of the screen has a tab called *CINAHL Headings*. When you click on this tab, you can enter a term of interest in the *Browse* field and select one of three options: *Term Begins With, Term Contains*, or *Relevancy Ranked* (which is the default). For example, if we entered *pain management* and then clicked on Browse, we would be shown the major subject headings relating to pain management; we could then search the database for any of the listed subject codes.

TIP Note that the keywords we used to illustrate this simplified search (pain management, child, nurse) would not be adequate for a comprehensive retrieval of studies relevant to our review question. For example, we would want to search for several additional terms (e.g., *pediatric*).

Title:	Nurses' Provision of Parental Guidance Regarding School-Aged Children's Postoperative Pain Management: A Descriptive Correlational Study
Authors:	He, Hong-Gu; Klainin-Yobas, Piyanee; Ang, Emily Neo Kim; Sinnappan, Rajammal; Pölkki, Tarja; Wang, Wenru
Affiliation:	Alice Lee Centre for Nursing Studies Department, Yong Loo Lin School of Medicine, National University of Singapore, Singapore; Clinical and Oncology Nursing, National University Hospital, Singapore; Division of Nursing, KK Women's and Children's Hospital, Singapore; Institute of Health Sciences, University of Oulu, Oulu, Finland
Source:	Pain Management Nursing (PAIN MANAGE NURS), Feb2015; 16(1): 40-50. (11p)
Publication Type:	Journal Article - research
Language:	English
Major Subjects:	Postoperative Pain – Prevention and Control – In Infancy and Childhood Parental Role Nurse Attitudes – Evaluation Parents – Education Pediatric Nursing
Minor Subjects:	Human; Multiple Linear Regression; Descriptive Research; Descriptive Statistics; Correlational Studies; Convenience Sample; T-Tests; Hospitals – Singapore; Singapore; Age Factors; Educational Status; Questionnaires; Adult; Child
Abstract:	Involving parents in children's pain management is essential to achieve optimal outcomes. Parents need to be equipped with sufficient knowledge and information. Only a limited number of studies have explored nurses' provision of parental guidance regarding the use of nonpharmacologic methods in children's pain management. This study aimed to examine nurses' perceptions of providing preparatory information and nonpharmacologic methods to parents, and how their demographics and perceived knowledge adequacy of these methods influence this guidance. A descriptive correlational study using questionnaire surveys was conducted to collect data from a convenience sample of 134 registered nurses working in seven pediatric wards of two public hospitals in Singapore. Descriptive statistics, independent-samples t test, and multiple linear regression were used to analyze the data. Most nurses provided various types of cognitive information to parents related to their children's surgery, whereas information about children's feelings was less often provided. Most nurses provided guidance to parents on positioning, breathing technique, comforting/reassurance, helping with activities of daily living, relaxation, and creating a comfortable environment. Nurses' provision of parental guidance on preparatory information and nonpharmacologic methods was significantly different between subgroups of age, education, parent or not, and perceived knowledge adequacy of nonpharmacologic methods. Nurses' perceived knowledge adequacy was the main factor influencing their provision of parental guidance. More attention should be paid to nurses who are younger, have less working experience, and are not parents. There is a need to educate nurses about nonpharmacologic pain relief methods to optimize their provision of parental guidance.
Journal Subset:	Blind Peer Reviewed; Core Nursing; Editorial Board Reviewed; Expert Peer Reviewed; Nursing; Peer Reviewed; USA
Special Interest:	Pain and Pain Management; Pediatric Care; Perioperative Care
ISSN:	1524-9042
MEDLINE info:	NLM UID: 100890606
Entry Date:	20150115
Revision Date:	20150710
DOI:	http://dx.doi.org.libraryproxy.griffith.edu.au/10.1016/j.pmn.2014.03.002
Accession No:	103873708

FIGURE 5.3 Example of a record from a CINAHL (Cumulative Index to Nursing and Allied Health Literature) search. (Abstract reprinted with permission from He H.G., Klainin-Yobas P., Ang E., Sinnappan R., Pölkki T., & Wang W. (2015). Nurses' provision of parental guidance regarding school-aged children's postoperative pain management: A descriptive correlational study. *Pain Management Nursing, 16*, 40–50.)

The MEDLINE Database and PubMed

The MEDLINE database was developed by the U.S. National Library of Medicine and is widely recognized as the premier source for bibliographic coverage of the biomedical literature. MEDLINE covers about 5,600 medical, nursing, and health journals published in about 70 countries and contains more than 28 million records dating back to the mid-1940s. In 1999, abstracts of systematic reviews from the Cochrane Collaboration became available through MEDLINE.

The MEDLINE database can be accessed through a commercial vendor, but it can be accessed for free through the PubMed website (http://www.ncbi.nlm.nih.gov/PubMed). This means that anyone, anywhere in the world with Internet access can search for journal articles, and thus PubMed is a lifelong resource. PubMed has excellent tutorials, including a 30-minute tutorial specifically for nurses (PubMed for Nurses). PubMed includes all references in the MEDLINE library plus additional references, such as those that have not yet been indexed.

On the Home page of PubMed, you can launch a basic search that looks for your keywords in text fields of the record. PubMed, like CINAHL, has an autocomplete feature that offers suggestions as you begin to enter your terms.

> **TIP** On the PubMed home page, you can also launch a Clinical Query search, which is a particularly useful tool for searching for evidence in the context of an EBP inquiry. Supplement A to this chapter on thePoint provides guidance for undertaking such a clinical query. 🛇

MEDLINE uses a controlled vocabulary called **MeSH** (Medical Subject Headings) to index articles. Indexers assign as many MeSH headings as appropriate to cover content and features of the article—typically 5 to 15 codes. You can learn about relevant MeSH terms by clicking on the "MeSH database" link on the Home page (under the heading *More Resources*). If, for example, we searched the MeSH database for "pain," we would find that Pain is a MeSH subject heading (a definition is provided) and there are 60 related categories—for example, "Cancer pain," "Back pain," and "Headache."

Each category has numerous subheadings, such as "Complications," "Etiology," and "Nursing."

If you begin with a keyword search, you can see how your term mapped onto MeSH terms by looking in the right-hand panel for a section labeled *Search Details*. For example, if we entered "children" as our keyword in the search field of the initial screen, Search Details would show us that PubMed searched for all references that have "child" or "children" in text fields of the database record, *and* it also searched for all references that had been coded "child" as a subject heading because "child" is a MeSH subject heading.

If we did a PubMed search of MEDLINE similar to the one we described earlier for CINAHL, we would find that a simple search for *pain management* would yield about 102,000 records; a search for *pain management AND child AND nurse* would yield nearly 700 records. We can place restrictions on the search using filters that are shown in the left sidebar of the screen. If we limited our search to entries with abstracts, written in English, and published in 2000 or later, the search would yield about 450 records. Thus, PubMed search yielded more references than the CINAHL search, in part because MEDLINE indexes more journals; another factor, however, is that in PubMed we could not limit the search to research articles because PubMed does not have a generic category that distinguishes research articles from nonresearch articles.

> **TIP** Here are the Search Details (the strategy and syntax) for the PubMed search just described: ("pain management"[MeSH Terms] OR ("pain"[All Fields] AND "management"[All Fields]) OR "pain management"[All Fields]) AND ("child"[MeSH Terms] OR "child"[All Fields]) AND ("nurses"[MeSH Terms] OR "nurses"[All Fields] OR "nurse"[All Fields]) AND (hasabstract[text] AND ("2000/01/01"[PDAT]: "3000/12/31"[PDAT]) AND English[lang])

From the Search Results page, we would then click on links to the citations that suggest a relevant article; this would bring up a new screen that provides the abstract for the article and further details. Figure 5.4 shows the full citation and abstract for the same study we located earlier in CINAHL. Beneath the abstract, the display presents the MeSH terms

Pain Manag Nurs. 2015 Feb;16(1):40-50. doi: 10.1016/j.pmn.2014.03.002. Epub 2014 Jun 21.

Nurses' provision of parental guidance regarding school-aged children's postoperative pain management: a descriptive correlational study.

He HG[1], Klainin-Yobas P[2], Ang EN[3], Sinnappan R[4], Pölkki T[5], Wang W[2].

Author information: 1 Alice Lee Centre for Nursing Studies Department, Yong Loo Lin School of Medicine, National University of Singapore, Singapore. Electronic address: nurhhg@nus.edu.sg. 2 Alice Lee Centre for Nursing Studies Department, Yong Loo Lin School of Medicine, National University of Singapore, Singapore. 3 Clinical and Oncology Nursing, National University Hospital, Singapore. 4 Division of Nursing, KK Women's and Children's Hospital, Singapore. 5 Institute of Health Sciences, University of Oulu, Oulu, Finland.

Abstract:

Involving parents in children's pain management is essential to achieve optimal outcomes. Parents need to be equipped with sufficient knowledge and information. Only a limited number of studies have explored nurses' provision of parental guidance regarding the use of nonpharmacologic methods in children's pain management. This study aimed to examine nurses' perceptions of providing preparatory information and nonpharmacologic methods to parents, and how their demographics and perceived knowledge adequacy of these methods influence this guidance. A descriptive correlational study using questionnaire surveys was conducted to collect data from a convenience sample of 134 registered nurses working in seven pediatric wards of two public hospitals in Singapore. Descriptive statistics, independent-samples t test, and multiple linear regression were used to analyze the data. Most nurses provided various types of cognitive information to parents related to their children's surgery, whereas information about children's feelings was less often provided. Most nurses provided guidance to parents on positioning, breathing technique, comforting/reassurance, helping with activities of daily living, relaxation, and creating a comfortable environment. Nurses' provision of parental guidance on preparatory information and nonpharmacologic methods was significantly different between subgroups of age, education, parent or not, and perceived knowledge adequacy of nonpharmacologic methods. Nurses' perceived knowledge adequacy was the main factor influencing their provision of parental guidance. More attention should be paid to nurses who are younger, have less working experience, and are not parents. There is a need to educate nurses about nonpharmacologic pain relief methods to optimize their provision of parental guidance.

PMID: 24957816   DOI: 10.1016/j.pmn.2014.03.002

MeSH Terms

- Child
- Female
- Humans
- Male
- Nursing Education Research
- Nursing Staff, Hospital/statistics & numerical data*
- Pain Management/nursing*
- Pain, Postoperative/prevention & control*
- Parent-Child Relations
- Parents/education*
- Postoperative Care/nursing*
- Professional-Family Relations*
- Singapore

FIGURE 5.4 Example of a record from a PubMed search. (Abstract reprinted with permission from He H.G., Klainin-Yobas P., Ang E., Sinnappan R., Pölkki T., & Wang W. (2015). Nurses' provision of parental guidance regarding school-aged children's postoperative pain management: A descriptive correlational study. *Pain Management Nursing, 16*, 40–50.)

that were indexed for this study. (Those marked with an asterisk, such as Pain Management/nursing, are MeSH subject headings that are a major focus of the article). As you can see, the MeSH terms are different than the subject headings for the same article in CINAHL. As with CINAHL, you can click on highlighted record entries (authors' names and MeSH terms) for possible new leads.

In the right panel of the screen for specific PubMed records, there is a list of *Similar Articles*, which is a useful feature once you have found a study that is a good exemplar of what you are seeking. Further down in the right panel, PubMed provides a list of any articles in the PubMed Central database that had cited this study. PubMed Central is a repository for full-text articles, so you could immediately download any of the articles that appeared in this list. You can also save articles that look pertinent to your review by clicking the button "Add to Favorites" at the top of the right panel.

A useful feature of PubMed is that it provides access to new research by including citations to forthcoming articles in many journals. The records for these not yet published articles have the tag "Epub ahead of print." McKeever et al. (2015) offer further suggestions for using PubMed for doing an exhaustive literature review.

> **TIP** Searching for qualitative studies can pose special challenges. Wilczynski et al. (2007) described optimal search strategies for qualitative studies in the CINAHL database. Flemming and Briggs (2006) compared three alternative strategies for finding qualitative research.

Google Scholar

Launched in 2004, Google Scholar (GS) has become an increasingly popular bibliographic search engine. GS includes articles in journals from scholarly publishers in all disciplines, as well as scholarly books, technical reports, and other documents. GS is accessible free of charge over the Internet. Like other bibliographic search engines, GS allows users to search by topic, by a title, and by author and uses Boolean operators and other search conventions. Like PubMed and CINAHL, GS has a *Cited By* feature for a descendancy search and a *Related Articles* feature to locate other sources with relevant content to an identified article. Because of its expanded coverage of material, GS can provide access to many free full-text publications.

Unlike other scholarly databases, GS does not order the retrieved references by publication date (i.e., most recent ones first). The ordering of records in GS is determined by an algorithm that puts most weight on the number of times a reference has been cited; this in turn means that older references are usually earlier on the list. Another disadvantage of GS is that the search filters are fairly limited.

In the field of medicine, GS has generated considerable controversy, with some arguing that it is of similar utility and quality to popular medical databases (Gehanno et al., 2013), and others urging caution in depending primarily on GS (e.g., Boeker et al., 2013; Bramer et al., 2013). Some have found that for quick clinical searches, GS returns more citations than PubMed (Shariff et al., 2013). The capabilities and features of GS may improve in the years ahead, but at the moment, it may be risky to depend on GS exclusively. For a full literature review, we think it is best to combine searches using GS with searches of other databases. We note, however, that GS has been of particular interest in efforts to retrieve the so-called *grey literature* (Haddaway et al., 2015).

> **TIP** For most reviews, other resources beyond bibliographic databases should be considered. Other sources include government reports, clinical trial registries (e.g., ClinicalTrials.gov), and records of studies that are in progress such as in NIH RePORTER, which is a searchable database of biomedical projects funded by the U.S. government.

Screening and Gathering References

Screening references for relevance is a multiphase process. The first screen is the title of the article itself. For example, suppose our study question was the one we presented earlier: *Among nurses working in hospitals, what characteristics of the nurses or their practice settings are associated with their management of children's pain?* The PubMed search for *pain management AND child AND nurse* yielded about 450 references in PubMed. The title of one article identified in this search was "Nurses' perceptions of caring for childbearing women who misuse opioids." Based on this title, we could conclude that this article (which was retrieved because the name of the journal in which it was published included the word "Child," one of our keywords) would provide no evidence about factors influencing nurses' pain management with children.

Once this initial screening is completed and the various search lists are also purged of duplicates, we would then examine the abstracts of the remaining references. When there is no abstract, or when the abstract is ambiguous as to its relevance to your review, it is usually necessary to screen the full article. During the screening, keep in mind that some articles judged to be not relevant for your primary question may be useful for a secondary question.

The next step is to retrieve the full text of references you think may have value for your review. If you are affiliated with an institution, you may have online access to most full-text articles, which you should download and file. If you are not so fortunate, more effort will be required to obtain the full-text articles. Consulting with a librarian is a good strategy.

The **open-access journal** movement is gaining momentum in healthcare publishing. Open-access journals provide articles free of charge online, regardless of any institutional subscriptions. Some journals have a hybrid format in which most articles are *not* open-access but some individual articles *are* designated as open-access. Bibliographic databases indicate which articles are open-access, and for these articles, the full text can be retrieved by clicking on a link. (In PubMed, the link to click on states "Free Article" or "Free PMC article.")

> **TIP** We provide links to open-access articles with content relevant to each chapter of this book in the Toolkit of the accompanying *Resource Manual*.

When an article is not available to you online, you may be able to access it by communicating with the lead author. Bibliographic databases usually provide an email address for lead authors. Another alternative is to go to *scholarly collaboration network* (SCN) websites such as *Research Gate* or *Academia.edu* and do a search for a particular author. Authors sometimes upload articles onto their profile for access by others. If an article has not been uploaded, these network sites provide a mechanism for you to send the author a message so that you can request an article to be sent to you directly.

Documentation in Literature Retrieval

If your goal is to "own" the literature, you will be using a variety of databases, keywords, subject headings, authors' names, and search strategies in an effort to pursue all leads. As you meander through the complex world of research information, you will likely lose track of your efforts if you do not document your actions from the outset.

It is advisable to use word processing, spreadsheet, or reference manager software to record your search strategies and search results. You should make note of information such as names of the databases searched; limits put on your search; specific keywords, subject headings, or authors used to direct the search; studies used to inaugurate a "Related Articles" or "descendancy" search; websites visited; links pursued; authors contacted to request further information or copies of articles not readily available; and any other information that would help you keep track of what you have done—including information about the dates your searches were undertaken. Part of your strategy usually can be documented by saving your search history from bibliographic databases. Completing a flow chart such as the one shown in Figure 5.2 is recommended if your goal is to publish a free-standing review.

By documenting your actions, you will be able to conduct a more efficient search—that is, you will not inadvertently duplicate a strategy you have already pursued. Documentation will also help you to assess what else needs to be tried—where to go next in your search. Finally, documenting your efforts is a step in ensuring that your literature review is reproducible.

EXTRACTING AND RECORDING INFORMATION

Once you have a set of useful source materials, you need a strategy for making sense of the information. If a literature review is fairly simple, it may be sufficient to jot down notes about key features of the studies under review and to use these notes as the basis for the synthesis.

Many literature reviews are sufficiently complex that a systematic process for extracting and recording information must be developed. In the past, researchers used paper-based data extraction forms to record information about each reference. The use of word processing or spreadsheet software is advantageous, however, because then the forms can be easily searched and sorted. We call them *data extraction forms* because, in a review, the "data" are the information from each study. The data extraction forms are the critical bridge between the information in the original research reports and the synthesis of evidence by reviewers.

An approach that is gaining in popularity is the creation of two-dimensional data collection forms (matrices or *evidence summary tables*) in which rows are used for individual studies and columns are used to insert relevant data about each study, such as sample characteristics, methodologic features, and results. Two-dimensional tables can provide insights into important "themes" in the data across studies.

Information to Extract

It is wise to record key information for each study in a systematic way. Regardless of what approach is used to record data, reviewers should decide in advance what information about each study is important. The key elements will vary from one review to the next, but you should have, as a goal, the creation of a file in which each study in the review is abstracted for a consistent set of features.

Box 5.1 presents a list of some elements that could be considered for your data extraction forms. Not all of these elements are needed for each review, and for other reviews additional elements are likely to be needed. Although many terms in this table may not be familiar to you yet, you will learn about them in later chapters.

Once you have decided on the elements you wish to use in your data extraction form, you should pilot test it with a sample of studies. If you discover later in the extraction process that other elements are needed, you would have to go back to every completed article to retrieve the new information.

TIP We encourage the use of two-dimensional data extraction forms, but if you prefer using a separate form to extract information for each study, an example is provided as a Word document in the Toolkit for this chapter that you can adapt.

Coding the Studies for Key Variables

In systematic reviews, the review team almost always develops coding systems to support statistical analyses of study findings. Coding may not be necessary in less formal reviews, but coding certain elements can be helpful in organizing the review, and so we offer some suggestions and an example.

We find it useful to code study findings for key variables (quantitative) or themes (qualitative). In our earlier example about factors affecting nurses' management of children's pain, nurses' characteristics are the independent variables and nurses' pain management behaviors are the dependent variables. By reading the retrieved articles, we find that several characteristics have been studied—nurses' knowledge about pain management, their nursing experience, demographic characteristics, and so on. We can assign codes to each type of factor. With regard to the dependent variable—nurses' pain management behaviors—some studies have focused on nurses' pain assessment, others have examined nurses' use of nonpharmacologic methods of pain relief, and so on. These outcome categories can also be coded. An example of a coding scheme is presented in Box 5.2—there are eight

| **BOX 5.1** | Information to Consider for Data Extraction in a Literature Review |

Source
- Citation
- Contact details of lead author

Methods
- Study design
  - Level of evidence
- Research tradition (qualitative)
- Longitudinal or cross-sectional
- Methods of bias control (e.g., blinding)
- Methods of enhancing trustworthiness (qualitative)

Participants
- Number of participants
  - Power analysis information
- Key characteristics of the sample
  - Age
  - Sex
  - Ethnicity/race
  - Socioeconomic
  - Diagnosis/disease
  - Comorbidities
- Country
- Method of sample selection
- Attrition (percent dropped out)

Intervention/Independent variable(s)
- Independent variable
  - Intervention or influence
  - Comparison
- Number of (intervention) groups
- Specific intervention (e.g., components of a complex intervention)
- Intervention fidelity

Outcomes/Dependent variables
- Outcomes (or phenomena in qualitative studies)
- Time points for outcome data collection
For each key outcome:
- Outcome definition
- Method of data collection (e.g., self-report, observation)
- Specific instrument (if relevant)
  - Reliability, validity information

Results
- Qualitative: Summary of major themes
- *Quantitative: for each outcome of interest*
- Summary of results
  - Effect size
  - *p* values
  - Confidence intervals
- Subgroup analyses

Evaluation
- Major strengths
- Major weaknesses
- Overall quality rating

Other
- Theoretical framework
- Funding source
- Key conclusions of the study authors

Broadly adapted from Table 7.3.a of the Cochrane Handbook for Systematic Reviews (Higgins & Green, 2011).

independent variable categories and five outcome categories.

The results of each study can then be coded. You can record these codes in data extraction forms, but we think it is also useful to note the codes in the margins of the articles themselves, so you can easily find the information. Figure 5.5, which presents an excerpt from the results section of the study by He et al. (2015), shows marginal coding of key variables. In this excerpt, we see

that the researchers reported that nurses' guidance to parents about pain management (Code E) varied by the nurses' age (Code 4), whether or not they had children of their own (Code 4), and their perceived knowledge about methods of pain relief (Code 1).

When reviews are more sharply focused than the one we have used as an example, coding may not be necessary or codes that are more fine-tuned could be used. For example, if our research

BOX 5.2 Substantive Codes for a Literature Review on Factors Affecting Nurses' Management of Children's Pain

CODES FOR NURSE CHARACTERISTICS ASSOCIATED WITH THEIR PAIN MANAGEMENT BEHAVIOR (INDEPENDENT VARIABLES)
1. Nurses' pain management knowledge or specialized pain training
2. Nurses' years of nursing experience
3. Nurses' pain attitudes and beliefs
4. Demographic nurse factors (e.g., age, sex, education, has own children)
5. Nurses' role/credential/status (e.g., RN, CNS, APN, NP)
6. Other nurse factors (e.g., self-efficacy, personal experience with pain)
7. Organizational factors (e.g., nurses' workload, organizational culture)
8. Participation in interventions to improve nurses' pain management skills

CODES FOR NURSES' PAIN MANAGEMENT BEHAVIORS (DEPENDENT VARIABLES)
A. Nurses' assessment of children's pain
B. Nurses' pain management—general strategies
C. Nurses' use of analgesics for pain management
D. Nurses' use of nonpharmacologic methods of pain management
E. Provision of guidance to parents about managing their child's pain

---

> With regard to nurses' provision of preparatory information scores, there was significant difference between nurses in the two age groups, with moderate ($\eta^2 = 0.06$) magnitude of the difference in the means (mean difference = −6; 95% confidence interval [CI], −10.1 to −1.9). There was significant difference in preparatory information scores between nurses with or without own child, with small ($\eta^2 = 0.05$) magnitude of the difference in the means (mean difference = −5.8; 95% CI, −9.6 to −2.0). There was significant
>
> E4 | difference in preparatory information scores between
> E4 | nurses who perceived having inadequate or adequate
> E1 | knowledge of nonpharmacologic methods, with large ($\eta^2 = 0.19$) magnitude of the difference in the means (mean difference = −10.5; 95% CI, −14.2 to −6.8).

FIGURE 5.5 Coded excerpt from the Results section of a research article: nurses' management of children's pain example. The codes in the margin, which here were entered as a comment on the pdf file, correspond to the codes explained in Box 5.2. Supplement B on thePoint discusses this excerpt and why additional codes would be required. **⑤** (Excerpt reprinted with permission from He H.G., Klainin-Yobas P., Ang E., Sinnappan R., Pölkki T., & Wang W. (2015). Nurses' provision of parental guidance regarding school-aged children's postoperative pain management: A descriptive correlational study. *Pain Management Nursing, 16,* 40–50.)

question focused explicitly on nurses' use of non-pharmacologic methods of pain relief (not about use of analgesics or pain assessment), the outcome categories might be specific nonpharmacologic approaches, such as distraction, guided imagery, music, massage, and so on. The point is to use codes to organize information in a way that facilitates retrieval and analysis. Further guidance on coding study findings is offered in Supplement B on thePoint. 🅢

Literature Review Summary Tables

As noted earlier, we recommend using two-dimensional tables (matrices) to extract and record information from the source documents because such tables directly support a thematic analysis of the retrieved evidence. For some literature reviews—for example, in a dissertation—such tables are sometimes included directly in the written product. In other words, these tables can serve not only as a data extraction tool, but also as a display of critical information in complex reviews.

As Box 5.1 suggests, the list of potential elements to be extracted from each study can be long. With two-dimensional tables for recording the extracted data, it may be advantageous to create multiple data extraction forms, so that the information can be conveniently displayed on your computer screen without having to scroll right and left. For example, separate forms can be used for source information, methods used, results, and evaluation.

Table 5.1 presents an example of one such matrix for extracting methodologic features of studies in a review. Such tables can be created in word processing or spreadsheet software. This table only shows one illustrative entry: the study by He et al. (2015), whose CINAHL and PubMed records were shown in Figures 5.3 and 5.4. Complete evidence summary tables would have a row for each study in the review. These tables can be electronically searched and sorted and re-sorted (e.g., by authors' names, year of publication, level of evidence, etc.). Although we have only included one entry in this table as an illustration, if this table listed 10 to 15 studies, we would be able to tell at a glance when

and where the studies had been done, what sampling methods had been used, and so on. The scrutiny of such tables can tell us not only what *has* been done but can also point to gaps or problems—for example, overreliance on nurses' self-reported pain management strategies rather than direct observation of nurses' behaviors.

Supplement B to this chapter on thePoint provides additional guidance about the use of evidence summary tables, together with more complete examples. 🅢

CRITICAL APPRAISAL OF THE EVIDENCE

In drawing conclusions about a body of research, reviewers must record not only factual information about studies—methodologic features and findings—but must also make judgments about the value of the evidence. This section discusses issues relating to the appraisal of studies in the review.

> **TIP** A distinction is sometimes made between a research *critique* and a *critical appraisal*. The latter term is favored by those focusing on the evaluation of evidence for nursing practice. The term *critique* is more often used when individual studies are being evaluated for their scientific merit—for example, when a manuscript is reviewed by two or more **peer reviewers** who make recommendations about publishing the paper, or when a person is preparing a literature review. In both critiques and appraisals, however, the point is to apply knowledge about research methods, theory, and substantive issues to draw conclusions about the validity and relevance of the findings.

Appraisals of Individual Studies

As traditionally defined, a research **critique** is an appraisal of the strengths and weaknesses of a study. A good critique identifies areas of adequacy and inadequacy in an unbiased manner. Literature reviews mainly concern the evaluation of a body of research evidence for a literature review, but we briefly offer some advice about appraisals of individual studies.

TABLE 5.1 • Example of an Evidence Summary Table for Methodologic Features of Relevant Studies

AUTHOR	YEAR	COUNTRY	DEPENDENT VARIABLES (WITH CODES)[a]	INDEPENDENT VARIABLES (WITH CODES)[a]	STUDY DESIGN	LEVEL OF EVIDENCE[b]	SAMPLE SIZE, CHARACTER-ISTICS	CHILD AGE	SAMPLING METHOD	DATA COLLECTION METHOD
He et al.	2015	Singapore	E: Nurses' provision of information regarding non-pharmacologic methods of pain management	1. Perceived knowledge of nonpharmacologic pain relief methods 2. Nursing experience 3. Demographic (age, education, having own child) 4. Nurses' role (staff nurse vs. more senior)	Descriptive correlational, cross-sectional	V	134 RNs in 7 pediatric wards of 2 hospitals	School-aged	Convenience	Questionnaire

[a]The codes for the independent and dependent variables are shown in Box 5.2.

[b]For this table, levels from the evidence hierarchy presented in Figure 2.2 in Chapter 2 were used—although this hierarchy is appropriate primarily for Therapy questions. Alternative hierarchies for different types of questions are described in Chapter 9.

We provide support for the critical appraisal of individual studies in several ways. First, suggestions for appraising relevant aspects of a study are included at the end of each chapter. Second, it can be illuminating to have a good model, and so Appendixes H and I of the accompanying *Resource Manual* include comprehensive appraisals of a quantitative and mixed methods study.

Third, we offer a set of key critical appraisal questions in this chapter, in Box 5.3 (quantitative studies) and Box 5.4 (qualitative studies). The second column in these two boxes lists appraisal questions, and the third column cross-references the more detailed appraisal guidelines in other chapters. Many questions may be too difficult for you to answer at this point, but your methodologic

	BOX 5.3 Guide to a Focused Critical Appraisal of Evidence Quality in a Quantitative Research Report	
SECTION OF THE REPORT	**CRITICAL APPRAISAL QUESTIONS**	**DETAILED GUIDELINES**
Method Research design	Was the most rigorous design used, given the purpose of the study? What was the level of evidence for the type of question asked—and is this level the highest possible? Were suitable comparisons made to enhance interpretability? Was the number of data collection points appropriate? Was the period of follow-up (if any) adequate? Did the design minimize threats to the internal validity of the study (e.g., was randomization and blinding used, was attrition minimized)? Did the design enhance the external validity and applicability of the study results? If there was an intervention, did it have a strong theoretical basis?	Box 9.1, page 201; Box 10.1, page 223 Box 31.1, page 720
Population and sample	Was the population identified? Was the sample adequately described? Was a good sampling design used to enhance the sample's representativeness of the population? Were sampling biases minimized? Was the sample size adequate? Was a power analysis used?	Box 13.1, page 274
Data collection and measurement	Were key variables operationalized using the best possible methods (e.g., interviews, observations)? Were clinically important and patient-centered outcomes measured? Did the data collection methods yield data that were reliable, valid, and responsive?	Box 14.1, page 291; Box 15.1, page 336
Procedures	If there was an intervention, was it rigorously developed and implemented? Did most participants allocated to the intervention group actually receive it? Were data collected in a manner that minimized bias?	Box 9.1, page 201; Box 10.1, page 223

BOX 5.3 Guide to a Focused Critical Appraisal of Evidence Quality in a Quantitative Research Report—Cont'd

SECTION OF THE REPORT	CRITICAL APPRAISAL QUESTIONS	DETAILED GUIDELINES
Results Data analysis	Were appropriate and powerful statistical methods used? Did the analysis help to control for confounding variables? Were Type I and Type II errors avoided or minimized? Were subgroup analyses undertaken to better understand the applicability of the results to different types of people?	Box 17.1, page 381 Box 18.1, page 408 Box 31.1, page 720
Findings	Were the findings adequately summarized? Was information about effect size and precision of estimates (confidence intervals) presented? Were findings reported in a manner that facilitates a meta-analysis, and with sufficient information needed for EBP?	Box 17.1, page 381
Discussion Interpretation of the findings	Were interpretations consistent with the study's limitations? Were causal inferences, if any, justified? Was the clinical significance of the findings discussed? Did the report address the generalizability and applicability of the findings?	Box 21.1, page 465
Summary Assessment	Despite any limitations, do the study findings appear to be valid—do you have confidence in the *truth value* of the results? Does the report inspire confidence about the types of people and settings for whom the evidence is applicable?	

and appraisal skills will improve as you progress through this book. The questions in these two boxes are relevant for a rapid critical appraisal that would be conducted as part of an EBP effort, as well as for appraisals for a literature review.

A few comments about these guidelines are worth noting. First, the questions in Boxes 5.3 and 5.4 mainly concern the *rigor* with which the researchers conducted their research. For example, there are no questions regarding ethical issues because—while extremely important—the researchers' handling of ethical concerns is unlikely to affect evidence quality.

Second, the questions in these two boxes call for a yes or no answer (although for some, the answer may be "Yes, *but...*"). In all cases, the desirable answer is "yes." A "no" suggests a possible limitation, and a "yes" suggests a likely strength. Therefore, the more "yeses" a study gets, the stronger its evidence is likely to be. These questions can thus cumulatively suggest a global assessment: a report with 10 "yeses" is likely to be superior to one with only 4.

Our simplified guidelines have shortcomings. In particular, they are generic despite the fact that appraisals cannot use a one-size-fits-all list of questions. Some questions that are relevant to, say, clinical trials do not make sense for descriptive studies. Thus, you need to use some judgment about whether the guidelines are appropriate in your situation.

BOX 5.4 Guide to a Focused Critical Appraisal of Evidence Quality in a Qualitative Research Report

SECTION OF THE REPORT	CRITICAL APPRAISAL QUESTIONS	DETAILED GUIDELINES
Method Research design/ research tradition	Is the identified research tradition congruent with the methods used to collect and analyze data? Was an adequate amount of time spent with study participants? Was there evidence of reflexivity in the design?	Box 22.1, page 490
Sample and setting	Was the group or population of interest adequately described? Were the setting and sample described in sufficient detail? Was a good method of sampling used to enhance information richness? Was the sample size adequate? Was saturation achieved?	Box 23.1, page 506
Data collection	Were appropriate methods used to gather data? Were data gathered through two or more methods to achieve triangulation? Were the data of sufficient depth and richness?	Box 24.1, page 526
Procedures	Do data collection and recording procedures appear appropriate? Were data collected in a manner that minimized bias?	Box 24.1, page 526
Enhancement of trustworthiness	Did the researchers use effective strategies to enhance the trustworthiness/integrity of the study? Was there "thick description" of the context, participants, and findings, and was it at a sufficient level to support transferability? Do the researchers' methodologic and clinical experience enhance confidence in the study findings and interpretations?	Box 26.1, page 580
Results Data analysis	Was the data analysis strategy compatible with the research tradition and with the nature and type of data gathered?	Box 25.1, page 553
Findings	Were findings effectively summarized, with good use of excerpts and strong supporting arguments? Did the analysis yield an insightful, provocative, authentic, and meaningful picture of the phenomenon under investigation?	Box 25.1, page 553
Theoretical integration	Were the themes or patterns logically connected to each other to form a convincing and integrated whole?	Box 25.1 page 553
Discussion Interpretation of the findings	Were the findings interpreted within an appropriate social or cultural context, and within the context of prior studies? Were interpretations consistent with the study's limitations? Did the report address the transferability and applicability of the findings?	Box 25.1, page 553
Summary Assessment	Do the study findings appear to be trustworthy—do you have confidence in the *truth* value of the results? Does the report inspire confidence about the types of people and settings for whom the evidence is applicable?	

Finally, there are questions in these guidelines for which there are no objective answers. Even experts sometimes disagree about what are the best methodologic strategies for a study.

> **TIP** Students may be asked to critically appraise a study to document their mastery of research concepts. Such appraisals may be expected to be comprehensive, covering substantive, theoretical, ethical, methodologic, and interpretive aspects. The Toolkit for this chapter offers more detailed lists of questions than are included in Boxes 5.3 and 5.4 for such comprehensive appraisals.

Evaluating a Body of Research

In reviewing the literature, you would not undertake a comprehensive critical appraisal of each study—but you would need to evaluate the evidence quality in each study so that you could aggregate appraisals across studies to draw conclusions about the overall body of evidence.

In preparing a literature review for a new study, the studies under review need to be assessed with an eye to answering some broad questions. First, to what extent do the cumulative findings accurately reflect the *truth* or, conversely, to what extent do methodologic flaws undermine the credibility of the evidence? Another important question to consider is: For which types of people does the evidence apply—that is, for whom is the evidence applicable?

The use of literature review matrices, as described in Supplement B (**S**), supports the analysis and evaluation of multiple studies. For example, if there is a column for sample size in the matrix (as in Table 5.1), one could readily see at a glance whether, for example, a lot of the evidence is from studies with small, unrepresentative samples.

> **TIP** Formal systems for *grading* a body of evidence have been developed and will be discussed in the chapter on systematic reviews (Chapter 30).

ANALYZING AND SYNTHESIZING INFORMATION

Once all the relevant studies have been retrieved, read, abstracted, and appraised, the information has to be analyzed and integrated. A literature review is not simply a summary of each previous study—it is a synthesis that features important patterns. As previously noted, doing a literature review is similar to doing a qualitative study, particularly with respect to the analysis of the data, which in this case is the information from the retrieved studies. In both, the focus is on identifying important *themes*.

A thematic analysis essentially involves detecting regularities, as well as inconsistencies and "holes." Several different types of themes can be identified, as described in Table 5.2. The reason we recommend using literature review summary tables can be seen by reading the list of possible themes and questions: it is easier to discern patterns by reading down the columns of the matrices than by flipping through a file of review forms or skimming through articles.

Clearly, it is not possible—even in lengthy freestanding reviews—to address all the questions in Table 5.2. Reviewers must decide which patterns to pursue. In preparing a review as part of a new study, you would need to determine which pattern is of greatest relevance for developing an argument and providing a context for the new research.

PREPARING A WRITTEN LITERATURE REVIEW

Writing literature reviews can be challenging, especially when voluminous information must be condensed into a few pages, as is typical for a journal article or proposal. We offer a few suggestions but acknowledge that skills in writing literature reviews develop over time.

Organizing the Review

Organization is crucial in a written review. Having an outline helps to structure the narrative's flow. If the review is complex, we recommend a written outline. The outline should list the main topics or

TABLE 5.2 • Thematic Possibilities for a Literature Review

NATURE OF THE THEME	QUESTIONS FOR THEMATIC ANALYSIS
Substantive	What does the pattern of evidence suggest? How much evidence is there? How consistent is the body of evidence across studies? How powerful are observed effects? How persuasive is the evidence? Has the clinical significance of the findings been assessed? What gaps are there in the body of evidence?
Methodologic	What types of research designs or approaches have predominated? What level of evidence is typical? What populations have been studied? Have certain groups been omitted from the research? What data collection methods have been used primarily? Are data typically of high quality? Overall, what are the methodologic strengths and deficiencies?
Theoretical	Which theoretical frameworks have been used—or has most research been atheoretical? How congruent are the frameworks?
Generalizability/ transferability	To what types of people and settings do the findings apply? Do findings vary for different types of people or settings?
Historical	Have there been substantive, methodologic, or theoretical trends over time? Is evidence getting better? When was most research conducted?
Researcher	Who has been doing the research, in terms of discipline, specialty area, and nationality? Do any of the researchers have a systematic program of research devoted to this topic?

themes to be discussed and the order of presentation. The important point is to have a plan before starting to write so that the review has a coherent progression of ideas. The goal is to structure the review in such a way that the presentation is logical, demonstrates meaningful thematic integration, and leads to a conclusion about the state of evidence on the topic.

Writing a Literature Review

It is beyond the scope of this book to offer detailed guidance on writing research reviews, but we offer a few comments on their content and style. Additional assistance is provided in books such as the ones by Fink (2020) and Galvan and Galvan (2017).

Content of the Written Literature Review

A written research review should provide readers with an objective, organized synthesis of evidence on a topic. A review should be neither a series of quotes nor a series of abstracts. The central tasks are to digest and critically evaluate the overall evidence so as to reveal the current state of knowledge—not simply to describe what researchers have done.

Although key studies may be described in some detail, it is seldom necessary to provide particulars for every reference. Studies with comparable findings often are summarized together.

Example of Grouped studies
Kayser et al. (2019) summarized findings from several studies in their introduction to a study of predictors of hospital-acquired pressure injuries: "In a review of 54 studies examining risk factors of pressure injuries...as many as 200 significant risk factors were identified (Coleman et al., 2015)...Examples of indirect risk factors studied include: incontinence, age, nutrition, diabetes, and vasopressor therapy."

The review should demonstrate that you have considered the cumulative worth of the body of research. The review should be as objective as possible. Studies that are at odds with your hypotheses should not be omitted, and the review should not ignore a study because its findings contradict other studies. Inconsistent results should be analyzed for insights into factors that might have led to discrepancies.

A literature review typically concludes with a concise summary of evidence on the topic and any gaps in the evidence. If the review is undertaken for a new study, this critical summary should demonstrate the need for the research and should clarify the basis for any hypotheses.

> **TIP** As you progress through this book, you will acquire proficiency in critically evaluating studies. We hope you will understand the *mechanics* of doing a review after reading this chapter, but you probably will not be ready to write a state-of-the-art review until you have gained more skills in research methods.

Style of a Research Review

Students preparing their first written research review often struggle with stylistic issues. Students sometimes accept research findings uncritically, perhaps reflecting a common misunderstanding about the conclusiveness of research. You should keep in mind that hypotheses cannot be proved or disproved by empirical testing, and no research question can be answered definitively in a single study. The issue is partly semantic: hypotheses are not proved; they are *supported* by research findings.

> **TIP** When describing study findings, you should use phrases suggesting that results are tentative, such as the following:
> - Several studies have *found*…
> - Findings thus far *suggest*…
> - The study results *support* the hypothesis that…
> - There *appears* to be good evidence that…

A related stylistic problem is the interjection of opinions into the review. The review should include opinions sparingly and should be explicit about their source. Reviewers' opinions do not belong in a literature review, except for assessments of study quality.

> **TIP** The Toolkit for this chapter in the accompanying *Resource Manual* includes a table with examples of several stylistic flaws, and suggests possible rewordings.

CRITICAL APPRAISAL OF RESEARCH LITERATURE REVIEWS

We conclude this chapter with some advice about appraising a literature review. It is often difficult to critique a research review because the author is almost invariably more knowledgeable about the topic than the readers. It is not usually possible to judge whether the author has included all relevant literature—although you may have suspicions if none of the citations are to recent articles. Several aspects of a review, however, are amenable to evaluation by readers who are not experts on the topic. Some suggestions for appraising written research reviews are presented in Box 5.5. (These questions could be used to review your own literature review as well.)

In assessing a literature review, the key question is whether it summarizes the current state of research evidence adequately. If the review is

---

BOX 5.5 Guidelines for Critically Appraising Literature Reviews

1. Is the review thorough—does it include all major studies on the topic? Does it include *recent* research (studies published within the previous 1-3 years)? Are studies from other related disciplines included, if appropriate?
2. Does the review rely mainly on primary source research articles?
3. Is the review merely a summary of existing work, or does it critically appraise and compare key studies? Does the review identify important trends and gaps in the literature?
4. Is the review well organized? Is the development of ideas clear?
5. Does the review use appropriate language regarding the tentativeness of prior findings? Is the review objective? Does the author paraphrase, or is there an overreliance on quotes from original sources?
6. If the review is part of a research report for a new study, does the review support the need for the study?
7. If it is a review designed to summarize evidence for clinical practice, does the review draw reasonable conclusions about practice implications?

written as part of an original research report, an equally important question is whether the review lays a solid foundation for the new study.

RESEARCH EXAMPLES OF LITERATURE REVIEWS

The best way to learn about the style and organization of a research literature review is to read reviews in nursing journals. We present excerpts from two reviews that were part of the introduction to journal articles about original studies.[a]

Literature Review From a Quantitative Research Report

Study: Evaluation of a person-centered, theory-based intervention to promote health behaviors (Worawong et al., 2018).

Statement of purpose: The purpose of this study was to test the effect of a behavioral, person-centered intervention (I) on physical activity and fruit and vegetable intake (Os) in community-living adults (P).

Literature review (excerpt): "Although many researchers have tested intervention effects on health behaviors, scholars continue to be challenged to develop stronger behavioral interventions to improve individuals' health (Desroches et al., 2013)… Scholars have tried to promote health behaviors, such as diet and activity, by focusing individuals on the need to prevent or minimize chronic illnesses (e.g., diabetes, Estabrooks et al., 2005; Guo, Chen, Whittemore, & Whitaker, 2016; or cardiovascular disease [CVD], Edelman et al., 2006; Parra-Medina et al. 2011; Sniehotta, Scholz, & Schwarzer, 2006). These approaches rest on the assumptions that individuals (a) value prevention highly, (b) perceive susceptibility to disease or its consequences, (c) perceive health behaviors as feasible, and (d) appreciate the connection between behaviors and clinical outcomes. However, these assumptions are not often valid as explained below.

People's motives for health behaviors can differ from those of researchers and clinicians. People can perceive

the distant risk of disease as less salient than their other life goals and may not initiate or sustain health behaviors (Carpenter, 2010; Segar, Eccles, & Richardson, 2008; Teixeira et al., 2012). Based on a systematic review, people engage in health behaviors to meet various proximal, short-term goals more so than to prevent a distal outcome such as disease (Rhodes, Quinlan, & Mistry, 2016). People may engage in physical activity or healthy eating to alter their moods in the short term or to look better in the long term (Bowen, Balbuena, Baetz, & Schwartz, 2013; Lauver, Worawong, & Olsen, 2008).

Thus, health behavior interventions could be strengthened by making them more patient-centered. This would involve customizing interventions on people's choices of health behaviors and on their motives, preferences, values, goals, beliefs, characteristics, or needs (Morgan & Yoder, 2012; Rhodes et al., 2016). Patient-centered interventions can be motivational and efficacious for improving diet, activity, and clinical status in the longer term (Greaves et al., 2011; Teixeira et al., 2012).

To strengthen behavioral interventions, researchers have tried to identify key components of successful dietary and activity interventions (Desroches et al., 2013; Pomerleau, Lock, Knai, & McKee, 2005). For example, interventions delivered face-to-face have been more efficacious than those without face-to-face contact on physical activity… and subsequent cardiovascular fitness… (Richards, Hillsdon, Thorogood, & Foster, 2013), as well as on maintenance of diet and activity behaviors (Fjeldsoe, Neuhaus, Winkler, & Eakin, 2011). Researchers need to identify what other components can contribute to interventions that are efficacious, feasible, acceptable, and cost-effective (Dombrowski, O'Carroll, & Williams, 2016; Teixeira et al., 2012)."

(Excerpt reprinted with permission from Worawong C., Borden M. J., Cooper K., Perez O., & Lauver D. (2018). Evaluation of a person-centered, theory-based intervention to promote health behaviors. *Nursing Research, 67,* 6-15.)

Literature Review From a Qualitative Research Report

Study: Understanding advanced prostate cancer decision-making utilizing an interactive decision tool (Jones et al., 2018)

Statement of purpose: The purposes of this study were to describe and understand the lived experiences

---

[a]Consult the full research reports for references cited within these excerpted literature reviews.

of patients with advanced prostate cancer and their decision partners who used an interactive decision aid (DecisionKEYS) in making informed, shared treatment decisions.

Literature review (excerpt): "Prostate cancer is the most commonly diagnosed cancer in men and the second leading cause of cancer deaths in the United States. In 2016, an estimated 180,890 men will be diagnosed with prostate cancer, and approximately 26,120 men will die of the disease (American Cancer Society, 2016). In a lifetime, approximately 14% of all men will be diagnosed with prostate cancer (National Cancer Institute, 2016)… There are numerous difficult decisions that patients with advanced prostate cancer must make, including treatment options, cost of care, and family involvement; however, over time, patients with advanced cancer often regret some past decisions (Brom et al., 2015; Christie et al., 2015; Mahal et al., 2015). Many factors may increase the likelihood that patients will not have complete information at the time it is needed in order to optimize decision making, for example, time constraints, forgetting to ask questions, and provider-patient miscommunication (Hillen et al., 2011; Lu et al., 2011; Shay & Lafata, 2015; Woods et al., 2013)…

Many patients with advanced prostate cancer struggle with treatment decisions… If patients and healthcare providers fail to engage in a systematic, informed, shared decision-making process (a collaborative process whereby patient and healthcare provider make a healthcare decision together, taking into account scientific/clinical evidence and the patient's/decision partner's values and preferences), there is a greater chance that the patient will be dissatisfied and regretful regarding the decisions that were made (Mahal et al., 2015; Poon, 2012; Weeks et al., 2012). Moreover, decision partners may become 'proxies' in interactions with healthcare providers, but they often misunderstand the patient's informational and decision needs (Longo & Slater, 2014).

Decision aids can help patients apply specific health information while actively participating in health-related decision making (O'Connor et al., 2009; Stacey et al., 2014)….Decision aids are most effective when they are tailored, interactive, collaborative, and focused on the priorities of the individual patient (Fowler et al., 2011; Jimbo et al., 2013; Ozanne et al., 2014; Sepucha et al., 2013; Stacey et al., 2014) but interactive decision aids are rarely implemented (Jimbo et al., 2013)."

(Excerpt reprinted with permission from Jones R., Hollen P., Wenzel J., Weiss G., Song D., Sims T., & Petroni G. (2018). Understanding advanced prostate cancer decision making utilizing an interactive decision aid. *Cancer Nursing, 41,* 2-10.)

SUMMARY POINTS

- A research **literature review** is a written synthesis of evidence on a research problem.
- Major steps in preparing a written research review include formulating a question, devising a search strategy, developing a plan to organize and document review activities, conducting a search, screening and retrieving relevant sources, extracting key data from the sources, appraising studies, analyzing aggregated information for important themes, and writing a synthesis.
- Research articles are the major focus of research reviews. Information in nonresearch references—e.g., case reports, editorials—may broaden understanding of a research problem but has limited utility in summarizing research evidence.
- A **primary source** is the description of a study prepared by the researcher who conducted it; a **secondary source** is a description of the study written by someone else. Literature reviews should be based on primary source material.
- Strategies for finding studies on a topic include the use of **bibliographic databases**, the *ancestry approach* (tracking down earlier studies cited in a reference list of a report), and the *descendancy approach* (using a pivotal study to search forward to subsequent studies that cited it.)
- Electronic searches of bibliographic databases are a key method of locating references. For nurses, the CINAHL and MEDLINE (via PubMed) databases are especially useful. Google Scholar is also a popular and free resource.
- In searching a database, users can perform a **keyword search** that looks for searcher-specified terms in text fields of a database record (or that *maps* keywords onto the database's subject codes) or they search according to **subject heading** codes themselves.

- Access to many journal articles is becoming easier through online resources, especially for articles available in an **open-access** format.
- References must be screened for relevance, and then pertinent information must be extracted for analysis. Two-dimensional *evidence summary tables* (matrices) facilitate the extraction and organization of data from the studies, as does a good coding scheme.
- A research **critique** (or **critical appraisal**) is a careful evaluation of a study's strengths and weaknesses. Critical appraisals for a research review tend to focus on the methodologic aspects and findings of retrieved studies.
- The analysis of information from a literature search involves the identification of important themes—regularities (and inconsistencies) in the information. Themes can take many forms, including substantive, methodologic, and theoretic themes.
- In preparing a written review, it is important to organize materials logically. The reviewers' role is to describe study findings, the dependability of the evidence, evidence gaps, and (in the context of a new study) contributions that the new study would make.

STUDY ACTIVITIES

Study activities are available to instructors on thePoint.

REFERENCES CITED IN CHAPTER 5

*Boeker, M., Vach, W., & Motschall, E. (2013). Google Scholar as replacement for systematic literature searches: Good relative recall and precision are not enough. *BMC Medical Research Methodology, 13*, 131.

*Bramer, W. M., Giustini, D., Kramer, B., & Anderson, P. (2013). The comparative recall of Google Scholar versus PubMed in identical searches for biomedical systematic reviews. *Systematic Reviews, 2*, 115.

Cooper, H. (2017). *Research synthesis and meta-analysis: A step-by-step approach* (5th ed.). Thousand Oaks, CA: Sage Publications.

Fink, A. (2020). *Conducting research literature reviews: From the Internet to paper* (5th ed.). Thousand Oaks, CA: Sage.

Flemming, K., & Briggs, M. (2006). Electronic searching to locate qualitative research: Evaluation of three strategies. *Journal of Advanced Nursing, 57*, 95–100.

Galvan, J. L.. & Galvan, M. (2017). *Writing literature reviews: A guide for students of the social and behavioral sciences* (7th ed.) New York: Routledge.

Garrard, J. (2017). *Health sciences literature review made easy: The matrix method* (5th ed.) Burlington, MA: Jones and Bartlett Publishers.

*Gehanno, J. F., Rollin, L., & Darmon, S. (2013). Is the coverage of Google Scholar enough to be used along for systematic reviews? *BMC Medical Informatics and Decision Making, 13*, 7.

Glaser, B. (1978). *Theoretical sensitivity*. Mill Valley, CA: The Sociology Press.

Gleason, K., Nazarian, S., & Dennison-Himmelfarb, C. (2018). Atrial fibrillation symptoms and sex, race, and psychological distress: A literature review. *Journal of Cardiovascular Nursing, 33*, 137–143.

*Grant, M., & Booth, A. (2009). A typology of reviews: An analysis of 14 review types and associated methodologies. *Health Information and Libraries Journal, 26*, 91–108.

Haddaway, N., Collins, A., Coughlin, D., & Kirk, S. (2015). *The role of Google Scholar in evidence reviews and its applicability to grey literature searching. *PLoS One, 10*, e0138237.

He, H. G., Klainin-Yobas, P., Ang, E., Sinnappan, R., Pölkki, T., & Wang W. (2015). Nurses' provision of parental guidance regarding school-aged children's postoperative pain management: A descriptive correlational study. *Pain Management Nursing, 16*, 40–50.

*Higgins, J., & Green, S., (Eds.). (2011). *Cochrane handbook for systematic reviews of interventions version 5.1*. Oxford: The Cochrane Collaboration.

**Jones, R., Hollen, P., Wenzel, J., Weiss, G., Song, D., Sims, T., & Petroni G. (2018). Understanding advanced prostate cancer decision making utilizing an interactive decision aid. *Cancer Nursing, 41*, 2–10.

Kayser, S., VanGilder, C., & Lachenbruch, C. (2019). Predictors of superficial and severe hospital-acquired pressure injuries: A cross-sectional study using the International Pressure Ulcer Prevalence™ survey. *International Journal of Nursing Studies, 89*, 46–52.

*McKeever, L., Nguyen, V., Peterson, S., Gomez-Perez, S., & Braunschweig, C. (2015). Demystifying the search button: A comprehensive PubMed search strategy for performing an exhaustive literature review. *Journal of Parenteral and Enteral Nutrition, 39*, 622–635.

Munhall, P. L. (2012). *Nursing research: A qualitative perspective* (5th ed.). Sudbury, MA: Jones & Bartlett.

*Shariff, S. Z., Bejaimal, S., Sontrop, J., Iansavichus, A., Haynes, R. B., Weir, M., & Garg, A. (2013). Retrieving clinical evidence: A comparison of PubMed and Google scholar for quick clinical searches. *Journal of Medical Internet Research*, *15*(8), e164.

Spradley, J. (1979). *The ethnographic interview*. New York: Holt Rinehart & Winston.

Wilczynski, N., Marks, S., Haynes, R. (2007). Search strategies for identifying qualitative studies in CINAHL. *Qualitative Health Research*, *17*, 705–710.

Worawong, C., Borden, M. J., Cooper, K. Perez, O., & Lauver, D. (2018). Evaluation of a person-centered, theory-based intervention to promote health behaviors. *Nursing Research*, *67*, 6–15.

A link to this open-access article is provided in the Toolkit for Chapter 5 in the **Resource Manual.** ⊗

**This journal article is available on thePoint *for this chapter.*

6 | Theoretical Frameworks

High-quality studies achieve a high level of *conceptual integration*. This means that the methods are appropriate for the research questions, the questions are consistent with existing evidence, and there is a plausible conceptual rationale for hypotheses to be tested or for the design of an intervention.

For example, suppose we hypothesized that a nurse-led smoking cessation intervention would result in reduced rates of smoking among patients with cardiovascular disease. Why would we make this prediction—what is our "theory" (our theoretical rationale) about how the intervention might change people's behavior? Do we predict that the intervention will change patients' knowledge? motivation? sense of control over their decision-making? Our view of how the intervention would "work"—what *mediates* the relationship between intervention receipt and the desired outcome—should guide the design of the intervention and the study.

In designing studies, researchers need to have a conceptualization of people's behaviors or characteristics, and how these affect or are affected by interpersonal, environmental, or biologic forces. In high quality research, a strong, defensible conceptualization is made explicit. This chapter discusses theoretical and conceptual contexts for nursing research problems.

THEORIES, MODELS, AND FRAMEWORKS

Many terms are used in connection with conceptual contexts for research, such as theories, models, frameworks, schemes, and maps. We offer guidance in distinguishing these terms but note that our definitions are not universal—indeed one confusing aspect of theory-related writings is that there is no consensus about terminology.

Theories

The term *theory* is used in many ways. For example, nursing instructors and students use the term to refer to classroom content, as opposed to the actual practice of performing nursing actions. In both lay and scientific usage, the term *theory* connotes an *abstraction*.

In research, the term theory is used differently by different authors. Classically, **theory** refers to an abstract generalization that explains how phenomena are interrelated. In this definition, a theory embodies at least two concepts that are related in a manner that the theory purports to explain. The purpose of traditional theories is to explain or predict phenomena.

Others, however, use the term *theory* less restrictively to refer to a broad representation that can thoroughly describe a phenomenon. Some authors refer to this type of theory as **descriptive theory**. Broadly speaking, descriptive theories are ones that describe or categorize characteristics of individuals, groups, or situations by abstracting common features observed across multiple manifestations. Descriptive theory plays an important role in qualitative studies. Qualitative researchers often strive to develop conceptualizations of phenomena that are grounded in actual observations. Descriptive theory is sometimes a precursor to predictive and explanatory theories.

Components of a Traditional Theory

Concepts are the basic building blocks of a theory. Classical theories comprise a set of propositions that indicate relationships among the concepts. Relationships are denoted by such terms as "is associated with," "varies directly with," or "is contingent on." The propositions form an interrelated deductive system. Theories provide a mechanism for logically deriving new statements from the original propositions.

Let us illustrate with the **Theory of Planned Behavior** (TPB; Ajzen, 2005), which is related to another theory called the *Theory of Reasoned Action* (Fishbein & Ajzen, 2010). TPB provides a framework for understanding people's behavior and its psychological determinants. A greatly simplified construction of the TPB consists of the following propositions:

1. Behavior that is volitional is determined by people's intention to perform that behavior.
2. Intention to perform or not perform a behavior is determined by three factors:
   - Attitudes toward the behavior (i.e., the overall evaluation of performing the behavior)
   - Subjective norms (i.e., perceived social pressure to perform or not perform the behavior)
   - Perceived behavioral control (i.e., the anticipated ease or difficulty of engaging in the behavior)
3. The relative importance of the three factors in influencing intention varies across behaviors and situations.

The concepts that form the basis of the TPB include *behaviors, intentions, attitudes, subjective norms*, and *perceived self-control*. The theory, which specifies the nature of the relationship among these concepts, provides a framework for generating hypotheses relating to health behaviors. For example, we might hypothesize that compliance with a medical regimen (the behavior) could be enhanced by changing people's attitudes toward compliance or by increasing their sense of control. The TPB has been used as the underlying theory for studying a wide range of health decision-making behaviors and in developing health-promoting interventions.

Example using the TPB

Shi et al. (2019) used the Theory of Planned Behavior to study factors influencing patient delay in seeking treatment among people with hemorrhoids in China.

TIP Links to websites devoted to theories and conceptual models mentioned in this chapter are listed in the Toolkit of the accompanying *Resource Manual* for you to click on directly

Levels of Theories

Theories differ in their level of generality and abstraction. The most common labels used in nursing for levels or scope of theory are *grand, middle-range*, and *micro* or *practice*.

Grand theories or *macrotheories* purport to describe and explain large segments of human experience. In nursing, several grand theories offer explanations of the whole of nursing and address the nature, goals, and mission of nursing practice, as distinct from the discipline of medicine. An example of a nursing theory that has been described as a grand theory is Parse's Humanbecoming Paradigm (Parse, 2014).

Theories of relevance to researchers are often more focused than grand theories. **Middle-range theories** attempt to explain such phenomena as decision-making, stress, comfort, and unpleasant symptoms. Middle-range theories are more specific and more amenable to empirical testing than grand theories (Peterson & Bredow, 2017). Literally dozens of middle-range theories have been developed by or used by nurses, a few of which we briefly describe in this chapter.

The least abstract level of theory is *practice theory* (sometimes called *situation-specific theory* or *micro theory*). Such theories are highly specific, narrow in scope, and have an action orientation. They are not always associated with research, although grounded theory studies can be a source of situation-specific theory (Peterson & Bredow, 2017).

Models

Conceptual models, *conceptual frameworks*, or *conceptual schemes* (we use the terms interchangeably) are a less formal means of organizing phenomena than theories. Like theories, conceptual models deal with abstractions (concepts) that are assembled by virtue of their relevance to a common theme. Conceptual models, however, lack the deductive system of propositions that purport to explain relationships among concepts. Conceptual models provide a perspective regarding interrelated phenomena but are more loosely structured than theories. Conceptual models can serve as springboards for generating hypotheses, but conceptual models in their entirety are not formally "tested." (In actuality, however, the terms *model* and *theory* are sometimes used interchangeably.)

The term *model* is often used in connection with a symbolic representation of a conceptualization. **Schematic models** (or *conceptual maps*), which are visual representations of some aspect of reality, use concepts as building blocks but with a minimal use of words. A visual or symbolic representation of a theory or conceptual framework often helps to express abstract ideas in a concise and accessible format.

Schematic models are common in both qualitative and quantitative research. Concepts and linkages among them are represented through the use of boxes, arrows, or other symbols. As an example, Figure 6.1 shows **Pender's Health Promotion Model**, which is a model for explaining and predicting the health-promotion component of lifestyle (Murdaugh et al., 2019). Such schematic models can be useful in succinctly communicating linkages among concepts.

Frameworks

A **framework** is the overall conceptual underpinnings of a study. Not every study is based on a formal theory or conceptual model, but every study has a framework—that is, a conceptual rationale. In a study based on a theory, the framework is a **theoretical framework**; in a study with roots in a conceptual model, the framework is a **conceptual framework**.

In most nursing studies, the framework is not an explicit theory or model, and sometimes the underlying conceptual rationale for the inquiry is not explained. Frameworks are often implicit, without being formally described. In studies without an articulated conceptual framework, it may be difficult to figure out what the researchers thought was "going on."

Sometimes researchers fail even to adequately describe key constructs at the conceptual level. The concepts in which researchers are interested are abstractions of observable phenomena, and our world view shapes how those concepts are defined and operationalized. Researchers should make clear the conceptual definition of their key variables, thereby providing information about the study's framework.

In most qualitative studies, the frameworks are part of the research tradition in which the study is embedded. For example, ethnographers usually begin their work within a theory of culture. The questions that most qualitative researchers ask and the methods they use to address those questions inherently reflect certain theoretical formulations.

TIP In recent years, *concept analysis* has become an important enterprise among students and nurse scholars, and several methods have been proposed for undertaking a concept analysis and clarifying conceptual definitions (e.g., Rodgers & Knafl, 2000; Walker & Avant, 2019). However, Bergdahl and Berterö (2016) have argued that concept analysis is not a suitable approach to theory development.

INDIVIDUAL
CHARACTERISTICS
AND EXPERIENCES

BEHAVIOR-SPECIFIC
COGNITIONS
AND AFFECT

BEHAVIORAL
OUTCOME

PERCEIVED
BENEFITS
OF ACTION

PERCEIVED
BARRIERS
TO ACTION

IMMEDIATE COMPETING
DEMANDS
(low control)
AND PREFERENCES
(high control)

PRIOR
RELATED
BEHAVIOR

PERCEIVED
SELF-EFFICACY

ACITIVITY-RELATED
AFFECT

COMMITMENT
TO A
PLAN OF ACTION

HEALTH-
PROMOTING
BEHAVIOR

PERSONAL
FACTORS
Biologic
Psychological
Sociocultural

INTERPERSONAL
INFLUENCES
(family, peers,
providers);
Norms: Support;
Models

SITUATIONAL
INFLUENCES
Options
Demand characteristics
Aesthetics

FIGURE 6.1 Pender's Health Promotion Model. (Retrieved from https://nolapender.weebly.com/critical-elements.html.)

Example of Developing a Conceptual Definition
Mollohan (2018) used Walker and Avant's eight-step concept analysis methods to conceptually define *dietary culture.* Mollohan searched and analyzed 67 relevant articles identified through multiple database and proposed the following: "Dietary culture can be defined as patterned group earing behaviors that are unconsciously influenced and socially organized" (p. E2).

THE NATURE OF THEORIES AND CONCEPTUAL MODELS

Theories and conceptual models have much in common, including their origin, general nature, purposes, and role in research. In this section,

we examine some characteristics of theories and conceptual models. We use the term *theory* in a broad sense, inclusive of conceptual models.

Origin of Theories and Models

Theories, conceptual frameworks, and models are not *discovered*; they are invented. Theory building depends not only on observable evidence but also on the originator's ingenuity in pulling facts together and organizing them. Theory construction is a creative enterprise that can be undertaken by anyone who is insightful, has a firm grounding in existing evidence, and is able to knit together evidence into an intelligible pattern.

Tentative Nature of Theories and Models

Theories and conceptual models cannot be proved—they represent a theorist's best effort to describe and explain phenomena. Today's flourishing theory may be discredited or revised tomorrow. This may happen if new evidence or observations undermine a previously accepted theory. Or, a new theory might integrate new observations into an existing theory to yield a more parsimonious or accurate explanation of a phenomenon.

Theories and models that are not congruent with a culture's values also may fall into disfavor over time. For example, certain psychoanalytic and structural social theories, which had broad support for decades, have come to be challenged as a result of changing views about women's roles. Theories are deliberately invented by humans, and so they are not free from human values, which can change over time.

The Role of Theories and Models

Theories allow researchers to integrate observations and facts into an orderly scheme. The linkage of findings into a coherent structure can make a body of evidence more useful.

In addition to summarizing, theories and models can guide a researcher's understanding of not only the *what* of natural phenomena but also the *why* of their occurrence. Theories often provide a basis for predicting phenomena. Prediction, in turn, has implications for influencing phenomena. A utilitarian theory has potential to bring about desirable changes in people's behavior or health outcomes. Thus, theories are an important resource for developing nursing interventions.

Theories and conceptual models help to stimulate research and the extension of knowledge by providing both direction and impetus. Thus, theories may serve as a springboard for advances in knowledge and the accumulation of evidence for practice.

Relationship Between Theory and Research

Theory and research have a reciprocal relationship. Theories are built inductively from observations, and research evidence is an excellent source for those observations. Concepts and relationships that are validated through research become the foundation for theory development. The theory, in turn, must be tested by subjecting deductions from it (hypotheses) to systematic inquiry. Thus, research plays a dual and continuing role in theory building. Theory guides and generates ideas for research; research assesses the worth of the theory and provides a foundation for new theories.

CONCEPTUAL MODELS AND THEORIES USED IN NURSING RESEARCH

Nurse researchers have used nursing and nonnursing frameworks to provide a conceptual context for their studies. This section briefly discusses several frameworks that have been found useful.

Conceptual Models and Theories of Nursing

Several nurses have formulated theories and models of nursing practice. These models offer formal explanations of what nursing is and what the nursing process entails. As Fawcett and DeSanto-Madeya (2013) have noted, four concepts are central to models of nursing: *human beings, environment, health,* and *nursing*. The various models, however, define these concepts differently, link them in diverse ways, and emphasize different relationships among them. Moreover, the models view different processes as being central to nursing.

The conceptual models were not developed primarily as a base for nursing research. Most models have had more impact on nursing education and practice than on research. Nevertheless, nurse researchers have been inspired by these conceptual models in formulating research questions and hypotheses. Two nursing models that have generated particular interest as a basis for research are briefly described.

Roy's Adaptation Model

In Roy's **Adaptation Model**, humans are viewed as biopsychosocial adaptive systems who cope with environmental change through the process of adaptation (Roy & Andrews, 2009). Within the human system, there are four subsystems: physiologic/physical, self-concept/group identity, role function, and interdependence. These subsystems constitute adaptive modes that provide mechanisms for coping with environmental stimuli and change. Health is viewed as both a state and a process of becoming integrated and whole that reflects the mutuality of persons and environment. The goal of nursing, according to this model, is to promote client adaptation. Nursing also regulates stimuli affecting adaptation. Nursing interventions usually take the form of increasing, decreasing, modifying, removing, or maintaining internal and external stimuli that affect adaptation. Roy's Adaptation Model has been the basis for several middle-range theories and dozens of studies.

Example Using Roy's Adaptation Model
Frank et al. (2017) were guided by Roy's Adaptation Model in their study of the effect of implementing a posttraumatic stress disorder screening tool for acute traumatically injured patients.

Orem's Self-Care Deficit Nursing Theory

Some basic concepts in Orem's **Self-Care Deficit Theory** include self-care, self-care deficit, and self-care agency (Orem et al., 2003). Self-care activities are what people do on their own behalf to maintain their life, health, and well-being. The ability to perform self-care is called self-care agency. Orem's universal self-care requisites to maintain health include air, food, water, elimination, activity and rest, solitude and social interaction, hazard prevention, and promotion of normality. Self-care deficit occurs when self-care agency is not adequate to meet a person's self-care demands. Orem's theory explains that patients need nursing care when their demands for self-care outweigh their abilities.

Example Using Orem's Theory
Using Orem's self-care deficit theory as her framework Treadwell (2017) explored depression among patients on dialysis. The researcher concluded that Orem's theory was appropriate for identifying depression and motivation for change, and for encouraging self-care practices with hemodialysis patients.

Other Models and Middle-Range Theories Developed by Nurses

In addition to conceptual models that are designed to describe and characterize the nursing process, nurses have developed middle-range theories and models that focus on more specific phenomena of interest to nurses. Examples of middle-range theories that have been used in research include:

- Beck's (2012) Theory of Postpartum Depression;
- Kolcaba's (2003) Comfort Theory;
- Symptom Management Model (Dodd et al., 2001);
- Theory of Transitions (Meleis et al., 2000);
- Peplau's (1997) Theory of Interpersonal Relations
- Swanson's (1991) Theory of Caring
- Reed's (1991) Self-Transcendence Theory
- Pender's Health Promotion Model (Murdaugh, Parsons, & Pender, 2019); and
- Mishel's Uncertainty in Illness Theory (1990).

The latter two are briefly described here.

The Health Promotion Model

Nola Pender's Health Promotion Model (HPM) focuses on explaining health-promoting behaviors, using a wellness orientation (Murdaugh et al., 2019). According to the model (see Figure 6.1), *health promotion* entails activities directed toward developing resources that maintain or enhance a person's well-being. The model embodies several theoretical propositions that can be used to develop interventions and to gain insight into health behaviors. For example, one HPM proposition is that people commit to behaviors from which they anticipate deriving valued benefits, and another is that perceived competence or self-efficacy relating to a given behavior increases the likelihood of performing it. Greater perceived self-efficacy is viewed as resulting in fewer perceived barriers to a health behavior. The model also incorporates interpersonal and situational influences on a person's commitment to health-promoting actions.

Example Using the HPM
Eren Fidanci et al. (2017) tested the effects of an intervention based on Pender's Health Promotion Model on the healthy life behaviors of obese children in Turkey.

Uncertainty in Illness Theory
Mishel's Uncertainty in Illness Theory (Mishel, 1990) focuses on the concept of uncertainty—a person's inability to determine the meaning of illness-related events. According to this theory, people develop subjective appraisals to assist them in interpreting the experience of illness and treatment. Uncertainty occurs when people are unable to recognize and categorize stimuli. Uncertainty results in the inability to obtain a clear conception of the situation, but a situation appraised as uncertain will mobilize individuals to use their resources to adapt to the situation. Mishel's theory as originally conceptualized was most relevant to patients in an acute phase of illness or in a downward illness trajectory, but it has been reconceptualized to include constant uncertainty in chronic or recurrent illness. Mishel's conceptualization of uncertainty, and her Uncertainty in Illness Scale, has been used in many nursing studies.

Example Using Uncertainty in Illness Theory
Shun et al. (2018) studied changes in patients' degree of uncertainty in relation to levels of symptom distress and unmet care needs among patients with recurrent hepatocellular carcinoma.

Other Models and Theories Used by Nurse Researchers

Many concepts of interest to nurse researchers are not unique to nursing, and so their studies are sometimes linked to frameworks that originated in other disciplines. Several of these alternative models have gained special prominence in the development of nursing interventions to promote health-enhancing behaviors. In addition to the previously described TPB, three nonnursing models or theories have often been used in nursing studies: Bandura's Social Cognitive Theory, Prochaska's Transtheoretical (stages of change) Model, and the Health Belief Model (HBM).

Bandura's Social Cognitive Theory
Social Cognitive Theory (Bandura, 1997, 2001), which is sometimes called **self-efficacy theory,** offers an explanation of human behavior using the concepts of self-efficacy and outcome expectations. Self-efficacy concerns people's belief in their own capacity to carry out particular behaviors (e.g., smoking cessation). Self-efficacy expectations influence the behaviors a person chooses to perform, their degree of perseverance, and the quality of the performance. Bandura identified four factors that influence a person's cognitive appraisal of self-efficacy: (1) their own mastery experience; (2) verbal persuasion; (3) vicarious experience; and (4) physiologic and affective cues, such as pain and anxiety. The role of self-efficacy has been studied in relation to numerous health behaviors (e.g., weight control, smoking).

TIP Bandura's self-efficacy construct is a key mediating variable in several theories discussed in this chapter. Self-efficacy has repeatedly been found to explain a significant amount of variation in people's behaviors *and* to be amenable to change. As a result, self-efficacy enhancement is often a goal in interventions designed to change people's health-related behaviors (Conn et al., 2001).

Example Using Social Cognitive Theory
Staffileno et al. (2018) evaluated a Web-based, culturally relevant lifestyle change intervention, with roots in Social Cognitive Theory, that targeted young African American women at risk for developing hypertension.

The Transtheoretical (Stages of Change) Model

The **Transtheoretical Model** (Prochaska et al., 2002; Prochaska & Velicer, 1997) has been the basis of numerous interventions designed to change people's problem behavior (e.g., alcohol abuse). The core construct around which other dimensions are organized is *stages of change*, which conceptualizes a continuum of *motivational readiness* to change dysfunctional behavior. The five stages of change are precontemplation, contemplation, preparation, action, and maintenance. Studies have shown that successful self-changers use different processes at each stage, suggesting the desirability of interventions that are individualized to the person's stage of readiness for change. The model incorporates a series of mediating variables, one of which is self-efficacy.

Example Using the Transtheoretical Model
Wen et al. (2019) tested the effectiveness of a Transtheoretical Model–based intervention on the self-management of people with an ostomy.

The Health Belief Model

The **Health Belief Model** (HBM; Becker, 1978) has become a popular framework in nursing studies focused on patient compliance and preventive healthcare practices. The model postulates that health-seeking behavior is influenced by a person's perception of a threat posed by a health problem and the value associated with actions aimed at reducing the threat. The major components of the HBM include perceived susceptibility, perceived severity, perceived benefits and costs, motivation, and enabling or modifying factors. Perceived susceptibility is a person's perception that a health problem is personally relevant or that a diagnosis is accurate. Even when one recognizes personal susceptibility, action will not occur unless the individual perceives the severity to be high enough to have serious implications. Perceived benefits are patients' beliefs that a given treatment will cure the illness or help prevent it, and perceived barriers include the complexity, duration, and accessibility of the treatment. Motivation is the desire to comply with a treatment. Among the modifying factors that have been identified are personality variables, patient satisfaction, and sociodemographic factors.

Example Using the HBM
Rakhshkhorshid et al. (2018) used concepts from the Health Belief Model in their study of the association of health literacy with breast cancer knowledge, perception, and screening behavior.

TIP A theoretical framework called the **Theoretical Domains Framework** (TDF) is being used increasingly in implementation science as a way to understand factors influencing the behaviors of healthcare professionals, as well as to facilitate the design of interventions. The TDF, which was developed by expert consensus, is a framework with 14 domains derived from 33 behavior-change theories (Michie et al., 2005).

Selecting a Theory or Model for Nursing Research

As we discuss in the next section, theory can be used by qualitative and quantitative researchers in various ways. A common challenge, however, is identifying an appropriate model or theory—a task made especially daunting because of the burgeoning number available. There are no rules for how this can be done, but there are two places to start—with the theory or model, or with the phenomenon being studied.

Readings in the theoretical literature often give rise to research ideas, so it is useful to become familiar with a variety of grand and middle-range theories. Several nursing theory textbooks provide good overviews of major nurse theorists (e.g., Alligood, 2018; Butts & Rich, 2018; Morse, 2017). Resources for learning more about middle-range theories include Smith and Liehr (2018) and Peterson and Bredow (2017).

S : The Supplement for this chapter on the **Point** includes a table that describes 11 nursing models that have been used by researchers. The Supplement also offers references for about 100 middle-range theories and models that have been used in nursing research, organized in broad domains (e.g., aging, mental health, pain).

If you begin with a research problem or topic and are looking for a theory, a good strategy is to examine the conceptual contexts of existing studies on a similar topic. You may find that several different theories have been used, and so the next step is to learn as much as possible about the most promising ones so that you can select a theory that is appropriate for your own study.

TIP Although it may be tempting to read about the features of a theory in a secondary source, it is best to consult a primary source and to rely on the most up-to-date reference because models are often revised as research accumulates. However, it is also a good idea to review studies that have used the theory so that you can judge how much empirical support the theory has received and how key variables were measured.

Many writers have offered advice on how to evaluate a theory for use in nursing practice and nursing research (e.g., Chinn & Kramer, 2018; Fawcett & DeSanto-Madeya, 2013; Smith & Parker, 2015). Box 6.1 presents some basic questions that can be asked in a preliminary assessment of a theory or model.

In addition to evaluating the general integrity of the model or theory, it is important to make sure that there is a proper "fit" between the theory and the research question to be studied. A critical issue is whether the theory has done a good job of explaining, predicting,

---

BOX 6.1 Some Questions for a Preliminary Assessment of a Model or Theory

Issue	Questions
Theoretical clarity	• Are key concepts defined, and are definitions clear? • Do all concepts "fit" within the theory? Are concepts used in the theory in a manner compatible with conceptual definitions? • Are schematic models helpful, and are they compatible with the text? Are schematic models needed but not presented? • Is the theory adequately explained? Are there ambiguities?
Theoretical complexity	• Is the theory sufficiently rich and detailed? • Is the theory overly complex? • Can the theory be used to explain or predict phenomena, or only to describe them?
Theoretical grounding	• Are the concepts identifiable in reality? • Is there a research basis for the theory? Is the basis a sound one?
Appropriateness of the theory	• Are the tenets of the theory compatible with nursing's philosophy? • Are key concepts within the domain of nursing?
Importance of the theory	• Could research based on this theory answer critical questions for nursing? • Will testing the theory contribute to nursing's evidence base?
General issues	• Are there other theories or models that would do a better job of explaining phenomena of interest? • Is the theory compatible with your world view?

or describing constructs that are key to your research problem. A few additional questions include the following:

- Has the theory been applied to similar research questions, and do the findings from prior research lend credibility to the theory's utility for research?
- Are the theoretical constructs in the model or theory readily operationalized? Do instruments of adequate quality exist?
- Is the theory compatible with your world view and with the world view implicit in the research question?

TESTING, USING, AND DEVELOPING A THEORY OR FRAMEWORK

In this section, we describe how theory is used by qualitative and quantitative researchers. We use the term *theory* broadly to include conceptual models and frameworks.

Theories and Qualitative Research

Theory is almost always present, either peripherally or centrally, in studies that are embedded in a qualitative research tradition such as ethnography, phenomenology, or grounded theory. These research traditions inherently provide an overarching framework that gives qualitative studies a theoretical grounding. However, different traditions involve theory in different ways.

Sandelowski (1993) made a useful distinction between **substantive theory** (conceptualizations of the target phenomenon under study) and theory that reflects a conceptualization of human inquiry. Some qualitative researchers insist on an atheoretical stance vis-à-vis the phenomenon of interest, with the goal of suspending a priori conceptualizations (substantive theories) that might bias their collection and analysis of data. For example, phenomenologists are in general committed to theoretical naiveté and explicitly try to hold preconceived views of the phenomenon in check. Nevertheless, they are guided in their inquiries by a philosophy of phenomenology that focuses their analysis on certain aspects of a person's lived experiences.

Ethnographers typically bring a strong cultural perspective to their studies, and this perspective shapes their initial fieldwork. Ethnographers often adopt one of two cultural theories: *ideational theories*, which suggest that cultural conditions stem from mental activity and ideas, or *materialistic theories*, which view material circumstances (e.g., resources, money, production) as the source of cultural developments.

The most prominent sociologic theory in grounded theory is **symbolic interaction** (or *interactionism*), which has three underlying premises (Blumer, 1986). First, humans act toward things based on the meanings that the things have for them. Second, the meaning of things arises out of the interaction humans have with other humans. Last, meanings are handled in, and modified through, an interpretive process in dealing with the things humans encounter. Despite having a theoretical umbrella, grounded theory researchers, like phenomenologists, attempt to hold prior substantive theory (existing knowledge and conceptualizations about the phenomenon) in abeyance until their own substantive theory begins to emerge.

Example of a Grounded Theory Study
Girardon-Perlini and Ângelo (2017) conducted a grounded theory study based on a symbolic interactionist framework to explore the experiences of rural families with relatives who had cancer. Their main category was "Caregiving to support the family world," which represented the family's strategies to reconcile care for the patient and care for family life.

The use of theory in qualitative studies has been the topic of some debate. Morse (2002) called for qualitative researchers to not be "theory ignorant but theory smart" (p. 296) and to "get over" their theory phobia. Morse (2004) elaborated by noting that qualitative research does not necessarily begin with holding in check all prior knowledge of the phenomenon under study. She suggested that if the boundaries of the concept of interest can be identified, a qualitative researcher can use these boundaries as a scaffold to inductively explore the attributes of the concept.

Some qualitative nurse researchers have adopted a perspective known as critical theory as their framework. **Critical theory** is a paradigm that involves a critique of society and societal processes and structures, as we discuss in Chapter 22.

Qualitative researchers sometimes use conceptual models of nursing as an interpretive framework, rather than as a guide for the conduct of a study. For example, some qualitative nurse researchers acknowledge that the philosophic roots of their studies lie in conceptual models of nursing developed by Newman, Parse, or Rogers.

One final note is that a systematic review of qualitative studies on a specific topic is another strategy leading to theory development. In metasyntheses (Chapter 30), qualitative studies on a topic are scrutinized to identify essential elements. The findings from different sources are then used for theory building.

Theories and Models in Quantitative Research

Quantitative researchers, like qualitative researchers, link research to theory or models in several ways. The classic approach is to test hypotheses deduced from an existing theory.

Testing an Existing Theory

Theories sometimes stimulate new studies. For example, a nurse might read about Pender's HPM (Figure 6.1), and the following type of reasoning might ensue: "If the HPM is valid, then I would expect that patients with osteoporosis who perceived the benefit of a calcium-enriched diet would be more likely to alter their eating patterns than those who perceived no benefits." Such a conjecture can serve as a starting point for testing the model.

In testing a theory or model, quantitative researchers deduce implications (as in the preceding example) and develop hypotheses, which are predictions about the way variables would be interrelated if the theory were sound. The hypotheses are then subjected to testing through systematic data collection and analysis.

The testing process involves a comparison between observed outcomes with those hypothesized. Through this process, a theory is continually subjected to potential disconfirmation. If studies repeatedly fail to disconfirm a theory, it gains support. Testing continues until pieces of evidence cannot be interpreted within the context of the theory but *can* be explained by a new theory that also accounts for previous findings. Theory-testing studies are most useful when researchers devise logically sound deductions from the theory, design a study that reduces the plausibility of alternative explanations for observed relationships, and use methods that assess the theory's validity under maximally heterogeneous situations so that potentially competing theories can be ruled out.

Researchers sometimes base a new study on a theory to explain earlier descriptive findings. For example, suppose several researchers had found that nursing home residents demonstrate greater levels of noncompliance with nursing staff around bedtime than at other times. These findings shed no light on underlying causes of the problem, and so suggest no way to improve it. Explanations rooted in theories of stress might be relevant in explaining the residents' behavior. By directly testing the theory in a study (i.e., deducing hypotheses derived from the theory), a researcher might be able to explain *why* bedtime is a vulnerable period for nursing home residents.

Researchers sometimes combine elements from two theories as a basis for generating hypotheses. In doing this, researchers need to be thoroughly knowledgeable about *both* theories to see if there is an adequate conceptual rationale for conjoining them. If underlying assumptions or conceptual definitions of key concepts are not compatible, the theories should not be combined (although perhaps elements of the two can be used to create a new conceptual framework with its own assumptions and definitions).

Tests of a theory increasingly are taking the form of testing theory-based interventions. If a theory is correct, it has implications for strategies to influence people's health-related attitudes or behavior and hence their health outcomes. The role of theory in the development of interventions is discussed at greater length in Chapter 28.

Example of a Theory-Based Intervention
Worawong et al. (2018), whose literature review was excerpted in the previous chapter, tested the effect of a person-centered intervention on physical activity and healthy nutrition in community-living adults. The intervention, which they called "Healthy You," was developed using integrated concepts from two theories—Self-Regulation Theory and Self-Determination Theory.

Using a Model or Theory as an Organizing Structure

Many researchers who cite a theory or model as their framework are not directly testing it, but rather using the theory as an organizational or interpretive tool. In such studies, researchers begin with a conceptualization of nursing (or stress, health beliefs, and so on) that is consistent with that of a model developer. The researchers *assume* that the model used as a framework is valid and proceed to conceptualize and operationalize constructs with the model in mind. Using models in this fashion can serve a valuable organizing purpose, but such studies do not address the issue of whether the theory itself is sound.

TIP The Toolkit with the accompanying *Resource Manual* offers some criteria for drawing conclusions about whether researchers were truly testing a theory or using a theory as an organizational or interpretive aid.

We should note that the framework for a quantitative study need not be a formal theory such as those described in the previous section. Sometimes quantitative studies are undertaken to further explicate constructs identified in grounded theory or other qualitative research.

Fitting a Problem to a Theory

Researchers sometimes develop a set of research questions or hypotheses and subsequently try to devise a theoretical context in which to frame them. Such an approach may in some case be worthwhile, but we caution that an after-the-fact linkage of theory to a problem does not always enhance a study. An important exception is when the researcher is struggling to make sense of findings and calls on an existing theory to help explain or interpret them.

If it is necessary to find a relevant theory or model after a research problem is selected, the search for such a theory must begin by first conceptualizing the problem on an abstract level. For example, take the following research question: "Do daily telephone conversations between a psychiatric nurse and a patient for 2 weeks after hospital discharge reduce rates of readmission by short-term psychiatric patients?" This is a relatively concrete research problem, but it might profitably be viewed within the context of reinforcement theory, a theory of social support, or a theory of crisis resolution. Part of the difficulty in finding a theory is that a single phenomenon of interest can be conceptualized in ways.

Fitting a problem to a theory after-the-fact should be done with circumspection. Although having a theoretical context can enhance the meaningfulness of a study, artificially linking a problem to a theory is not the route to scientific utility. If a conceptual model is really linked to a problem, then the design of the study, decisions about what to measure and how to measure it, and the interpretation of the findings *flow* from that conceptualization.

TIP If you begin with a research question and then subsequently identify a theory or model, be willing to adapt or augment your original research problem as you gain greater understanding of the theory.

Developing a Framework in a Quantitative Study

Novice researchers may think of themselves as unqualified to develop a conceptual scheme of their own. But theory development depends less on research experience than on powers of observation, grasp of a problem, and knowledge of prior research. Nothing prevents a creative and astute person from formulating an original conceptual framework for a study. The framework may not be a full-fledged theory, but it should place the issues of the study into some broader perspective.

The basic intellectual process underlying theory development is induction—that is, reasoning from particular observations and facts to broader generalizations. The inductive process involves integrating what one has experienced or learned into an organized scheme. For quantitative research, the observations used in the inductive process usually are findings from other studies. When patterns of relationships among variables are derived in this fashion, one has the makings of a theory that can be put to a more rigorous test. The first step in the development of a framework, then, is to formulate a generalized scheme of relevant concepts that is firmly grounded in the research literature.

Let us use as an example a study question identified in Chapter 4, namely, What is the effect of humor on stress in patients with cancer? (See the problem statement in Box 4.2). In undertaking a literature review, we find that researchers and reviewers have suggested a myriad of complex relationships among such concepts as humor, social support, stress, coping, appraisal, immune function, and neuroendocrine function on the one hand and various health outcomes (pain tolerance, mood, depression, health status, and eating and sleeping disturbances) on the other (e.g.,

Christie and Moore, 2005). While there is a fair amount of research evidence for the existence of these relationships, it is not clear how they all fit together. Without some kind of "map" of what might be going on, it could be challenging to design a strong study—we might, for example, not measure all the key variables or we might not undertake an appropriate analysis. And, if our goal is to design a humor therapy, we might struggle in developing a strong intervention in the absence of a framework.

The conceptual map in Figure 6.2 represents an attempt to put the pieces of the puzzle together for a study involving a test of a humor intervention to improve health outcomes for patients with cancer. According to this map, stress is affected by a cancer diagnosis and treatment both directly and indirectly, through the person's appraisal of the situation. That appraisal, in turn, is affected by the patient's coping skills, personality factors, and available social supports (factors that themselves are interrelated). Stress and physiological function (neuroendocrine and immunologic) have reciprocal relationships.

Note that we have not yet put in a "box" for humor in Figure 6.2. How do we think humor might operate? If we see humor as having

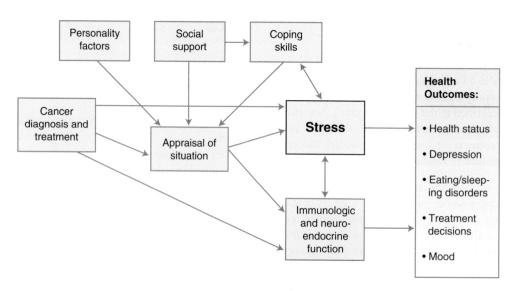

FIGURE 6.2 Conceptual Model of Stress and Health Outcomes in Patients with Cancer.

primarily a direct effect on physiologic response, we would place humor near the bottom and draw an arrow from the box to immune and neuroendocrine function. But perhaps humor reduces stress because it helps a person cope (i.e., its effects are primarily psychological). Or maybe humor will affect the person's appraisal of the situation. Alternatively, a nurse-initiated humor therapy might have its effect primarily because it is a form of social support. Each conceptualization has a different implication for the design of the intervention and the study. To give but one example, if the humor therapy is viewed primarily as a form of social support, then we might want to compare our intervention with an alternative intervention that involves the presence of a comforting nurse (another form of social support), without any special effort at including humor.

This type of inductive conceptualization based on existing research is a useful means of providing theoretical grounding for a study. Of course, our research question in this example could have been addressed within the context of an existing conceptualization, such as the psychoneuroimmunology (PNI) framework of McCain et al. (2005), but hopefully our example illustrates how developing an original framework can inform researchers' decisions and strengthen the study. Havenga et al. (2014) offer additional tips on developing a model.

TIP We strongly encourage you to draw a conceptual map before launching an investigation based on either an existing theory or your own inductive conceptualization—even if you do not plan to formally test the entire model or present the model in a report. Such maps are valuable heuristic devices in planning a study.

Example of Developing a New Model

Hoffman et al. (2017) developed and tested a rehabilitation program for lung cancer patients. The intervention was based on their own model, which represented a synthesis of two theories, the Transitional Care Model and the Theory of Symptom Self-Management.

CRITICAL APPRAISAL OF FRAMEWORKS IN RESEARCH REPORTS

It is often challenging to critically appraise the theoretical context of a published research report—or its absence—but we offer a few suggestions.

In a qualitative study in which a grounded theory is developed and presented, you probably will not be given enough information to refute the proposed theory because only evidence supporting it is presented. You can, however, assess whether the theory seems logical, whether the conceptualization is insightful, and whether the evidence in support of it is persuasive. In a phenomenologic study, you should look to see if the researcher addressed the philosophical underpinnings of the study. The researcher should briefly discuss the philosophy of phenomenology upon which the study was based.

Critiquing a theoretical framework in a quantitative report is also difficult, especially because you are not likely to be familiar with a range of relevant theories and models. Some suggestions for evaluating the conceptual basis of a quantitative study are offered in the following discussion and in Box 6.2.

The first task is to determine whether the study does, in fact, have a theoretical or conceptual framework. If there is no mention of a theory, model, or framework, you should consider whether the study's contribution is weakened by this absence. In some cases, the research may be so pragmatic that it does not really need a theory to enhance its utility. If, however, the study involves evaluating a complex intervention or testing hypotheses, the absence of a formally stated theoretical framework or rationale suggests conceptual fuzziness.

If the study does have an explicit framework, you must ask whether the particular framework is appropriate. You may not be able to challenge the researcher's use of a particular theory, but you can assess whether the link between the problem and the theory is genuine. Did the researcher present a convincing rationale for the framework used? Do the hypotheses flow from the theory? Will the findings contribute to the validation of the theory? Did the researcher

> **BOX 6.2**   Guidelines for Critically Appraising Theoretical and Conceptual Frameworks in a Research Article
>
> 1. Did the report describe an explicit theoretical or conceptual framework for the study? If not, does the absence of a framework detract from the usefulness or significance of the research?
> 2. Did the report adequately describe the major features of the theory or model so that readers could understand the study's conceptual basis?
> 3. Does the theory or model fit the research problem? Would a different framework have been more appropriate?
> 4. If there is an intervention, was there a cogent theoretical basis or rationale for how the intervention was expected to "work" to produce desired outcomes?
> 5. Was the theory or model used as a basis for generating hypotheses, or was it used as an organizational or interpretive framework? Was this appropriate?
> 6. Did the research problem and hypotheses (if any) naturally flow from the framework, or did the purported link between the problem and the framework seem contrived? Were deductions from the theory logical?
> 7. Were concepts adequately defined, and in a way that is consistent with the theory? If there was an intervention, were intervention components consistent with the theory?
> 8. Was the framework based on a conceptual model of nursing or on a model developed by nurses? If it was borrowed from another discipline, is there adequate justification for its use?
> 9. Did the framework guide the study methods? For example, was the appropriate research tradition used if the study was qualitative? If quantitative, did the operational definitions correspond to the conceptual definitions?
> 10. Did the researcher tie the study findings back to the framework in the Discussion section? Did the findings support or challenge the framework? Were the findings interpreted within the context of the framework?

interpret the findings within the context of the framework? If the answer to such questions is no, you may have grounds for criticizing the study's framework, even though you may not be able to articulate how the conceptual basis of the study could be improved.

RESEARCH EXAMPLES

Throughout this chapter, we have mentioned studies that were based on various conceptual and theoretical models. This section presents more detailed examples of the linkages between theory and research from the nursing research literature—one from a quantitative study and the other from a qualitative study.

Research Example From a Quantitative Study: The Health Promotion Model

Study: The relationship between religiosity and health-promoting behaviors in pregnant women (Cyphers et al., 2017)

Statement of purpose: The purpose of the study was to examine the relationship between religiosity and health-promoting behaviors of women at Pregnancy Resource Centers (PRCs).

Theoretical framework: The Health Promotion Model (HPM, Figure 6.1) was the guiding framework for the study: "The…HPM, a middle-range theory based on expectancy-value theory and Social Cognitive Theory, provides a holistic, multidimensional framework for exploring a person's health-promoting behavior… Religiosity had not been previously studied with the HPM, but as religiosity can be considered a personal factor…, it was included in this research study" (p. 1430).

Method: The study was conducted in eastern Pennsylvania. The researchers sampled 86 pregnant women who visited PRCs, which are community centers that offer Christian, faith-based approaches to care. Study participants completed an anonymous questionnaire in a private area of the PRC. The questionnaire was used to gather data on pregnancy intention, religiosity, health-promoting behaviors, services used at the PRC, and demographics.

Key findings: The researchers found that women who attended more classes at the centers reported more frequent health-promoting behaviors. Religiosity, attendance at religious services, and a scale measuring "satisfaction with surrender to God" were also found to be associated with higher health-promoting behavior scores. These variables included personal factors, behavior-specific cognitions, and interpersonal factors of Pender's model.

Research Example From a Qualitative Study: A Grounded Theory

Study: Follow the yellow brick road: Self-management by adolescents and young adults after a stem cell transplant (Morrison et al., 2018)

Statement of purpose: The purpose of the study was to understand the process adolescents and young adults use to manage their care after a stem cell transplant, and to explore self-management facilitators, barriers, processes, and behaviors.

Theoretical framework: A grounded theory approach was chosen to explore the psychosocial processes that adolescents and young adults use in managing their care. The authors noted that "Grounded theory is an ideal methodology for studying complex social and psychological actions and processes. Data gathered are rich and detailed including participants' views, actions, intentions, feelings, and life structures and the context in which they are occurring" (p. 348).

Method: Data were collected through in-depth interviews with 17 adolescents and young adults (AYA) who underwent a stem cell transplant between the ages of 13 and 25. In addition, caregivers of 13 of the AYA participants were interviewed to gain a deeper understanding of how AYA care is managed after the transplant. Interviews, which lasted about an hour, were digitally recorded and transcribed for analysis. Data collection and data analysis occurred concurrently, and data collection continued until saturation occurred.

Key findings: AYA and caregiver interviewer data were integrated into one framework that was developed inductively. The metaphor of Dorothy's journey in the *Wizard of Oz* was applied after theoretical brainstorming by the research team was completed. Figure 6.3 provides a graphical depiction of their framework. Key concepts include "at the mercy of transplant" (the tornado), "education and instructions" (the yellow brick road), and "inner strength" (the Great and Powerful Oz).

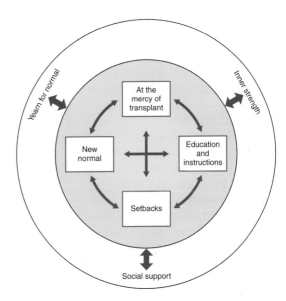

FIGURE 6.3 A grounded theory of the self-management process of adolescents and young adults after a stem cell transplant. Process starts with "At the mercy of transplant" and proceeds through the cycle. Adolescents/young adults may skip setbacks and proceed to new normal, or they may revert back to another stage and repeat the cycle. Yearn for normal, inner strength, and social support influence and are influenced by the context of SCT and self-management. (Adapted with permission from Morrison C., Martsolf D., Borich A., Coleman K., Ramirez P., Wehrkamp N., Pai A. (2018). Follow the yellow brick road: Self-management by adolescents and young adults after a stem cell transplant. *Cancer Nursing, 41,* 347–358.)

SUMMARY POINTS

- High-quality research requires *conceptual integration*, one aspect of which is having a defensible theoretical rationale for the study. Researchers demonstrate conceptual clarity by delineating a theory, model, or framework on which the study is based.

- A **theory** is a broad characterization of phenomena. As classically defined, a theory is an abstract generalization that systematically explains relationships among phenomena. **Descriptive theory** thoroughly describes a phenomenon.

- Concepts are the basic components of a theory. Classically defined theories consist of a set of propositions about the interrelationships among concepts, arranged in a logical system that permits new statements (hypotheses) to be deduced from them.
- **Grand theories** (*macrotheories*) attempt to describe large segments of the human experience. **Middle-range theories** (e.g., Pender's HPM) are specific to certain phenomena (e.g., stress, uncertainty in illness).
- Concepts are also the basic elements of **conceptual models**, but concepts are not linked in a logically ordered deductive system. Conceptual models, like theories, provide context for nursing studies.
- The goal of theories and models in research is to make findings meaningful, to integrate knowledge into coherent systems, to stimulate new research, and to explain phenomena and relationships among them.
- **Schematic models** (or **conceptual maps**) are graphic, theory-driven representations of phenomena and their interrelationships using symbols or diagrams and a minimal use of words.
- A **framework** is the conceptual underpinning of a study, including an overall rationale and conceptual definitions of key concepts. In qualitative studies, the framework often springs from distinct research traditions.
- Several conceptual models and grand theories of nursing have been developed. The concepts central to models of nursing are *human beings, environment, health*, and *nursing*. Two major conceptual models of nursing used by researchers are Roy's **Adaptation Model** and Orem's **Self-Care Deficit Theory**.
- Nonnursing models used by nurse researchers include Bandura's **Social Cognitive Theory**, Prochaska's **Transtheoretical Model**, and Becker's **Health Belief Model**.
- In some qualitative research traditions (e.g., phenomenology), the researcher avoids existing **substantive theories** of the phenomenon under study, but there is a rich theoretical underpinning associated with the tradition itself.

- Some qualitative researchers specifically seek to develop *grounded theories*—data-driven explanations to account for phenomena under study through inductive processes.
- In the classical use of theory, researchers test hypotheses deduced from an existing theory. An emerging trend is the testing of theory-based interventions.
- In both qualitative and quantitative studies, researchers sometimes use a theory or model as an organizing framework or an interpretive tool.
- Researchers sometimes develop a problem, design a study, and *then* look for a conceptual framework; such an after-the-fact selection of a framework usually is less compelling than a more systematic application of a particular theory.
- Even in the absence of a formal theory, quantitative researchers can inductively weave together the findings from prior studies into a conceptual scheme that provides methodologic and conceptual direction to the inquiry.

STUDY ACTIVITIES

Study activities are available to instructors on thePoint.

REFERENCES CITED IN CHAPTER 6

Ajzen, I. (2005). *Attitudes, personality and behavior* (2nd ed.). New York: McGraw Hill.

Alligood, M. R. (2018). *Nursing theorists and their work* (9th ed.). St. Louis, MO: Elsevier.

Bandura, A. (1997). *Self-efficacy: The exercise of control*. New York: W. H. Freeman.

Bandura, A. (2001). Social cognitive theory: An agentic perspective. *Annual Review of Psychology, 52*, 1–26.

Beck, C. T. (2012). Exemplar: Teetering on the edge: A second grounded theory modification. In Munhall, P. L. (Ed.), *Nursing research: A qualitative perspective* (5th ed.) (pp. 257–284). Sudbury, MA: Jones & Bartlett Learning.

Becker, M. (1978). The health belief model and sick role behavior. *Nursing Digest, 6*, 35–40.

Bergdahl, E., & Berterö, C. (2016). Concept analysis and the building blocks of theory: Misconceptions regarding theory development. *Journal of Advanced Nursing, 72*, 2558–2566.

Blumer, H. (1986). *Symbolic interactionism: Perspective and method*. Berkeley: University of California Press.

Butts, J., & Rich, K. (2018). *Philosophies and theories for advanced nursing practice* (3rd ed.). Burlington, MA: Jones & Bartlett.

Chinn, P., & Kramer, M. (2018). *Knowledge development in nursing: Theory and process* (10th ed.). St. Louis: Mosby.

Christie, W., & Moore, C. (2005). The impact of humor on patients with cancer. *Clinical Journal of Oncology Nursing, 9*, 211–218.

Conn, V. S., Rantz, M. J., Wipke-Tevis, D. D., & Maas, M. L. (2001). Designing effective nursing interventions. *Research in Nursing & Health, 24*, 433–442.

*Cyphers, N., Clements, A., & Lindseth, G. (2017). The relationship between religiosity and health-promoting behaviors in pregnant women. *Western Journal of Nursing Research, 39*, 1429–1446.

Dodd, M., Janson, S., Facione, N., Fawcett, J., Froelicher, E. S., Humphreys, J., … Taylor, D. (2001). Advancing the science of symptom management. *Journal of Advanced Nursing, 33*, 668–676.

Eren Fidanci, B., Akbayrak, N., & Arslan, F. (2017). Assessment of a health promotion model on obese Turkish children. *Journal of Nursing Research, 25*, 436–446.

Fawcett, J., & DeSanto-Madeya, S. (2013). *Contemporary nursing knowledge: Analysis and evaluation of nursing models and theories* (3rd ed.). Philadelphia: F.A. Davis Company.

Fishbein, M., & Ajzen, I. (2010). *Predicting and changing behavior: The reasoned action approach*. New York, NY: Psychology Press.

Frank, C., Schroeter, K., & Shaw, C. (2017). Addressing traumatic stress in the acute traumatically injured patient. *Journal of Trauma Nursing, 24*, 78–84.

*Girardon-Perlini, N., & Ângelo, M. (2017). The experience of rural families in the face of cancer. *Revista Brasileira Enfermagem, 70*, 550–557.

Havenga, Y., Poggenpoel, M., & Myburgh, C. (2014). Developing a model: An illustration. *Nursing Science Quarterly, 27*, 149–156.

Hoffman, A., Brintnall, R., Given, B., von Eye, A., Jones, L., & Brown, J. (2017). Using perceived self-efficacy to improve fatigue and fatigability in postsurgical lung cancer patients. *Cancer Nursing, 40*, 1–12.

Kolcaba, K. (2003). *Comfort theory and practice*. New York: Springer Publishing Co.

*McCain, N. L., Gray, D. P., Walter, J. M., & Robins, J. (2005). Implementing a comprehensive approach to the study of health dynamics using the psychoimmunology paradigm. *Advances in Nursing Science, 28*, 320–332.

Meleis, A. I., Sawyer, L. M., Im, E., Hilfinger Messias, D., & Schumacher, K. (2000). Experiencing transitions: An emerging middle-range theory. *Advances in Nursing Science, 23*, 12–28.

*Michie, S., Johnston, M., Abraham, C., Lawton, R., Parker, S., & Walker, A. (2005). Making psychological theory useful for implementing evidence-based practice: A consensus approach. *Quality & Safety in Health Care, 14*, 26–33.

Mishel, M. H. (1990). Reconceptualization of the uncertainty in illness theory. *Image: Journal of Nursing Scholarship, 22*, 256–262.

Mollohan, E. A. (2018). Dietary culture: A concept analysis. *Advances in Nursing Science, 41*, E1–E12.

**Morrison, C., Martsolf, D., Borich, A., Coleman, K., Ramirez, P., Wehrkamp, N., … Pai, A. (2018). Follow the yellow brick road: Self-management by adolescents and young adults after a stem cell transplant. *Cancer Nursing, 41*, 347–358.

Morse, J. M. (2002). Theory innocent or theory smart? *Qualitative Health Research, 12*, 295–296.

Morse, J. M. (2004). Constructing qualitatively derived theory. *Qualitative Health Research, 14*, 1387–1395.

Morse, J. M. (2017). *Analyzing and conceptualizing the theoretical foundations of nursing*. New York: Springer Publishing Company.

Murdaugh, C., Parsons, M. A., & Pender, N. J. (2019). *Health promotion in nursing practice* (8th ed.). Upper Saddle River, NJ: Pearson.

Orem, D., Taylor, S., Renpenning, K., & Eisenhandler, S. (2003). *Self-care theory in nursing: Selected papers of Dorothea Orem*. New York: Springer.

Parse, R. R. (2014). *The humanbecoming paradigm: A transformational worldview*. Pittsburgh, PA: A Discovery International Publication.

Peplau, H. E. (1997). Peplau's theory of interpersonal relations. *Nursing Science Quarterly, 10*, 162–167.

Peterson, S. J., & Bredow, T. S. (2017). *Middle range theories: Applications to nursing research* (4th ed.). Philadelphia: Lippincott Williams & Wilkins.

Prochaska, J. O., Redding, C. A., & Evers, K. E. (2002). The transtheoretical model and stages of changes. In Lewis, F. M. (Ed.), *Health behavior and health education: Theory, research and practice* (pp. 99–120). San Francisco: Jossey Bass.

Prochaska, J. O., & Velicer, W. F. (1997). The transtheoretical model of health behavior change. *American Journal of Health Promotion, 12*, 38–48.

Rakhshkhorshid, M., Navaee, M., Nouri, N., & Safarzaii, F. (2018). The association of health literacy with breast cancer knowledge, perception and screening behavior. *European Journal of Breast Health, 14*, 144–147.

Reed, P. G. (1991). Toward a nursing theory of self-transcendence. *Advances in Nursing Science, 13*, 64–77.

Rodgers, B.,, & Knafl, K.,. (Eds.). (2000). *Concept development in nursing: Foundations, techniques, and applications* (2nd ed.). Philadelphia: Saunders.

Roy, C., Sr., & Andrews, H. (2009). *The Roy adaptation model* (3rd ed.). Upper Saddle River, NJ: Pearson.

Sandelowski, M. (1993). Theory unmasked: The uses and guises of theory in qualitative research. *Research in Nursing & Health, 16*, 213–218.

Shi, Y., Yang, D., Chen, S., Wang, S., Li, H., Ying, J., ... Sun, J. (2019). Factors influencing patient delay in individuals with haemorrhoids: A study based on theory of planned behavior and common sense model. *Journal of Advanced Nursing, 75*(5), 1018–1028.

Shun, S., Chou, Y., Chen, C., & Yang, J. (2018). Change of uncertainty in illness and unmet care needs in patients with recurrent hepatocellular carcinoma during active treatment. *Cancer Nursing, 41*, 279–289.

Smith, M. J., & Liehr, P. (2018). *Middle-range theory for nursing* (4th ed.). New York, NY: Springer Publishing Co.

Smith, M. C., & Parker, M. (2015). *Nursing theories and nursing practice* (4th ed.). Philadelphia: F.A. Davis.

Staffileno, B., Tangney, C., & Fogg, L. (2018). Favorable outcomes using an eHealth approach to promote physical activity and nutrition among you African American women. *Journal of Cardiovascular Disease, 33*, 62–71.

Swanson, K. M. (1991). Empirical development of a middle-range theory of caring. *Nursing Research, 40*, 161–166.

Treadwell, A. A. (2017). Examining depression in patients on dialysis. *Nephrology Nursing Journal, 44*, 295–307.

Walker, L. O., & Avant, K. C. (2019). *Strategies for theory construction in nursing* (6th ed.). Upper Saddle River, NJ: Prentice Hall.

Wen, S., Li, J., Wang, A., Lv, M., Li, H., Lu, Y., & Zhang, J. (2019). Effects of transtheoretical-model-based intervention on the self-management of patients with an ostomy: A randomised controlled trial. *Journal of Clinical Nursing, 28*(9–10), 1936–1951.

Worawong, C., Borden, M. J., Cooper, K. Perez, O., & Lauver, D. (2018). Evaluation of a person-centered, theory-based intervention to promote health behaviors. *Nursing Research, 67*, 6–15.

A link to this open-access article is provided in the Toolkit for Chapter 6 in the **Resource Manual**. ✪

This journal article is available on thePoint *for this chapter.*

7 | Ethics in Nursing Research

Researchers who conduct studies with human being or animals must do so ethically. Ethical demands can be challenging because they sometimes conflict with the goal of producing rigorous evidence. This chapter discusses major ethical principles for conducting research.

ETHICS AND RESEARCH

The obligation for ethical conduct with human study participants may strike you as self-evident, but ethics have not always been given adequate attention. Historical examples of ethical transgressions are abundant, as described in the chapter Supplement on the book's website. 🟢

Codes of Ethics

Human rights violations in the name of science have led to the development of various **codes of ethics**. The *Nuremberg Code*, developed after Nazi crimes were made public in the Nuremberg trials, was an international effort to establish ethical standards. The *Declaration of Helsinki*, another international set of ethical principles regarding human experimentation, was adopted in 1964 by the World Medical Association and was most recently revised in 2013.

Most disciplines (e.g., psychology, medicine) have established their own ethical codes. In nursing, the American Nurses Association

(ANA) issued *Ethical Guidelines in the Conduct, Dissemination, and Implementation of Nursing Research* (Silva, 1995). The ANA, which declared 2015 the Year of Ethics, published a revised *Code of Ethics for Nurses with Interpretive Statements*, a document that includes principles that apply to nurse researchers. In Canada, the Canadian Nurses Association published a revised version of *Ethical Research Guidelines for Registered Nurses* in 2017. In Australia, three nursing organizations collaborated to develop the *Code of Ethics for Nurses in Australia* (2018). Additionally, the International Council of Nurses (ICN) developed the *ICN Code of Ethics for Nurses*, which was most recently revised in 2012.

Government Regulations for Protecting Study Participants

Governments throughout the world fund research and establish rules for adhering to ethical principles. For example, Health Canada created the *Tri-Council Policy Statement: Ethical Conduct for Research Involving Humans* as the guidelines to protect study participants in all types of research, most recently revised in 2014. In Australia, the National Health and Medical Research Council issued the *National Statement on Ethical Conduct in Human Research,* updated in 2018.

In the United States, the National Commission for the Protection of Human Subjects of Biomedical and Behavioral Research adopted a code of ethics in 1978. The commission issued the *Belmont Report*, which provided a model for many disciplinary guidelines. Regulations affecting research sponsored by the U.S. government, including studies supported by the National Institute of Nursing Research (NINR), are based on the Belmont Report. The U.S. Department of Health and Human Services (DHHS) has issued ethical regulations that have been codified as Title 45 Part 46 of the Code of Federal Regulations (45 CFR 46). These regulations were revised most recently in 2018.

TIP Many useful websites are devoted to research ethics. Several websites are listed in the Toolkit of the accompanying *Resource Manual*, for you to click on directly.

Ethical Dilemmas in Conducting Research

Research that violates ethical principles is rarely done to be cruel, but usually reflects a conviction that knowledge is important and beneficial in the long run. There are situations in which participants' rights and study demands are in direct conflict, posing **ethical dilemmas** for researchers. Here are examples of research problems in which the desire for rigor conflicts with ethical considerations:

1. *Research question:* Does a new medication improve mobility in patients with Parkinson disease?
   Ethical dilemma: The best way to test the effectiveness of an intervention is to administer the intervention to some participants but withhold it from others to see if differences between the groups emerge. However, if the intervention is untested (e.g., a new drug), the group receiving the intervention may be exposed to potentially hazardous side effects. On the other hand, the group *not* receiving the drug may be denied a beneficial treatment.
2. *Research question:* Are nurses equally empathic in their care of male and female patients in the intensive care unit (ICU)?

   Ethical dilemma: Ethics require that participants be aware of their role in a study. Yet if the researcher informs nurse participants that their empathy in treating male and female ICU patients will be scrutinized, will their behavior be "normal"? If the nurses' usual behavior is altered because of the known presence of research observers, then the findings will be misleading.
3. *Research question:* How do parents cope if a child has a terminal illness?
   Ethical dilemma: To answer this question, the researcher may need to probe into parents' psychological state at a vulnerable time; such probing could be painful or traumatic. Yet knowledge of the parents' coping mechanisms might help to design effective ways of addressing parents' stress and grief.
4. *Research question:* What is the process by which adult children adapt to the day-to-day stresses of caring for a parent with Alzheimer's disease?
   Ethical dilemma: Sometimes, especially in qualitative studies, a researcher may get so close to participants that they become willing to share "secrets" and privileged information. Interviews can become confessions—sometimes of unseemly or illegal behavior. In this example, suppose a woman admitted to physically abusing her mother—how does the researcher respond to that information without undermining a pledge of confidentiality? And, if the researcher divulges the information to authorities, how can a pledge of confidentiality be given in good faith to other participants?

As these examples suggest, researchers are sometimes in a bind. They want to develop good evidence, but they must also protect human rights. Another dilemma can arise if nurse researchers are confronted with conflict of interest situations, in which their expected behavior as researchers conflicts with their expected behavior as nurses (e.g., deviating from a research protocol to give assistance to a patient). It is precisely because of such dilemmas that codes of ethics have been developed to guide researchers' efforts.

ETHICAL PRINCIPLES FOR PROTECTING STUDY PARTICIPANTS

The *Belmont Report* articulated three broad principles on which standards of ethical conduct in research in the United States are based: beneficence, respect for human dignity, and justice. We briefly discuss these principles and then describe procedures researchers adopt to comply with them.

Beneficence

Beneficence imposes a duty on researchers to maximize benefits and minimize harm. Human research should be intended to produce benefits for participants or—a more common situation—for others. This principle covers multiple aspects.

> **TIP** The increased involvement of patients and lay people in the development of research questions and protocols has been viewed as an especially ethical approach to research conduct. As noted by Domecq et al. (2014), "there is an overarching ethical mandate for patient participation in research as a manifestation of the 'democratization' of the research process" (p. 1).

The Right to Freedom From Harm and Discomfort

Researchers have an obligation to avoid, prevent, or minimize harm (*nonmaleficence*) in research with humans. Participants should not be subjected to unnecessary risks of harm or discomfort, and their participation must be essential to achieving societally important aims that could not otherwise be realized. In research with humans, *harm* and *discomfort* can be physical (e.g., injury, fatigue), emotional (e.g., stress, fear), social (e.g., diminished social support), or financial (e.g., loss of wages). Ethical researchers must use strategies to minimize all types of harms and discomforts, even ones that are temporary.

Research should be conducted by qualified people, especially if potentially dangerous procedures are used. Ethical researchers must be prepared to terminate a study if they suspect that continuation would result in injury or undue distress to participants. When a new medical procedure or drug is being tested, prior experimentation with animals or tissue cultures is advisable.

Protecting human beings from physical harm may be straightforward, but psychological consequences are often subtle. For example, participants may be asked questions about their personal weaknesses, fears, or concerns. Such queries might lead people to reveal very personal information. The point is not that researchers should refrain from asking questions but that they need to be aware of the intrusion on people's psyches.

The need for sensitivity may be greater in qualitative studies, which often involve in-depth exploration of personal topics. Extensive probing may expose deep-seated anxieties that participants had previously repressed. Qualitative researchers must be vigilant in anticipating potential ethical challenges.

The Right to Protection From Exploitation

Study involvement should not place participants at a disadvantage or expose them to damages. Participants need to be assured that their participation, or information they provide, will not be used against them. For example, people divulging illegal drug use should not fear exposure to criminal authorities.

Study participants enter into a special relationship with researchers, and this relationship should never be exploited. Exploitation may be overt and malicious (e.g., sexual exploitation, commercial use of donated blood) but might be more elusive. For example, suppose people agreed to participate in a study requiring 30 minutes of their time, but the time commitment was actually 2 hours. In such a situation, the researcher might be accused of exploiting the researcher–participant relationship.

Because nurse researchers may have a nurse–patient (in addition to a researcher–participant) relationship, special care may be required to avoid exploiting that bond. Patients' consent to participate in a study may result from their understanding of the researcher's role as *nurse*, not as *researcher*.

In qualitative research, psychological distance between researchers and participants often declines as the study progresses. The emergence of a pseudotherapeutic relationship is not uncommon, which can heighten the risk that exploitation could occur inadvertently (Eide & Kahn, 2008). On the other hand, qualitative researchers often are in a better position than quantitative researchers to *do good*, rather than just to avoid doing harm.

Example of Therapeutic Research Experiences
Some of the participants in Beck et al.'s (2015) study on secondary traumatic stress among certified nurse-midwives told the researchers that writing about the traumatic births they had attended was therapeutic for them. One participant wrote, "I think it's fascinating how little respect our patients and coworkers give to the traumatic experiences we suffer. It is healing to be able to write out my experiences in this study and actually have researchers interested in studying this topic."

Respect for Human Dignity

Respect for human dignity is the second ethical principle in the *Belmont Report*. This principle includes the right to self-determination and the right to full disclosure.

The Right to Self-Determination

Humans should be treated as autonomous agents. **Self-determination** means that prospective participants can voluntarily decide whether to take part in a study, without risk of prejudicial treatment. It also means that people have the right to ask questions, to refuse to give information, and to withdraw from the study.

A person's right to self-determination includes freedom from **coercion**, which involves threats of penalty for failing to participate in a study or excessive rewards for agreeing to participate. Protecting people from coercion requires careful thought when the researcher is in a position of authority or influence over potential participants, as is often the case in a nurse–patient relationship. The issue of coercion may require scrutiny even when there is not a preestablished relationship. For example, a generous monetary incentive (or **stipend**) offered to encourage participation among an economically disadvantaged group (e.g., the homeless) might be considered mildly coercive because such incentives might pressure prospective participants into cooperation.

The Right to Full Disclosure

People's right to make informed, voluntary decisions about study participation requires full disclosure. **Full disclosure** means that the researcher has fully described the study, the right to refuse participation, the researcher's responsibilities, and likely risks and benefits. The right to self-determination and the right to full disclosure are the two major elements of *informed consent*, discussed later in this chapter.

Full disclosure can, however, create biases and sample recruitment problems. Suppose we were testing the hypothesis that high school students with a high rate of absenteeism are more likely to be substance abusers than students with good attendance. If we approached potential participants and fully explained the study purpose, some students likely would refuse to participate, and nonparticipation would be selective; those least likely to volunteer might well be substance abusing students—the group of primary interest. Moreover, by knowing the research question, those who *do* participate might not give candid responses. In such a situation, full disclosure could undermine the study.

A technique that is sometimes used in such situations is **covert data collection** (*concealment*), which is the collection of data without participants' knowledge and consent. This might happen, for example, if a researcher wanted to observe people's behavior in real-world settings and worried that doing so openly would affect the behavior of interest. Researchers might choose to obtain the information through concealed methods, such as by videotaping with hidden equipment or observing while pretending to be engaged in other activities. Covert data collection may in some cases be acceptable if risks are negligible and participants' right to privacy has not been violated. Covert data collection is least likely to be ethically tolerable if the study is focused on sensitive aspects of people's behavior, such as drug use or sexual conduct.

A more controversial technique is the use of **deception**, which involves deliberately withholding information about the study or providing participants with false information. For example, in studying high school students' use of drugs, we might describe the research as a study of students' health practices, which is a mild form of misinformation.

Deception and concealment are problematic ethically because they interfere with people's right to make informed decisions about personal costs and benefits of participation. Some people argue that deception is never justified. Others, however, believe that if the study involves minimal risk to participants and if there are anticipated benefits to society, then deception may be justified as a means of enhancing the validity of the findings.

Another issue that has emerged in this era of electronic communication concerns data collection over the Internet. For example, some researchers analyze the content of messages posted to social media sites. The issue is whether such messages can be treated as research data without permission and informed consent. Some researchers believe that messages posted electronically are in the public domain and can be used without consent for research purposes. Others, however, feel that standard ethical rules should apply in cyberspace research and that researchers must carefully protect the rights of those who participate in "virtual" communities. Guidance for the ethical conduct of health research on the Internet is offered by Ellett et al. (2004) and Heilferty (2011).

Justice

The third broad principle articulated in the *Belmont Report* concerns justice, which includes participants' right to fair treatment and their right to privacy.

The Right to Fair Treatment
One aspect of justice concerns the equitable distribution of benefits and burdens of research. Participant selection should be based on study requirements and not on a group's vulnerability.

Participant selection has been a key ethical issue historically, with researchers sometimes selecting groups with lower social standing (e.g., prisoners) as participants. The principle of justice imposes special obligations toward individuals who are unable to protect their own interests (e.g., dying patients) to ensure that they are not exploited.

Distributive justice also imposes duties to not discriminate against individuals or groups who may benefit from research. During the 1980s and 1990s, it became evident that women and minorities were being unfairly excluded from many clinical studies in the United States. This led to the promulgation of regulations requiring that researchers who seek funding from the National Institutes of Health (NIH) include women and minorities as participants. The regulations also require researchers to examine whether clinical interventions have differential effects (e.g., whether benefits are different for men than for women), although this provision has had limited adherence (Polit & Beck, 2009, 2013).

The fair treatment principle covers issues other than participant selection. The right to fair treatment means that researchers must treat people who decline to participate (or who withdraw from the study) in a nonprejudicial manner; that they must honor all agreements with participants; that they demonstrate respect for the beliefs and lifestyles of people from different backgrounds or cultures; that they give participants access to research staff for desired clarification; and that they treat participants courteously and tactfully at all times.

The Right to Privacy
Research with humans involves intrusions into personal lives. Researchers should ensure that their research is not more intrusive than it needs to be and that participants' privacy is maintained. Participants have the right to expect that their data will be kept in strict confidence.

Privacy issues have become especially salient in the U.S. healthcare community since the passage of the Health Insurance Portability and Accountability Act of 1996 (HIPAA), which articulates federal standards to protect patients' health information. In response to the HIPAA legislation, the

U.S. Department of Health and Human Services issued the regulations *Standards for Privacy of Individually Identifiable Health Information.*

> **TIP** Some information relevant to HIPAA compliance is presented in this chapter, but you should confer with organizations that are involved in your research (if they are covered entities) regarding their practices and policies relating to HIPAA provisions. Here is a website that provides information about the implications of HIPAA for health research: https://privacyruleandresearch.nih.gov.

PROCEDURES FOR PROTECTING STUDY PARTICIPANTS

Now that you are familiar with fundamental ethical principles in research, you need to understand procedures that researchers use to adhere to them.

Risk/Benefit Assessments

One strategy that researchers use to protect participants is to conduct a **risk/benefit assessment.** Such an assessment is designed to evaluate whether the benefits of participating in a study are in line with the costs, be they financial, physical, emotional, or social—i.e., whether the *risk/benefit ratio* is acceptable. A summary of risks and benefits should be communicated to recruited individuals so that they can evaluate whether it is in their best interest to participate. Box 7.1 summarizes some potential costs and benefits of research participation.

> **TIP** The Toolkit in the accompanying *Resource Manual* includes a Word document with the factors in Box 7.1 arranged in worksheet form for you to complete in doing a risk/benefit assessment. By completing the worksheet, it may be easier for you to envision opportunities for "doing good" and to avoid possibilities of doing harm.

BOX 7.1 Potential Benefits and Risks of Research to Participants

Major potential benefits to participants

- Access to a potentially beneficial intervention that might otherwise be unavailable
- Comfort in being able to discuss their situation or problem with a friendly, objective person
- Increased knowledge about themselves or their conditions, either through opportunity for introspection and self-reflection or through direct interaction with researchers
- Escape from normal routine
- Satisfaction that information they provide may help others with similar conditions
- Direct monetary or material gains through stipends or other incentives

Major potential risks to participants

- Physical harm, including unanticipated side effects
- Discomfort, fatigue, or boredom
- Emotional distress as a result of self-disclosure, introspection, discomfort with strangers, fear of repercussions, anger, or embarrassment at the questions being asked
- Social risks, such as the risk of stigma, adverse effects on personal relationships, loss of status
- Loss of privacy
- Loss of time
- Monetary costs (e.g., for transportation, child care, time lost from work)

The risk/benefit ratio should take into account whether risks to participants are commensurate with benefits to society. A broad guideline is that the degree of risk by participants should never exceed the potential humanitarian benefits of the evidence to be gained. Thus, the selection of a significant topic that has the potential to improve patient care is the first step in ensuring that research is ethical. Gennaro (2014) has written eloquently about this issue.

All research involves some risks, but risk is sometimes small. **Minimal risk** is defined as risks no greater than those ordinarily encountered in daily life or during routine procedures. When the risks are not minimal, researchers must proceed with caution, taking every step possible to diminish risks and maximize benefits.

In quantitative studies, most details of the study usually are spelled out in advance, and so a reasonably accurate risk/benefit assessment can be developed. Qualitative studies, however, usually evolve as data are gathered, and so it may be difficult to assess all risks at the outset. Qualitative researchers must remain sensitive to potential risks throughout the study.

Example of Ongoing Vigilance and Assessment
Stormorken et al. (2017) studied factors impacting the illness trajectory of postinfectious fatigue syndrome (PIFS) following an outbreak of *Giardia lamblia* in Norway. Recognizing that interviewing people with PIFS could trigger painful emotional reactions, the interviewers were vigilant for signs of emotional distress (e.g., crying) and asked participants if they wanted to terminate the interview. Invariably, participants renewed their consent to continue, "as they wished to complete their story of living with the condition" (p. 6).

One potential benefit to participants is monetary. Stipends offered to prospective participants are rarely viewed as an opportunity for financial gain, but there is ample evidence that stipends are useful incentives to participant recruitment and retention (Edwards et al., 2009). Financial incentives are especially effective when the group under study is difficult to recruit, when the study is time-consuming or tedious, or when participants incur study-related costs (e.g., for child care or transportation). Stipends can range from $1 to hundreds of dollars, but many are in the $25 to $75 range.

TIP In evaluating the anticipated risk/benefit ratio of a study design, you might want to consider how comfortable *you* would feel about being a study participant.

Informed Consent and Participant Authorization

A particularly important procedure for safeguarding participants is to obtain their informed consent. **Informed consent** means that participants have adequate information about the research, comprehend that information, and can consent to or decline participation voluntarily. This section discusses procedures for obtaining informed consent and for complying with HIPAA rules regarding accessing patients' health information.

The Content of Informed Consent

Fully informed consent typically involves communicating the following pieces of information to participants:

1. *Participant status.* Prospective participants need to understand the distinction between *research* and *treatment*. They should be told which healthcare activities are routine and which are implemented specifically for the study. They also should be informed that data they provide will be used for research purposes.
2. *Study goals.* The overall goals of the research should be stated, in lay rather than technical terms. The use to which the data will be put should be described.
3. *Type of data.* Prospective participants should be told what type of data (e.g., self-reports, laboratory tests) will be collected.
4. *Procedures.* Prospective participants should be given a description of the data collection procedures and procedures to be used regarding any innovative treatment.
5. *Nature of the commitment.* Participants should be told the expected time commitment at each point of contact and the number of contacts within a given time frame.

6. *Sponsorship.* Information on who is sponsoring or funding the study should be noted; if the research is part of an academic requirement, this information should be shared.

7. *Participant selection.* Prospective participants should be told how they were selected for recruitment and how many people will be participating.

8. *Potential risks.* Foreseeable risks (physical, psychological, social, or economic) or discomforts should be communicated, as well as efforts that will be made to minimize risks. The possibility of unforeseeable risks should be discussed, if appropriate. If injury is possible, treatments that will be made available to participants should be described. When risks are more than minimal, prospective participants should be encouraged to seek advice before consenting.

9. *Potential benefits.* Specific benefits to participants, if any, should be described, as well as possible benefits to others.

10. *Alternatives.* If appropriate, participants should be told about alternative procedures or treatments that might be advantageous to them.

11. *Compensation.* If stipends or reimbursements are to be paid (or if treatments are offered without any fee), these arrangements should be discussed.

12. *Confidentiality pledge.* Prospective participants should be assured that their privacy will be protected. If anonymity can be guaranteed, this should be stated.

13. *Voluntary consent.* Researchers should indicate that participation is strictly voluntary and that failure to volunteer will not result in any penalty or loss of benefits.

14. *Right to withdraw and withhold information.* Prospective participants should be told that, after consenting, they have the right to withdraw from the study or to withhold any specific piece of information. Researchers may need to describe circumstances under which researchers would terminate the study.

15. *Contact information.* The researcher should tell participants whom they could contact in the event of questions, comments, or complaints.

In qualitative studies, especially those requiring repeated contact with participants, it may be difficult to obtain meaningful informed consent at the outset. Qualitative researchers do not always know in advance how the study will evolve. Because the research design emerges during data collection, researchers may not know the exact nature of the data to be collected, what the risks and benefits to participants will be, or how much of a time commitment they will be expected to make. Thus, in a qualitative study, consent is often viewed as an ongoing, transactional process, sometimes called **process consent**. In process consent, the researcher continually renegotiates the consent, allowing participants to play a collaborative role in making decisions about ongoing participation.

Example of Process Consent
Coombs et al. (2017) studied the decision-making processes that influence transitions in care when approaching the end of life. Terminally ill patients and family members were interviewed when they were recruited for the study and then again 3 to 4 months later. Written consent was obtained before the first interview, and then a process consent model was adopted.

Comprehension of Informed Consent

Consent information is typically presented to prospective participants while they are being recruited, either orally or in writing. Written notices should not, however, take the place of spoken explanations, which provide opportunities for elaboration and for participants to question and "screen" the researchers.

Because informed consent is based on a person's evaluation of the potential risks and benefits of participation, the information must not only be communicated but understood. Researchers may have to play a "teacher" role in conveying consent information. They should use simple language and avoid technical terms whenever possible. Written statements should be consistent with the participants' reading levels. For participants from a general population (e.g., patients in a hospital), statements should be at about the seventh or eighth grade reading level.

TIP Innovations to improve understanding of consent are being developed. Nishimura et al. (2013) did a systematic review of 54 of them.

For some studies, especially those involving more than minimal risk, researchers need to ensure that prospective participants understand what participation will entail. This might involve testing participants' comprehension of informed consent material before deeming them eligible. Such efforts are especially warranted with participants whose native tongue is not the same as the researchers or who have cognitive impairments (Fields & Calvert, 2015; Simpson, 2010).

Example of Ensuring Comprehension in Informed Consent

Zhang et al. (2018) tested a nurse case-managed intervention to reduce substance abuse among homeless gay/bisexual men and transgender women. All participants signed written informed consent forms. Participants were later asked to repeat critical aspects of the design and study procedures, to confirm their cognitive capacity and their understanding of key consent provisions.

Documentation of Informed Consent

Researchers usually document informed consent by having participants sign a **consent form**. In the United States, federal regulations for studies funded by the government require written consent of participants, except under certain circumstances. When the study does not involve an intervention and data are collected anonymously—or when existing data from records or specimens are used without linking identifying information to the data—regulations requiring written informed consent usually do not apply. HIPAA legislation is explicit about the type of information that must be eliminated from patient records for the data to be considered **de-identified**, as we illustrate in the Toolkit.

The consent form should contain all the information essential to informed consent. Prospective participants (or their *legally authorized representatives*) should have ample time to review the document before signing it. The consent form should also be signed by the researcher, and a copy should be retained by both parties.

TIP In developing a consent form, the following suggestions might prove helpful:
1. Organize the form coherently so that prospective participants can follow the logic of what is being communicated. If the form is complex, use headings as an organizational aid.
2. Use a large enough font so that the form can be easily read, and use spacing that avoids making the document appear too dense. Make the form attractive and inviting.
3. In general, simplify. Avoid technical terms if possible, and if they are needed, include definitions.
4. Assess the form's reading level by using a **readability formula** to ensure an appropriate level for the group under study. There are several such formulas, including the Flesch Reading Ease score and Flesch–Kincaid grade level score (Flesch, 1948). Microsoft Word provides Flesch readability statistics.
5. Test the form with people similar to those who will be recruited, and ask for feedback.

In certain circumstances (for example, with non–English-speaking participants), researchers have the option of presenting the full information orally and then summarizing essential information in a **short form**. If a short form is used, however, the oral presentation must be witnessed by a third party and the witness's signature must appear on the short consent form. The signature of a third-party witness is also advisable in studies involving more than minimal risk, even when a comprehensive consent form is used.

When the primary means of data collection is through self-administered questionnaires, some researchers do not obtain written informed consent because they assume **implied consent** (i.e., that the return of the completed questionnaire reflects voluntary consent to participate). In such situations, researchers often provide an *information sheet* that contains all the elements of an informed consent form but does not require a signature. An example of such an information sheet used in a study of Cheryl Beck (an author of this book) is presented in Figure 7.1. The numbers in the margins of this figure correspond to the types of information for informed consent outlined earlier.

Principal Investigator: Cheryl Tatano Beck, DNSc, CNM, FAAN
Study Title: Impact of Traumatic Childbirth on Mothers' Experiences Caring for Their Children

1   <u>Introduction</u> You are invited to participate in a research study so that we can better understand the impact of traumatic childbirth on mothers' experiences interacting with and caring for their infants and older children.

2   **Why is this study being done?** For decades now researchers have studied the long term effects that postpartum depression can have on mother-infant interactions and child development. Much less attention has focused on the possible effects of posttraumatic stress on mother-infant interaction and attachment and children's emotional and cognitive development. The purpose of this study is to help understand the experiences of mothers who have had a traumatic birth and how this may impact their interactions with their infants and older children.

3   **What are the study procedures? What will I be asked to do?** If you agree to take part in this survey you will be asked to complete (1) a participant Profile Form which includes questions about yourself such as your age, education, and type of delivery, and (2) to describe in as much detail as you wish your
4   experiences of caring for and interacting with your infant and any older children you may have. Depending on how in depth you write about your experiences, participation in the study could take between 30- 60
5   minutes. Your participation will be anonymous and you will not be contacted again in the future. You will not be paid for being in this study.

8   **What are the risks or inconveniences of the study?** We believe there are no known risks associated with this research study; however, if you become anxious remembering your traumatic childbirth please know you can stop participating in the study. You do not have to complete the study. One possible inconvenience to you may be the time it takes to complete this survey.

9   **What are the benefits of the study?** You may not directly benefit from this research; however, we hope your participation in this survey will help health care professionals provide better care to mothers who have experienced a traumatic childbirth.

11 **Will I receive payment for participation? Are there costs to participate?** There are no costs and you will not be paid to be in this study.

12 **How will my personal information be protected?** The following procedures will be used to protect the confidentiality of your data. The researchers will keep all study records indefinitely in a locked file in a secure location. Research records will be labeled with a code. The code will be derived from a sequential 3 digit number that reflects how many people have enrolled in the study. All electronic files (e.g., database, spreadsheet, etc.) will be password protected. Any computer hosting such files will also have password protection to prevent access by unauthorized users. Only the members of the research staff will have access to the passwords. At the conclusion of this study, the researchers may publish their findings. Information will be presented in summary format and you will not be identified in any publications or presentations.

> "We will do our best to protect the confidentiality of the information we gather from you but we cannot guarantee 100% confidentiality. Your confidentiality will be maintained to the degree permitted by the technology used. Specifically, no guarantees can be made regarding the interception of data sent via the Internet by any third parties."

You should also know that the UConn Institutional Review Board (IRB) and Research Compliance Services may inspect study records as part of its auditing program, but these reviews will only focus on the researchers and not on your responses or involvement. The IRB is a group of people who review research studies to protect the rights and welfare of research participants.

13 **Can I stop being in the study and what are my rights?** You do not have to be in this study if you do not want to. If you agree to be in the study, but later change your mind, you may drop out at any time. There
14 are no penalties or consequences of any kind if you decide that you do not want to participate.

15 **Whom do I contact if I have questions about the study?** Take as long as you like before you make a decision. We will be happy to answer any question you have about this study. If you have further questions about this project or if you have a research-related problem, you may contact the principal investigator, (Dr. Cheryl Beck, 860-xxx-xxx). If you have any questions concerning your rights as a research subject, you may contact the University of Connecticut Institutional Review Board (IRB) at 860-xxx-xxxx

FIGURE 7.1 Example of an information sheet for study participants (University of Connecticut template).

TIP The Toolkit in the accompanying *Resource Manual* includes several informed consent forms and information sheets as Word documents that can be adapted for your use. Most universities now offer templates for consent forms.

Authorization to Access Private Health Information

Under HIPAA regulations in the United States, a covered entity such as a hospital can disclose *individually identifiable health information* (IIHI) from its records if the patient signs an authorization. The authorization can be incorporated into the consent form, or it can be a separate document. Using a separate authorization form may be advantageous to protect the patients' confidentiality because the form does not need to provide detailed information about the study purpose. If the research purpose is not sensitive, or if the entity is already cognizant of the study purpose, an integrated form may suffice. The authorization, whether obtained separately or as part of the consent form, must include the following: (1) who will receive the information; (2) what type of information will be disclosed; and (3) what further disclosures the researcher anticipates.

Confidentiality Procedures

Study participants have the right to expect that data they provide will be kept in strict confidence. Participants' right to privacy is protected through various confidentiality procedures.

Anonymity

Anonymity, the most secure means of protecting confidentiality, occurs when the researcher cannot link participants to their data. For example, if questionnaires were distributed to a group of nursing home residents and were returned without any identifying information, responses would be anonymous. As another example, if a researcher reviewed hospital records from which all identifying information had been expunged, anonymity would

protect participants' right to privacy. Whenever it is possible to achieve anonymity, researchers should strive to do so.

Example of Anonymity
Wilson et al. (2019) conducted a study of nurses' views on legalizing assisted dying in New Zealand. A sample of 475 nurses responded to an anonymous online survey.

Confidentiality in the Absence of Anonymity

When anonymity is not possible, other confidentiality procedures are needed. A promise of **confidentiality** is a pledge that any information participants provide will not be reported in a manner that identifies them and will not be accessible to others. This means that research information should not be shared with strangers nor with people known to participants (e.g., relatives, doctors, other nurses), unless participants give explicit permission to do so.

Researchers can take a number of steps to ensure that a **breach of confidentiality** does not occur, including the following:

- Obtain identifying information (e.g., name, address) from participants only when essential.
- Assign an **identification** (ID) **number** to each participant and attach the ID number rather than other identifiers to actual data forms.
- Maintain identifying information in a locked file.
- Restrict access to identifying information to only a few people on a need-to-know basis.
- Enter identifying information onto computer files that are encrypted.
- Destroy identifying information as quickly as practical.
- Make research personnel sign confidentiality pledges if they have access to identifying information.
- Report research information in the aggregate; if information for an individual is reported, disguise the person's identity, such as through the use of a fictitious name.

TIP Researchers who plan to collect data from participants multiple times (or who use multiple forms that need to be linked) do not have to forego anonymity. A technique that has been successful is to have participants themselves generate an ID number. They might be instructed, for example, to use the first three letters of their mother's middle names and their birth year as their ID code (e.g., FRA1983). This code would be put on every form so that forms could be linked, but researchers would not know participants' identities.

Qualitative researchers may need to take extra steps to safeguard participants' privacy. Anonymity is rarely possible in qualitative studies because researchers typically become closely involved with participants. Moreover, because of the in-depth nature of qualitative studies, there may be a greater invasion of privacy than is true in quantitative research. Researchers who spend time in the home of a participant may, for example, have difficulty segregating the public behaviors that the participant is willing to share from private behaviors that unfold during data collection. A final issue concerns disguising participants in reports. Because the number of participants is small, qualitative researchers need to take special precautions to safeguard identities. This may mean more than simply using a fictitious name. Qualitative researchers may have to slightly distort identifying information or provide broad descriptions. For example, a 49-year-old antique dealer with ovarian cancer might be described as "a middle-aged cancer patient who was a shop owner" to avoid identification that could occur with the more detailed description.

Example of Confidentiality Procedures in a Qualitative Study

Strandås et al. (2019) conducted a focused ethnography to gain a deeper understanding of nurse–patient relationships in Norwegian public home care. Participants (who were observed interacting with nurses and were also interviewed) received information about the researchers and the study, including rights to withdraw. Oral informed consent was obtained from patients who were included in observations. Data were anonymized by removing names and locations and by changing some details. Interview transcripts and audiotapes were kept in locked files.

Certificates of Confidentiality

In some situations, confidentiality can create tensions between researchers and legal or other authorities, especially if participants engage in criminal activity (e.g., substance abuse). To avoid the possibility of forced, involuntary disclosure of sensitive research information (e.g., through a court order or subpoena), researchers in the United States can apply for a **Certificate of Confidentiality** from the National Institutes of Health (Lutz et al., 2000; Wolf et al., 2015). Any research that involves the collection of personally identifiable, sensitive information is potentially eligible for a Certificate. Information is considered sensitive if its release might damage participants' financial standing, employability, or reputation. Information about a person's mental health, as well as genetic information, is also considered sensitive. A Certificate allows researchers to refuse to disclose identifying information on study participants in any civil, criminal, administrative, or legislative proceeding at the federal, state, or local level.

A Certificate of Confidentiality helps researchers to achieve their research objectives without threat of involuntary disclosure and can be helpful in recruiting participants. Researchers who obtain a Certificate should inform prospective participants about this valuable protection in the consent form and should state any planned exceptions to those protections. For example, a researcher might decide to voluntarily comply with state child abuse reporting laws even though the Certificate would prevent authorities from punishing researchers who chose not to comply.

Example of Obtaining a Certificate of Confidentiality

Mallory and Hesson-McInnis (2013) pilot tested an HIV (human immunodeficiency virus) infection prevention intervention with incarcerated and other high-risk women. The women were asked about various sensitive topics, and so the researchers obtained a Certificate of Confidentiality.

Debriefings, Communications, and Referrals

Researchers can show their respect—and proactively minimize emotional risks—by carefully attending to the nature of their interactions with participants. For example, researchers should always be gracious and polite, should phrase questions tactfully, and should be considerate with regard to cultural and linguistic diversity.

Researchers can also use formal strategies to communicate respect for participants' well-being. For example, it is sometimes useful to offer **debriefing** sessions after data collection is completed to permit participants to ask questions or air complaints. Debriefing is especially important when the data collection has been stressful or when ethical guidelines had to be "bent" (e.g., if any deception was used in explaining the study).

Example of Debriefing

Payne (2013) evaluated the effectiveness of a diabetes support group for indigenous women in Australia. Information was obtained before and after implementing the support group. At the end of the study "A final group debriefing was implemented for ethical closure" (p. 41).

It is also thoughtful to communicate with participants after the study is completed, to let them know that their participation was appreciated. Researchers sometimes offer to share study findings with participants once the data have been analyzed (e.g., by emailing them a summary). The National Academies in the United States (2018) has published guidance on returning individual results to participants.

Finally, in some situations, researchers may need to assist study participants by referring them to appropriate health, social, or psychological services.

Example of Referrals

Mwalabu et al. (2017) studied factors influencing the sexual and reproductive healthcare experiences of female adolescents in Malawi with perinatally acquired HIV. In-depth interviews were conducted with 42 young women. Provisions were made to refer the young women to support services if they became distressed.

Treatment of Vulnerable Groups

Adherence to ethical standards is often straightforward, but additional procedures may be required to protect special **vulnerable groups**. Vulnerable populations may be incapable of giving fully informed consent (e.g., cognitively impaired people) or may be at risk of unintended side effects because of their circumstances (e.g., pregnant women). Researchers interested in studying high-risk groups should understand guidelines governing informed consent, risk/benefit assessments, and acceptable research procedures for such groups. Research with vulnerable groups should be undertaken only when the risk/benefit ratio is low or when there is no alternative (e.g., studies of prisoners' health behaviors require inmates as participants).

Among the groups that nurse researchers should consider vulnerable are the following:

- *Children.* Legally and ethically, children do not have competence to give informed consent, so the informed consent of their parents or legal guardians must be obtained. It is appropriate, however—especially if the child is at least 7 years old—to obtain the child's assent as well. **Assent** refers to the child's agreement to participate. If the child is mature enough to understand basic informed consent information, it is advisable to obtain written consent from the child and the parent, as evidence of respect for the child's right to self-determination. Recent research suggests that children at the age of 12 years are competent to give consent (Hein et al., 2015). The U.S. government has issued special regulations (Code of Federal Regulations, 2009, Subpart D) for additional protections of children as study participants.

TIP Crane and Broome (2017) have prepared a systematic review on the ethical aspects of research participation from the perspective of participating children and adolescents.

- *Mentally or emotionally disabled people.* Individuals whose disability makes it impossible for them to weigh the risks and benefits of participation (e.g., people who are in a coma) also cannot legally or ethically provide informed consent. In such cases, researchers should obtain the written consent of a legal guardian. If possible, informed consent or assent from participants themselves should be sought as a supplement to a guardian's consent. NIH guidelines stipulate that studies involving people whose autonomy is compromised by disability should focus directly on their condition.

- *Severely ill or physically disabled people.* For patients who are very ill, it might be prudent to assess their ability to make reasoned decisions about study participation. For certain disabilities, special procedures for obtaining consent may be required. For example, with deaf participants, the entire consent process may need to be in writing. For people who have a physical impairment preventing them from writing or for participants who cannot read, alternative procedures for documenting informed consent (e.g., video recording consent proceedings) should be used.

- *The terminally ill.* Terminally ill people seldom expect to benefit personally from participating in research, and so the risk/benefit ratio needs to be carefully assessed. Researchers must take steps to ensure that the care and comfort of terminally ill participants are not compromised.

- *Institutionalized people.* Prudence is required in recruiting institutionalized people because their dependence on healthcare personnel may make them feel pressured into participating; they may believe that their treatment would be jeopardized by failure to cooperate. Prison inmates, who have lost autonomy in many spheres of activity, may also feel constrained in their ability to withhold consent. The U.S. government has issued specific regulations for the protection of prisoners as study participants (see Code of Federal Regulations, 2009, Subpart C). Researchers studying institutionalized groups need to emphasize the voluntary nature of participation.

- *Pregnant women.* The U.S. government has issued additional requirements governing research with pregnant women and fetuses (Code of Federal Regulations, 2009, Subpart B). These requirements reflect a desire to safeguard both the pregnant woman, who may be at heightened physical and psychological risk, and the fetus, who cannot give informed consent. The regulations stipulate that a pregnant woman cannot be involved in a study unless its purpose is to meet the health needs of the pregnant woman and risks to her and the fetus are minimized or there is only a minimal risk to the fetus.

Example of Research With a Vulnerable Group
Culbert and Williams (2018) developed a culturally adapted medication adherence intervention for prisoners living with HIV in Indonesia. The cultural adaptation was based on an ethnographic appraisal of the target group. The intervention was pilot tested in two prisons in Jakarta. Participation was voluntary, and participants were selected equitably without prison staff involvement.

Researchers need to proceed with extreme caution in conducting research with people who fall into two or more vulnerable categories (e.g., incarcerated youth).

External Reviews and the Protection of Human Rights

Researchers, who have a commitment to their research, may not be objective in their risk/benefit assessments or in their plans to protect participants' rights. Because a biased self-evaluation is possible, the ethical dimensions of a study normally should be subjected to external review.

Most institutions where research is conducted have formal committees for reviewing proposed research plans. These committees are sometimes called *human subjects committees, ethical advisory boards,* or *research ethics committees.* In the United States, the committee usually is called an **Institutional Review Board (IRB)**; in Canada, it is called a **Research Ethics Board (REB)**.

TIP You should find out early what an institution's requirements are regarding ethics, in terms of its forms, procedures, and review schedules. It is wise to allow a generous amount of time for negotiating with IRBs, which may require modifications and re-review.

Institutional Review Boards

In the United States, federally sponsored studies are subject to strict guidelines for evaluating the treatment of human participants. Before undertaking such a study, researchers must submit research plans to the IRB and must also go through formal training on ethical conduct and a certification process.

The duty of the IRB is to ensure that the proposed plans meet federal requirements for ethical research. An IRB can approve, require modifications to, or disapprove the proposed plans. The main requirements governing IRB decisions may be summarized as follows (Code of Federal Regulations, 2009, §46.111):

- Risks to participants are minimized.
- Risks to participants are reasonable in relation to anticipated benefits, if any, and the importance of the knowledge that may reasonably be expected to result.
- Selection of participants is equitable.
- Informed consent will be sought, as required, and appropriately documented.
- Adequate provision is made for monitoring the research to ensure participants' safety.
- Appropriate provisions are made to protect participants' privacy and confidentiality of the data.
- When a vulnerable group is involved, appropriate additional safeguards are included to protect the rights and welfare of participants.

Example of Institutional Review Board Approval
Dzikowicz and Carey (2019) evaluated the possible relationship between QRS-T angle (a measure of repolarization heterogeneity and potentially a predictor of poor ventricular health) and blood pressure during exercise among on-duty firefighters. The study was approved by the IRB of the State University of New York.

Many studies require a full IRB review at a meeting with a majority of IRB members present. An IRB must have five or more members, at least one of whom is not a researcher (e.g., a lawyer or someone from the patient population). One IRB member must be a person who is not affiliated with the institution and is not a family member of an affiliated person. To protect against potential biases, the IRB cannot comprise entirely men, women, or members from a single profession.

For certain research involving no more than minimal risk, the IRB can use expedited review procedures, which do not require a meeting. In an **expedited review**, a single IRB member (usually the IRB chairperson) carries out the review. An example of research that qualifies for an expedited IRB review is minimal-risk research "…employing survey, interview, oral history, focus group, program evaluation, human factors evaluation, or quality assurance methodologies" (Code of Federal Regulations, 2009, §46.110).

Federal regulations also allow certain types of research in which there are no apparent risk to participants to be exempt from IRB review. The website of the Office for Human Research Protections, in its policy guidance section, includes decision charts designed to clarify whether a study is exempt.

TIP Researchers seeking a Certificate of Confidentiality must first obtain IRB approval, which is a prerequisite for the Certificate. Applications for the Certificate should be submitted at least 3 months before participants are expected to enroll in the study.

Data and Safety Monitoring Boards

In addition to IRBs, researchers in the United States may have to communicate information about ethical aspects of their studies to other groups. For example, some institutions have established separate **Privacy Boards** to review researchers' compliance with provisions in HIPAA, including review of authorization forms and requests for waivers.

For researchers evaluating interventions in clinical trials, NIH also requires review by a **data and safety monitoring board** (DSMB). The purpose of a DSMB is to oversee the safety of participants, to promote data integrity, and to review accumulated outcome data on a regular basis to evaluate whether study protocols should be altered or the study stopped altogether. Members of a DSMB are selected based on their clinical, statistical, and methodologic expertise. The degree of monitoring by the DSMB should be proportionate to the degree of risk involved. Slimmer and Andersen (2004) offer suggestions on developing a DSM plan. Artinian et al. (2004) provided good descriptions of their data and safety monitoring plan for a study of a nurse-managed telemonitoring intervention and discussed how IRBs and DSMBs differ.

Building Ethics Into the Design of the Study

Researchers need to give thought to ethical requirements while planning a study and should ask themselves whether intended safeguards are sufficient. They must continue their vigilance throughout the course of the study as well, because unforeseen ethical dilemmas may arise. Of course, first steps in doing ethical research include asking clinically important questions and using rigorous methods—it can be construed as unethical to do poorly designed research because it would be a poor use of participants' time. Another issue concerns dissemination: it can be considered unethical and wasteful of people's time to not communicate research findings to others.

The remaining chapters of the book offer advice on how to design studies that yield high-quality evidence for practice. Methodologic decisions about rigor, however, must be made within the context of ethical requirements. Box 7.2 presents examples of questions that might be posed in thinking about ethical aspects of study design.

TIP After study procedures have been developed, researchers should evaluate those procedures to determine if they meet ethical requirements. Box 7.3 later in this chapter provides guidelines that can be used for such a self-evaluation.

OTHER ETHICAL ISSUES

In discussing ethical issues relating to the conduct of nursing research, we have given primary consideration to the protection of human participants. Two other ethical issues also deserve mention: the treatment of animals in research and research misconduct.

 BOX 7.2 Examples of Questions for Building Ethics into the Design of a Study

RESEARCH DESIGN
- Will participants be assigned fairly to different treatment groups?
- Will the study setting minimize participants' discomfort or anxiety?

INTERVENTION
- Is the intervention designed to maximize benefits and minimize harms?
- Under what conditions could the intervention be withdrawn or altered?

SAMPLE
- Is the population under study defined so as to minimize the risk that certain types of people (e.g., women, minorities) will be excluded or underrepresented?
- Will potential participants be recruited into the study equitably and without the use of coercion?

DATA COLLECTION
- Will respondent burden be minimized? Will participants' time be used efficiently?
- Will procedures for ensuring confidentiality of data be adequate?
- Will data collection staff be trained to be courteous, respectful, and caring?

REPORTING
- Will participants' identities be adequately protected?

Ethical Issues in Using Animals in Research

Some nurse researchers work with animal subjects. Despite opposition to such research by animal rights activists, researchers in health fields likely will continue to use animals to explore physiologic mechanisms and interventions that could pose risks to humans.

Ethical considerations are clearly different for animals and humans: the concept of *informed consent* is not relevant for animal subjects. Guidelines have been developed governing treatment of animals in research. In the United States, the Public Health Service has issued a policy statement on the humane care and use of laboratory animals. The guidelines articulate nine principles for the proper treatment of animals used in biomedical and behavioral research. These principles cover such issues as alternatives to using animals, pain and distress in animal subjects, researcher qualifications, use of appropriate anesthesia, and conditions for euthanizing animals. In Canada, researchers who use animals in their studies must adhere to the policies and guidelines of the Canadian Council on Animal Care (CCAC) as articulated in their *Guide to the Care and Use of Experimental Animals.* Holtzclaw and Hanneman (2002) noted several important considerations in the use of animals in nursing research, and Osier et al. (2016) discussed the use of animal models in genomic nursing research.

Example of Research With Animals
Kupferschmid and Therrien (2018) investigated the time trajectory of age-dependent sickness responses over 5 days in adult and aged male Brown-Norway rats. Animals were housed individually in a temperature-controlled room and allowed free access to food and water. The University of Michigan Animal Care and Use Committee approved all procedures.

Research Misconduct

Ethics in research involves not only the protection of human and animal subjects but also protection of the public trust. The issue of **research misconduct** has received greater attention in recent years as incidents of researcher fraud and misrepresentation have come to light. Currently, the agency in the United States responsible for overseeing efforts to improve research integrity and for handling allegations of research misconduct is the Office of Research Integrity (ORI). Researchers seeking funding from NIH must demonstrate that they have received training on research integrity and the responsible conduct of research.

Research misconduct is defined by U.S. Public Health Service regulation (42 CFR Part 93.103) as "fabrication, falsification, or plagiarism in proposing, performing, or reviewing research, or in reporting research results." To be construed as misconduct, there must be a significant departure from accepted practices in the research community, and the misconduct must have been committed intentionally and knowingly. *Fabrication* involves making up data or study results. *Falsification* involves manipulating research materials, equipment, or processes; it also involves changing or omitting data or distorting results. *Plagiarism* involves the appropriation of someone's ideas, results, or words without giving due credit, including information obtained as a reviewer of research proposals or manuscripts.

Example of Research Misconduct
In 2015, the U.S. ORI ruled that a researcher engaged in scientific misconduct in a study supported by the NINR. The researcher falsified and fabricated data that were reported in five publications and three grant applications submitted to the NINR.

Although the official definition focuses on only three types of misconduct, there is widespread agreement that research misconduct covers many other issues including improprieties of authorship, poor data management, conflicts of interest, inappropriate financial arrangements, failure to comply with governmental regulations, and unauthorized use of confidential information.

Research integrity is an important concern in nursing. Habermann et al. (2010) studied 1,645 research coordinators' experiences with research misconduct in their clinical environments. More than 250 coordinators, most of them nurses, said they had firsthand knowledge of research misconduct that included protocol violations, consent violations, fabrication, falsification, and financial conflicts of interest. Fierz et al. (2014) concluded that research misconduct in nursing science "not only compromises scientific integrity by distorting empirical evidence, but it might endanger patients" (p. 271).

CRITICAL APPRAISAL OF ETHICS IN RESEARCH

Guidelines for critically appraising the ethical aspects of a study are presented in Box 7.3. Members of an ethics committee should be provided with sufficient information to answer all these questions. Research journal articles, however, do not always include detailed information about ethics because of space constraints. Thus, it is not always possible to evaluate researchers' adherence to ethical guidelines, but we offer a few suggestions for considering a study's ethical aspects.

Many research reports acknowledge that study procedures were reviewed by an IRB or ethics committee, and some journals require such statements. When a report specifically mentions a formal review, it is usually safe to assume that a group of concerned people did a conscientious review of the study's ethical issues.

You can also come to some conclusions based on a description of the study methods. There may be sufficient information to judge, for example, whether participants were subjected to harm or discomfort. Reports do not always state whether informed consent was secured, but you should be alert to situations in which the data could not have been gathered as described if participation were purely voluntary (e.g., if data were gathered unobtrusively).

In thinking about ethical issues, you should also consider who the study participants were. For example, if a study involved vulnerable groups, there should be more information about protective procedures. You might also need to consider who the study participants were *not*. For example, there has been considerable concern about the omission of certain groups (e.g., minorities) from clinical research.

It is often difficult to determine whether the participants' privacy was safeguarded unless the

BOX 7.3 Guidelines for Critically Appraising the Ethical Aspects of a Study

1. Was the study approved and monitored by an Institutional Review Board, REB, or other similar ethics review committee?
2. Were participants subjected to any physical harm, discomfort, or psychological distress? Did the researchers take appropriate steps to remove, prevent, or minimize harm?
3. Did the benefits to participants outweigh any potential risks or actual discomfort they experienced? Did the benefits to society outweigh the costs to participants?
4. Was any type of coercion or undue influence used to recruit participants? Did they have the right to refuse to participate or to withdraw without penalty?
5. Were participants deceived in any way? Were they fully aware of participating in a study and did they understand the purpose and nature of the research?
6. Were appropriate informed consent procedures used? If not, were there valid and justifiable reasons?
7. Were adequate steps taken to safeguard participants' privacy? How was confidentiality maintained? Were Privacy Rule procedures followed (if applicable)? Was a Certificate of Confidentiality obtained? If not, *should* one have been obtained?
8. Were vulnerable groups involved in the research? If yes, were special precautions used because of their vulnerable status?
9. Were groups omitted from the inquiry without a justifiable rationale, such as women (or men), minorities, or older people?

researcher mentions pledges of confidentiality or anonymity. A situation requiring special scrutiny arises when data are collected from two related people, such as a husband/wife or parent/child, who are interviewed either jointly or separately (Forbat & Henderson, 2003; Haahr et al., 2014). For example, researchers may struggle with asking one person probing questions after having been given confidential information about the issue by the other.

RESEARCH EXAMPLES

Two research examples that highlight ethical issues are presented in the following sections.

Research Example From a Quantitative Study

Study: Using simulated family presence to decrease agitation in older hospitalized delirious patients (Waszynski et al., 2018).

Study purpose: The purpose of this study was to examine the effect of simulated family presence through prerecorded video messages on the agitation level of delirious, acutely agitated hospitalized patients.

Research methods: A total of 111 hospitalized patients in an inner-city trauma center experiencing delirium participated in the study. Participants were assigned, at random, to one of three groups. One group viewed a 1-minute family video message, the second group viewed a 1-minute nature video, and the third group had usual care without a video. Patients' level of agitation before, during, and after the intervention was measured.

Ethics-related procedures: The study was approved and monitored by the IRBs of Hartford Healthcare and the researchers' university, in accordance with the Code of Ethics of the World Medical Association. Because all participants were delirious, informed consent was obtained from a legally appointed representative or next of kin. Informed consent was also obtained from members of the family who participated in the creation of the family video message. The principal investigator assessed each patient for delirium and obtained verbal assent. Assent was obtained by asking participants if the researcher could return later

that day—if and when the patient felt "out of sorts"—to show a video. An independent observer rated each family video message as positive, neutral, or negative; the vast majority were rated as positive with an encouraging message.

Key findings: A significantly greater proportion of participants in the family video group (94%) experienced a reduction in agitation from pre-intervention to during the intervention than those viewing the nature video (70%) or those in usual care (30%).

Research Example From a Qualitative Study

Study: The changing nature of relationships between parents and healthcare providers when a child dies in the pediatric intensive care unit (Butler et al., 2018).

Study purpose: The purpose of the study was to explore bereaved parents' interactions with healthcare providers when a child dies in the pediatric intensive care unit.

Study methods: The researchers used a grounded theory approach. Data for the study were gathered through in-depth interviews with 26 bereaved parents from four pediatric ICUs. The interviews, which lasted between 1.5 and 2.5 hours, were mostly undertaken in the participants' homes and were audio-recorded.

Ethics-related procedures: The study was approved by human research ethics committees in the relevant facilities. Participants signed written informed consent forms, and verbal consent was reaffirmed throughout the interview process. The interviews were conducted with parents either individually or jointly, at their request. The researchers, who were conscious of the highly sensitive nature of the research, paid significant attention to the parents' psychological well-being. The consent form identified the strong likelihood of emotional distress, to enhance the parents' ability to make an informed decision about their participation. The researchers also encouraged the parents to take breaks during the interview and to call upon personal coping strategies. The interviewer, in preparing for this project, took a bereavement counseling course, to be able to offer support following the interview during debriefing. The researchers offered further support in a follow-up telephone call. Social workers were available for on-going follow-up if required.

Key findings: The researchers identified a three-phase process that they described as "Transitional togetherness." In phase 1, "Welcoming expertise," the focus was on the child's medical needs. In phase 2, "Becoming a team" involved working collaboratively with providers. Finally, in the "Gradually disengaging" phase, the parents expressed a desire for the relationship with providers to continue after the child's death.

SUMMARY POINTS

- Researchers sometimes face **ethical dilemmas** in designing studies that are rigorous *and* ethical. **Codes of ethics** have been developed to guide researchers.
- Three major ethical principles from the *Belmont Report* are incorporated into most guidelines: beneficence, respect for human dignity, and justice.
- **Beneficence** involves the performance of some good and the protection of participants from physical and psychological harm and exploitation.
- **Respect for human dignity** involves participants' **right to self-determination**, which means they are free to control their own actions, including voluntary participation.
- **Full disclosure** means that researchers have fully divulged participants' rights and the risks and benefits of the study. When full disclosure could bias the results, researchers sometimes use **covert data collection** (the collection of information without the participants' knowledge or consent) or **deception** (providing false information).
- **Justice** includes the **right to fair treatment** and the **right to privacy**. In the United States, privacy has become a major issue because of the Privacy Rule regulations that resulted from the Health Insurance Portability and Accountability Act (HIPAA).
- Various procedures have been developed to safeguard study participants' rights. For example, researchers can conduct a **risk/benefit**

assessment in which the potential benefits of the study to participants and society are weighed against the risks.

- **Informed consent** procedures, which provide prospective participants with information needed to make a reasoned decision about participation, normally involve signing a **consent form** to document voluntary and informed participation.
- In qualitative studies, consent may need to be continually renegotiated with participants as the study evolves, through **process consent** procedures.
- Privacy can be maintained through **anonymity** (wherein not even researchers know participants' identities) or through formal **confidentiality procedures** that safeguard the information participants provide. Researchers must guard against a **breach of confidentiality**.
- U.S. researchers can seek a **Certificate of Confidentiality** that protects them against the forced disclosure of confidential information (e.g., by a court order).
- Researchers sometimes offer **debriefing** sessions after data collection to provide participants with more information or an opportunity to air complaints.
- **Vulnerable groups** require additional protection. These people may be vulnerable because they are unable to make a truly informed decision about study participation (e.g., children); because of diminished autonomy (e.g., prisoners); or because circumstances heighten the risk of physical or psychological harm (e.g., pregnant women).
- External review of the ethical aspects of a study by an ethics committee or **Institutional Review Board (IRB)** is often required by the agency funding the research and the organization from which participants are recruited.
- In studies in which risks to participants are minimal, an **expedited review** by a single member of the IRB may be substituted for a full board review; in cases in which there are no anticipated risks, the research may be exempted from review.
- Researchers need to give careful thought to ethical requirements throughout the study's

planning and implementation and to ask themselves continually whether safeguards for protecting humans are sufficient.

- Ethical conduct in research involves not only protection of the rights of human and animal subjects, but also efforts to maintain high standards of integrity and avoid such forms of **research misconduct** as *plagiarism, fabrication* of results, or *falsification* of data.

STUDY ACTIVITIES

Study activities are available to instructors on the Point.

REFERENCES CITED IN CHAPTER 7

Artinian, N., Froelicher, E., & Wal, J. (2004). Data and safety monitoring during randomized controlled trials of nursing interventions. *Nursing Research, 53*, 414–418.

Beck, C. T., LoGiudice, J., & Gable, R. K. (2015). A mixed methods study of secondary traumatic stress in certified nurse-midwives: Shaken belief in the birth process. *Journal of Midwifery and Women's Health, 60*, 16–23.

Butler, A., Hall, H., & Copnell, B. (2018). The changing nature of relationships between parents and healthcare providers when a child dies in the paediatric intensive care unit. *Journal of Advanced Nursing, 74*, 89–99.

*Coombs, M., Parker, R., & de Vries, K. (2017). Managing risk during care transitions when approaching end of life: A qualitative study of patients' and health care professionals' decision making. *Palliative Medicine, 31*, 617–624.

Crane, S., & Broome, M. (2017). Understanding ethical issues of research participation from the perspective of participating children and adolescents: A systematic review. *Worldviews on Evidence-Based Nursing, 14*, 200–209.

Culbert, G., & Williams, A. (2018). Cultural adaptation of a medication adherence intervention with prisoners living with HIV in Indonesia. *Journal of the Association of Nurses in AIDS Care, 29*, 454–465.

*Domecq, J., Prutsky, G., Elraiyah, T., Wang, Z., Nabhan, M., Shippee, N., ... Murad, M. H. (2014). Patient engagement in research: A systematic review. *BMC Health Services Research, 14*, 89.

**Dzikowicz, D., & Carey, M. (2019). Widened QRS-T angle may be a measure of poor ventricular stretch during exercise among on-duty firefighters. *Journal of Cardiovascular Nursing, 34*(3), 201-207.

*Edwards, P., Roberts, I., Clarke, M., Diguiseppi, C., Wentz, R., Kwan, I., ... Pratap, S. (2009). Methods to increase response to postal and electronic questionnaires. *Cochrane Database of Systematic Reviews*, MR000008.

Eide, P., & Khan, D. (2008). Ethical issues in the qualitative researcher-participant relationship. *Nursing Ethics, 15*, 199–207.

Ellett, M., Lane, L., & Keffer, J. (2004). Ethical and legal issues of conducting nursing research via the Internet. *Journal of Professional Nursing, 20*, 68–74.

*Fields, L., & Calvert, J. (2015). Informed consent procedures with cognitively impaired patients: A review of ethics and best practices. *Psychiatry and Clinical Neurosciences, 69*, 462–471.

Fierz, K., Gennaro, S., Dierickx, K., Van Achtenberg, T., Morin, K., & DeGeest, S. (2014). Scientific misconduct: Also an issue in nursing science? *Journal of Nursing Scholarship, 46*, 271–280.

Flesch, R. (1948). New readability yardstick. *Journal of Applied Psychology, 32*, 221–223.

Forbat, L., & Henderson, J. (2003). "Stuck in the middle with you": The ethics and process of qualitative research with two people in an intimate relationship. *Qualitative Health Research, 13*, 1453–1462.

Gennaro, S. (2014). Conducting important and ethical research. *Journal of Nursing Scholarship, 46*, 2.

Haahr, A., Norlyk, A., & Hall, E. (2014). Ethical challenges embedded in qualitative research interviews with close relatives. *Nursing Ethics, 21*, 6–15.

*Habermann, B., Broome, M., Pryor, E., Ziner, K. W. (2010). Research coordinators' experiences with scientific misconduct and research integrity. *Nursing Research, 59*, 51–57.

Heilferty, C. M. (2011). Ethical considerations in the study of online illness narratives. *Journal of Advanced Nursing, 67*, 945–953.

*Hein, I., DeVries, M., Troost, P., Meynen, G., Van Goudoever, J., & Lindauer, R. (2015). Informed consent instead of assent is appropriate in children from the age of twelve: Policy implications of new findings on children's competence to consent in clinical research. *BMC Medical Ethics, 16*, 76.

Holtzclaw, B. J., & Hanneman, S. (2002). Use of non-human biobehavioral models in critical care nursing research. *Critical Care Nursing Quarterly, 24*, 30–40.

Kupferschmid, B., & Therrien, B. (2018). Spatial learning responses to lipopolysaccharide in adults and aged rats. *Biological Research for Nursing, 20*, 32–39.

Lutz, K. F., Shelton, K., Robrecht, L., Hatton, D., & Beckett, A. (2000). Use of certificates of confidentiality in nursing research. *Journal of Nursing Scholarship, 32*, 185–188.

Mallory, C., & Hesson-McInnis, M. (2013). Pilot test results of an HIV prevention intervention for high-risk women. *Western Journal of Nursing Research, 35*, 313–329.

*Mwalabu, G., Evans, C., & Redsell, S. (2017). Factors influencing the experience of sexual and reproductive healthcare for female adolescents with perinatally-acquired HIV. *BMC Women's Health, 17*, 125.

*National Academies of Sciences, Engineering & Medicine (2018). *Returning individual research results to participants: Guidance for a new research paradigm.* Washington, DC: National Academies.

*Nishimura, A., Carey, J., Erwin, P., Tilburt, J., Murad, M., & McCormick, J. (2013). Improving understanding in the research informed consent process: A systematic review of 54 interventions tested in randomized control trials. *BMC Medical Ethics, 14,* 28.

Osier, N., Pham, L., Savarese, A., Sayles, K., & Alexander, S. (2016). Animal models in genomic research: Techniques, applications, and roles for nurses. *Applied Nursing Research, 32,* 247–256.

Payne, C. (2013). A diabetes support group for Nywaigi women to enhance their capacity for maintaining physical and mental wellbeing. *Contemporary Nurse, 46,* 41–45.

Polit, D. F., & Beck, C. T. (2009). International gender bias in nursing research, 2005–2006: A quantitative content analysis. *International Journal of Nursing Studies, 46,* 1102–1110.

Polit, D. F., & Beck, C. T. (2013). Is there still gender bias in nursing research? An update. *Research in Nursing & Health, 36,* 75–83.

Silva, M. C. (1995). *Ethical guidelines in the conduct, dissemination, and implementation of nursing research.* Washington, DC: American Nurses Association.

Simpson, C. (2010). Decision-making capacity and informed consent to participate in research by cognitively impaired individuals. *Applied Nursing Research, 23,* 221–226.

Slimmer, L., & Andersen, B. (2004). Designing a data and safety monitoring plan. *Western Journal of Nursing Research, 26,* 797–803.

*Stormorken, E., Jason, L., & Kirkevold, M. (2017). Factors impacting the illness trajectory of post-infectious fatigue syndrome. *BMC Public Health, 17,* 952.

Strandås, M., Wackerhausen, S., & Bondas, T. (2019). The nurse-patient relationship in the new public management era, in public home care: A focused ethnography. *Journal of Advanced Nursing, 75*(2), 400–411.

Waszynski, C., Milner, K., Staff, I., & Molony, S. (2018). Using simulated family presence to decrease agitation in older hospitalized delirious patients: A randomized controlled trial. *International Journal of Nursing Studies, 77,* 154–161.

Wilson, M., Oliver, P., & Malpas, P. (2019). Nurses' views on legalizing assisted dying in New Zealand: A cross-sectional study. *International Journal of Nursing Studies, 89,* 116–124.

*Wolf, L. E., Patel, M., Williams-Tarver, B., Austin, J., Dame, L., & Beskow, L. (2015). Certificates of confidentiality: Protecting human subject research data in law and practice. *Journal of Law, Medicine, and Ethics, 43,* 594–609.

Zhang, S., Shoptaw, S., Reback, C., Yadav, K., & Nyamathi, A. (2018). Cost-effective way to reduce stimulant-abuse among gay/bisexual men and transgender women. *Public Health, 154,* 151–160.

*A link to this open-access journal article is provided in the Toolkit for Chapter 7 in the **Resource Manual**. ✪

**This journal article is available on thePoint for this chapter.

8 | Planning a Nursing Study

Advance planning is required for all research. This chapter provides advice for planning qualitative and quantitative studies.

TOOLS AND CONCEPTS FOR PLANNING RIGOROUS RESEARCH

This section discusses key methodologic concepts and tools in meeting the challenges of doing rigorous research.

Inference

Inference is an integral part of doing and evaluating research. An **inference** is a conclusion drawn from the study evidence, taking into account the methods used to generate that evidence. Inference is the attempt to come to conclusions based on limited information, using logical reasoning processes.

Inference is necessary because researchers use proxies that "stand in" for the things that are fundamentally of interest. A sample of participants is a proxy for an entire population. A study site is a proxy for all relevant sites in which the phenomena of interest could unfold. A control group that does not receive an intervention is a proxy for what would happen to those receiving the intervention if they did not receive it.

Researchers face the challenge of using methods that yield persuasive evidence in support of inferences they wish to make.

Reliability, Validity, and Trustworthiness

Researchers want their inferences to correspond with the *truth*. Research cannot contribute evidence to guide clinical practice if the findings are biased or fail to represent the experiences of the target group. Consumers of research need to assess the quality of a study's evidence by evaluating the conceptual and methodologic decisions the researchers made, and those who do research must strive to make decisions that result in high-quality evidence.

Quantitative researchers use several criteria to assess the rigor of a study, sometimes referred to as its **scientific merit**. Two especially important criteria are reliability and validity. **Reliability** refers to the accuracy and consistency of information obtained in a study. The term is most often associated with the methods used to measure variables. For example, if a thermometer measured Alan's temperature as 98.1°F 1 minute and as 102.5°F the next minute, the reliability of the thermometer would be suspect.

Validity is a more complex concept that broadly concerns the *soundness* of the study's evidence—whether the findings are unbiased and well grounded. Like reliability, validity is a key criterion for evaluating methods to measure variables. In this context, the validity question is whether the methods are really measuring the concepts that they purport to measure. Is a self-reported measure of depression *really* measuring depression? Or is it measuring something else, such as loneliness? Researchers strive for solid conceptualizations of research variables and valid methods to operationalize them.

Validity is also relevant with regard to inferences about the effect of the independent variable on the dependent variable. Did a nursing intervention *really* bring about improvements in patients' outcomes—or were other factors responsible for patients' progress? Researchers make numerous methodologic decisions that influence this type of study validity. Yet another validity question concerns whether the evidence can validly be extrapolated to people who did not participate in the study.

Qualitative researchers use different criteria (and different terminology) in evaluating a study's quality. Qualitative researchers pursue methods of enhancing the **trustworthiness** of the study evidence (Lincoln & Guba, 1985). Trustworthiness encompasses several dimensions—credibility, transferability, confirmability, dependability, and authenticity—which are described in Chapter 26.

Credibility, an especially important aspect of trustworthiness, is achieved to the extent that the research methods inspire confidence that the results and interpretations are truthful. Credibility can be enhanced in various ways, but one strategy merits early discussion because it has implications for the design of all studies, including quantitative ones. **Triangulation** is the use of multiple sources or referents to draw conclusions about what constitutes the truth. In a quantitative study, this might mean using multiple measures of an outcome variable to see if predicted effects are consistent. In a qualitative study, triangulation might involve trying to reveal the complexity of a phenomenon by using multiple means of data collection to converge on the truth (e.g., having in-depth discussions with participants, as well as watching their behavior in natural settings). Or, it might involve triangulating the interpretations of multiple researchers working

together as a team. Nurse researchers are increasingly triangulating across paradigms—that is, integrating both qualitative and quantitative data in a **mixed methods study** to enhance the validity of the conclusions (Chapter 27).

> **Example of Triangulation**
> Bower et al. (2018) conducted an exploratory study of nurses' decision-making when they are interrupted during administration of medication in the pediatric intensive care unit (PICU). During their fieldwork, the researchers conducted in-depth interviews with PICU nurses and made observations during medication administration.

Nurse researchers need to design their studies in such a way that the reliability, validity, and trustworthiness of their studies are maximized. This book offers advice on how to do this.

Bias

A **bias** is an influence that produces a distortion or error. Bias can threaten a study's validity and trustworthiness and is a major concern in designing a study. Bias can result from factors that need to be considered in planning a study. These include the following:

- *Participants' lack of candor.* Sometimes people distort their behavior or statements—consciously or subconsciously—to present themselves in the best light.
- *Researcher subjectivity.* Investigators may distort inferences in the direction of their expectations or in line with their own experiences—or they may unintentionally communicate their expectations to participants and thereby induce biased responses.
- *Sample imbalances.* The sample itself may be biased; for example, if a researcher studying abortion attitudes included only members of right-to-life (or pro-choice) groups in the sample, the results would be distorted.
- *Faulty methods of data collection.* Inadequate methods of capturing concepts can lead to biases; for example, a flawed measure of patient satisfaction with nursing care may exaggerate or underestimate patients' concerns.

- *Inadequate study design.* A researcher may structure the study in such a way that an unbiased answer to the research question cannot be achieved.
- *Flawed implementation.* Even a well-designed study can sustain biases if the study protocols are not carefully implemented.

A researcher's job is to reduce or eliminate bias to the extent possible, to establish mechanisms to detect or measure it when it exists, and to take known biases into account in interpreting study findings. The job of consumers is to scrutinize methodologic decisions to reach conclusions about whether biases undermined the study evidence.

Unfortunately, bias can seldom be avoided totally because the potential for its occurrence is pervasive. Some bias is haphazard. **Random bias** (or *random error)* is essentially "noise" in the data. When error is random, distortions are as likely to bias results in one direction as the other. **Systematic bias**, on the other hand, is consistent and distorts results in a single direction. For example, if a scale consistently measured people's weights as being 2 pounds heavier than their true weight, there would be systematic bias in the data on weight.

Researchers adopt a variety of strategies to eliminate or minimize bias and strengthen study rigor. Triangulation is one such approach, the idea being that multiple sources of information or points of view can help counterbalance biases and offer avenues to identify them. Methods that quantitative researchers use to combat bias often involve research control.

Research Control

Quantitative researchers usually make efforts to control aspects of the study. **Research control** typically involves holding constant other influences on the dependent variable so that the true relationship between the independent and dependent variables can be understood. In other words, research control attempts to eliminate contaminating factors that might obscure the relationship between the variables of central interest.

Contaminating factors—called **confounding** (or **extraneous) variables**—can best be illustrated with an example. Suppose we were studying whether urinary incontinence (UI) affects depression. Prior evidence suggests a link, but the question is whether UI itself (the independent variable) contributes to higher levels of depression, or whether other factors account for the relationship between UI and depression. We need to design a study to control other determinants of depression that are also related to the independent variable, UI.

One confounding variable in this situation is age. Levels of depression tend to be higher in older people; people with UI tend to be older than those without this problem. In other words, perhaps age is the *real* cause of higher depression in people with UI. If age is not controlled, then any observed relationship between UI and depression could be caused by UI or by age.

Three possible explanations might be portrayed schematically as follows:

1. UI → depression
2. Age → UI → depression
3.

The arrows here symbolize a causal mechanism or an influence. In Model 1, UI directly affects depression, independent of any other factors. In Model 2, UI is a **mediating variable**—the effect of age on depression is *mediated* by UI. According to this representation, age affects depression *through* the effect that age has on UI. In Model 3, both age and UI have separate effects on depression and age also increases the risk of UI. Some research is specifically designed to test paths of mediation and multiple causation, but in the present example, age is extraneous to the research question. We want to design a study so that the first explanation can be tested. Age must be controlled if our goal is to explore the validity of Model 1, which posits that, no matter what a person's age, having UI makes a person more vulnerable to depression.

How can we impose such control? There are several ways (Chapter 10), but the general principle is that confounding variables must be *held constant*. The confounding variable must somehow be handled so that, in the context of the study, it is not related to the independent variable or the outcome. As an example, let us say we wanted to compare the average scores on a depression scale for those with and without UI. We would want to design a study in such a way that the ages of those in the UI and non-UI groups are comparable, even though, in general, the groups are not comparable in terms of age.

By exercising control over age, we would have more confidence in explaining the relationship between UI and depression. The world is complex: many variables are interrelated in complicated ways. When studying a problem in a quantitative study, it is difficult to examine this complexity directly; researchers analyze only a few relationships at a time. The value of the evidence in quantitative studies is often related to how well researchers controlled confounding influences. In the present example, we identified one variable (age) that could affect depression, but dozens of others might be relevant (e.g., social support, self-efficacy). Researchers need to isolate the independent and dependent variables in which they are interested and then identify confounding variables that need to be controlled.

 Confounding variables need to be controlled only if they are simultaneously related to both the dependent and independent variables, as explained in the Supplement to this chapter on thePoint.

Research control is a critical tool for managing bias and enhancing validity in quantitative studies. Sometimes, however, too much control can introduce bias. If researchers tightly control the ways in which key study variables are manifested, the true nature of those variables may be obscured. In studying phenomena that are poorly understood or whose dimensions have not been clarified, a qualitative approach that allows flexibility and exploration is more appropriate.

Randomness

For quantitative researchers, bias reduction often involves **randomness**—having features of the study established by chance rather than by researcher preference. When people are selected at random to participate in the study, for example, each person in the initial pool has an equal probability of being selected—which means that there are no systematic biases in the sample's makeup. Similarly, if participants are assigned randomly to groups that will be compared (for example intervention and "usual care" groups), then there would be no systematic biases in the groups' composition. Randomness is a compelling method of controlling confounding variables and reducing bias.

Example of Randomness
Van der Meulen et al. (2018) tested a protocol that involved screening with the Distress Thermometer and Problem List for patients with head and neck cancer. A total of 110 patients were assigned, at random, to either the Distress Thermometer intervention or to usual care. The two groups were then compared in terms of cancer worry, depressive symptoms, and quality of life.

Qualitative researchers almost never consider randomness a desirable tool. Qualitative researchers tend to use information obtained early in the study in a purposeful (nonrandom) fashion to guide their inquiry and to pursue information-rich sources that can help them expand or refine their conceptualizations. Researchers' judgments are viewed as indispensable vehicles for uncovering the complexities of phenomena of interest.

Reflexivity

Qualitative researchers do not use research control or randomness, but they are as interested as quantitative researchers in discovering the truth about human experience. Qualitative researchers often rely on reflexivity to guard against personal bias in making judgments. **Reflexivity** is the process of reflecting critically on the self and of analyzing and recording personal values that could affect data collection and interpretation.

Schwandt (2007) has described reflexivity as having two aspects. The first concerns an acknowledgment that the researcher is part of the setting or context under study. The second involves self-reflection about one's own biases, preferences, and fears about the research. Qualitative researchers are encouraged to explore these issues, to be reflexive about decisions made during the inquiry, and to note their reflexive thoughts in personal journals. As Patton (2015) noted, "To excel in qualitative inquiry requires keen and astute self-awareness" (p. 71).

Reflexivity can be a useful tool in quantitative as well as qualitative research. Self-awareness and introspection can enhance the quality of any study.

Example of Reflexivity

Currie and Szabo (2019) explored parents' perspectives on caring for a child with a rare disease. Reflexivity played an important role in the analysis and interpretation of their interview data with 15 parents: "Data were analyzed considering reflexivity throughout the process…The interpretation is a process of cocreation between the researcher and the participant through reinterpretation and reflection" (p. 97).

Generalizability and Transferability

Nurses increasingly rely on evidence from research in their clinical practice. Evidence-based practice is based on the assumption that study findings are not unique to the people, places, or circumstances of the original research (Polit & Beck, 2010).

Generalizability is a criterion used in quantitative studies to assess the extent to which findings can be applied to people and settings beyond those used in a study. How do researchers enhance the generalizability of a study? First and foremost, they must design studies strong in reliability and validity. There is no point in wondering whether results are generalizable if they are not accurate or valid. In selecting participants, researchers must also give thought to the types of people to whom the results might be generalized—and then select participants in such a way that the sample reflects the population of interest. If a study is intended to have implications for male and female patients, then men and women should be included as participants. Several chapters in this book describe strategies for enhancing generalizability.

Qualitative researchers do not specifically aim for generalizability, but they do want to generate knowledge that could be useful in other situations. Lincoln and Guba (1985), in their influential book on naturalistic inquiry, discussed the concept of **transferability**, the extent to which qualitative findings can be transferred to other settings, as an aspect of a study's trustworthiness. An important mechanism for promoting transferability is the amount of rich descriptive information qualitative researchers provide about study contexts. Transferability in qualitative research is discussed in Chapter 26.

TIP Researchers are increasingly paying attention to the *applicability* of their findings—that is, the extent to which findings can be applied to individuals or small subgroups. We discuss this issue at length in Chapter 31.

Stakeholder Engagement

There is growing agreement within the healthcare community that greater **stakeholder** engagement is needed in all phases of research, beginning in the planning phase—or even earlier, during the identification of a research problem. Proponents of stakeholder involvement during the planning and implementation of health research argue that it enhances the relevance and transparency of the research and accelerates the adoption of research evidence in practice.

TIP In Europe, advocates often use the term **patient and public involvement (PPI)**. In the United States, the Patient-Centered Outcomes Research Institute (PCORI) was established in 2010 to fund research that can help patients make better healthcare choices, and patients play a role in guiding the research agenda.

Although patients have been identified as key stakeholders, researchers can consider involving others in planning a study. Concannon et al. (2012) developed a taxonomy to guide researchers in this new era of stakeholder-engaged research and proposed this definition of "engagement" of stakeholders: "A bi-directional relationship between the stakeholder and the researcher that results in informed decision-making about the selection, conduct, and use of research" (p. 986). They created a framework called the 7Ps to aid in the identification of stakeholders: Patients and the public; providers (e.g., nurses, physicians); purchasers; payers; policy makers; product makers; and principal investigators. Researchers need to identify key stakeholders and determine how best to involve them in the planning process.

OVERVIEW OF RESEARCH DESIGN FEATURES

A study's research design spells out the basic strategies that researchers adopt to develop evidence that is accurate and interpretable. The research design incorporates some of the most important methodologic decisions that researchers make, particularly in quantitative studies.

Table 8.1 describes seven design features that need to be considered in planning a quantitative study; several are also pertinent in qualitative studies. These features include:

● whether or not there will be an *intervention*;
● how confounding variables will be *controlled*;
● whether *blinding* will be used to avoid biases;
● what the *relative timing* for collecting data on dependent and independent variables will be;
● what types of *comparisons* will be made to enhance interpretability;
● what the *location* of the study will be; and
● what *timeframes* will be adopted.

This section discusses the last three features because they are relevant in planning both qualitative and quantitative studies. Chapters 9 and 10 elaborate on the first four.

TABLE 8.1 • Key Research Design Features in Quantitative Studies

FEATURE	KEY QUESTIONS	DESIGN OPTIONS
Intervention	Will there be an intervention? What will the intervention entail? What specific design will be used?	Experimental (randomized controlled trial), quasi-experimental, nonexperimental (observational) design
Control over confounding variables	How will confounding variables be controlled? Which confounding variables will be controlled?	Matching, homogeneity, blocking, crossover, randomization, statistical control
Blinding (masking)	From whom will critical information be withheld to avoid bias?	Open versus closed study; single-blind, double-blind (with blinded groups specified)
Relative timing	When will information on independent and dependent variables be collected—looking backward or forward?	Retrospective, prospective design
Comparisons	What type of comparisons will be made to illuminate key processes or relationships? What is the nature of the comparison?	Within-subject design, between-subject design, mixed design, external comparisons
Location	Where will the study take place?	Single site versus multisite; in the field vs. controlled setting
Timeframes	How often will data be collected? When, relative to other events, will data be collected?	Cross-sectional, longitudinal design; repeated measures design

Note: Many terms in this table are explained in subsequent chapters.

TIP Design decisions affect the integrity of your findings. These decisions may influence whether you receive funding (if you seek financial support) or whether your findings will be published (if you submit to a journal). Therefore, a great deal of care and thought should go into these decisions during the planning phase.

Comparisons

In most quantitative (and some qualitative) studies, researchers incorporate comparisons into their design to provide a context for interpreting results. Most quantitative research questions involve either an explicit or an implicit comparison. For example, if our research question asks what is the effect of massage on anxiety in hospitalized patients, the implied comparison is massage versus no massage, which is the independent variable.

Researchers can structure their studies to make various types of comparison, the most common of which are as follows:

1. *Comparison between two or more groups.* For example, if we were studying the emotional consequences of having a mastectomy, we might compare the emotional status of women who had a mastectomy with that of women with breast cancer who did not have a mastectomy. Or, we might compare those receiving a special intervention with those receiving "usual care." In a qualitative study, we might compare mothers and fathers with respect to their experience of having a child diagnosed with leukemia.

2. *Comparison of one group's status at two or more points in time.* For example, we might want to compare patients' levels of stress before and after introducing a procedure to reduce pre-operative stress. Or we might want to compare coping processes among caregivers of patients with AIDS early and later in the caregiving experience.

3. *Comparison of one group's status under different circumstances.* For example, we might compare people's heart rates during two different types of exercise.

4. *Comparison based on relative rankings.* If, for example, we hypothesized a relationship between the pain level and degree of hopefulness in patients with cancer, we would be asking whether those with high levels of pain felt less hopeful than those with low levels of pain. This research question involves a comparison of those with different rankings—higher versus lower—on both variables.

5. *Comparison with external data.* Researchers may compare their results with those from other studies or with **norms** (standards from a large and representative sample). This type of comparison often supplements rather than replaces other comparisons. In quantitative studies, this approach is useful primarily when the dependent variable is measured with a reliable, well-accepted method (e.g., blood pressure readings, scores on a respected measure of depression).

Example of Using Comparative Data From External Sources
Dias et al. (2018) studied the health status of bereaved parents during the first 6 months after their child's death. They used measures of health and well-being for which national comparative data were available, which enabled them to compare their participants' outcomes with national norms for adults in the United States.

Research designs for quantitative studies can be categorized based on the type of comparisons that are made. Studies that compare different people (as in examples 1 and 4) are **between-subjects designs**. Sometimes, however, it is preferable to make comparisons for the *same* participants at different times or under difference circumstances, as in examples 2 and 3. Such designs are **within-subjects designs**. When two or more groups of people are followed over time, the design is sometimes called a **mixed design** because comparisons can be both within groups over time or between different groups at a given point in time.

Comparisons provide a context for interpreting the findings. In example 1 regarding the emotional status of women who had a mastectomy, it would be difficult to know whether the women's emotional state was worrisome without comparing it with that of others—or comparing it to their state at an earlier time (for example, prior to diagnosis). In designing a study, quantitative researchers choose comparisons that will best illuminate answers to the research question.

Qualitative researchers sometimes plan to make comparisons when they undertake an in-depth study, but comparisons are rarely their primary focus. Nevertheless, patterns emerging in the data often suggest that certain comparisons have rich descriptive value.

> **TIP** Try not to make design decisions single-handedly. Seek the advice of faculty or colleagues; patient input may also be desirable. Once you have made design decisions, consider writing out a rationale for your choices and sharing it with others to see if they can suggest improvements. A worksheet for documenting design decisions is available in the Toolkit of the accompanying *Resource Manual*.

Research Location

An important planning task is to identify sites for the study. In some situations the study site is a "given," as might be the case for a clinical study conducted in a hospital or institution with which researchers are affiliated, but in other studies the identification of an appropriate site involves considerable effort. The closer the setting is to the "real world," the more relevant the evidence is likely to be to clinical practice (Chapter 31).

Planning the study location involves two types of activities—selecting the site or sites and gaining access to them. Although some of the issues we discuss here are of particular relevance to qualitative researchers working in the field, many quantitative studies also need to attend to these matters in planning a project, especially in intervention studies.[*]

Site Selection

The primary consideration in site selection is whether the site has people with the behaviors, experiences, or characteristics of interest. The site must also have a sufficient *number* of these kinds of people and adequate *diversity* or mix of people to achieve research goals. In addition, the site must be

one in which access to participants will be granted. Both methodologic goals (e.g., ability to impose needed controls) and ethical requirements (e.g., ability to ensure privacy and confidentiality) need to be achieved in the chosen site.

Researchers sometimes must decide *how many* sites to include. Having multiple sites is advantageous for enhancing the generalizability of the study findings, but multisite studies are complex and challenging. Multiple sites are a good strategy when several coinvestigators from different institutions are working together on a project.

Site visits to potential sites and clinical field-work are useful to assess the "fit" between what the researcher needs and what the site has to offer. During site visits, the researcher makes observations and converses with key gatekeepers or stakeholders in the site to better understand its characteristics and constraints. Buckwalter et al. (2009) have noted particular issues of concern when working in sites that are "unstable" research environments, such as critical care units or long-term care facilities.

Gaining Entrée

Researchers must gain entrée into the sites deemed suitable for the study. If the site is an entire community, a multitiered effort of gaining acceptance from gatekeepers may be needed. For example, it may be necessary to enlist the cooperation first of community leaders and subsequently of administrators and staff in specific institutions (e.g., domestic violence organizations) or leaders of specific groups (e.g., support groups).

Because establishing *trust* is a central issue, gaining entrée requires strong interpersonal skills, as well as familiarity with the site's customs and language. Researchers' ability to gain the gate-keepers' trust can best occur if researchers are candid about research requirements and express genuine interest in and concern for people in the site. Gatekeepers are most likely to be cooperative if they believe that there will be direct benefits to them or their constituents.

Information to help gatekeepers make a decision about granting access usually should be put in writing, even if the negotiation takes place in person.

An information sheet should cover the following points: (1) the purpose and significance of the research; (2) why the site was chosen; (3) what the research would entail (e.g., study timeframes, how much disruption there might be, what resources are required); (4) how ethical guidelines would be maintained, including how results would be reported; and (5) what the gatekeeper or others at the site have to gain from cooperating in the study. Figure 8.1 presents an example of a letter of inquiry for gaining entrée into a facility.

Gaining entrée may be an ongoing process of establishing relationships and rapport with people at the site, including prospective informants. The process might involve *progressive entry*, in which certain privileges are negotiated at first and then are subsequently expanded. Ongoing communication with gatekeepers between the time that access is granted and the start-up of the study is recommended—this may be a lengthy period if funding requests are involved. It is not only courteous to keep people informed, it may

---

Ms. Wendy Smith, R.N.
Family Birth Place
General Hospital
Hartford, CT

Dear Ms. Smith:

I am the Principal Investigator of a study whose primary goal is to improve the detection of postpartum depression in Hispanic mothers. The study will involve testing a standard Spanish version of the Postpartum Depression Screening Scale (PDSS). Postpartum depression is a cross-cultural mental illness that can have devastating effects for 10%–15% of new mothers and their families. It has been estimated that up to 50% of all cases go undetected. Non–English-speaking women in this country may be even more disadvantaged and isolated in their environments and may thus be at even higher risk for depression than English-speaking women, and thus effective screening with a valid instrument may be especially important.

Your hospital would be a desirable site for this research because of the high percentage of Hispanic women who deliver at your Family Birth Place. The research would require a sample of 75 Hispanic mothers 18 years of age or older who have given birth within the past 3 months. Each mother would complete the PDSS-Spanish Version and would participate in a diagnostic interview for *DSM-IV* depressive disorders, conducted by a female Hispanic psychologist. If a woman is diagnosed with postpartum depression, she would be referred for psychiatric follow-up. Each mother would be given a gift certificate for $25.00 for participating in the study.

If feasible, I would like to approach the 75 Hispanic women to invite them to participate in the study soon after delivery, while they are on the postpartum unit. The mothers would be recruited by a Hispanic research assistant who is an RN. Prospective participants will be asked to sign an informed consent form, which will be available in both English and Spanish (whichever language version participants prefer). Confidentiality will be strictly maintained. No name or identifying information will be written on any of the data collection forms. All data will be kept in a locked file cabinet in my office at the University of Connecticut.

Results of the study will be presented at research conferences and in a nursing research journal. The study findings will provide you with a more complete picture of your own Hispanic population and the percentage suffering from postpartum depression. A Spanish version of the PDSS will be made available for your use for screening Hispanic mothers at your hospital.

If it is possible, I would like to schedule an appointment with you so that we can discuss the possibility of my conducting this research on your unit.

Sincerely,
Cheryl Tatano Beck, DNSc, CNM, FAAN
Professor

FIGURE 8.1 Sample letter of inquiry for gaining entrée into a research site (fictitious).

prove critical to the project's success because circumstances (and leadership) at the site can change.

Timeframes

Research designs designate when, and how often, data will be collected. In many studies, data are collected at one point in time. For example, patients might be asked on a single occasion to describe their health-promoting behaviors. Some designs, however, call for multiple contacts with participants, often to assess changes over time. Thus, in planning a study, researchers must decide on the number of data collection points needed to address the research question properly. The research design also designates *when*, relative to other events, data will be collected. For example, the design might call for weight measurements 4 and 8 weeks after an exercise intervention.

Designs can be categorized in terms of study timeframes. The major distinction, for both qualitative and quantitative researchers, is between cross-sectional and longitudinal designs.

Cross-Sectional Designs

Cross-sectional designs involve the collection of data once: the phenomena under study are captured at a single time point. Cross-sectional studies are appropriate for describing the status of phenomena or for describing relationships at a fixed point in time. For example, we might be interested in examining whether psychological symptoms in women going through menopause correlate contemporaneously with physiologic symptoms.

Example of a Cross-Sectional Study
Van Hoek et al. (2019) studied the influence of demographic factors, resilience, and stress-reducing activities on the academic outcomes of undergraduate nursing students. Data were gathered at a single point in time from 554 Belgian nursing students.

Inferences about causal relationships are tricky when cross-sectional designs are used. For example, we might test the hypothesis, using cross-sectional data, that a determinant of excessive alcohol consumption is low impulse control, as measured by a psychological test. When both alcohol consumption and impulse control are measured concurrently, however, it is difficult to know which variable influenced the other, if either.

Cross-sectional data can best be used to infer time sequence under two circumstances: (1) when a cogent theoretical rationale guides the analysis or (2) when evidence or logic indicates that one variable preceded the other. For example, in a study of the effects of low birth weight on morbidity in school-aged children, it is clear that birth weight came first.

Cross-sectional studies can be designed to permit inferences about processes evolving over time, but such designs are weaker than longitudinal ones. Suppose, for example, we were studying changes in children's health promotion activities between the ages of 10 and 13 years. One way to study this would be to interview children at the age of 10 years and then 3 years later at the age of 13 years—a longitudinal design. On the other hand, we could use a cross-sectional design by interviewing *different* children of ages 10 and 13 years and then comparing their responses. If 13-year-olds engaged in more health-promoting activities than 10-year-olds, we might infer that children improve in making healthy choices as they age. To make this kind of inference, we would have to assume that the older children would have responded like the younger ones had they been questioned 3 years earlier, or, conversely, that 10-year-olds would report more health-promoting activities if they were questioned again 3 years later. Such a design, which involves a comparison of multiple age cohorts, is sometimes called a *cohort comparison design*.

Cross-sectional studies are economical but inferring changes over time with such designs is problematic. In our example, 10- and 13-year old children may have different attitudes toward health promotion, independent of maturation. Rapid social and technologic changes make it risky to assume that differences in the behaviors or traits of different age groups are the result of time passing rather than of cohort differences. In cross-sectional studies designed to explore change, there are often alternative explanations for the findings—and that is precisely what good research design tries to avoid.

Example of a Cross-Sectional Study With Inference of Change Over Time

Hladek et al. (2018) studied the feasibility of using sweat to measure cytokines in older adults (aged 65+) compared with those in younger adults (aged 18-40 years). Higher concentrations of TNF-α and IL-10 were observed in older adults, consistent with the hypothesis that cytokines increase with age.

Longitudinal Designs

A study in which researchers collect data at more than one point in time *over an extended period* is a **longitudinal design**. There are four situations in which a longitudinal design is appropriate:

1. *Studying time-related processes.* Some research questions specifically concern phenomena that evolve over time (e.g., wound healing).
2. *Determining time sequences.* It is sometimes important to establish how phenomena are sequenced. For example, if it is hypothesized that infertility affects depression, then it would be important to ascertain that the depression did not precede the fertility problem.
3. *Assessing changes over time.* Some studies examine whether changes have occurred over time. For example, an intervention study might examine both short-term and long-term changes in health outcomes. A qualitative study might explore the evolution of grieving in the spouses of palliative care patients.
4. *Enhancing research control.* Quantitative researchers sometimes collect data at multiple points to enhance the interpretability of the results. For example, when two groups are being compared with regard to the effects of alternative interventions, the collection of preintervention data allows the researcher to assess group comparability initially.

There are several types of longitudinal designs. Most involve collecting data from one group of participants multiple times, but others involve different samples. **Trend studies**, for example, are investigations of a specific phenomenon using different samples from the same population over time (e.g., every 2 years). Trend studies permit researchers to examine patterns and rates of change and to predict future developments. Many trend studies document trends in public health issues, such as smoking, obesity, and so on.

Example of a Trend Study

Neaigus et al. (2017) studied trends in HIV and hepatitis C virus risk behaviors among people who inject drugs in New York City. The team examined changes from 2005 to 2009 and to 2012. Significant trends in risk behaviors included a decline in unsafe syringe source, but an increase in vaginal or anal sex without condoms.

In a more typical longitudinal study, the *same* people provide data at two or more points in time. Longitudinal studies of general (nonclinical) populations are sometimes called **panel studies**. The term *panel* refers to the sample of people providing data. Because the same people are studied over time, researchers can examine diverse patterns of change (e.g., those whose health improved or deteriorated). Panel studies are intuitively appealing as an approach to studying change, but they are expensive.

Example of a Panel Study

Many national governments sponsor large-scale panel studies whose data have been analyzed by nurse researchers. For example, Davis et al.(2018) used data from the Australian Longitudinal Study on Women's Health to examine the relationship between parity and long-term weight gain over a 16-year period.

Follow-up studies are undertaken to examine the subsequent development of individuals who have a specified condition or who have received a specific treatment. For example, patients who have received a special nursing intervention may be followed to ascertain long-term effects. Or, in a qualitative study, patients interviewed shortly after a diagnosis of prostate cancer may be followed to assess their experiences after treatment decisions have been made.

Example of a Qualitative Follow-Up Study

Hansen et al. (2017) followed-up, over a 6-month period, the family members caring for patients with terminal hepatocellular carcinoma as patients approached the end of life. The caregivers were interviewed monthly.

In some longitudinal studies, called **cohort studies**, a group of people (the cohort) is tracked over time to see if subsets with exposure to different factors diverge in terms of subsequent outcomes. For example, in a cohort of women, those with or without a history of childbearing could be tracked to examine differences in rates of ovarian cancer. This type of study, sometimes called a *prospective study,* is discussed in Chapter 9.

Longitudinal studies are appropriate for studying the trajectory of a phenomenon over time, but a major problem is **attrition**—the loss of participants after initial data collection. Attrition is problematic because those who drop out of the study often differ in systematic ways from those who continue to participate, resulting in potential biases and difficulty in generalizing to the original population. The longer the interval between data collection points, the greater the risk of attrition and resulting biases.

In longitudinal studies, researchers make decisions about the number of data collection points and the intervals between them. When change or development is rapid, numerous time points at short intervals may be needed to document it. Researchers interested in outcomes that may occur years after the original data collection must use longer-term follow-up—*or* use **surrogate outcomes**. For example, in evaluating the effectiveness of a smoking cessation intervention, the main outcome of interest might by lung cancer incidence or age at death, but the researcher would likely use subsequent smoking (e.g., 3 months after the intervention) as the surrogate outcome.

Repeated Measures Designs

Studies with multiple points of data collection are sometimes described as having a **repeated measures design**, which usually signifies a study in which data are collected three or more times. Longitudinal studies, such as follow-up and cohort studies, sometimes use a repeated measures design.

Repeated measures designs, however, can also be used in studies that are essentially cross-sectional. For example, a study involving the collection of postoperative patient data on vital signs hourly over a 6-hour period would not be described as longitudinal because the study does not involve an extended time perspective. Yet, the design could be characterized as repeated measures. Researchers are especially likely to use the term *repeated measures design* when they use a repeated measures approach to statistical analysis (see Chapter 18).

Example of a Repeated Measures Design

Krause-Parello et al. (2018) studied the effects of an animal-assisted intervention on hospitalized veterans receiving palliative care. Blood pressure, heart rate, and salivary cortisol were measured before, immediately after, and again 30 minutes after the intervention.

TIP In making design decisions, you will need to balance various considerations, such as time, cost, ethics, and study rigor. Try to understand your "upper limits" before finalizing your design. That is, what is the *most* money that can be spent on the project? What is the *maximum amount* of time available for conducting the study? What is the limit of acceptability with regard to attrition? These limits often eliminate some design options. With these constraints in mind, the central focus should be on designing a study that maximizes the rigor or trustworthiness of the study.

PLANNING DATA COLLECTION

In planning a study, researchers must select methods to gather their research data. This section provides an overview of various methods of data collection for qualitative and quantitative studies.

Overview of Data Collection and Data Sources

A broad array of data collection methods can be used in research. In some cases, researchers may be able to use data from existing sources, such as records. Most often, however, researchers collect new data, and one key planning decision concerns the types of data to gather. Three approaches have been used most frequently by nurse researchers: self-reports, observation, and biophysiologic measures.

Self-Reports (Patient-Reported Outcomes)

A good deal of information can be gathered by questioning people directly, a method known as **self-report**. In the medical literature, self-reports are often called **patient-reported outcomes** or **PROs**, but some self-reports are not about patients (e.g., self-reports about nurses' burnout) and some are not *outcomes* (self-reports about prior hospitalizations). Most nursing studies involve self-report data. The unique ability of humans to communicate verbally makes direct questioning a particularly important part of nurse researchers' data collection repertoire.

Self-reports are versatile. If we want to know what people think, believe, or plan to do, the most efficient approach is to ask them. Self-reports can yield information that would be impossible to gather by other means. Behaviors can be observed but only if participants engage in them publicly. Furthermore, observers can observe only those behaviors occurring at the time of the study. Through self-reports, researchers can gather *retrospective data* about events occurring in the past or information about behaviors in which people plan to engage in the future. Self-reports can also capture psychological attributes such as motivation or resilience.

Nevertheless, verbal report methods have some weaknesses. The most serious issue concerns their validity and accuracy: Can we be sure that people feel or act the way they say they do? We all have a tendency to present ourselves positively, and this may conflict with the truth. Researchers who gather self-report data should recognize this limitation and take it into consideration when interpreting the results.

Example of a Study Using Self-Reports

Beattie et al. (2019) explored the perceptions of healthcare providers on workplace violence perpetrated by clients. The data came from in-depth group and one-on-one interviews with nurses and other healthcare staff in Australia.

Self-report methods depend on respondents' willingness to share personal information. **Projective techniques** are sometimes used to obtain data about people's psychological states indirectly. Projective techniques present participants with a stimulus of low structure, permitting them to "read in" and describe their interpretations. The Rorschach (inkblot) test is an example of a projective technique. Other projective methods encourage self-expression through the construction of a product (e.g., drawings). The assumption is that people express their needs, motives, and emotions by working with or manipulating materials. Projective methods are used by nurse researchers mainly in studies exploring sensitive topics with children.

Example of a Study Using Projective Methods

Anderson and Tulloch-Reid (2019) investigated the experiences of adolescents with diabetes living in Jamaica. Participants took part in group interviews and were also asked to draw pictures representing their experiences.

Observation

An alternative to self-reports is **observation** of study participants. Observation can be done directly through the human senses or with technical apparatus, such as video equipment, X-rays, and so on. Observational methods can be used to gather information about a wide range of phenomena, such as: (1) people's characteristics and conditions (e.g., patients' sleep–wake state); (2) verbal communication (e.g., nurse–patient dialogue); (3) nonverbal communication (e.g., facial expressions); (4) activities and behavior (e.g., geriatric patients' self-grooming); (5) skill attainment (e.g., diabetic patients' skill in testing their urine); and (6) environmental conditions (e.g., architectural barriers in nursing homes).

Observation in healthcare settings is an important data-gathering strategy. Nurses are in an advantageous position to observe, relatively unobtrusively, the behaviors of patients, their families, and hospital staff. Moreover, nurses may, by training, be especially sensitive observers.

Observational methods are especially useful when people are unaware of their own behavior (e.g., manifesting preoperative symptoms of anxiety), when people are embarrassed to report activities (e.g., aggressive actions), when behaviors are emotionally laden (e.g., grieving), or when people cannot describe their actions (e.g., young children). A shortcoming of observation is potential behavior distortions when participants are aware of being observed—a problem called **reactivity**. Reactivity can be eliminated if observations are made without people's knowledge, through concealment—but this may pose ethical concerns. Another problem is **observer biases**. Several factors (e.g., prejudices, emotions, fatigue) can undermine objectivity. Observational biases can be minimized through careful training.

> **Example of a Study Using Observation**
> Vittner et al. (2018) studied whether skin-to-skin contact between parents and stable preterm infants alleviates parental stress while also supporting mother–father–infant relationships. Parent–infant interactions were examined via video-recorded observations, in which levels of synchrony and responsiveness were recorded.

Biophysiologic Measures/Biomarkers

Many clinical studies rely on the use of **biophysiologic measures** or biomarkers. **Biomarkers** are objective, quantifiable characteristics of biological processes (Strimbu & Tavel, 2010). Biophysiologic and physical variables typically are measured using specialized technical instruments and equipment. Because such equipment is available in healthcare settings, the costs of these measures to nurse researchers may be small or nonexistent.

A major strength of biophysiologic measures is their objectivity. Nurse A and nurse B, reading from the same spirometer output, are likely to record the same forced expiratory volume (FEV) measurements. Furthermore, two different spirometers are likely to produce the same FEV readouts. Another advantage of physiologic measurements is the relative precision they normally offer. By *relative*, we are implicitly comparing physiologic instruments with measures of psychological

phenomena, such as self-report measures of anxiety or pain. Biophysiologic measures usually yield data of exceptionally high quality.

> **Example of a Study Using Biomarkers**
> Imes et al. (2019) studied factors associated with endothelial function in older adults with obstructive sleep apnea and cardiovascular disease. The variables examined included body mass index, blood pressure, and several cholesterol values.

Records

Most researchers create original data for their studies, but sometimes they take advantage of information available in **records**. Electronic health records and other records constitute rich data sources to which nurse researchers may have access. Research data obtained from records are advantageous because they are economical: the collection of original data can be time-consuming and costly. Also, records avoid problems stemming from people's reaction to study participation.

On the other hand, when researchers are not responsible for collecting data, they may be unaware of the records' limitations and biases, such as the biases of *selective deposit* and *selective survival*. If the available records are not the entire set of all possible such records, researchers must question how representative existing records are. Many record keepers *intend* to maintain an entire universe of records but may not succeed. Careful researchers should attempt to learn what biases might exist. Gregory and Radovinsky (2012) have suggested some strategies for enhancing the reliability of data extracted from medical records, and Dziadkowiec et al. (2016) have described a method of "cleaning" data extracted from electronic health records.

Other difficulties also may be relevant. Sometimes records have to be verified for their authenticity or accuracy, which may be difficult if the records are old. In using records to study trends, researchers should be alert to possible changes in record-keeping procedures. Another problem is the increasing difficulty of gaining access to institutional records. Thus, although records may be plentiful and inexpensive, they should not be used without paying attention to potential problems.

> **TIP** Nurse researchers are increasingly using information from "Big Data" sources, such as large administrative databases or *registries*. Registries are collections of large amounts of data about a particular disease or patient population, such as trauma or cancer registries. Talbert and Sole (2013) and Gephart et al. (2018) have written about doing research with large databases.

Example of a Study Using Records
Pressler et al. (2018) studied the symptoms, nutrition, and pressure ulcer status among older women with heart failure in relation to their return to the community from a skilled nursing facility. The data were collected from the electronic medical records.

Dimensions of Data Collection Approaches

Data collection methods vary along three key dimensions: structure, researcher obtrusiveness, and objectivity. In planning a study, researchers make decisions about where on these dimensions the data collection methods should fall.

Structure

In structured data collection, information is gathered from participants in a comparable, prespecified way. Most self-administered questionnaires are structured: They include a fixed set of questions, usually with predesignated response options (e.g., agree/disagree). Structured methods give participants limited opportunities to qualify their answers or to explain the meaning of their responses. By contrast, qualitative studies rely mainly on unstructured methods of data collection.

Structured methods often take considerable effort to develop, but they yield data that are relatively easy to analyze because the data can be readily quantified. Structured methods are not appropriate for an in-depth examination of a phenomenon,

however. Consider the following two methods of asking people about their levels of stress:

Structured. During the past week, would you say you felt stressed:

1. rarely or none of the time,
2. some or a little of the time,
3. occasionally or a moderate amount of the time, or
4. most or all of the time?

Unstructured. How stressed or anxious have you been this past week? Please tell me about any tensions and stresses you experienced.

The structured question allows us to compute what percentage of respondents felt stressed most of the time but provides no information about the circumstances of the stress. The unstructured question allows for deeper and more thoughtful responses but may not be useful for people who are not good at expressing themselves; moreover, the resulting data are more difficult to analyze.

Researcher Obtrusiveness

Data collection methods differ in the degree to which people are aware of the data-gathering process. If people know they are under scrutiny, their behavior and responses may not be "normal," and distortions can undermine the value of the research. When data are collected unobtrusively, however, ethical problems may emerge.

Study participants are most likely to distort their behavior and their responses to questions under certain circumstances. Researcher obtrusiveness is likely to be most problematic when (1) a program is being evaluated and participants have a vested interest in the evaluation outcome; (2) participants engage in socially unacceptable or unusual behavior; (3) participants have not complied with medical and nursing instructions; and (4) participants are the type of people who have a strong need to "look good." When researcher obtrusiveness is unavoidable under these circumstances, researchers should make an effort to put participants at ease, to emphasize the importance of candor, and to adopt a nonjudgmental demeanor.

Objectivity

Objectivity refers to the degree to which two independent researchers can arrive at similar "scores" or make similar observations regarding concepts of interest. Objectivity is a mechanism for avoiding biases. Some data collection approaches require more subjective judgment than others. Researchers with a positivist orientation usually strive for a reasonable amount of objectivity. In research based on the constructivist paradigm, however, the subjective judgment of investigators is considered essential for understanding human experiences.

Developing a Data Collection Plan

In planning a study, researchers make decisions about the type and amount of data to collect. Several factors, including costs, must be weighed, but a key goal is to identify the kinds of data that will yield accurate, valid, and trustworthy information for addressing the research question.

Most researchers face the issue of balancing information needs against the risk of overburdening participants. In many studies, more data are collected than are needed or analyzed. Although it is better to have adequate data than to have unwanted omissions, minimizing *participant burden* should be an important goal. Specific guidance on data collection plans is offered in Chapter 14 for quantitative studies and Chapter 24 for qualitative studies.

ORGANIZATION OF A RESEARCH PROJECT

Studies typically take many months to complete and longitudinal studies require years of work. During the planning phase, it is a good idea to make preliminary estimates of how long various tasks will require. Having deadlines helps to restrict tasks that might otherwise continue indefinitely, such as a literature review.

Chapter 3 presented a sequence of steps that quantitative researchers follow in a study. The steps represented an idealized conception: the research process rarely follows a neatly prescribed sequence of procedures, even in quantitative studies. Decisions made in one step, for example, may require alterations in a previous activity. For example, sample size decisions may require rethinking how many sites are needed. Nevertheless, preliminary time estimates are valuable. In particular, it is important to have a sense of how much total time the study will require and when it will begin.

> **TIP** We could not suggest even approximations for the percentage of time that should be spent on each task. Some projects need many months to recruit participants, whereas other studies can rely on an existing group. Clearly, not all steps are equally time-consuming.

Researchers sometimes develop visual timelines to help them organize a study. These devices are especially useful if funding is sought because the schedule helps researchers to understand when and for how long staff support is needed (e.g., for transcribing interviews). This can best be illustrated with an example, in this case of a hypothetical quantitative study.

Suppose a researcher was studying the following problem: Is a woman's decision to have an annual mammogram related to her perceived susceptibility to breast cancer? Using the organization of steps outlined in Chapter 3, here are some of the tasks that might be undertaken:[a]

1. The researcher is concerned that many older women do not get mammograms regularly. Her specific *research question* is whether mammogram practices are different for women with different perceptions about their susceptibility to breast cancer.
2. The researcher *reviews the research literature* on breast cancer, mammography use, and factors affecting mammography decisions.

---

[a]This is only a partial list of tasks and is designed to illustrate the flow of activities; the flow in this example is more orderly than would ordinarily be true.

3. The researcher does *clinical fieldwork* by discussing the problem with nurses and other healthcare professionals in various clinical settings and by having informal discussions with women in a support group for breast cancer patients.

4. The researcher *seeks theories* and models for her problem. She finds that the Health Belief Model is relevant, which helps her to develop a conceptual definition of susceptibility to breast cancer.

5. Based on the framework, the following *hypothesis is developed*: Women (P) who perceive themselves as susceptible to breast cancer (I) are more likely than other women (C) to get an annual mammogram (O).

6. The researcher adopts a nonexperimental, cross-sectional, between-subjects *research design.* Her comparison strategy will be to compare women with different rankings on a measure of susceptibility to breast cancer. She designs the study to control the confounding variables of age, marital status, and health insurance status. Her research site will be Pittsburgh.

7. There is no *intervention* in this study and so this step is unnecessary.

8. The researcher designates that the *population* of interest is women between the ages of 50 and 65 years living in Pittsburgh who have not been previously diagnosed as having any form of cancer.

9. The researcher will recruit 250 women living in Pittsburgh as her *research sample*; they are identified at random using a procedure known as *random-digit dialing,* and so she does not need to gain entrée into any institution.

10. *Research variables will be measured* by self-report; the independent variable (perceived susceptibility), dependent variable (mammogram history), and confounding variables will be measured by asking participants a series of questions.

11. The Institutional Review Board (IRB) at the researcher's institution is asked to review the plans to ensure that the study *adheres to ethical standards.*

12. *Plans for the study are finalized*: the methods are reviewed by colleagues with clinical and methodologic expertise and by the IRB; the data collection instruments are pretested; and interviewers who will collect the data are trained.

13. *Data are collected* by means of telephone interviews with women in the research sample.

14. *Data are prepared for analysis* by coding them and entering them onto a computer file.

15. *Data are analyzed* using statistical software.

16. The results indicate that the hypothesis is supported; however, the researcher's *interpretation* must take into consideration that many women who were asked to participate declined to do so.

17. The researcher presents an early report on her findings and interpretations at a conference of Sigma Theta Tau International. She subsequently publishes the report in the *International Journal of Nursing Studies.*

18. The researcher seeks out clinicians to discuss how the study findings can be *used in practice.*

The researcher plans to conduct this study over a 2-year period; Figure 8.2 presents a hypothetical schedule. Many steps overlap or are undertaken concurrently; some steps are projected to involve little time, whereas others require months of work. (The Toolkit in the accompanying *Resource Manual* includes Figure 8.2 as a Word document for you to adapt.)

In developing a schedule, several considerations should be kept in mind, including methodologic expertise and the availability of funding. In the present example, if the researcher needed financial support to pay for the cost of interviewers, the timeline would need to be expanded to accommodate the time required to prepare a proposal and await the funding decision. It is also important to consider the practical aspects of performing the study, which were not noted in the preceding section. Securing permissions, hiring staff,

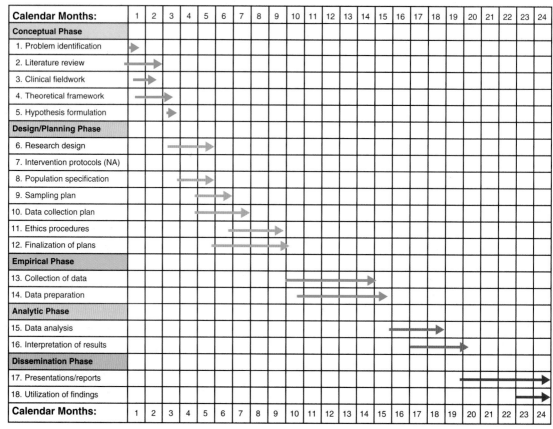

Calendar Months:	1	2	3	4	5	6	7	8	9	10	11	12	13	14	15	16	17	18	19	20	21	22	23	24
Conceptual Phase																								
1. Problem identification																								
2. Literature review																								
3. Clinical fieldwork																								
4. Theoretical framework																								
5. Hypothesis formulation																								
Design/Planning Phase																								
6. Research design																								
7. Intervention protocols (NA)																								
8. Population specification																								
9. Sampling plan																								
10. Data collection plan																								
11. Ethics procedures																								
12. Finalization of plans																								
Empirical Phase																								
13. Collection of data																								
14. Data preparation																								
Analytic Phase																								
15. Data analysis																								
16. Interpretation of results																								
Dissemination Phase																								
17. Presentations/reports																								
18. Utilization of findings																								
Calendar Months:	1	2	3	4	5	6	7	8	9	10	11	12	13	14	15	16	17	18	19	20	21	22	23	24

FIGURE 8.2 Project timeline (in months) for a hypothetical study of women's mammography decisions.

and holding meetings are all time-consuming, but necessary, activities.

In large-scale studies—especially studies in which there is an intervention—it is wise to undertake a **pilot study**. A pilot study is a trial run designed to test planned methods and procedures. Results and experiences from pilot studies help to inform many of decisions for larger projects. We discuss the important role of pilot studies in Chapter 29.

Individuals differ in the kinds of tasks that appeal to them. Some people enjoy the preliminary phase, which has an intellectual component; others are more eager to collect the data, which is more interpersonal. Researchers should, however, allocate a sensible amount of time to do justice to each activity.

TIP Getting organized for a study has many dimensions beyond having a timeline. Two important issues concern having the right team and mix of skills for a research project, and developing plans for hiring and monitoring research staff (Nelson & Morrison-Beedy, 2008).

CRITICAL APPRAISAL OF THE PLANNING ASPECTS OF A STUDY

Researchers typically do not describe the planning process or problems that arose during the study in journal articles. Thus, there is typically little that readers can do to critically appraise the researcher's planning efforts. What *can* be appraised, of course, are the outcomes of the planning—that is, the methodologic decisions themselves. Guidelines for critically appraising those decisions are provided throughout this book.

Readers can, however, be alert to a few things relating to research planning. First, evidence of careful conceptualization provides a clue that the project was well planned. If a conceptual map is presented (or implied) in the report, it means that the researcher had a "road map" that facilitated planning.

Second, readers can consider whether the researcher's plans reflect adequate attention to concerns about evidence-based practice. For example, was the comparison group strategy designed to reflect a realistic practice concern? Was the setting one that maximizes potential for the generalizability of the findings? Did the timing of data collection correspond to clinically important milestones? Was the intervention sensitive to the constraints of a typical practice environment?

Finally, a report might provide clues about whether the researcher devoted sufficient time and resources in preparing for the study. For example, if the report indicates that the study grew out of earlier research on a similar topic, or that the researcher had previously used the same instruments, or had completed other studies in the same setting, this suggests that the researcher was not plunging into unfamiliar waters. Unrealistic planning can sometimes be inferred from a discussion of sample recruitment. If the report indicates that the researcher was unable to recruit the originally hoped-for number of participants, or if recruitment took months longer than anticipated, this suggests that the researcher may not have done adequate homework during the planning phase.

RESEARCH EXAMPLE

In this section, we describe a pilot study and the "lessons learned" by the researchers. This is a good example of the importance of strong advance planning for a study.

Study: Recruitment of older African American males for depression research: Lessons learned (Bryant et al., 2014)

Purpose: The purpose of the article was to describe the setbacks and lessons learned in a pilot study aimed at exploring the signs and symptoms of depression experienced by older African American men.

Methods: The researchers sought to recruit a sample of about 20 African American men aged 60 years and older over a 3 to 4-month recruitment period. The men were to have been interviewed to learn how they recognize, express, and describe their depression. Initial recruitment was through flyers distributed to community clinics and physicians' offices serving the target group. The colorful flyers included photos and a description of the study and contact information.

Findings: Nine months into recruitment, only one person had inquired about participation in the study, and that person was deemed ineligible. This recruitment failure prompted members of the team to solicit feedback from university community liaisons and a local community development group. The advisers thought the study was important, but noted that the researchers faced numerous recruitment barriers, such as the likelihood that older black men would not easily trust outsiders and might believe that they are too strong to be depressed. The advisers also provided valuable feedback about the recruitment flier and other aspects of the study design.

Conclusions: The researchers concluded that their "failure to recruit participants can be ascribed to a number of missteps: non-culturally relevant recruitment materials, a failure to build trust and engage community coalitions beforehand, (and) the use of ineffective strategies to address the stigma associated with mental illness" (p. 4). They noted that the lessons learned would hopefully facilitate future recruitment efforts for mental health research involving black men.

SUMMARY POINTS

- Researchers face numerous challenges in planning a study, including the challenge of designing a study that is strong with respect to reliability and validity (quantitative studies) or trustworthiness (qualitative studies).

- **Reliability** refers to the accuracy and consistency of information obtained in a study. **Validity** is a more complex concept that broadly concerns the *soundness* of the study's evidence—that is, whether the findings are cogent and well grounded.

- **Trustworthiness** in qualitative research encompasses several different dimensions, including dependability, confirmability, authenticity, transferability, and credibility.

- **Credibility** is achieved to the extent that the research methods engender confidence in the truth of the data and in the researchers' interpretations. **Triangulation**, the use of multiple sources or referents to draw conclusions about what constitutes the truth, is one approach to enhancing credibility.

- A **bias** is an influence that distorts study results. **Systematic bias** results when a bias operates in a consistent direction.

- In quantitative studies, **research control** is used to *hold constant* outside influences on the outcome variable so that its relationship to the independent variable can be better understood. Researchers use various strategies to control **confounding variables,** which are extraneous to the study aims and can obscure understanding.

- In quantitative studies, a powerful tool to eliminate bias is **randomness**—having certain features of the study established by chance rather than by researchers' intentions.

- **Reflexivity,** the process of reflecting critically on the self and of scrutinizing personal values that could affect interpretation, is an important tool in qualitative research.

- **Generalizability** in a quantitative study concerns the extent to which findings can be applied to people or settings other than the ones used in the research. **Transferability** is the extent to which qualitative findings can be transferred to other settings.

- During the planning phase, researchers need to consider the extent to which key **stakeholders** will be involved in the research and who the key stakeholders are.

- In planning a study, researchers make many design decisions, including whether to have an intervention, how to control confounding variables, what type of comparisons will be made, where the study will take place, and what the study timeframes will be.

- Quantitative researchers often incorporate comparisons into their designs to enhance interpretability. In **between-subjects designs**, different groups of people are compared. **Within-subjects designs** involve comparisons of the same people at different times or under different circumstances, and **mixed designs** involve both types of comparison.

- Site selection for a study often requires **site visits** to evaluate suitability and feasibility. Gaining entrée into a site involves developing and maintaining trust with gatekeepers.

- **Cross-sectional designs** involve collecting data at one point in time, whereas **longitudinal designs** involve data collection two or more times over an extended period.

- **Trend studies** have multiple points of data collection with different samples from the same population. **Panel studies** gather data from the same people, usually from a general population, more than once. In a **follow-up study,** data are gathered two or more times from a well-defined group (e.g., those with a particular health problem). In a **cohort study**, a cohort of people is tracked over time to see if subsets with different exposures to risk factors differ in terms of subsequent outcomes.

- A **repeated measures design** typically involves collecting data three or more times, either in a longitudinal fashion or in rapid succession over a shorter timeframe.

- Longitudinal studies are typically expensive and time-consuming, and have risk of **attrition** (loss of participants over time) but are essential for illuminating time-related phenomena.

- Researchers also develop a **data collection plan**. In nursing, the most widely used methods are self-report, observation, biophysiological measures, and existing records.

- **Self-report** data (sometimes called **patient-reported outcomes** or **PROs**) are obtained by directly questioning people. Self-reports are versatile and powerful but a drawback is the potential for respondents' deliberate or inadvertent misrepresentations.
- A wide variety of human activity and traits are amenable to direct **observation**. Observation is subject to **observer biases** and distorted participant behavior (**reactivity**).
- **Biophysiologic measures** (**biomarkers**) tend to yield high-quality data that are objective and valid.
- Existing **records** and documents are an economical source of research data, but two potential biases in records are *selective deposit* and *selective survival.*
- Data collection methods vary in terms of structure, researcher obtrusiveness, and objectivity, and researchers must decide on these dimensions in their plan.
- Planning efforts should include the development of a timeline that provides estimates of when important tasks will be completed.

STUDY ACTIVITIES

Study activities are available to instructors on thePoint.

REFERENCES CITED IN CHAPTER 8

Anderson, M., & Tulloch-Reid, M. (2019). "You cannot cure it, just control it": Jamaican adolescents living with diabetes. *Comprehensive Child and Adolescent Nursing, 42*(2), 109–123.

Beattie, J., Griffiths, D., Innes, K., & Morphet, J. (2019). Workplace violence perpetrated by clients of health care: A need for safety and trauma-informed care. *Journal of Clinical Nursing, 28*, 116–124.

Bower, R., Coad, J., Manning, J., & Pengelly, T. (2018). A qualitative, exploratory study of nurses' decision-making when interrupted during medication administration within the paediatric intensive care unit. *Intensive & Critical Care Nursing, 44*, 11–17.

*Bryant, K., Wicks, M., & Willis, N. (2014). Recruitment of older African American males for depression research: Lessons learned. *Archives of Psychiatric Nursing, 28*, 17–20.

*Buckwalter, K., Grey, M., Bowers, B., McCarthy, A., Gross, D., Funk, M., & Beck, C. (2009). Intervention research in highly unstable environments. *Research in Nursing & Health, 32*, 110–121.

*Concannon, T., Meissner, P., Grunbaum, J., McElwee, N., Guise, J. M., Santa, J., … Leslie, L. (2012). A new taxonomy for stakeholder engagement in patient-centered outcomes research. *Journal of General Internal Medicine, 27*, 985–991.

Currie, G., & Szabo, J. (2019). "It is like a jungle gym, and everything is under consideration": The parent's perspective of caring for a child with a rare disease. *Child: Care, Health and Development, 45*, 96–103.

Davis, D., Brown, W., Foureur, M., Nohr, E., & Xu, F. (2018). Long-term weight gain and risk of overweight in parous and nulliparous women. *Obesity, 26*, 1072–1077.

Dias, N., Brandon, D., Haase, J., & Tanabe, P. (2018). Bereaved parents' health status during the first 6 months after their child's death. *American Journal of Hospice & Palliative Care, 35*, 829–839.

*Dziadkowiec, O., Callahan, T., Ozkaynak, M., Reeder, B., & Welton, J. (2016). Using a data quality framework to clean data extracted from the electronic health record: A case study. *EGEMS, 4*, 1201.

Gephart, S., Davis, M., & Shea, K. (2018). Perspectives on policy and the value of nursing science in a Big Data era. *Nursing Science Quarterly, 31*, 78–81.

*Gregory, K. E., & Radovinsky, L. (2012). Research strategies that result in optimal data collection from the patient medical record. *Applied Nursing Research, 25*, 108–116.

Hansen, L., Rosenkranz, S., Wherity, K., & Sasaki, A. (2017). Living with hepatocellular carcinoma near the end of life: Family caregivers' perspectives. *Oncology Nursing Forum, 44*, 562–570.

Hladek, M., Szanton, S., Cho, Y., Lai, C., Sacko, C., Roberts, L., & Gill, J. (2018). Using sweat to measure cytokines in older adults compared to younger adults. *Journal of Immunological Methods, 454*, 1–5.

**Imes, C., Baniak, L., Choi, J., Luyster, F., Morris, J., Ren, D., & Chasens, E. (2019). Correlates of endothelial function in older adults with untreated obstructive sleep apnea and cardiovascular disease. *Journal of Cardiovascular Nursing, 34*, E1–E7.

Krause-Parello, C., Levy, C., Holman, E., & Kolassa, J. (2018). Effects of VA facility dog on hospitalized veterans seen by a palliative care psychologist. *American Journal of Hospice & Palliative Care, 35*, 5–14.

Lincoln, Y. S., & Guba, E. G. (1985). *Naturalistic inquiry.* Newbury Park, CA: Sage.

Neaigus, A., Reilly, K., Jenness, S., Hagan, H., Wendel, T., Gelpi-Acosta, C., & Marshall, D. (2017). Trends in HIV and HVC risk behaviors and prevalent infection among people who inject drugs in New York City, 2005-2012. *Journal of Acquired Immune Deficiency Syndromes, 75,* S325–S332.

*Nelson, L. E., & Morrison-Beedy, D. (2008). Research team training: moving beyond job descriptions. *Applied Nursing Research, 21,* 159–164.

Patton, M. Q. (2015). *Qualitative research & evaluation methods* (4th ed.). Thousand Oaks, CA: Sage.

Polit, D. F., & Beck, C. T. (2010). Generalization in qualitative and quantitative research: Myths and strategies. *International Journal of Nursing Studies, 47,* 1451–1458.

Pressler, S., Jung, M., Titler, M., Harrison, J., & Lee, K. (2018). Symptoms, nutrition, pressure ulcers, and return to community among older women with heart failure at skilled nursing facilities. *Journal of Cardiovascular Nursing, 33,* 22–29.

Schwandt, T. (2007). *The Sage dictionary of qualitative inquiry* (3rd ed.). Thousand Oaks, CA: Sage.

*Strimbu, K., & Tavel, J. (2010). What are biomarkers? *Current Opinion in HIV & AIDS, 5,* 463–366.

Talbert, S., & Sole, M. L. (2013). Too much information: Research issues associated with large databases. *Clinical Nurse Specialist, 27,* 73–80.

Van Hoek, G., Portzky, M., & Franck, E. (2019). The influence of sociodemographic factors, resilience and stress-reducing activities on academic outcomes of undergraduate nursing students: A cross-sectional research study. *Nurse Education Today, 72,* 90–96.

Van der Meulen, I., May, A., Koole, R., & Ros, W. (2018). A distress thermometer intervention for patients with head and neck cancer. *Oncology Nursing Forum, 45,* E14–E32.

Vittner, D., McGrath, J., Robinson, J., Lawhon, G., Cusson, R., Eisenfeld, L., … Cong, X. (2018). Increase in oxytocin from skin-to-skin contact enhances development of parent-infant relationship. *Biological Research for Nursing, 20,* 54–62.

*A link to this open-access article is provided in the Toolkit for Chapter 8 in the **Resource Manual.**

**This journal article is available on thePoint for this chapter.*

Part 3

DESIGNING AND CONDUCTING QUANTITATIVE STUDIES TO GENERATE EVIDENCE FOR NURSING

9 | Quantitative Research Design

GENERAL DESIGN ISSUES

This chapter describes options for designing quantitative studies. We begin by discussing several broad issues.

Causality

Several types of research questions are relevant to evidence-based nursing practice—questions about interventions (Therapy); Diagnosis and assessment; Prognosis; Etiology (causation) and prevention of harm; Description; and Meaning or process. Questions about meaning or process call for qualitative approaches (Chapter 22). Questions about diagnosis or assessment, as well as questions about the status quo of health-related situations, are typically descriptive. Many research questions, however, are about *causes* and *effects:*

- Does a telephone therapy intervention (I) for patients diagnosed with prostate cancer (P) *cause* improvements in their decision-making skills (O)? (Therapy question)
- Do birthweights less than 1,500 g (I) *cause* developmental delays (O) in children (P)? (Prognosis question)
- Does a high-carbohydrate diet (I) *cause* cognitive impairment (O) in the elderly (P)? (Etiology [causation]/prevention of harm question)

Causality is a hotly debated issue, and yet we all understand the general concept of a **cause**. For example, we understand that lack of sleep *causes* fatigue and that high caloric intake *causes* weight gain.

Most phenomena have multiple causes. Weight gain, for example, can be the effect of high caloric consumption, but many other factors can cause weight gain. Causes of health-related phenomena usually are not *deterministic*, but rather are *probabilistic*—that is, the causes increase the probability that an effect will occur. For example, there is ample evidence that smoking is a cause of lung cancer, but not everyone who smokes develops lung cancer, and not everyone with lung cancer has a history of smoking.

The Counterfactual Model

While it might be easy to grasp what researchers mean when they talk about a *cause*, what exactly is an **effect**? Shadish et al. (2002), who wrote a seminal book on research design and causal inference, explained that a good way to grasp the meaning of an effect is to conceptualize a counterfactual. In a research context, a **counterfactual** is what would have happened *to the same people* exposed to a causal factor if they *simultaneously* were *not* exposed to the causal factor. An effect is the difference between what actually did happen with the exposure and what would have happened without it. A counterfactual clearly can never be realized, but it is a good model to keep in mind in designing a study to answer cause-probing questions. As Shadish and colleagues noted, "A central task for all cause-probing research is to create reasonable approximations to this physically impossible counterfactual" (p. 5).

Criteria for Causality

Several writers have proposed criteria for establishing a *cause-and-effect relationship*. Three criteria are attributed to 19th-century philosopher John Stuart Mill:

1. *Temporal:* A cause must precede an effect in time. If we test the hypothesis that smoking causes lung cancer, we need to show that cancer occurred *after* smoking commenced.
2. *Relationship:* An *empirical relationship* between the presumed cause and the presumed effect must exist. In our example, an association between smoking and cancer must be found— i.e., that a higher percentage of smokers than nonsmokers get lung cancer.
3. *No confounders:* The relationship cannot be explained as being *caused by a third variable*. Suppose that most smokers lived in urban environments. The relationship between smoking and lung cancer might then reflect an underlying causal link between the environment and lung cancer.

Additional criteria were proposed by Bradford-Hill (1965)—precisely as part of the discussion about the causal link between smoking and lung cancer. Two of Bradford-Hill's criteria foreshadow the importance of meta-analyses, techniques for which had not been developed when the criteria were proposed. The criterion of *coherence* involves having similar evidence from multiple sources, and the criterion of *consistency* involves having similar levels of statistical relationship in several studies. Another important criterion is *biologic plausibility*, that is, evidence from laboratory or basic physiologic studies that a causal pathway is credible.

Causality and Research Design

Researchers testing hypotheses about casual relationships seek to provide persuasive evidence that these various criteria have been met. Some research designs are better at revealing cause-and-effect relationships than others. True experimental designs are the best possible designs for illuminating causal relationships, but it is not always possible to use such designs.

Design Terminology

Research design terms can be confusing because there is inconsistency among writers. Also, design terms used by medical researchers are often different from those used by social scientists. Early nurse researchers got research training in social science fields such as psychology before doctoral training became available in nursing schools, and so social scientific terms have prevailed in the nursing literature.

Nurses interested in establishing an evidence-based practice must comprehend studies from many disciplines. We use both medical and social science terms in this book. The first column of Table 9.1 shows design terms used by social scientists and the second shows corresponding terms used by medical researchers.

EXPERIMENTAL DESIGN

A basic distinction in quantitative research design is between experimental and nonexperimental research. In an **experiment** (typically called a **randomized controlled trial, RCT**), researchers are active agents, not simply observers. Early physical scientists learned that although observation is valuable, complexities in nature often made it difficult to disentangle relationships. This problem was addressed by isolating phenomena and controlling the conditions under which they occurred. The 20th century witnessed the acceptance of experimental methods by researchers interested in human physiology and behavior.

Controlled experiments are considered the *gold standard* for yielding reliable evidence about causes and effects. Experimenters can be relatively confident in the veracity of causal relationships because

TABLE 9.1 • Research Design Terminology in the Social Scientific and Medical Literature

SOCIAL SCIENTIFIC TERM	MEDICAL RESEARCH TERM
Experiment, true experiment, experimental study	Randomized controlled trial, randomized clinical trial, RCT
Quasi-experiment, quasi-experimental study	Controlled clinical trial; clinical trial without randomization
Nonexperimental study; correlational study	Observational study
Retrospective study	Case–control study
Prospective nonexperimental study	Cohort study
Group or condition (e.g., experimental or control group/ condition)	Group or arm (e.g., intervention or control arm)
Experimental group	Treatment or intervention group
Dependent variable	Outcome or endpoint

they are observed under controlled conditions and meet the criteria for causality. Hypotheses are never *proved* by scientific methods, but RCTs offer the most convincing evidence about whether one variable has a casual effect on another.

A true experimental or RCT design is characterized by the following properties:

- *Manipulation:* the researcher *does* something to at least some participants—there is some type of intervention
- *Control:* the researcher introduces controls, including devising a counterfactual approximation—usually, a control group that does not receive the intervention
- *Randomization:* the researcher assigns participants to a control or experimental condition on a random basis

Design Features of True Experiments

Researchers have many options in designing an experiment. We begin by discussing several features of experimental designs.

Manipulation: The Experimental Intervention

Manipulation involves *doing* something to study participants. Experimenters manipulate the independent variable by administering a **treatment** (or **intervention** [I]) to some people and withholding it from others (C), or by administering alternative treatments to two or more groups. Experimenters deliberately *vary* the independent variable (the presumed cause) and observe the effect on the outcome (O)—which is sometimes referred to as an **endpoint** in the medical literature.

For example, suppose we hypothesized that gentle massage is an effective pain relief strategy for nursing home residents (P). The independent variable, receipt of gentle massage, can be manipulated by giving some patients the massage intervention (I) and withholding it from others (C). We would then compare pain levels (O) in the two groups to see if receipt of the intervention resulted in group differences in average pain levels.

In designing RCTs, researchers make many decisions about what the experimental condition entails. To get a fair test, the intervention should be appropriate to the problem, consistent with a theoretical rationale, and of sufficient intensity and duration that effects might reasonably be expected. The full nature of the intervention must be delineated in formal **intervention protocols** that spell out exactly what the treatment is. Here are some questions intervention researchers need to address:

- What *is* the intervention, and how does it differ from usual methods of care?
- What is the dosage or intensity of the intervention?

- Over how long a period will the intervention be administered, how frequently will it be administered, and when will the treatment begin (e.g., 2 hours after surgery)?
- Who will administer the intervention? What are their credentials? What type of special training will they need?
- Under what conditions will the intervention be withdrawn or altered?

The goal in most RCTs is to have an identical intervention for all people in the treatment group. For example, in most drug studies, those in the experimental group are given the exact same ingredient, in the same dose, administered in exactly the same manner. There has, however, been a growing interest in **tailored interventions** or **patient-centered interventions** (PCIs), whose purpose is to enhance treatment efficacy by taking people's characteristics into account (Lauver et al., 2002). In tailored interventions, each person receives an intervention customized to certain characteristics, such as demographic traits (e.g., gender) or cognitive factors (e.g., reading level). Behavioral interventions based on the Transtheoretical (Stages of change) Model (Chapter 6) usually are PCIs because the intervention is tailored to fit people's readiness to change their behavior. Some evidence suggests that tailored interventions can be effective (e.g., Richards et al., 2007), but special challenges face those conducting PCI research (Beck et al., 2010).

> **TIP** Although PCIs are not universally standardized, they are administered according to well-defined procedures; intervention agents are trained in making systematic decisions about who should get which type of treatment.

Manipulation: The Control Condition

Evidence about relationships requires a comparison. If we were to supplement the diet of premature infants (P) with a special nutrient (I) for 2 weeks, their weight (O) at the end of 2 weeks would tell us nothing about treatment effectiveness. At a bare minimum, we would need to compare posttreatment weight with pretreatment weight to

determine if, at least, their weight had increased. But let us assume that we find an average weight gain of 1 pound. Does this gain support the conclusion that the nutrition supplement (the independent variable) caused weight gain (the outcome)? No, it does not. Babies normally gain weight as they mature. Without a control group—a group that does *not* receive the supplement (C)—it is hard to separate the effects of maturation from those of the treatment.

The term **control group** refers to a group of participants whose performance on an outcome is used to evaluate the performance of the treatment group on the same outcome. Researchers with training in the social sciences use the term "group" or "condition" (e.g., the control group or control condition), but medical researchers often use the term "arm," as in the "intervention arm" or the "control arm" of the study.

The control condition is a proxy for an ideal counterfactual. Researchers have choices about what to use as the counterfactual. Possibilities for the counterfactual include the following:

1. An alternative intervention; for example, participants could receive alternative therapies for pain, such as music versus massage.
2. Standard methods of care—i.e., the usual procedures used to care for patients. This is the most typical control condition in nursing studies.
3. A **placebo** or pseudointervention presumed to have no therapeutic value; for example, in drug studies, some patients get the experimental drug and others get an innocuous substance. Placebos are used to control for the nonpharmaceutical effects of drugs, such as extra attention. There can, however, be **placebo effects**—changes in the outcome attributable to the placebo condition—because of participants' expectations of benefits or harms.

Example of a Placebo Control Group

Saad and an interprofessional team (2018) tested the effect of vitamin D supplementation in children with autism spectrum disorder (ASD). They randomly assigned 109 children with ASD to receive vitamin D or a placebo for 4 months.

4. Sometimes researchers use an **attention control group** when they want to rule out the possibility that intervention effects are caused by the special attention given to those receiving the intervention, rather than by the actual treatment itself. The idea is to separate the "active ingredients" of the treatment from the "inactive ingredient" of special attention.

Example of an Attention Control Group
Doering and Dogan (2018) did a pilot test of an intervention for postpartum sleep and fatigue. Participants were randomized to the theory-guided intervention that focused on self-management or to an attention control group that received general information about healthy eating and sleep.

5. Different doses or intensities of treatment wherein all participants get some type of intervention, but the experimental group gets an intervention that is richer, more intense, or longer. This approach is attractive when there is a desire to analyze **dose-response effects**, i.e., to test whether larger doses are associated with larger benefits, or whether a smaller (and less costly or burdensome) dose would suffice.

Example of an Alternative Dose Design
Breneman and an interdisciplinary team (2019) studied the effect of two moderate-intensity walking programs with low-dose versus high-dose energy expenditure on night-to-night variability in sleep among older women. Participants were randomized to one of the programs.

6. **Wait-list control group,** with delayed treatment; the control group eventually receives the full intervention after all outcomes are assessed.

In terms of inferential conclusiveness, the best test is between two conditions that are as different as possible, as when the experimental group gets a strong treatment and the control group gets no treatment. Ethically, the wait-list approach (number 6) is appealing, but may be hard to do pragmatically. Testing two competing interventions (number 1) also has ethical appeal but runs the risk of ambiguous results if both interventions are moderately effective. This option is,

however, the preferred approach in **comparative effectiveness research (CER)**, which strives to produce evidence that is especially useful for clinical decision-making. CER is described in Chapters 11 and 31.

Some researchers combine several comparison strategies. For example, they might test two alternative treatments (option 1) against a placebo (option 3). The use of three or more comparison groups is often attractive but adds to the cost and complexity of the study.

Example of a Three-Group Randomized Design
Özkan and Zincir (2017) tested the effect of reflexology on the spasticity and muscular function of children with cerebral palsy. Children were randomized to a reflexology group, a placebo group (sham reflexology), or a control group (no intervention).

The control group decision should be based on an underlying conceptualization of how the intervention might "cause" the intended effect and should also reflect what needs to be controlled. For example, if attention control groups are being considered, there should be an underlying conceptualization of the construct of "attention" (Gross, 2005).

Researchers need to carefully spell out their control group strategy. In research reports, researchers sometimes say that the control group got "usual care" without explaining what usual care entailed. In drawing on evidence for practice, nurses need to understand exactly what happened to study participants in different conditions. Barkauskas et al. (2005) and Shadish et al. (2002) offer useful advice about developing a control group strategy.

Randomization

Randomization (also called **random assignment** or **random allocation**) involves assigning participants to treatment conditions at random. *Random* means that participants have an equal chance of being assigned to any group. If people are placed in groups randomly, there is no systematic bias in the groups with respect to preintervention attributes that are potential confounders that could affect outcomes.

Randomization Principles. The purpose of random assignment is to approximate the ideal—but impossible—counterfactual of having the same people exposed to two or more conditions simultaneously. For example, suppose we wanted to study the effectiveness of a contraceptive counseling program for multiparous women (P) who wish to avoid another pregnancy (O). Two groups of women are included—one will be counseled (I) and the other will not (C). Women in the sample are likely to be diverse in terms of age, marital status, income, and so on. Any of these characteristics could affect a woman's contraceptive use, independent of whether she receives counseling. We need to have the "counsel" and "no counsel" groups equal with respect to confounding traits to assess the impact of counseling on subsequent pregnancies. Random assignment of people to one group or the other is designed to perform this equalization function.

Although randomization is the preferred method for equalizing groups, there is no *guarantee* that the groups will be equal. The risk of unequal groups is high when sample size is small. For example, with a sample of only 10—5 men and 5 women—it is possible that all 5 men would be assigned to one group and all 5 women to the other. The likelihood of getting markedly unequal groups is reduced as the sample size increases.

You may wonder why we do not consciously control characteristics that are likely to affect the outcome through **matching**. For example, if matching were used in the contraceptive counseling study, we could ensure that if there were a married, 38-year-old woman with three children in the experimental group, there would be a married, 38-year-old woman with three children in the control group. To match effectively, however, we must know the characteristics that are likely to affect the outcome, but this knowledge is often imperfect. Even if we knew the relevant traits, the complications of matching on more than two or three confounders simultaneously are prohibitive. With random assignment, *all* personal characteristics—age, income, health status, and so on— are likely to be equally distributed in all groups. Over the long run, randomized groups tend to be counterbalanced with respect to an infinite number of biologic, psychological, economic, and social traits.

Basic Randomization. The most straightforward randomization procedure for a two-group design is to simply allocate each person as they enroll into a study on a random basis—for example, by flipping a coin. If the coin comes up "heads," a participant would be assigned to one group; if it comes up "tails," he or she would be assigned to the other group. This type of randomization, with no restrictions, is sometimes called *complete randomization*. Each successive person has a 50-50 chance of being assigned to the intervention group. The problem with this approach is that large imbalances in group size can occur, especially when the sample size is small. For example, with a sample of 10 subjects, there is only a 25% probability that perfect balance (5 per group) would result. In other words, three times out of four, the intervention and control groups would be of unequal size, by chance alone. This method is not recommended with sample sizes less than 200 (Lachin et al., 1988).

Researchers often want treatment groups of equal size or with predesignated proportions. *Simple randomization* involves starting with a known sample size, and then prespecifying the proportion of subjects who will be randomly allocated to different treatment conditions. To illustrate simple randomization, suppose we were testing two interventions to reduce the anxiety of children who are about to undergo tonsillectomy. One intervention involves giving structured information about the surgical team's activities (procedural information); the other involves structured information about what the child will feel (sensation information). A third control group receives no special intervention. We have a sample of 15 children, and 5 will be randomly assigned to each group.

Before widespread availability of computers, researchers used a **table of random numbers** to randomize. A small portion of such a table is shown in Table 9.2. In a table of random numbers, any digit from 0 to 9 is equally likely to follow any

TABLE 9.2 • Small Table of Random Digits

46	85	05	23	26	34	67	75	83	00	74	91	06	43	45
69	24	89	34	60	45	30	50	75	21	61	31	83	18	55
14	01	33	17	92	59	74	76	72	77	76	50	33	45	13
56	30	38	73	15	16	**52**	06	96	76	11	65	49	98	93
81	30	44	85	85	68	65	22	73	76	92	85	25	58	66
70	28	42	43	26	79	37	59	52	20	01	15	96	32	67
90	41	59	36	14	33	52	12	66	65	55	82	34	76	41
39	90	40	21	15	59	58	94	90	67	66	82	14	15	75
88	15	20	00	80	20	55	49	14	09	96	27	74	82	57
45	13	46	35	45	59	40	47	20	59	43	94	75	16	80
70	01	41	50	21	41	29	06	73	12	71	85	71	59	57
37	23	93	32	95	05	87	00	11	19	92	78	42	63	40
18	63	73	75	09	82	44	49	90	05	04	92	17	37	01
05	32	78	21	62	20	24	78	17	59	45	19	72	53	32
95	09	66	79	46	48	46	08	55	58	15	19	02	87	82
43	25	38	41	45	60	83	32	59	83	01	29	14	13	49
80	85	40	92	79	43	52	90	63	18	38	38	47	47	61
81	08	87	70	74	88	72	25	67	36	66	16	44	94	31
84	89	07	80	02	94	81	03	19	00	54	10	58	34	36

other digit. Going in any direction from any point in the table produces a random sequence.

In our example, we would number the 15 children from 1 to 15, as shown in column 2 of Table 9.3, and then draw numbers between 01 and 15 from the random number table. To find a random starting point, you can close your eyes and let your finger fall at some point on the table. For this example, assume that our starting point is at number 52, bolded in Table 9.2. We can move in any direction from that point, selecting numbers that fall between 01 and 15. Let us move to the right, looking at two-digit combinations. The number to the right of 52 is 06. The person whose number is 06, Alexander, is assigned to group I. Moving along, the next number within our range is 11. (To find numbers in the desired range, we bypass numbers between 16 and 99.) Violet, whose number is 11, is also assigned to group I. The next three numbers are 01, 15, and 14. Thus, Alaine, Christopher, and Paul are assigned to group I. The next five numbers between 01 and 15 in the table are used to assign five children to group II, and the remaining five are put into group III. Note that numbers often reappear in the table before

TABLE 9.3 • Example for Random Assignment Procedure

CHILD'S NAME	NUMBER	GROUP ASSIGNMENT
Alaine	01	I
Kristina	02	III
Julia	03	III
Lauren	04	II
Grace	05	II
Alexander	06	I
Norah	07	III
Cormac	08	III
Ronan	09	II
Cullen	10	III
Violet	11	I
Maren	12	II
Leo	13	II
Paul	14	I
Christopher	15	I

the task is completed. For example, the number 15 appeared four times during this randomization. This is normal because the numbers are random.

We can look at the three groups to see if they are similar for one discernible trait, gender. We started out with eight girls and seven boys. Randomization did a fairly good job of allocating boys and girls similarly across the three groups: there are 2, 3, and 3 girls and 3, 2, and 2 boys in groups I through III, respectively. We must hope that other characteristics (e.g., age, initial anxiety) are also well distributed in the randomized groups. The larger the sample, the stronger the likelihood that the groups will be balanced on all factors that could affect the outcome.

Researchers usually assign participants proportionately to groups being compared. For example, a sample of 300 participants in a two-group design would generally be allocated 150 to the treatment group and 150 to the control group. If there were three groups, there would be 100 per group. It is also possible (and sometimes desirable ethically) to have a different allocation. For example, if an especially promising treatment were developed, we could assign 200 to the treatment group and 100 to the control group. Such an allocation does, however, make it more difficult to detect treatment effects at statistically significant levels—or, to put it another way, the overall sample size must be larger to attain the same level of statistical reliability.

Computerized resources are available for free on the Internet to help with randomization (e.g., www.randomizer.org, which has a useful tutorial). Standard statistical software packages (e.g., SPSS or SAS) can also be used.

TIP There is considerable confusion—even in research methods textbooks—about random assignment versus random sampling. Randomization is a *signature* of an experimental design. If participants are not randomly allocated to conditions, then the design is not a true experiment. Random *sampling*, by contrast, is a method of selecting people for a study (see Chapter 13). Random sampling is *not* a signature of an experiment. In fact, most RCTs do *not* involve random sampling.

Randomization Procedures. The success of randomization depends on two factors. First, the allocation process should be truly random. Second, there must be strict adherence to the randomization schedule. The latter can be achieved if the allocation is *unpredictable* (for both participants and those enrolling them) and *tamperproof*. Random assignment should involve **allocation concealment** that prevents those who enroll participants from knowing upcoming assignments, to avoid potential biases. As an example, if the person doing the enrollment knew that the next person would be assigned to a promising intervention, he or she might defer enrollment until a needier patient enrolled.

Several methods of allocation concealment have been devised, several of which involve developing a randomization schedule before the study begins. This is advantageous when people do not enter a study simultaneously, but rather on a *rolling enrollment* basis. One method is to have *sequentially numbered, opaque sealed envelopes (SNOSE)* containing assignment information. Participants entering the study receive the next envelope in the sequence (for procedural suggestions, see Doig & Simpson, 2005). The gold standard approach is to have treatment allocation performed by an agent unconnected with enrollment and communicated to researchers by telephone or e-mail. Herbison et al. (2011) found, however, that trials with a SNOSE system had a comparable risk of bias as trials with centralized randomization.

TIP Downs et al. (2010) offer recommendations for avoiding practical problems in implementing randomization.

Timing of randomization is important. Study eligibility—whether a person meets the criteria for inclusion—should be ascertained before randomization. If **baseline data** (preintervention data on outcomes) are collected, this should occur before randomization to rule out any possibility that knowledge of the group assignment might distort baseline measurements. Randomization should occur as closely as possible to the intervention start-up, to increase the likelihood that participants will actually receive the condition to

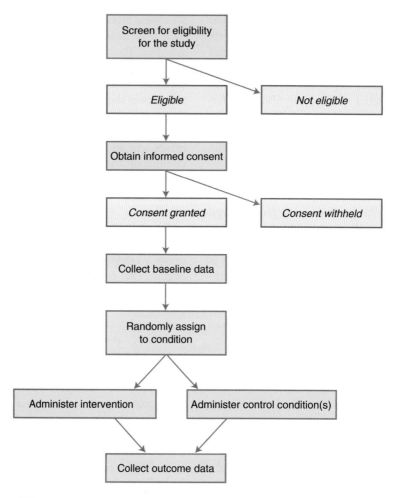

FIGURE 9.1 Sequence of steps in a standard two-arm randomized design.

which they have been assigned. Figure 9.1 illustrates the sequence of steps that occurs in most RCTs, including the timing for obtaining informed consent.

> **TIP** Some studies use **quasi-randomization**, which is a method of allocating participants in a manner that is not strictly random. For example, participants may be assigned to groups on an alternating basis (every other person to a group) or based on whether their birthdate is an odd or even number. These are not true methods of randomization.

Randomization Variants. Simple or complete randomization is used in many nursing studies, but variants of randomization offer advantages in terms of ensuring group comparability or minimizing certain biases. These variants include the following:

- **Stratified randomization,** in which randomization occurs separately for distinct subgroups (e.g., males and females);
- **Permuted block randomization,** in which people are allocated to groups in small, randomly sized blocks to ensure a balanced distribution in each block;

- **Urn randomization,** in which group balance is continuously monitored and the allocation probability is adjusted when an imbalance occurs (i.e., the probability of assignment becomes higher for the condition with fewer participants);
- **Randomized consent,** in which randomization occurs prior to obtaining informed consent (also called a **Zelen design**);
- **Partial randomization,** in which only people without a strong treatment preference are randomized—sometimes called **partially randomized patient preference (PRPP)**; and
- **Cluster randomization,** which involves randomly assigning clusters (e.g., hospitals) rather than people to different treatment groups.

S: These and other randomization variants are described in greater detail in the Supplement to Chapter 9 on thePoint.

Blinding or Masking

People usually want things to turn out well. Researchers want their ideas to work, and they want their hypotheses supported. Participants want to be helpful and want to present themselves in a positive light. These tendencies can lead to biases because they can affect what participants do and say (and what researchers ask and perceive) in ways that distort the truth.

A procedure called **blinding** (or **masking**) is often used in RCTs to prevent biases stemming from *awareness*. Blinding involves concealing information from participants, data collectors, care providers, intervention agents, or data analysts to enhance objectivity and minimize **expectation bias**. For example, if participants are not aware of whether they are getting an experimental drug or a placebo, then their outcomes cannot be influenced by their expectations of its efficacy. Blinding typically involves disguising or withholding information about participants' status in the study (e.g., whether they are in the experimental or control group) but can also involve withholding information about study hypotheses or baseline performance on outcomes.

Lack of blinding can result in several types of bias. **Performance bias** refers to systematic differences in the care provided to members of different groups of participants, apart from any intervention. For example, those delivering an intervention might treat participants in groups differently (e.g., with greater attentiveness), apart from the intervention itself. Efforts to avoid performance bias usually involve blinding participants and the agents who deliver treatments. **Detection** (or **ascertainment**) bias, which concerns systematic differences between groups in how outcome variables are measured, verified, or recorded, is addressed by blinding those who collect the outcome data or, in some cases, those who analyze the data.

Unlike allocation concealment, blinding is not always possible. Drug studies often lend themselves to blinding but many nursing interventions do not. For example, if the intervention were a smoking cessation program, participants would know whether they were receiving the intervention, and the interventionist would be aware of who was in the program. However, it is usually possible, and desirable, to mask participants' treatment status from people collecting outcome data and from clinicians providing normal care.

> **TIP** Blinding may not be necessary if subjectivity in measuring the outcome is low. For example, participants' ratings of pain are susceptible to biases stemming from their own or data collectors' awareness of treatment group status. Hospital readmission and length of hospital stay, on the other hand, are less likely to be affected by people's awareness.

When blinding is not used, the study is an *open study*, in contrast to a *closed study*. When blinding is used with only one group of people (e.g., study participants), it is sometimes called a **single-blind study**. When it is possible to mask with two groups (e.g., those delivering an intervention and those receiving it), it is sometimes called **double blind**. However, recent guidelines recommend that researchers not use these terms without explicitly stating which groups were blinded because the term "double blind" has been used to refer to many different combinations of blinded groups (Moher et al., 2010).

The term *blinding*, though widely used, has been criticized because of possible pejorative connotations. The American Psychological Association, for example, has recommended using masking instead. Medical researchers appear to prefer *blinding* unless the people in the study have vision impairments (Schulz et al., 2002). Most nurse researchers use the term *blinding* rather than *masking* (Polit et al., 2011).

Example of an Experiment With Blinding

George et al. (2018) conducted a multicenter RCT to evaluate an oral health program initiated by midwives to improve oral health and birth outcomes for pregnant women. Data collectors and study investigators were blinded to whether participants were in the intervention or control group.

Specific Experimental Designs

Some popular experimental designs are described in this section. We illustrate some of them using design notation from a classic monograph (Campbell & Stanley, 1963). In this system, R means random assignment; O represents outcome measurements; and X stands for exposure to the intervention. Each row designates a different group. (Supplement A to Chapter 10 on thePoint provides more detail about various designs using this notation).

Basic Experimental Designs

Earlier in this chapter, we described a study that tested the effect of gentle massage on pain in nursing home residents. This example illustrates a simple design that is sometimes called a **posttest-only design** (or *after-only design*) because data on the outcome are collected only once—after randomization and completion of the intervention. Here is the notation for this design, which shows that both groups are randomized (R), but only the first group gets the intervention (X):

R   X   O
R   O

A second basic design involves collecting baseline data, like the design in Figure 9.1. Suppose

we hypothesized that convective airflow blankets are more effective than conductive water-flow blankets in cooling critically ill febrile patients. Our design involves assigning patients to the two blanket types (the independent variable) and measuring the outcome (body temperature) twice, before and after the intervention. Here is a diagram for this design:

R O_1 X O_2
R O_1 O_2

This design allows us to examine whether one blanket type is more effective than the other in *reducing* fever; with this design researchers can examine *change*. This design is a **pretest–posttest design** (*before–after design*), which are mixed designs: analyses can examine both differences *between* groups and changes *within* groups over time. Some pretest–posttest designs include data collection at multiple postintervention points, i.e., *repeated measures designs*. These basic designs can be "tweaked" in various ways—for example, the design could involve comparison of three or more groups.

Example of a Pretest–Posttest Experimental Design

Ng and Wong (2018) studied the effects of a home-based palliative program on the quality of life, symptom burden, functional status, and satisfaction with care of patients with end-stage heart failure. The outcomes for patients in the intervention and control groups were measured at baseline, and at 4 and 6 weeks after discharge from the hospital.

Factorial Design

Most experimental designs involve manipulating only one independent variable, but it is possible to manipulate two or more variables simultaneously. Suppose we wanted to compare two therapies for premature infants: tactile versus auditory stimulation. We also want to learn if the daily *amount* of stimulation (15, 30, or 45 minutes) affects infants' progress. The outcomes are measures of infant development (e.g., weight gain). Figure 9.2 illustrates the structure of this RCT.

This **factorial design** allows us to address three research questions:

1. Does auditory stimulation have a more beneficial effect on premature infants' weight gain than tactile stimulation, or vice versa?
2. Is amount of stimulation (independent of type) related to infants' weight gain?
3. Is auditory stimulation most effective when linked to a certain dose and tactile stimulation most effective when coupled with a different dose?

The third question shows the strength of factorial designs: they permit us to test not only **main effects** (effects from the manipulated variables, as in questions 1 and 2) but also **interaction effects** (effects from combining treatments). Our results may indicate that 30 minutes of auditory stimulation is the most beneficial treatment. We could not have learned this by conducting two separate studies that manipulated one independent variable and held the second one constant.

In factorial experiments, participants are randomly assigned to a specific combination of conditions. In our example (Figure 9.2), infants would be assigned randomly to one of six **cells**—i.e., six treatment conditions. The two independent variables in a factorial design are the **factors**. Type of stimulation is factor A, and amount of daily exposure is factor B. Level 1 of factor A is auditory and level 2 is tactile. When describing the dimensions of the design, researchers refer to the number of **levels**. The design in Figure 9.2 is a 2 × 3 design: two levels in factor A times three

levels in factor B. Factorial experiments with more than two factors are rare.

Example of a Factorial Design
Adams et al. (2017) used a factorial design in their study of strategies to increase adults' physical activity. In their 2 × 2 design, one factor was type of goal setting strategy (adaptive versus static goals for number of steps per day) and the other factor was timing of rewards (immediate versus delayed). The outcome was number of steps walked per day.

Crossover Design

Thus far, we have described RCTs in which different people are randomly assigned to different conditions. For instance, in the previous example, infants who received auditory stimulation were not the same infants as those who received tactile stimulation. A **crossover design** involves exposing the same people to more than one condition. This within-subjects design has the advantage of ensuring the highest possible equivalence among participants exposed to different conditions—the groups being compared are equal with respect to age, weight, and so on because they are composed of the same people.

Because randomization is a signature of an experiment, participants in a crossover design must be randomly assigned to different *orderings* of treatments. For example, if a crossover design were used to compare the effects of auditory and tactile stimulation on infant development, some infants would be randomly assigned to receive auditory stimulation first, and others would be assigned to receive tactile stimulation first. When there are three or more conditions to which participants will be exposed, the procedure of **counterbalancing** can be used to rule out ordering effects. For example, if there were three conditions (A, B, C), participants would be randomly assigned to one of six counterbalanced orderings:

A, B, C	A, C, B
B, C, A	B, A, C
C, A, B	C, B, A

Type of stimulation

		Auditory A1		Tactile A2	
Daily dose	15 min. B1	A1	B1	A2	B1
	30 min. B2	A1	B2	A2	B2
	45 min. B3	A1	B3	A2	B3

FIGURE 9.2 Example of a 2 × 3 factorial design.

Although crossover designs are powerful, they are inappropriate for certain research questions because of possible **carry-over effects**. When people are exposed to two different conditions, they may be influenced in the second condition by their experience in the first one. Drug studies, for example, rarely use a crossover design because drug B administered *after* drug A is not necessarily the same treatment as drug B administered *before* drug A. When carry-over effects are a potential concern, researchers often have a **washout period** in between the treatments (i.e., a period of no treatment exposure).

Example of a Crossover Design
Reddy and an interprofessional team (2018) used a randomized crossover design with a sample of patients with type 1 diabetes to test the effect of different exercise routines on sleep and nocturnal hypoglycemia.

TIP New experimental designs are emerging in response to growing interest in personalized health care. Several of these designs, such as **N-of-1 trials** and **adaptive trials** are discussed in Chapter 31, which focuses on the applicability and relevance of research evidence.

Strengths and Limitations of Experiments

In this section, we explore why experimental designs are held in high esteem and examine some limitations.

Experimental Strengths

Experimental designs are the gold standard for testing interventions because they yield strong evidence about intervention effectiveness. Experiments offer greater corroboration than other approaches that, *if* the independent variable (e.g., diet, drug, teaching approach) is varied, *then* certain consequences to the outcomes (e.g., weight loss, recovery, learning) will ensue. The great strength of RCTs, then, lies in the confidence with which causal relationships can be inferred. Through the controls imposed

by manipulation, comparison, and randomization, alternative explanations can be discredited. It is because of this strength that meta-analyses of RCTs, which integrate evidence from multiple experiments, are at the pinnacle of evidence hierarchies for Therapy questions (Figure 2.2 of Chapter 2).

Experimental Limitations

Despite the benefits of experiments, they also have limitations. First, constraints—which we discuss later in this chapter—often make an experimental approach impractical or impossible.

TIP Shadish et al. (2002) described 10 situations that are especially conducive to randomized experiments; these are summarized in a table in the Toolkit.

Experiments are sometimes criticized for their artificiality, which partly stems from the requirements for comparable treatment within randomized groups, with strict adherence to protocols. In ordinary life, by contrast, we interact with people in nonformulaic ways. A related concern is that the rigidity of the research process can undermine translation into real-world settings, an issue we address in Chapter 31.

Problems also emerge when participants "opt out" of the intervention. Suppose, for example, that we randomly assigned patients with HIV to a support group intervention or to a control group. Intervention subjects who elect not to participate in the support groups, or who participate infrequently, are in a "condition" that looks more like the control condition than the experimental one. The treatment is diluted through nonparticipation, and it may be difficult to detect treatment effects, no matter how effective it might otherwise have been.

Another potential problem is the **Hawthorne effect**, which is caused by people's expectations. The term is derived from a series of experiments conducted at the Hawthorne plant of the Western Electric Corporation in which various environmental conditions, such as light and working hours, were varied to test their effects on worker productivity. Regardless of what change was introduced, that is, whether the light was made better or worse, productivity increased. Knowledge of being in the study (not just knowledge of being in a particular group) appears to have affected people's behavior, obscuring the effect of the intervention.

In sum, despite the superiority of RCTs for testing causal hypotheses, they have several limitations, some of which may make them difficult to apply to real clinical problems. Nevertheless, with the growing demand for strong evidence for practice, experimental designs are increasingly being used to test the effects of nursing interventions.

QUASI-EXPERIMENTS

Quasi-experiments, sometimes called *controlled trials without randomization* in the medical literature, involve an intervention, but they lack randomization, the signature of a true experiment. Some quasi-experiments even lack a control group. The signature of a quasi-experimental design, then, is an intervention in the absence of randomization.

Quasi-Experimental Designs

We describe a few widely used quasi-experimental designs in this section, and for some we use the schematic notation introduced earlier.

Nonequivalent Control Group Designs
The **nonequivalent control group pretest–posttest design** (sometimes called a *controlled before–after design* in the medical literature) involves two groups of participants, for whom outcomes are measured before and after the intervention. For example, suppose we wished to study the effect of a new chair yoga intervention for older people. The intervention is being offered to everyone at a community senior center, and randomization is not workable. For comparative purposes, we collect outcome data at a different senior center that is not instituting the intervention. Data on health-related quality of

life are collected from both groups at baseline and again 10 weeks after implementing the intervention. Here is a schematic representation of this design:

$$O_1 \qquad X \qquad O_2$$
$$O_1 \qquad \qquad O_2$$

The top line represents those receiving the intervention (X) at the experimental site and the second row represents the group at the comparison site. This diagram is identical to the experimental pretest–posttest design depicted earlier *except* there is no "R"—participants have not been randomized to groups. The quasi-experimental design is weaker because *it cannot be assumed that the experimental and comparison groups are initially equivalent.* Because there is no randomization, quasi-experimental comparisons provide a weaker counterfactual than experimental comparisons. The design is nevertheless strong because baseline data allow us to assess whether patients in the two centers had similar quality of life scores at the outset. If the two groups are similar, on average, at baseline, we could be relatively confident inferring that posttest differences in outcomes were the result of the yoga intervention. If quality of life scores are different initially, however, it will be difficult to interpret posttest differences. Note that in quasi-experiments, the term **comparison group** is used in lieu of *control group* to refer to the group with whom the treatment group is compared.

Now suppose we had been unable to collect baseline data:

$$X \qquad \qquad O$$
$$\qquad \qquad O$$

This design has a major flaw. We no longer have information about initial equivalence of people in the two senior centers. If quality of life in the experimental center is higher than that in the control site at posttest, can we conclude that the intervention *caused* improved quality of life? An alternative explanation for posttest differences is that the people in the two centers differed at the outset. This *nonequivalent control group posttest-only design* is a much weaker quasi-experimental design.

Example of a Nonequivalent Control Group Pretest–Posttest Design

Takahashi and an interprofessional team (2018) used a quasi-experimental design to test the effectiveness of community-based interventions to reduce harmful alcohol consumption in rural Kenya. Problem drinkers in one village got the brief intervention with motivational talks, those in another village got the intervention without the talks, and those in a third village received only general health information. Alcohol consumption was measured at baseline and follow-up.

In lieu of using a contemporaneous comparison group, researchers sometimes use a **historical comparison group**. That is, comparison data are gathered from other people *before* implementing the intervention. Even when the people are from the same institutional setting, however, it is risky to assume that the two groups are comparable, or that the environments are comparable except for the new intervention. The possibility remains that something other than the intervention could account for observed differences in outcomes.

Example of a Historical Comparison Group

Barta et al. (2017) studied the reconviction rates of driving-under-the-influence (DUI) offenders who participated in an intensive supervision program that included prerelease psycho-education and close postrelease supervision. Their rates of reconviction were compared with those of an historical comparison group of 302 DUI offenders.

Time Series Designs

In the designs just described, a control group was used but randomization was not, but some quasi-experiments have neither. Suppose that a hospital implemented rapid response teams (RRTs) in its acute care units. Administrators want to examine the effects on patient outcomes (e.g., unplanned ICU admissions, mortality rate). For the purposes of this example, assume no other hospital could serve as a good comparison. One comparison that can be made is a before–after contrast. If RRTs were to be implemented in January, the mortality rate (for example) during the 3 months before

RRTs could be compared with the mortality rate during the subsequent 3-month period. The schematic representation of such a study is:

$$O_1 \qquad X \qquad O_2$$

This one-group pretest–posttest design seems straightforward, but it has several weaknesses. What if either of the 3-month periods is atypical, apart from the innovation? What about the effects of other policy changes inaugurated during the same period? What about the effects of external factors that influence mortality, such as a flu outbreak? This design cannot control these factors.

In our RRT example, the design could be modified so that some alternative explanations for changes in mortality could be ruled out. One such design is the **time series design** (or *interrupted time series design*). In a time series, data are collected over an extended period during which an intervention is introduced, as in this diagram:

$$O_1 \quad O_2 \quad O_3 \quad O_4 \quad X \quad O_5 \quad O_6 \quad O_7 \quad O_8$$

Here, O_1 through O_4 represent four separate instances of preintervention outcome measurement, X is the introduction of the intervention, and O_5 through O_8 represent four posttreatment measurements. In our example, O_1 might be the number of deaths in January through March in the year before the new RRT system, O_2 the number of deaths in April through June, and so forth. After RRTs are introduced, data on mortality are collected for four consecutive 3-month periods, giving us observations O_5 through O_8.

Even though the time series design does not eliminate all interpretive challenges, the extended time period strengthens our ability to attribute change to the intervention. Figure 9.3 demonstrates why this is so. The line graphs (*A and B*) in the figure show two possible outcome patterns for eight mortality observations. The vertical dotted line in the center represents the introduction of the RRT system. Patterns *A* and *B* both reflect a feature common to time series studies—fluctuation from one data point to another. These fluctuations are normal. One would not expect that, if 480 patients died in a hospital in 1 year, the deaths would be spaced evenly with 40 per month. It is precisely because of these fluctuations that the one-group pretest–posttest design, with only one observation before and after the intervention, is so weak.

Let us compare the interpretations for the outcomes shown in Figure 9.3. In both patterns A and B, mortality decreased between O_4 and O_5, immediately after RRTs were implemented. In B, however, the number of deaths rose at O_6 and continued to rise at O_7. The decrease at O_5 looks similar to other apparently haphazard fluctuations in mortality. In A, on the other hand, the number of deaths decreased at O_5 and remained relatively low for subsequent observations. There may well be other explanations for a change in the mortality rate, but the time series design permits us to rule out the possibility that the data reflect unstable measurements of deaths at only two points in time. If we had used a simple pretest–posttest design, it would have been analogous to obtaining the measurements at O_4 and O_5 of Figure 9.3 only.

The outcomes in both A and B are the same at these two time points. The broader time perspective leads us to draw different conclusions about the effects of RRTs. Nevertheless, the absence of a comparison group means that the design does not yield an ideal counterfactual.

Example of a Time Series Design

Norman et al. (2017) tested the effect of a multimodal educational intervention designed to reduce the unnecessary use of urinary catheters in hospital patients at a large teaching hospital. Incidence of urinary catheterizations was measured monthly for over 3 years; the monthly incidence declined after the intervention.

One drawback of a time series design is that many data points—100 or more—are recommended for a traditional analysis (Shadish et al., 2002), and the analysis tends to be complex. Nurse researchers have, however, begun to use a versatile approach called **statistical process control (SPC)** to assess effects when they have collected data sequentially over a period of time before and

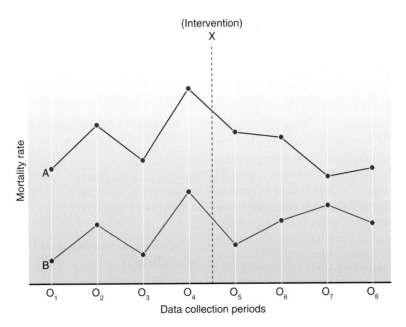

FIGURE 9.3 Two possible time series outcome patterns for quarterly mortality data.

after implementing a practice change (Polit & Chaboyer, 2012). Time series designs with SPC analyses are important in *quality improvement (QI)* projects because randomization is rarely possible in QI (see Chapter 12).

A particularly powerful quasi-experimental design results when the time series and nonequivalent control group designs are combined. In the example just described, a time series nonequivalent control group design would involve collecting data over an extended period from both the hospital introducing the RRTs and another similar hospital not implementing the system. Information from another comparable hospital would make any inferences regarding the effects of RRTs more convincing because other external factors influencing the trends (e.g., a flu outbreak) would likely be similar in both cases.

Numerous variations on the simple time series design are possible. For example, additional evidence regarding the effects of a treatment can be achieved by instituting the treatment at several different points in time, strengthening the treatment over time, or instituting the treatment at one point in time and then withdrawing it at a later point, sometimes with reinstitution.

Other Quasi-Experimental Designs

Earlier in this chapter, we mentioned the PRPP design. Those without a strong treatment preference are randomized, but those *with* a preference are given the condition they prefer and are followed up as part of the study. The two randomized groups are part of the true experiment, but the two groups who get their preference are part of a quasi-experiment. This type of design can yield valuable information about the kind of people who prefer one condition over another and may help persuade people to participate in a study. However, evidence of treatment effectiveness is weak in the quasi-experimental segment because the people who elected a certain treatment likely differ from those who opted for the alternative—and these preintervention differences, rather than the alternative treatments, could account for observed differences in outcomes. Yet, evidence

from the quasi-experiment could usefully support or qualify evidence from the experimental portion of the study.

Example of a PRPP Design

Chalmers and an interprofessional team (2018) are assessing the feasibility of providing a psychosocial assessment via telehealth (versus face-to-face) to adolescents and young adults receiving treatment for cancer. The trial is using a PRPP design—participants with strong preferences are being given the assessment in the manner they chose and those without a preference are being randomized.

Another quasi-experimental approach—sometimes embedded within a true experiment—is a **dose–response** design in which the outcomes of those receiving different doses of an intervention (not as a result of randomization) are compared. For example, in lengthy interventions, some people attend more sessions or get more intensive treatment than others. The rationale for a quasi-experimental dose–response analysis is that if a larger dose corresponds to better outcomes, the results provide supporting evidence that the treatment caused the outcome. The difficulty, however, is that people tend to get different treatment doses because of differences in motivation, physical function, or other characteristics that could be the true cause of outcome differences. Nevertheless, dose–response evidence may yield useful information.

Example of a Dose–Response Analysis

Smith et al. (2018) implemented an online resilience training program. The analysis tested a dose–response effect—that is, whether the amount of time spent in the training program affected the amount of change in participants' resilience.

Quasi-Experimental and Comparison Conditions

Researchers using a quasi-experimental approach should develop intervention protocols that document what the interventions entail. Researchers need to be especially careful in understanding and documenting the counterfactual. In the case of nonequivalent control group designs, this means understanding the conditions to which the comparison group is exposed (e.g., activities at the senior center without the yoga intervention in our example). In time series designs, the counterfactual is the conditions existing before implementing the intervention, and these should be understood. Blinding should be used, to the extent possible—indeed, this may be more feasible in a quasi-experiment than in an RCT.

Strengths and Limitations of Quasi-Experiments

A major strength of quasi-experiments is that they are practical. In clinical settings, it may be impossible to conduct true experimental tests of nursing interventions. Strong quasi-experimental designs introduce some research control when full experimental rigor is not possible.

Another advantage of quasi-experiments is that patients are not always willing to relinquish control over their treatment condition. Indeed, people are increasingly unwilling to volunteer to be randomized in clinical trials (Vedelø & Lomborg, 2011). Quasi-experimental designs, because they do not involve random assignment, are likely to be acceptable to a broader group of people. This, in turn, has positive implications for the generalizability of the results—but the problem is that the evidence may be less conclusive.

Researchers using quasi-experimental designs should realize their weaknesses and take them into account in interpreting results. When a quasi-experimental design is used, there usually are **rival hypotheses** competing with the intervention as explanations for the results. (This issue relates to *internal validity*, discussed in Chapter 10.) Take as an example the case in which we administer a special diet to frail nursing home residents to assess its effects on weight gain. If we use no comparison group or a nonequivalent control group and then observe a weight gain, we must ask: Is it *plausible* that some other factor caused the gain? Is it *plausible* that pretreatment differences between the intervention and comparison groups resulted in differential gain? Is it *plausible* that the elders on average gained weight because the frailest patients died? If the answer is "yes" to such questions, then inferences about the causal effect of the intervention are weakened. The plausibility of any particular rival explanation typically cannot be known unequivocally, but nevertheless a careful *plausibility analysis* should be undertaken. We describe how to do this in Supplement B of Chapter 10.🅢

> **TIP** The *Journal of Clinical Epidemiology* has published an excellent 13-paper series on quasi-experimental designs. Examples include papers by Geldsetzer and Fawzi (2017) and Bärnighausen et al. (2017).

NONEXPERIMENTAL/ OBSERVATIONAL RESEARCH

Many research questions—including ones seeking to establish causal relationships—cannot be addressed with an experimental or quasi-experimental design. For example, at the beginning of this chapter we posed this Prognosis question: Do birthweights less than 1,500 g *cause* developmental delays in children? Clearly, we cannot manipulate birthweight, the independent variable. One way to answer this question is to compare developmental outcomes for two groups of infants—babies with birthweights above and below 1,500 g. When researchers do not intervene by manipulating the independent variable, the study is **nonexperimental**, or, in the medical literature, **observational**.

Most nursing studies are nonexperimental because most human characteristics (e.g., weight, lactose intolerance) cannot be manipulated. Also, many variables that could *technically* be manipulated cannot be manipulated ethically. For example, if we were studying the effect of prenatal care on infant mortality, it would be unethical to provide such care to one group of pregnant women while deliberately depriving women in a randomized control group. We would need to locate naturally occurring groups of pregnant women who had or had not received prenatal care, and then compare their birth outcomes. The problem, however, is that the two groups of women are likely to differ in terms of other characteristics, such as age, education, and income, any of which individually or in combination could affect infant mortality, independent of prenatal care. Nevertheless, many nonexperimental studies explore cause-and-effect relationships when an experimental design is not possible.

Correlational Cause-Probing Research

When researchers study the effect of a potential *cause* that they cannot manipulate, they use **correlational designs** to examine relationships between variables. A **correlation** is a relationship or association between two variables, that is, a tendency for variation in one variable to be related to variation in another. For example, in human adults, height and weight are correlated because there is a tendency for taller people to weigh more than shorter people.

As mentioned earlier, one criterion for causality is that an empirical relationship (correlation) between variables must be demonstrated. It is risky, however, to infer causal relationships in correlational research. A famous research dictum is relevant: *correlation does not prove causation.* The mere existence of a relationship between variables is not enough to conclude that one variable caused the other, even if the relationship is strong. In experiments, researchers directly control the independent variable; the experimental treatment can be administered to some and withheld from others, and the two groups can be equalized through randomization with respect to everything except the independent variable. In correlational research, investigators do not control the independent variable, which often has already occurred. Groups being compared often differ in ways that affect outcomes of interest—that is, there are usually confounding variables. Although correlational studies are inherently weaker than experimental

studies in confirming causal relationships, different designs offer differing degrees of supportive evidence.

Retrospective Designs

Studies with a **retrospective design** are ones in which a phenomenon existing in the present is linked to phenomena that occurred in the past. The signature of a retrospective study is that the researcher begins with the dependent variable (the effect) and then examines whether it is correlated with one or more previously occurring independent variables (potential causes).

Most early studies of the smoking–lung cancer link used a retrospective **case–control design**, in which researchers began with a group of people who had lung cancer (*cases*) and another group who did not (*controls*). The researchers then looked for differences between the two groups in antecedent circumstances or behaviors, such as smoking.

In designing a case–control study, researchers try to identify controls without the disease or condition who are as similar as possible to the cases on key confounding variables (e.g., age, gender). Researchers sometimes use matching or other techniques to control for confounding variables. To the degree that researchers can demonstrate comparability between cases and controls regarding confounding traits, inferences regarding the presumed cause of the disease are enhanced. The difficulty, however, is that the two groups are almost never totally comparable on factors influencing the outcome. Grimes and Schulz (2005) offer guidance on identifying controls for case–control studies.

Example of a Case–Control Design
Yuan et al. (2018) studied risk factors for death among patients with severe stroke. A total of 188 patients who died of stroke at a university hospital in China were the cases; 188 stroke survivors from the same neurological ICU were randomly selected as the controls. Clinical characteristics of the two groups were compared.

Not all retrospective studies can be described as using a case–control design. Sometimes researchers use a retrospective approach to identify risk factors for different *amounts* of an outcome rather than "caseness." For example, a retrospective design might be used to identify factors predictive of the length of time new mothers breastfed their infants. Such a design often is intended to understand factors that *cause* women to make different breastfeeding decisions (i.e., an Etiology question).

Many retrospective studies are cross-sectional, with data on both the dependent and independent variables collected at a single point in time. In such studies, data for the independent variables often are based on recollection (retrospection)—or the researchers "assume" that the independent variables occurred before the outcome. One problem, however, is that recollection can be biased by subsequent events or memory lapses.

Example of a Retrospective Design

Como (2018) used cross-sectional data in a retrospective study designed to identify factors predictive of perceived physical and mental health among people with chronic heart failure. The independent variables included self-efficacy, health literacy, and medication adherence.

Prospective Nonexperimental Designs

In correlational studies with a **prospective design** (called a **cohort design** in medical circles), researchers start with a presumed cause and then go forward in time to the presumed effect. For example, in prospective lung cancer studies, researchers start with a cohort of adults (P) that includes smokers (I) and nonsmokers (C), and then compare the two groups in terms of subsequent lung cancer incidence (O). The best design for Prognosis questions, and for Etiology questions when randomization is impossible, is a cohort design. A particularly strong design for Prognosis questions is an **inception cohort design**, which involves the study of a group assembled at a common time early in a health disorder or exposure to a putative "cause" of an outcome (e.g., immediately after a traumatic brain injury), and then followed thereafter to assess the outcomes.

Prospective studies are more costly than retrospective studies, in part because prospective studies require at least two rounds of data collection. A lengthy follow-up period may be needed before the outcome of interest occurs, as is the case in prospective studies of cigarette smoking and lung cancer. Also, prospective designs require large samples if the outcome of interest is rare. Another issue is that in a good prospective study, researchers take steps to confirm that all participants are free from the effect (e.g., the disease) at the time the independent variable is measured, and this may be difficult or expensive to do. For example, in prospective smoking/lung cancer studies, lung cancer may be present initially but not yet diagnosed.

Despite these issues, prospective studies are considerably stronger than retrospective studies. Any ambiguity about whether the presumed cause occurred before the effect is resolved in prospective research if the researcher has confirmed the initial absence of the effect. In addition, samples are more likely to be representative, and investigators may be able to impose controls to rule out competing explanations for the results.

TIP The term "prospective" is not synonymous with "longitudinal." Although most nonexperimental prospective studies *are* longitudinal, prospective studies are not *necessarily* longitudinal. Prospective means that information about a possible cause is obtained prior to information about an effect. RCTs are inherently prospective because researchers introduce the intervention and then determine its effect. An RCT that collected outcome data 1 hour after an intervention would be prospective, but not longitudinal.

Some prospective studies are exploratory. Researchers sometimes measure a wide range of possible "causes" at one point in time (e.g., foods consumed), and then examine an outcome of interest at a later point (e.g., a cancer diagnosis). Such studies are usually more convincing than retrospective studies if it can be determined that the outcome was not present initially because time sequences are clear. They are not, however, as powerful as prospective studies that involve specific *a priori* hypotheses and the comparison of cohorts known to differ on a presumed cause. Researchers doing exploratory retrospective or prospective studies are sometimes accused of going on "fishing expeditions" that can lead to erroneous conclusions because of spurious or idiosyncratic relationships in a particular sample of participants.

Example of a Prospective Nonexperimental Study
Ndosi and an interprofessional team (2018) studied the prognosis of infected diabetic foot ulcers. Clinical information was obtained for the patients 12 months after they required antibiotic therapy. The researchers studied factors relating to ulcer healing, such as having single versus multiple ulcers and perfusion grades >2.

Natural Experiments

Researchers are sometimes able to study the outcomes of a **natural experiment** in which a group exposed to a phenomenon with potential health consequences is compared with a nonexposed group. Natural experiments are nonexperimental because the researcher does not intervene, but they are called "natural *experiments*" if people are affected essentially at random. For example, the psychological well-being of people living in a community struck with a natural disaster (e.g., a volcanic eruption) could be compared with the well-being of people living in a similar but unaffected community to assess the toll exacted by the disaster (the independent variable).

Example of a Natural Experiment
Dotson et al. (2016) studied whether the administration of calcium was associated with adverse outcomes in critically ill patients receiving parenteral nutrition. Outcomes such as in-hospital mortality and acute respiratory failure were studied before and after a calcium gluconate shortage, which created the opportunity for this natural experiment.

Path Analytic Studies

Researchers interested in testing theories of causation using nonexperimental data often use a technique called **path analysis** (or similar *causal modeling* techniques). Using sophisticated statistical procedures, researchers test a hypothesized causal chain among a set of independent variables, mediating variables, and a dependent variable. Path analytic procedures allow researchers to test whether nonexperimental data conform sufficiently to the underlying model to justify causal inferences. Path analytic studies can be done within the context of both cross-sectional and longitudinal designs, the latter providing a stronger basis for causal inferences because of the ability to verify time sequences.

Example of a Path Analytic Study
Lau et al. (2018) tested a causal model to explain early breastfeeding initiation. Their path analysis tested hypothesized causal pathways between mode of birth, labor duration, NICU admission, and early skin-to-skin contact and early breastfeeding initiation, the outcome.

Descriptive Research

Descriptive research is a second broad class of nonexperimental research. The purpose of descriptive studies is to observe, describe, and document a situation as it naturally occurs. Sometimes descriptive studies are a starting point for hypothesis generation or theory development.

Descriptive Correlational Studies

Some research problems are cast in noncausal terms. We may ask, for example, whether men are less likely than women to seek assistance for depression, not whether configurations of sex chromosomes *caused* differences in health behavior. Unlike other types of correlational research—such as the cigarette smoking and lung cancer investigations—the aim of **descriptive correlational research** is to describe relationships among variables rather than to support inferences of causality.

Example of a Descriptive Correlational Study
Rosenzweig et al. (2019) conducted a descriptive correlational study to examine the relationship between financial toxicity (out-of-pocket treatment expenses) and quality of life and cancer-related distress in women with metastatic breast cancer.

Studies designed to address Diagnosis/assessment questions—i.e., whether a tool or procedure yields accurate assessment or diagnostic information about a condition or outcome—often involve descriptive correlational designs—although sometimes two procedures or tools are tested against each other for accuracy in RCTs.

Univariate Descriptive Studies

The aim of some descriptive studies is to describe the frequency of occurrence of a behavior or condition, rather than to study relationships. **Univariate descriptive studies** are not necessarily focused on a single variable. For example, a researcher interested in women's experiences during menopause might gather data about the frequency of various symptoms and the use of medications to alleviate symptoms. The study involves multiple variables, but the primary purpose is to describe the status of each, not to study correlations among them.

Two types of descriptive study come from the field of epidemiology. **Prevalence studies** are done to estimate the prevalence rate of some condition (e.g., a disease or a behavior, such as smoking) at a particular point in time. Prevalence studies rely on cross-sectional designs in which data are obtained from the population at risk of the condition. The researcher takes a "snapshot" of the population at risk to determine the extent to which the condition is present. The formula for a **prevalence rate** (PR) is:

$$\frac{\text{Number of cases with the condition or disease}}{\text{Number in the population at risk of being a case}} \times K$$

K is the number of people for whom we want to have the rate established (e.g., per 100 or per 1,000 population). When data are obtained from a sample, the denominator is the size of the sample, and the numerator is the number of cases identified with the condition. If we sampled 500 adults living in a community, administered a measure of depression, and found that 80 people met the criteria for clinical depression, then the estimated prevalence rate of clinical depression would be 16 per 100 adults in that community.

Incidence studies estimate the frequency of *new* cases. Longitudinal designs are needed to estimate incidence because the researcher must first establish who is at risk of becoming a new case—that is, who is free of the condition at the outset. The formula for an **incidence rate** (IR) is:

$$\frac{\begin{array}{c}\text{Number of new cases with the condition or} \\ \text{disease over a given time period}\end{array}}{\begin{array}{c}\text{Number in the population at risk of being a} \\ \text{case (free of the condition at the outset)}\end{array}} \times K$$

Continuing with our previous example, suppose in July 2019 we found that 80 in a sample of 500 people were clinically depressed (PR = 16 per 100). To determine the 1-year incidence rate, we would reassess the sample in July 2020. Suppose that, of the 420 previously deemed *not* to be clinically depressed in 2018, 21 were now found to meet the criteria for depression. In this case, the estimated 1-year incidence rate would be 5 per 100 ([21 ÷ 420] × 100 = 5).

Prevalence and incidence rates can be calculated for subgroups of the population (e.g., for men versus women). When this is done, it is possible to calculate another important descriptive index. **Relative risk** is an estimated risk of "caseness" in one group compared with another. Relative risk is computed by dividing the rate for one group by the rate for another. Suppose we found that the 1-year incidence rate for depression was 6 per 100 women and 4 per 100 men. Women's relative risk for developing depression over the 1-year period would be 1.5; that is, women would be estimated to be 1.5 times more likely to develop depression than men. Relative risk (discussed in Chapter 17) is an important index in assessing the contribution of risk factors to a disease or condition.

Example of a Prevalence Study

Wong et al. (2018) used data from three large private hospitals in Australia to estimate the prevalence of the use of peripheral intravenous cannulae in hospital wards.

TIP The quality of studies that test hypothesized causal relationship is heavily dependent on design decisions—that is, how researchers design their studies to rule out competing explanations for the outcomes. Methods of enhancing the rigor of such studies are described in the next chapter. The quality of descriptive studies, by contrast, depends more on having a good sample (Chapter 13) and strong measures (Chapter 15).

Strengths and Limitations of Correlational Research

The quality of a study is not necessarily related to its approach; there are many excellent nonexperimental studies as well as flawed RCTs. Nevertheless, nonexperimental correlational studies have several drawbacks if causal explanations are sought.

Limitations of Correlational Research

Relative to experimental and quasi-experimental research, nonexperimental studies are weak in their ability to support causal inferences. In correlational studies, researchers work with preexisting groups that were not formed at random, but rather through **self-selection**. A researcher doing a correlational study cannot assume that groups being compared were similar before the occurrence of the hypothesized cause—i.e., the independent variable. Preexisting differences may be a plausible alternative explanation for any group differences on the outcome variable.

The difficulty of interpreting correlational findings stems from the fact that, in the real world, behaviors and characteristics are interrelated (correlated) in complex ways. An example may help to clarify the problem. Suppose we conducted a cross-sectional study that examined the relationship between level of depression in cancer patients and their level of social support (i.e., assistance and emotional support from others). We hypothesize that social support (the independent variable) affects levels of depression (the outcome). Suppose we find that the patients with weak social support are significantly more depressed than patients with strong support. We could interpret this finding to mean that patients' emotional state is influenced by the adequacy of their social supports. This relationship is diagrammed in Figure 9.4A. Yet, there are alternative explanations. Perhaps a third variable influences *both* social support and depression, such as the patients' marital status. It may be that having a spouse is a powerful influence on how depressed cancer patients feel *and* on the quality of their social support. This set of relationships is diagrammed in Figure 9.4B. In this scenario, social support and depression are correlated simply because marital status affects both. A third possibility is reversed causality (Figure 9.4C). Depressed patients with cancer may find it more difficult to elicit needed support from others than patients who are more cheerful or amiable. In this interpretation, the person's depression causes

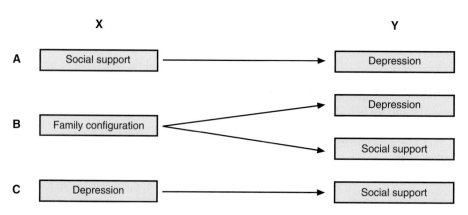

FIGURE 9.4 Alternative explanations for relationship between depression and social support in patients with cancer.

the amount of received social support, and not the other way around. Thus, interpretations of most correlational results should be considered tentative, particularly if the research has no theoretical basis and if the design is cross-sectional.

Strengths of Correlational Research

Earlier, we discussed constraints that limit the application of experimental designs. Correlational research will continue to play a crucial role in nursing research because many interesting problems cannot be addressed any other way.

Correlational research is often efficient in that it may involve collecting a large amount of data about a problem. For example, it would be possible to collect extensive information about the health histories and eating habits of a large number of individuals. Researchers could then examine which health problems were associated with which diets and could discover a large number of interrelationships in a relatively short amount of time. By contrast, an experimenter looks at only a few variables at a time. One experiment might manipulate foods high in cholesterol, whereas another might manipulate salt, for example.

Finally, correlational research is often strong in realism. Unlike many experimental studies, correlational research is seldom criticized for its artificiality.

TIP It can be useful to design a study with several relevant comparisons. In nonexperimental studies, multiple comparison groups can be effective in dealing with self-selection, especially if groups are chosen to address competing biases. For example, in case–control studies of potential causes of lung cancer, cases would be people with lung cancer, one comparison group could be people with a different lung disease, and a second could be those with no pulmonary disorder.

DESIGNS AND RESEARCH EVIDENCE

Evidence for nursing practice depends on descriptive, correlational, and experimental research. There is often a progression to evidence expansion that begins with rich description, including description from qualitative research. In-depth qualitative research may suggest causal links that could be the focus of controlled quantitative research. For example, Colón-Emeric et al. (2006) explored communication patterns among the medical and nursing staff in relation to information flow in two sites. Their findings suggested that a "chain of command" type communication style may limit clinicians' ability to provide high-quality care. The study suggests possibilities for interventions—and indeed, Colon-Emeric et al. (2013) tested an intervention designed to improve nursing home staff's communication and problem solving. Thus, although qualitative studies are low on the standard evidence hierarchy for *confirming* causal connections, they serve an important function in stimulating ideas.

Correlational studies also play a role in developing evidence for causal inferences. Retrospective case–control studies may pave the way for more rigorous (but more expensive) prospective studies. As the evidence base builds, conceptual models may be developed and tested using path analytic designs and other theory-testing strategies. These studies can provide hints about how to structure an intervention, who can most profit from it, and when it can best be instituted.

Different questions relating to causality (Therapy, Prognosis, Etiology) have different evidence hierarchies for ranking designs according to the risk of bias, as we show in Table 9.4, which augments the evidence hierarchy presented in Figure 2.2 (Chapter 2). For Therapy questions (and some Etiology questions), experimental designs are the gold standard (Level II), superseded only by systematic reviews of RCTs on level-of-evidence scales (Level I). On the next rung of the hierarchy for Therapy questions are quasi-experimental designs (and even at this rung, some designs have a lower risk of bias than others). Further down the hierarchy are observational and qualitative studies, which tend not to be strong in corroborating causal hypotheses.

For Prognosis questions, by contrast, randomization to groups is not possible (e.g.,

TABLE 9.4 • Level of Evidence Rankings for Different Cause-Probing Research Questions

LEVEL	TYPE OF QUESTION	
	THERAPY/INTERVENTION AND ETIOLOGY (CAUSATION)/ PREVENTION OF HARM[a]	PROGNOSIS
I	Systematic review of RCTs[b]	Systematic review of nonexperimental studies
II	Randomized controlled trial	Prospective cohort study
III	Quasi-experimental study	Path analytic/theory-based study
IV	Systematic review of nonexperimental studies	Retrospective/case–control study
V	Nonexperimental/observational study a. Prospective cohort study b. Path analytic/theory-based study c. Retrospective case/control study d. Descriptive correlational study	Descriptive correlational study
VI	Metasynthesis of qualitative studies	Metasynthesis of qualitative studies
VII	Qualitative study	Qualitative study
VIII	Nonresearch source	Nonresearch source

[a]RCTs and quasi-experimental designs can sometimes be used for Etiology (causation)/prevention of harm questions (e.g., the effect of salt intake on blood pressure levels). If intervening is not possible (e.g., testing smoking as a cause of lung cancer), the level of evidence rankings would be the same as for Prognosis questions.

[b]Systematic reviews (Level I) sometimes include RCTs and quasi-experimental studies.

for the question of whether low birthweight causes developmental delays). In the hierarchy for Prognosis questions, the best design for an individual study is a prospective cohort design. Path analytic studies with longitudinal data and a strong theoretical basis can also be powerful. Retrospective case–control studies are relatively weak in addressing questions about causality. Systematic reviews of multiple prospective studies, together with support from theories or biophysiologic research, represent the strongest evidence for these types of question.

In terms of Etiology questions, RCTs are sometimes feasible (e.g., Does low salt intake cause reductions in blood pressure levels?). For such questions, the hierarchy is the same as that for Therapy questions. Many important Etiology questions will never be answered using evidence from RCTs, however. A good example is the Etiology question of whether smoking causes lung cancer. Despite the inability to randomize people to smoking and nonsmoking groups, few people doubt that this causal connection exists. Thinking about the criteria for causality discussed early in this chapter, there is abundant evidence that smoking cigarettes is correlated with lung cancer and, through prospective studies, that smoking precedes lung cancer. Researchers have been able to control for, and thus rule out, other possible "causes" of lung cancer. There has been a great deal of consistency and coherence in the findings, and the criterion of biologic plausibility has been met through basic physiologic research.

TIP Some early studies found that evidence from experimental and observational studies often do not yield the same results. The relationship between "causes" and "effects" was found to be stronger in nonexperimental studies than in randomized studies. However, other studies have found that well-designed observational studies do not overestimate the magnitude of effects in comparison with RCTs, especially when the criteria for participating in the study are similar (e.g., Concato et al., 2000).

CRITICAL APPRAISAL OF QUANTITATIVE RESEARCH DESIGNS

The research design used in a quantitative study strongly influences the quality of its evidence, and so should be carefully scrutinized. Researchers' design decisions have more of an impact on study quality than any other methodologic decision when the research question is about causal relationships.

Actual designs and some control techniques (randomization, blinding, allocation concealment) were described in this chapter, and the next chapter explains in greater detail specific strategies for enhancing research control. The guidelines in Box 9.1 are the first of two sets of questions to help you in critically appraising quantitative research designs.

BOX 9.1 Guidelines for Critically Appraising Quantitative Research Designs

1. What type of question (Therapy, Prognosis, etc.) was being addressed in this study? Is the research question cause-probing, i.e., does it concern a hypothesized causal relationship between the independent and dependent variables?
2. What would be the strongest design for the research question? How does this compare to the design actually used?
3. Was there an intervention or treatment? Was the intervention adequately described? Was the control or comparison condition adequately described? Was an experimental or quasi-experimental design used?
4. If the study was an RCT (a true experiment), what specific design was used? Was this design appropriate?
5. In RCTs, what type of randomization was used? Were randomization procedures adequately explained and justified? Was allocation concealment confirmed?
6. If the design was quasi-experimental, what specific quasi-experimental design was used? Was there adequate justification for deciding not to randomize participants to treatment conditions? Did the report provide evidence that any groups being compared were equivalent prior to the intervention?
7. If the design was nonexperimental, was the study inherently nonexperimental? If not, is there adequate justification for not manipulating the independent variable? What specific nonexperimental design was used? If a retrospective design was used, is there good justification for not using a prospective design? What evidence did the report provide that any groups being compared were similar with regard to important confounding characteristics?
8. What types of comparisons were specified in the design (e.g., before–after? between groups?) Did these comparisons adequately illuminate the relationship between the independent and dependent variables? If there were no comparisons, or faulty comparisons, how did this affect the study's integrity and the interpretability of the results?
9. Was the study longitudinal? Was the timing of the collection of data appropriate? Was the number of data collection points reasonable?
10. Was blinding/masking used? If yes, who was blinded—and was this adequate? If not, was there a justifiable rationale for failure to mask? Was the intervention a type that could raise participants' expectations that, in and of themselves, could affect the outcomes?

RESEARCH EXAMPLES

In this section we present descriptions of an experimental, quasi-experimental, and nonexperimental study.

Research Example of an RCT

Study: Nonnutritive sucking, oral breast milk, and facilitated tucking relieve preterm infant pain during heel-stick procedures (Peng et al., 2018).

Statement of Purpose: The purpose of this study was to compare the effects of alternative strategies to reduce the pain of preterm infants during heel-stick procedures.

Treatment Groups: In this trial, there were three treatment groups. Preterm infants received either (1) combined nonnutritive sucking + oral expressed breast milk, (2) nonnutritive sucking + breast milk + facilitated tucking, or (3) routine care. Those in the control group received position support and gentle touch. For those receiving breast milk, infants were orally fed expressed milk through a syringe 2 minutes before the heel stick.

Method: A sample of 109 preterm infants (gestational age 39-37 weeks) needing procedural heel sticks were randomly assigned to one of the three conditions. Infants were excluded if they had a condition that might influence their responses to pain (e.g. a congenital anomaly). Random assignment was carried out by a blinded statistician, who used a block randomization procedure. Heel sticks by a senior nurse were used to collect infants' blood. The time for heel-stick procedures was controlled at 2 minutes in all three conditions. The heel sticks occurred over eight phases: phase 1 (baseline without stimuli), phases 2 and 3 (the second and third minutes during the procedures), and phases 4 to 8 (recovery, a 10-minute period starting when the nurse finished collecting blood and left the infant). During all 8 phases, the infants' reactions were video recorded. Infant pain was scored by a research assistant from the videos at 1-minute intervals. The research assistant was blinded to the study purpose and the infants' clinical information.

Key Findings: The combined use of sucking + breast milk—with or without tucking—was found to have reduced preterm infants' pain during heel-stick procedures. Adding facilitated tucking helped infants recover from pain.

Research Example of a Quasi-Experimental Study

Study: Thyroid cancer patients receiving an interdisciplinary team-based care approach (ITCA-ThyCa) appear to display better outcomes (Henry et al., 2018)

Statement of Purpose: The purpose of the study was to evaluate the effects of a special Interdisciplinary Team-based Care Approach (ITCA) for thyroid cancer patients.

Treatment Groups: Adult patients with a biopsy indicating confirmed or highly suspicious thyroid cancer at the Jewish General Hospital in Montreal, Canada, received the special ITCA intervention. The approach included a dedicated nurse who had a central, integrative role in an interdisciplinary team that included surgery, endocrinology, pharmacy, dietetics, social work, and community supports. The ITCA also included regularly scheduled team meetings to promote service coordination and continuity of care. The comparison group comprised patients having undergone a thyroidectomy at the McGill University Health Centre, a facility with similar sociodemographic and clinical profiles and medical approach as those in the intervention hospital. The comparison group received care as usual.

Method: The researchers initially sought to use a randomized design but discovered that patients were too distressed to provide consent while they were waiting for surgery, and so they opted for a nonequivalent control group design. A total of 200 patients (122 in the intervention group and 78 in the comparison group) participated and completed various patient-reported assessments that measured patient satisfaction and general well-being at the end of the study.

Key Findings: The intervention and comparison group members were similar demographically and clinically. Patients in the ITCA group had higher levels of well-being and fewer physical and practical concerns than patients in the comparison group at the posttest. Those in the intervention group were also more satisfied with their care and were more likely to recommend their hospital.

Research Example of a Correlational Study

Study: Dementia-related restlessness: Relationship to characteristics of persons with dementia and family caregivers (Regier & Gitlin, 2018)

Statement of Purpose: The purpose of the study was to examine the relationship of dementia-related restlessness to patient outcomes and to caregiver well-being.

Method: The study participants in this cross-sectional study were 569 caregivers of persons with moderate-stage dementia who had one or more behavioral disturbances. Caregivers were included if they lived with the person with dementia, provided at least 4 hours of daily care, and reported that the patient exhibited boredom, sadness, anxiety, agitation, or restlessness. Caregivers completed questionnaires that included measures of their perceptions of the patients' neuropsychiatric symptoms (including restlessness), pain, and functional capacity. Measures of the caregivers' level of burden, depression, and caregiver mastery were also incorporated into the questionnaires. The team also had scores for the person with dementia's score on a measure of cognition. The analysis involved examining correlations among the various variables.

Key Findings: Nearly 65% of the dementia caregivers reported restlessness as a symptom. Persons with restlessness had significantly higher pain scores, were more likely to be on behavioral medications, and had more neuropsychiatric symptoms than those without restlessness. Caregivers of patients with restlessness reported greater burden and depression.

SUMMARY POINTS

- Many quantitative nursing studies aim to facilitate inferences about *cause-and-effect relationships.*
- One criterion for causality is that the cause must precede the effect. Two other criteria are that a relationship between a presumed cause (independent variable) and an effect (dependent variable) exists and cannot be explained as being caused by other (confounding) variables.
- In an idealized model, a **counterfactual** is what would have happened to the same people simultaneously exposed *and* not exposed to a causal factor. The *effect* is the difference between the two. The goal of research design is to find a good approximation to the idealized (but impossible) counterfactual.
- **Experiments** (or **randomized controlled trials, RCTs**) involve **manipulation** (the researcher manipulates the independent variable by introducing a **treatment** or **intervention**); control (including use of a **control group** that does not receive the intervention and represents the comparative counterfactual); and **randomization/random assignment** (with people allocated to experimental and control groups at random so that they are equivalent at the outset).
- Participants in the experimental group usually all get the same intervention as delineated in formal protocols, but some studies involve **patient-centered interventions (PCIs)** that are *tailored* to meet individual needs or characteristics.
- Researchers can expose the control group to various conditions, including no treatment; an alternative treatment; standard treatment ("usual care"); a **placebo** or pseudointervention; different doses of the treatment; or a *delayed treatment* (for a **wait-list** group).
- Random assignment is done by methods that give every participant an equal chance of being in any group, such as by flipping a coin or using a **table of random numbers**. Randomization is the most reliable method for equalizing groups on all characteristics that could affect study outcomes. Randomization should involve **allocation concealment** that prevents foreknowledge of upcoming assignments.
- Several variants to simple randomization exist, such as **permuted block randomization**, in which randomization is done for blocks of people—for example, 6 or 8 at a time, in randomly selected block sizes.
- **Blinding** (or **masking**) is often used to avoid biases stemming from participants' or research agents' awareness of group status or study hypotheses. In **double-blind studies,** two groups (e.g., participants and investigators) are blinded.
- Many specific experimental designs exist. A **posttest-only** (*after-only*) **design** involves collecting data after an intervention only. In a

pretest–posttest (*before–after*) **design**, data are collected both before and after the intervention, permitting an analysis of change.

- **Factorial designs,** in which two or more independent variables are manipulated simultaneously, allow researchers to test both **main effects** (effects from manipulated independent variables) and **interaction effects** (effects from combining treatments).

- In a **crossover design**, subjects are exposed to more than one condition, administered in a randomized order, and thus they serve as their own controls.

- Experimental designs are the *gold standard* because they come closer than any other design in meeting criteria for inferring causal relationships.

- **Quasi-experimental designs** (*trials without randomization*) involve an intervention but lack randomization. Strong quasi-experimental designs incorporate features to support causal inferences.

- The **nonequivalent control group pretest–posttest design** involves using a nonrandomized **comparison group** and the collection of pre-treatment data so that initial group equivalence can be assessed.

- In a **time series design**, information on the dependent variable is collected multiple times before and after the intervention in a single group. The extended time period for data collection enhances the ability to attribute change to the intervention.

- Other quasi-experimental designs include non-randomized **dose–response analyses** and the nonrandomized **arms** of a **partially randomized patient preference** (**PRPP**) design (i.e., groups with strong preferences).

- In evaluating the results of quasi-experiments, it is important to ask whether it is plausible that factors other than the intervention caused or affected the outcomes (i.e., whether there are credible **rival hypotheses** for explaining the results).

- **Nonexperimental** (or **observational**) **research** includes **descriptive research**—studies that summarize the status of phenomena—and **correlational** studies that examine relationships among variables but involve no manipulation of independent variables (often because they *cannot* be manipulated).

- Designs for cause-probing correlational studies include **retrospective (case–control) designs** (which look back in time for antecedent causes of "caseness" by comparing **cases** that have a disease or condition with controls who do not); **prospective (cohort) designs** (studies that begin with a presumed cause and look forward in time for its effect); **natural experiments** (in which a group is affected by a random event, such as a disaster); and **path analytic studies** (which test causal models developed on the basis of theory).

- **Descriptive correlational studies** describe how phenomena are interrelated without invoking a causal explanation. **Univariate descriptive studies** examine the frequency or average value of variables.

- Descriptive studies include **prevalence studies** that document the **prevalence rate** of a condition at one point in time and **incidence studies** that document the frequency of *new* cases, over a given time period. When the **incidence rates** for two subgroups are estimated, researchers can compute the **relative risk** of "caseness" for the two.

- The primary weakness of correlational studies for cause-probing questions is that they can harbor biases, such as **self-selection** into groups being compared.

STUDY ACTIVITIES

Study activities are available to instructors on thePoint.

REFERENCES CITED IN CHAPTER 9

*Adams, M., Hurley, J., Todd, M., Bhuiyan, N., Jarrett, C., Tucker, W., … Angadi, S. (2017). Adaptive goal setting and financial incentives: a 2 × 2 factorial randomized controlled trial to increase adults' physical activity. *BMC Public Health, 17*, 286.

Barkauskas, V. H., Lusk, S. L., Eakin, B. L. (2005). Selecting control interventions for clinical outcome studies. *Western Journal of Nursing Research, 27,* 346–363.

Bärnighausen, T., Tugwell, P., Røttingen, J., Shemilt, I., Rockers, P., Geldsetzer, P., … Atun, R. (2017). Quasi-experimental study design series—paper 4: uses and value. *Journal of Clinical Epidemiology, 89,* 4–11.

Barta, W., Fisher, V., & Hynes, P. (2017). Decreased reconviction rates of DUI offenders with intensive supervision and home confinement. *American Journal of Drug & Alcohol Abuse, 43,* 742–746.

*Beck, C., McSweeney, J., Richards, K., Robertson, P., Tsai, P., & Souder, E. (2010). Challenges in tailored intervention research. *Nursing Outlook, 58,* 104–110.

Bradford-Hill, A. (1965). The environment and disease: association or causation. *Proceedings of the Royal Society of Medicine, 58,* 295–300.

Breneman, C., Kline, C., West, D., Sui, X., Porter, R., Bowyer, K., … Wang, X. (2019). The effect of moderate-intensity exercise on nightly variability in objectively measured sleep parameters among older women. *Behavioral Sleep Medicine, 17,* 459–469.

Campbell, D. T., & Stanley, J. C. (1963). *Experimental and quasi-experimental designs for research.* Chicago: Rand McNally.

*Chalmers, J., Sansom-Daly, U., Patterson, P., McCowage, G., & Anazodo, A. (2018). Psychosocial assessment using telehealth in adolescents and young adults with cancer: a partially randomized patient preference pilot study. *JMIR Research Protocols, 7,* e168.

*Colón-Emeric, C., Ammarell, N, Bailey, D., Corazzini, K., Lekan-Rutledge, D., Piven, M., … Anderson, R. A. (2006). Patterns of medical and nursing staff communication in nursing homes. *Qualitative Health Research, 16,* 173–188.

*Colón-Emeric, C., McConnell, E., Pinheiro, S., Corazzini, K., Porter, K., Earp, K., … Anderson, R. A. (2013). CONNECT for better fall prevention in nursing homes. *Journal of the American Geriatric Society, 61,* 2150–2159.

**Como, J. M. (2018). Health literacy and health status in people with chronic heart failure. *Clinical Nurse Specialist, 32,* 29–42.

*Concato, J., Shah, N., & Horwitz, R. (2000). Randomized, controlled trials, observational studies, and the hierarchy of research designs. *New England Journal of Medicine, 342,* 1887–1892.

Doering, J., & Dogan, S. (2018). A postpartum sleep and fatigue intervention feasibility pilot study. *Behavioral Sleep Medicine, 16,* 185–201.

Doig, G., & Simpson, F. (2005). Randomization and allocation concealment: a practical guide for researchers. *Journal of Critical Care, 20,* 187–191.

Dotson, B., Larabell, P., Patel, J., Wong, K., Qasem, L., Arthur, W., … Tennenberg, S. (2016). Calcium administration is associated with adverse outcomes in criticall ill patients receiving parenteral nutrition: results from a natural experiment created by a calcium gluconate shortage. *Pharmacotherapy, 36,* 1185–1190.

Downs, M., Tucker, K., Christ-Schmidt, H., & Wittes, J. (2010). Some practical problems in implementing randomization. *Clinical Trials, 7,* 235–245.

Geldsetzer, P., & Fawzi, W. (2017). Quasi-experimental study design series—paper 2: complementary approaches to advancing global health knowledge. *Journal of Clinical Epidemiology, 89,* 12–16.

*George, A., Dahlen, H., Blinkhorn, A., Ajwani, S., Bhole, S., Ellis, S., … Johnson, M. (2018). Evaluation of a midwifery initiated oral health-dental service program to improve oral health and birth outcomes for pregnant women: a multi-centre randomised controlled trial. *International Journal of Nursing Research, 82,* 49–57.

Grimes, D., & Schulz, K. (2005). Compared to what? Finding controls for case-control studies. *The Lancet, 365,* 1429–1433.

Gross, D. (2005). On the merits of attention control groups. *Research in Nursing & Health, 28,* 93–94.

Henry, M., Frenkiel, S., Chartier, G., Payne, R., MacDonald, C., Black, M., … Hier, M. (2018). Thyroid cancer patients receiving an interdisciplinary team-based care approach (ITCA-ThyCa) appear to display better outcomes: program evaluation results indicating a need for further integrated care and support. *Psycho-oncology, 27,* 937–945.

Herbison, P., Hay-Smith, J., & Gillespie, W. (2011). Different methods of allocation to groups in randomized trials are associated with different levels of bias. A meta-epidemiological study. *Journal of Clinical Epidemiology, 64,* 1070–1075.

Lachin, J. M., Matts, J., & Wei, L. (1988). Randomization in clinical trials: conclusions and recommendations. *Controlled Clinical Trials, 9,* 365–374.

Lau, Y., Tha, P., Ho-Lim, S., Wong, L., Lim, P., Citra Nurfarah, B., & Shorey, S. (2018). An analysis of the effects of intrapartum factors, neonatal characteristics, and skin-to-skin contact on early breastfeeding initiation. *Maternal & Child Nutrition, 14*(1).

Lauver, D. R., Ward, S. E., Heidrich, S. M., Keller, M. L., Bowers, B. J., Brennan, P. F., Kirchhoff, K. T., & Wells, T. J. (2002). Patient-centered interventions. *Research in Nursing & Health, 25,* 246–255.

*Moher, D., Hopewell, S., Schulz, K. F., Montori, V., Gotzsche, P., Devereaux, P., … Altman, D. G. (2010). CONSORT 2010 explanation and elaboration: updated guidelines for reporting parallel-group randomised trials. *BMJ, 340,* c869.

Ndosi, M., Wright-Hughes, A., Brown, S., Backhouse, M., Lipsky, B., Bhogal, M., … Nelson, E. (2018). Prognosis of the infected diabetic foot ulcer: a 12-month prospective observational study. *Diabetic Medicine, 35,* 78–88.

Ng, A., & Wong, F. (2018). Effects of a home-based palliative heart failure program on quality of life, symptom burden, satisfaction and caregiver burden: a randomized controlled trial. *Journal of Pain and Symptom Management, 55,* 1–11.

Norman, R., Ramsden, R., Ginty, L., & Sinha, S. (2017). Effect of a multimodal educational intervention on use of urinary catheters in hospitalized individuals. *Journal of the American Geriatric Society, 65,* 2679–2684.

Özkan, F., & Zincir, H. (2017). The effect of reflexology upon spasticity and function among children with cerebral palsy who received physiotherapy: three group randomised trial. *Applied Nursing Research, 36*, 128–134.

Peng, H., Yin, T., Yang, L., Wang, C., Chang, Y., Jeng, M., & Liaw, J. (2018). Non-nutritive sucking, oral breast milk, and facilitated tucking relieve pretern infants pain during heel-stick procedures: a prospective, randomized controlled trial. *International Journal of Nursing Studies, 77*, 162–170.

Polit, D. F., & Chaboyer, W. (2012). Statistical process control in nursing research. *Research in Nursing & Health, 35*, 82–93.

Polit, D., Gillespie, B., & Griffin, R. (2011). Deliberate ignorance: a systematic review of the use of blinding in nursing clinical trials. *Nursing Research, 61*, 9–16.

Reddy, R., El Youssef, J., Winters-Stone, K., Branigan, D., Leitschuh, J., Castle, J., & Jacobs, P. (2018). The effect of exercise on sleep in adults with type 1 diabetes. *Diabetes, Obesity & Metabolism, 20*, 443–447.

Regier, N., & Gitlin, L. (2018). Dementia-related restlessness: relationship to characteristics of persons with dementia and family caregivers. *International Journal of Geriatric Psychiatry, 33*, 185–192.

Richards, K., Enderlin, C., Beck, C., McSweeney, J., Jones, T., & Robertson, P. (2007). Tailored biobehavioral interventions: a literature review and synthesis. *Research and Theory for Nursing Practice, 21*, 271–285.

*Rosenzweig, M., West, M., Matthews, J., Stokan, M., Yoojin Kook, Y., Gallups, S., & Diergaarde, B. (2019). Financial toxicity among women with metastatic breast cancer. *Oncology Nursing Forum, 46*, 83–91.

Saad, K., Abdel-Rahman, A., Elserogy, Y., Al-Altram, A., El-Houfey, A., Othman, H., … Abdel-Salam, A. (2018). Randomized controlled trial of vitamin D supplementation in children with autism spectrum disorder. *Journal of Child Psychology and Psychiatry, 59*, 20–29.

Schulz, K. F., Chalmers, I., & Altman, D. G. (2002). The landscape and lexicon of blinding in randomized trials. *Annals of Internal Medicine, 136*, 254–259.

Shadish, W. R., Cook, T. D., & Campbell, D. T. (2002). *Experimental and quasi-experimental designs for generalized causal inference.* Boston: Houghton Mifflin.

*Smith, B., Shatté, A., Perlman, A., Siers, M., & Lynch, W. (2018). Improvements in resilience, stress, and somatic symptoms following online resilience training: a dose-response effect. *Journal of Occupational and Environmental Medicine, 60*, 1–5.

Takahashi, R., Wilunde, C., Magutah, K., Mwaura-Tenambergen, W., Atwoli, L., & Perngparn, U. (2018). Evaluation of alcohol screening and community-based brief interventions in rural western Kenya: a quasi-experimental study. *Alcohol and Alcoholism, 53*, 121–128.

Vedelø, T. W., & Lomborg, K. (2011). Reported challenges in nurse-led randomised controlled trials: an integrative review of the literature. *Scandinavian Journal of the Caring Sciences, 25*, 194–200.

Wong, K., Cooper, A., Brown, J., Boyd, L., & Levinson, M. (2018). The prevalence of peripheral intravenous cannulae and pattern of use: a point prevalence in a private hospital setting. *Journal of Clinical Nursing, 27*, e363–e367.

Yuan, M., Li, F., Fang, Q., Wang, W., Peng, J., Qin, D., Wang, X., & Liu, G. (2018). Research on the cause of death for severe stroke patients. *Journal of Clinical Nursing, 27*, 450–460.

A link to this open-access article is provided in the Toolkit for Chapter 9 in the Resource Manual. ✪

**This journal article is available on thePoint *for this chapter.*

10 | Rigor and Validity in Quantitative Research

VALIDITY AND INFERENCE

This chapter describes strategies for controlling sources of bias in quantitative studies. Many of these strategies strengthen inferences that can be made about cause-and-effect relationships.

Validity and Validity Threats

In designing a study, it is useful to anticipate factors that could undermine the **validity** of inferences. Shadish, Cook, and Campbell (2002) define validity in the context of research design as "the approximate truth of an inference" (p. 34). For example, inferences that a *cause* results in a hypothesized *effect* are valid to the extent that researchers can marshal strong supporting evidence. Validity is always a matter of degree, not an absolute.

Validity is a property of an inference, not of a research design, but design elements profoundly affect the inferences that can be made. **Threats to validity** are reasons that an inference could be wrong. When researchers introduce design features to minimize potential threats, the validity of the inference about relationships under study is strengthened.

Types of Validity

Shadish and colleagues (2002) proposed a taxonomy that identified four types of validity and cataloged dozens of validity threats. This chapter describes the taxonomy and summarizes major threats, but we urge researchers to consult this seminal work for further guidance.

The first type of validity, **statistical conclusion validity**, concerns the validity of inferences that there truly is an empirical relationship, or correlation, between the presumed cause and the effect. The researcher's job is to provide strong evidence that an observed relationship is *real*.

Internal validity concerns the validity of inferences that, given that an empirical relationship exists, it is the independent variable, rather than something else, that caused the outcome. Researchers must develop strategies to rule out the plausibility that some factor other than the independent variable accounts for the observed relationship.

Construct validity involves the validity of inferences "from the observed persons, settings, and cause-and-effect operations included in the study to the constructs that these instances might represent" (p. 38). One aspect of construct validity concerns the degree to which an intervention is a good representation of the underlying construct that was theorized as having the potential to cause beneficial outcomes. Another issue concerns whether the measures of the outcomes are good operationalizations of the constructs for which they are intended.

External validity concerns whether inferences about observed relationships will hold over variations in persons, setting, or time. External validity, then, relates to the generalizability of inferences—a critical concern for evidence-based nursing practice.

These four types of validity and their associated threats are discussed in this chapter. Many validity threats result from inadequate control over confounding variables, and so we briefly review methods of controlling confounders associated with participants' characteristics.

Controlling Confounding Participant Characteristics

This section describes six methods of controlling participant characteristics—characteristics that could compete with the independent variable as the cause of an outcome.

Randomization

As noted in Chapter 9, randomization is the most effective method of controlling individual characteristics. The function of randomization is to secure comparable groups—i.e., to equalize groups with respect to confounding variables. A distinct advantage of random assignment, compared with other strategies, is that it can control *all* possible sources of confounding variation, *without any conscious decision about which variables need to be controlled.*

Crossover

Randomization within a crossover design is an especially powerful method of ensuring equivalence between groups being compared—participants serve as their own controls. Moreover, fewer participants usually are needed in such a design. Fifty people exposed to two treatments in random order yield 100 data points (50 × 2); 50 people randomly assigned to two different groups yield only 50 data points (25 × 2). Crossover designs are not appropriate for all studies, however, because of possible carry-over effects: people exposed to two different conditions may be influenced in the second condition by their experience in the first.

Homogeneity

When randomization and crossover are not feasible, alternative methods of controlling confounding

characteristics are needed. One method is to use only people who are homogeneous with respect to confounding variables. Suppose we were testing the effectiveness of a physical fitness program on the cardiovascular functioning of elders. In our quasi-experimental design, elders from two different nursing homes are recruited, with elders in one of them receiving the intervention. If gender were a key confounding variable—and if the two nursing homes had different proportions of men and women—we could control gender by using only men (or only women) as participants.

The price of homogeneity is that research findings cannot be generalized to types of people who did not participate in the study. If the physical fitness intervention were found to have beneficial effects on the cardiovascular status of a sample of women 65 to 75 years of age, its usefulness for improving the cardiovascular status of men in their 80s would require a separate study. Indeed, one criticism of this approach is that researchers sometimes exclude people who are extremely ill, which means that the findings cannot be generalized to those who may be most in need of interventions.

Example of Control Through Homogeneity
Bang and colleagues (2018) used a nonequivalent control group design to test the effects of a health promotion program with nursing student mentors on the psychological health of elementary school children in Korea. Several variables were controlled through homogeneity, including the children's age (all in grades 4-6) and socioeconomic background (all children were considered "vulnerable"), and all were getting social services in community centers.

TIP The principle of homogeneity is often used to control (hold constant) *external* factors known to influence outcomes. For example, it may be important to collect outcome data at the same time of the day for all participants if time could affect the outcome (e.g., fatigue). As another example, it may be desirable to maintain **constancy of conditions** in terms of data collection locale—e.g., interviewing all respondents in their homes, rather than some in their places of work, because context can influence responses to questions.

Stratification/Blocking

Another approach to controlling confounders is to include them in the research design through stratification. To pursue our example of the physical fitness intervention with gender as the confounding variable, we could use a *randomized block design* in which men and women are assigned separately to treatment groups. This approach can enhance the likelihood of detecting differences between our experimental and control groups because the effect of the blocking variable (gender) on the outcome is eliminated. In addition, if the blocking variable is of interest substantively, researchers have the opportunity to study differences in the subgroups created by the stratifying variable (e.g., men versus women).

Matching

Matching (also called **pair matching**) involves using information about people's characteristics to create comparable groups. If matching were used in our physical fitness example and age and gender were the confounding variables, we would match a person in the intervention group with one in the comparison group with respect to age and gender.

Matching is often problematic: to use matching, researchers must know the relevant confounders in advance. Also, it is difficult to match on more than two or three variables. This problem is sometimes addressed with a sophisticated matching technique, called **propensity matching.** This method, which requires some statistical sophistication, involves the creation of a **propensity score** that captures the conditional probability of exposure to a treatment given various preintervention characteristics. Members of the groups being compared (either in an observational or quasi-experimental study) can then be matched on the propensity score (Qin et al., 2008). Both conventional and propensity matching are most easily implemented when there is a large pool of potential comparison group participants from which good matches to treatment group members can be selected. Nevertheless, matching as the primary control technique should be used only when other, more powerful procedures are not feasible.

Sometimes, as an alternative to matching, researchers use a **balanced design** with regard to key confounders. In such situations, researchers attempt only to ensure that the groups being compared have similar proportional representation on confounding variables, rather than matching on a one-to-one basis. For example, if gender and age were the two variables of concern, we would strive to ensure that the same percentage of men and women were in the two groups and that the average age was comparable. Such an approach is less cumbersome than matching but has similar limitations. Nevertheless, both matching and balancing are preferable to failing to control participant characteristics at all.

Example of Control Through Matching

Fehlberg and an interdisciplinary team (2017) used a case–control design to study associations between hyponatraemia, sodium depletion, and the risk of falls in hospitalized patients. Data were collected in four hospitals from 699 adult patients who fell and 1,189 matched controls who did not. Up to two controls with similar length of stay who were on the same nursing unit at the time the case fell were selected. Low serum sodium levels were found to be strongly associated with falls.

Statistical Control

Another method of controlling confounding variables is through statistical analysis rather than research design. A detailed description of powerful **statistical control** mechanisms will be postponed until Chapter 19, but we will explain underlying principles with a simple illustration of a procedure called **analysis of covariance (ANCOVA).**

In our physical fitness example, suppose we used a nonequivalent control group design with elders from two nursing homes, and resting heart rate was an outcome. Individual differences in heart rate in the sample would be expected—that is, heart rate would vary from one person to the next. The research question is, "Can some of the differences in heart rate be attributed to program participation?" We know that differences in heart rate are also related to other traits, such as age. In Figure 10.1, the large circles represent the total amount of variation for resting heart rate. A certain amount

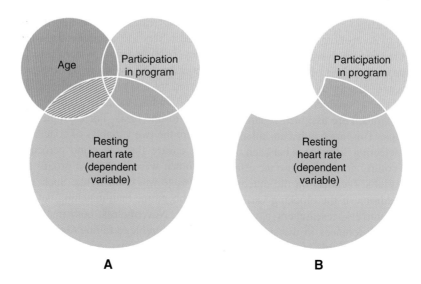

FIGURE 10.1 Schematic diagram illustrating principles of analysis of covariance conceptually.

of variation can be explained by a person's age, depicted as the small circle on the left in Figure 10.1A. Other variation may be explained by participation or nonparticipation in the program, represented as the small circle on the right. The two small circles (age and program participation) overlap, indicating a relationship between the two. In other words, people in the physical fitness group are, on average, either older or younger than those in the comparison group. Age should be controlled; otherwise, we could not determine whether postintervention differences in resting heart rate are due to differences in age or program participation.

Analysis of covariance statistically removes the effect of confounding variables on the outcome. In the illustration, the portion of heart rate variability attributable to age (the hatched area of the large circle in A) is removed through ANCOVA. Figure 10.1B shows that the final analysis tests the effect of program participation on heart rate *after removing the effect of age*. By controlling heart rate variability resulting from age, we get a more accurate estimate of the effect of the program on heart rate. Note that even after removing variability due to age, there is still individual variation not associated with the program treatment—the bottom half of the large circle in B. This means that the study

can probably be improved by controlling additional confounders, such as gender, smoking history, and so on. ANCOVA and other sophisticated procedures can control multiple confounding variables.

Example of Statistical Control
Abbasi and colleagues (2018) tested the effectiveness of e-learning versus an educational booklet (or usual care without any intervention) on the childbirth self-efficacy of pregnant women. The researchers compared the scores of women in the three groups on a childbirth self-efficacy measure after the intervention, statistically controlling for baseline values on the same measure.

TIP Confounding participant characteristics that need to be controlled vary from one study to another, but we can offer some guidance. The best variable is the outcome variable itself, measured before the independent variable occurs. In our physical fitness example, controlling preprogram measures of cardiovascular functioning would be a good choice. Major demographic variables (e.g., age, race/ethnicity, education) and health indicators are usually good candidates for statistical control. Confounding variables that correlate with the outcomes should be identified through a literature review.

Evaluation of Control Methods

Table 10.1 summarizes benefits and drawbacks of the six control mechanisms. Randomization is the most effective method of managing confounding variables—that is, of approximating the ideal but unattainable counterfactual discussed in Chapter 9—because it tends to cancel out individual differences on all possible confounders. Crossover designs are a useful supplement to randomization but are not always appropriate. The remaining alternatives have common disadvantages: Researchers must know in advance the relevant confounding variables and can rarely control all of them. To use homogeneity, stratify, match, or perform ANCOVA,

TABLE 10.1 • Methods of Control Over Participant Characteristics

METHOD	BENEFITS	LIMITATIONS
Randomization	• Controls all preintervention confounding variables • Does not require advance knowledge of which variables need to be controlled	• Constraints (ethical, practical) on which variables can be manipulated • Possible artificiality of conditions • Resistance to being randomized by many people
Crossover	• If done with randomization, very strong approach: subjects serve as their own controls and thus are perfectly "matched"	• Cannot be used if there are possible carry-over effects from one condition to the next • History threat may be relevant if external factors change over time
Homogeneity	• Easy to achieve in all types of research • Could enhance interpretability of relationships	• Limits generalizability • Requires knowledge of which variables to control • Range restriction could lower statistical conclusion validity
Stratification/ blocking	• Enhances the ability to detect and interpret relationships • Offers opportunity to examine stratifying variable as an independent variable	• Usually restricted to a few stratifying variables • Requires knowledge of which variables to control
Matching	• Enhances ability to detect and interpret relationships • May be easy if there is a large "pool" of potential available comparison subjects	• Usually restricted to a few matching variables (except with propensity matching) • Requires knowledge of which variables to match • May be difficult to find comparison group matches, especially if there are more than two matching variables
Statistical control	• Enhances ability to detect and interpret relationships • Relatively economical means of controlling several confounding variables	• Requires knowledge of which variables to control, as well as measurement of those variables • Requires some statistical sophistication

researchers must know which variables need to be measured and controlled. Yet, when randomization is impossible, the use of any of these strategies is better than no control strategy.

STATISTICAL CONCLUSION VALIDITY

One criterion for establishing causality is demonstrating that there is a relationship between the independent and dependent variable. Statistical methods are used to support inferences about whether relationships exist. Researchers can make design decisions that protect against reaching false statistical conclusions. Shadish and colleagues (2002) discussed nine threats to statistical conclusion validity. We focus here on three especially important threats.

Low Statistical Power

Detecting existing relationships among variables requires **statistical power**. Adequate statistical power can be achieved in various ways, the most straightforward of which is to use a sufficiently large sample. When small samples are used, statistical power tends to be low, and the analyses may fail to show that the independent and dependent variables are related—*even when they are*. Power and sample size are discussed in Chapters 13 and 18.

Another aspect of a powerful design concerns how the independent variable is defined. Both statistically and substantively, results are clearer when differences between groups being compared are large. Group differences on the outcomes can be enhanced by maximizing differences on the independent variable. Conn and colleagues (2001) offered good suggestions for enhancing the power and effectiveness of nursing interventions. Note that strengthening group differences is easier in RCTs than in nonexperimental research. In experiments, investigators can devise treatment conditions that are as distinct as money, ethics, and practicality permit.

Another aspect of statistical power concerns maximizing **precision**, which is achieved through accurate measuring tools, controls over

confounding variables, and powerful statistical methods. Precision can best be explained with an example. Suppose we were studying the effect of admission into a nursing home on depression by comparing people who were or were not admitted. Depression varies from one elderly person to another for various reasons. We want to isolate—as precisely as possible—variation in depression attributable to a person's entry into a nursing home. The following ratio expresses what we wish to assess in this example:

$$\frac{\text{Variability in depession}}{\text{due to nursing home admission}}$$
$$\frac{}{\text{Variability in depression due to other factors}}$$
$$\text{(e.g., age, pain, medical condition)}$$

This ratio, greatly simplified here, captures the essence of many statistical tests. We want to make variability in the numerator (the upper half) as large as possible relative to variability in the denominator (the lower half), to evaluate precisely the relationship between nursing home admission and depression. The smaller the variability in depression due to confounding variables (e.g., age, pain), the easier it will be to detect differences in depression between elders who were or were not admitted to a nursing home. Thus, reducing variability caused by confounders can increase statistical conclusion validity. As a purely hypothetical illustration, we will attach some numeric values[*] to the ratio as follows:

$$\frac{\text{Variability due to nursing home admission}}{\text{Variability due to all confounding variables}} = \frac{10}{4}$$

If we can make the bottom number smaller, say by changing it from 4 to 2, we will have a more precise estimate of the effect of nursing home admission on depression, relative to other influences. Control mechanisms such as those described earlier help to reduce variability caused by extraneous variables. We illustrate this by continuing our example, singling out age as a key confounding variable. Total variability in levels of depression

---

[*]You should not be concerned with how these numbers can be obtained. Analytic procedures are explained in Chapter 18.

can be conceptualized as having the following components:

Total variability in depression = Variability due to nursing home admission + Variability due to age + Variability due to other confounding variables

This equation can be taken to mean that part of the reason why elders differ in depression is that some were admitted to a nursing home and others were not; some were older and some were younger; and other factors (e.g., pain) also affect depression.

One way to increase precision in this study would be to control age, thereby removing the variability in depression that results from age differences. We could do this, for example, by restricting age to elders younger than 80 years, thereby reducing the variability in depression due to age. As a result, the effect of nursing home admission on depression becomes greater, relative to the remaining variability. Thus, this design decision (homogeneity) enabled us to get a more precise estimate of the effect of nursing home admission on level of depression (although, of course, this limits generalizability). Research designs differ in the sensitivity with which effects under study can be detected statistically. Lipsey (1990) has prepared a good guide to enhancing the sensitivity of research designs.

Restriction of Range

The control of extraneous variation through homogeneity is easy to use and can help to clarify the relationship between key research variables, but it can be risky. Not only does this approach limit generalizability, it can sometimes undermine statistical conclusion validity. When the use of homogeneity restricts the range of values on the outcome variable, relationships between the outcome and the independent variable will be *attenuated* and may therefore lead to the erroneous conclusion that the variables are unrelated. For example, if *everyone* in the sample had a depression score of 50, scores would be unrelated to age, nursing home admission, and so on.

In our example, we suggested limiting the sample of nursing home residents to people younger than 80 years to reduce variability in the denominator. Our aim was to enhance the variability in depression scores attributable to nursing home admission, relative to depression variability due to other factors. But what if few elders younger than 80 years were depressed? With limited variability, relationships cannot be detected. Therefore, in designing a study, you should consider whether there will be sufficient variability to support the statistical analyses envisioned. The issue of *floor effects* and *ceiling effects*, which involve range restrictions at the lower and upper end of a measure, respectively, is discussed later in this book.

Unreliable Implementation of a Treatment

The strength of an intervention—and statistical conclusion validity—can be undermined if an intervention is not as powerful in reality as it is "on paper." **Intervention fidelity** (or **treatment fidelity**) concerns the extent to which the implementation of an intervention is faithful to its plan. There is growing interest in intervention fidelity and considerable advice on how to achieve it (e.g., Bova et al., 2017; Rixon et al., 2016).

Interventions can be weakened by various factors, which researchers can often influence. One issue concerns whether the intervention is similar from one person to the next. Usually, researchers strive for constancy of conditions in implementing a treatment because lack of standardization adds extraneous variation. Even in tailored, patient-centered interventions, there are protocols, though different protocols are used with different people. Using the notions just described, when standard protocols are not followed, variability due to the intervention (i.e., in the numerator) can be suppressed, and variability due to other factors (i.e., in the denominator) can be inflated, possibly leading to the erroneous conclusion that the intervention was ineffective. This suggests the need for some standardization, the use of procedures manuals, thorough training of personnel, and vigilant monitoring (e.g., observing delivery of the intervention) to ensure that the intervention is being implemented as planned—and that control group members have not gained access to the intervention.

Assessing whether the intervention was delivered as intended may need to be supplemented with efforts to ensure that the intervention was *received* as intended. This may involve a **manipulation check** to assess whether the treatment was perceived in an expected manner. For example, if we were testing the effect of soothing versus jarring music on anxiety, we might want to learn whether participants themselves perceived the music as soothing and jarring. Another aspect of treatment fidelity for behavior change interventions concerns the concept of enactment (Bellg et al., 2004). *Enactment* refers to participants' performance of the treatment-related skills, behaviors, and cognitive strategies in relevant real-life settings.

Example of Attention to Intervention Fidelity

Morrison and colleagues (2017) described strategies for enhancing and evaluating intervention fidelity, using as an illustration the efforts used in a multisite RCT for adults with multiple sclerosis. Their approach included audiotaping intervention classes, auditing computer exercises completed by participants, and monitoring class attendance.

Treatment adherence can be another problem. It is not unusual for those in the intervention group to elect not to participate fully in the treatment—for example, they may stop going to treatment sessions. Researchers should take steps to encourage participation among those in the treatment group. This might mean making the intervention as enjoyable as possible, offering incentives, and reducing burden in terms of data collection (Polit & Gillespie, 2010). Nonparticipation in an intervention is rarely random. Researchers should document which people got what amount of treatment so that individual differences in "dose" can be examined in the analysis or interpretation of results.

> **TIP** Except for small-scale studies, every study should have a **procedures manual** that delineates the protocols and procedures for implementation. The Toolkit section of the accompanying *Resource Manual* provides a model table of contents for such a procedures manual. The Toolkit also includes a model checklist to monitor delivery of an intervention through direct observation of intervention sessions.

INTERNAL VALIDITY

Internal validity refers to the extent to which it is possible to make an inference that the independent variable, rather than another factor, truly had a causal effect on the outcome. We infer from an effect to a cause by eliminating other potential causes. The control mechanisms reviewed earlier are strategies for improving internal validity. If researchers do not manage confounding variation, the conclusion that the outcome was caused by the independent variable is open to challenge.

Threats to Internal Validity

Experiments possess a high degree of internal validity because manipulation and random assignment allows researchers to rule out most alternative explanations for the results. Researchers who use quasi-experimental or correlational designs must contend with competing explanations of what caused the outcomes. Major threats to internal validity are examined in this section.

Temporal Ambiguity

One criterion for inferring a causal relationship is that the cause must precede the effect. In RCTs, researchers create the independent variable and then observe subsequent performance on an outcome, so establishing temporal sequencing is never a problem. In correlational studies, however, it may be unclear whether the independent variable preceded the dependent variable, or vice versa—and this is especially true in cross-sectional studies.

Selection

Selection (self-selection) encompasses biases resulting from preexisting differences between groups. When individuals are not assigned to groups randomly, the groups being compared are seldom completely equivalent. Differences on the outcomes could then reflect initial group differences rather than the effect of the independent variable. For example, if we found that men who were overweight were more likely to be depressed than men who were not overweight, it would be impossible to conclude that the two groups differed in depression *because* of their weight. The problem of selection is reduced if researchers can collect data on participants' characteristics before the occurrence of the independent variable. In our example, if we could measure men's level of depression *before* they became overweight, then the study could be designed to control earlier levels of depression. Selection bias is the most problematic and frequent threat to internal validity in studies not using an experimental design.

History

The **history threat** concerns the occurrence of external events that take place concurrently with the independent variable and that can affect the outcomes. For example, suppose we were studying the effectiveness of an outreach program to encourage pregnant women in rural areas to improve health practices (e.g., smoking cessation, prenatal care). The program might be evaluated by comparing the average birth weight of infants born in the 12 months before the outreach program with the average birth weight of those born in the 12 months after the program was introduced, using a time series design. However, suppose that 1 month after the new program was launched, a well-publicized TV program about the importance of healthy lifestyles during pregnancy was aired. Infants' birth weight might now be affected by both the intervention and the messages in the TV program, and it would be difficult to disentangle the two effects.

In a true experiment, history is not as likely to be a threat to a study's internal validity because we can often assume that external events are as likely to affect the intervention group as the control group. When this is the case, group differences on the dependent variables represent effects over and above those created by outside factors. There are, however, exceptions. For example, when a crossover design is used, an event external to the study may occur during the first half (or second half) of the experiment, and so treatments would be contaminated by the effect of that event. That is, some people would receive treatment A with the event and others would receive treatment A without it, and the same would be true for treatment B.

Selection biases sometimes interact with history to compound the threat to internal validity. For example, if the comparison group is different from the treatment group, then the characteristics of the members of the comparison group could lead them to have different intervening experiences, thereby introducing both history and selection biases into the design.

Maturation

In a research context, **maturation** refers to processes occurring during the study as a result of the passage of time rather than as a result of the independent variable. Examples of such processes include physical growth, emotional maturity, and fatigue. For instance, if we wanted to evaluate the effects of a sensorimotor program for developmentally delayed children, we would have to consider that progress occurs in these children even without special assistance. A one-group pretest–posttest design is highly susceptible to this threat.

Maturation is often a relevant consideration in health research. Maturation does not refer just to aging but rather to any change that occurs as a function of time. Thus, maturation in the form of wound healing, postoperative recovery, and other bodily changes could be a rival explanation for the independent variable's effect on outcomes.

Mortality/Attrition

Mortality is the validity threat that arises from attrition in groups being compared. If different kinds of people remain in the study in one group versus another, then these differences, rather than the independent variable, could account for observed differences on the outcomes. Severely ill patients might drop out of an experimental condition because it is too demanding, or they might drop out of the control group because they see no advantage to participating. In a prospective cohort study, there may be differential attrition between groups being compared because of death, illness, or geographic relocation. Attrition bias can also occur in single-group quasi-experiments if those dropping out of the study are a biased subset that makes it look like a change in average values resulted from a treatment.

The risk of attrition is especially great when the length of time between points of data collection is long. A 12-month follow-up of participants, for example, tends to produce higher rates of attrition than a 1-month follow-up (Polit & Gillespie, 2009). In clinical studies, the problem of attrition may be especially acute because of patient death or disability.

If attrition is random (i.e., those dropping out of a study are comparable to those remaining in it), then there would not be bias. However, attrition is rarely random. In general, the higher the rate of attrition, the greater the likelihood of bias.

TIP In longitudinal studies, attrition may occur because researchers cannot locate participants, not because they dropped out of the study. An effective strategy for **tracing** people is to obtain **contact information** from participants at each point of data collection. Contact information should include the names, addresses, telephone numbers, and email addresses of two to three people with whom the participant is close (e.g., siblings)—people who could provide information if participants moved. A sample contact information form is provided in the Toolkit of the accompanying *Resource Manual*.

Testing and Instrumentation

Testing refers to the effects of taking a pretest on people's performance on a posttest. It has been found, particularly in studies of attitudes, that the mere act of collecting data from people changes them. Suppose a sample of nursing students completed a questionnaire about attitudes toward assisted suicide. We then teach them about various arguments for and against assisted suicide, outcomes of court cases, and the like. Then we give them the same attitude measure and observe whether their attitudes have changed. The problem is that the first questionnaire might sensitize students, resulting in attitude changes regardless of whether instruction follows. If a comparison group is not used, it may be impossible to segregate the effects of the instruction from the pretest effects. Sensitization, or testing, problems are more likely to occur when people are exposed to controversial or novel material in the pretest.

A related threat is **instrumentation**. This bias reflects changes in measuring instruments or methods of measurement between two points of data collection. For example, if we used one measure of stress at baseline and a revised measure at follow-up, any differences might reflect changes in the measuring tool rather than the effect of an independent variable. Instrumentation effects can occur even if the same measure is used. For example, if the measuring tool yields more accurate measures on a second administration (e.g., if data collectors are more experienced) or less accurate measures the second time (e.g., if participants become bored and answer haphazardly), then these differences could bias the results.

Internal Validity and Research Design

Quasi-experimental and correlational studies are especially susceptible to threats to internal validity. Table 10.2 lists specific designs that are *most* vulnerable to the threats just described—but it should not be assumed that threats are irrelevant in designs not listed. Each threat represents an alternative explanation that competes with the independent variable as a cause of the outcome. The aim of a strong research design is to rule out competing explanations.

An experimental design normally rules out most rival hypotheses, but even in RCTs, researchers must exercise caution. For example, if there is treatment infidelity or contamination between treatments, then history might be a rival explanation for any group differences (or lack of differences). Mortality can be a salient threat in true experiments. Because the experimenter does things differently with the experimental and control groups, people in the groups may drop out of the study differentially. This is particularly apt to happen if the experimental treatment is painful or inconvenient or if the control condition is boring or bothersome. When this happens, participants remaining in the study may differ from those who left, thereby nullifying the initial equivalence of the groups. In short, researchers should consider how best to guard against and detect all possible threats to internal validity, no matter what design is used. Supplement A to this chapter on thePoint

TABLE 10.2 • Research Designs and Threats to Internal Validity

THREAT	DESIGNS MOST SUSCEPTIBLE
Temporal ambiguity	Case–control
	Other retrospective/cross-sectional studies
Selection	Nonequivalent control group (especially, posttest-only)
	Case–control
	"Natural" experiments with two groups
	Time series, if the population undergoes a change
History	One-group pretest–posttest
	Time series
	Prospective cohort
	Crossover
Maturation	One-group pretest–posttest
Mortality/attrition	Prospective cohort
	Longitudinal studies (experimental and observational)
	One-group pretest–posttest
Testing	All pretest–posttest designs
Instrumentation	All pretest–posttest designs

provides more detailed information about internal validity threats for specific experimental and quasi-experimental designs.

> **TIP** Traditional evidence hierarchies or level of evidence scales (e.g., Figure 2.2), rank evidence sources almost exclusively based on the risk of internal validity threats.

Internal Validity and Data Analysis

The best strategy for enhancing internal validity is to use a strong research design that includes control mechanisms and design features discussed in this chapter. Even when this is possible (and, certainly, when this is *not* possible), it is advisable to conduct analyses to assess the nature and extent of biases. When biases are detected, the information can be used to interpret the substantive results. Moreover, in some cases, biases can be statistically controlled.

Researchers need to be self-critics. They need to consider fully and objectively the types of biases that could have arisen—and then systematically search for evidence of their existence (while hoping, of course, that no evidence can be found). To the extent that biases can be ruled out or controlled, the quality of causal evidence will be strengthened.

Selection biases should always be examined. Typically, this involves comparing groups on pretest measures, when pretest data have been collected. For example, if we were studying depression in women who gave birth to a baby by cesarean delivery versus those who gave birth vaginally, selection bias could be assessed by comparing depression scores in these two groups during or before the pregnancy. If there are significant predelivery differences, then any postdelivery differences would have to be interpreted with initial differences in mind (or with differences controlled). In designs with no pretest measure of the outcome, researchers should assess selection biases by comparing groups with respect to key background variables, such as age, health status, and so on.

Whenever the research design involves multiple points of data collection, researchers should analyze attrition biases. This is typically achieved by comparing those who did and did not complete the study on baseline measures of the outcome or on other baseline characteristics.

Example of Assessing Internal Validity Threats
Uhm and Kim (2019) used a quasi-experimental design to study the effectiveness of a mother–nurse partnership program on the outcomes for mothers and infants in a pediatric cardiac intensive care unit. They tested for selection bias and found significant differences in the intervention and comparison group with respect to several baseline variables (e.g., preoperative NICU care), and these were controlled statistically using ANCOVA in the main analyses. There was no attrition in either group.

When people withdraw from an intervention study, researchers are in a dilemma about whom to "count" as being "in" a condition. One approach is a **per-protocol analysis**, which includes members in a treatment group only if they actually received the treatment. Such an analysis is problematic, however, because not receiving the treatment involves self-selection that can undo initial group comparability. This type of analysis will almost always be biased toward finding positive treatment effects. The "gold standard" approach is to use an **intention-to-treat analysis**, which involves keeping participants who were randomized in the groups to which they were assigned even if they drop out (Polit & Gillespie, 2009, 2010). An intention-to-treat analysis may yield an underestimate of the effects of a treatment if many participants did not actually get the assigned treatment—but may better reflect what would happen in the real world. One difficulty with an intention-to-treat analysis is that it is often difficult to obtain outcome data for people who have dropped out of a treatment, but there are strategies for estimating outcomes for those with missing data, as we discuss in Chapter 20.

Example of an Intention-to-treat Analysis
Zhang and colleagues (2018) explored the effect of suction pressure generated by a breast pump on mothers' onset of lactation and milk supply after cesarean birth. Mothers were randomly assigned to a high-pressure group, a low-pressure group, or a control group. The researchers, who used an intention-to-treat analysis, found that high-pressure pumping boosted the timing of the onset of lactation.

In a crossover design, history is a potential threat both because an external event could differentially affect people in different treatment orderings and because the different orderings are in themselves a kind of differential history. *Substantive* analyses of the data involve comparing outcomes under treatment A versus treatment B. The analysis of bias, by contrast, involves comparing participants in the different orderings (e.g., A then B versus B then A). Significant differences between the two orderings are evidence of an **ordering bias**.

In summary, efforts to enhance the internal validity of a study should not end once the design strategy has been put in place. Researchers should seek additional opportunities to understand (and possibly to correct) the various threats to internal validity that can arise.

Ⓢ Supplement B to this chapter on thePoint provides guidance on how to do a **plausibility analysis** to assess your design for internal validity threats when randomization is not possible, as well as other strategies for strengthening internal validity in quasi-experimental and case–control designs.

CONSTRUCT VALIDITY

Researchers conduct a study with specific exemplars of treatments, outcomes, settings, and people, which are stand-ins for broad constructs. Construct validity involves inferences from study particulars to the higher-order constructs that they are intended to represent. Constructs are the means for linking the operations used in a study to mechanisms for translating the resulting evidence into practice. If studies contain construct errors, the evidence may be misleading.

Enhancing Construct Validity

The first step in fostering construct validity is a careful explication of the treatment, outcomes, setting, and population constructs of interest; the next step is to select instances that match those constructs as closely as possible. Construct validity is further cultivated when researchers assess the match between the exemplars and the constructs and the degree to which any "slippage" occurred.

Construct validity has most often been a concern to researchers in connection with the measurement of outcomes, an issue we discuss in Chapter 15. There is a growing interest, however, in the careful conceptualization and development of theory-based interventions in which the treatment itself has strong construct validity (see Chapter 28). It is just as important for the independent variable (whether it be an intervention or something not amenable to manipulation) to be a strong instance of the construct of interest as it is for the measured outcome to have strong correspondence to the outcome construct. In nonexperimental research, researchers do not create and manipulate the hypothesized cause, so ensuring construct validity of the independent variable is often difficult.

Shadish and colleagues (2002) broadened the concept of construct validity to cover persons and settings as well as outcomes and treatments. For example, some nursing interventions specifically target groups that are characterized as "disadvantaged," but there is not always agreement on how this term is defined and operationalized. Researchers select specific people to represent the construct of a disadvantaged group about which inferences will be made, and so it is important that the specific people are good exemplars of the underlying construct. The construct "disadvantaged" must be carefully delineated before a sample is selected. Similarly, if a researcher is interested in such settings as "immigrant neighborhoods" or "school-based clinics," these are constructs that require careful description and the selection of good exemplars that match those constructs.

Threats to Construct Validity

Threats to construct validity are reasons that inferences from a particular study exemplar to an abstract construct could be erroneous. Such a threat could occur if the operationalization of the construct fails to incorporate all the relevant characteristics of the underlying construct or if it includes extraneous content—both of which are instances of a mismatch. Shadish and colleagues (2002) identified 14 threats to construct validity (their Table 3.1) and several additional threats specific to case–control designs (their Table 4.3). Among the most noteworthy threats are the following:

1. *Reactivity to the study situation.* Participants may behave in a particular manner because they are aware of their role in a study (the Hawthorne effect). When people's responses reflect, in part, their perceptions of study participation, those perceptions become an unwanted part of the treatment construct under study. Strategies to reduce this problem include blinding, the use of outcome measures not susceptible to

reactivity (e.g., from hospital records), and the use of preintervention strategies to satisfy participants' desire to look competent or please the researcher.

Example of a Possible Hawthorne Effect
Bhimani (2016) evaluated the effect of a series of strategies designed to reduce work-related musculoskeletal nursing injuries. A 50% reduction in injuries was found, but Bhimani noted that the Hawthorne effect likely contributed to the decline in injury rates.

2. *Researcher expectancies.* A similar threat stems from the researcher's influence on participant responses through subtle (or not-so-subtle) communication about desired outcomes. When this happens, the researcher's expectations become part of the treatment construct that is being tested. Blinding can reduce this threat, but another strategy is to make observations to detect verbal or behavioral signals of research staff's expectations and correct them.

3. *Novelty effects.* When a treatment is new, participants and research agents alike might alter their behavior. People may be either enthusiastic or skeptical about new methods of doing things. Results may reflect reactions to the novelty rather than to the intrinsic nature of an intervention, and so the intervention construct is clouded by novelty content.

4. *Compensatory effects.* In intervention studies, *compensatory equalization* can occur if health care staff or family members try to compensate for the control group members' failure to receive a perceived beneficial treatment. The compensatory goods or services are then part of the construct description of study conditions. *Compensatory rivalry* is a related threat arising from the control group members' desire to demonstrate that they can do as well as those receiving a special treatment.

5. *Treatment diffusion or contamination.* Alternative treatment conditions can become blurred, which can impede good construct descriptions of the independent variable. This may occur when participants in a control group condition receive services similar to those in the

treatment condition. More often, blurring occurs when those in a treatment condition essentially put themselves into the control group by dropping out of the intervention. This threat can also occur in nonexperimental studies. For example, in case–control comparisons of smokers and nonsmokers, care must be taken during screening to ensure that participants are appropriately categorized (e.g., some people may consider themselves nonsmokers even though they smoke regularly, but only on weekends).

Construct validity requires careful attention to what we *call* things (i.e., construct labels) so that appropriate construct inferences can be made. Enhancing construct validity in a study requires careful thought before a study is undertaken, in terms of a well-considered explication of constructs, and requires poststudy scrutiny to assess the degree to which a match between operations and constructs was achieved.

EXTERNAL VALIDITY

External validity concerns the extent to which it can be inferred that relationships observed in a study hold true over variations in people, conditions, and settings. External validity has emerged as a major concern in an EBP world in which there is an interest in generalizing evidence from tightly controlled research settings to real-world clinical practice settings.

External validity questions may take several different forms. We may ask whether relationships observed in a study sample can be generalized to a larger population—for example, whether results from a smoking cessation program found effective with pregnant teenagers in Boston can be generalized to pregnant teenagers throughout the United States. Other external validity questions are about generalizing to types of people, settings, or treatments unlike those in the research (Polit & Beck, 2010). For example, can findings about a pain reduction treatment in a study of Australian women be generalized to men in Canada? Sometimes new studies are needed to answer questions about external validity, but external validity often can be enhanced by researchers' design decisions.

Enhancements to External Validity

One aspect of external validity concerns the *representativeness* of the participants used in the study. For example, if the sample is selected to be representative of a population to which the researcher wishes to generalize the results, then the findings can more readily be applied to that population (Chapter 13). Similarly, if the settings in which the study occurs are representative of the clinical settings in which the findings might be applied, then inferences about relevance in those other settings can be strengthened.

An important concept for external validity is *replication*. Multisite studies are powerful because more confidence in the generalizability of the results can be attained if findings are replicated in several sites—particularly if the sites are different on important dimensions (e.g., size, nursing skill mix, and so on). Studies with a diverse sample of participants can test whether study results are replicated for subgroups of the sample—for example, whether benefits from an intervention apply to men *and* women. Systematic reviews are a crucial aid to external validity precisely because they illuminate the consistency of results in studies replicated with different groups and settings.

Threats to External Validity

In the previous chapter, we discussed *interaction effects* that can occur in a factorial design when two treatments are simultaneously manipulated. The interaction question is whether the effects of treatment A hold (are comparable) for all levels of treatment B. Conceptually, questions regarding external validity are similar to this interaction question. Threats to external validity concern ways in which relationships between variables might interact with or be moderated by variations in people, settings, time, and conditions. Shadish and colleagues (2002) described several threats to external validity, such as the following two:

1. *Interaction between relationship and people.* An effect observed with certain types of people might not be observed with other types of people. A common complaint about RCTs is that many people are excluded—not because

they would not benefit from the treatment, but because they cannot provide needed research data (e.g., cognitively impaired patients, non-English speakers) or because they would not allow the "best test" of the intervention (e.g., they have complex comorbidities).

2. *Interaction between causal effects and treatment variation.* An innovative treatment might be effective because it is paired with other elements, and sometimes those elements are intangible—e.g., an enthusiastic project director. The same "treatment" could never be fully replicated, and thus different results might be obtained in subsequent tests.

Shadish and colleagues (2002) noted that moderators of relationships are the norm, not the exception. With interventions, it is normal for a treatment to "work better" for some people than for others. We address this issue in Chapter 31.

TRADEOFFS AND PRIORITIES IN STUDY VALIDITY

Quantitative researchers strive to design studies that are strong with respect to all four types of study validity. Sometimes, efforts to increase one type of validity also benefit another type. In many instances, however, addressing one type of validity increases threats to others.

For example, suppose we were scrupulous in maximizing intervention fidelity in an RCT. Our efforts might include strong training of staff, careful monitoring of intervention delivery, and steps to maximize participants' adherence to treatment. Such efforts would have positive effects on statistical conclusion validity because the treatment was made powerful. Internal validity would be enhanced if attrition biases were minimized. Intervention fidelity would also improve the construct validity of the treatment because the content delivered and received would better match the underlying construct. But what about external validity? All of the actions undertaken to ensure that the intervention is strong, construct-valid, and administered according to plan are not consistent with the realities of clinical settings. People are not normally paid to adhere to treatments; nurses are not monitored and corrected to ensure that they are following a script; training in the use of new protocols is usually brief; and so on.

This example illustrates that researchers need to give careful thought to how design decisions may affect various types of study validity. Of particular concern are tradeoffs between internal and external validity.

Internal Validity and External Validity

Tension between the goals of achieving internal validity and external validity is pervasive. Many control mechanisms that are designed to rule out competing explanations for hypothesized cause-and-effect relationships make it difficult to infer that the relationships hold true in uncontrolled real-life settings.

Internal validity was long considered the "sine qua non" of experimental research (Campbell & Stanley, 1963). The rationale was this: If there is insufficient evidence that an intervention really caused an effect, why worry about generalizing the results? This high priority given to internal validity, however, is somewhat at odds with the current emphasis on evidence-based practice. A reasonable question might be: If study results cannot be generalized to real-world clinical settings, who *cares* if an intervention is effective? Clearly, both internal and external validity are important to building an evidence base for nursing practice.

There are several "solutions" to the conflict between internal and external validity. The first (and most prevalent) approach is to emphasize one and sacrifice the other. Most often, it is external validity that is sacrificed. For example, external validity is not even considered in ranking evidence in level of evidence scales (Chapter 2).

A second approach is to use a phased series of studies. In the earlier phase, there are tight controls, strict intervention protocols, and stringent criteria for including people in the RCT. Such studies are **efficacy studies**. Once the intervention has been deemed to be effective under tightly controlled conditions in which internal validity was the priority, it is tested with larger samples in multiple sites under less restrictive conditions, in **effectiveness studies** that emphasize external validity.

A third approach is to compromise. There has been recent interest in promoting designs that aim to achieve a balance between internal and external validity in a single intervention study. We describe such *pragmatic clinical trials* in Chapter 31, a new chapter that discusses the *applicability* of research findings.

Prioritization and Design Decisions

It is impossible to avoid all possible threats to study validity. By understanding the various threats, however, you can pinpoint the tradeoffs you are willing to make to achieve study goals. Some threats are more worrisome than others in terms of likelihood of occurrence and dangers to inferences you would like to make. Moreover, some threats are costlier to avoid than others. Resources available for a study must be allocated to address the most important validity issues. For example, with a fixed budget, you need to decide whether it is better to increase the size of the sample and hence power (statistical conclusion validity) or to use the money on efforts to reduce attrition (internal validity).

The point is that you should make conscious decisions about how to structure a study to address validity concerns. Every design decision has both a "payoff" and a cost in terms of study integrity.

TIP A useful strategy is to create a matrix that lists various design decisions in the first column (e.g., randomization, crossover design), and then use the next four columns to identify the potential impact of those options on the four types of study validity. The Toolkit section of the accompanying *Resource Manual* includes a model matrix as a Word document for you to use and adapt.

CRITICAL APPRAISAL OF STUDY VALIDITY

In critically appraising a research report to evaluate its potential contribution to nursing practice, it is crucial to make judgments about the extent to which threats to validity were minimized— or, at least, assessed and taken into consideration

in interpreting the results. The guidelines in Box 10.1 ⊗ focus on validity-related issues to further help you to appraise quantitative research designs. Together with the guidelines in the previous chapter, they are likely to be the core of a critical evaluation of the evidence that quantitative studies yield. From an EBP perspective, it is important to remember that drawing inferences about causal relationships relies not only on how high up on the evidence hierarchy a study is (Figure 2.2), but also, for any given level of the hierarchy, how successful the researcher was in managing study validity and balancing competing validity demands.

RESEARCH EXAMPLE

We conclude this chapter with an example of a study in which careful attention was paid to many aspects of study validity. The design being used in this research is explained more fully in Chapter 31.

Study: Using SMART design to improve symptom management among cancer patients (Sikorskii et al., 2017).

Statement of purpose: The purpose of the study, which was still in progress when the article about the study protocol was written, was to evaluate the efficacy of a Sequential Multiple Assignment Randomized Trial (SMART) of interventions to improve symptom management among patients with cancer.

Treatment groups: The study is testing two evidence-based practices: reflexology and meditative (mindfulness) practices. Dyads of solid tumor cancer patients and their caregivers are initially assigned to one of these interventions, which is offered in the patients' homes, or to a control group of usual care. After 4 weeks, intervention group dyads that show little improvement in fatigue are rerandomized to either continuing in the original intervention or adding the alternative intervention.

Method: The researchers are using a design that addresses many validity concerns. Randomization (both initially and at rerandomization) is being done using a computer minimization algorithm that is designed to balance the arms for the patient's site of cancer (e.g., breast, lung, colon), stage of cancer, and

BOX 10.1 Guidelines for Critically Appraising Design Elements and Study Validity in Quantitative Studies

1. Was there adequate statistical power? Did the manner in which the independent variable was operationalized create strong contrasts that enhanced statistical power? Was precision enhanced by controlling confounding variables? If hypotheses were not supported (e.g., a hypothesized relationship was not found), is it possible that statistical conclusion validity was compromised and the results are wrong?
2. In intervention studies, did the researchers attend to intervention fidelity? For example, were staff adequately trained? Was the implementation of the intervention monitored? Was attention paid to both the delivery and receipt of the intervention?
3. What evidence does the report provide that selection biases were eliminated or minimized? What steps were taken to control confounding participant characteristics that could affect the equivalence of groups being compared? Were these steps adequate?
4. To what extent did the research design rule out the plausibility of other threats to internal validity, such as history, attrition, maturation, and so on? What are your overall conclusions about the internal validity of the study?
5. Were there any major threats to the construct validity of the study? In intervention studies, was there a good match between the underlying conceptualization of the intervention and its operationalization? Was the intervention confounded with extraneous content, such as researcher expectations? Was the setting or site a good exemplar of the type of setting envisioned in the conceptualization?
6. Was the context of the study sufficiently described to enhance its capacity for external validity? Were the settings or participants representative of the types to which results were designed to be generalized?
7. Overall, did the researcher appropriately balance validity concerns? Was attention paid to certain types of threats (e.g., internal validity) at the expense of others (e.g., external validity)?

type of treatment. (See Supplement to Chapter 9 for information about this type of randomization.) The researchers estimated how large a sample was needed to achieve adequate power for statistical conclusion validity, using a procedure called power analysis (Chapter 13).

Additional study validity efforts: For dyads in the reflexology group, caregivers are trained by a study reflexologist. For dyads in the meditative group, both the patient and the caregiver are trained by a study meditation provider. All intervention agents are being carefully trained and monitored. Patients and caregivers in all groups are interviewed twice by telephone, at baseline and then at study week 12. The interviewers are blinded to the dyad's group assignments. The interviewers gather information about patients' fatigue, pain, depression, and anxiety using instruments known to be of high quality. A study coordinator calls patients weekly to ask about their

symptoms and also asks caregivers in the intervention groups about the number of sessions conducted with the patients. Although the analysis was not yet undertaken when this paper was written, the researchers plan to control statistically for demographic and baseline clinical characteristics. The researchers are implementing extensive procedures to ensure intervention fidelity. For example, both the intervention agents and the caregivers must achieve proficiency in their therapies. The caregivers' enactment of the therapies is being monitored. The researchers plan to undertake an attrition analyses to compare the characteristics of those who do or do not drop out of the study.

Conclusions: When the paper was written, the researchers had enrolled 150 of the 430 dyads they planned to enroll. Forty dyads of the 150 have been rerandomized. The researchers acknowledged that the recruitment of dyads is challenging.

SUMMARY POINTS

- Study validity concerns the extent to which appropriate inferences can be made. **Threats to validity** are reasons that an inference could be wrong. A key function of quantitative research design is to rule out validity threats.
- Control over confounding participant characteristics is key to managing many validity threats. The best control method is randomization to treatment conditions, which effectively controls all confounding variables—especially in the context of a crossover design.
- When randomization is not possible, other control methods include **homogeneity** (the use of a homogeneous sample to eliminate variability on confounding characteristics); blocking or stratifying, as in the case of a *randomized block design*; **pair matching** participants on key variables to make groups more comparable (or by using **propensity matching**, which involves matching on a **propensity score** for each participant); **balancing** groups to achieve comparability; and **statistical control** to remove the effect of a confounding variable statistically (e.g., through **analysis of covariance**).
- Homogeneity, stratifying, matching, and statistical control share two disadvantages: Researchers must know in advance which confounding variables to control, and they can rarely control all of them.
- Four types of validity affect the rigor of a quantitative study: statistical conclusion validity, internal validity, construct validity, and external validity.
- **Statistical conclusion validity** concerns the validity of the inference that a relationship between variables really exists.
- Threats to statistical conclusion validity include low **statistical power** (the ability to detect true relationships among variables); low **precision** (the exactness of the relationships revealed after controlling confounding variables); and factors that weaken the operationalization of the independent variable.

- **Intervention** (or **treatment**) **fidelity** concerns the extent to which the implementation of a treatment is faithful to its plan. Intervention fidelity is enhanced through standardized treatment protocols, careful training of intervention agents, monitoring of the delivery and receipt of the intervention, **manipulation checks,** and steps to promote **treatment adherence** and avoid **contamination of treatments**.
- **Internal validity** concerns the inference that outcomes were caused by the independent variable, rather than by confounding factors. Threats to internal validity include temporal ambiguity (lack of clarity about whether the presumed cause preceded the outcome); **selection** (preexisting group differences); **history** (the occurrence of external events that could affect outcomes); **maturation** (changes resulting from the passage of time); **mortality** (effects attributable to attrition); **testing** (effects of a pretest); and **instrumentation** (changes in the way data are gathered).
- Internal validity can be enhanced through judicious design decisions but can also be addressed analytically (e.g., through an analysis of selection or attrition biases). When people withdraw from a study, an **intention-to-treat analysis** (analyzing outcomes for all people in their original treatment conditions) is preferred to a **per-protocol analysis** (analyzing outcomes only for those who received the full treatment) for maintaining the integrity of randomization.
- **Construct validity** concerns inferences from the particular exemplars of a study (e.g., the specific treatments, outcomes, and settings) to the higher-order constructs that they are intended to represent. The first step in fostering construct validity is a careful explication of those constructs.
- Threats to construct validity can occur if the operationalization of a construct fails to incorporate all relevant characteristics of the construct, or if it includes extraneous content. Examples of such threats include *subject reactivity, researcher expectancies, novelty effects, compensatory effects*, and *treatment diffusion*.

- **External validity** concerns inferences about the extent to which study results can be generalized—i.e., whether relationships observed in a study hold true over variations in people, settings, time, and treatments. External validity can be enhanced by selecting *representative* people and settings and through replication.
- Researchers need to prioritize and recognize tradeoffs among the various types of validity, which sometimes compete with each other. Tensions between internal and external validity are especially prominent. One solution has been to begin with a study that emphasizes internal validity (**efficacy studies**) and then if a causal relationship can be inferred, to undertake **effectiveness studies** that emphasize external validity.

STUDY ACTIVITIES

Study activities are available to instructors on thePoint.

REFERENCES CITED IN CHAPTER 10

Abbasi, P., Mohammed-Alizadeh, S., & Mirghafourvand, M. (2018). Comparing the effect of e-learning and educational booklet on the childbirth self-efficacy: A randomized controlled clinical trial. *Journal of Maternal-Fetal & Neonatal Medicine, 31*, 633–650.

*Bang, K., Kim, S., Song, M., Kang, K., & Jeong, Y. (2018). The effects of a health promotion program using urban forests and nursing student mentors on the perceived and psychological health of elementary school children in vulnerable populations. *International Journal of Environmental Research and Public Health, 15*, 1977.

*Bellg, A., Borrelli, B., Resnick, B., Hecht, J., Minicucci, D., et al. (2004). Enhancing treatment fidelity in health behavior change studies: Best practices and recommendations from the NIH Behavior Change Consortium. *Health Psychology, 23*, 443–451.

Bhimani, R. (2016). Prevention of work-related musculoskeletal injuries in rehabilitation nursing. *Rehabilitation Nursing, 41*, 326–335.

Bova, C., Jaffarian, C., Crawford, S., Quintos, J., Lee, M., & Sullivan-Bolyai, S. (2017). Intervention fidelity: Monitoring drift, providing feedback, and assessing the control condition. *Nursing Research, 66*, 54–59.

Campbell, D. T., & Stanley, J. C. (1963). *Experimental and quasi-experimental designs for research.* Chicago: Rand McNally.

Conn, V. S., Rantz, M. J., Wipke-Tevis, D. D., & Maas, M. L. (2001). Designing effective nursing interventions. *Research in Nursing & Health, 24*, 433–442.

*Fehlberg, E., Lucero, R., Weaver, M., McDaniel, A., Chandler, A., Richey, P., … Shorr, R. (2017). Associations between hyponatraemia, volume depletion and the risk of falls in US hospitalised patients. *BMJ Open, 7*, e017045.

Lipsey, M. W. (1990). *Design sensitivity: Statistical power for experimental research.* Newbury Park, CA: Sage.

**Morrison, J., Becker, H., & Stuifbergen, A. (2017). Evaluation of intervention fidelity in a multisite clinical trial in persons with multiple sclerosis. *Journal of Neuroscience Nursing, 49*, 344–348.

Polit, D. F., & Beck, C. T. (2010). Generalization in qualitative and quantitative research: Myths and strategies. *International Journal of Nursing Studies, 47*, 1451–1458.

Polit, D. F., & Gillespie, B. (2009). The use of the intention-to-treat principle in nursing clinical trials. *Nursing Research, 58*, 391–399.

Polit, D. F., & Gillespie, B. (2010). Intention-to-treat in randomized controlled trials: Recommendations for a total trial strategy. *Research in Nursing & Health, 33*, 355–368.

*Qin, R., Titler, M., Shever, L., & Kim, T. (2008). Estimating effects of nursing intervention via propensity score analysis. *Nursing Research, 57*, 444–452.

*Rixon, L., Baron, J., McGale, N., Lorencatto, F., Francis, J., & Davies, A. (2016). Methods used to address fidelity of receipt in health intervention research: A citation analysis and systematic review. *BMC Health Services Research, 16*, 663.

Shadish, W. R., Cook, T. D., & Campbell, D. T. (2002). *Experimental and quasi-experimental designs for generalized causal inference.* Boston: Houghton Mifflin Co.

Sikorskii, A., Wyatt, G., Lehto, R., Victorson, D., Badger, T., & Pace, T. (2017). Using SMART design to improve symptom management among cancer patients: A study protocol. *Research in Nursing & Health, 40*, 501–511.

Uhm, J., & Kim, H. (2019). Impact of the mother-nurse partnership programme on mother and infant outcomes in paediatric cardiac intensive care unit. *Intensive & Critical Care Nursing, 50*, 79–87.

Zhang, F., Yang, Y., Bai, T., Sun, L., Sun, M., Shi, X., … Xia, H. (2018). Effect of pumping pressure on onset of lactation after caesarean section: A randomized controlled study. *Maternal & Child Nutrition, 14*, (1).

A link to this open-access journal article is provided in the Toolkit for Chapter 10 in the **Resource Manual.** ✖

**This journal article is available on* thePoint *for this chapter.*

11 | Specific Types of Quantitative Research

All quantitative studies can be categorized as experimental, quasi-experimental, or nonexperimental in design. This chapter describes types of research that vary in study purpose rather than research design. The first two types (clinical trials and evaluations) involve interventions, but methods for each have evolved separately because of their disciplinary roots. Clinical trials are associated with health care and medicine, and evaluation research is associated with the fields of education, social work, and public policy. There is overlap in approaches, but to acquaint you with relevant terms, we discuss each separately. Later sections of this chapter describe comparative effectiveness research, outcomes research, survey research, and several other types relevant to nursing.

CLINICAL TRIALS

Clinical trials are studies designed to assess clinical interventions. Many nurse researchers are involved in clinical trials, often as members of interprofessional teams.

Phases of a Clinical Trial

In medical and pharmaceutical research, clinical trials often adhere to a planned sequence of studies—often a series of four phases, as follows:

Phase I occurs after initial development of the drug or therapy and is designed primarily to establish safety and tolerance and to determine optimal dose. This phase typically involves small-scale studies using simple designs, such as a one group pretest–posttest design. The focus is on developing the best possible (and safest) treatment.

Phase II involves gathering preliminary evidence about the intervention's practicability. During this phase, researchers assess the feasibility of launching a rigorous test, seek evidence that the treatment holds promise, and identify refinements to improve the intervention. This phase, a pilot test of the treatment, may be designed either as a small-scale experiment or as a quasi-experiment. Pilot tests of interventions are described in Chapter 29.

> **Example of an Early Phase Clinical Trial**
> Heyland and colleagues (2018) described a protocol for a Phase II trial of two alternative approaches to partnering with family members in the care of critically ill long-stay ICU patients. A total of 150 families were randomly assigned to a control group or to one of the two approaches of supporting families in shared decision-making (50 per group).

Phase III is a full test of the intervention—a randomized controlled trial (RCT) with randomization to treatment groups under controlled conditions. The goal of this phase is to develop evidence about treatment *efficacy*—i.e., whether the treatment is more efficacious than usual care (or an alternative counterfactual). Adverse effects are also monitored. Phase III RCTs often involve a fairly large sample of participants, sometimes selected from multiple sites to ensure that findings are not unique to a single setting. Phase III (and Phase IV) efforts may also examine the cost-effectiveness of the intervention.

Example of a Multisite Phase III RCT

Watson and colleagues (2018) undertook a Phase III cluster RCT to assess the postdischarge outcomes (functional status and quality of life) of children hospitalized in 31 medical centers. A total of 1,360 ventilated children were randomly assigned to either a nurse-implemented goal-directed sedation protocol or to usual care.

Phase IV trials are studies of the *effectiveness* of an intervention in a general population. The emphasis is on the external validity of an intervention that has shown promise of efficacy under controlled (but often artificial) conditions.

TIP Researchers should record their trials in a **clinical trials registry**. These registries provide transparency about research and offer information for accessing the trial. Most registries are searchable online (e.g., by disease, location of the trial). The largest registry is ClinicalTrials.gov; another important registry is the International Clinical Trials Registry of the World Health Organization. Some journals refuse to publish reports of trials unless they have been registered. Protocols for clinical trials are often registered before the study gets underway.

Superiority, Noninferiority, and Equivalence Trials

The vast majority of RCTs are **superiority trials,** in which researchers hypothesize that the intervention is "superior" to (more effective than) the control condition. Standard statistical analysis does not permit a straightforward testing of the null hypothesis, i.e., the hypothesis that the effects of two treatments are comparable. Yet,

there are circumstances in which it is desirable to test whether a new (and perhaps less costly or less painful) intervention results in similar outcomes to a standard intervention. In a **noninferiority trial**, the goal is to assess whether a new intervention is no worse than a reference treatment (typically, the standard of care). Other trials are called **equivalence trials,** in which the goal is to test the hypothesis that the outcomes from two interventions are equal. In a noninferiority trial, it is necessary to specify in advance the smallest margin of inferiority on a primary outcome (e.g., 1%) that would be tolerated to accept the hypothesis of noninferiority. In equivalence trials, a *tolerance* must be established for the nonsuperiority of one treatment over the other, and the statistical test is two-sided—meaning that equivalence is accepted if the two are not different (in either direction) by no more than the specified tolerance. Both noninferiority and equivalence trials require statistical sophistication and very large samples to ensure statistical conclusion validity. Further information is provided by Christensen (2007) and Piaggio et al. (2012).

Example of an Equivalence Trial

Makenzius and colleagues (2017) conducted an equivalence trial to test whether women with incomplete abortion seeking postabortion care in a low-resource area in Kenya had the same outcomes when misoprostol was administered by midwives compared with administration by physicians. A total of 810 women were randomized. The results indicated that treatment by midwives was equally effective, safe, and accepted by the patients.

TIP In a traditional Phase III trial, it may take months to recruit and randomize a sufficiently large sample and years to draw conclusions about efficacy (i.e., after all data have been collected and analyzed). In a **sequential clinical trial**, experimental data are continuously analyzed as they become available, and the trial can be stopped when the evidence is strong enough to support a conclusion about the intervention's efficacy. More information about sequential trials is provided by Bartroff et al. (2013).

Pragmatic Clinical Trials

One problem with traditional Phase III RCTs is that, in efforts to enhance internal validity in support of a causal inference, the designs are so tightly controlled that their relevance to real-life applications can be questioned. Concern about this situation has led to a call for **pragmatic** (or *practical*) **clinical trials**, in which researchers strive to maximize external validity with minimal negative effect on internal validity (Glasgow et al., 2005). Pragmatic clinical trials address practical questions about the benefits and risks of an intervention as they would unfold in routine clinical practice. We elaborate on pragmatic clinical trials in Chapter 31.

EVALUATION RESEARCH

Evaluation research focuses on developing information needed by decision-makers about whether to adopt, modify, or abandon a program, practice, procedure, or policy. Patton (2015) distinguishes *research* and *evaluation,* stating that "research has as its primary purpose contributing to knowledge, and evaluation has as its primary purpose informing action," (p. 86). However, evaluations often generate knowledge that can be used in other settings. Concepts from evaluation research are embedded in many efforts to test health care interventions.

Evaluations often try to answer broader questions than whether a program is effective—for example, they may involve efforts to improve the program or to learn how the program actually "works" in practice. Evaluations sometimes address *black box questions*—that is, what specifically is it about a multifaceted program that is driving observed effects? Good resources for learning more about evaluation research include the books by Patton (2012) and Rossi and colleagues (2019).

> **TIP** Evaluations can be threatening. Even though the focus of most evaluations is on a nontangible entity (e.g., a program), it is *people* who implement it. People may think that they, or their work, are being evaluated and may feel that their jobs or reputation are at stake. Thus, evaluation researchers need to have more than methodologic skills—they need to be adept in interpersonal relations.

Evaluation Components

Evaluations may involve several components to answer a range of questions, as we describe in this section.

Process/Implementation Analyses

A **process** or **implementation analysis** provides descriptive information about the manner in which a program gets implemented and how it actually functions. A process analysis typically addresses questions such as the following: Does the program operate the way its designers intended? How does the program differ from traditional practices? What were the barriers to its implementation? What do staff and clients like most/least about the program?

A process analysis may be undertaken with the aim of improving a program (a *formative evaluation*). In other situations, the purpose of the process analysis is primarily to describe a program carefully so that it can be replicated—or so that people can understand why the program was or was not effective in meeting its objectives. In either case, a process analysis involves an in-depth examination of the operation of a program, often requiring the collection of both qualitative and quantitative data. Process evaluations sometimes overlap with efforts to monitor intervention fidelity.

> **Example of a Process Analysis**
> Boersma and colleagues (2017) undertook a process analysis during the implementation of an intervention called the Veder contact method (which combines elements from psychosocial interventions with theatrical and poetic communication) in nursing home care. The process analysis involved group and individual interviews with multiple stakeholders.

Outcome and Impact Analyses

Evaluations may focus on whether a program or policy is meeting its objectives. The intent of such evaluations is to help people decide whether the program should be continued or replicated. Some evaluation researchers distinguish between an outcome analysis and an impact analysis. An **outcome analysis** (or *outcome evaluation*) simply documents the extent to which the goals of the program are attained, that is, the extent to which positive outcomes occur. For example, a program may be designed to encourage women in a poor rural community to obtain prenatal care. In an outcome analysis, the researchers might document the percentage of pregnant women who had obtained prenatal care, the average month in which prenatal care was begun, and so on, and perhaps compare this information to preintervention community data.

An **impact analysis** assesses a program's **net impacts**—impacts that can be attributed to the program, over and above effects of a counterfactual (e.g., standard care). Impact analyses use an experimental or strong quasi-experimental design because their aim is to facilitate causal inferences about program effects. In our example, suppose that the program to encourage prenatal care involved having nurses make home visits to women in rural areas to explain the benefits of early care. If the visits could be made to pregnant women randomly assigned to the program, the outcomes of the group of women receiving the home visits could be compared with those not receiving them to assess the intervention's net impacts—for example, the percentage *increase* in receipt of prenatal care among the experimental group relative to the control group.

Example of an Impact Analysis

Račić and colleagues (2017) tested the impact of interprofessional diabetes education on the knowledge of nursing, medical, and dental students. Students were randomized to interprofessional versus uniprofessional education. Those in the interprofessional education group had significantly higher knowledge scores and self-assessments of teamwork skills.

Cost/Economic Analyses

New programs are often expensive to implement, and existing programs also may be costly. In our current situation of spiraling health care costs, evaluations (and clinical trials) may include a **cost analysis** (**economic analysis**) to examine whether program benefits outweigh the monetary costs. Administrators make decisions about resource allocations for health services based not only on whether something "works," but also on whether it is economically viable. Cost analyses are typically done in connection with impact analyses and Phase III clinical trials, that is, alongside rigorous tests of a program's or intervention's efficacy.

Two types of economic analysis are cost–benefit and cost-effectiveness analyses:

- **Cost–benefit analysis,** in which monetary estimates are established for both costs and benefits. One difficulty, however, is that it is sometimes difficult to quantify benefits of health services in monetary terms. There is also controversy about methods of assigning dollar amounts to the value of human life.
- **Cost-effectiveness analysis,** which is used to compare health outcomes and resource costs of alternative interventions. Costs are measured in monetary terms, but outcome effectiveness is not. Such analyses estimate what it costs to produce impacts on outcomes that cannot easily be valued in dollars, such as quality of life. Without information on monetary benefits, however, such research may face challenges in persuading decision-makers to make changes.

Example of a Cost-Effectiveness Analysis

Mervin and colleagues (2018) undertook a cost-effectiveness analysis of using PARO, a therapeutic robotic seal used to reduce agitation and medication use among patients with dementia. The analysis was based on data from a cluster randomized trial of 28 long-term care facilities in Australia.

Cost–utility analyses are a third type of economic analysis. This approach is preferred when morbidity and mortality are outcomes of interest or when quality of life is a major concern. An index called the **quality-adjusted life year** (**QALY**) is an important outcome indicator in cost–utility analyses. As a measure of disease burden, QALY includes both the quality and quantity of life lived. One QALY equates to 1 year in perfect health; zero QALY is associated with death.

Example of a Cost–Utility Analysis

Heslin and an interprofessional team (2017) conducted a cost–utility analysis in the context of an RCT that tested an intervention to improve health and reduce substance use in people with severe mental illness, compared with standard care. One outcome in their analysis was QALY at 12 and 15 months after baseline.

In doing economic analyses, researchers must think about possible short-term costs (e.g., clients' days of work missed within 6 months) and long-term costs (e.g., lost years of productive work life). Often the cost analyst examines economic gains and losses from different accounting perspectives—for example, for the target group; the hospitals implementing the program; taxpayers; and society as a whole. Distinguishing these different perspectives is crucial if a program effect is a loss for one group (e.g., taxpayers) but a gain for another (e.g., the target group).

Nurse researchers are increasingly becoming involved in cost analyses—although Cook and colleagues (2017) recently found many deficiencies in the quality of economic evaluations in nursing research in the United States. A useful resource for further guidance is the internationally acclaimed textbook by Drummond and colleagues (2015).

> **TIP** Among those planning an evidence-based practice improvement, the costs of an innovation may be a concern. A key question might be whether there is the potential for **return on investment (ROI),** that is, whether the innovation might save money (or at least be cost neutral) in the long run, relative to the time and resources that will be expended to implement it in routine practice.

Realist Evaluations

Some nurse researchers have begun to undertake **realist evaluations,** which constitute a theory-driven approach to evaluating programs—especially complex programs or interventions. The realist approach acknowledges that interventions are not always effective for everyone, because people are diverse and embedded in complicated social and cultural contexts. In a realist evaluation, consideration is given to the theoretical mechanisms underlying the effects of an intervention. The focus is on understanding why certain groups benefitted from an intervention while others did not benefit.

Pawson and Tilley (1997), who are key proponents of realist evaluations, argued that to be useful to decision-makers, evaluators need to identify "What works for whom and under what circumstances?" rather than simply, "Does this work?"

Realist evaluations are not undertaken with a prescribed set of methods; decisions about design, data collection, and analysis are guided by the types of data needed to answer the evaluation questions and test the initial program theory. Most often, realist evaluations involve the collection of both quantitative and qualitative data, and qualitative approaches play an especially important role.

> **Example of a Realist Evaluation**
> Kerr and colleagues (2018) used a realist evaluation framework in their mixed-methods study of a program to facilitate transition from children's services to adult services for young adults with life-limiting conditions.

> **TIP** Health technology assessments (HTAs) are systematic evaluations of the effects of health technologies and interventions. HTA is a form of health policy research that examines the health and social consequences of the application of technology. A central goal of such evaluations is to provide policy-makers with evidence on policy alternatives. Ramacciati (2013) has written a useful review about health technology assessments in nursing.

COMPARATIVE EFFECTIVENESS RESEARCH

Comparative effectiveness research (CER) involves direct comparisons of two or more health interventions. Like realist approaches, CER seeks insights into which intervention works best, for which patients. CER has emerged as a major force in health research; disappointment with some of the methods favored for evidence-based practice—especially the strong reliance on tightly controlled RCTs with placebo comparators—has led to the development of new ideas, new models, and new methods of research that fall within the umbrella of comparative effectiveness research.

In the United States, CER gained ground in the early 2000s and the impetus crystallized with the publication of a report by the Institute of Medicine (IOM) in 2009. The IOM, which proposed initial priorities for comparative effectiveness research, defined CER as: "the generation and synthesis of evidence that compares the benefits and harms of alternative methods to prevent, diagnose, treat, and monitor a clinical condition or to improve the delivery of care. The purpose of CER is to assist consumers clinicians, purchasers, and policy makers to make informed decisions that will improve health care at both the individual and population level" (Chapter 2, p. 41).

Another major stimulus for CER in the United States was the creation of the independent nonprofit organization called the **Patient-Centered Outcomes Research Institute** (**PCORI**), which was authorized by the U.S. Congress in 2010. PCORI specifically sponsors comparative effectiveness research—in fact, CER is sometimes referred to as **patient-centered outcomes research**. PCORI funds research that is designed to help patients select the health care options that best meet their needs. CER studies often incorporate outcomes that are especially important to patients and their caregivers. The standard outcomes used in medical research (e.g., blood pressure, mortality) are increasingly being supplemented by outcomes in which patients have a strong interest, such as functional limitations, quality of life, and experiences with care. Barksdale and colleagues (2014) have described the relevance of PCORI to nursing, including funding opportunities.

Designs for CER vary widely. Some studies are RCTs involving a comparison of two or more active (nonplacebo) treatments. Some CER projects, however, are observational studies using data from large databases, such as patient registries. Comparative effectiveness research is described at greater length in Chapter 31, which focuses on methods to enhance the applicability of research to individual patients in real-world clinical settings.

Example of Comparative Effectiveness Research

In 2017, PCORI awarded $14 million to an interprofessional team led by a nurse researcher (Huong Nguyen) for a 15-site project called "A non-inferiority comparative effectiveness trial of home-based palliative care in older adults (HomePal)". The project, which will compare home-based palliative care with in-person or video consultation, is expected to be completed in 2024. (https://www.pcori.org/research-results/2017/comparing-home-based-palliative-care-person-or-video-consultation).

HEALTH SERVICES AND OUTCOMES RESEARCH

Health services research is the broad interdisciplinary field that studies how organizational structures and processes, social factors, and personal behaviors affect access to health care, the cost and quality of health care, and, ultimately, people's health and well-being.

Outcomes research, a subset of health services research, comprises efforts to understand the end results of the structures and processes of health care and to assess the effectiveness of health care services. While evaluation research focuses on a specific program or policy, outcomes research is a more global assessment of the value of health care services. In nursing, outcomes research addresses the question, "What effect does nursing have on patient outcomes?" Outcomes research seeks evidence about the nursing profession's contribution to care.

Outcomes research represents a response to the increasing demand from policy-makers, insurers, and the public to justify care practices and systems in terms of costs and improved patient outcomes. Outcomes research reflects a shift in emphasizing outcome-based health care (what do health care staff *accomplish*?) rather than task-based health care (what do health care staff *do* for patients?). The focus of outcomes research in the 1980s and 1990s was predominantly on patient health status and costs associated with medical care, but there is a growing interest in studying broader patient outcomes and an awareness that nursing practice can play a role in quality improvement and health care safety, despite the many challenges.

TIP Interest in improving care quality and documenting key health outcomes has led to several initiatives in nursing. For example, the Quality and Safety Education for Nurses (QSEN) project is part of the effort to transform the quality of nursing care by strengthening the competencies of nurses (Sherwood & Barnsteiner, 2012).

Although many nursing studies examine patient outcomes, specific efforts to appraise and document the impact of nursing care—as distinct from the care provided by the overall health care system—are less common. A major obstacle is *attribution*—that is, linking patient outcomes to specific nursing actions, distinct from the actions of other members of the health care team. Outcomes research has used a variety of traditional nonexperimental designs and methodologic strategies (primarily quantitative ones) but is also developing new methods.

Models of Health Care Quality

In appraising quality in nursing services, various factors need to be considered. Donabedian (1987), whose pioneering efforts created a framework for outcomes research, emphasized three factors: structure, process, and outcomes. The underpinning of this framework is that good structures will support good processes, which in turn will result in desirable patient outcomes. The *structure* of care refers to broad organizational features. For example, structure can be appraised in terms of such attributes as size and range of services. *Processes* involve aspects of clinical management, decision-making, and clinical interventions (e.g., discharge planning). *Outcomes* refer to the specific clinical end results of patient care, such as quality of life and functional status. Mitchell and co-authors (1998) noted that "the emphasis on evaluating quality of care has shifted from structures (having the right things) to processes (doing the right things) to outcomes (having the right things happen)" (p. 43).

Several modifications to Donabedian's framework for appraising health care quality have been proposed. One noteworthy framework is the Quality Health Outcomes Model developed by the American Academy of Nursing (Mitchell et al., 1998). This model is less linear and more dynamic than Donabedian's original framework and takes client and system characteristics into account. This model does not link actions and processes directly to outcomes. Rather, the effects of actions are seen as mediated by client and system characteristics. This model and others like it are increasingly used as the conceptual framework for studies that evaluate quality of care (Baernholdt et al., 2018; Mitchell & Lang, 2004). Another quality framework has been developed with specific

reference to nursing performance: the Nursing Care Performance Framework or NCPF (Dubois et al., 2013). Outcomes research usually focuses on various linkages within such models, rather than on testing the overall model.

Structure of Care

Several studies have examined the effect of nursing structures on various patient outcomes. Numerous indicators of structure of relevance to nursing care have been identified. For example, nurse staffing levels, nursing skill mix, nursing staff experience, nursing care hours per patient, and continuity of nurse staffing are structural variables that have been found to correlate with patient outcomes. These structural variables can be reliably measured, and data for these variables are generally routinely available.

Efforts have been made to measure a more complex structural variable, nurses' practice environments. The most well-known measure, which has been translated into several languages, is the Nursing Work Index-Revised (NWI-R, Aiken & Patrician, 2000), particularly its Practice Environment Scale (Lake, 2002). Warshawsky and Havens (2011) have documented that the use of the NWI-R has grown across clinical settings and countries.

> **Example of Research on Structure of Care**
> Zhu and colleagues (2018) studied the relationships between a hospital's Magnet status and nurse staffing levels on temporal trends in hospitals' performance on measures of patients' hospital experiences.

Nursing Processes and Actions

To demonstrate nurses' effects on health outcomes, nurses' clinical actions and behaviors must be described and documented. Examples of nursing process variables include nurses' problem-solving; clinical decision-making; clinical competence; and specific activities or interventions (e.g., communication, touch, ambulation assistance).

The work that nurses do has been documented in classification systems and taxonomies. Several research-based classification systems of nursing interventions have been developed, refined, and tested. Among the most prominent are the Nursing Diagnoses Taxonomy of the North American Nursing Diagnosis Association or NANDA (NANDA International, 2018) and the Nursing Intervention Classification or NIC developed at the University of Iowa (Butcher et al., 2018). NIC consists of more than 400 interventions, and each is associated with a definition and a detailed set of activities that a nurse undertakes to implement the intervention.

Patient Risk Adjustment

Patient outcomes vary not only because of the care they receive, but also because of differences in patient conditions and comorbidities. Adverse outcomes can occur no matter what nursing intervention is used. Thus, in evaluating the effects of nursing actions on outcomes, there needs to be some way of taking into account patients' risks for poor outcomes or the mix of risks in a caseload.

Risk adjustments have been used in many nursing outcomes studies. These studies typically adopt global measures of patient risks or patient acuity, such as the Acute Physiology and Chronic Health Evaluation (APACHE I, II, III, or IV) system for critical care environments. Wheeler (2009) has discussed the pros and cons of the different versions of the system.

Example of Outcomes Research With Risk Adjustment
Lee and colleagues (2017) studied the relationship between nurse workload/staffing ratios (structural indicators) on hospital survival (the outcome) in critically ill patients. The analysis used APACHE III to adjust for the patients' severity of illness. The researchers found that patients exposed to high workload-to-nurse ratios for 1 day or more had lower odds of survival.

Nursing-Sensitive Outcomes

Understanding the link between patient outcomes and nursing actions is critical in making improvements to nursing quality. Outcomes of relevance to nursing can be defined in terms of physical or physiologic function (e.g., heart rate, blood pressure), psychological function (e.g., comfort, satisfaction with care), or health behaviors (e.g., self-care, exercise). Outcomes may be either temporary (e.g., postoperative body temperature) or longer-term (e.g., return to employment). Furthermore, outcomes may be the end results to individual patients receiving care or to broader units such as a family or a community.

Nursing-sensitive outcomes are patient outcomes that improve if there is greater quantity or quality of nurses' care (Burston et al., 2013; Doran, 2011). Examples include pressure ulcers, falls, and intravenous infiltrations. Several nursing-sensitive outcome classification systems have been developed. The American Nurses Association has developed a database of such outcomes, the National Database of Nursing Quality Indicators or NDNQI (Montalvo, 2007). Also, the Nursing-Sensitive Outcomes Classification (NOC) has been developed by nurses at the University of Iowa College of Nursing to complement the Nursing Intervention Classification (Moorhead et al., 2018).

Example of Outcomes Research With Nursing-Sensitive Outcomes
Backhaus and colleagues (2017) studied the relationship between nurse staffing (the presence of nurses with a baccalaureate education) and outcomes such as patient falls and pressure ulcer incidence for residents in Dutch long-term care facilities.

Challenges in Outcomes Research

The nursing profession faces several challenges in efforts to document the effects of nursing practice on patient outcomes. As noted by Jones (2016), "empirical evidence to support the unique contribution to quality outcomes is currently lacking" (p. 1). One challenge is that nursing care is more difficult to conceptualize and measure than medical actions. Nursing interventions are often more diffuse than medical interventions—for example, nursing surveillance does not involve a single discrete act, or even a single nurse.

Perhaps for this reason, nursing-sensitive indicators have tended not to be endorsed by bodies that legislate and make policy relating to health care quality. For example, in the United States, consensus standards for measures of quality need the endorsement of the National Quality Forum (NQF). As of this writing, the NQF has endorsed only 15 new nursing-sensitive indicators out of the 150 potential measures that were submitted to the NQF for review, and it has not endorsed any such indicators since 2004. Examples of NQF-approved nursing outcome indicators include falls prevalence, pressure ulcer prevalence, and restraint prevalence (NQF, 2004). Further research documenting the link between nursing actions and patient outcomes may eventually lead to a greater appreciation of nursing's important role in improving health outcomes.

Another challenge is developing and validating nursing-sensitive *process* variables (Heslop & Lu, 2014; Jones, 2016). Efforts are needed to identify and measure the active ingredients of nursing care. The National Quality Forum endorsed only three nursing-sensitive process indicators—all of them relating to smoking cessation counseling for three different disease populations. Clearly, the full scope of nursing practice is not captured in these three NQF indicators.

Dubois and colleagues (2013) have urged the nursing profession to develop better conceptualizations of nursing care performance. Dubois and others (2017) have recently identified a set of indicators that "have sufficient breadth and depth to capture the whole spectrum of nursing care" (p. 3154), and they envision their effort as setting the stage for new initiatives in operationalizing nursing care performance.

One other challenge deserves mention, and that is the difficulty of ensuring full documentation of nursing actions. Reliable nurse process measures that can be assessed for their impact on patient outcomes require comprehensive documentation. The documentation burden for nurses is traditionally high, and the introduction of electronic health records does not necessarily decrease that burden or produce more comprehensive documentation (Bilyeu & Eastes, 2013; Cutugno et al., 2015).

SURVEY RESEARCH

A **survey** is designed to obtain information about the prevalence, distribution, and interrelations of phenomena within a population. Political opinion polls are examples of surveys. When a survey involves a sample, as is usually the case, it may be called a **sample survey** (as opposed to a **census**, which covers an entire population). Survey research relies on participants' **self-reports**—participants respond to a series of questions posed by investigators. Surveys, which yield quantitative data primarily, may be cross-sectional or longitudinal (e.g., panel studies). Surveys are especially appropriate for answering Description questions, but longitudinal surveys are also used to address Etiology and Prognosis questions. The quality of evidence from surveys for descriptive and correlational purposes is highly dependent on the quality of the sample used (Chapter 13) and the quality of the data collected (Chapter 15).

Survey research is flexible: it can be applied to many populations; it can focus on a wide range of topics; and its information can be used for many purposes. Information obtained in most surveys, however, tends to be relatively superficial: surveys rarely probe deeply into human complexities.

Any information that can reliably be obtained by direct questioning can be gathered in a survey, although surveys include mostly questions that require brief responses (e.g., yes/no, always/sometimes/never). Surveys often focus on what people do: what they eat, how they care for their health, and so forth. In some instances, the emphasis is on what people plan to do—for example, health screenings they plan to have done—or what they have done in the past.

Survey data can be collected in various ways. The most respected method is through **personal interviews** (or *face-to-face interviews*), in which interviewers meet in person with respondents. Personal interviews tend to be costly because they involve a lot of personnel time. Nevertheless, personal interviews are regarded as the best method of collecting survey data because of the quality of information they yield and because refusal rates tend to be low.

Example of a Survey With Personal Interviews
Mutiso and colleagues (2018) conducted a community household survey to investigate patterns of mental illness and stigma in two settings (an urban slum and a rural community) in Kenya. Household members from the selected communities were sampled and completed an in-person interview that included a measure of neuropsychiatric status.

Telephone interviews are less costly than in-person interviews, but respondents may be uncooperative (or difficult to reach) on the telephone. Telephoning can be an acceptable method of collecting data if the interview is short, specific, and not too personal or if researchers have had prior personal contact with respondents. For example, some researchers conduct in-person interviews in clinical settings at baseline and then conduct follow-up interviews on the telephone. Telephone interviews may be difficult for certain groups of respondents, including the elderly, who may have hearing problems.

Questionnaires, unlike interviews, are self-administered. Respondents read the questions and then give their answers in writing. Respondents differ in their reading levels and in their ability to communicate in writing, so care must be taken in a questionnaire to word questions clearly and simply. Questionnaires are economical but are not appropriate for surveying certain populations (e.g., children). In survey research, questionnaires can be distributed in person in clinical settings or through the mail (sometimes called a *postal survey*), but are increasingly being distributed over the Internet. Further guidance on mailed and web-based surveys is provided in Chapter 14.

Example of a Mailed Survey
Miyashita and colleagues (2018) mailed questionnaires to caregivers of family members who had died in palliative care units and home hospices in Japan. The post-bereavement questionnaires included questions about the perceived benefits and stresses of participating in the survey.

Survey researchers are using new technologies to assist in data collection. Most major telephone surveys now use **computer-assisted telephone interviewing (CATI)**, and some in-person surveys use **computer-assisted personal interviewing**

(CAPI) with laptop computers. Both procedures involve developing computer programs that present interviewers with the questions to be asked on the monitor; interviewers then enter coded responses directly onto a computer file. CATI and CAPI surveys, although costly, greatly facilitate data collection and improve data quality because there is less opportunity for interviewer error.

Audio-CASI or **ACASI** (*computer-assisted self-interview*) technology is an approach for giving respondents more privacy than is possible in an interview (e.g., when asking about drug abuse) and is useful for populations with literacy problems (Brown et al., 2013; Jones, 2003). With audio-CASI, respondents sit at a computer and listen to questions over headphones. Respondents enter their responses directly onto the keyboard, without the interviewer seeing the responses. This approach is also being extended to surveys with tablets and smartphones.

Example of Audio-CASI
Lor and Bowers (2017) tested the feasibility of a culturally and linguistically adapted audio-CASI with helper assistance for collecting health data from Hmong older adults. Participants found the interface user-friendly, but they confirmed that a helper was necessary during the survey process.

There are many excellent resources for learning more about survey research, including the classic books by Fowler (2014) and Dillman et al. (2014).

OTHER TYPES OF RESEARCH

The majority of quantitative studies that nurse researchers have conducted are the types described thus far in this chapter or in Chapter 9, but nurse researchers have pursued other specific types of research. In this section, we provide a brief description of some of them. The Supplement for this chapter on thePoint provides more details about each type. **S**

- **Translational research.** Translational research (sometimes called *translation science*) is an interdisciplinary field that involves systematic efforts to convert basic research knowledge into practical applications to enhance human well-being.

- **Implementation research.** The goal of implementation research is to solve problems in the implementation of health care improvements, such as new programs, policies, or practices.
- **Secondary analysis.** Secondary analyses involve the use of data from a previous study (or from large databases) to test hypotheses or answer questions that were not initially envisioned. Secondary analyses often are based on quantitative data from a large data set (e.g., from national surveys), but secondary analyses of data from qualitative studies have also been undertaken (Beck, 2019). Several websites for locating publicly available datasets are provided in the Toolkit of the accompanying *Resource Manual.* 🔀
- **Needs assessments.** Researchers conduct needs assessments to understand the needs of a group, community, or organization. The aim of such studies is to assess the need for special services or to see if standard services are meeting the needs of intended beneficiaries.
- **Delphi surveys.** Delphi surveys were developed as a tool for short-term forecasting. The technique involves a panel of experts who are asked to complete several rounds of questionnaires focusing on their judgments about a topic of interest. Multiple iterations are used to achieve consensus.

- **Replication studies.** Researchers sometimes undertake a replication study, which is an explicit attempt to see if findings obtained in one study can be duplicated in another setting.
- **Methodologic studies.** Nurse researchers have undertaken many methodologic studies, which are aimed at gathering evidence about strategies of conducting high-quality, rigorous research.

CRITICAL APPRAISAL OF STUDIES DESCRIBED IN THIS CHAPTER

It is difficult to provide guidance on critically appraising the types of studies described in this chapter because they are so varied and because many of the fundamental methodologic issues that require an appraisal concern the overall design. Guidelines for appraising design-related issues were presented in the previous two chapters.

Box 11.1 offers a few specific questions for appraising the kinds of research included in this chapter. Separate guidelines for appraising economic evaluations, which are technically complex, are offered in the Toolkit section of the accompanying *Resource Manual.* 🔀

BOX 11.1 Some Guidelines for Critically Appraising Studies Described in Chapter 11

1. Does the study purpose match the study design? Was the best possible design used to address the study purpose?
2. If the study was a clinical trial, was adequate attention paid to developing a strong, carefully conceived intervention? Was the intervention adequately pilot tested?
3. If the study was a clinical trial or evaluation, was there an effort to understand how the intervention was implemented (i.e., a process-type analysis)? Were the financial costs and benefits assessed? If not, should they have been?
4. If the study was an evaluation, to what extent do the study results serve the practical information needs of key decision-makers or intended users?
5. If the study was outcomes research, were nursing-sensitive indicators used? Were the hypothesized linkages (e.g., between nursing structures and outcomes or nursing processes and outcomes) cogent in terms of the potential to illuminate nursing's unique contribution to care?
6. If the study was a survey, was the most appropriate method used to collect the data (i.e., in-person interviews, telephone interviews, or mail or Internet questionnaires)?

RESEARCH EXAMPLE

This section describes a set of related studies that stemmed from a clinical trial.

Background: Dr. Claire Rickard has undertaken a series of studies in Australia relating to the replacement of peripheral intravenous catheters. The main study, which was based on results from smaller clinical trials (Rickard et al., 2010; Van Donk et al., 2009), was a large, multisite RCT that included a cost-effectiveness analysis. The study also required some methodologic work. Data from the parent study have been used in secondary analyses.

Phase III randomized equivalence trial: Rickard and colleagues (2012) hypothesized that patients who had intravenous catheters replaced when clinically indicated would have equivalent rates of phlebitis and complications (e.g., bloodstream infections), but a reduced number of catheter insertions, compared with patients whose catheters were removed according to the standard guideline of every 3 days. Adults with expected catheter use of more than 4 days were recruited into the trial. A sample of 3,283 adults from three hospitals were randomized to clinically indicated catheter replacement or to third daily routine replacement. The equivalence margin was set to 3%. Consistent with the hypothesis of equivalence, phlebitis was found to occur in 7% of the patients in both groups. No serious adverse events relating to the two insertion protocols were observed.

Cost-effectiveness study: A cost-effectiveness study was also undertaken in connection with the RCT (Tuffaha et al., 2014). The team collected data on resource use and associated costs. Patients in the "clinically indicated" group used significantly fewer catheters. The mean dwell time for catheters in situ on Day 3 was 99 hours when replaced as clinically indicated, compared with 70 hours when routinely replaced. The cost analysis concluded that the incremental net monetary benefit of clinically indicated replacement was approximately $8 per patient.

Methodologic substudy: As described in a review paper (Ray-Barruel, Polit, Murfield & Rickard, 2014), Rickard and her team developed and tested a new method to reliably measure the incidence of phlebitis in the RCT.

Secondary analyses: Wallis and a team of colleagues (2014) used data from the trial in a secondary analysis. Data from all 3,283 patients were used to explore risk factors for peripheral intravenous catheter (PIVC) failure. The researchers found that some of the factors that predicted phlebitis were modifiable (e.g., large diameter PIVC, ward insertion versus insertion by operating room staff), but others were not (e.g., women were at higher risk). In a separate secondary analysis of the trial data, Webster and colleagues (2015) studied risk factors for postinfusion phlebitis.

SUMMARY POINTS

- **Clinical trials** to assess the effectiveness of clinical interventions can unfold in a series of phases. Features of the intervention are finalized in *Phase I. Phase II* involves seeking opportunities for refinements and preliminary evidence of feasibility and efficacy. *Phase III* is a full experimental test of treatment *efficacy*. In *Phase IV*, researchers focus primarily on generalized *effectiveness*.

- Most trials are **superiority trials**, in which researchers hypothesize that an intervention will result in better outcomes than the counterfactual. In a **noninferiority trial**, the goal is to test whether a new intervention is no worse than a reference treatment. In **equivalence trials**, the goal is to test the hypotheses that the outcomes from two treatments are equal, within a specified level of tolerance.

- **Evaluation research** assesses the effectiveness of a program, policy, or procedure and often involves several components. **Process** or **implementation analyses** describe the process by which a program gets implemented and how it functions in practice. **Outcome analyses** describe the status of outcomes after the introduction of a program. **Impact analyses** test whether a program caused **net impacts** on key outcomes, relative to a counterfactual. **Cost (economic) analyses** assess whether the monetary costs of a program are outweighed by benefits and include **cost–benefit analyses, cost-effectiveness analyses,** and **cost–utility**

analyses. Realist evaluations constitute a theory-driven approach to evaluating programs; the theoretical mechanisms underlying the effects of an intervention are a key concern.

- **Comparative effectiveness research (CER)** involves direct comparisons of clinical and public health interventions to gain insights into which work best for which patients—as well as which have greater risks of harm. The **Patient-Centered Outcomes Research Institute (PCORI)** is a major funder of CER.

- **Outcomes research** (a subset of **health services research**) examines the quality and effectiveness of health care and nursing services. Models of health care and nursing quality typically encompass several broad concepts, including *structure* (factors such as nursing skill mix); *process* (e.g., nursing actions); client risk factors (e.g., illness severity, comorbidities); and *outcomes*. In nursing, researchers often focus on the effects of nursing structure and processes on **nursing-sensitive outcomes**—patient outcomes that benefit from greater quantity or quality of nurse care (e.g., patient falls, pressure ulcers).

- **Survey research** involves gathering data about people's characteristics, behaviors, and intentions by asking them questions. One survey method is through **personal interviews**, in which interviewers meet respondents face-to-face and question them. **Telephone interviews** are less costly but are inadvisable if the interview is long or if questions are sensitive. **Questionnaires** are self-administered (i.e., questions are read by respondents, who then give written responses) and are usually distributed by mail or over the Internet.

- Other specific types of research include the following: **translational research** (which involves systematic efforts to convert basic research knowledge into practical applications); **implementation research** (in which researchers seek methods to improve the implementation of innovative program, policies, or interventions); **secondary analysis** (in which researchers analyze previously collected data); **needs assessments** (which are designed to understand and document the needs of a group or community);

Delphi surveys (which involve several rounds of questioning with an expert panel to achieve consensus); **replication studies** (which duplicate prior studies to test whether results can be repeated); and **methodologic studies** (in which the focus is to develop and test methodologic tools or strategies).

STUDY ACTIVITIES

Study activities are available to instructors on the Point.

REFERENCES CITED IN CHAPTER 11

Aiken, L., & Patrician, P. (2000). Measuring organizational traits of hospitals: The revised nursing work index. *Nursing Research, 49*, 146–153.

*Backhaus, R., van Rossum, E., Verbeek, H., Halfens, R., Tan, F., Capezuti, E., & Hamers, J. (2017). Relationship between the presence of baccalaureate-education RNs and quality of care: A cross-sectional study in Dutch long-term care facilities. *BMC Health Services Research, 17*, 53.

Baernholdt, M., Dunton, N., Hughes, R., Stone, P., & White, K. (2018). Quality measures: A stakeholder analysis. *Journal of Nursing Care Quality, 33*, 149–156.

*Barksdale, D., Newhouse, R., & Miller, J. (2014). The Patient-Centered Outcomes Research Institute (PCORI): Information for academic nursing. *Nursing Outlook, 62*, 192–200.

Bartroff, J., Lai, T. L., & Shih, M. (2013). *Sequential experimentation in clinical trials*. New York: Springer.

Beck, C. T. (2019). *Secondary qualitative data analysis in the health and social sciences*. New York: Routledge.

Bilyeu, P., & Eastes, L. (2013). Use of the electronic medical record for trauma resuscitations: How does this impact documentation completeness? *Journal of Trauma Nursing, 20*, 166–168.

Boersma, P., van Weert, J., van Meijel, B., & Droes, R. (2017). Implementation of the Veder contact method in daily nursing home care for people with dementia: A process analysis according to the RE-AIM framework. *Journal of Clinical Nursing, 26*, 436–455.

*Brown, J., Swartzendruber, A., & DuClemente, R. (2013). Application of audio computer-assisted self-interviews to collect self-reported health data: An overview. *Caries Research, 47*, S40–S45.

Burston, S., Chaboyer, W., & Gillespie, B. (2013). Nurse-sensitive indicators suitable to reflect nursing care quality: A review and discussion of the issues. *Journal of Clinical Nursing, 23*, 1785–1793.

Butcher, H., Bulechek, G., Dochterman, J. M., & Wagner, C. (2018). *Nursing interventions classification (NIC)* (7th ed.). St. Louis: Elsevier.

Christensen, E. (2007). Methodology of superiority vs. equivalence trials and non-inferiority trials. *Journal of Hepatology, 46,* 947–954.

Cook, W., Morrison, M., Eaton, L., Theodore, B., & Doorenbos, A. (2017). Quantity and quality of economic evaluations in U.S. Nursing research, 1997–2015: A systematic review. *Nursing Research, 66,* 28–39.

Cutugno, C., Hozak, M., Fitzsimmons, D., & Ertogan, H. (2015). Documentation of preventive nursing measures in the elderly trauma patient: Potential financial impact and the health record. *Nursing Economic$, 33,* 219–226.

Dillman, D. A., Smyth, J., & Christian, L. (2014). *Internet, phone, mail, and mixed-mode surveys: The tailored design method* (4th ed.). New York: John Wiley.

Donabedian, A. (1987). Some basic issues in evaluating the quality of health care. In Rinke, L. T. (Ed.), *Outcome measures in home care* (Vol. 1, pp. 3–28). New York: National League for Nursing.

Doran, D., (Ed.). (2011). *Nursing outcomes: State of the science* (2nd ed.). Sudbury, MA: Jones & Bartlett.

Drummond, M., Sculpher, M., Claxton, G., Stoddart, G., & Torrance, G. (2015). *Methods for the economic evaluation of health care programs* (4th ed.). Oxford: Oxford Medical Publications.

Dubois, C., D'Amour, D., Brault, I., Dallaire, C., Dery, J., Duhous, A., … Zufferey, A. (2017). Which priority indicators to use to evaluate nursing care performance? A discussion paper. *Journal of Advanced Nursing, 73,* 3154–3167.

*Dubois, C., D'Amour, D., Pomey, M., Girard, F., & Brault, I. (2013). Conceptualizing performance of nursing care as a prerequisite for better measurement: A systematic and interpretive review. *BMC Nursing, 12,* 7.

Fowler, F. J. (2014). *Survey research methods* (5th ed.). Thousand Oaks, CA: Sage.

Glasgow, R.E., Magid, D., Beck, A., Ritzwoller, D., & Estabrooks, P. (2005). Practical clinical trials for translating research to practice: Design and measurement recommendations. *Medical Care, 43* 551–557.

*Heslin, M., Patel, A., Stahl, D., Gardner-Sood, P., Mushore, M., Smith, S., … Gaughran, E. (2017). Randomised controlled trial to improve health and reduce substance use in established psychosis (IMPaCT): Cost effectiveness of integrated psychosocial health promotion. *BMC Psychiatry, 17,* 407.

*Heslop, L., & Lu, S. (2014). Nursing-sensitive indicators: A concept analysis. *Journal of Advanced Nursing, 70,* 2469–2482.

*Heyland, D., Davidson, J., Skrobik, Y., des Ordons, A., Van Scoy, L. Day, A, … Marshall, A. (2018). Improving partnerships with family members of ICU patients: Study protocol for a randomized controlled trial. *Trials, 19,* 3.

*Institute of Medicine of the National Academies (2009). *Initial priorities for comparative effectiveness research.* Washington, DC: IOM.

Jones, R. (2003). Survey data collection using audio computer-assisted self-interview. *Western Journal of Nursing Research, 25,* 349–358.

*Jones, T. (2016). Outcome measurement in nursing: Imperatives, ideals, history, and challenges. *The Online Journal of Issues in Nursing, 21,* 2.

Kerr, H., Price, J., Nicholl, H., & O'Halloran, P. (2018). Facilitating transition from children's to adult services for young adults with life-limiting conditions (TASYL): Programme theory developed from a mixed methods realist evaluation. *International Journal of Nursing Research, 86,* 125–138.

Lake, E. T. (2002). Development of the practice environment scale of the Nursing Work Index. *Research in Nursing & Health, 25,* 176–188.

*Lee, A., Cheung, Y., Joynt, G., Leung, C., Wong, W., & Gomersall, C. (2017). Are high nurse workload/staffing ratios associated with decreased survival in critically ill patients? *Annals of Intensive Care, 7,* 46.

Lor, M., & Bowers, B. (2017). Feasibility of audio-computer-assisted self-interviewing with color coding and helper assistance (ACASI-H) for Hmong older adults. *Research in Nursing & Health, 40,* 360–371.

*Makenzius, M., Oguttu, M., Klingberg-Allvin, M., Gemzell-Danielsson, K., Odero, T., & Faxelid, E. (2017). Post-abortion care with misoprostol—equally effective, safe and accepted when administered by midwives compared to physicians: A randomised controlled equivalence trial in a low-resource setting in Kenya. *BMJ Open, 7,* e016157.

Mervin, M., Moyle, W., Jones, C., Murfield, J., Draper, B., Beattie, E., … Thalib, L. (2018). The cost-effectiveness of using PARO, a therapeutic robotic seal, to reduce agitation and medication use in dementia. *Journal of the American Medical Directors Association, 19,* 619–622.

Mitchell, P., Ferketich, S., & Jennings, B. (1998). Quality health outcomes model. *Image: The Journal of Nursing Scholarship, 30,* 43–46.

Mitchell, P., & Lang, N. (2004). Framing the problem of measuring and improving healthcare quality: Has the Quality Health Outcomes Model been useful? *Medical Care, 42,* II4–11.

Miyashita, M., Aoyama, M., Yoshida, S., Yamada, Y., Abe, M., Yahagihara, K, … Nakahata, M. (2018). The distress and benefit to bereaved family members of participating in a post-bereavement survey. *Japanese Journal of Clinical Oncology, 48,* 135–143.

*Montalvo, I. (2007). The National Database of Nursing Quality Indicators® (NDNQI®). *The Online Journal of Issues in Nursing, 12* (3).

Moorhead, S., Johnson, M., Maas, M., & Swanson, E. (2018). *Nursing Outcomes Classification (NOC): Measurement of health outcomes* (6th ed.). St. Louis: Elsevier.

Mutiso, V., Musyimi, C., Tomita, A., Loeffen, L., Burns, J., & Nditei, D. (2018). Epidemiological patterns of mental disorders and stigma in a community household survey in urban slum and rural settings in Kenya. *International Journal of Social Psychiatry, 64,* 120–129.

NANDA International (2018). *NANDA International Nursing Diagnoses: Definitions and classification, 2018–2020* (11th ed.). Oxford: Wiley-Blackwell.

*National Quality Forum (2004). *National voluntary consensus standards for nursing-sensitive care: An initial performance set. A consensus report.* Washington, DC: National Quality Forum.

Patton, M. Q. (2012). *Essentials of utilization-focused evaluation.* Thousand Oaks, CA: Sage.

Patton, M. Q. (2015). *Qualitative research and evaluation methods* (4th ed.). Thousand Oaks, CA: Sage.

Pawson, R., & Tilley, N. (1997). *Realistic evaluation.* London: Sage.

Piaggio, G., Elbourne, D., Pocock, S., Evans, S., Altman, D. (2012). Reporting of noninferiority and equivalence randomized trials: Extension of the CONSORT 2010 statement. *Journal of the American Medical Association, 308,* 2594–2604.

Račić, M., Joksimović, B., Cicmil, S., Kusmuk, S., Ivković, N., Hadzivuković, N., … Dubravac, M. (2017). The effects of interprofessional diabetes education on the knowledge of medical, dentistry, and nursing students. *Acta Medica Academica, 46,* 145–154.

Ramacciati, N. (2013). Health technology assessment in nursing: A literature review. *International Nursing Review, 60,* 23–30.

Ray-Barruel, G., Polit, D., Murfield, J., & Rickard, C. M. (2014). Infusion phlebitis assessment measures: A systematic review. *Journal of Evaluation in Clinical Practice, 20,* 191–202.

*Rickard, C. M., McCann, D., Munnings, J., & McGrail, M. (2010). Routine resite of peripheral intravenous devices every 3 days did not reduce complications compared with clinically indicated resite. *BMC Medical, 8,* 53.

Rickard, C. M., Webster, J., Wallis, M., Marsh, N., McGrail, M., French, V., … Whitby, M. (2012). Routine versus clinically indicated replacement of peripheral intravenous catheters: A randomised controlled equivalence trial. *The Lancet, 380,* 1066–1074.

Rossi, P., Lipsey, M., & Henry, G. (2019). *Evaluation: A systematic approach* (8th ed.). Thousand Oaks, CA: Sage.

Sherwood, G., & Barnsteiner, J. (2012). *Quality and safety in nursing: A competence approach to improving outcomes.* Ames, Iowa: Wiley-Blackwell.

Tuffaha, H. W., Rickard, C. M., Webster, J., Marsh, N., Gordon, L., Wallis, M., & Scuffham, P. (2014). Cost-effectiveness of clinically indicated versus routine replacement of peripheral intravenous catheters. *Applied Health Economics and Health Policy, 12,* 51–58.

Van Donk, P., Rickard, C. M., McGrail, M., & Doolan, G. (2009). Routine replacement versus clinical monitoring of peripheral intravenous catheters in a regional hospital in the home program. *Infection Control and Hospital Epidemiology, 30,* 915–917.

Wallis, M., McGrail, M., Webster, J., Marsh, N., Gowardman, J., Playford, E., & Rickard, C. M. (2014). Risk factors for peripheral intravenous catheter failure: A multivariate analysis of data from a randomized controlled trial. *Infection Control and Hospital Epidemiology, 35,* 63–68.

*Warshawsky, N. E., & Havens, D. (2011). Global use of the Practice Environment Scale of the Nursing Work Index. *Nursing Research, 60,* 17–31.

Watson, R., Asaro, L., Hertzog, J., Sorce, L., Kachmar, A., Dervan, L., … Curley, M. (2018). Long-term outcomes after protocolized sedation vs usual care in ventilated pediatric patients. *American Journal of Respiratory & Critical Care Medicine, 197,* 1457–1467.

*Webster, J., McGrail, M., Marsh, N., Wallis, M., Ray-Barruel, G., & Rickard, C. (2015). Postinfusion phlebitis: Incidence and risk factors. *Nursing Research and Practice, 2015,* 691934.

Wheeler, M. M. (2009). APACHE: An evaluation. *Critical Care Nursing Quarterly, 32,* 46–48.

**Zhu, J., Dy, S., Wenzel, J., & Wu, A. (2018). Association of Magnet status and nurse staffing with improvements in patient experience with hospital care, 2008-2015. *Medical Care, 56,* 111–120.

*A link to this open-access journal is provided in the Toolkit for Chapter 11 in the **Resource Manual.** ✪

This journal article is available on thePoint **for this chapter.*

12 | Quality Improvement and Improvement Science

The improvement of healthcare services and patient outcomes is a goal shared by all health disciplines. Several forces converged around the turn of the century that led to the emergence of new endeavors and lines of inquiry relating specifically to healthcare improvement. Quality improvement (QI) and improvement science are rapidly evolving and are still in their early stages of development, leaving abundant opportunity for nurses to participate as leaders in this field. This chapter highlights a few key features of quality improvement initiatives; we urge you to consult other references (e.g., Finkelman, 2018; Hughes, 2008) for more comprehensive presentations.

QUALITY IMPROVEMENT BASICS

In this section, we describe how quality improvement (QI) differs from research, discuss the QI movement, and review basic features of QI.

Quality Improvement Versus Research

A decade ago, there was a lot of discussion in nursing journals about the differences and similarities between quality improvement, research, and evidence-based practice (EBP) projects. All three have a lot in common, notably the use of systematic methods of solving health problems with an overall aim of fostering improvements in health care. Often, the methods used overlap: patient data and statistical analysis—sometimes combined with analysis of qualitative data—are also used in all three.

Although the definitions proposed for QI, research, and EBP are distinct, it is not always easy to distinguish them in real-world projects; as a result, there is sometimes confusion. **Quality improvement** has been defined by the U.S. Centers for Medicare and Medicaid Services (CMS) as "an assessment, conducted by or for a QI organization, of a patient care problem for the purpose of improving patient care through peer analysis, intervention, resolution of the problem, and follow-up" (CMS, 2003, Chapter 16). Under the code of U.S. Federal Regulations, *research* is defined as a "systematic investigation, including research development, testing and evaluation, designed to develop or contribute to generalizable knowledge" (U.S. Code of Federal Regulations). EBP projects are efforts to translate "best evidence" into protocols to guide the actions of healthcare staff to maximize good outcomes for clients.

Shirey and colleagues (2011) created a comparison chart describing the similarities and differences of the three types of efforts across 20 dimensions. For some dimensions, the differences noted in the chart continue to be relevant—for example, whether approval from an Institutional Review Board or ethics committee is needed. Most QI efforts (as well as EBP projects) are not subject to the regulations protecting human subjects in research, and patient informed consent is typically not obtained. As noted by Morris and Dracup (2007), a key difference between research and QI concerns how patients are exposed to risk—in QI projects, risks are usually minimal.

For other dimensions, however, differences between QI and research are becoming less clear-cut than suggested in Shirey et al.'s comparison chart. Take, for example, the dimension "Expectations for knowledge dissemination." In the past, the expectation for QI was that results would be internally disseminated; publication in professional journals was not considered necessary. In fact, a decade ago, many people considered publication in a professional journal a criterion for classifying something as "research," rather than as QI or EBP, but this is no longer the case. Not only are many QI projects now described in professional journals, but several journals are now devoted specifically to improvement activities.

A related dimension on which QI, EBP, and research were compared by Shirey and colleagues (2011) is the generalizability of the knowledge gained from the project. Their chart stated that knowledge from QI is not generalizable—it is specific to the organization in which the QI is undertaken, which is consistent with limited publication of QI results. However, the growing interest in healthcare improvement has led to efforts to inspire more systematic, rigorous, theoretical, and replicable improvement activity—in short, to develop and advance **improvement science** (Marshall et al., 2015). Increasingly, improvement researchers are developing their own base of QI evidence. Systematic reviews of QI evidence are being published and will facilitate **evidence-based quality improvement** (**EBQI**).

Example of a Review of a Quality Improvement Strategy

Phelan and colleagues (2017) conducted a review to identify key factors contributing to the successful implementation and sustainability of QI projects that promoted the early mobilization of patients in intensive care units. The researchers identified and critically appraised 13 articles. They identified several factors in the success of QI projects, including strong leadership, interdisciplinary team collaboration, and the use of strategies to overcome barriers to implementation.

The Impetus for Improvement in Health care

In 1999, the U.S. Institute of Medicine (IOM) published an influential report, *To Err Is Human*, which highlighted the large number of deaths in the United States attributable to medical errors—nearly 100,000 deaths annually. Two years later, IOM (2001) published another report, *Crossing the Quality Chasm*, which outlined six goals to address quality problems, sometimes referred to by the acronym **STEEEP** (Finkelman, 2018):

1. *Safe.* Avoiding injuries to patients from the care intended to help them
2. *Timely.* Reducing waits and harmful delays
3. *Effective.* Providing services based on knowledge (i.e., evidence-based) and avoiding the provision of services not likely to benefit patients
4. *Efficient.* Avoiding waste of resources and energy
5. *Equitable.* Providing care that does not vary in quality because of patients' personal characteristics
6. *Patient-centered.* Providing care that is respectful of individual patient preferences and ensuring that patient values guide clinical decisions

Yet another IOM report, *Health Professions Education: A Bridge to Quality*, was published in 2003. The expert panel that prepared this report identified five core competencies for healthcare professionals to reach a desired level of quality of care: (1) providing patient-centered care, (2) working in interprofessional teams, (3) employing EBP, (4) applying quality improvement, and (5) using information technology.

These and other IOM "Quality Chasm" reports have galvanized diverse sectors of the healthcare system (e.g., providers, policy-makers, the public) and various healthcare disciplines with a sense of urgency to address quality problems. Perspectives on responsibility for quality health care began to shift from healthcare administrators to *all* healthcare providers. Bataldon and Davidoff (2007) proposed defining quality improvement as "the combined and unceasing efforts of everyone—healthcare professionals, patients and their families, researchers, payers, planners and educators—to make changes that will lead to better patient outcomes (health), better system performance (care), and better professional development (learning)" (p. 2).

Features of Quality Improvement and Improvement Science

Quality improvement projects typically have as their primary goal the swift attainment of positive change in a healthcare service. QI projects are practical and are often focused on a specific problem identified in a local context. Quality improvement can also involve an ongoing process in which interprofessional teams collaborate to improve systems and processes, with the goals of reducing waste, increasing efficiency, and increasing satisfaction. The ongoing nature of such efforts is integral to a quality management philosophy called **continuous quality improvement** (**CQI**). CQI encourages members of healthcare teams to continuously ask such questions as, "How are we doing?" and "Can we do this better?" (National Learning Consortium, 2013).

Several features characterize many QI projects. For example, the intervention or protocol for an improvement project can change as it is being evaluated to incorporate new ideas and insights— unlike what occurs in quantitative studies. Another feature is that QI projects are designed to achieve an improvement that is sustainable. Typically, QI projects are interprofessional, involving a team with diverse perspectives on a problem.

> **TIP** The Agency for Healthcare Research and Quality (AHRQ) in the United States offers training in a teamwork system (TeamSTEPPS) designed to improve communication and teamwork skills and eliminate barriers to quality and safety.

The field of healthcare improvement is an emergent one characterized by debate and differences of opinion. In particular, there have been discussions about whether improvement efforts can be simultaneously practical (aimed at producing change in local contexts) and scientific (aimed at producing knowledge that is more generalizable) (Portela et al., 2015). The dividing line is increasingly blurry, and our view is that QI will inevitably serve both purposes.

Marshall and colleagues (2015) are among a growing group of advocates promoting improvement science as a distinct discipline. They have argued that improvement science "aims to generate local wisdom and generalizable or transferable knowledge with robust, well established research methods applied in highly pragmatic ways" (p. 419). They have noted—as have many other commentators—that QI projects are often methodologically weak, relying on poor strategies and unverified data to reach conclusions. They called for the adoption of a more scientific approach to healthcare improvement and for increased efforts to draw on and contribute to theories of how change happens in complex adaptive systems. Others have noted the importance of carefully studying the role of contextual factors on quality improvement initiatives (Coles et al., 2017).

> **TIP** A Delphi survey was conducted (by a team that included nurses) with experts in seven European countries to arrive at a consensus definition of *improvement science*. The definition is closely aligned with the aims articulated in IOM's Quality Chasm reports (i.e., STEEEP): "The generation of knowledge to cultivate change and deliver person-centered care that is safe, effective, efficient, equitable and timely. It improves patient outcomes, health system performance and population health" (Skela-Savič, 2017).

Despite great enthusiasm for improvement initiatives, QI teams are often confronted with numerous challenges. For example, Tappen and colleagues (2017) described several critical barriers to implementing a widely publicized change initiative in long-term care settings (INTERACT). Major barriers included the magnitude and complexity of the change, leadership instability, competing demands, stakeholder resistance, scarce resources, and technical problems.

Nursing and Improvement Science

Seidl and Newhouse (2012) have argued that "quality improvement skills and engagement are central to nurses' responsibility in healthcare settings" (p. 299). Indeed, quality improvement is one of the six core competencies identified by the Quality and Safety Education for Nurses (QSEN) project. (The six QSEN core competencies directly map to the five competencies identified in the 2003 IOM report on healthcare education, with the exception of the additional QSEN competency category for *safety*).

Nurses are being encouraged to not only participate in QI efforts but also to play a lead role. As Johnson (2012) observed, "Who better to lead the effort to improve healthcare delivery and outcomes than the professionals delivering the majority of health care…?" (p. 113). To play such a role, nurses must learn new skills and become familiar with new tools—which we hope to facilitate in this chapter.

Indeed, nurses have been prominent in several organizations devoted to QI. For example, the Improvement Science Research Network (ISRN) is a group whose mission is to accelerate interprofessional improvement science in a systems context. ISRN was funded by the National Institutes of Nursing Research, beginning in 2009 with a grant to researchers at the University of Texas. As another example, a leading and cutting-edge organization in improvement science, the Institute for Healthcare Improvement (IHI), had (at the time of this writing) several nurses on its staff, including two vice presidents.

Nurses have worked on QI teams within local healthcare organizations and have also been involved in several large-scale improvement projects. The Robert Wood Johnson Foundation (RWJF) has been an especially strong supporter of nurses' efforts in this area. For example, the QSEN project was funded by the foundation, and the Nursing Alliance for Quality Care was started in 2010 with support from RWJF. An important quality initiative, called Transforming Care at the Bedside (TCAB), was implemented by the foundation in collaboration with the IHI. The TCAB initiative developed, tested, and disseminated a process for empowering nurses to take the lead in improving the quality of patient care on medical-surgical units. TCAB-related projects have been undertaken in several countries.

Example of a TCAB Project
Lavoie-Tremblay and colleagues (2017) described the impact of a TCAB program on the healthcare team's effectiveness and on patient safety and patient experience. The program was implemented in 8 units in a multihospital academic health science center in Montreal, Canada. Improvements on several outcomes were observed (e.g., a reduced rate of vancomycin-resistant Enterococcus).

Types of Quality Improvement Interventions

Efforts to improve quality and safety in healthcare organizations have involved a wide variety of approaches to achieving positive change. Ting and colleagues (2009) have identified eight types of QI intervention:

1. *Provider education.* Many QI projects involve teaching members of healthcare teams about how best to manage particular situations or conditions. Educational interventions might involve workshops, the distribution of educational material, or other forms of educational outreach.

Example of a Provider Education Quality Improvement Project
Policicchio and Dontje (2018) undertook a QI project designed to improve the knowledge and skills of community health workers on an American Indian reservation relating to the management of diabetes. Training was provided in six face-to-face sessions.

2. *Provider reminders.* QI projects sometimes involve the development of reminders or decision support materials designed to prompt healthcare professionals to undertake some action. The reminders can be paper-based or electronic.

Example of Reminders to Nurses in a Quality Improvement Project
Hassan and colleagues (2017) designed a QI intervention (the MOVIN' project) to promote nurse-led mobilization of intubated critically ill patients. Initial strategies focused on educating nurses, but the team subsequently introduced a series of visual reminders, which resulted in a large increase in mobilization.

3. *Audit and feedback.* This approach to QI involves providing a summary of clinical performance delivered by individual healthcare providers or units back to those providers. The feedback is often accompanied by recommended targets or benchmarks.

Example of the Use of Audits in Quality Improvement

DiLibero and colleagues (2018) carried out a quality improvement initiative designed to improve the accuracy of delirium assessments of neuroscience patients. The QI project involved education of all nurses in a new neuroscience intermediate unit (NIMU) in an urban academic medical and trauma center. The project also involved the use of nurse champions who completed several audits and provided real-time feedback on delirium assessment accuracy.

4. *Patient education.* Quality improvement efforts sometimes involve interventions designed to increase patients' understanding of specific prevention or treatment strategies.
5. *Promotion of patient self-management.* Other QI initiatives develop resources to promote patient self-management and compliance with recommended treatment plans. This approach sometimes involves providing patients with access to resources that support their day-to-day decisions.
6. *Patient reminders.* QI initiatives sometimes involve developing methods (e.g., phone calls, text messages) to encourage patients to keep appointments or to adhere to self-care regimens.

Example of a Patient-Focused Quality Improvement Initiative

Downey and colleagues (2017) implemented a QI project to reduce the risks of misuse and abuse of opioid medications in a primary care practice. The QI intervention involved having adult patients who were prescribed a long-term schedule II medication for chronic pain sign a patient agreement that described provider and patient responsibilities; patients had to agree to random urine screens and a prescription monitoring program. Significant improvements were observed for both patient and provider behaviors.

7. *Structural changes and case management programs.* QI efforts may involve structural changes, such as the creation of case management systems or disease management teams. Systems can be implemented to coordinate diagnosis, treatment, and follow-up.

Example of a Care Coordination Quality Improvement Initiative

Gallo de Moraes and colleagues (2018) implemented and tested a QI initiative within an academic medical center that involved expanding the presence of primary services at rapid response team activations. They found that the intervention led to transfers to higher levels of care and changes in code status but did not reduce hospital length of stay.

8. *Financial incentives, regulation, and policy.* QI projects sometimes involve financial incentives offered to clinicians for performing certain care processes or achieving specific outcomes.

Example of a Financial Incentive Quality Improvement Program

Rhodes and colleagues (2015) described an incentive pay plan for advanced practice nurses that was designed to promote job satisfaction, decrease turnover, and improve care quality and clinical productivity. The institution had an increase in patient visits following implementation of the program.

Ting and colleagues (2009) have pointed out that, based on systematic reviews, these QI strategies have typically yielded small to modest effects. Like other commentators, they advocated for a more thoughtful approach to QI: "One important reason for the generally poor performance of these established quality improvement interventions is that they are often lifted off the shelf with little thought to the degree that the selected solution matches the target quality problem" (p. 1968). Similarly, Shojania and Grimshaw (2005) have noted that "the choices of particular interventions lack compelling theories predicting their success or informing specific features of their development" (p. 148). Ting et al. have also observed that the limited impact of QI interventions could reflect inattention to mediating factors and to contextual factors related to the implementation setting.

TIP For many years, the concept known as The Triple Aim was a popular way to conceptualize the optimization of health system performance. The Triple Aim guided health system improvement in three dimensions of performance simultaneously: improving the health of populations, enhancing patients' experience of care, and reducing costs. In 2014, Bodenheimer and Sinsky urged the inclusion of a fourth dimension, resulting in The Quadruple Aim: the improvement of the work life of healthcare providers. Thus, some QI projects now involve efforts to improve the wellbeing and satisfaction of clinicians and other health staff as a path to improving patient care.

QUALITY IMPROVEMENT MODELS

Quality improvement projects typically are based on one of several general models to guide processes and activities. We briefly review four prominent models and provide examples of QI projects linked to these models in which nurses have played a role.

The Lean Approach

Many quality improvement initiatives in healthcare use process improvement methods adapted from industry. The **Lean approach,** also called the *Toyota Production System*, is an important example. Lean thinking has been used in industry and health care in efforts to achieve improved quality and efficiency at lower costs (Institute for Healthcare Improvement, 2005). A major feature of Lean is that it strives to eliminate three types of waste: (1) unnecessary actions, waiting, overproduction; (2) unevenness and variability in product or in flow of information; and (3) unreasonableness of a process for a person's (or equipment's) capability. The goal of a Lean process is to eliminate non–value-added steps, to identify what "value" means to customers (patients) and to serve customers' needs.

Lean approaches generally focus on an entire system or process—for example, from the time a patient enters a healthcare setting to the time the patient leaves. Lean thinking involves systematically analyzing steps in the process of providing a

care service and rethinking the process to make it more efficient. Flow diagrams are used to critically analyze processes to look for inefficiencies, redundancies, and opportunities to improve workflow. The goal is continuous improvement and standardization of work practices. In nursing and health care, the Lean approach has been used to improve patient flow in clinical areas (e.g., in the emergency department, in the operating room) and to reduce waiting times (Johnson et al., 2012).

Example of a Lean Quality Improvement Project
Kieran and an interdisciplinary team (2017) used Lean methods to improve drug round efficiency, reduce interruptions, and reduce the time to complete oral drug rounds.

Failure Mode and Effect Analysis

The **Failure Mode and Effect Analysis (FMEA)** is a systematic approach to identifying and preventing problems and failures *before* they occur. FMEA is used to assess complex processes using a standardized approach, with the aim of identifying factors that carry a risk of causing harm. Like Lean, the FMEA process has its origins in industry. In the United States, The Joint Commission (which accredits and certifies hospitals and other healthcare organizations) introduced the FMEA model in 2001. Accredited facilities are required to conduct at least one FMEA-type project each year.

TIP Worksheets and templates for an FMEA analysis (and for other QI analyses) are widely available online. The Toolkit for this chapter in the accompanying *Resource Manual* includes links to many relevant websites. A particularly useful resource is the Institute for Healthcare Improvement's (2017) "QI Essential Toolkit."

A FMEA project involves a review of the following: Failure modes (What could go wrong?), failure causes (Why would the failure happen?), and failure effects (What would be the consequences of a failure?). The analysis of processes for possible failure allows healthcare teams to prevent them by making proactive corrections, rather than waiting for adverse events to occur. DeRosier and coauthors (2002) described the use of FMEA in the U.S. Department of Veterans Affairs Center for Patient Safety as a five-step process:

1. Define the FMEA topic in a high-risk or high-vulnerability area
2. Assemble an interdisciplinary team
3. Graphically describe the process under consideration using process flow diagrams
4. Conduct a hazard analysis, listing all possible failure modes for each part of the process under examination
5. Develop a description of action for each failure mode cause and identify outcome measures

Example of a Failure Mode and Effect Analysis
An interdisciplinary team led by Yakov (2018) used FMEA to explore high restraint use in a high-acuity inpatient psychiatric unit. The team observed patient and staff overstimulation between 4 and 7 pm, which contributed to behavioral escalations. The team implemented sensory reduction improvements to prevent excessive restraint use.

Six Sigma

The **Six Sigma** approach was developed by the Motorola Corporation in the 1980s (Pysdek & Keller, 2014). "Sigma" refers to the Greek letter (σ), which is used as the representation of a statistical index of variation—the standard deviation (Chapter 17). When a product or process is almost perfect, there is minimum variation; the boundaries for performance are three standard deviations above and below an average—that is, six sigmas. The Six Sigma standard is 3.4 problems (e.g., medication errors) per million "opportunities."

The Six Sigma model uses a systematic framework to understand and improve performance. The model involves five steps (DMAIC): Define, measure, analyze, improve, and control. The goal is to improve outputs by minimizing variation, which is assessed using *control charts* with data collected multiple times before and after QI changes are made. Six Sigma methods have been widely adopted in quality improvement efforts, often used jointly with other methods such as Lean

(sometimes called Lean Six Sigma) or Plan-Do-Study-Act (PDSA)/Plan-Do-Check-Act (PDCA), which we discuss next.

Example of a Six Sigma Project
An interdisciplinary team of stakeholders (e.g., nurses, physicians, rehabilitation specialists) used a Six Sigma approach to reducing the risk of patient falls in an academic medical center in Saudi Arabia (Kuwaiti & Subbarayalu, 2017). The five-step DMAIC process was adopted using various QI tools. The fall rate was reduced by over 70% after implementing improvement strategies.

Plan-Do-Study-Act

The most widely used QI model in health care is **Plan-Do-Study-Act (PDSA)**, which is sometimes referred to as **Plan-Do-Check-Act (PDCA)**. The PDSA cycle, part of the IHI's Model for Improvement, was originally introduced by Deming and Shewhart as a framework for CQI in business and manufacturing (Hughes, 2008). Typically, PDSA relies on multiple **rapid cycles** of investigating and acting on a problem. The idea underpinning rapid cycle improvement is to first try an improvement strategy on a small scale to see how well it works and then modify it and try it again until there is confidence in the effectiveness of the change.

Deming used the acronym FOCUS along with PDSA to guide process improvements:

- **F:** Find a process with opportunity for improvement
  - Finding a process typically involves brainstorming, reviewing information about trends and events, and preparing an *opportunity statement* that identifies the key issue and its importance.
- **O:** Organize a team that understands the process
  - Key stakeholders in the process from all relevant disciplines need to be identified, and representatives need to be recruited.
- **C:** Clarify current knowledge about the process
  - Current best practices should be examined by doing a literature review. Also, current workflow in the institution is often analyzed by creating flowchart diagrams, which can help identify why the current process might be problematic.

- **U:** Understand causes of variation or poor quality
  - In this step, the team examines why variations exist or why current practices deviate from best practices.
- **S:** Select a part of the process to improve
  - The last step is to consider what specific aspects of a problem will be addressed.

As shown in Figure 12.1, these five steps lead to PDSA cycles. PDSA allows the QI team to test improvement strategies in a controlled manner, to measure results of these strategies, and to drive further improvements. The PDSA/PDCA process involves the following:

1. **Plan:** The QI team initially works on developing explicit strategies or interventions to address the problem identified during the FOCUS work. During this phase, the team also develops a plan for data collection and identifies key measures that will be used to assess improvement. Baseline (pre-QI intervention) data typically are collected during this phase.

2. **Do:** The team then implements the process improvement and collects data on key outcomes to assess whether improvement occurred. In a PDSA cycle, each improvement is tested on a fairly small scale.

3. **Study/Check:** Data from the trial run are analyzed to see if a positive change occurred.

4. **Act:** If the QI project resulted in improved outcomes, the team considers how best to sustain (and perhaps disseminate) the practice change. If no improvements were observed, or were modest, the team would work through the PDSA/PSCA model again, starting with decisions on what changes to make next.

Ideally, multiple PDSA cycles are used in fairly quick succession (rapid cycle), with the easiest changes made early in the initiative, and more difficult ones tested later.

> **TIP** The U.S. Agency for Healthcare Research and Quality (AHRQ) offers PDSA worksheets and other tools and resources for QI projects (http://www.innovations.ahrq.gov/content.aspx?id=2398).

FIGURE 12.1 The FOCUS-PDSA (Plan-Do-Study-Act) Model.

Example of a PDSA Project

Timmons and colleagues (2017) used PDSA cycles to develop and implement a nurse-driven protocol to decrease rates of catheter-associated urinary tract infections (CAUTIs). They noted that the PDSA framework "allowed for assessing changes in catheter dwell time during project implementation and refining the protocol as needed before implementing it throughout the hospital" (p. 105). Average catheter dwell times decreased by 11% following the intervention.

TIP Root cause analyses are often undertaken by looking globally at factors that contribute to a quality problem. In some QI initiatives, however, separate root cause analyses are undertaken for *each* occurrence of a problem. For example, Ouslander and an interdisciplinary team (2016) conducted a study that involved having a root cause analysis completed each time a patient was transferred from a skilled nursing facility to an acute care hospital.

SPECIFIC QUALITY IMPROVEMENT TOOLS AND METHODS

Quality improvement projects often involve the use of many of the same designs, methods, measures, and procedures that are used in research studies. Yet, tools and methods that are distinctive to QI have been developed. Some of these tools are especially useful in the planning stage. Most of these tools can be used in any of the QI models just described.

Quality improvement Planning Tools: Root Cause Analysis

During the planning of QI initiatives, a major issue is the identification of a problem on which to focus. This is likely to involve informal discussions with key stakeholders, brainstorming, a review of institutional trends, a search for relevant evidence, and the creation of flowcharts and process maps.

Once a problem or process has been selected for improvement, the QI team usually tries to investigate the *causes* of the problem. It is difficult to develop solutions to institutional problems without understanding the underlying factors contributing to it. QI teams often undertake what is called a **root cause analysis (RCA)** that involves efforts to identify underlying process deficiencies (Haxby & Shuldham, 2018). RCA can involve the use of various tools and processes; only a few of which will be described here.

The 5 Whys

One tool for identifying the root cause of a problem is a process called the "**5 Whys**." Figure 12.2 (available as a worksheet in the Toolkit ✳) shows a template for a 5-whys analysis. The process begins by identifying the specific problem, then asking why the problem happens. If the answer fails to get to the underlying cause, "Why" is asked again. The process may be completed in fewer than five rounds of "Whys" or may require additional probing. Here is an example (Chambers et al., 2014):

Problem: Patient falls while toileting.

1. Why do patients fall while toileting? → *Because nurses do not stay in the bathroom with their patients.*
2. Why don't nurses stay in the bathroom with patients? → *Because patients don't understand that a nurse should stay with them.*
3. Why don't patients understand why a nurse should stay? → *Because they don't know that they might be unstable and that nurses can prevent them from falling if they stay in the room.*
4. Why don't patients know this? → *Because nurses have not explained this safety precaution to them.*
5. Why don't nurses explain this safety precaution to them? → *Because current training and practice do not address this strategy.*

Some advice for carrying out the 5 Whys properly includes the following: (1) Focus on the process, not on people—do not be tempted to arrive at a root cause that is "human error" or "Mary's fault," (2) distinguish causes from symptoms, (3) identify successive causes step-by-step without jumping to

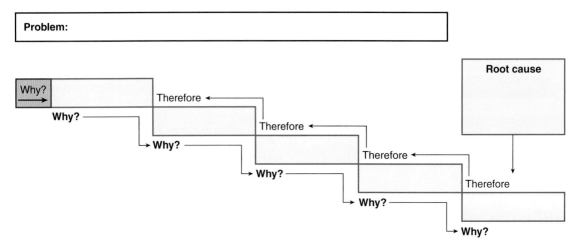

FIGURE 12.2 Template for a 5-whys analysis.

conclusions, and (4) continue asking "Why" until you identify the root cause, the elimination of which will minimize the risk that the problem will recur.

Fishbone Analysis

Another tool for root cause analyses is called a **fishbone analysis**, which may be undertaken alongside the 5-Whys process. A fishbone analysis uses a *fishbone diagram* (also called a *cause-and-effect diagram* or an *Ishikawa diagram*) to visualize causal processes and identify opportunities for improvement (Phillips & Simmonds, 2013).

As shown in Figure 12.3, the "head" of the fishbone, at the tip of the diagram, specifies the "effect," which is the problem under consideration. Each "bone" represents a broad category that can be used to identify potential causes of the problem. Commonly used categories are: (1) people (which could be healthcare staff, patients, family members, and so on); (2) equipment; (3) environmental factors; (4) processes/methods; (5) materials; and (6) management (Johnson, 2012). However, additional categories (e.g., regulations) might be relevant or fewer categories might be needed, depending on the problem.

TIP The fishbone diagram template shown in Figure 12.3 is included in the Toolkit for this chapter in the *Resource Manual*. The Toolkit also includes an example of a completed fishbone diagram.

The diagram facilitates discussion—usually in interdisciplinary brainstorming sessions that encourage collaboration—and provides a tool for detecting a wide range of possible causes of a problem. The group collaboratively should identify the category headings, and each main category should be explored in detail. The goal is to illuminate causal factors for which the healthcare staff might find solutions that they had not previously considered.

Example of Using a Fishbone Diagram
Powell and colleagues (2016) undertook a QI initiative to reduce unplanned extubations in the neonatal intensive care unit (NICU). Their rapid-cycle PDSA project involved creating a fishbone diagram in the Plan step, which helped them identify six opportunities for improvement. Changes were rolled out in two phases and resulted in a significant reduction in the rate of unplanned extubations.

Pareto Charts

Sometimes QI teams graph the "root causes" of a problem on a **Pareto chart** that shows graphically the distribution of factors contributing to the targeted problem. Vilfredo Pareto, an Italian economist, observed that about 80% of the "effects" (occurrences of a problem) come from 20% of the causes—this is the so-called *80-20 rule*. Pareto charts are designed to visually portray the "vital

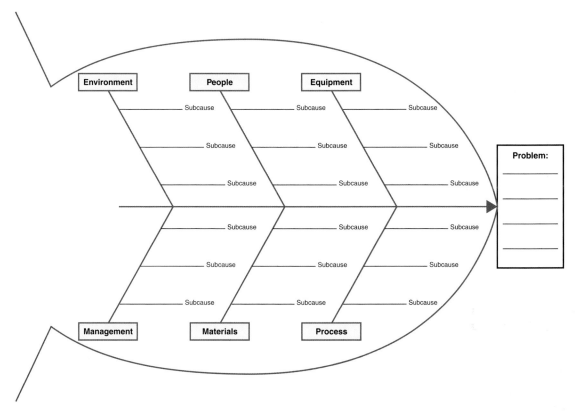

FIGURE 12.3 Template for a fishbone analysis diagram.

few" causes against the "trivial many" causes. Pareto diagrams are useful when there are many possible courses of action, and the QI team wants to select ones that will yield the best improvement benefit. These charts, in other words, can be a good priority-setting tool (Chambers et al., 2014).

Pareto charts have a series of bars on the horizontal axis, each of which represents an identified cause of (or factor in) a problem (Figure 12.4). Frequencies (number of times a given cause resulted in the problem) are on the left vertical axis; the right vertical axis portrays cumulative percentages. The "causes" (bars) are arranged from left to right in decreasing order of frequency. A dot associated with each bar is added, and then the dots are connected to show cumulative percentages with successive causal factors. In the fictitious example in Figure 12.4, nearly 80% of patient falls occurred while patients were engaged in four activities.

Example of a Quality Improvement Project Using Pareto Charts

Merkel and colleagues (2014) undertook a QI project using the PDSA model to reduce unplanned extubations (UEs) in the NICU. Causes of unplanned extubations were analyzed using Pareto charts. They found that patient care procedures (e.g., suctioning, repositioning), patient movement, and loose tape/adhesive failure accounted for 70% to 80% of the UEs.

TIP   Pareto charts can be created within Microsoft Excel and other spreadsheet programs.

Designs for Quality Improvement Projects

Most QI projects use simple designs that tend to be at risk of bias and misinterpretation. Conducting projects within real-world healthcare settings

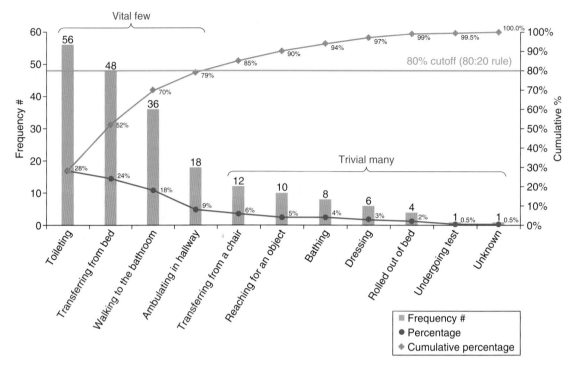

FIGURE 12.4 Example of a (fictitious) Pareto chart.

makes it challenging to use strong designs, but those who are promoting a more rigorous approach (i.e., those advocating for *improvement science*) are urging QI teams to consider stronger designs.

Randomized controlled trials (RCTs) are rare in the field of QI, but they do exist. Portela and colleagues (2015) have noted that RCTs are especially suitable when an improvement intervention is being considered for widespread use based on early evidence.

Example of a Quality Improvement Randomized Controlled Trial

A publicly available QI program called INTERACT (INTErventions to Reduce Acute Care Transfers) focuses on improving the identification and management of acute changes of nursing home residents to avoid hospitalizations. A team that included a nurse researcher conducted a randomized implementation trial of the INTERACT program in 85 nursing homes (Kane et al., 2017).

Most QI teams, however, rely on quasi-experimental designs to test the effectiveness of changes to systems or processes of care. Before–after designs, which measure changes to key outcomes after implementing a QI intervention, are especially common, but they are notably weak designs. They do not, for example, take into account secular trends in the population or the outcomes.

The nonequivalent control group design, which would involve comparisons with an institution not implementing the QI intervention, is a much stronger design option. Portela and colleagues (2015) have noted that it may be challenging to find a suitable comparison but also warned not to select a comparison site solely on superficial structural characteristics such as size or location: "The choice of relevant characteristics should be made based on anticipated hypotheses concerning the mechanisms of changes involved in the intervention and the contextual influences on how they work (e.g., ...organizational culture)" (p. 348).

Time series type designs are especially useful for sorting out the effects of seasonal or cyclical trends from QI intervention effects. Time series designs involve the collection of outcome data over an extended time period, with multiple measurements before and after introducing an intervention. Traditional time series studies require enormous sample sizes, but an option pursued by many QI projects is the use of **statistical process control (SPC)**. SPC is often associated with the Six Sigma approach to QI but is also used in other improvement models. SPC uses **control charts** to map variation in the outcome of interest over time, typically using data from existing health records (Polit & Chaboyer, 2012).

Figure 12.5 presents an example of an SPC control chart used in a nurse-led quality improvement project. Gillespie and colleagues (2019) implemented a training intervention designed to improve nontechnical skills (communication, teamwork, decision-making) in surgical teams. Surgical teams were observed and assigned a score on a measure of proficiency in nontechnical skills (NOTECS) for about 25 weeks before the intervention and 20 to 25 weeks after the intervention. Figure 12.5 plots the mean scores for one of the four surgical teams who received the QI intervention—the cardiac team. Even without training in SPC methods, it is easy to see in this graph that noteworthy improvements in nontechnical skills were observed after the intervention was introduced. These improvements, according to SPC rules, were statistically significant.

SPC is a complex topic that requires understanding fundamental statistical principles. The

FIGURE 12.5 Example of an statistical process control (SPC) chart plotting mean scores on a measure of nontechnical skills (NOTECS) over a 25-week preintervention period and a 20-week postintervention period for cardiac teams. (Adapted with permission from Gillespie, B., Harbeck, E., Kang, E., Steel, C., Fairweather, N., Pamwatwanich, K., & Chaboyer, W. Effects of a brief team training program on surgical teams' nontechnical skills: An interrupted time-series design. *Journal of Patient Safety.* doi:10.1097/PTS.0000000000000361.)

Supplement to this chapter on thePoint provides a basic overview of SPC for those with some statistical knowledge.🅢

Example of a Quality Improvement Project Using Statistical Process Control
Brown and an interprofessional team (2016) tested a nurse-driven QI intervention to improve the timeliness of corticosteroid administration to pediatric patients with acute asthma in the emergency department. They used statistical process control to examine time to administration over a 12-month period before the intervention and 12-months after it was implemented.

Quality Improvement and Measurement

Quality improvement relies on the ability of the team to assess whether the QI effort yielded a positive change. Measurement of healthcare performance variables is integral to quality improvement—indeed, it is sometimes said that measures *drive* improvement.

In the United States, the National Quality Forum (NQF) plays a critical role in endorsing performance measures for quality improvement efforts. Each measure in the NQF portfolio is carefully assessed, using four criteria: the importance of the measure to healthcare quality; its scientific soundness, based on evidence of the measure's reliability and validity (see Chapter 15); the usability and relevance of the measure to intended users; and the feasibility of collecting data on the measure without undue burden.

The NQF has endorsed measures in five categories, building on the Donabedian (1987) framework discussed in Chapter 11 in connection with outcomes research. The five categories are:

• *Process measures* that capture whether an action was completed or appropriate steps were taken and followed correctly;
• *Structural measures* that reflect the conditions in which providers care for their patients (e.g., staffing);
• *Outcome measures* that capture the actual results of care (these are usually the measures that providers are most interested in improving);

• *Patient experience measures* that capture patients' perspectives on their care; and
• *Composite measures* that combine multiple performance measures.

TIP As noted in Chapter 11, NQF has been slow to endorse nursing-sensitive measures, but that situation is likely to change as more nurses play leadership roles in QI initiatives.

Increasingly, data for QI projects are being retrieved from electronic health records (EHRs). However, several commentators have expressed concerns about the challenges of using EHR data, including the extensive time needed to document actions and outcomes, the failure of EHRs to include some relevant quality measures, the structure of the EHR, presentational challenges, problems of missing data, and problems in the availability of resources to guide data extraction (Baernholdt et al., 2018; Samuels et al., 2015). It can be expected that considerable progress in making EHRs more responsive to QI needs will occur in the future. One promising trend is the growing interest in data visualization to convey complex information (Caban & Gotz, 2015; Monsen et al., 2015).

TIP Many QI projects use mixed-methods designs that involve collecting both qualitative and quantitative data. Qualitative methods are especially well-suited during the planning phase and during the "Act" phase when the QI team must consider what to do next.

CRITICAL APPRAISAL OF QUALITY IMPROVEMENT STUDIES

Box 12.1 offers several questions for critically appraising quality improvement reports. Due to page constraints in journals, the reports may not provide rich description of all aspects of a QI project. In particular, many QI reports do not provide a lot of detail about the tools they used to identify root causes of the problem being targeted, focusing instead on the interventions they introduced and

BOX 12.1 Guidelines for Critically Appraising Quality Improvement Studies

1. Was the nature and significance of the problem adequately described? Was the purpose of the QI initiative clear?
2. Did the project draw on existing evidence about solutions to similar problems? Was the initiative linked to a theory of change?
3. Who was on the QI team? Was interprofessional collaboration an important aspect of the project?
4. What methods were used to identify the root causes of the problem? Were those methods adequate?
5. What model of QI was used (e.g., Lean, PDSA)? Was it used appropriately?
6. What specific QI interventions were implemented? Were the interventions sufficiently described so that others could reproduce them?
7. What research design was used to assess the effects of the QI changes? Did the design rule out alternative explanations for the findings (i.e., was there good internal validity)? If statistical process control was used, were there enough data points before and after the intervention?
8. What outcome measures were used to assess the effects of the QI effort? Were these measures appropriate, and was there evidence that the measures were of good quality?
9. Were the results clearly explained? Was the interpretation of the results consistent with the rigor of the methods used?
10. Did the report discuss any limitations to the generalizability of the QI study?

what they learned in efforts to evaluate the intervention. However, the authors should ideally offer a rationale (a theoretical explanation) for why they believed the intervention would lead to improved outcomes, and this rationale should guide the interpretation of the results.

As with research studies, the design of QI projects should be scrutinized to assess internal validity, as well as construct and statistical conclusion validity. Ideally, the report would provide fairly detailed information about the context so that readers could assess whether a similar quality improvement strategy could work in their setting.

RESEARCH EXAMPLE

This section describes a quality improvement project that was under the leadership of a nurse educator.

Study: Reducing CBC clotting rates in the neonatal patient care areas (McCoy, Tichon, & Narvey, 2016)

Background: In the Health Science Center in Winnipeg, Canada, bedside nurses were required to perform capillary blood sampling of infants in the NICU and Intermediary Care Nursery. The nurses then sent the blood samples to the lab for analysis. However, if the sample was clotted, the lab was unable to perform the complete blood count (CBC) analysis, and the nurses then had to draw another blood sample. The nurses became frustrated because they realized that their rate of clotting was high. The nurse educator at the center decided to undertake a system-wide analysis and a rapid-cycle QI project.

The QI initiative: The QI team included the nurse educator, patient care managers, two staff members from the laboratory, and a product representative from the company supplying lancets and blood collecting tubes. They began by mapping out the blood draw process and then undertaking a root cause analysis of this process (the team's process map is included in the Toolkit for this chapter ⊗). Over the next 3 years, several interventions were introduced with the primary goal of reducing clotting rates in the two neonatal patient care areas, from the 30% observed at the outset to 7% to 10% of blood samples.

PDSA cycles: The team used the PDSA model to continuously improve the process of bedside blood draws. Four rapid PDSA cycles were undertaken. McCoy et al.'s article spelled out actions undertaken in each phase of the four cycles (their figure is presented in the Toolkit ⊗). Here are a few highlights from the first cycle, which began in May 2012 and was completed by December 2012:

- *Plan.* Nursing and laboratory staff developed a plan to address potential contributing factors. The team determined that it would be more appropriate to focus an intervention on collection methods and nurses' skills, rather than investigating the transport process for sending blood samples to the lab.
- *Do.* Educational sessions with "hands-on" practice were developed and offered to nurses and information posters were prepared.
- *Study.* Representatives from the manufacturer came to observe nurses' bedside collection methods and provided feedback. Regular data collection of CBC clotting began.
- *Act.* Lab staff informed the team that further education and hands-on training was needed to affect positive change, together with ongoing monitoring of CBC clotting rates. This led to cycle 2 of the PDSA.

Results: The rate of clotting was reduced from 30% at the outset of the QI initiative to 14% after cycle 4. The authors wrote that "the CBC clotting rates continued to decrease over time due to the integration of a multi-faceted educational plan into biannual education days designed for current staff nurses, as well as into the orientation plan for newly hired and student nurses" (p. 1).

SUMMARY POINTS

- **Quality improvement (QI)** in health care is the collaborative effort of healthcare professionals to make changes that will improve patient outcomes and result in better system performance.
- **Improvement science** is the discipline devoted to the systematic and rigorous generation and evaluation of evidence to cultivate positive change in healthcare processes and outcomes.
- Research is considered distinct from QI projects, but distinctions are becoming blurred because QI is no longer considered exclusively a "local" enterprise. QI projects are increasingly being reported in journals, and the evidence from QI studies is the focus of systematic reviews—with

an eye to facilitating the use of **evidence-based quality improvement (EBQI)** in other settings.

- In the United States, the IOM's *Quality Chasm* reports galvanized interest in making systematic healthcare improvements and in adopting a quality management philosophy called **continuous quality improvement (CQI)** that encourages ongoing scrutiny of quality. Nurses are playing an increasingly important role in improvement science.
- Various types of QI interventions have been implemented, including provider education, provider reminders, provider feedback, patient education, patient reminders, patient supports for self-management, case management and care coordination, and financial incentives.
- Several quality improvement models, many originating in industry, have been used in healthcare initiatives. The **Lean approach** (also known as the *Toyota Production System*) strives to eliminate waste, inefficiencies, and redundancies. The goal is continuous improvement and the standardization of work practices.
- The **Failure Mode and Effect Analysis (FMEA)** model is a systematic approach to identifying and preventing problems before they occur. A FMEA project seeks answers to such question as: What could go wrong? Why would a failure occur? And What could be the consequences of a failure?
- **Six Sigma** is an approach designed to standardize processes and reduce variation. The model involves five steps (DMAIC): Define, measure, analyze, improve, and control.
- The most widely used QI model in health care is called **Plan-Do-Study-Act (PDSA)** (or **Plan-Do-Check-Act [PDCA]**), which involves multiple **rapid cycles** of improvements and testing. The PDSA cycles are guided by **FOCUS** steps: Find a process for improvement, Organize a team, Clarify current knowledge about the process, Understand causes of variation or poor quality, and Select a part of the process to improve.
- During the planning phase of a QI study, the team can use a variety of tools, such as flowcharts, process maps, and methods for doing a **root cause analysis (RCA)**. RCA involves efforts to review and understand underlying process deficiencies.

- One tool for an RCA is called the **5 Whys,** which probes for fundamental reasons for a problem by asking "Why" multiple times in response to the answers to previous "Whys."
- Another RCA tool is a **fishbone analysis** that seeks to portray diagrammatically all potential causes of a problem on a chart that resembles a fish skeleton.
- Causes of a problem can be graphed on a **Pareto chart** that visually portrays the causes of a problem in descending order of occurrence. Pareto charts can facilitate prioritizing QI efforts; the so-called *80-20 rule* articulates the expectation that about 80% of a problem is attributable to about 20% of the causes.
- Many QI studies use weak before–after designs that are at risk to various biases and confounders. One of the strongest designs for QI is the time series design, which is often used with an analytic strategy called **statistical process control (SPC).**
- SPC involves the use of **control charts** that map variation in the outcome of interest over time, with many points of data collection before and after introducing the QI intervention.
- Although QI projects can involve the collection of both qualitative and quantitative data, performance measures play a key role in QI projects, and increasingly those performance measures are being extracted from electronic health records (EHRs).

STUDY ACTIVITIES

Study activities are available to instructors on thePoint

REFERENCES CITED IN CHAPTER 12

Baernholdt, M., Dunton, N., Hughes, R., Stone, P., & White, K. (2018), Quality measures: A stakeholder analysis. *Journal of Nursing Care Quality, 33*, 149–156.

*Batalden, P., & Davidoff, F. (2007). What is "quality improvement" and how can it transform healthcare? *Quality and Safety in Healthcare, 16*, 2–3.

*Bodenheimer, T., & Sinsky, C. (2014). From triple to quadruple aim: Care of the patient requires care of the provider. *Annals of Family Medicine, 12*, 573–576.

*Brown, K., Iqbal, S., Sun, S., Fritzeen, J., Chamberlain, J., & Mullan, P. (2016). Improving timeliness for acute asthma care for paediatric ED patients using a nurse-driven intervention: An interrupted time series analysis. *BMJ Quality Improvement Reports, 5*, u216506.w5621.

Caban, J., & Gotz, D. (2015). Visual analytics in healthcare—opportunities and research challenges. *Journal of the American Medical Informatics Association, 22*, 260–262.

Centers for Medicare & Medicaid Services. (2003). *Quality improvement organization manual.* Downloaded December 30, 2018, Retrieved from https://www.cms.gov/Regulations-and-Guidance/Guidance/Manuals/Downloads/qio110c16.pdf.

Chambers, C., Petrie, J., Lindsie, S., & Makic, M. B. (2014). How to use quality improvement processes to implement evidence-based practice. In Fink, R., Oman, K., & Makic, B. B. (Eds.). *Research & evidence-based practice manual* (3rd ed. pp. 37–48). Aurora, CO: University of Colorado Hospital Authority.

*Coles, E., Wells, M., Maxwell, M., Harris, F., Anderson, J., Gray, N., … McGillivray, S. (2017). The influence of contextual factors on healthcare quality improvement initiatives: What works, for whom and in what setting? *Systematic Reviews, 6*, 168.

*DeRosier, J., Stalhandske, E., Bagian, J., & Nudell, T. (2002). Using health care Failure Mode and Effect Analysis: The VA National Center for Patient Safety's prospective risk analysis system. *The Joint Commission Journal on Quality Improvement, 27*, 248–267.

DiLibero, J., DeSanto-Madya, S., Dottery, R., Sullivan, L., & O'Donoghue, S. (2018). Improving the accuracy of delirium assessments in neuroscience patients. *Dimensions of Critical Care Nursing, 37*, 27–34.

Donabedian, A. (1987). Some basic issues in evaluating the quality of health care. In Rinke, L. T. (Ed.), *Outcome measures in home care* (Vol. I, pp. 3–28). New York: National League for Nursing.

*Downey, E., Pan, W., Harrison, J., Poza-Juncal, E., & Tanabe, P. (2017). Implementation of a Schedule II patient agreement for opioids and stimulants in an adult primary care practice. *Journal of Family Medicine and Primary Care, 6*, 52–57.

Finkelman, A. (2018). *Quality improvement: A guide for integration in nursing.* Burlington, MA: Jones & Bartlett.

Gallo de Moraes, A., O'Horo, J., Sevilla-Berrios, R., Iacovella, G., Lenhertz, A., Schmidt, J., … Jensen, J. (2018). Expanding the presence of primary services at rapid response team activations: A quality improvement project. *Quality Management in Health Care, 27*, 50–55.

Gillespie, B., Harbeck, E., Kang, E., Steel, C., Fairweather, N., Pamwatwanich, K., & Chaboyer, W. (2019). Effects of a brief team training program on surgical teams' nontechnical skills: An interrupted time-series design. *Journal of Patient Safety.* doi:10.1097/PTS.0000000000000361.

Hassan, A., Rajamani, A., Fitzsimons, F. (2017). The MOVIN' project (mobilisation of ventilated intensive care patients at Nepean): A quality improvement project based on the principles of knowledge translation to promote nurse-led mobilization of critically ill ventilated patients. *Intensive & Critical Care Nursing, 42*, 36–43.

Haxby, E., & Shildham, C. (2018). How to undertake a root cause analysis investigation to improve patient safety. *Nursing Standard, 32*, 41–46.

*Hughes, R. G. (2008). Tools and strategies for quality improvement and patient safety. In Hughes, R. G. (Ed.). *Patient safety and quality: An evidence-based handbook for nurses*. Rockville, MD: Agency for Healthcare Research and Quality.

Institute for Healthcare Improvement. (2005). *Going Lean in health care*. Cambridge, MA: IHI.

*Institute for Healthcare Improvement. (2017). *Quality essentials Toolkit*. Cambridge, MA: IHI.

*Institute of Medicine. (1999). *To err is human: Building a safer health system*. Washington, DC: National Academies Press.

*Institute of Medicine. (2001). *Crossing the quality chasm: A new health system for the 21st century*. Washington, DC: National Academies Press.

Institute of Medicine. (2003). *Health professions education: A bridge to quality*. Washington, DC: National Academies Press.

Johnson, J. (2012). Quality improvement. In Sherwood, G. & Barnsteiner, J. (Eds.), *Quality and safety in nursing: A competency approach to improving outcomes* (pp. 113–132). New York: John Wiley & Sons.

Johnson, J. E., Smith, A., & Mastro, K. (2012). From Toyota to the bedside: Nurses can lead the Lean way in health care reform. *Nursing Administration Quarterly, 36*, 234–242.

Kane, R., Huckfeldt, P., Tappen, R., Engstrom, G., Rojido, C., Newman, D., … Ouslander, J. (2017). Effects of an intervention to reduce hospitalizations from nursing homes: A randomized implementation trial of the INTERACT program. *Journal of the American Medical Association Internal Medicine, 177*, 1257–1264.

Kieran, M., Cleary, M., DeBrun, A., & Igoe, A. (2017). Supply and demand: Application of Lean Six Sigma methods to improve drug round efficiency and release nurse time. *International Journal for Quality in Health Care, 29*, 803–809.

Kuwaiti, A. A., & Subbarayalu, A. V. (2017). Reducing patients' falls rate in an academic medical center (AMC) using Six Sigma "DMAIC" approach. *International Journal of Health Care Quality Assurance, 30*, 373–384.

Lavoie-Tremblay, M., O'Connor, P., Biron, A., Lavigne, G., Fréchette, J., & Briand, A. (2017). The effects of the Transforming Care at the Bedside Program on perceived team effectiveness and patient outcomes. *Health Care Management, 36*, 10–20.

Marshall, M., Pronovost, P., & Dixon-Woods, M. (2015). Promotion of improvement as science. *The Lancet, 381*, 419–421.

*McCoy, J., Tichon, T., & Narvey, M. (2016). Reducing CBC clotting rates in the neonatal patient care areas. *BMC Quality Improvement Reports, 5*, u215456.w4946.

*Merkel, L., Beers, K., Lewis, M., Stauffer, J., Mujsce, D., & Kresch, M. (2014). Reducing unplanned extubations in the NICU. *Pediatrics, 133*, e1367–e1372.

Monsen, K., Peterson, J., Mathiason, M., Kim, E., Lee, S., Chi, C., & Pieczkiewicz, D. (2015). Data visualization techniques to showcase nursing care quality. *Computers, Informatics, Nursing, 33*, 417–426.

*Morris, P. E., & Dracup, K. (2007). Quality improvement or research? The ethics of hospital oversight. *American Journal of Critical Care, 16*, 424–426.

*National Learning Consortium (2013). *Continuous quality improvement (CQI) strategies to optimize your practice*. Washington, DC: NLC.

*Ouslander, J., Naharci, I., Engstrom, G., Shutes, J., Wolf, D., Rojido, M, … Newman, D. (2016). Hospital transfers of skilled nursing facility (SNF) patients within 48 hours and 30 days after SNF admission, *Journal of the American Medical Directors Association, 17*, 839–845.

Phelan, S., Lin, F., Mitchell, M., & Chaboyer, W. (2017). Implementing early mobilization in the intensive care unit: An integrative review. *International Journal of Nursing Studies, 77*, 91–105.

*Phillips, J., & Simmonds, L. (2013). Using fishbone analysis to investigate problems. *Nursing Times, 109*, 18–20.

Policicchio, J., & Dontje, K. (2018). Diabetes training for community health workers on an American Indian reservation. *Public Health Nursing, 35*, 40–47.

Polit, D., & Chaboyer, W. (2012). Statistical process control in nursing research. *Research in Nursing & Health, 35*, 82–93.

*Portela, M., Pronovost, P., Woodcock, T., Carter, P., & Dixon-woods, M. (2015). How to study improvement interventions: A brief overview of possible study types. *BMJ Quality & Safety, 24*, 325–336.

Powell, B., Gilbert, E., & Volsko, T. (2016). Reducing unplanned extubations in the NICU using Lean methodology. *Respiratory Care, 61*, 1567–1572.

Pyzdek, T., & Keller, P. (2014). *The Six Sigma handbook* (4th ed.). New York: McGraw Hill.

Rhodes, C., Bechtle, M., & McNett, M. (2015). An incentive pay plan for advanced practice registered nurses: Impact on provider and organizational outcomes. *Nursing Economic$, 33*, 125–131.

Samuels, J., McGrath, R., Fetzer, S., Mittal, P., & Bourgoine, D. (2015). Using the electronic health record in nursing research: Challenges and opportunities. *Western Journal of Nursing Research, 37*, 1284–1294.

Seidl, K., & Newhouse, R. (2012). The intersection of evidence-based practice with 5 quality improvement methodologies. *Journal of Nursing Administration, 42*, 299–304.

Shirey, M., Hauck, S., Embree, J., Kinner, T., Schaar, G., Phillips, L., … McCool, I. (2011). Showcasing differences between quality improvement, evidence-based practice, and research. *Journal of Continuing Education in Nursing, 42*, 57–68.

Shojania, K., & Grimshaw, J. (2005). Evidence-based quality improvement: The state of the science. *Health Affairs, 24*, 138–150.

*Skela-Savič, B., MacRae, R., Lillo-Crespo, M., & Rooney, K. (2017). The development of a consensus definition for healthcare improvement science (HIS) in seven European countries. *Zdravstveno Varstvo, 56*, 82–90.

Tappen, R., Wolf, D., Rahemi, Z., Engstrom, G., Rojido, C., Shutes, J., & Ouslander, J. (2017). Barriers and facilitators to implementing a change initiative in long-term care using the INTERACT® quality improvement program. *Health Care Management, 36*, 219–230.

**Timmons, B., Vess, J., & Conner, B. (2017). Nurse-driven protocol to reduce indwelling catheter dwell time: A healthcare improvement initiative. *Journal of Nursing Care Quality, 32*, 104–107.

*Ting, H., Shojania, K., Montori, V., & Bradley, E. (2009). Quality improvement: Science and action. *Circulation, 119*, 1962–1974.

United States Code of Federal Regulations, 45CFR 46.102 (d). http://www.hhs.gov/ohrp/humansubjects/guidance/45cfr46. Accessed July 23, 2019.

Yakov, S., Birur, B., Bearden, M., Aguilar, B., Ghelani, K., & Fargason, R. (2018). Sensory education on the general milieu of a high-acuity inpatient psychiatric unit to prevent use of physical restraints: A successful open quality improvement trial. *Journal of the American Psychiatric Nurses Association, 24*, 133–144.

A link to this open-access journal is provided in the Toolkit for Chapter 12 in the **Resource Manual.**

**This journal article is available on thePoint for this chapter.*

13 | Sampling in Quantitative Research

Researchers almost always obtain data from samples. In testing the efficacy of a new fall prevention program for hospital patients, for example, researchers reach conclusions without testing it with *every* hospitalized patient worldwide, or even with every patient in a specific hospital. But researchers must be careful not to draw conclusions based on a flawed sample.

Quantitative researchers seek to select samples that will allow them to achieve statistical conclusion validity and to generalize their results beyond the sample used. They develop a **sampling plan** that specifies in advance how participants are to be selected and how many to include. Qualitative researchers, by contrast, make sampling decisions during the course of data collection and use different criteria to evaluate sampling adequacy. This chapter discusses sampling for quantitative studies.

BASIC SAMPLING CONCEPTS

We begin by reviewing some terms associated with sampling—terms that are used primarily (but not exclusively) in quantitative research.

Populations

A **population** (the "P" of PICO questions) is the entire aggregation of cases in which a researcher is interested. For instance, if we were studying American nurses with doctoral degrees, the population could be defined as all U.S. citizens who are registered nurses (RNs) and who have a PhD, DNSc., DNP, or other doctoral-level degree. Other possible populations might be all patients who had cardiac surgery at Memorial Hospital in 2019, all women with irritable bowel syndrome in Sweden, or all children in Canada with cystic fibrosis. Populations are not restricted to humans. A population might consist of all blood samples at a particular laboratory. Whatever the basic unit, the population comprises the aggregate of the elements of interest.

It is sometimes useful to distinguish between target and accessible populations. The **accessible population** is the aggregate of cases that conform to designated criteria *and* that are accessible for a study. The **target population** is the aggregate of cases about which the researcher would like to generalize. A target population might consist of all diabetic people in California, but the accessible population might consist of all patients with diabetes being treated at clinics in Los Angeles. Researchers usually sample from an accessible population and hope to generalize to a target population.

> **TIP** Many quantitative researchers fail to identify their target population or to discuss the generalizability of the results. Evidence for nursing practice must come from research that is relevant to particular clinical populations. Thus, the population of interest needs to be carefully considered in planning and reporting a study.

Eligibility Criteria

Researchers must specify criteria that define who is in the population. Consider the population, American nursing students. Does this population include students in all types of nursing programs? Do foreign students enrolled in American nursing programs qualify? Researchers must indicate the exact criteria by which it could be decided whether an individual would or would not be classified as a member of the population. The criteria that specify population characteristics are the **eligibility criteria** or **inclusion criteria**. Sometimes, a population is also defined in terms of characteristics that people must *not* possess (i.e., **exclusion criteria**). For example, the population may be defined to exclude people who do not speak English.

In thinking about ways to define the population, it is important to consider whether the resulting sample is likely to be a good exemplar of the population construct in which you are interested. A study's construct validity is enhanced when there is a good match between the eligibility criteria and the population construct.

Of course, eligibility criteria for a study often reflect considerations other than substantive concerns. Eligibility criteria may reflect one or more of the following:

- *Costs.* Some criteria reflect cost constraints. For example, when non–English-speaking people are excluded, this likely does not mean that researchers are uninterested in non-English speakers, but rather that they cannot afford to hire translators or multilingual staff.
- *Practical constraints.* Sometimes, there are other practical constraints, such as difficulty including people from rural areas, people who are hearing impaired, and so on.
- *People's ability to participate in a study.* The health condition of some people may preclude their participation. For example, people with cognitive impairments, who are in coma, or who are in an unstable medical condition may need to be excluded.

- *Design considerations.* As noted in Chapter 10, it is sometimes advantageous to define a homogeneous population, as a means of controlling confounding variables.

The criteria used to define a population for a study have implications for the interpretation and generalizability of the findings. In fact, a growing concern about the sampling plans for randomized controlled trials (RCTs) is that researchers often use exclusion criteria that make it impossible to apply the results to the people who are most in need of the intervention (e.g., excluding people with a comorbidity). Exclusion criteria may reflect a desire to strengthen internal validity, at the expense of external validity, as we discuss in Chapter 31.

Example of Inclusion and Exclusion Criteria

Warren and Kent (2019) studied the impact of a bowel management protocol on clinician's compliance and patient outcomes (e.g., incidence of constipation and diarrhea) among patients in cardiac intensive care. Patients had to have a length of stay of more than 72 hours in intensive care and be older than 18 years. There were numerous exclusion criteria, such as a history of bowel or gastric surgery, a spinal cord injury, a stoma in situ, and intestinal obstruction.

Samples and Sampling

Sampling is the process of selecting cases to represent an entire population, to permit inferences about the population. A **sample** is a subset of population **elements**, which are the most basic units about which data are collected. In nursing research, elements most often are humans.

Samples and sampling plans vary in quality. *Two key considerations in assessing a sample in a quantitative study are its representativeness and size.* A **representative sample** is one whose key characteristics closely approximate those of the population. If the population in a study of patients is 50% male and 50% female, then a representative sample would have a similar gender distribution. If the sample is not representative of the population, the study's external validity and construct validity are at risk.

Certain sampling methods are less likely to result in biased samples than others, but a representative sample can never be guaranteed. Researchers operate under conditions in which error is possible. Quantitative researchers strive to minimize errors and, when possible, to estimate their magnitude.

Sampling designs are classified as either probability sampling or nonprobability sampling. **Probability sampling** involves random selection of elements. In probability sampling, researchers can specify the probability that an element of the population will be included in the sample. Greater confidence can be placed in the representativeness of probability samples. In **nonprobability samples**, elements are selected by nonrandom methods. There is no way to estimate the probability that each element has of being included in a nonprobability sample, and every element usually does *not* have a chance for inclusion.

Strata

Sometimes, it is useful to think of populations as consisting of subpopulations or **strata**. A stratum is a mutually exclusive segment of a population, defined by one or more characteristics. For instance, suppose our population was all RNs in the United Kingdom. This population could be divided into three strata based on gender (male, female, other). Or, we could specify two age strata: nurses younger than 40 years or nurses 40 years or older. Strata are often used in sample selection to enhance the sample's representativeness. Using strata in the sampling design can also facilitate the analysis of data for subgroups, to see if results differ for people with different characteristics.

Staged Sampling

Samples are sometimes selected in multiple phases, in what is called **multistage sampling**. In the first stage, large units (such as hospitals or nursing homes) are selected. Then, in the next stage, smaller units (e.g., individuals) are sampled. In staged sampling, it is possible to combine probability and nonprobability sampling. For example, the first stage could involve the deliberate (nonrandom) selection of study sites. Then, people within the selected sites could be selected through random procedures.

Sampling Bias

Researchers seldom have the resources to study all members of a population. It is possible to obtain fairly accurate information from a sample, but data from samples *can* be erroneous. Finding 100 people willing to participate in a study may be easy, but it is often hard to select 100 people who are an unbiased subset of the population. **Sampling bias** refers to the systematic overrepresentation or underrepresentation of a population subgroup on a characteristic relevant to the research question.

As an example of consciously biased selection, suppose we were investigating patients' responsiveness to nurses' touch and decide to recruit the first 50 patients meeting eligibility criteria. We decide, however, to omit Mr. Z from the sample because he has been hostile to nursing staff. Mrs. X, who has just lost her spouse, is also bypassed. These decisions to exclude certain people do not reflect bona fide eligibility criteria. Such decisions can lead to bias because responsiveness to nurses' touch (the outcome variable) may be affected by patients' feelings about nurses or their emotional state.

Sampling bias often occurs unconsciously, however. If we were studying nursing students and systematically interviewed every 10th student who entered the nursing school library, the sample would be biased in favor of library-goers, even if we are conscientious about including every 10th student regardless of age, gender, or other traits.

TIP Internet surveys are attractive because they can be distributed to geographically dispersed people. However, there is an inherent bias in such surveys, unless the population is defined as people who have easy access to, and comfort with, computers and the Internet.

Sampling bias is partly a function of population homogeneity. If population elements were all identical on key attributes, then any sample would be as good as any other. Indeed, if the population were completely homogeneous—exhibited no variability at all—then a *single* element would be sufficient. For many physiologic attributes, it may be safe to assume reasonably high homogeneity. For example, the blood in a person's veins is relatively homogeneous and so a single blood sample is adequate. For most human attributes, however, homogeneity is the exception rather than the rule. Age, stress, resilience—all these attributes reflect human heterogeneity. When variation occurs in the population, then similar variation should be reflected, to the extent possible, in a sample.

NONPROBABILITY SAMPLING

Nonprobability sampling is less likely than probability sampling to produce representative samples. Despite this fact, the vast majority of studies in nursing and other health disciplines rely on nonprobability samples.

Convenience Sampling

Convenience sampling entails using the most conveniently available people as participants. For example, a nurse who conducts a study of teenage risk-taking by recruiting students from a local youth organization is relying on a convenience sample. The problem with convenience sampling is that those who participate might be atypical of the population with regard to critical variables.

Sometimes, researchers seeking people with certain characteristics place an ad in a newspaper, put up signs in clinics, or post messages on online social media. These "convenient" approaches are subject to bias because people who respond to posted notices likely differ from those who do not volunteer or do not see the notices.

Snowball sampling (also called *network sampling* or *chain sampling*) is a variant of convenience sampling. With this approach, early sample members (called **seeds**) are asked to refer other people who meet the eligibility criteria. This approach is often used when the population involves people who might otherwise be difficult to identify (e.g., people who have recurrent nightmares).

Convenience sampling is the weakest form of sampling. In heterogeneous populations, no other sampling approach faces a greater risk of sampling bias. Yet, convenience sampling is the most commonly used method in many disciplines.

> **Example of a Convenience Sample**
> Dev et al. (2019) studied variation in the barriers to compassion across healthcare disciplines in New Zealand. The researchers recruited a convenience sample of 1,700 nurses, physicians, and medical students.

> **TIP** Rigorous methods of sampling *hidden populations*, such as the homeless or injection drug users, are emerging. Because standard probability sampling is inappropriate for such hidden populations, a method called **respondent-driven sampling (RDS)**, a variant of snowball sampling, has been developed. RDS, unlike traditional snowballing, allows the assessment of relative inclusion probabilities based on mathematical models (Magnani et al., 2005). Further information about the RDS approach is provided by McCreesh et al (2012, 2013).

Quota Sampling

A **quota sample** is one in which the researcher identifies population strata and determines how many participants are needed from each stratum. By using information about population characteristics, researchers can ensure that diverse segments are represented in the sample, in the proportion in which they occur in the population.

Suppose we were interested in studying nursing students' attitudes toward working with AIDS patients. The accessible population is a nursing school with 500 undergraduate students; a sample

TABLE 13.1 • Numbers and Percentages of Students in Strata of a Population, Convenience Sample, and Quota Sample

STRATA	POPULATION	CONVENIENCE SAMPLE	QUOTA SAMPLE
Male	100 (20%)	5 (5%)	20 (20%)
Female	400 (80%)	95 (95%)	80 (80%)
Total	500 (100%)	100 (100%)	100 (100%)

of 100 students is desired. The easiest procedure would be to distribute questionnaires in classrooms through convenience sampling. Suppose, however, that we suspect that male and female students have different attitudes. A convenience sample might result in too many men or too many women. Table 13.1 presents fictitious data showing the gender distribution for the population (column 2) and for a convenience sample (column 3). In this example, the convenience sample underrepresents men. We can, however, establish "quotas" so that the sample includes the appropriate number of cases from both strata. The far-right column of Table 13.1 shows the number of men and women required for a quota sample.

You may better appreciate the dangers of sampling bias with a concrete example. Suppose a key question for study participants was, "Would you be willing to work on a unit that cared exclusively for AIDS patients?" The number and percentage of students in the population who would respond "yes" are shown in the first column of Table 13.2. We would not know these values—they are shown to illustrate a point. Within the population, men are more likely than women to say they would work on a unit with AIDS patients, yet men were underrepresented in the convenience sample. As a result, population and sample values on this key question are discrepant: Nearly twice as many students in the population (20%) are favorable toward working with AIDS patients than we would conclude based on results from the convenience sample (11%). The quota sample does a better job of reflecting the views of the population (19%). In actual research situations, the distortions from a convenience

TABLE 13.2 • Students Willing to Work on an AIDS Unit, in the Population, Convenience Sample, and Quota Sample

	POPULATION	CONVENIENCE SAMPLE	QUOTA SAMPLE
Willing males (number)	28	2	6
Willing females (number)	72	9	13
Total number of willing students	100	11	19
Total number of all students	500	100	100
Percentage willing	20%	11%	19%

sample may be smaller than in this example but could be larger as well.

Stratification should be based on variables that would reflect important differences in the outcome, such as gender in our fictitious example. Variables such as age, ethnicity, gender, education, and medical diagnosis may be good stratifying variables.

Procedurally, quota sampling is like convenience sampling. The people in any subgroup are a convenience sample from that population stratum. For example, the initial sample of 100 students in Table 13.1 constituted a convenience sample from the population of 500. In the quota sample, the 20 men are a convenience sample of the 100 men in the population. Quota sampling can share similar weaknesses as convenience sampling. For instance, if a researcher is required by a quota sampling plan to interview 10 men between the ages of 65 and 80 years, a trip to a nursing home might be the most convenient method of obtaining participants. Yet this approach would fail to represent older men living independently in the community.

Despite its limitations, quota sampling is a major improvement over convenience sampling. Quota sampling does not require sophisticated skills or a lot of effort. Many researchers who use a convenience sample could profitably use quota sampling.

> **Example of a Quota Sample**
> Butler et al. (2017) studied the relationship between smoking in the home and lung cancer worry and perceived risk. They recruited a sample of 515 homeowners in Kentucky. They used quota sampling to ensure that half of the sample had a smoker in the home and half did not.

Consecutive Sampling

Consecutive sampling involves recruiting *all* the people from an accessible population who meet the eligibility criteria over a specific time interval or for a specified sample size. For example, in a study of ventilated-associated pneumonia in intensive care unit (ICU) patients, if the accessible population were patients in an ICU of a specific hospital, a consecutive sample might consist of all eligible patients admitted to that ICU over a 6-month period. Or it might be the first 250 eligible patients admitted to the ICU, if 250 were the targeted sample size.

Consecutive sampling is a far better approach than sampling by convenience, especially if the sampling period is sufficiently long to deal with potential biases that reflect seasonal or other time-related fluctuations. When all members of an accessible population are invited to participate in a study over a fixed time period, the risk of bias is greatly reduced. Consecutive sampling is often a good choice for a sampling design when there is "rolling enrollment" into a contained accessible population.

> **Example of a Consecutive Sample**
> Madi and Clinton (2018) studied pain and its effects on the functional ability of children treated for cancer. They recruited a consecutive sample of 62 children being treated at the Children's Cancer Center of Lebanon.

Purposive Sampling

Purposive sampling uses researchers' knowledge about the population to make selections. Researchers might decide purposely to select people who are judged to be particularly knowledgeable about the issues under study, for example, as in the case of a Delphi survey. A drawback is that this approach may not result in a typical or representative sample. Purposive sampling is sometimes used to good advantage in two-staged sampling. For example, sites can first be sampled purposively, with efforts made to select sites that reflect divergent population characteristics; then people can be sampled from the sites in some other fashion, such as by using consecutive sampling.

Example of Purposive Sampling
Hewitt and Cappiello (2015) conducted a Delphi survey of nurse experts to identify the essential competencies in American nursing education for prevention and care related to unintended pregnancy. Purposive sampling was used to recruit 100 panelists representing all 50 U.S. states.

Evaluation of Nonprobability Sampling

Except for some consecutive samples, nonprobability samples are rarely representative of the population. When every element in the population does not have a chance of being included in the sample, it is likely that some segment of it will be systematically underrepresented. When there is sampling bias, the results could be misleading, and efforts to generalize to a broader population could be misguided.

Nonprobability samples will continue to predominate, however, because of their practicality. Probability sampling requires time, skill, and resources, so using a probability approach might not be an option. Convenience sampling without explicit efforts to enhance representativeness, however, should be avoided. We would argue that quantitative researchers would do better at achieving representative samples for generalizing to a population if they had an approach that was more purposeful (Polit & Beck, 2010).

Quota sampling is a semipurposive sampling strategy that is far superior to convenience sampling because it seeks to ensure sufficient representation within key strata of the population. Another purposive strategy for enhancing generalizability is deliberate multisite sampling. For instance, a convenience sample could be obtained from two communities known to differ socioeconomically, so that the sample would reflect the experiences of both lower- and middle-class participants. In other words, if the population is known to be heterogeneous, you should take steps to capture important variation in the sample.

Even in one-site studies in which convenience sampling is used, researchers can make an effort to explicitly add cases to correspond more closely to population traits. For example, if half the population

is known to be male, then the researcher can check to see if approximately half the sample is male and then use outreach to recruit more males if they are underrepresented.

Quantitative researchers using nonprobability samples must be cautious about the inferences they make, especially if they do not make efforts to deliberately (purposively) enhance representativeness. Purposive approaches, although not usually held in high esteem in quantitative research, can be used to great advantage to improve the relevance of research evidence to real-world clinical settings.

PROBABILITY SAMPLING

Probability sampling involves the random selection of elements from a population. **Random sampling** involves a selection process in which each element in the population has an equal, independent chance of being selected. Probability sampling is a complex, technical topic; books such as those by Thompson (2012) offer further guidance for advanced students.

TIP Random sampling should not be (but often is) confused with random assignment, which was described in connection with experimental designs (Chapter 9). Random assignment is the process of allocating people to different treatment conditions at random. Random *assignment* is unrelated to how people in an RCT were selected in the first place. Indeed, random sampling is rarely used in RCTs.

Simple Random Sampling

The most basic probability sampling is **simple random sampling**. Researchers using simple random sampling establish a **sampling frame**, the technical name for the list of elements from which the sample will be randomly chosen. If nursing students at the University of Connecticut were the accessible population, then a roster of those students would be the sampling frame. If the sampling unit were 300-bed or larger hospitals in Taiwan, then a list of all such hospitals would be the sampling frame. Sometimes a population is defined in terms of an existing sampling frame. For example, if we wanted to use a voter registration list as a sampling frame, we would have to define the community population as residents who had registered to vote.

Once a sampling frame has been developed, elements are numbered consecutively. A table of random numbers or computer software would then be used to draw a random sample of the desired size. An example of a sampling frame for a population of 50 people is shown in Table 13.3. Assume we wish to randomly sample 20 people. We could find a starting place in a random numbers table by blindly placing our finger at some point on the page to find a 2-digit combination between 01 and 50. For this example, suppose that we began with the first 2-digit number in the random number table of Table 9.2 (p. 182), which is 46, the person corresponding to that number, D. Abraham, is the first person selected to participate in the study. Number 05, H. Edelman, is the second selection, and number 23, J. Yepsen, is the third. This process would continue until 20 participants were chosen. The selected elements are circled in Table 13.3.

A sample selected randomly in this fashion is unbiased. Although there is no guarantee that a random sample will be representative, random selection ensures that differences in the attributes of the sample and the population are purely a function of chance. The probability of selecting an unrepresentative sample decreases as the size of the sample increases.

Simple random sampling tends to be laborious. Developing a sampling frame, numbering all elements, and selecting elements are time-consuming chores, particularly if the population is large. In actual practice, simple random sampling is used infrequently because it is relatively inefficient. Furthermore, it is not always possible to get a listing of every element in the population, so other methods are often required.

Example of a Simple Random Sample

Boamah et al. (2018) studied the relationship between perceptions of nurse managers' transformational leadership behaviors on the one hand and nurses' job satisfaction and patient safety outcomes on the other. A random sample of 378 acute care nurses in Ontario participated in a survey.

TABLE 13.3 • Sampling Frame for Simple Random Sampling Example

No.	Name	No.	Name
1.	N. Alexander	26.	C. Ball
2.	D. Brady	27.	L. Chodos
3.	D. Carroll	28.	K. DiSanto
4.	M. Dakes	29.	B. Eddy
5.	H. Edelman	30.	J. Fishon
6.	L. Forester	31.	R. Griffin
7.	J. Galt	32.	B. Hebert
8.	L. Hall	33.	C. Joyce
9.	R. Ivry	34.	S. Kane
10.	A. Janosy	35.	C. Lace
11.	J. Kettlewell	36.	M. Montanari
12.	L. Lack	37.	B. Nicolet
13.	B. Mastrianni	38.	T. Opitz
14.	K. Nolte	39.	J. Portnoy
15.	N. O'Hara	40.	G. Queto
16.	T. Piekarz	41.	A. Ryan
17.	J. Quint	42.	S. Singleton
18.	M. Riggi	43.	L. Tower
19.	M. Solomons	44.	V. Vaccaro
20.	S. Thompson	45.	B. Wilmot
21.	C. VanWagner	46.	D. Abraham
22.	R. Walsh	47.	V. Brusser
23.	J. Yepsen	48.	O. Crampton
24.	M. Zimmerman	49.	R. Davis
25.	A. Arnold	50.	C. Eldred

Stratified Random Sampling

In **stratified random sampling**, the population is first divided into two or more homogeneous strata (e.g., based on gender), from which elements are selected at random. Unlike quota sampling, stratified random sampling requires that a person's status in a stratum be known before making selections, which can be problematic. Patient listings or organizational directories may contain information for meaningful stratification, but many lists do not.

The most common procedure for drawing a stratified random sample is to group together elements belonging to a stratum and to select the desired number of elements randomly. To illustrate, suppose that the list in Table 13.3 consisted of 25 men (numbers 1 through 25) and 25 women (numbers 26 through 50). Using gender as the stratifying variable, we could guarantee a sample of 10 men and 10 women by randomly sampling 10 numbers from the first half of the list and 10 from the second half. As it turns out, simple random sampling did result in 10 people being chosen from each half-list, but this was purely by chance. It would not have been unusual to draw, say, 8 names from one half and 12 from the other. Stratified sampling can guarantee the appropriate representation of different population segments.

Stratification usually divides the population into unequal subpopulations. For example, if the person's race were used to stratify the population of US citizens, the subpopulation of white people would be larger than that of nonwhite people. In **proportionate stratified sampling,** participants are selected in proportion to the size of the population stratum. If the population was students in a nursing school that had 20% African American, 20% Hispanic, 10% Asian, and 50% white students, then a proportionate stratified sample of 100 students, with race/ethnicity as the stratifier, would draw 20, 20, 10, and 50 students from the respective strata.

Proportionate sampling may result in insufficient numbers for making comparisons between strata. In our example, it would be risky to draw conclusions about Asian nursing students based on only 10 cases. For this reason, researchers may use **disproportionate sampling** when comparisons are sought between strata of greatly unequal size. In our example, the sampling proportions might be altered to select 20 African American, 20 Hispanic, 20 Asian, and 40 white students. This design would ensure more adequate coverage of Asian nurses. When disproportionate sampling is used, however, it is necessary to make an adjustment to arrive at the best estimate of *overall* population values. This adjustment, called **weighting**, is a simple mathematic computation described in textbooks on sampling.

Stratified random sampling enables researchers to sharpen a sample's representativeness. Stratified sampling, however, may be impossible if information on the critical variables is unavailable. Furthermore, a stratified sample requires even more labor and effort than simple random sampling because the sample must be drawn from multiple enumerated listings.

Example of Stratified Random Sampling
Willgerodt et al. (2018) sought to describe the school nursing workforce. They used survey data from 1,062 public schools in the United States. The sample of schools was selected using a stratified random design, with stratification based on region, urban/rural status, and school level.

Multistage Cluster Sampling

For many populations, it is impossible to obtain a listing of all elements. For example, the population of full-time nursing students in Canada would be difficult to list and enumerate for the purpose of drawing a random sample. Large-scale surveys almost never use simple or stratified random sampling; they usually rely on multistage sampling, beginning with clusters.

Cluster sampling involves selecting broad groups (clusters), rather than selecting individuals, as the first stage of a multistage approach. For a sample of nursing students, we might first draw a random sample of nursing schools and then draw a sample of students from the selected schools. The usual procedure for selecting samples from a general population in the United States is to sample successively such administrative units as census tracts, then households, and then household members. The resulting design can be described in terms of the number of stages (e.g., three-stage sampling). Clusters can be selected by simple or stratified methods. For instance, in selecting nursing schools, we could stratify on geographic region.

For a specified number of cases, multistage sampling tends to be less accurate than simple or stratified random sampling. Yet, multistage sampling is more practical than other types of probability sampling, particularly when the population is large and widely dispersed.

Example of Multistage Sampling
Abdolaliyan et al. (2017) explored the determinants of weight-control self-efficacy among pregnant women in Isfahan, Iran. The researchers first randomly sampled two health centers from each of five districts in Isfahan. Then, the medical records of 20 pregnant women from the health centers were randomly selected, and these women were invited to participate in the study.

Systematic Sampling

Systematic sampling involves selecting every *k*th case from a list, such as every 10th person on a patient listing or every 25th person on a student roster. When this sampling method is applied to a sampling frame, an essentially random sample can be drawn, using the following procedure.

The desired sample size is established at some number (*n*). The size of the population must be known or estimated (*N*). By dividing *N* by *n*, a sampling interval (*k*) is established. The **sampling interval** is the standard distance between sampled elements. For instance, if we wanted a sample of 200 from a population of 40,000, then our sampling interval would be as follows:

$$k = \frac{40,000}{200} = 200$$

In other words, every 200th element on the list would be sampled. The first element should be selected randomly. Suppose that we randomly selected number 73 from a random number table. People corresponding to numbers 73, 273, 473, and so on would be sampled.

Systematic sampling yields essentially the same results as simple random sampling but involves less work. Problems can arise if a list is arranged in such a way that a certain type of element is listed at intervals coinciding with the sampling interval. For instance, if every 10th nurse listed in a nursing staff roster was a head nurse and the sampling interval was 10, then head nurses would either always or never be included in the sample. Problems of this type are rare, fortunately. Systematic sampling can also be applied to lists that have been stratified.

TIP Systematic sampling is sometimes used to sample every *k*th person entering a store or leaving a hospital. In such situations, unless the population is narrowly defined as all those people entering or leaving, the sample is essentially a sample of convenience.

Example of a Systematic Sample
Abera et al. (2017) investigated Ethiopian students' intention to use condoms. Systematic sampling was used to select students at a large high school. The total source population was 3,674. When divided by the desired sample size (442), the sampling interval was found to be 8. The first student was randomly selected.

Evaluation of Probability Sampling

Probability sampling is the best method of obtaining representative samples. If all the elements in a population have an equal probability of being selected, then the resulting sample is likely to do a good job of representing the population. Another advantage is that probability sampling allows researchers to estimate the magnitude of sampling error. **Sampling error** refers to differences between sample values (e.g., the average age of the sample) and population values (the average age of the population).

The drawback of probability sampling is its impracticality. It is typically not possible to select a probability sample, unless the population is narrowly defined—and if it *is* narrowly defined, probability sampling might be "overkill." Probability sampling is the preferred and most respected method of obtaining sample elements but is often unfeasible.

TIP The quality of the sampling plan is of particular importance in survey research, because the purpose of surveys is to obtain information about the prevalence or average values for a population. All national surveys, such as the National Health Interview Survey in the United States, use probability samples. Probability samples are almost never used in intervention studies.

SAMPLE SIZE IN QUANTITATIVE STUDIES

Quantitative researchers typically identify how large a sample they need at the outset of a study. A procedure called **power analysis** (Cohen, 1988) can be used to estimate sample size needs, but some statistical knowledge is needed before this procedure can be explained. In this section, we offer guidelines to beginning researchers; advanced students can read about power analysis in Chapter 18 or in a sampling or statistics textbook (e.g., Polit, 2010).

Sample Size Basics

There are no simple formulas that can tell you how large a sample you will need in study, but as a general recommendation, you should use as large a sample as possible. The larger the sample, the more representative of the population it is likely to be. Every time researchers calculate a percentage or an average based on sample data, they are estimating a population value. Larger samples yield smaller sampling errors.

Let us illustrate this with an example of monthly aspirin consumption in a nursing home (Table 13.4). The population consists of 15 residents whose aspirin consumption averages 16.0 aspirins per month, as shown in the top row of the table. We drew 8 simple random samples—two each with sample sizes of 2, 3, 5, and 10. Each sample average represents an estimate of the population average (here, 16.0). With a sample size of two, our estimate might have been wrong by as many as eight aspirins (sample 1B, average of 24.0), which is 50% greater than the population value. As the sample size increases, the averages get closer to the true population value, *and the differences in the estimates between samples A and B get smaller as well.* As sample size increases, the probability of getting a deviant sample diminishes. Large samples provide an opportunity to counterbalance atypical values. In the absence of a power analysis, the safest procedure is to obtain data from as large a sample as is feasible.

Large samples are no assurance of accuracy, however. When nonprobability sampling is used, even large samples can harbor bias. A famous example is

TABLE 13.4 • Comparison of Population and Sample Values and Averages: Nursing Home Aspirin Consumption Example

NUMBER OF PEOPLE IN GROUP	GROUP	INDIVIDUAL DATA VALUES (NUMBER OF ASPIRINS CONSUMED, PRIOR MONTH)	AVERAGE
15	Population	2, 4, 6, 8, 10, 12, 14, 16, 18, 20, 22, 24, 26, 28, 30	16.0
2	Sample 1A	6, 14	10.0
2	Sample 1B	20, 28	24.0
3	Sample 2A	16, 18, 8	14.0
3	Sample 2B	20, 14, 26	20.0
5	Sample 3A	26, 14, 18, 2, 28	17.6
5	Sample 3B	30, 2, 26, 10, 4	14.4
10	Sample 4A	22, 16, 24, 20, 2, 8, 14, 28, 20, 4	15.8
10	Sample 4B	12, 18, 8, 10, 16, 6, 28, 14, 30, 22	16.4

the 1936 American presidential poll conducted by the magazine *Literary Digest*, which predicted that Alfred Landon would defeat Franklin D. Roosevelt by a landslide. About 2.5 million people participated in this poll. Biases resulted from the fact that this large sample was drawn from telephone directories and automobile registrations during a depression year when only the affluent (who preferred Landon) had a car or telephone. Thus, a large sample cannot correct for a faulty sampling design, but a large non-probability sample is preferable to a small one.

Most nursing studies use samples of convenience, and many are based on samples that are too small to provide an adequate test of research hypotheses. Research reports often offer no justification for sample size. When samples are too small, quantitative researchers run the risk of gathering data that will not support their hypotheses, *even when their hypotheses are correct*, thereby undermining statistical conclusion validity.

Factors Affecting Sample Size Requirements in Quantitative Research

The number of participants needed in a study is affected by various factors, including effect size, homogeneity of the population, cooperation and attrition, and subgroup analysis.

Effect Size
Power analysis builds on the concept of an **effect size**, which expresses the strength of relationships among research variables. If there is reason to expect that the independent and dependent variables are strongly correlated, then a relatively small sample may be adequate to reveal the relationship statistically. Typically, however, nursing interventions have moderate effects. When there is no a priori reason for believing that relationships are strong, then small samples are risky.

Homogeneity of the Population
If the population is relatively homogeneous, a small sample may be adequate. The greater the variability, the greater is the risk that a small sample will not adequately capture the full range of variation. For most nursing studies, it is probably best to assume a fair degree of heterogeneity.

Cooperation and Attrition
In most studies, not everyone invited to participate in a study agrees to do so. Therefore, in developing a sampling plan, it is good to begin with a realistic, evidence-based estimate of the percentage of people likely to cooperate. Thus, if your targeted sample size is 200 but you expect a 50% refusal rate, you would have to recruit about 400 eligible people.

In longitudinal studies, the number of participants usually declines over time. Attrition is most likely to occur if the time lag between data collection points is great, if the population is mobile, or if the population is at risk of death or disability. Participants might be less likely to drop out if they have an ongoing relationship with the researchers, but it is rarely 0%. Thus, in estimating sample size needs, attrition needs to be considered.

Attrition problems are not restricted to longitudinal studies. People who initially agree to cooperate in a study may be subsequently unable or unwilling to participate for various reasons, such as death, deteriorating health, early discharge, or simply a change of heart. Researchers should expect participant loss and recruit accordingly.

> **TIP** Polit and Gillespie (2009) found, in a sample of over 100 nursing RCTs, that the average participant loss was 12.5% for studies with follow-up data collection between 31 and 90 days after baseline and 18% when the final data collection was more than 6 months after baseline.

Subgroup Analyses
Researchers sometimes wish to test hypotheses not only for an entire population but for subgroups. For example, suppose we were interested in assessing whether a structured exercise program is effective in improving infants' motor skills. We might also want to test whether the intervention is more effective for certain infants (e.g., low-birthweight versus normal-birthweight infants). When a sample is divided to test for **subgroup effects**, the sample must be large enough to support analyses with subsets of the sample.

IMPLEMENTING A QUANTITATIVE SAMPLING PLAN

This section provides some practical guidance about implementing a sampling plan.

Steps in Sampling in Quantitative Studies

The steps to be undertaken in drawing a sample vary somewhat from one sampling design to the next, but a general outline of procedures can be described.

1. *Identify the population.* You should begin with a clear idea about the population to which you would like to generalize your results. Unless you have extensive resources, you are unlikely to have access to the full target population, so you will also need to identify the population that is accessible to you. Researchers sometimes *begin* by identifying an accessible population and then decide how best to characterize the target population.
2. *Specify the eligibility criteria.* The criteria for eligibility should then be spelled out. The criteria should be as specific as possible with regard to characteristics that might exclude potential participants (e.g., extremes of poor health, inability to read English). The criteria might lead you to redefine the target population.
3. *Specify the sampling plan.* Next, you must decide the method of drawing the sample and how large it will be. If you can perform a power analysis to estimate the needed number of participants, we highly recommend that you do so. Similarly, if probability sampling is a viable option, that option should be exercised. If you are not in a position to do either, we recommend using as large a sample as possible and taking steps to build representativeness into the design (e.g., by using quota or consecutive sampling).
4. *Recruit the sample.* The next step is to recruit prospective participants (after any needed institutional permissions have been obtained) and ask for their cooperation. Issues relating to participant recruitment are discussed next.

Sample Recruitment

Recruiting people to participate in a study typically involves two major tasks: identifying eligible candidates and persuading them to participate. Researchers must consider the best sources for recruiting potential participants. Researchers must ask such questions as, Where do large numbers of people matching my population construct live or obtain care? Will I have direct access, or will I need to work through gatekeepers? Will there be sufficiently large numbers in one location, or will multiple sites be necessary? During the recruitment phase, it may be necessary to create a **screening instrument**, which is a brief form that allows researchers to determine whether a prospective participant meets the study's eligibility criteria.

The next task involves gaining the cooperation of people who have been deemed eligible. There is considerable evidence that the percentage of people willing to cooperate in clinical trials and surveys is declining, and so it is critical to have an effective recruitment strategy.

> **TIP** Technological innovations have made it possible to "buy" research samples for certain kinds of studies. Participants can be recruited through specialized crowdsourcing platforms, such as Amazon's Mechanical Turk (Buhrmester et al., 2011). For example, Arora et al. (2016) explored the intuitions of non–health professionals regarding resource allocation and rationing decisions in the neonatal intensive care unit (NICU), using a sample of 119 respondents from Mechanical Turk. Another innovation in recruiting for clinical trials involves the creation of a large pool of potential participants who may be selected at random for different trials, called a *cohort multiple randomized controlled trials design* (Richards et al., 2014).

A lot of recent methodologic research in health fields has focused on strategies for effective recruitment. Researchers have found that rates of cooperation can often be enhanced by means of the following: face-to-face recruitment; multiple contacts and requests; monetary and nonmonetary incentives; brief data collection; inclusion of questions perceived as having high relevance to participants; assurances of anonymity; and endorsement of the study by a respected person or institution. Researchers have also anticipated recruitment benefits from the involvement of patients in the research process, but the evidence about the success of such efforts is mixed (Brett et al., 2014).

The Supplement to Chapter 13 on the**Point** offers more detailed guidance on recruitment and retention strategies, with special emphasis on clinical trials and surveys. The Toolkit of the accompanying *Resource Manual* includes examples of recruitment materials.

Participant recruitment often proceeds at a slower pace than researchers anticipate. This makes it useful to develop contingency plans for recruiting more people, should the initial plan prove overly optimistic. For example, a contingency plan might involve relaxing the eligibility criteria, identifying another institution through which participants could be recruited, offering incentives to make participation more attractive, or lengthening the recruitment period. When such plans are developed at the outset, it reduces the likelihood that you will have to settle for a less-than-desirable sample size.

Generalizing From Samples

Ideally, the sample is representative of the accessible population, and the accessible population is representative of the target population. By using a strong sampling plan, researchers can be reasonably confident that the first part of this ideal has been realized. The second part of the ideal entails greater risk. Are diabetic patients in Boston representative of diabetic patients in the United States? Researchers must exercise judgment in assessing the degree of similarity.

The best advice is to be realistic and conservative and to ask challenging questions: Is it reasonable to assume that the accessible population is representative of the target population? In what ways might they differ? How would such differences affect the conclusions? If differences are great, it would be prudent to specify a more restricted target population to which the findings could be meaningfully generalized.

Interpretations about the generalizability of findings can be strengthened by comparing sample characteristics with population characteristics, when this is possible. Published information about the characteristics of many populations may be available to help in evaluating sampling bias. For example, if you were studying low-income children in Chicago, you could obtain information on the Internet about salient characteristics (e.g., race/ethnicity, age

distribution) of low-income American children from the U.S. Bureau of the Census. Population characteristics could then be compared with sample characteristics and differences taken into account in interpreting the findings.

> **Example of Comparing Sample and Population Characteristics**
> Griffin, Polit, and Byrne (2008) conducted a survey of over 300 pediatric nurses, whose names had been randomly sampled from a list of 9,000 nurses. Demographic characteristics of the sample (e.g., gender, race/ethnicity, education) were compared to characteristics of a nationally representative sample of nurses.

We encourage further reading on the important topic of sampling. For example, Sousa et al. (2004) have provided suggestions for drawing conclusions about whether a convenience sample is representative of the population. Greenhouse et al. (2008) described an approach for making what they call "generalizability judgments" from clinical trial data. Sen et al. (2016) proposed a multitrait metric to explore how a study's eligibility criteria affect its generalizability.

CRITICAL APPRAISAL OF SAMPLING PLANS

In coming to conclusions about the quality of evidence that a study yields, you should carefully scrutinize the sampling plan. If the sample is too small or likely to be biased, the findings may be misleading or just plain wrong.

You should consider two issues in your appraisal of a study's sampling plan. The first is whether the researcher adequately described the sampling strategy. Reports of nursing studies have been found to be deficient in their descriptions of sampling plans (e.g., Suhonen et al., 2015). Ideally, research reports should include a description of the following:

- The type of sampling approach used (e.g., convenience, simple random)
- The study population and eligibility criteria for sample selection
- The number of participants and a rationale for the sample size, including whether a power analysis was performed

- A description of the main characteristics of sample members (e.g., age, gender, medical condition, and so forth) and, ideally, of the population
- The number and characteristics of potential participants who declined to participate in the study and/or who did not participate in later rounds of data collection

If the description of the sample is insufficient, you may not be able to come to conclusions about whether the researcher made good sampling decisions. And, if the description is incomplete, it will be difficult to know whether the evidence is of use in your clinical practice.

Sampling plans should be scrutinized with respect to their effects on the construct, internal, external, and statistical conclusion validity of the study. If a sample is small, statistical conclusion validity may be undermined. If the eligibility criteria are restrictive, this could benefit internal validity—but possibly to the detriment of construct and external validity.

You will never know for sure if a study sample adequately represents the population, but if the sampling design is weak or if the sample size is small, there is reason to suspect some bias. When researchers adopt a sampling plan in which the risk for bias is high, they should take steps to estimate the direction and degree of this bias so that readers can draw informed conclusions.

Even with a rigorous sampling plan, the sample may be biased if not all people invited to participate in a study agree to do so—which is almost always the case. If certain segments of the population refuse to participate, then a biased sample can result, even when probability sampling is used. Research reports should provide information about **response rates** (i.e., the number of people participating in a study relative to the number of people sampled) and about possible **nonresponse bias** (sometimes called *response bias*), which reflects differences between participants and those who declined to participate. In longitudinal studies, attrition bias should be reported.

One of your jobs in appraising studies is to come to conclusions about the reasonableness of generalizing the findings from the researcher's sample to the accessible population and from the accessible population to a target population. If the sampling plan is flawed, it may be risky to generalize the findings without replicating the study with another sample.

Box 13.1 presents some guiding questions for critically appraising the sampling plan of a quantitative research report. ⚙️

BOX 13.1 Guidelines for Critically Appraising Quantitative Sampling Plans

1. Was the study population identified and described? Were eligibility criteria specified? Were the sample selection procedures clearly delineated?
2. Do the sample and population specifications (eligibility criteria) support an inference of construct validity with regard to the population construct?
3. What type of sampling plan was used? Was the sampling plan one that could be expected to yield a representative sample? Would an alternative sampling plan have yielded a better sample?
4. If sampling was stratified, was a useful stratification variable selected? If a consecutive sample was used, was the time period long enough to address seasonal or temporal variation? In a multisite study, were sites selected in a manner that improved representativeness?
5. How were people recruited into the sample? Does the method suggest potential biases? Were strategies used to strengthen recruitment?
6. Is it likely that some factor other than the sampling plan (e.g., a low response rate, recruitment difficulties) affected the representativeness of the sample?
7. Are possible sample biases or other sampling deficiencies identified by the researchers?
8. Are key characteristics of the sample described (e.g., average age, percent female)?
9. Is the sample size sufficiently large to enhance statistical conclusion validity? Was the sample size justified on the basis of a power analysis or other rationale?
10. Does the sample support inferences of external validity? To whom can the study results reasonably be generalized?

RESEARCH EXAMPLE

In this section, we describe in some detail the sampling plan of a quantitative nursing project.

Studies: Several studies using a dataset created by Dr. Barbara A. Mark.

Purpose: With funding from National Institute of Nursing Research (NINR), Dr. Mark launched a large multisite study called the Outcomes Research in Nursing Administration Project-II (ORNA-II). The overall purpose was to investigate relationships of hospital context and structure on the one hand and patient, nurse, and organization outcomes on the other. Data from this project have been used in numerous studies, four of which are cited here.

Design: The study design was prospective and correlational.

Sampling plan: Sampling was multistaged. In the first stage, 146 acute care hospitals were randomly selected from a list of hospitals accredited by The Joint Commission on Accreditation of Health Organizations. To be included, hospitals had to have at least 99 licensed beds. Hospitals were excluded if they were federal, for-profit, or psychiatric facilities. Then, from each selected hospital, two medical, surgical, or medical-surgical units were selected to participate in the study. Units were excluded if they were critical care, pediatric, obstetric, or psychiatric units. Among hospitals with only two eligible units, both participated. Among hospitals with more than two eligible units, an on-site study coordinator selected two to participate. Ultimately, 281 nursing units in 143 hospitals participated in the study. Data from each hospital were gathered in three rounds of data collection over a 6-month period. On each participating unit, all RNs with more than 3 months of experience on that unit were asked to complete questionnaires. The response rates were 75% of nurses at time 1 (4,911 nurses), 58% at time 2 (3,689 nurses), and 53% at time 3 (3,272 nurses). Patients were also invited to participate at time 3. Ten patients on each unit were randomly selected to fill out a questionnaire. Patients were included if they were 18 years of age or older, had been hospitalized for at least 48 hours, were able to speak and read English, and were not scheduled for immediate discharge. A total of 2,720 patients participated; the response rate was 91%.

Some key findings:

- Using data from the ORNA-II project, Bacon, Lee, and Mark (2015) found that when work complexity increased, nurses' participation in decision-making decreased.
- In an analysis focusing on errors, Hughes et al. (2012) found that nurses in Magnet hospitals were more likely to communicate about errors and participate in error-related problem solving than those in non–Magnet hospitals.
- Gates and Mark (2012) found a positive relationship between racial/ethnic workplace diversity among nurses and nurses' job satisfaction.
- In an analysis of medication errors, nursing units with a strong learning climate were found to have fewer errors (Chang & Mark, 2011).

SUMMARY POINTS

- **Sampling** is the process of selecting a portion of the **population,** which is an entire aggregate of cases, for a study. An **element** is the most basic population unit about which information is collected—usually humans in nursing research.
- **Eligibility criteria** are used to establish population characteristics and to determine who can participate in a study—either who can be included (**inclusion criteria**) or who should be excluded (**exclusion criteria**).
- Researchers usually sample from an **accessible population** but should identify the **target population** to which they would like to generalize their results.
- In quantitative studies, a key quality criterion for a sample is its **representativeness**—the extent to which the sample is similar to the population and free from bias. **Sampling bias** refers to the systematic overrepresentation or underrepresentation of some segment of the population.
- Methods of **nonprobability sampling** (wherein elements are selected by nonrandom methods) include convenience, quota, consecutive, and purposive sampling. Nonprobability sampling designs are practical but usually have strong potential for bias.

- **Convenience sampling** uses the most readily available or convenient group of people for the sample. **Snowball sampling** is a type of convenience sampling in which referrals for potential participants are made by those already in the sample.
- **Quota sampling** divides the population into homogeneous **strata** (subpopulations) to ensure representation of subgroups; within each stratum, people are sampled by convenience.
- **Consecutive sampling** involves taking *all* of the people from an accessible population who meet the eligibility criteria over a specific time interval or for a specified sample size.
- In **purposive sampling**, elements are handpicked to be included in the sample based on the researcher's knowledge about the population.
- **Probability sampling** designs, which involve the random selection of elements from the population, yield more representative samples than nonprobability designs and permit estimates of the magnitude of **sampling error**.
- **Simple random sampling** involves the random selection of elements from a **sampling frame** that enumerates all population elements. **Stratified random sampling** divides the population into homogeneous strata from which elements are selected at random, either *proportionately* relative to the size of the subgroup in the population or *disproportionately* to ensure an adequate sample size for small subgroups.
- **Cluster sampling** involves sampling of large units. In **multistage random sampling,** there is a successive, multistaged selection of random samples from larger units (clusters) to smaller units (individuals) by either simple random or stratified random methods.
- **Systematic sampling** is the selection of every *k*th case from a list. By dividing the population size by the desired sample size, the researcher establishes the **sampling interval,** which is the standard distance between the selected elements.
- In quantitative studies, researchers ideally should use a **power analysis** to estimate **sample size** needs. Large samples are preferable to small ones because larger samples enhance statistical

conclusion validity and tend to be more representative, but even large sample do not *guarantee* representativeness.
- The recruitment of study participants is increasingly challenging. **Response rates** are often low, which can lead to a biased sample and to problems reaching the desired sample size.

STUDY ACTIVITIES

Study activities are available to instructors on thePoint.

REFERENCES CITED IN CHAPTER 13

*Abdolaliyan, N., Shahnazi, H., Kzemi, A., & Hasanzadeh, A. (2017). Determinants of the self-efficacy of physical activity for maintaining weight during pregnancy. *Journal of Education and Health Promotion, 6*, 93.

*Abera, H., Tamiru, F., & Kibret, G. (2017). Intention toward condom use and it associated factors among students of Debre Work Senior Secondary and Preparatory School, East Gojjam Zone, Amhara Region, Ethiopia. *HIV/AIDS, 9*, 137–143.

*Arora, C., Savulescu, J., Maslen, H., Seigelid, M., & Wilkinson, D. (2016). The Intensive Care Lifeboat: A survey of lay attitudes to rationing dilemmas in neonatal intensive care. *BMC Medical Ethics, 17*, 69.

**Bacon, C., Lee, S., & Mark, B. (2015). The relationships between work complexity and nurses' participation in decision making in hospitals. *Journal of Nursing Administration, 45*, 200–205.

Boamah, S., Spence Laschinger, H., Wong, C., & Clarke, S. (2018). Effect of transformational leadership on job satisfaction and patient safety outcomes. *Nursing Outlook, 66*, 180–189.

*Brett, J., Staniszewska, S., Mockford, C., Herron-Marx, S., Hughes, J., Tysall, C., & Suleman, R. (2014). Mapping the impact of patient and public involvement on health and social care research: A systematic review. *Health Expectations, 17*, 637–650.

Buhrmester, M., Kwang, T., & Gosling, S. (2011). Amazon's Mechanical Turk: A new source of inexpensive, yet high-quality data? *Perspectives on Psychological Science, 6*, 3–5.

*Butler, K., Rayens, M., Wiggins, A., Rademacher, K., & Hahn, E. (2017). Association of smoking in the home with lung cancer worry, perceived risk, and synergistic risk. *Oncology Nursing Forum, 44*, E55–E63.

*Chang, Y., & Mark, B. A. (2011). Effects of learning climate and registered nurse staffing on medication errors. *Nursing Research, 60*, 32–39.

Cohen, J. (1988). *Statistical power analysis for the behavioral sciences* (2nd ed.). Hillsdale, NJ: Lawrence Erlbaum Associates.

Dev, V., Fernando, A., Kirby, J., & Consedine, N. (2019). Variation in the barriers to compassion across healthcare training and disciplines: A cross-sectional study of doctors, nurses, and medical students. *International Journal of Nursing Studies, 90*, 1–10.

*Gates, M. G., & Mark, B. A. (2012). Demographic diversity, value congruence, and workplace outcomes in acute care. *Research in Nursing & Health, 35*, 265–276.

*Greenhouse, J., Kaizar, E., Kelleher, K., Seltman, H., & Gardner, W. (2008). Generalizing from clinical trial data. *Statistics in Medicine, 27*, 1801–1813.

Griffin, R., Polit, D., & Byrne, M. (2008). Nurse characteristics and inferences about children's pain. *Pediatric Nursing, 34*, 297–305.

Hewitt, C., & Cappiello, J. (2015). Essential competencies in nursing education for prevention and care related to unintended pregnancy. *Journal of Obstetric, Gynecologic, & Neonatal Nursing, 44*, 69–76.

Hughes, L., Chang, Y., & Mark, B. (2012). Quality and strength of patient safety climate on medical-surgical units. *Journal of Nursing Administration, 42*, S27–S36.

Madi, D., & Clinton, M. (2018). Pain and its impact on the functional ability of children treated at the Children's Cancer Center of Lebanon. *Journal of Pediatric Nursing, 39*, e11–e20.

Magnani, R., Sabin, K., Saidel, T., & Heckathorn, D. (2005). Review of sampling hard-to-reach and hidden populations for HIV surveillance. *AIDS, 19*, S67–S72.

*McCreesh, N., Copas, A., Seeley, J., Johnston, L., Sonnenberg, P., Hayes, R. J., … White, R. (2013). Respondent-driven sampling: Determinants of recruitment and a method to improve point estimation. *PLoS One, 8*, e78402.

*McCreesh, N., Frost, S., Seeley, J., Katongole, J., Tarsh, M., Ndunguse, R., & White, R. G. (2012). Evaluation of respondent-driven sampling. *Epidemiology, 23*, 138–147.

Polit, D. F. (2010). *Statistics and data analysis for nursing research* (2nd ed.). Upper Saddle River, NJ: Pearson.

Polit, D. F., & Beck, C. T. (2010). Generalization in qualitative and quantitative research: Myths and strategies. *International Journal of Nursing Studies, 47*, 1451–1458.

Polit, D. F., & Gillespie, B. (2009). The use of the intention-to-treat principle in nursing clinical trials. *Nursing Research, 58*, 391–399.

*Richards, D. A., Ross, S., Robens, S., & Borglin, G. (2014). The DiReCT study—Improving recruitment into clinical trials: A mixed methods study investigating the ethical acceptability, feasibility and recruitment yield of cohort multiple randomised controlled trials design. *Trials, 15*, 398.

*Sen, A., Chakrabarti, S., Goldstein, A., Wang, S., Ryan, P., & Weng, C. (2016). GIST 2.0: A scalable multi-trait metric for quantifying population representativeness of individual clinical studies. *Journal of Biomedical Informatics, 63*, 325–336.

Sousa, V., Zauszniewski, J., & Musil, C. (2004). How to determine whether a convenience sample represents the population. *Applied Nursing Research, 17*, 130–133.

Suhonen, R., Stolt, M., Katajisto, J., & Leino-Kilpi, H. (2015). Review of sampling, sample and data collection procedures in nursing research. *Scandinavian Journal of the Caring Sciences, 29*, 843–858.

Thompson, S. K. (2012). *Sampling* (3rd ed.). New York: John Wiley.

Warren, D., & Kent, B. (2019). Determining the impact of a bowel management protocol on patients and clinicians' compliance in cardiac intensive care. *Journal of Clinical Nursing, 28*, 89–103.

Willgerodt, M., Brock, D., & Maughan, E. (2018). Public school nursing practice in the United States. *Journal of School Nursing, 34*, 232–244.

A link to this open-access article is provided in the Toolkit for Chapter 13 in the Resource Manual. ✸

**This journal article is available on thePoint for this chapter.*

14 | Data Collection in Quantitative Research

Quantitative researchers typically collect data that are highly structured. The goal is to achieve consistency for each variable, in an effort to reduce biases and facilitate analysis. Major methods of collecting structured data are discussed in this chapter.

DEVELOPING A DATA COLLECTION PLAN

Data collection plans for quantitative studies ideally yield accurate, valid, and meaningful data. This is a challenging goal, requiring considerable effort to achieve. Steps in developing a data collection plan are described in this section. A flowchart illustrating a typical sequence of steps in a data collection plan is available in the Toolkit of the accompanying *Resource Manual.* ✖

Identifying Data Needs

Researchers usually begin by identifying the types of data needed for their study. In quantitative studies, researchers need data for several of the following purposes:

1. *Testing hypotheses, addressing research questions.* Researchers must include one or more measures of all key variables.

TIP Researchers sometimes cannot measure the "real" outcomes in which they are interested. For example, mortality is an important clinical outcome, but it is rarely used in nursing research because it is too distal. When there are impediments to using a desired ultimate outcome, researchers use **surrogate outcomes**. Surrogate outcomes are not important clinical events (e.g., malnutrition), but they *predict* such events (e.g., nonuse of nutritional supplements). Although the use of surrogate outcomes is inevitable in clinical research, potential problems have been noted (e.g., Fleming & Powers, 2012; Weintraub et al., 2015).

2. *Describing the sample.* Information is usually gathered about demographic and health characteristics of sample members. We advise gathering data about participants' age, gender, race or ethnicity, and education or income. This information is critical in understanding the population to whom findings can be generalized. If the sample includes participants with a health problem, data on the nature of that problem should be gathered (e.g., severity, time since diagnosis).

TIP Asking demographic questions in the right way is more difficult than you might think. The Toolkit of the *Resource Manual* includes guidelines and a demographic form that you can adapt.

3. *Controlling confounding variables.* Some approaches to controlling confounding variables require measuring them. For example, researchers must gather data for variables that will be statistically controlled.

4. *Analyzing potential biases.* Data for testing potential biases should be collected. For example, researchers should gather information that can shed light on selection or attrition biases.

5. *Understanding subgroup effects.* It is often desirable to answer research questions for key subgroups of participants. For example, we may wish to know if an intervention for pregnant women is equally effective for primiparas and multiparas. In such a situation, we would need to collect data about participants' childbearing history.

6. *Assessing treatment fidelity.* In intervention studies, it is useful to gather data on whether the intended treatment was actually received.

7. *Assessing costs.* In intervention studies (and in some quality improvement projects), information about costs and monetary benefits of alternative interventions is useful.

8. *Documenting administrative features.* Administrative data often need to be gathered (e.g., dates of data collection, participants' contact information).

The list of possible data needs may seem daunting, but many categories overlap. For example, participant characteristics for sample description are often used for analyzing bias, controlling confounders, or creating subgroups. If resource constraints make it impossible to collect data for the full range of variables, then researchers must prioritize data needs.

Selecting Types of Measures

After data needs have been identified, a data collection method (e.g., self-report) must be selected for each variable. It is common to combine methods (self-reports, observations, biomarkers, records) in a single study.

Data collection decisions must be guided by ethical considerations (e.g., whether covert data collection is warranted), cost constraints, availability of assistants to help with data collection, and other issues discussed in the next section. Data collection is often the costliest and lengthiest part of a study, and so compromises about the type or amount of data collected must sometimes be made.

Selecting and Developing Instruments

After making preliminary data collection decisions, researchers search for **instruments** to measure study variables (or determine whether data are available in existing records). Potentially useful data collection instruments then need to be assessed. The primary consideration is conceptual relevance: Does the instrument correspond to your conceptual definition of the variable? Another important criterion is whether the instrument will yield high-quality data. Approaches to evaluating data quality are discussed in Chapter 15. Additional factors that may affect decisions in selecting an instrument are as follows:

1. *Resources.* Resource constraints sometimes prevent the use of the highest-quality instruments. There may be direct costs (e.g., some instruments must be purchased), but the biggest expense is likely to be compensation for data collectors if you cannot collect data single-handedly. In such a situation, the instrument's length may affect its practicability. The use of costly methods may mean that you will be forced to cut costs elsewhere (e.g., using a smaller sample), so data collection expenses must be estimated.

2. *Population appropriateness.* Instruments must be chosen with the characteristics of the target population in mind. Participants' age and literacy levels are especially important. If there is concern about participants' reading skills, the *readability* of a prospective instrument should be assessed. If participants include members of minority groups, you should strive to find instruments that are culturally appropriate. If non–English-speaking participants are included in the sample, then the selection of an instrument may be based on the availability of a translated version.

3. *Norms and comparisons.* It may be desirable to select an instrument that has relevant norms. **Norms** indicate the "normal" values

on the measure for a specified population, and thus offer a useful comparison. Also, it may be advantageous to select an instrument because it was used in other similar studies, which could facilitate interpretation of study findings.

4. *Clinical significance.* As we discuss in Chapter 21, efforts are increasingly being made to identify thresholds for clinically significant change on outcome measures. It might be beneficial to select an instrument for which such thresholds have been established (i.e., measures for which a *minimal important change* benchmark is available).

5. *Administration issues.* Some instruments have special requirements. For example, measuring the developmental status of children may require the skills of a professional psychologist. Some instruments require stringent conditions with regard to administration time limits, privacy, and so on. In such a case, requirements for obtaining valid measures must match attributes of the research setting.

6. *Reputation.* Two measures of the same construct may differ in the reputation they enjoy among specialists in a field, even if they are comparable with regard to data quality. Thus, it may be useful to seek the advice of people with experience using the instruments. Also, some instruments have been evaluated by special expert panels. For example, the U.S. Agency for Healthcare Research and Quality maintains a National Quality Measures Clearinghouse with recommended measures that are especially useful for outcomes research and quality improvement projects (https://www.qualitymeasures. ahrq.gov/). As another example, the COMET Initiative is an effort to standardize outcome measures used in randomized controlled trials (Williamson, 2017).

If existing instruments are not suitable for some variables, you may be faced with either adapting an instrument or developing a new one. Creating a new instrument should be a last resort, especially for novice researchers, because it is challenging to develop accurate and valid measuring tools (see Chapter 15).

If you locate a suitable instrument, your next step likely will be to obtain the authors' permission to use it. Instruments that have been developed under a government grant are often in the public domain, but when in doubt, it is best to obtain permission. By contacting the instrument's author, you can also request more information about the instrument and its quality. (A sample letter requesting permission to use an instrument is in the Toolkit. ✖)

TIP In finalizing decisions about instruments, you may need to consider tradeoffs between data quality and data quantity (i.e., how much data are collected). If compromises have to be made, it is preferable to forego quantity: long data collection instruments tend to depress participant cooperation.

Pretesting the Data Collection Package

Researchers who develop a new instrument usually subject it to rigorous **pretesting** so that it can be evaluated and refined. Even when the data collection plan involves existing instruments, however, it is wise to conduct a pretest with a small sample of people (usually 10-15) who are similar to actual participants.

One purpose of a pretest is to see how much time it takes to administer the entire instrument package. Time estimates are often required for informed consent purposes, for developing a budget, and for assessing participant burden. Pretests (especially pretests of self-report instruments) can serve many other purposes, including the following:

- Identifying parts of the instrument that are hard for participants to read or understand
- Identifying questions that participants find objectionable or offensive
- Assessing whether the sequencing of questions or instruments is sensible
- Evaluating the training needs of data collectors
- Evaluating whether the measures yield data with sufficient variability

With regard to the last purpose, researchers need to ensure that there is adequate variation on key variables. For example, in a study of the link between depression and a miscarriage, depression would be compared for women who had or had not experienced a miscarriage. If the entire pretest sample looked very depressed (or not at all depressed), however, it would be advisable to pretest a different measure of depression because the original measure might not be sufficiently sensitive to detect varying levels of depression.

Example of Pretesting

Emelonye and colleagues (2017) conducted surveys with women, their spouses, and midwives to learn about barriers inhibiting the use of spousal presence for childbirth pain relief in Nigeria. All three instruments were pretested. The researchers sought "feedback on potential difficulties with the questionnaires, such as ambiguity of words, misinterpretation of questions, inability to answer questions, sensitivity of questions and any other perceived problems" (p. 570).

Developing Data Collection Forms and Procedures

After finalizing the instruments, researchers face several administrative tasks, such as developing various forms (e.g., screening forms to assess eligibility, informed consent forms, records of attempted contacts with participants). It is prudent to design forms that are attractively formatted, legible, and inviting to use; they should also be designed to ensure confidentiality. For example, identifying information (e.g., name, address) should be recorded on a page that can be detached and kept separate from other data.

TIP Whenever possible, try to avoid reinventing the wheel. It is seldom necessary to start from scratch—not only in developing instruments but also in creating forms, training materials, and protocols. Ask seasoned researchers if they have materials you could borrow or adapt.

In most quantitative studies, researchers develop **data collection protocols** that spell out procedures to be used in data collection. These protocols describe such things as the following:

- Conditions for collecting the data (e.g., Can others be present during data collection? Where must data collection occur?)
- Specific requirements for collecting the data (e.g., sequencing instruments, recording information)

- Answers to questions participants might ask (i.e., answers to FAQs). Examples of such questions include the following: How will information from this study be used? How did you get my name? How long will this take? Who will have access to this information? Can I see the study results? Whom can I contact if I have a complaint? Will I be paid or reimbursed for expenses?
- Procedures to follow if a participant becomes distraught, or for any other reason cannot complete the data collection process.

Researchers also need to decide how to actually gather, record, and manage their data. Technological advances continue to offer new options, some of which we discuss later in the chapter. Suggestions about new technology for data collection are offered by Coons et al. (2015), Schick-Makaroff and Molzahn (2015), and Udtha et al. (2015).

TIP Document all major actions and decisions as you develop and implement your data collection plan. You may need the information later when you write your research report, request funding for a follow-up study, or help other researchers with a similar study.

STRUCTURED SELF-REPORT INSTRUMENTS

The most widely used data collection method by nurse researchers is structured self-reports, which involve formal instruments. The instrument is an **interview schedule** when questions are asked orally in face-to-face or telephone interviews. It is called a **questionnaire** or an SAQ (self-administered questionnaire) when respondents complete the instrument themselves, either in a paper-and-pencil format or on a computer. This section discusses the development and administration of structured self-report instruments.

Types of Structured Questions

Structured self-report instruments consist of a set of questions (often called **items**) in which the wording of both the questions and, in most cases,

response options is predetermined. Participants are asked to respond to the same questions, in the same order, and with a fixed set of response alternatives. Researchers developing structured instruments must carefully attend to the content, form, and wording of questions.

Open- and Closed-ended Questions

Instruments vary in degree of structure through different combinations of open-ended and closed-ended questions. **Open-ended questions** allow people to respond in their own words, in narrative fashion. The question, "What was your biggest challenge after your surgery?" is an example of an open-ended question. In questionnaires, respondents are asked to give a written reply to open-ended items, and so adequate space must be provided to permit a full response. Interviewers are expected to quote oral responses verbatim.

Closed-ended (or *fixed-alternative*) **questions** offer response options, from which respondents choose the one that most closely matches their answer. The alternatives may range from a simple *yes* or *no* ("Have you smoked a cigarette today?") to complex expressions of opinion or behavior.

Both open- and closed-ended questions have certain strengths and weaknesses. Good closed-ended items are often difficult to construct but easy to administer and, especially, to analyze. With closed-ended questions, researchers need only to tabulate the number of responses to each alternative to gain descriptive insights. The analysis of open-ended items is more difficult and time-consuming. The usual procedure is to develop categories and code open-ended responses into the categories. That is, researchers essentially transform open-ended responses to fixed categories in a post hoc fashion so that tabulations can be made.

Closed-ended items are more efficient than open-ended questions: respondents can answer more closed- than open-ended questions in a given amount of time. In questionnaires, participants may be less willing to compose written responses than to check off a response alternative. Closed-ended items are also preferred if respondents cannot express themselves well verbally. Furthermore,

some questions are less intrusive in closed form than in open form. Take the following example:

1. What was your family's total annual income last year?
2. In what range was your family's total annual income last year?
   - ☐ 1. Under $50,000,
   - ☐ 2. $50,000 to $99,999, or
   - ☐ 3. $100,000 or more.

The second question gives respondents greater privacy than the open-ended question and is less likely to go unanswered.

A drawback of closed-ended questions is the risk of failing to include important response options. Such omissions can lead to inadequate understanding of the issues or to outright error if respondents choose an alternative that misrepresents their position. Another issue is that closed-ended items tend to be superficial. Open-ended questions allow for a richer and fuller perspective on a topic, if respondents are verbally expressive and cooperative. Some of this richness may be lost when researchers tabulate answers they have categorized, but direct excerpts from open-ended responses can be valuable in imparting the flavor of the replies. Finally, some people object to being forced to choose from response options that do not exactly reflect their opinions.

Decisions about the mix of open- and closed-ended questions are based on such considerations as the sensitivity of the questions, respondents' verbal ability, and the amount of time available. Combinations of both types can be used to offset the strengths and weaknesses of each. Questionnaires typically use closed-ended questions primarily, to minimize respondents' writing burden. Interview schedules, on the other hand, tend to be more variable in their mixture of these two question types.

Specific Types of Closed-Ended Questions

The analytic advantages of closed-ended questions are often compelling. Various types of closed-ended questions, illustrated in Table 14.1, are described here.

- **Dichotomous questions** require respondents to make a choice between two response alternatives, such as yes/no. Dichotomous questions are most useful for gathering factual information.

TABLE 14.1 • Examples of Closed-Ended Questions

QUESTION TYPE	EXAMPLE
1. Dichotomous question	Have you ever been pregnant? 1. Yes 2. No
2. Multiple-choice question	How important is it to you to avoid a pregnancy at this time? 1. Extremely important 2. Very important 3. Somewhat important 4. Not important
3. Rank-order question	People value different things in life. Below is a list of things that many people value. Please indicate their order of importance to you by placing a "1" beside the most important, "2" beside the second-most important, and so on. _____ Career achievement/work _____ Family relationships _____ Friendships, social interactions _____ Health _____ Money _____ Religion
4. Forced-choice question	Which statement most closely represents your point of view? 1. What happens to me is my own doing. 2. Sometimes I feel I don't have enough control over my life.
5. Rating question	On a scale from 0 to 10, where 0 means "extremely dissatisfied" and 10 means "extremely satisfied," how satisfied were you with the nursing care you received during your hospitalization? 0 1 2 3 4 5 6 7 8 9 10 Extremely Extremely dissatisfied satisfied

- **Multiple-choice questions** offer three or more response alternatives. Graded alternatives are preferable to dichotomous items for attitude questions because researchers get more information (intensity as well as direction of opinion).
- **Rank-order questions** ask respondents to rank concepts on a continuum, such as most to least important. Respondents are asked to assign a 1 to the concept that is most important, a 2 to the concept that is second in importance, and so

on. Rank-order questions can be useful, but some respondents misunderstand them so good instructions are needed. Rank-order questions should involve 10 or fewer rankings.
- **Forced-choice questions** require respondents to choose between two statements that represent polar positions.
- **Rating scale questions** ask respondents to evaluate something on an ordered dimension. Rating questions are typically on a **bipolar scale**, with

The next question is about things that may have happened to you personally. Please indicate how recently, if ever, these things happened to you:

	Yes, within past 12 mo	Yes, 2–3 years ago	Yes, more than 3 years ago	No, never
a. Has someone ever yelled at you all the time or put you down on purpose?	1	2	3	4
b. Has someone ever tried to control your every move?	1	2	3	4
c. Has someone ever threatened you with physical harm?	1	2	3	4
d. Has someone ever hit, slapped, kicked, or physically harmed you?	1	2	3	4

FIGURE 14.1 Example of a checklist (matrix question).

end points specifying opposite extremes on a continuum. The end points and sometimes intermediary points along the scale are verbally labeled. The number of gradations or points along the scale can vary but is preferably an odd number, such as 5, 7, 9, or 11, to allow for a neutral midpoint. (In the example in Table 14.1, the rating question has 11 points, numbered 0-10.)

- **Checklists** include multiple questions with the same response options. A checklist is a two-dimensional matrix in which questions are listed on one dimension (usually vertically) and response options are listed on the other. Checklists are relatively efficient and easy to understand but are difficult to communicate orally, so they are used more often in SAQs than in interviews. Figure 14.1 presents an example of a checklist.
- **Visual analog scales** (**VASs**) are used to measure subjective experiences, such as pain, dyspnea, or fatigue. The VAS is a straight line, the end anchors end points of which are labeled as the extreme limits of the sensation or feeling being measured. People are asked to mark a point on the line corresponding to the amount of sensation experienced. Traditionally, the VAS line is 100 mm in length, which facilitates the derivation of a score from 0 to 100 through simple measurement by simply measuring the distance from one end of the scale to the person's

FIGURE 14.2 Example of a visual analog scale.

mark on the line. An example of a VAS is shown in Figure 14.2 (there is also one available in the Toolkit ⊗).

Researchers sometimes collect information about activities and dates using an **event history calendar** (Martyn & Belli, 2002; Vanhoutte & Nazroo, 2016). Such calendars are matrixes that plot time on one dimension (usually horizontally) and events or activities on the other. The person recording the data (either the participant or an interviewer) draws lines to indicate the stop and start dates of the specified events or behaviors. Event history calendars are especially useful in collecting information about the occurrence and sequencing of events retrospectively. Data quality about past occurrences is enhanced because the calendar helps participants relate the timing of some events to the timing of others. An example of an event history calendar is included in the Toolkit of the *Resource Manual*. ⊗

An alternative to collecting event history data retrospectively is to ask participants to maintain information in an ongoing structured **diary** over a specified time period. This approach is often used to collect quantitative information about sleeping, eating, exercise behavior, or symptom experiences.

> **Example of a Structured Diary**
> Rhéaume and Mullen (2018) studied the effect of long work hours and shift work on nurses' cognitive errors and performance. The nurses recorded information about their sleep patterns in sleep diaries.

Composite Scales and Other Structured Self-Reports

Multi-item composite scales are an important type of structured self-report. A **scale** yields a numeric score that places respondents on a continuum with respect to an attribute, much like a scale for measuring people's weight. Scales are used to discriminate quantitatively among people with different attitudes, symptoms, conditions, and needs. In the medical literature, a self-report scale completed by patients is typically called a **patient-reported outcome (PRO)**.

Likert-Type Summated Rating Scales

A widely used scaling technique is the **Likert scale**, named after the psychologist Rensis Likert. A traditional Likert scale consists of several declarative items that express a viewpoint on a topic. Respondents are asked to indicate the degree to which they agree or disagree with the opinion expressed in the item.

Table 14.2 illustrates a six-item Likert-type scale for measuring attitudes toward condom use. Likert-type scales often have more than six items; our example simply illustrates key features. After respondents complete a Likert scale, their responses are scored. Typically, agreement with positively worded statements and disagreement with negatively worded ones are assigned higher scores (see Chapter 16, however, regarding problems in including both positive and negative items on a scale). The first statement in Table 14.2 is positively worded; agreement indicates a favorable attitude

toward condom use. Thus, a higher score would be assigned to those agreeing with this statement than to those disagreeing. With five response options, we would give a score of 5 to those strongly agreeing, 4 to those agreeing, and so forth. The responses of two hypothetical respondents are shown by a check or an X; item scores are shown in far-right columns. Person 1, who agreed with the first statement, has an item score of 4, whereas person 2, who strongly disagreed, has a score of 1. The second statement is negatively worded, and so scoring is reversed—a 1 is assigned to those who strongly agree, and so on. This reversal is needed so that a high score consistently reflects positive attitudes toward condom use. A person's total score is computed by adding together individual item scores. Such scales are often called **summated rating scales** because of this feature. The total scores of both respondents are shown at the bottom of Table 14.2. The scores reflect a much more positive attitude toward condom use for person 1 (score = 26) than person 2 (score = 11).

The summation feature of such scales makes it possible to finely discriminate among people with different viewpoints. A single question from our scale would allow people to be put in only five categories. A six-item scale, such as the one in Table 14.2, permits finer gradation—from a minimum possible score of 6 (6 × 1) to a maximum possible score of 30 (6 × 5).

Summated rating scales can be used to measure a wide array of attributes. The bipolar scale is not always on an agree/disagree continuum—it might be always/never, likely/unlikely, and so on. Constructing a good summated rating scale requires considerable skill and work. Chapter 16 describes the steps involved in developing and testing such scales.

> **Example of a Likert Scale**
> Romisher and colleagues (2018) used a 20-item Likert scale to measure nurses' attitudes, knowledge, and practice in the care of infants with neonatal abstinence syndrome (NAS). Here is an example of an item measuring attitudes: "I find dealing with mothers of infants with NAS to be stressful or upsetting." Responses were on a 5-point scale: *strongly agree, agree, neither agree nor disagree, disagree,* and *strongly disagree.*

TABLE 14.2 • Example of a Likert Scale

SCORING DIRECTION[a]	ITEM	RESPONSES[b]					SCORE	
		SA	A	?	D	SD	PERSON 1 (✓)	PERSON 2 (×)
+	1. Using a condom shows you care about your partner.	✓				×	4	1
−	2. My partner would be angry if I talked about using condoms.			×		✓	5	3
−	3. I wouldn't enjoy sex as much if my partner and I used condoms.		×		✓		4	2
+	4. Condoms are a good protection against AIDS and other sexually transmitted diseases.			✓	×		3	2
+	5. My partner would respect me if I insisted on using condoms.	✓				×	5	1
−	6. I would be too embarrassed to ask my partner about using a condom.		×			✓	5	2
	Total score						26	11

[a]Researchers would not indicate the direction of scoring on a Likert scale administered to study participants. The scoring direction is indicated in this table for illustrative purposes only.

[b]SA, strongly agree; A, agree; ?, uncertain; D, disagree; SD, strongly disagree.

TIP Most nurse researchers use existing scales rather than developing their own. Some websites for finding scales are noted in the Toolkit. Another place to look for existing instruments is in the Health and Psychosocial Instruments (HaPI) database. Systematic reviews of instruments for specific constructs also appear in the healthcare literature. For example, Casal and colleagues (2017) reviewed instruments that measure breastfeeding attitudes, knowledge, and support.

Cognitive and Neuropsychological Tests

Nurse researchers sometimes assess or study cognitive functioning. Several different types of **cognitive tests** are available. For example, *intelligence tests* evaluate a person's global ability to solve problems and *aptitude tests* measure potential for achievement. Nurse researchers are most likely to use ability tests in studies of high-risk groups, such as low-birthweight children.

Some cognitive tests are specially designed to assess neuropsychological functioning among people with potential cognitive impairments, such as the Mini-Mental Status Examination (MMSE). These tests capture varying types of competence, such as the ability to concentrate and the ability to remember. A good source for learning more about ability tests is the book by the Buros Institute (2017), which is updated every 3 years.

> **Example of a Study Assessing Neuropsychological Function**
> Frain and Chen (2018) tested the effectiveness of an intervention for improving cognitive function in older adults with mild cognitive impairment living with HIV. The researchers used the Montreal Cognitive Assessment test to measure cognitive function before and after the intervention.

Other Types of Structured Self-Reports

Nurse researchers sometimes use other types of structured self-report methods. A brief description of these data collection methods is offered here; we include further information in the Supplement to this chapter on thePoint $\textbf{S}$.

- **Semantic differential (SD) scales** are a technique for measuring attitudes—an alternative to Likert scales. With the SD, respondents are asked to rate concepts (e.g., dieting, exercise) on a series of *bipolar adjectives*, such as good/bad, effective/ineffective, important/unimportant.
- **Q sorts** present participants with a set of cards on which statements are written. Participants are asked to sort the cards along a specified dimension, such as most helpful/least helpful, never true/always true.
- **Vignettes** are brief descriptions of events or situations (fictitious or actual) to which respondents are asked to react and provide information about how they would handle the situation described.
- **Ecological momentary assessments** involve repeated assessments of people's current behaviors, feelings, and experiences in real time, within their natural environment, using contemporary technologies such as text messaging.

Questionnaires Versus Interviews

In developing data collection plans, researchers must decide whether to collect self-report data through interviews or questionnaires. Each method has advantages and disadvantages.

Advantages of Questionnaires

Self-administered questionnaires, which can be distributed in person, by mail, or over the Internet, offer some advantages, such as the following:

- *Cost.* Questionnaires, relative to interviews, are much less costly. Distributing questionnaires to groups (e.g., nursing home residents) is inexpensive and expedient. And, with a fixed amount of funds or time, a larger and more geographically diverse sample can be obtained with mailed or Internet questionnaires than with interviews.
- *Anonymity.* Unlike interviews, questionnaires offer the possibility of complete anonymity. A guarantee of anonymity can be crucial in obtaining candid responses to sensitive questions. Anonymous questionnaires often result in a higher proportion of responses revealing socially undesirable viewpoints or traits than interviews.
- *Interviewer bias.* The absence of an interviewer ensures that there will be no interviewer bias. Interviewers ideally are neutral agents through whom questions and answers are passed. Studies have shown, however, that this ideal is difficult to achieve. Respondents and interviewers interact as humans, and this interaction can affect responses.

Internet data collection is especially economical and can yield a dataset directly amenable to analysis, without requiring someone to enter data onto a file; the same is also true for computer-assisted personal and telephone interviews—CAPI and CATI. Internet surveys also provide opportunities for providing participants with customized feedback and prompts that can minimize missing responses.

Advantages of Interviews

It is true that interviews are costly, prevent anonymity, and bear the risk of interviewer bias. Nevertheless, interviews are considered superior to questionnaires for most research purposes because of the following advantages:

- *Response rates.* Response rates tend to be high in face-to-face interviews. People are less likely to refuse to talk to an interviewer who seeks their cooperation than to ignore a mailed questionnaire or an email. A well-designed interview study normally achieves response rates in the vicinity of 80% to 90%, whereas mailed and Internet questionnaires typically achieve response rates of less than 50%. Because nonresponse is not random, low response rates can introduce bias. However, if questionnaires are personally distributed—e.g., to patients in a clinic—reasonably good response rates often can be achieved (🅢 The Supplement to Chapter 13 on thePoint describes strategies to enhance response rates in mail and Internet surveys).

- *Audience.* Many people cannot fill out a questionnaire. Examples include young children and blind or illiterate individuals. Interviews, on the other hand, are feasible with most people. An important drawback for Internet questionnaires is that not everyone has access to computers or uses them regularly—but this problem is declining.

- *Clarity.* Interviews offer some protection against ambiguous or confusing questions. Interviewers can provide needed clarifications. With questionnaires, misinterpreted questions can go undetected.

- *Depth of questioning.* Information obtained from questionnaires tends to be more superficial than from interviews, largely because questionnaires usually contain mostly closed-ended items. Furthermore, interviewers can enhance the quality of self-report data through *probing*, a topic we discuss later in this chapter.

- *Missing information.* Respondents are less likely to give "don't know" responses or to leave a question unanswered in an interview than on a questionnaire.

- *Supplementary data.* Face-to-face interviews can yield additional data through observation. Interviewers can observe and assess respondents' level of understanding, degree of cooperativeness, living conditions, and so forth. Such information can be useful in interpreting responses.

Some advantages of face-to-face interviews also apply to telephone interviews. Long or detailed interviews or ones with sensitive questions are not well suited to telephone administration, but for relatively brief instruments, telephone interviews are economical and tend to yield higher response rates than mailed or Internet questionnaires.

Designing Structured Self-Report Instruments

We discussed major steps for developing structured self-report instruments earlier in this chapter, but a few additional considerations should be mentioned. For example, related constructs should be clustered into *modules* or areas of questioning. For example, an interview schedule may consist of a module on demographic information, another on health symptoms, and a third on health-promoting activities.

Thought needs to be given to sequencing modules, and questions within modules, to arrive at an order that is psychologically meaningful and encourages candor. The schedule should begin with questions that are interesting and not too sensitive. Whenever both general and specific questions about a topic are included, general questions should be placed first to avoid "coaching."

Instruments should be prefaced by introductory comments about the nature and purpose of the study. In interviews, introductory information is communicated by the interviewer, who typically follows a script. In questionnaires, the introduction takes the form of a **cover letter** (or cover email). The introduction should be carefully constructed because it is the earliest point of contact with potential respondents. An example of a cover letter for a mailed questionnaire is presented in Figure 14.3. (This cover letter is included in the Toolkit for you to adapt. ✲)

Dear Mr. O'Hara,

    We are doing a study to understand how men who are nearing retirement age (55-65 years old) manage their health. This study, sponsored by the National Institutes of Health, will enable health care providers to better meet the needs of men in your age group. Would you please assist us by completing the enclosed questionnaire? Your input is needed to give an accurate picture of men's health.

    Your name was selected at random from a list of residents in your area. The questionnaire is completely anonymous, so we hope you will feel comfortable giving your honest opinions. If you have concerns about any questions, feel free to contact me by e-mail (dfp1@grifuni.edu) or by phone (518-587-3994).

    The questionnaire should only take about 10 minutes of your time. A postage-paid return envelope is enclosed for your convenience. Please return your questionnaire by May 12. In appreciation for your help, I am enclosing $2.

    Your participation in the study is completely voluntary. By returning your booklet, you will be consenting to participate in the study. Thank you in advance for your assistance.

                                                    Sincerely,
                                                  Denise F. Polit, Ph.D.
                                                    Professor

FIGURE 14.3 Example of a cover letter for a mailed questionnaire. This cover letter could be readily adapted for an email message inviting people to participate in a web-based survey.

When a first draft of the instrument is in reasonably good order, it should be reviewed by experts in questionnaire construction, by substantive content area specialists, and by someone capable of detecting spelling mistakes or grammatical errors. When feedback is incorporated into the instrument, it can then be pretested.

In the remainder of this section, we offer some specific suggestions for designing high-quality self-report instruments. Additional guidance is offered in the books by Fowler (2014) and Bradburn and colleagues (2007).

Tips for Wording Questions

We all are accustomed to asking questions, but the proper phrasing of questions for a study is not easy. In wording questions, researchers should keep four important considerations in mind.

1. *Clarity.* Questions should be worded clearly and unambiguously. This is usually easier said than done. Respondents do not always have the same mind-set as the researchers.

2. *Ability of respondents to give information.* Researchers need to consider whether respondents can be expected to understand the question or are qualified to provide meaningful answers.

3. *Bias.* Questions should be worded in a manner that minimizes the risk of response bias.

4. *Sensitivity.* Researchers should strive to be courteous, considerate, and sensitive to respondents' circumstances, especially when asking questions of a private nature.

Here are some specific suggestions with regard to these four considerations:

• Clarify in your own mind the information you are seeking. The question, "When do you usually eat your evening meal?" might elicit such responses as "around 6 pm," or "when my son gets home from soccer practice," or "when I feel like cooking." The question itself contains no words that are difficult, but the question is unclear because the researcher's intent is not apparent.

- Avoid jargon or technical terms (e.g., edema) if lay terms (e.g., swelling) are equally appropriate. Use words that are simple enough for the *least* educated sample members.
- Do not assume that respondents will be aware of, or informed about, issues in which you are interested—and avoid giving the impression that they *ought* to be informed. Questions on complex issues can be worded in such a way that respondents will be comfortable admitting ignorance (e.g., "Many people have not read about factors that increase the risk of diabetes. Do you happen to know of any risk factors?"). Another approach is to preface a question by a short explanation about terminology or issues.
- Avoid leading questions that suggest a particular answer. A question such as, "Do you agree that nurse-midwives play an indispensable role in the health team?" is not neutral.
- State a range of alternatives within the question itself when possible. For instance, the question, "Do you like to get up early on weekends?" is more suggestive of the "right" answer than "Do you prefer to get up early or to sleep late on weekends?"
- For questions that ask about socially undesirable behavior (e.g., excessive drinking), closed-ended questions may be preferred. It is easier to check off having engaged in socially disapproved actions than to verbalize those actions in response to open-ended questions. When controversial behaviors are presented as options, respondents are more likely to believe that their behavior is commonplace, and admissions of such behavior become less awkward.
- Impersonal wording of questions is sometimes useful in encouraging honesty. For example, compare these two statements with which respondents might be asked to agree or disagree: (1) "I am dissatisfied with the nursing care I received during my hospitalization," (2) "The quality of nursing care in this hospital is unsatisfactory." A respondent might feel more comfortable admitting dissatisfaction with nursing care in the less personally worded second question.

Tips for Preparing Response Options
If closed-ended questions are used, researchers also need to develop response alternatives. Below are some suggestions for preparing them.

- Response options should cover all significant alternatives. If respondents are forced to choose from options provided by researchers, the available options should be reasonably inclusive. As a precaution, researchers often have a final response option with a phrase such as "Other—please specify."
- Alternatives should be mutually exclusive. The following categories for a question on a person's age are *not* mutually exclusive: 30 years or younger, 30 to 50 years, or 50 years or older. People who are exactly 30 or 50 would qualify for two categories.
- Response options should be ordered rationally. Options often can be placed in order of decreasing or increasing favorability, agreement, or intensity (e.g., strongly agree, agree, etc.). When options have no "natural" order, alphabetic ordering can avoid leading respondents to a particular response (e.g., see the rank-order question, Table 14.1).
- Response options should be brief. One sentence or phrase for each option is usually sufficient to express a concept. Response alternatives should be about equal in length.

Tips for Formatting an Instrument
The appearance and layout of an instrument may seem a matter of minor administrative importance. Yet, a poorly designed format can have substantive consequences if respondents (or interviewers) become confused, miss questions, or answer questions they should have omitted. The format is especially important in questionnaires because respondents cannot ask for help. The following suggestions may be helpful in laying out an instrument:

- Do not compress questions into too small a space. An extra page of questions is better than a form that appears dense and confusing and that provides inadequate space for responses to open-ended questions.

- Set off the response options from the question or stem. Response alternatives are often aligned vertically (see Table 14.1).
- Give care to formatting **filter questions**, which route respondents through different sets of questions depending on their responses. In interview schedules, **skip patterns** instruct interviewers to skip to a specific question for a given response (e.g., SKIP TO Q10). In SAQs, skip instructions can be confusing. It is often better to put questions appropriate to a subset of respondents apart from the main series of questions, as illustrated in Box 14.1, part B. An important advantage of CAPI, CATI, audio-CASI, and Internet surveys is that skip patterns are built into the computer program, leaving no room for human error.
- Avoid forcing all respondents to go through inapplicable questions in an SAQ. Suppose question 2 in Box 14.1, part B had been worded as

follows: "If you are a member of the American Nurses Association, for how long have you been a member?" Nonmembers may not be sure how to handle this question and may be annoyed at having to read irrelevant material.

Administering Structured Self-Report Instruments

Administering interview schedules and questionnaires involves different issues and skills.

Collecting Interview Data

The quality of interview data relies on interviewer proficiency. Interviewers for large survey organizations receive extensive training. Although we cannot cover all the principles of good interviewing, we can identify some major issues. Additional guidance can be found in Fowler (2014).

A primary task of interviewers is to put respondents at ease so that they feel comfortable in expressing their views honestly. Interviewers should always be punctual (if an appointment has been made), courteous, and friendly. Interviewers should strive to appear unbiased and to create an atmosphere that encourages candor. All opinions of respondents should be accepted as natural; interviewers should not express surprise, disapproval, or even approval.

BOX 14.1 Examples of Formats for a Filter Question

A. **Interview Format**
1. Are you currently a member of the American Nurses Association?
   ❏ 1. Yes
   ❏ 2. No (SKIP TO Q3)
2. For how many years have you been a member?
   _____ YEARS
3. Do you subscribe to any nursing journals?
   ❏ 1. Yes
   ❏ 2. No
B. **Questionnaire Format**
1. Are you currently a member of the American Nurses Association?
   ❏ 1. Yes
   ❏ 2. No
      2. If yes: For how many years have you been a member?
         _____ Years
3. Do you subscribe to any nursing journals?
   ❏ 1. Yes
   ❏ 2. No

Example of Well-Trained Interviewers
Nyamathi and colleagues (2015) gathered data relating to the risk for incarceration among homeless young adults. The baseline interview was "administered by the research staff well trained in confidential data collection, which included respecting each individual as a person, not judging the participant on reported behaviors, and in administering the questionnaire in a private location" (p. 803).

Interviewers should follow question wording in the interview schedule precisely. Interviewers should not offer spontaneous explanations of what questions mean. Repetition of a question is usually adequate to dispel misunderstandings, especially if the instrument has been pretested. Interviewers should not read questions mechanically. A natural, conversational tone is essential in building rapport, and this tone is impossible to achieve if interviewers are not thoroughly familiar with the questions.

When closed-ended questions have lengthy response alternatives or when a series of questions has the same response options, interviewers should hand respondents a **show card** that lists the options. People cannot be expected to remember detailed unfamiliar material and may choose the last response option if they cannot recall earlier ones. (An example of a show card is included in the Toolkit ⊗).

Interviewers record answers to closed-ended items by checking or circling the appropriate alternative, but responses to open-ended questions must either be written out in full or recorded for later transcription. Interviewers should not paraphrase or summarize respondents' replies.

Obtaining complete, relevant responses to questions is not always easy. Respondents may reply to seemingly straightforward questions with partial answers. Some may say, "I don't know" to avoid giving their opinions on sensitive topics, or to stall while they think. In such cases, the interviewers' job is to **probe**. The purpose of a probe is to elicit more useful information than respondents volunteered initially. A probe can take many forms. Sometimes it involves repeating the question and sometimes it is a long pause intended to communicate to respondents that they should continue. It may be necessary to encourage a more complete response to open-ended questions by using a nondirective supplementary question, such as, "How is that?" Interviewers must be careful to use only *neutral* probes that do not influence the content of a response. Box 14.2 gives examples of neutral, nondirective probes used by professional interviewers to stimulate more complete responses to questions. The ability to probe well is perhaps the greatest test of an interviewer's skill. To know when to probe and which probe to use, interviewers must understand the purpose of each question. (The Toolkit for Chapter 14 ⊗ has material relating to interviewer training.)

Guidelines for telephone interviews are essentially the same as those for face-to-face interviews, but additional effort usually is required to build

BOX 14.2 Examples of Neutral, Nondirective Probes

- Is there anything else?
- Go on.
- Are there any other reasons?
- How do you mean?
- Could you please tell me more about that?
- Would you tell me what you have in mind?
- There are no right or wrong answers; I'd just like to get your thinking.
- Could you please explain that?
- Could you please give me an example?

rapport over the telephone. In both cases, interviewers should strive to make the interview a pleasant and satisfying experience in which respondents come to understand that the information they are providing is valued.

Example of a Telephone Survey Interview
Pisu and an interprofessional team (2018) conducted a telephone survey of 1,457 older adults with cancer. The purpose of the study was to identify factors that contributed to the participants' health-related quality of life.

Collecting Questionnaire Data through In-Person Distribution

Questionnaires can be distributed by personal delivery, through the mail, and over the Internet on various devices. The most convenient procedure is to distribute questionnaires to a group of people who complete the instrument at the same time. This approach has the obvious advantages of maximizing the number of completed questionnaires and allowing respondents to ask questions. Group administrations may be possible in some clinical and educational settings.

Researchers can also hand out questionnaires to individual respondents. Personal contact has a positive effect on response rates, and researchers can answer questions. Individual distribution of questionnaires in clinical settings is often inexpensive and efficient.

Example of Personal Distribution of Questionnaires
Pölkki and colleagues (2018) distributed questionnaires to 178 parents whose infants were being treated in Finnish neonatal intensive care units. The questionnaires asked about the parent's use of nonpharmacologic methods of managing their infants' procedural pain.

Collecting Questionnaire Data Through the Mail

For surveys of a broad population, questionnaires can be mailed. A *mail* (or *postal*) *survey* approach is cost-effective for reaching geographically dispersed respondents, but it tends to yield low response rates, often lower than 50%. The risk of bias in such cases is great. Response rates can be affected by how the questionnaires are designed and mailed. The recommended procedure is to include a stamped, addressed return envelope.

> **TIP** People are more likely to complete a mailed questionnaire if they are encouraged to do so by someone whose name they recognize. If possible, obtain an endorsement of a well-known person or write the cover letter on the stationery of a respected organization, such as a university.

Follow-up reminders are critical in improving response rates for mailed and Internet questionnaires. This involves additional mailings urging nonrespondents to complete and return their forms. Follow-up reminders should be sent about 5 to 10 days after the initial mailing. Sometimes reminders simply involve a postcard of encouragement to nonrespondents, but it may be necessary to send another questionnaire because many nonrespondents will have misplaced or discarded the original. With anonymous questionnaires, researchers may not be able to distinguish respondents and nonrespondents for the purpose of sending follow-up letters. In such a situation, the best procedure is to send out a follow-up notice to everyone, thanking those who have already answered and asking others to cooperate (see Example of a Reminder Postcard for a Mailed Questionnaire in the Toolkit ⊗). Dillman and colleagues (2014) offer excellent advice regarding mail, Internet, and telephone surveys.

Example of Mailed Questionnaires
Etingen and colleagues (2018) studied the relationships between pain interference and psychosocial well-being among veterans with spinal cord injuries/disorders (SCI/D). Questionnaires were mailed to a national sample of veterans with SCI/D who received prior year Veterans Affairs healthcare.

Collecting Questionnaire Data via the Internet

The Internet provides an economical means of distributing questionnaires. Internet surveys appear to be a promising approach for accessing groups of people interested in specific topics.

Surveys can be administered through the Internet in several ways. One method is to design a questionnaire in a word processing program, as for mailed questionnaires. The file with the questionnaire is then attached to an email message and distributed. Respondents can complete the questionnaire and return it as an email attachment or print it and return it by mail or fax. This method may be problematic if respondents have trouble opening attachments or if they use a different word processing program. Surveys sent via email also run the risk of not getting delivered to the intended party, either because email addresses have changed or because the email messages are blocked by security filters.

Increasingly, researchers collect data through **web-based surveys**. This approach requires researchers to have a website on which the survey is placed or to use survey platforms such as Survey Monkey (http://www.surveymonkey.com/) or Qualtrics (www.qualtrics.com/). Respondents typically access the website by clicking on a hypertext link. For example, respondents may be invited to participate in the survey through an email message that includes the link to the survey or they may be invited to participate when they enter a website related in content to the survey (e.g., the website of a cancer support organization).

Web-based forms often can be programmed to include interactive features. By having dynamic features, respondents can receive as well as give information—a feature that can increase motivation to participate. For example, respondents can be given information about their own responses (e.g., how they scored on a scale) or aggregated information about responses from previous participants. A major advantage of web-based surveys is that the data are directly amenable to analysis.

Example of a Web-Based Survey
Rosman and colleagues (2019) used a national web-based registry of women with peripartum cardiomyopathy to study the women's psychosocial adjustment and quality of life.

TIP When sending out an email invitation, avoid using the word "survey" or "questionnaire" in the subject line—these words tend to discourage people from opening the email. There is some evidence that the best time to send out email invitations is Monday mornings.

Internet surveys have proliferated. They are inexpensive and can reach a broad audience. However, samples are almost never representative, and response rates tend to be low—even lower than mailed questionnaires. Several references are available to help researchers who wish to launch an Internet survey. For example, the books by Dillman et al. (2014), Tourangeau et al. (2013), and Callegaro et al. (2015) provide useful information. In the nursing literature, Cope (2014) and McPeake and colleagues (2014) have offered advice about electronic surveys.

A project funded by the National Institutes of Health offers another option for gathering patient-reported outcomes over the Internet. The Patient-Reported Outcomes Measurement Information System (**PROMIS®**) initiative (Cella et al., 2010) makes it possible to measure a broad range of patient-reported outcomes online, using measures that have been rigorously developed and tested. Examples of patient outcomes in PROMIS® include those in the physical health domain (e.g., fatigue, physical functioning, sleep disturbance), in the mental health domain (e.g., anxiety, depression, anger), and in the social health domain (e.g., social support). Measures are available for both

adult and pediatric populations and can be administered online and scored, with normed information provided instantly. A link is available in the Toolkit. ⊗

Example of a Study Using PROMIS®
Hanish and Han (2018) studied sleep outcomes in adolescents with PAX6 haploinsufficiency. Study participants completed two PROMIS® scales—the sleep-related impairment and sleep disturbance scales.

Evaluation of Structured Self-Reports

Structured self-reports are a powerful data collection method. They are versatile and yield information that can be readily analyzed statistically. Structured questions can be carefully worded and rigorously pretested. On the other hand, structured questions tend to be more superficial than questions in unstructured interviews.

Structured self-reports are susceptible to the risk of various **response biases**—some of which can also occur with unstructured self-reports. Respondents may give biased answers in reaction to the interviewers' behavior or appearance, for example. Perhaps the most pervasive problem is people's tendency to present a favorable image of themselves. **Social desirability response bias** refers to the tendency of some individuals to misrepresent themselves by giving answers that are congruent with prevailing social values. This problem is often difficult to combat. Subtle, indirect, and delicately worded questioning sometimes can help to minimize this response bias. Creating a nonjudgmental atmosphere and providing anonymity also encourage frankness. In an interview situation, interviewer training is essential.

Some response biases, called **response sets**, are most commonly observed in composite scales. **Extreme responses** are a bias reflecting consistent selection of extreme alternatives (e.g., "strongly agree"). These extreme responses distort the findings because they do not necessarily reflect the most intense feelings about the phenomenon under study, but rather capture a trait of the respondent.

Some people have been found to agree with statements regardless of content. Such people are called **yea-sayers**, and the bias is known as the **acquiescence response set**. A less common problem is the opposite tendency for other individuals, called **nay-sayers**, to disagree with statements independently of question content.

Researchers who construct scales should try to eliminate or minimize response set biases. If an instrument or scale is being developed for use by others, evidence should be gathered to demonstrate that the scale is sufficiently free from response biases to measure the critical variable.

STRUCTURED OBSERVATION

Structured observation is used to record behaviors, interactions, and events in a systematic way. Structured observation involves using formal instruments and protocols that specify what to observe, how long to observe it, and how to record information. Although observations often focus on patients or their caretakers, observations are also used to record the behaviors of nurses and other healthcare professionals, especially in quality improvement studies.

Methods of Recording Structured Observations

Researchers recording structured observations often use either a checklist or a rating scale. Both types of record-keeping instruments are designed to produce numeric information.

Category Systems and Checklists

Structured observation often involves constructing a category system to classify observed phenomena. A **category system** represents a method of capturing consistently the qualitative behaviors and events transpiring in the observational setting.

Some category systems are constructed so that *all* observed behaviors within a specified domain (e.g., speech) can be classified into one and only one category. In such an exhaustive system, the categories are mutually exclusive.

> **Example of Exhaustive Categories**
> Shabani and colleagues (2016) used a crossover design to test the effects of music therapy on premature infants' pain responses from blood sampling. The infants' sleep–wake states, which were recorded every 15 seconds, were coded into one of six mutually exclusive categories (deep sleep, active sleep, drowsy, quiet alert, active alert, and crying).

When all behaviors of a certain type (e.g., verbal exchanges) are observed and recorded, researchers usually need to carefully define categories so that observers know when one behavior ends and a new one begins. The assumption in using such a category system is that behaviors, events, or actions that are allocated to a particular category are equivalent to every other behavior, event, or action in that same category.

Another approach is to develop a system in which only certain behaviors (which may or may not occur) are recorded. For example, if we were studying autistic children's aggressive behavior, we might specify categories such as "strikes another child" or "kicks/hits walls or floor." In such a category system, many behaviors—all the ones that are nonaggressive—would not be classified. Such nonexhaustive systems may be adequate, but one risk is that resulting data might be difficult to interpret. Problems may arise if a large number of behaviors are not categorized or if long segments of the observation sessions do not involve the target behaviors. In such situations, investigators should record the amount of time in which the target behaviors occurred, relative to the total time under observation.

> **Example of Nonexhaustive Categories**
> Dey and colleagues (2017) studied the mistreatment of women by healthcare providers—including nurses—during childbirth in India. Trained observers recorded the presence of six types of mistreatment on a checklist (e.g., physical abuse, verbal abuse, abandonment, etc.). Provider behaviors that were not abusive (e.g., supportive behaviors) were not recorded.

A good category system requires the careful definition of behaviors or characteristics to be observed. Each category must be explained carefully so that observers have unambiguous criteria for identifying the occurrence of a specified phenomenon. Even with detailed definitions of categories, virtually all category systems require observer inference, to a greater or lesser degree. For instance, coding providers' behaviors as abusive in the study mentioned in the previous example (i.e., the Dey et al. (2017) study of the care of women during childbirth) would require considerable inference, even with good training materials.

Category systems are the basis for a **checklist**, which is the instrument observers use to record observed phenomena. The checklist is usually formatted with behaviors or events from the category system listed vertically on the left and space for recording the frequency, duration, or intensity of behavior occurrences on the right. With nonexhaustive category systems, the behaviors of interest, which may or may not be manifested, are listed on the checklist. The observer's tasks are to watch for instances of these behaviors and to record their occurrence.

With exhaustive checklists, the observers' task is to place all behaviors in only one category for each element. By **element**, we refer to either a unit of behavior, such as a sentence in a conversation, or a specified time interval. To illustrate, suppose we were studying the problem-solving behavior of a group of public health staff discussing an intervention for the homeless. Our category system involves eight categories: (1) seeks information, (2) gives information, (3) describes problem, (4) offers suggestion, (5) opposes suggestion, (6) supports suggestion, (7) summarizes, and (8) miscellaneous. Observers would be required to classify every group member's contribution—using, for example, each sentence as the element—into one of these eight categories.

Another approach with exhaustive systems is to categorize relevant behaviors at regular time intervals. For example, in a category system for infants' motor activities, the researcher might use 10-second time intervals as the element; observers would categorize infant movements within 10-second periods.

Rating Scales

An alternative to a checklist for recording structured observations is a **rating scale** that requires observers to rate a phenomenon along a descriptive continuum that is typically bipolar. Observers may be required to rate behaviors or events at specified intervals throughout the observational period (e.g., every 5 minutes). Alternatively, observers may rate entire events or transactions after observations are completed. Postobservation ratings require observers to integrate a number of activities and to judge which point on a scale most closely fits their interpretation of the situation. For example, suppose we were observing children's behavior during a scratch test for allergies. After each session, observers might be asked to rate the children's overall anxiety during the procedure on a graphic rating scale such as the following:

Rate how calm or nervous the child appeared to be during the procedure:

1	2	3	4	5	6	7
Extremely calm			Neither calm nor nervous			Extremely nervous

TIP Observational rating scales are sometimes incorporated into structured interviews. For example, in a study of the health problems of 4,000 low-income families, interviewers were asked to rate the safety of children's home environment with regard to potential health hazards on a 5-point scale, from completely safe to extremely unsafe (Polit et al., 2007).

Rating scales can also be used as an extension of checklists, wherein observers record not only the occurrence of a behavior but also rate some qualitative aspect of it, such as its intensity. When rating scales are coupled with a category scheme, considerable information about a phenomenon can be obtained, but it places a large burden on observers, particularly if there is extensive activity.

Example of Observational Ratings
Mitchell and colleagues (2016) conducted a clinical trial to assess the effectiveness of alternative pain-relief treatments (e.g., noninvasive electrical stimulation at acupuncture points) for neonates during routine heelsticks. Infant pain was measured using the Premature Infant Pain Profile (PIPP), a widely used measure that incorporates both observers' ratings of infant behaviors and physiological indicators (e.g., heart rate).

In the PIPP system, observers watch an infant for 30 seconds and score certain behaviors, such as *eye squeeze* and *behavioral state*. Table 14.3 shows the PIPP rating system for the four observer-rated behaviors.

> **TIP** It is often advisable to spend some time with participants before observations and data recording begin. Having a warm-up period helps to relax people, especially if audio or video equipment is being used and can be helpful to observers (for example, if participants have a strong accent or speech patterns to which they must adjust).

Constructing Versus Borrowing Structured Observational Instruments

Compared to the abundance of books that provide guidance in developing self-report instruments, there are relatively few resources for healthcare researchers who want to design their own observational instruments. Yoder and colleagues (2018) provide one resource for observational measurements of behavior.

As with self-report instruments, however, we encourage you to search for an available observational instrument, rather than creating one yourself. The use of an existing instrument saves considerable work and time and facilitates cross-study comparisons. The best source for existing instruments is recent research literature on the study topic. For example, if you were conducting an observational study of infant pain, a good place to begin would be to read recent research on this topic to learn how infant pain was operationalized.

Sampling for Structured Observations

Researchers must decide when, and for how long, structured observations will be undertaken. Observations are typically done for a specific amount

TABLE 14.3 • Observer-Rated Categories for the Premature Infant Pain Profile (PIPP)

INDICATOR	OBSERVATION[a]	POINTS
Behavioral state	Active/awake, eyes open, facial movements	0
	Quiet/awake, eyes open, no facial movements	1
	Active/sleep, eyes closed, facial movements	2
	Quiet/sleep, eyes closed, no facial movements	3
Brow bulge	None (<9% of time)	0
	Minimum (10%-39% of time)	1
	Moderate (40%-69% of time)	2
	Maximum (>70% of time)	3
Eye squeeze	None (<9% of time)	0
	Minimum (10%-39% of time)	1
	Moderate (40%-69% of time)	2
	Maximum (>70% of time)	3
Nasolabial furrow	None (<9% of time)	0
	Minimum (10%-39% of time)	1
	Moderate (40%-69% of time)	2
	Maximum (>70% of time)	3

Adapted with permission from Stevens, B., et al. (1996). Premature Infant Pain Profile: Development and initial validation. *Clinical Journal of Pain, 12*, 13–22.

[a]Observations are made in a 15-second baseline period and in a 30-second period immediately after a painful event.

of time, and the amount of time is standardized across participants. Sampling may be needed to obtain representative examples of behaviors. *Observational sampling* concerns the selection of behaviors or activities to be observed, not the selection of participants.

With **time sampling**, researchers select time periods during which observations occur. The time frames may be selected systematically (e.g., 60 seconds at 5-minute intervals) or at random. For example, suppose we were studying mothers' interactions with their children in a clinic. During a 30-minute observation period, we sample moments to observe, rather than observing continuously. Let us say that observations are made in 2-minute segments. If we used systematic sampling, we would observe for 2 minutes, then cease observing for a prespecified period, say 3 minutes. With this scheme, a total of six 2-minute observations would be made for each dyad. A second approach is to sample 2-minute periods at random from the total of 15 such periods in a half hour; a third is to use all 15 periods. Decisions about the length and number of periods for creating a good sample must be consistent with research aims. In establishing time units, a key consideration is determining a psychologically meaningful time frame. Pretesting with different sampling plans is advisable.

> **Example of Time Sampling**
> Teipel and an interprofessional team (2017) undertook a multidimensional behavior assessment of people with dementia living in nursing homes in Germany. The researchers used Dementia Care Mapping (DCM), a standardized observation of residents' well-being (e.g., behaviors of aggression, pacing, restlessness). DCM was conducted every 5 minutes.

Event sampling uses integral behavior sets or events for observation. Event sampling requires that the investigator either have knowledge about the occurrence of events or be in a position to wait for (or arrange) their occurrence. Examples of integral events suitable for event sampling include nurses' shift changes and cast removals of pediatric patients. This approach is preferable to time sampling when events of interest are widely spaced in time. When phenomena of interest are frequent, time sampling can enhance the representativeness of observed behaviors.

> **Example of Event Sampling**
> Saxton and Cahill (2017) tested a quality improvement intervention designed to decrease interruptions during medication administration. The outcomes included time spent on medication occurrences and number of interruptions. A trained observer, using an observational instrument and a stopwatch, observed medication administration (the event), from the nurses' retrieval of medication to administration of the drug.

Technical Aids in Observations

A wide array of technical devices is available for recording behaviors and events, making analysis or categorization at a later time possible. When the target behavior is auditory (e.g., verbal interactions), recordings can be used to obtain a permanent record. Technologic advances have vastly improved the quality, sensitivity, and unobtrusiveness of recording equipment. Auditory recordings can also be analyzed using speech software to obtain objective quantitative measures of certain features (e.g., volume, pitch).

Video recording can be used when permanent visual records are desired. Video records can capture complex behaviors that might elude on-the-spot observers. Videos make it possible to check coders' accuracy and are useful in observer training. Finally, cameras are often less obtrusive than a human observer. Video records have a few drawbacks, some of which are technical, such as lighting requirements, lens limitations, and so on. Sometimes the camera angle can present a lopsided view of an event. Also, some participants may be self-conscious in front of a video camera. Still, for many applications, visual records offer unparalleled opportunities to expand the scope of observational studies. Haidet and colleagues (2009) offer valuable advice on improving data quality of video-recorded observations.

There is a growing technology for assisting with the encoding and recording of observations. For example, some equipment and software permit observers to enter observational data directly into a computer as the observation occurs, and in some cases, the equipment can record physiologic data concurrently.

Example of Using Equipment

Pecanac and colleagues (2015) described the use of handheld technology to capture continuous observations of behavior, which they referred to as *timed event sequential data*. The technology, which could be used to capture both patients' and nurses' behaviors, can address such questions as "When does this behavior occur? How long does the behavior last?" (p. 67). They illustrated with a study designed to answer the question: "What are the frequency, duration, and sequence of nursing care related to mobilizing older patients in acute care settings?" (p. 68).

Structured Observations by Nonresearch Observers

The observations discussed thus far are undertaken by research team members. Sometimes, however, researchers ask people not connected with the research to provide structured data, based on their observations of others. This method has much in common (in terms of format and scoring) with self-report instruments; the primary difference is that the person answering questions is asked to describe the behaviors of *another* person. For example, mothers might be asked to describe their children's behavior problems.

Obtaining observational data from nonresearchers is economical compared with using trained observers. For example, observers might have to watch children for hours or days to capture the nature and intensity of behavior problems, whereas parents or teachers could do this readily. Some behaviors might never lend themselves to outsider observation because they occur in private situations.

On the other hand, such methods may have the same problems as self-reports (e.g., response set biases) in addition to observer bias. Observer bias may in some cases be extreme, such as may happen when parents provide information about their children. Nonresearch observers are typically not trained, and interobserver agreement usually cannot be assessed. Thus, this approach has some problems but will continue to be used because, in many cases, there are no alternatives.

Example of Observations by Nonresearch Personnel

Cui and colleagues (2018) investigated the relationship between maternal and paternal physical abuse of their children and the children's behavior problems in China. Mothers completed the Child Behavior Checklist for their children (average age = 12.3 years) as a measure of the children's externalizing and internalizing behaviors.

Evaluation of Structured Observation

Structured observation is an important data collection method, particularly for recording aspects of people's behaviors when they are incapable of reliable self-report. Observational methods are particularly valuable for gathering data about infants and children, older people who are confused or agitated, or people whose communication skills are impaired.

Observations, like self-reports, are vulnerable to biases. One source of bias comes from those being observed. Participants may distort their behaviors in the direction of "looking good." They may also behave atypically because of their awareness of being observed (*reactivity*), or their shyness in front of strangers or a camera.

Biases can also reflect observers' perceptual errors. To make and record observation in a completely objective fashion is challenging. The risk of bias is especially great when a high degree of observer inference is required.

Several types of observational bias may occur. With **assimilatory biases**, observers distort observations in the direction of identity with previous inputs. This bias would have the effect of miscategorizing information in the direction of regularity and orderliness. Assimilation to the observer's expectations and attitudes also occurs.

With regard to rating scales, the **halo effect** is the tendency of observers to be influenced by one characteristic in judging other, unrelated characteristics. For example, if we had a positive general impression of a person, we might rate that person as intelligent and dependable simply because these traits are positively valued. Ratings may reflect observers' personality. The **error of leniency** is the tendency for observers to rate everything positively, and the **error of severity** is the contrasting tendency to rate too harshly.

The careful pretesting of checklists and rating scales and the thorough training of observers are essential in minimizing biases. Training should include practice sessions in which the comparability of observers' classifications and ratings is assessed. That is, two or more independent observers should watch a trial situation and observational coding should then be compared. *Interrater reliability* of structured observations is described in the next chapter.

> **TIP** People being observed are less likely to behave typically if they think they are being appraised. Even positive cues (such as nodding approval) should be avoided because approval may induce repetition of a behavior that might not otherwise have occurred.

BIOMARKERS

As defined by the Biomarker Working Group at the National Institutes of Health (2001), a **biomarker** is "a characteristic that is objectively measured and evaluated as an indicator of normal biological processes, pathogenic processes, or pharmacologic response to a therapeutic intervention" (p. 90). Examples of biomarkers include routine clinical measurements (e.g., blood pressure) and complex laboratory tests of blood, other body fluids, and tissue.

Settings in which nurses work are typically filled with a wide variety of technical instruments for measuring physiologic functions. Nurse researchers have used biomarkers for a wide variety of purposes. Examples include studies of basic biophysiologic processes, explorations of the ways in which nursing actions and interventions affect physiologic outcomes, and studies of the correlates of physiologic functioning in patients with health problems. Corwin and Ferranti (2016) have urged nurse researchers to integrate biomarkers into their studies to be "better able to precisely tailor and test nursing interventions" (p. 293).

It is beyond the scope of this book to describe the many kinds of biomarkers available to nurse researchers. Our goals are to present an overview of biophysiologic measures, to illustrate their use in research and to note considerations in decisions to use them.

Types of Biomarkers

Physiologic measurements are either in vivo or in vitro. **In vivo measurements** are performed directly in or on living organisms. Examples include measures of oxygen saturation, blood pressure, and body temperature. An **in vitro measurement**, by contrast, is performed outside the organism's body, for example, measuring serum potassium concentration in the blood.

In vivo instruments have been developed to measure all bodily functions, and technologic improvements continue to advance our ability to measure biophysiologic phenomena more accurately, conveniently, and rapidly than ever before.

> **Example of a Study With In Vivo Measures**
> Burrai and colleagues (2019) tested the effects of listening to live singing in patients undergoing hemodialysis. The singing intervention was associated with improvements in patients' systolic and diastolic blood pressure.

With in vitro measures, data are gathered by extracting physiologic material from people and submitting it for laboratory analysis. Usually, labs establish a *reference range* of normal values for each measurement, which helps in interpreting the results. Several classes of laboratory analysis have been used by nurse researchers, including chemical measurements (e.g., measures of potassium levels), microbiologic measures (e.g., bacterial counts), cytologic *or* histologic measures (e.g., tissue biopsies), and genetic testing. Laboratory analyses of blood and urine samples are the most frequently used in vitro measures in nursing investigations.

> **Example of a Study With In Vitro Measures**
> Rieder and colleagues (2019) tested salivary biomarkers of the sympathetic nervous system and hypothalamic–pituitary–adrenal axis function as predictors of maternal stress among mothers under community criminal justice supervision.

Selecting a Biomarker

The most basic issue in selecting a biomarker is whether it will yield good information about key research variables. In some cases, researchers need to consider whether the variable should be measured by observation or self-report instead of (or in addition to) using biophysiologic equipment. For example, stress could be measured by asking people questions (e.g., using the State-Trait Anxiety Inventory), by observing their behavior during exposure to stressful stimuli, or by measuring heart rate, blood pressure, or levels of adrenocorticotropic hormone in urine samples.

TIP There has been considerable debate in the medical community about the use of biomarkers as surrogates for clinical end points in clinical trials. A critical issue is whether treatment effects on a biomarker reliably predict treatment effects on end points that are more clinically meaningful (Fleming & Powers, 2012).

Several other considerations should be kept in mind in selecting a biophysiologic measure. Some key questions include the following:

- Is the necessary equipment or laboratory analysis readily available to you?
- Will you have difficulty obtaining permission from an Institutional Review Board or other institutional authority?
- Is a single measure of the outcome sufficient, or are multiple measures needed for a reliable estimate? If the latter, what burden does this place on participants?
- Are your measures likely to be influenced by reactivity (participants' awareness of their status)?
- Are you thoroughly familiar with safety precautions, such as grounding procedures?

Evaluation of Biomarkers

Biophysiologic measures offer the following advantages to nurse researchers:

- Biomarkers are accurate and precise compared with psychological measures (e.g., self-report measures of anxiety).
- Biomarkers are objective. Two nurses reading from the same sphygmomanometer are likely to obtain the same blood pressure measurements, and two different sphygmomanometers are likely to produce the same readouts. Patients cannot easily distort measurements of biophysiologic functioning.

- Biophysiologic instruments provide valid measures of targeted variables: thermometers can be depended on to measure temperature and not blood volume, and so forth. For self-report and observational measures, it is more difficult to be certain that the instrument is really measuring the target concept.

Biomarkers also have a few disadvantages:

- The cost of collecting some types of biophysiologic data may be low or nonexistent, but when laboratory tests are involved, they may be more expensive than other methods (e.g., assessing smoking status by means of cotinine assays versus self-report).
- The measuring tool may affect the variables it is attempting to measure. The presence of a sensing device, such as a transducer, located in a blood vessel partially blocks that vessel and, hence, alters the pressure–flow characteristics being measured.
- Energy must often be applied to the organism when taking the biophysiologic measurements; caution must be exercised to avoid the risk of damaging cells by high-energy concentrations.
- Laboratory protocols can vary between independent research labs and clinical or commercial labs, and these differences can lead to variations in results.
- Normed values of biological markers are often based on information from Caucasian males, and normal values may vary by sex, age, race, and ethnicity.

The difficulty in choosing biomarkers for nursing studies lies not in their shortage nor in their inferiority to other methods. Indeed, they are plentiful, often highly reliable and valid, and extremely useful in clinical nursing studies. Care must be exercised, however, in selecting instruments or laboratory analyses with regard to practical, ethical, medical, and technical considerations.

PHYSICAL PERFORMANCE TESTS

Patients' abilities and skills are sometimes measured with **performance tests**. For example, the 6-Minute Walk Test (6MWT) is a widely used measure of physical functioning for patients with various cardiovascular, respiratory, or neurologic diseases or those in need of surgical or rehabilitative intervention. The measure is the distance walked in a 6-minute period, sometimes involving the use of a treadmill. Many other physical performance tests have been devised to measure such attributes as balance, mobility, endurance, and flexibility.

Example of Performance Testing

In a randomized controlled trial, Xueyu and colleagues (2017) tested the effect of a low-intensity exercise intervention for older adults with chronic heart failure. The study outcomes included the patients' performance on the 6-Minute Walk Test and the Timed Up-and-Go Test.

DATA EXTRACTED FROM RECORDS

In many nursing studies—and, especially, in quality improvement projects and outcomes research—at least some study data come from existing records. Electronic health records (EHRs) can be a good source of data for many studies. Even though data from records are "available," that does not mean that researchers can put them to use without a careful plan.

Medical records from electronic databases are easier and more efficient to search than paper-based records. Worster and Haines (2004) have noted, however, that electronic databases may be less accurate because of possible clerical errors if transcription is involved.

Researchers using either paper or electronic records must develop means of extracting data on key variables in a manner that enhances accuracy and consistency. Extracted data can be recorded on data collection forms that are either paper-based or computerized (e.g., in spreadsheets). Worster and Haines (2004) have suggested some useful strategies to enhance data quality when extracting data from medical records:

- Data abstractors should be carefully trained;
- Abstractors should be blinded to study hypotheses;
- Inclusion and exclusion criteria for the records to be abstracted should be explicit;

- The variables of interest should be carefully defined, and, if relevant, the possible range of values should be communicated (e.g., on a measure that should be coded 1 or 0, a 2 would be out of range);
- Unambiguous guidelines about how to deal with missing data should be established at the outset;
- Clear-cut rules should be established about how to deal with conflicting data (i.e., when there are two or more versions of the same variable in the database);
- Data abstractors should be told from the start that their work will be checked for accuracy; and
- The accuracy of the abstraction should, indeed, be verified in random samples of records.

Gregory and Radovinsky (2012) offer some additional advice about extracting high-quality data from medical records and provide examples of data collection forms and coding guidelines. Additional guidance on using data from EHRs in nursing studies is offered by Samuels et al. (2015) and Seaman et al. (2017).

IMPLEMENTING A DATA COLLECTION PLAN

Data quality in a quantitative study is affected by both the data collection plan and how the plan is implemented.

Selecting Research Personnel

An important decision concerns who will actually collect the research data. In small studies, the lead researcher usually collects the data personally, but in large studies this is not feasible. When data are collected by others, it is important to select appropriate people. In general, they should be neutral agents—their characteristics or behavior should not affect the data. Here are some considerations to keep in mind when selecting research personnel:

- *Experience.* Research staff ideally have had relevant prior experience (e.g., prior interviewing experience). If this is not feasible, look for people who can readily acquire needed skills (e.g., interviewers should have good verbal and social skills).

- *Congruence with sample characteristics.* If possible, data collectors should match participants with respect to racial or cultural background and gender. The greater the sensitivity of the questions, the greater the desirability of congruence.
- *Unremarkable appearance.* Extremes of appearance should be avoided. For example, data collectors should not dress very casually (e.g., in tee shirts) nor formally (e.g., in designer clothes). Data collectors should not wear anything that conveys their political, social, or religious views.
- *Personality.* Data collectors should be pleasant (but not effusive), sociable (but not overly chatty), and nonjudgmental (but not unfeeling). The goal is to have nonthreatening data collectors who can put participants at ease.

In some situations, researchers cannot select research personnel. For example, the data collectors may be staff nurses employed at a hospital. Training of the data collection staff is particularly important in such situations. When researchers collect their own data, they should self-monitor their demeanor and prepare for their role with care.

Training Data Collectors

Depending on prior experience, training needs to cover both general procedures (e.g., how to probe in an interview) and ones specific to the study (e.g., how to ask a particular question or how to categorize a behavior). Complex projects may require several days of training. The lead researcher is usually the best person to develop training materials and to conduct the training.

Data collection protocols usually are a good foundation for a **training manual**. The manual normally includes background materials (e.g., the study aims), general instructions, specific instructions, and copies of all data forms.

TIP A table of contents (TOC) for a training manual for a self-report study is included in the Toolkit of the *Resource Manual*. Models for some sections in this TOC (a section on avoiding interviewer bias and another on how to probe) are also in the Toolkit. If you are collecting self-report data yourself, you should learn techniques of professional interviewing.

Training often includes demonstrations of high-quality fictitious data collection sessions, performed live or on video. Training may involve having trainees do trial runs of data collection (*mock interviews*) in front of the trainers to demonstrate their understanding of the instructions. Thompson and colleagues (2005) provide additional tips about the training of research personnel.

Another issue concerns blinding. Ideally, the data collectors would be blinded to study hypotheses and to participants' membership in groups being compared. Data collectors should understand the study *variables* and the *population* but not researchers' expectations.

Example of Data Collector Training
In a two-wave panel study of the health of 4,000 low-income families, Polit and co-researchers (2007) trained about 100 interviewers in four research sites. Training sessions lasted 3 days, including a half day of training on the use of CAPI. Several trainees were not hired because they did not show good interviewing skills in the mock interviews.

CRITICAL APPRAISAL OF STRUCTURED METHODS OF DATA COLLECTION

Researchers make many decisions about data collection methods and procedures that can affect data quality and hence overall study quality. These decisions should be critically appraised in evaluating the study's evidence, to the extent possible. The guidelines in Box 14.3 (which is also found in the Toolkit ✖) focus on broad issues relating to the design and implementation of a data collection plan. Note, however, that data collection procedures are often not thoroughly described in research reports, owing to space constraints in journals. A full appraisal of data collection plans is seldom feasible.

A second set of critical appraisal guidelines is presented in Box 14.4 (which is also found in the Toolkit ✖). These questions focus on specific methods of collecting data in quantitative studies. Further guidance on drawing conclusions about data quality is provided in the next chapter.

BOX 14.3 Guidelines for Critically Appraising Data Collection Plans in Quantitative Studies

1. Was the collection of structured data (versus unstructured data) consistent with study aims?
2. Were appropriate methods used to collect the data (self-report, observation, etc.)? Was triangulation of different methods used appropriately? Should additional data collection methods have been used?
3. Was the right amount of data collected? Were data collected to address the varied needs of the study? Were *too much* data collected, resulting in high participant burden; if so, how might this have affected data quality?
4. Did the researcher select good instruments, in terms of congruence with underlying constructs, data quality, reputation, efficiency, and so on? Were new instruments developed without a justifiable rationale?
5. Were data collection instruments adequately pretested?
6. Did the report provide sufficient information about data collection procedures?
7. Who collected the data? Were data collectors judiciously chosen, with traits that were likely to enhance data quality?
8. Was the training of data collectors described? Was the training adequate? Were steps taken to improve data collectors' ability to produce high-quality data, or to monitor their performance?
9. Where and under what circumstances were data gathered? Was the setting for data collection appropriate?
10. Were other people present during data collection? Could the presence of others have resulted in biases?
11. Were data collectors blinded to study hypotheses or to participants' group status?

BOX 14.4 Guidelines for Critically Appraising Structured Data Collection Methods

1. If self-report data were collected, did the researcher make good decisions about the specific method used to solicit self-report information (e.g., a mix of open- and closed-ended questions, use of composite scales, and so on)?
2. Was the instrument package adequately described in terms of conceptual appropriateness, reading level of the questions, length of time to complete it, and so on?
3. Was the mode of obtaining the self-report data appropriate (e.g., in-person interviews, mailed questionnaires, web-based questionnaires)?
4. Were self-report data gathered in a manner that promoted high-quality and unbiased responses (e.g., in terms of privacy, efforts to put respondents at ease, etc.)?
5. If observational methods were used, did the report adequately describe the specific constructs that were observed?
6. Was a category system or rating system used to record observations? Was the category system exhaustive? How much inference was required of the observers? Were decisions about exhaustiveness and degree of observer inference appropriate?
7. What methods were used to sample observational units? Was the sampling approach a good one—that is, did it likely yield a representative sample of behavior?
8. To what degree were observer biases controlled or minimized?
9. Were biomarkers used in the study, and was this appropriate? Did the researcher appear to have the skills necessary for proper interpretation of biomarkers?
10. Were performance measures used in the study, and was this appropriate?
11. Were data extracted from records? If so, were appropriate steps taken to ensure high-quality data?

RESEARCH EXAMPLE

In the study described next, a variety of data collection approaches were used to measure study variables.

Study: Predicting children's response to distraction from pain (Dr. Ann McCarthy and Dr. Charmaine Kleiber, Principal Investigators, NINR grant 1-R01-NR005269)

Statement of purpose: Drs. McCarthy and Kleiber developed and tested an intervention to train parents as coaches to distract their children during insertion of an intravenous (IV) catheter. The overall study purpose was to test the effectiveness of the intervention in reducing children's pain and distress, to identify factors that predicted which children benefitted from the distraction, and to identify characteristics of parents who were successful in distracting their children.

Design: In this multisite clinical trial, 542 parents were randomly assigned to an intervention group or a usual-care control group. Their children, aged 4 to 10 years, were scheduled to undergo an IV insertion for a diagnostic medical procedure. Parents in the intervention group received 15 minutes of training regarding effective methods of distraction before the child's IV insertion.

Data collection plan: The researchers collected a wealth of data both prior to and following the intervention and IV procedure, using self-reports, observations, and biomarkers. The data collection plan included using formal instruments to measure sample characteristics, to assess key child outcomes, to measure factors they hypothesized would predict the intervention's effectiveness, to capture characteristics of the IV procedure, and to evaluate treatment fidelity. The researchers undertook a thorough literature review to identify factors influencing children's responses to a painful procedure and developed a conceptual model that guided their data collection efforts. Before proceeding with the full-scale study, the instruments were pretested (Kleiber & McCarthy, 2006). The pretest was used to assess whether the instruments were understandable and to evaluate the quality of data they would yield. Because of the extensiveness of their data collection plan, we describe only a few specific measures here.

Self-report instruments: Both parents and children provided self-report data. For example, the Oucher scale was used as a self-report measure of children's pain. Children also reported their level of anxiety on a visual analog scale. Another self-report instrument (Child Behavioral Style Scale) measured children's coping style, using a vignette-type approach with four stressful scenarios. Parents completed self-administered questionnaires that incorporated scales to measure parenting style (Parenting Dimensions Inventory) and anxiety (State-Trait Anxiety Inventory). They also completed instruments that describe children's temperament (Dimensions of Temperament Survey).

Observational instruments: A research assistant video recorded the parent and the child during their time in the treatment room. Video files were entered into a computerized video editing program and divided into 10-second intervals for analysis. The authors coded the parents' behavior in terms of the quality and frequency of distraction coaching, using an observational instrument that the researchers carefully developed, the Distraction Coaching Index (Kleiber et al., 2007). The videos were also used to code the children's level of distress, using the Observation Scale of Behavioral Distress.

Biomarkers: Children's stress was measured using salivary cortisol levels. Children chewed a piece of sugarless gum as a salivary stimulant. After discarding the gum, the children spat saliva into a collection tube. Each child provided four salivary cortisol samples: before IV insertion, 20 minutes after IV insertion, and two home samples to assess baseline cortisol levels. Care was taken to ensure the integrity of the samples and to control conditions under which they were obtained (McCarthy et al., 2009).

Key findings: Reports on the results of the intervention indicated that parents in the intervention group had significantly higher scores than those in the control group for distraction coaching frequency and quality (Kleiber et al., 2007); children with the highest level of distraction coaching had the lowest levels of distress (McCarthy et al., 2010). In another analysis, McCarthy and colleagues (2011) compared behavioral distress and baseline salivary cortisol levels for children with and without attention-deficit/hyperactivity disorder (ADHD). Hanrahan et al. (2012) developed a predictive model to predict children's risk of distress. McCarthy et al. (2014) explored the effects of three different doses of the distraction intervention for children at high and medium risks for distress. Ersig and colleagues (2017) examined genomic variation associated with children's pain, anxiety, and distress using data from this study.

SUMMARY POINTS

- Quantitative researchers develop a **data collection plan** before they begin to collect their data. For structured data, researchers use formal data collection **instruments** that place constraints on those collecting data and those providing them.

- An early step in developing a data collection plan is the identification and prioritization of data needs. Then, measures of the variables must be located. The selection of existing instruments should be based on such factors as conceptual suitability, data quality, population appropriateness, cost, and reputation.

- Even when existing instruments are used, the instruments should be **pretested** to assess length, clarity, and overall adequacy.

- Structured self-report instruments, which are sometimes referred to as **patient-reported outcomes** or PROs, can include open- and closed-ended questions. **Open-ended questions** permit respondents to reply in narrative fashion, whereas **closed-ended** (*fixed-alternative*) **questions** offer **response options** from which respondents must choose.

- Types of closed-ended questions include (1) **dichotomous questions**, which require a choice between two options (e.g., yes/no), (2) **multiple-choice questions**, which offer a range of alternatives, (3) **rank-order questions**, in which respondents are asked to rank concepts on a continuum, (4) **forced-choice questions**, which require respondents to choose between two competing options, (5) **rating questions**, which ask respondents to make graded ratings along a bipolar dimension, (6) **checklists** that include several questions with the same response format, and (7) **visual analog scales (VASs)**, which are continua used to measure subjective experiences such as fatigue. **Event**

history calendars and *diaries* are used to capture data about the occurrence of events.

- Composite psychosocial **scales** are multiquestion self-report tools for measuring the degree to which individuals possess or are characterized by target attributes. Traditional **Likert scales (summated rating scales)** comprise a series of statements (**items**) about a phenomenon (e.g., abortions). Respondents rate their reaction to the item along a *bipolar continuum* (e.g., strongly agree/disagree). A total score is computed by summing item scores, each of which is scored for the intensity and direction of favorability expressed.

- Other self-report methods include **semantic differentials**, which consist of a set of bipolar rating scales on which respondents indicate reactions toward a phenomenon; **Q sorts**, in which people sort a set of card statements into piles according to specified criteria; **vignettes,** which are descriptions of an event or situation to which respondents are asked to react; and **ecological momentary assessments**, which involve repeated assessments of people's current behaviors or experiences in real time.

- Structured self-report instruments are administered either orally (via **interview schedules**) or in written form (**questionnaires**). Questionnaires are less costly and time-consuming than interviews and offer the possibility of anonymity. Interviews have higher response rates, are suitable for a wider variety of people, and tend to yield richer data than questionnaires.

- Data quality in interviews depends on interviewers' interpersonal skills. Interviewers must put respondents at ease and build rapport and need to **probe** skillfully for additional information when respondents give incomplete responses.

- Group administration is the most economical way to distribute questionnaires. Another approach is to mail them. Self-administered questionnaires (SAQs) can be distributed via the Internet, most often as a **web-based survey** that is accessed through a hypertext link. Questionnaires, especially those distributed over the Internet, tend to have low **response rates**, which can result in bias. Techniques such as **follow-up reminders** and good **cover letters** increase response rates to questionnaires.

- Structured self-reports are vulnerable to the risk of biases. **Response set biases** reflect the tendency of some people to respond to questions in characteristic ways, independently of content. Common response sets include **social desirability**, **extreme response**, and **acquiescence** (**yea-saying**).
- Methods of **structured observation** impose limits on what observers watch for and record, to enhance the accuracy and consistency of observations and to obtain an adequate representation of phenomena of interest.
- **Checklists** are used in observations to record the occurrence, frequency, duration, or intensity of designated behaviors, events, or actions. Checklists are based on **category systems** for encoding observed phenomena into discrete categories. When using **rating scales**, observers rate phenomena along a dimension that is typically bipolar (e.g., passive/aggressive).
- In collecting observational data, observers use different sampling approaches. **Time sampling** involves specifications of the duration and frequency of observational periods and inter-session intervals. **Event sampling** selects integral behaviors or events of a special type for observation.
- Observational methods are an excellent way to operationalize some constructs but are subject to various biases. The greater the degree of observer inference, the more likely that distortions will occur.
- **Biomarkers** comprise **in vivo measurements** (those performed within or on living organisms, such as blood pressure measurement) and **in vitro measurements** (those performed outside the organism's body, such as blood tests).
- Biomarkers are objective, accurate, and precise, but care must be taken in using such measures with regard to practical, technical, and ethical considerations.
- Physical **performance tests** are sometimes used to gather outcome data relating to patients' physical functioning.
- Data for research or quality improvement projects are increasingly drawn from medical records, especially electronic health records

(EHRs). The extraction of records data requires the development of explicit rules and procedures.
- When researchers cannot collect the data without assistance, they should select data collection staff with care and devote resources to formally train them.

STUDY ACTIVITIES

Study activities are available to instructors on thePoint.

REFERENCES CITED IN CHAPTER 14

Biomarker Definitions Working Group. (2001). Biomarkers and surrogate endpoints: Preferred definitions and conceptual framework. *Clinical Pharmacology & Therapeutics, 69*, 89–95.

Bradburn, N., Sudman, S., & Wansink, B. (2007). *Asking questions: The definitive guide for questionnaire design* (2nd ed.). San Francisco: Jossey Bass.

Buros Institute, Carlson, J., Geisinger, K., & Jonson, J. (Eds.). (2017). *The 20th mental measurements yearbook*. Lincoln, NE: The Buros Institute.

Burrai, F., Lupi, R., Luppi, M., Micheluzzi, V., Donati, G., Lamanna, G., & Raghaven, R. (2019). Effects of listening to live singing in patients undergoing hemodialysis. *Biological Research for Nursing, 21*, 30–38.

Callegaro, M., Manfreda, K., & Vehovar, V. (2015). *Web survey methodology*. Thousand Oaks, CA: Sage.

Casal, C., Lei, A., Young, S., & Tuthill, E. (2017). A critical review of instruments measuring breastfeeding attitudes, knowledge, and social support. *Journal of Human Lactation, 33*, 21–47.

*Cella, D., Riley, W., Stone, A., Rothrock, N., Reeve, B., Yount, S., … PROMIS Cooperative Group . (2010). The Patient-Reported Outcomes Measurement Information System (PROMIS) developed and tested its first wave of adult self-reported health outcome item banks. *Journal of Clinical Epidemiology, 63*, 1179–1194.

*Coons, S., Eremenco, S., Lundy, J., O'Donohue, P., O'Gorman, H., & Malizia, W. (2015). Capturing patient-reported outcome (PRO) data electronically: The past, present, and promise of ePRO measurement in clinical trials. *The Patient, 8*, 301–309.

Cope, D. (2014). Using electronic surveys in nursing research. *Oncology Nursing Forum, 41*, 681–682.

Corwin, E., & Ferranti, E. (2016). Integration of biomarkers to advance precision nursing interventions for family research across the lifespan. *Nursing Outlook, 64*, 292–298.

Cui, N., Deatrick, J., & Liu, J. (2018). Maternal and paternal physical abuse: Unique and joint associations with child behavioral problems. *Child Abuse & Neglect, 76*, 524–532.

*Dey, A., Shakya, H., Chandurkar, D., Kuman, S., Das, A., Anthony, J., … Raj, A. (2017). Discordance in self-report and observation data on mistreatment of women by providers during childbirth in Uttar Pradesh, India. *Reproductive Health, 14*, 149.

Dillman, D., Smyth, J., & Christian, L. M. (2014). *Internet, phone, mail, and mixed-mode surveys: The tailored design method* (4th ed.). New York: John Wiley & Sons.

Emelonye, A., Pitkaaho, T., Aregbesola, A., & Vehvilainen-Julkunen, K. (2017). Barriers to spousal contribution to childbirth pain relief in Nigeria. *International Nursing Review, 64*, 568–575.

Ersig, A., Schutte, D., Standley, J., Leslie, J., Zimmerman, B., Kleiber, C., … McCarthy, A. (2017). Relationship of genetic variants with procedural pain, anxiety, and distress in children. *Biological Research for Nursing, 19*, 339–349.

Etingen, B., Miskevics, S., & LaVela, S. (2018). The relationship between pain interference and psychosocial well-being among veterans with spinal cord injuries/disorders. *Journal of Neuroscience Nursing, 50*, 48–55.

*Fleming, T., & Powers, J. (2012). Biomarkers and surrogate endpoints in clinical trials. *Statistics in Medicine, 31*, 2973–2984.

Fowler, F. J. (2014). *Survey research methods* (5th ed.). Thousand Oaks, CA: Sage.

*Frain, J., & Chen, L. (2018). Examining the effectiveness of a cognitive intervention to improve cognitive function in a population of older adults living with HIV. *Therapeutic Advances in Infectious Disease, 5*, 19–28.

*Gregory, K., & Radovinsky, L. (2012). Research strategies that result in optimal data collection from the patient medical record. *Applied Nursing Research, 25*, 108–116.

*Haidet, K. K., Tate, J., Divirgilio-Thomas, D., Kolanowski, A., & Happ, M. (2009). Methods to improve reliability of video-recorded behavioral data. *Research in Nursing & Health, 32*, 465–474.

Hanish, A., & Han, J. (2018). Delayed onset of sleep in adolescents with PAX6 haploinsufficiency. *Biological Research for Nursing, 20*, 237–243.

*Hanrahan, K., McCarthy, A. M., Kleiber, C., Ataman, K., Street, W., Zimmerman, M., & Ersig, A. (2012). Building a computer program to support children, parents, and distraction during healthcare interventions. *Computers, Informatics, Nursing, 30*, 554–561.

Kleiber, C., & McCarthy, A. M. (2006). Evaluating instruments for a study on children's responses to a painful procedure when parents are distraction coaches. *Journal of Pediatric Nursing, 21*, 99–107.

Kleiber, C., McCarthy, A. M., Hanrahan, K., Myers, L., & Weathers, N. (2007). Development of the Distraction Coaching Index. *Children's Health Care, 36*, 219–235.

Martyn, K., & Belli, R. (2002). Retrospective data collection using event history calendars. *Nursing Research, 51*, 270–274.

*McCarthy, A. M., Hanrahan, K., Kleiber, C., Zimmerman, M. B., Lutgendorf, S., & Tsalikian, E. (2009). Normative salivary cortisol values and responsivity in children. *Applied Nursing Research, 22*, 54–62.

*McCarthy, A. M., Hanrahan, K., Scott, L., Zemblidge, N., Kleiber, C., & Zimmerman, M. (2011). Salivary cortisol responsivity to an intravenous catheter insertion in children with attention-deficit/hyperactivity disorder. *Journal of Pediatric Psychology, 36*, 902–910.

*McCarthy, A. M., Kleiber, C., Hanrahan, K., Zimmerman, M., Westhus, N., & Allen, S. (2010). Impact of parent-provided distraction on child responses to an IV insertion. *Children's Health Care, 39*, 125–141.

McCarthy, A. M., Kleiber, C., Hanrahan, K., Zimmerman, M., Westhus, N., & Allen, S. (2014). Matching doses of distraction with child risk for distress during a medical procedure. *Nursing Research, 63*, 397–407.

McPeake, J., Bateson, M., O'Neill, A. (2014). Electronic surveys: How to maximise success. *Nurse Researcher, 21*, 24–26.

Mitchell, A. J., Hall, R., Golianu, B., Yates, C., Williams, D., Chang, S., & Janwaljeet, J. (2016). Does noninvasive electrical stimulation of acupuncture points reduce heelstick pain in neonates? *Acta Paediatrica, 105*, 1434–1439.

*Nyamathi, A., Reback, C., Salem, B., Zhang, S., Shoptaw, S., Branson, C., & Leake, B. (2015). Correlates of self-reported incarceration among homeless gay and bisexual stimulant-using young adults. *Western Journal of Nursing Research, 37*, 799–811.

Pecanac, K., Doherty-King, B., Yoon, J., Brown, R., & Schiefelbein, T. (2015). Using timed event sequential data in nursing research. *Nursing Research, 64*, 67–71.

Pisu, M., Azuero, A., Halilova, K., Williams, C., Kenzik, K., Kvale, E., … Rocque, G. (2018). Most impactful factors on the health-related quality of life of a geriatric population with cancer. *Cancer, 124*, 596–605.

Polit, D. F., London, A. S., & Martinez, J. M. (2007). *The health of poor urban women*. New York: MDRC.

Pölkki, T., Korhonen, A., & Laukkala, H. (2018). Parents' use of nonpharmacologic methods to manage procedural pain in infants. *Journal of Obstetric, Gynecologic, & Neonatal Nursing, 47*, 43–51.

Rhéaume, A., & Mullen, J. (2018). The impact of long work hours and shift work on cognitive errors in nurses. *Journal of Nursing Management, 26*, 26–32.

**Rieder, J., Goshin, L., Sissoko, D., Kleshchova, O., & Weierich, M. (2019). Salivary biomarkers of parenting stress in mothers under community criminal justice supervision. *Nursing Research, 68*, 48–56.

Romisher, R., Hill, D., & Cong, X. (2018). Neonatal abstinence syndrome: Exploring nurses' attitudes, knowledge, and practice. *Advances in Neonatal Care, 18*, E3–E11.

Rosman, L., Salmoirago-Blotcher, E., Cahill, J., & Sears, A. (2019). Psychosocial adjustment and quality of life in patients with peripartum cardiomyopathy. *Journal of Cardiovascular Nursing, 34*, 20–28.

Samuels, J., McGrath, R., Fetzer, S., Mittal, P., & Bourgoine, D. (2015). Using the electronic health record in nursing research: Challenges and opportunities. *Western Journal of Nursing Research, 37*, 1284–1294.

Saxton, R., & Cahill, R. (2017). Impact of no-interruption intervention on safety and efficiency. *Journal of Nursing Care Quality, 32*, 281–284.

*Schick-Makaroff, K., & Molzahn, A. (2015). Strategies to use tablet computers for collection of electronic patient-reported outcomes. *Health and Quality of Life Outcomes, 13*, 2.

Seaman, J., Evans, A., Sciulli, A., Barnato, A., Sereika, S., & Happ, M. (2017). Abstracting ICU nursing care quality from the electronic health record. *Western Journal of Nursing Research, 39*, 1271–1288.

*Shabani, F., Nayeri, N., Karimi, R., Zarei, K., & Chehrazi, M. (2016). Effects of music therapy on pain responses induced by blood sampling in premature infants. *Iranian Journal of Nursing and Midwifery Research, 21*, 391–396.

Stevens, B., Joshnston, C., Petryshen, P., & Taddio, A. (1996). Premature Infant Pain Profile: Development and initial validation. *Clinical Journal of Pain, 12*, 13–22.

*Teipel, S., Heine, C., Hein, A., Kruger, F., Kutschke, A., Kernebeck, S., … Kirste, T. (2017). Multidimensional assessment of challenging behaviors in advanced stages of dementia in nursing homes—The inside DEM framework. *Alzheimer's & Dementia, 8*, 36–44.

*Thompson, A., Pickler, R., & Reyna, B. (2005). Clinical coordination of research. *Applied Nursing Research, 18*, 102–105.

Tourangeau, R., Conrad, F., & Couper, M. (2013). *The science of web surveys.* New York: Oxford University Press.

Udtha, M., Nomie, K., Yu, E., & Sanner, J. (2015). Novel and emerging strategies for longitudinal data collection. *Journal of Nursing Scholarship, 47*, 152–160.

*Vanhoutte, B., & Nazroo, J. (2016). Life-history data. *Public Health Research & Practice, 26*, e2631630.

*Weintraub, W., Lüscher, T., & Pocock, T. (2015). The perils of surrogate endpoints. *European Heart Journal, 36*, 2212–2218.

*Williamson, P., Altman, D., Bagley, H., Barnes, K., Blazeby, J., Brookes, S., … Young, B. (2017). The COMET Handbook: Version 1.0. *Trials, 18*(Suppl. 3), 280.

*Worster, A., & Haines, T. (2004). Advanced statistics: Understanding medical record review (MRR) studies. *Academic Emergency Medicine, 11*, 187–192.

Xueyu, L., Hao, Y., Shunlin, X., Rongbin, L., & Yuan, G. (2017). Effects of low-intensity exercise in older adults with chronic heart failure during the transitional period from hospital to home in China: A randomized controlled trial. *Research in Gerontological Nursing, 10*, 121–128.

Yoder, P., Lloyd, B., & Symons, F. (2018). *Observational measurement of behavior* (2nd ed.). Baltimore: Paul H. Brooks Publishing Co.

*A link to this open-access article is provided in the Toolkit for Chapter 14 in the **Resource Manual**. ✪

**This journal article is available on the Point *for this chapter.*

15 | Measurement and Data Quality

In quantitative studies, an ideal data collection procedure is one that measures a construct accurately, soundly, and with precision. Biomarkers are better at attaining these goals than self-report or observational methods, but no method is flawless. In this chapter, we discuss criteria for evaluating the quality of data obtained through formal measurements. A more detailed presentation of statistical issues in measurement is provided in Polit and Yang (2016). We begin by discussing principles of measurement.

MEASUREMENT

Quantitative researchers obtain data through the measurement of constructs. **Measurement** involves assigning numbers to represent the amount of an attribute present in a person or object. Attributes are not constant: They vary from day to day or from one person to another. Variability is capable of a numeric expression signifying *how much* of an attribute is present. The purpose of assigning numbers is to distinguish people with different amounts of the attribute.

Rules and Measurement

Measurement involves assigning numbers according to rules. *Rules* promote consistency and interpretability. The rules for measuring temperature, weight, and other physical attributes are familiar to us. Rules for measuring constructs such as nausea or quality of life, however, must be invented. Whether the data are collected by observation, self-report, or some other method, researchers must specify criteria for assigning numeric values to the characteristic of interest. Researchers create a **measure** of a construct when they invent rules to quantify it. Measures yield **scores**—numeric values that communicate *how much* of an attribute is present or whether it is present at all.

Rules for measuring constructs should be evaluated to see if they are *good* rules. The rules must yield quantitative information that accurately corresponds to different amounts of the targeted trait. New measurement rules reflect hypotheses about how attributes vary. The adequacy of the hypotheses—the worth of the measures—needs to be assessed empirically.

Advantages of Measurement

What exactly does measurement accomplish? Consider how disadvantaged clinicians would be without measurements. For example, what if there were no measures of body temperature or blood pressure? A major strength of measurement is that it removes subjectivity. Because measurement is based on explicit rules, resulting information tends to be objective—it can be independently verified. Two people measuring a person's weight using the same scale would likely get identical results. Most measures incorporate mechanisms for minimizing subjectivity.

Measurement also makes it possible to obtain reasonably precise information. Instead of describing Alex as "rather tall," we can depict him as being 6 feet 3 inches tall.

Finally, measurement is a language of communication. Numbers are less vague than words. If a researcher reported that the average temperature of a sample of patients was "high," different readers might interpret the sample's physiologic state differently. However, if the researcher reported an average temperature of 99.8°F, there would be no ambiguity.

Theories of Measurement

Psychometrics is a field of inquiry concerned with the theory and methods of psychological measurement. Health measurement has been strongly influenced by psychometrics, although differences in aims and conceptualizations are emerging. When new measures are developed and tested, researchers often say that they are undertaking a *psychometric assessment.*

Within psychometrics (and health measurement), two theories of measurement have been influential. **Classical test theory (CTT)** is a theory of measurement that has been dominant until fairly recently. CTT has been used as a basis for developing multi-item measures of health constructs and is also appropriate for conceptualizing all types of measurements (e.g., biomarkers). An alternative measurement theory (**item response theory or IRT**) is gaining in popularity, as discussed in Chapter 16. Unlike CTT, IRT is an appropriate measurement framework only for multi-item scales and tests.

Errors of Measurement

Procedures for obtaining measurements, as well as the objects being measured, are susceptible to influences that can alter the resulting data. Some biasing influences can be controlled or minimized, but such efforts are rarely completely successful.

Instruments that are not perfectly accurate yield measurements containing some error. Within classical test theory, an **observed** (or **obtained**) **score** can be conceptualized as having two parts—an error component and a true component. This can be written as follows:

$$\text{Obtained score} = \text{True score} \pm \text{Error}$$

or

$$X_O = X_T \pm X_E$$

The first term in the equation is an observed score—for example, a score on an anxiety scale. X_T is the value that would be obtained with an infallible measure. The **true score** is hypothetical—it can never be known because measures are *not* infallible. The final term is the **error of measurement**. The difference between true and obtained scores results from factors that distort the measurement.

When researchers measure an attribute, they are also "measuring" attributes that are not of interest. The true score component is what they wish to isolate; the error component is a composite of other factors that are also being measured, contrary to their wishes. We illustrate with an exaggerated example. Suppose a researcher measured the weight of 10 people on a spring scale. As participants step on the scale, the researcher places a hand on their shoulders and applies pressure. The resulting measures (the X_Os) will be biased upward because scores reflect both actual weight (X_T) and pressure (X_E). Errors of measurement are problematic because their value is unknown and because they often are variable. In this example, the amount of pressure applied likely would vary from one person to the next. In other words, the proportion of true score component in an obtained score varies from one person to the next.

Many factors contribute to errors of measurement. Some errors are random while others are systematic, reflecting *bias*. Common sources of measurement error include the following:

1. *Transient personal factors.* A person's score can be influenced by such personal states as fatigue or mood. In some cases, such factors directly affect the measurement, as when anxiety affects pulse rate measurement. In other cases, personal factors alter scores by influencing people's motivation to cooperate, act naturally, or do their best.

2. *Situational contaminants.* Scores can be affected by the conditions under which they are produced. A participant's awareness of an observer's presence (reactivity) is one source of bias. Environmental factors, such as temperature, lighting, and time of day, are potential sources of measurement error.

3. *Response set biases.* Relatively enduring characteristics of people can interfere with accurate measurements. Response sets such as social desirability or acquiescence are potential biases in self-report measures (Chapter 14).

4. *Administration variations.* Alterations in the methods of collecting data from one person to the next can result in score variations unrelated to variations in the target attribute. For example, if some physiologic measures are taken before a feeding and others are taken after a feeding, then measurement errors can potentially occur.

5. *Instrument clarity.* If the directions on an instrument are poorly understood, then scores may be affected. For example, questions in a self-report instrument may be interpreted differently by different respondents, leading to a distorted measurement of the variable.

6. *Item sampling.* Errors can be introduced as a result of the sampling of items used in the measure. For example, a nursing student's score on a 100-item test of critical care nursing knowledge will be influenced by *which* 100 questions are included. A person might get 94 questions correct on one test but 92 right on another similar test.

TIP The Toolkit section of Chapter 15 of the *Resource Manual* includes suggestions for enhancing data quality and minimizing measurement error in quantitative studies.

Major Types of Measures

Measurements can vary in a number of ways. For example, measurements can vary in terms of information source (i.e., self-reports, observation), complexity (e.g., a visual analog scale or a multidimensional scale with dozens of items), and type of scores they yield (e.g., continuous scores, categorical scores). Some measures are *generic*—that is, broadly applicable across different clinical or nonclinical populations; other measures are *specific*—that is, designed for use with specific groups of people. For example, there are self-efficacy scales that are generic, but there are many disease-specific self-efficacy scales (e.g., for diabetes or asthma).

Static and Adaptive Measures

Multi-item measures can be either static or adaptive. A **static measure** is administered in a comparable manner for everyone being measured. For a static composite scale, people complete an entire set of items and then are scored based on responses to all items. Most health-related measures are static. As an example, a widely used generic measure of depression is called the Center for Epidemiologic Studies Depression Scale, the CES-D (Radloff, 1977). Total scores on the full CES-D rely on responses to the same 20 questions for everyone. Static scales are used to illustrate many key measurement concepts in this book.

An **adaptive measure**, by contrast, involves using responses to early questions to guide the selection of subsequent questions. Dynamic adaptive measures are becoming popular as a way to obtain precise information about an attribute with minimum respondent burden. Adaptive testing has its origin in measurement advances from item response theory. *Item banks* with hundreds of items have been created for broad health topics, such as physical function, pain, and sleep disturbance. The most important example of item banking is PROMIS® (Patient-Reported Outcomes Measurement Information System), developed with support from the U.S. National Institutes of Health (Cella et al., 2007). An approach called **computerized adaptive testing (CAT)** uses these item banks to create measurements that are tailored to individuals. With such tailoring, the set of items used to measure a construct can be different for each person. Despite item differences, cross-person comparisons can be made because the testing places people along a dimension of interest.

Reflective Scales and Formative Indexes

An important distinction is whether a multi-item measure is formative or reflective, which concerns the nature of the relationship between a construct and the measure of the construct. Constructs are not directly observable—they must be inferred by the effects they have on observables, such as responses to items on a patient-reported outcome (PRO) or behaviors witnessed and recorded on an observational scale. Most health scales are **reflective scales**: the items are viewed as *reflections* of the construct. For example, on the CES-D, it is presumed that a person's underlying level of depression *causes* her or him to respond in a certain way to the items about sleep disturbance, sadness, and on. The items on a reflective scale share a common cause—in this example, level of depression. Items on reflective scales are expected to be interrelated, because they all reflect (are caused by) the construct.

Not all multi-item instruments, however, are reflective. A multi-item measure can be conceptualized as having items that "cause" or define the attribute (rather than being the effect of the attribute). Such measures are called **formative measures**. Several writers advocate using the term *scale* for multi-item reflective measures, and the term **index** for multi-item formative measures (DeVellis, 2017; Streiner, 2003). A formative index involves constructs that are *formed* by its components, rather than causing them.

A good illustration of a formative index is the Holmes–Rahe Social Readjustment Scale, which is a measure of stress. Psychiatrists Holmes and Rahe studied whether stressful life events might cause illness and devised an index that asked patients to indicate which of 43 life events they had experienced in the previous year (Holmes & Rahe, 1967). Examples of life event items include death of a spouse, pregnancy, and change in residence. The life events are assigned different weights or "life change units" (e.g., 100 for death of a spouse, 20 for a change in residence), and the units are then added together. The sum of life change units defines the construct of stressful life events. The items are not the "effect" of the construct—for example, having high stress does not "cause" the death of a spouse or a residential move.

Because the items on an index are not *caused* by an underlying construct, they are not necessarily intercorrelated. In fact, items with modest correlations that capture different aspects of an attribute are desired in a formative index. Many screening tools are formative and are comprised of components that independently predict an outcome.

The development of reflective scales and formative indexes is necessarily different. For example, because the items on a formative index define the attribute, the specific items matter very much. If the item "I had crying spells" on the CES-D scale was removed, for example, the other 19 items could carry most of the burden of measuring depression. But if the item "Death of a spouse" was removed from the Holmes–Rahe index, the score would misrepresent the stress levels of people who had lost a spouse. Another consequence of having noncorrelated items on a formative index is that some of the standard assessment methods associated with CTT are not appropriate, as we explain later in this chapter.

TIP Formative indexes are seldom created using standard psychometric approaches. Formative indexes are sometimes developed within the field of **clinimetrics**, which is devoted to the development of measures of clinical phenomena. Polit and Yang (2016) have written a chapter on clinimetrics in their measurement book.

MEASUREMENT PROPERTIES: AN OVERVIEW

In making decisions about measuring constructs, careful researchers select instruments that are known to be psychometrically sound—that is, ones that have good **measurement properties.** Psychometricians have traditionally focused on two measurement properties—reliability and validity. Measurement experts in health disciplines, however, have taken a broader view.

A Measurement Taxonomy

A working group based in the Netherlands used a Delphi-type approach with a panel of health measurement experts to identify key measurement properties and to develop a taxonomy and definitions of those properties. The result was the creation of **COSMIN**, the **Co**nsensus-based **S**tandards for the selection of health **M**easurement **In**struments (Mokkink et al., 2010b, 2010a; Terwee et al., 2012) (Information about COSMIN can be accessed at http://www.cosmin.nl). Polit and Yang (2016), building on the groundbreaking COSMIN work, made small modifications to the taxonomy to more clearly incorporate a time perspective. A graphic depiction of the Polit–Yang measurement taxonomy is shown in Figure 15.1.

In this taxonomy, there are four measurement property domains. Two are cross-sectional, addressing the quality of measurements at one point in time. These cross-sectional domains are *reliability* and *validity*, the properties used for decades by psychometricians. Two other domains in the taxonomy concern longitudinal measurement—the quality of measurements capturing changes over time. These two domains are called the *reliability of change scores* and *responsiveness*. New measures that are likely to be used to measure a construct at a single point *and* to measure how scores on the construct change over time ideally would be evaluated for all four measurement properties. The taxonomy also incorporates another concept—interpretability—that has relevance for both point-in-time scores and change scores.

FIGURE 15.1 A taxonomy of measurement properties.

For each measurement property, researchers can estimate **measurement parameters** that quantify the degree to which scores on a measure have desirable attributes. These estimates are the means by which conclusions can be drawn about an instrument's quality, for a particular population and application. ⊗

TIP The Toolkit for Chapter 15 in the *Resource Manual* includes a summary table that specifies measurement parameters that are relevant under different scenarios.

The four measurement property domains and the two interpretability aspects correspond to six key measurement questions, which we illustrate with an example. Suppose we were testing the effects of a nurse-led support program for family caregivers of patients with dementia, and one of our outcome variables was depression. Suppose that we found that a caregiver in the intervention group had a score of 20 on the CES-D at baseline (high level of depression) and a score of 15 (less depression) at a 6-month follow-up. Six questions we could ask, corresponding to the elements in the measurement taxonomy, are as follows:

1. *Reliability:* Is the score of 20 at baseline the right score for this person—is it a dependable score value?
2. *Validity:* Is the scale truly measuring the construct depression, or is it measuring something else?
3. *Interpretation of a score:* What does a score of 20 *mean?* Is it high or low?
4. *Reliability of change:* Is the change from 20 to 15 a *real* change, or does it merely reflect random fluctuations in measurement?
5. *Responsiveness:* Does the change from 20 to 15 correspond to a commensurate improvement in degree of depression?
6. *Interpretation of a change score:* What does a 5-point improvement *mean?* Is the improvement large enough to be considered clinically significant?

This chapter describes the four domains in the measurement taxonomy. Issues relating to interpretation are discussed in Chapters 16 and 21.

TIP Nurse researchers have mainly followed standard psychometric approaches to assessing measurement properties, which means that most of their efforts have focused on reliability and validity. Longitudinal measurement properties have not been given much scrutiny, but changes are likely in light of the influential COSMIN work.

Measurement and Statistics

Assessments of measurement properties require some statistical knowledge. In this chapter, we mainly describe principles rather than statistical details. However, because several measurement properties rely on the calculation of a statistical index called a correlation coefficient, we must briefly explain this index before proceeding.

We have pointed out that researchers seek to detect and explain relationships among phenomena. For example, is there a relationship between patients' gastric acidity levels and their degree of stress? The **correlation coefficient** is a tool for quantitatively describing the magnitude and direction of a relationship between two variables. The most widely used correlation coefficient is called **Pearson's r**.

Two variables that are obviously related are people's height and weight. Tall people tend to be heavier than short people. We would say that there was a **perfect relationship** if the tallest person in a population were the heaviest, the second tallest person were the second heaviest, and so forth. Correlation coefficients summarize how perfect a relationship is. The possible values for a correlation coefficient range from −1.00 through .00 to +1.00. If height and weight were perfectly correlated, the correlation coefficient expressing this relationship would be +1.00. Because the relationship exists but is not perfect, the correlation coefficient is in the vicinity of +.50 or +.60 (which would typically be written as .50 and .60). The relationship between height and weight is a **positive relationship** because *increases* in height tend to be associated with *increases* in weight.

When two variables are totally unrelated, the correlation coefficient equals zero. One might expect that women's height is unrelated to their intelligence. Tall women are as likely to perform well on IQ tests as short women. The correlation coefficient summarizing such a relationship would presumably be in the vicinity of .00.

Correlation coefficients running from .00 to −1.00 express **inverse** or **negative relationships**. When two variables are inversely related, increases in one variable are associated with *decreases* in the second variable. Suppose that there is an inverse relationship between people's age and the amount of sleep they get. This means that, on average, the older the person, the fewer the hours of sleep. If the relationship were perfect (e.g., if the oldest person in a population slept the fewest hours, and so on), the correlation coefficient would be −1.00. In actuality, the relationship between age and sleep is probably modest—in the vicinity of −.15 or −.20. A correlation coefficient of this magnitude describes a weak relationship: older people *tend* to sleep fewer hours and younger people *tend* to sleep more, but nevertheless some younger people sleep few hours, and some older people sleep a lot.

Correlation coefficients are important in evaluating the quality of measuring instruments.

RELIABILITY

The reliability of a quantitative measure is a major criterion for assessing its quality. **Reliability**, broadly speaking, is the extent to which scores are free from measurement error. However, from an operational perspective, an extended definition is more useful. Adapting slightly from COSMIN, we offer this definition:

- Reliability is the extent to which scores for people *who have not changed* are the same for repeated measurements, under several situations: repetition on different occasions, by different persons, on different versions of a measure, or in the form of different items on a multi-item instrument (internal consistency).

In other words, reliability concerns consistency—the *absence* of variation—in measuring a stable attribute for an individual. All types of

reliability assessment involve a *replication* to evaluate the extent to which scores for a stable trait are the same. Assessments to evaluate consistency require a heterogeneous sample of people, because the role of a reliable measure is to allow people to be distinguished from one another.

In our taxonomy shown in Figure 15.1, as well as in the COSMIN taxonomy, the cross-sectional reliability domain encompasses three components: reliability, internal consistency, and measurement error. We briefly discuss each component and describe the measurement parameters corresponding to each component.

Reliability

The first component within the broad reliability domain is simply called reliability. It covers four different approaches to reliability assessment, including:

- **test–retest reliability:** administration of the same measure to the same people on two occasions (repetition over occasions),
- **interrater reliability:** measurements by two or more raters using the same instrument (repetition over persons),
- **intrarater reliability:** measurements by the same rater on two or more occasions (repetition over occasions), and
- **parallel test reliability:** measurements of the same attribute using alternate versions of the same instrument, with the same people (repetition over versions).

Assessments of reliability involve the calculation of a statistic broadly called a **reliability coefficient**, sometimes symbolized as R. These coefficients, calculated from sample data, are estimates of how reliable the scores are. Different types of coefficients are used in different situations, but they typically range from a low of .00 (signifying no reliability) to a high of 1.00 and are thus like correlation coefficients, but not negative in value. The higher the coefficient, the more reliable the scores. Perfect reliability—a coefficient of 1.00—is virtually impossible to obtain, but it is the goal.

Test–Retest Reliability

In **test–retest reliability**, replication takes the form of administering a measure to the same people twice. The assumption is that for traits that have not changed, any differences in people's scores on the two testings reflect measurement error. When score differences across waves are small, reliability is high. This type of reliability is sometimes called *stability* or *reproducibility*—the extent to which scores can be reproduced on repeated administrations.

To illustrate, suppose we were interested in the test–retest reliability of a 16-item self-esteem scale. Self-esteem is a fairly stable attribute that does not fluctuate much from day to day; we would expect a reliable measure of it to yield consistent scores on two occasions. To assess the instrument's reliability, we administer the scale 2 weeks apart. Fictitious data for this example are shown in Table 15.1 for a sample of 10 people (in a real assessment, the sample would be larger). In general, differences in scores on the two testings are not large. The person who scored highest at time 1 (participant 3) also scored highest at time 2, for example.

TABLE 15.1 • Fictitious Data for 2-Week Test–Retest Reliability of Self-Esteem Scale

PARTICIPANT NUMBER	TIME 1	TIME 2	
1	55	57	
2	49	46	
3	78	74	
4	37	35	
5	44	46	
6	50	56	
7	58	55	
8	62	66	
9	48	50	
10	67	63	ICC = .95

ICC = intraclass coefficient.

When a measure yields continuous scores, as in this example, the preferred reliability parameter for test–retest reliability is the **intraclass correlation coefficient** or **ICC**. It is beyond the scope of this book to explain how the ICC is computed, but in our example, the value of the ICC is .95.[1] ICCs can be computed in major statistical software packages, such as the Statistical Software for the Social Sciences or SPSS.

> **TIP** Many nurse researchers compute a Pearson's *r* as the reliability estimate in retest situations. However, measurement experts consider Pearson's correlation inappropriate for estimating reliability (e.g., DeVet et al., 2011), even though the values of the ICC and *r* are usually close. In our example of self-esteem scores, the value of the Pearson's *r* coefficient is also .95.

Test–retest reliability can be assessed with virtually all measures, including biomarkers, observational measures, performance tests, 1-item measures (e.g., visual analog scales, single demographic questions), formative indexes, and reflective scales. Nevertheless, retest reliability assessment can be problematic. One issue is that many traits *do* change over time, independently of the measure's stability. Attitudes, knowledge, skills, and so on can be modified by experiences between testings—and true change would make a measure look less reliable than it actually is. For this reason, a major issue in retest reliability assessment is finding the right interval between testings.

Another issue is that people's responses on a second administration can be influenced by their memory of initial responses. Such memory interference, called a *carryover effect*, could result in spuriously high reliability coefficients. Another difficulty is that people may actually change *as a result of* the first administration. Finally, people may not be as careful using the same instrument

---

[1] ICCs can be computed using several different formulas. As explained more fully in Polit and Yang (2016), a main distinction is between what is called ICC for agreement versus ICC for consistency. In our example in Table 15.1, the reliability estimate is .951 for $ICC_{Consistency}$ and .956 for $ICC_{Agreement}$ Researchers reporting the value of ICC should state which ICC was calculated.

a second time. If they find the process boring on the second occasion, then responses could be haphazard, resulting in a spuriously low estimate of reliability. Other complications relating to retest reliability assessments, and strategies to deal with them, have been described by Polit (2014).

The myriad problems of retest reliability assessment led some psychometricians to discourage using the test–retest approach (e.g., Nunnally & Bernstein, 1994). Healthcare researchers, however, have disagreed with this viewpoint and have emphasized retest reliability. Nurse researchers have often pursued standard psychometric methods, and so those who have developed new scales have not always estimated test–retest reliability; we hope this will change in the years ahead.

Example of Test–Retest Reliability
Thoyre and colleagues (2018) developed a parent-report instrument to measure feeding problems in their young children, the Pediatric Eating Assessment Tool (PediEAT). In their psychometric assessment of the measure with 567 parents, the researchers found that the 2-week retest reliability was .95.

TIP Many reflective scales and formative indexes contain two or more **subscales**, each of which measures distinct but related concepts (e.g., a measure of fatigue might include subscales for mental and physical fatigue). The reliability of each subscale should be assessed. If subscale scores are summed for a total score, the scale's overall reliability is also computed.

Interrater and Intrarater Reliability

When observers make scoring judgments to measure a construct, a key source of measurement error can stem from the person making the measurements. This is a familiar situation for observational instruments (e.g., scales to measure agitation in nursing home residents), and for some biophysiologic measurements (e.g., skinfold measurement) and performance tests (balance tests). In such situations, it is important to evaluate how reliably the measurements reflect attributes of the person being rated rather than attributes of the raters. Developers

of new observational measures need to know if their instruments are capable of yielding reliable scores with trained observers. And, users of such measures need to know whether they can reliably apply the measure, and how much training is needed to achieve adequate reliability.

A typical approach is to undertake an **interrater** (or *interobserver*) **reliability** assessment, which involves having two or more observers independently applying the instrument with the same people. Then, the observers' scores are compared to see if the scores are consistent across raters.

A less frequently used approach—but one that is appropriate in many clinical situations—is an **intrarater reliability** assessment in which the *same* rater makes the measurements on two or more occasions, blinded to the ratings assigned previously. Intrarater reliability is an index of self-consistency. It is analogous to retest reliability, except that the focus in retest situations is the consistency of the person *being measured*, and intrarater reliability concerns the consistency of the person *making the measurements*. Like retest reliability, intrarater reliability assessments require a carefully selected interval between testings.

Estimates of inter- or intrarater reliability can be obtained by computing an ICC if the measurements yield continuous scores. In other situations, however, observers are asked to *classify* their observations into categories. When ratings are categorical, one procedure is to calculate the **proportion of agreement**, using the following equation:

$$\frac{\text{Number of agreements}}{\text{Number of agreements} + \text{disagreements}}$$

This formula unfortunately tends to overestimate agreements because it fails to account for agreement by chance. If a behavior were coded for absence versus presence, observers would agree 50% of the time by chance alone. A widely used statistic in this situation is Cohen's **kappa**, which adjusts for chance agreement. Values of kappa usually range from .00 to 1.00. Different standards have been proposed for acceptable levels of kappa, but there is some agreement that a value of .60 is minimally acceptable, and that values of .75 or higher are very good.

Example of Interrater Reliability
Coleman and colleagues (2018) developed and evaluated a new pressure ulcer risk assessment instrument, the Pressure Ulcer Risk Primary or Secondary Evaluation Tool (PURPOSE T). Assessments using the instrument were undertaken simultaneously by ward nurses and expert nurses for evaluating 230 patients. When the instrument was used to dichotomize patients as "at risk" versus "not at risk," the proportion of agreement was .93 and the kappa value was .81.

Parallel Test Reliability

Multi-item *parallel tests* (or *alternative-form tests*) are not common in healthcare measurement, but there are a few examples. For instance, the latest version of the Mini-Mental State Examination (MMSE-2), a measure of cognitive impairment, has alternate forms (Folstein et al., 2010). Parallel tests can be created by randomly sampling two sets of items from an item pool. If the two tests are truly parallel, then they are replicates whose true scores are identical. Having measures that are parallel is useful when researchers expect to make measurements in a fairly short period of time and want to avoid carryover biases. Similar to test–retest reliability, **parallel test reliability** involves administration of the parallel tests to the same people and then estimating a reliability parameter, which would be the ICC.

Interpretation of Reliability Coefficients

Reliability coefficients are important indicators of an instrument's quality. Unreliable measures reduce statistical power and affect statistical conclusion validity. If data fail to support a hypothesis, one possibility is that the instruments were unreliable—not necessarily that the expected relationship does not exist.

For group-level comparisons, reliability coefficients in the vicinity of .70 may be adequate (especially for subscales), but coefficients of .80 or greater are desirable. By group-level comparisons, we mean when researchers compare scores of groups, such as males versus females or experimental versus control participants. The reliability coefficients for measures used for making decisions about individuals ideally should be .90 or better. For instance, if a score was used to make decisions about a patient's eligibility

for a special intervention, then the test's reliability would be of critical importance.

Reliability coefficients have a special interpretation that relates to the decomposition of observed scores into error and true score components. Suppose we administered a scale that measures hopefulness to 50 patients with cancer. The scores would vary from one person to another—some people would be more hopeful than others. Some variability in scores is true variability, reflecting real individual differences in hopefulness; some variability, however, is measurement error. Thus,

$$V_O = V_T + V_E$$

where V_O = observed total variability in scores,
V_T = true variability,
V_E = variability owing to error

A reliability coefficient is directly associated with this equation. *Reliability is the proportion of true variability to the total obtained variability,* or

$$R = \frac{V_T}{V_O}$$

If, for example, the reliability coefficient were .85, then 85% of the variability in obtained scores would represent true individual differences, and 15% would reflect extraneous fluctuations. Looked at in this way, it should be clear why instruments with reliability lower than .70 are risky to use.

Factors Affecting Reliability

Several factors under researchers' control can affect the value of reliability coefficients. With observational scales, for example, reliability can be improved with greater clarity in explaining the underlying construct during observer training.

A measure's reliability is related to the heterogeneity of the sample with which it is tested. The more homogeneous the sample (i.e., the more similar their scores), the lower the reliability coefficient will be. This is because instruments are designed to measure differences among those being measured. If the sample is homogeneous, then it is more difficult for the instrument to discriminate reliably among those who possess varying degrees of the attribute. For example, suppose that the self-esteem scores shown in Table 15.1 were changed for two individuals. If participant 3 (the high scorer) had scores of 58 and 54 (rather than 78 and 74) and if participant 4 (the low scorer) had scores of 57 and 55 (rather than 37 and 35), the ICC would be .85 rather than .95 because now the range of scores is smaller (44-67 versus 37-78).

An important thing to keep in mind in computing or interpreting reliability coefficients within the CTT framework—or in selecting an instrument for use in a study—is that *reliability is not a fixed property of an instrument*. For a given measure, reliability will vary from one population to another or from one situation to another. It is better to think of reliability as a property of a particular set of scores than as a property of a measure itself. Users of an instrument need to consider how similar their population is to the population used to estimate reliability parameters. If the populations are similar, then the reliability estimate calculated by the scale developer is probably a reasonably good index of the instrument's accuracy in the new research. But if the population is very different, new estimates of reliability should be computed.

Internal Consistency

Another component within the reliability domain of the measurement taxonomy (Figure 15.1) is **internal consistency**. Our reliability definition supports including internal consistency within the reliability domain: Reliability is the extent to which scores for patients who have not changed are the same for repeated measurements. For internal consistency, replication involves people's responses to multiple items during a single administration. Whereas reliability estimates described in the previous section assess a measure's degree of consistency across time, raters, and versions of a measure, internal consistency captures consistency across items.

Single items are often inadequate for measuring a construct—indeed, the low reliability of single items is the reason for constructing multi-item scales. In responding to an item, people are influenced not only by the underlying construct but also by idiosyncratic reactions to the words.

By sampling multiple items with various wordings, item irrelevancies are expected to cancel each other out. An instrument is said to be internally consistent to the extent that its items measure the same trait.

The most widely used statistic for evaluating internal consistency is **coefficient alpha** (or **Cronbach's alpha**). Coefficient alpha estimates the extent to which different subparts of an instrument (i.e., items) are reliably measuring the critical attribute, and greater internal consistency is obtained with a set of items that are highly intercorrelated. Coefficient alpha can be interpreted like other reliability coefficients: the normal range of values is between .00 and +1.00, and higher values reflect better internal consistency. Coefficients of .80 or higher are considered especially desirable. It is beyond the scope of this text to explain computations of coefficient alpha, but information is available in measurement textbooks (e.g., Polit & Yang, 2016). Most standard statistical software such as SPSS can be used to calculate alpha.

An important feature of internal consistency is that the value of coefficient alpha is partly a function of the scale's length. To improve internal consistency, more items tapping the same construct should be added.

Internal consistency has been the most widely reported aspect of reliability assessment among nurse researchers. Its popularity reflects the fact that it is economical (it requires only one administration) and is a means of assessing an important source of measurement error in psychosocial instruments, the sampling of items.

Internal consistency is a relevant measurement property only for multi-item reflective scales, however. It is *not* relevant for formative indexes, which are comprised of items that are not necessarily intercorrelated. For formative indexes, only retest reliability should be estimated. For most multi-item reflective scales (whether they are self-report scales or observational scales), both internal consistency and retest reliability should be assessed by the scale developer. Users of an existing scale should also compute coefficient alpha with data from their research sample.

Example of Internal Consistency Reliability
Radwin and colleagues (2019) developed and tested a scale to measure nurses' and other healthcare providers' patient-centered care. Three subscales were evaluated for internal consistency, and the values of coefficient alpha ranged from .94 to .98.

TIP Reliability estimates vary according to the procedures used to obtain them. A scale's test–retest reliability coefficient (ICC) should not be expected to be the same or even similar in value to an internal consistency estimate (alpha).

Measurement Error

Measurement error is another component within the reliability domain of our taxonomy. The concepts of measurement error and reliability are inextricably connected: unless a reliability coefficient is 1.0 (which is virtually never the case), measurement error is present. Yet, measurement error statistics yield information that reliability coefficients do not provide. For example, measurement error statistics can be used to estimate the precision of a continuous score—that is, the range within which the true score probably lies.

The Standard Error of Measurement

The most widely used index of measurement error is the **standard error of measurement (SEM).** The SEM can be thought of as quantifying "typical error" on a measure. It is an index that can be computed in connection with estimates of either reliability (e.g., test–retest reliability) or internal consistency.

Reliability coefficients, which typically range from .00 to 1.00, are not in the units of measurement associated with the actual measure. A reliability coefficient is a *relative* index that varies from sample to sample and across populations. SEMs, by contrast, are in the measurement units of the instrument. The SEM for a body weight would be in pounds (or grams), and the SEM for a scale such as the CES-D would be in the units of points on the CES-D scale. SEMs are more stable than reliability coefficients and not as affected by sample homogeneity.

The SEM can be estimated using one of several formulas. A popular and easy formula involves taking the square root of 1 minus the reliability coefficient $(1 - R)$ and multiplying that value by an index of how variable the sample scores are.[2] (R could be either the ICC estimate from a test–retest analysis or alpha from an internal consistency analysis). Unfortunately, the SEM is not computed in many major software packages, which might explain why it is not more routinely reported in instrument development papers.

For the self-esteem scores shown in Table 15.1, the SEM is 2.65 at time 1 and 2.49 at time 2. Knowing the value of the SEM allows us to state the probability that a person's true score lies within a certain range. For example, participant 1 had a score of 55 at time 1. Knowing that the SEM is 2.65, we could state that there is a 95% probability that his or her true score at time 1 was between about 50 and 60 (i.e., roughly twice the SEM on either side of the obtained score).

Limits of Agreement

An alternative index of measurement error is the **limits of agreement (LOA)**, derived from work done by Bland and Altman (1986). *Bland–Altman plots* are widely used by medical researchers to examine aspects of both the reliability and validity of measures but are seldom used by psychometricians or nurse researchers. A Bland–Altman plot is a useful device for visually interpreting and differentiating random measurement error and systematic error (bias) in retest or interrater assessments when scores are continuous.

Like the SEM, the LOA provides information about the precision of scores. Limits of agreement are easy to compute[3] but are not routinely calculated in standard statistical software packages such as SPSS. For the self-esteem scores in Table 15.1, the limits of agreement are about +7.0 around a difference score (i.e., the difference between time 1

---

[2]Specifically, this formula for the SEM is: $\text{SEM} = \text{SD}\sqrt{1 - R}$.

[3]Limits of agreement can be computed using output from a paired *t*-test analysis. For 95% confidence, the LOA is 1.96 times the standard deviation of difference between the test and retest scores.

and time 2 scores). This means that any difference in a person's score that is greater than 7 is beyond what we would expect for measurements of a stable trait. None of the score differences in Table 15.1 is greater than 7. A Bland–Altman plot showing the LOA for the data in Table 15.1 is presented in the Toolkit of the accompanying *Resource Manual.* ✖

Example of Measurement Error Information
Ambrosio and colleagues (2016) evaluated the six-item Satisfaction with Life Scale (SLS-6) in a population of patients with Parkinson disease. Using data from 324 patients from five countries, the researchers calculated the SEM to be 3.48.

TIP Measurement error is routinely estimated for multi-item measures developed with item response theory (IRT) methods. Indeed, estimating measurement error typically replaces efforts to estimate internal consistency or reliability. One problem with measurement error in CTT measures is that the estimate is the same for everyone in a sample, whereas IRT models estimate measurement error for each individual. In computer-adaptive tests, a "stopping rule" is established at a desired level of precision (i.e., for a maximum allowable amount of measurement error), and the stopping rule dictates how many items each respondent completes.

VALIDITY

A second domain in the taxonomy of measurement properties is validity. In measurement, **validity** is the degree to which an instrument is measuring the construct it purports to measure. When researchers develop a scale to measure *resilience,* they need to be sure that the resulting scores validly reflect this construct and not something else, such as self-efficacy, hope, or perseverance. Assessing the validity of abstract constructs requires a careful conceptualization of the construct—as well as conceptualization of what the construct is *not.*

Like reliability, validity has different aspects and assessment approaches. As shown in Figure 15.1, the three major components within the validity domain are content and face validity, criterion

validity, and construct validity. Unlike reliability, however, an instrument's validity is difficult to gauge. There are no equations that can easily be applied to the scores of a resilience scale to estimate how good a job the scale is doing in measuring the critical variable. Validation is an evidence-building enterprise, in which the goal is to assemble sufficient evidence from which validity can be inferred. The greater the amount of evidence supporting validity, the more sound the inference.

TIP Reliability and validity are not totally independent properties of an instrument. A measuring device that is unreliable cannot be valid. An instrument cannot validly measure an attribute if it is inconsistent.

Content and Face Validity

Face validity refers to whether the instrument *looks* like it is measuring the target construct. Although face validity is not considered strong evidence of validity, it is helpful for a measure to have face validity if there is evidence of other types of validity. Face validity can be important if patients' resistance to being measured reflects the view that the scale is not relevant to their problems or situations. One reason for developing disease-specific measures, in fact, is that general measures sometimes lack face validity.

Example of Face Validity
Bikker and colleagues (2017) developed and tested the Consultation and Relational Empathy (CARE) instrument, using patients' responses for 943 consultations with sexual health nurses. Face validity of CARE was assessed by counting the number of "not applicable" and missing values for the 10 CARE items and by examining the patients' ratings of how important the items were for capturing the nurses' empathy.

Content validity may be defined as the extent to which an instrument's content adequately captures the construct—that is, whether an instrument has an appropriate sample of items for the construct being measured. It is increasingly recognized that evaluating and enhancing a measure's content validity is a critical early step in enhancing the construct validity of an instrument. If the content of an instrument is a good reflection of a construct, then the instrument has a greater likelihood of achieving its measurement objectives.

Content validation typically involves consultations with a panel of experts. Three issues are pertinent: relevance, comprehensiveness, and balance.

- *Relevance.* An assessment for relevance involves feedback on the relevance of individual items and the overall set of items. For each item, one needs to know: Is this item relevant to the construct or to a specific dimension of the construct? Another consideration is whether the items have relevance for the target population.
- *Comprehensiveness.* The flip side of asking experts about the relevance of items is to ask them if there are notable omissions. To be content valid, a measure should encompass the full complexity of the construct.
- *Balance.* An instrument that is content valid represents the domains of the construct in a balanced manner. In a multi-item scale, a sufficient number of items are needed for each dimension to ensure high internal consistency of subscales.

Researchers designing a new instrument should begin with a thorough conceptualization of the construct. Such a conceptualization might be based on rich firsthand knowledge, an exhaustive literature review, consultation with experts, and in-depth conversations with members of the target population. Specific advice about applying qualitative methods to content validity efforts was offered by Brod and colleagues (2009).

Example of Using Qualitative Data to Enhance Content Validity

Olsen and colleagues (2018) developed the Risk Engagement and Protection Survey (REPS), a measure of fathers' attitudes toward child injury protection and risk engagement. The initial items were developed based on in-depth interviews with 32 fathers in a grounded theory study.

An instrument's content validity is necessarily based on judgment. There are various approaches to assessing content validity using an expert panel, but nurse researchers have been in the forefront in developing an approach that involves the calculation of a **content validity index (CVI)**.

At the item level, a common procedure is to have experts rate items on a 4-point scale of relevance. There are several variations of labeling the 4 points, but the scale used most often is as follows: 1 = *not relevant*, 2 = *somewhat relevant*, 3 = *quite relevant*, and 4 = *highly relevant*. Then, for each item, the **item CVI (I-CVI)** is computed as the number of experts giving a rating of 3 or 4, divided by the number of experts—that is, the proportion in agreement about relevance. For example, an item rated as "quite" or "highly" relevant by 4 out of 5 experts would have an I-CVI of .80, which is considered an acceptable value. Items with an I-CVI below .78 should be carefully scrutinized and either revised or discarded.

There are two approaches to calculating **scale CVIs (S-CVIs)**, and unfortunately instrument development papers do not always indicate which approach was used (Polit & Beck, 2006). The approach we recommend is to compute the S-CVI by averaging all the I-CVIs. We suggest a value of .90 for the S-CVI/Averaging as the standard for establishing excellent content validity (Polit et al., 2007). Content validation should be done with at least three experts, but a larger group is preferable. Further guidance is offered in Chapter 16.

Example of Using a Content Validity Index

Egger-Rainer (2018) developed a scale called the Epilepsy Monitoring Unit Comfort Questionnaire. Nine experts evaluated the content validity of the scale. Based on I-CVI values <.78, many items were reworded or discarded. The S-CVI for 38 remaining items was .90.

Criterion Validity

Criterion validity is the extent to which the scores on an instrument are a good reflection of a "gold standard"—that is, a criterion considered an ideal measure of the construct. Not all measures can be validated using a criterion approach, because there is not always a gold standard to use.

One might reasonably ask: If there is an established criterion, why do we need the focal measure at all—why not simply use the gold standard?

Reasons for creating a new measure include: (1) the expense of administering the gold standard measure is too high, (2) the criterion is burdensome, (3) there are risks or discomfort in using the gold standard, and (4) the criterion is not routinely available in a clinical setting.

A requirement for criterion validation is the availability of a reliable criterion with which measures on the focal instrument can be compared, which is not always the case. For example, it would be difficult to identify a criterion for such attributes as patients' satisfaction with care or quality of life. When a criterion is unavailable, construct validation approaches must be used.

Criterion validation involves testing an implicit hypothesis that the focal measure yields score information that is as good as that obtained from the criterion. This means that scores on the two are hypothesized to be correlated. When such a hypothesis is upheld through formal testing, users gain some assurance that the measure will support appropriate inferences regarding the attribute in question when used with the target population in a similar context.

One type of criterion validity, **concurrent validity,** is assessed when the measurements of the criterion and the new instrument occur at the same time. In such a situation, the implicit hypothesis is that the new measure is an adequate substitute for a contemporaneous criterion. In **predictive validity**, the focal measure is tested against a criterion that is measured in the future. Screening scales are often tested against some future criterion—the occurrence of the phenomenon for which a screening tool is sought.

A broad array of statistical procedures can be used to test whether the criterion validity hypothesis is supported by data from a relevant sample. The choice of statistics depends on whether the focal measure and the criterion are measured as a continuous score value or as categorical ones. Three situations are especially common.

Criterion Validity With a Continuous Measure and a Continuous Criterion

The first situation is when both the focal measure being tested and the criterion are continuous scores.

For example, suppose we were assessing the criterion validity of a 2-minute walk test as a measure of functional performance, and we used the well-established 6-minute walk test as the criterion. In this situation, we would obtain measures of both tests from a sample of patients and compute a Pearson's r (the correlation coefficient) between the two sets of scores. The higher the value of r, the better the evidence of criterion validity.

> **Example of Concurrent Validity Using Correlations**
>
> Bowen and colleagues (2017) developed and tested a new performance-based instrument, the Physical and Cognitive Performance Test for Assisted Living Facilities (PCPT ALF). A sample of residents from assisted living facilities completed the PCPT ALF and two gold standard measures, the Barthel Index and Functional Independence Measure. Correlations exceeded .72, supporting the conclusion of criterion validity for the new measure.

Criterion Validity With a Dichotomous Measure and a Dichotomous Criterion

When both the focal measure and the criterion are dichotomous, several statistical methods can be used but, most often, methods of assessing **diagnostic accuracy** are applied. **Sensitivity** is the ability of a measure to identify a "case" correctly, that is, to screen in or diagnosis a condition correctly. A measure's sensitivity is its rate of yielding "true positives." **Specificity** is the measure's ability to identify noncases correctly, that is, to screen *out* those without the condition. Specificity is an instrument's rate of yielding "true negatives." Of course, to evaluate an instrument's sensitivity and specificity, researchers need a reliable and valid criterion of "caseness" against which scores on the instrument can be assessed.

To illustrate, suppose we wanted to evaluate the validity of adolescents' self-reports about smoking, and we asked 100 teenagers whether they had smoked a cigarette in the previous 24 hours. The gold standard for nicotine consumption is cotinine levels in a body fluid, so we performed a urinary cotinine assay. We use the results to dichotomize the adolescents as positive (>200 ng/mL)

TABLE 15.2 • Example Illustrating Sensitivity, Specificity, and Likelihood Ratios

SELF-REPORTED SMOKING	URINARY COTININE LEVEL (CRITERION)		
	POSITIVE (>200 NG/ML)	NEGATIVE (<200 NG/ML)	TOTAL
Yes	Cell A: true positives 30	Cell B: false positives 5	35 (A + B)
No	Cell C: false negatives 10	Cell D: true negatives 55	65 (C + D)
Total	40 (A + C)	60 (B + D)	100 (A + B + C + D)

Sensitivity: A ÷ (A + C) = .75
Specificity: D ÷ (B + D) = .92
Positive predictive value (PPV): A ÷ (A + B) = .86
Negative predictive value (NPV): D ÷ (C + D) = .85
Likelihood ratio-positive (LR+): Sensitivity ÷ (1 − Specificity) = 9.04
Likelihood ratio-negative (LR−): (1 − Sensitivity) ÷ Specificity = 0.27

or negative for smoking. Some fictitious data are shown in Table 15.2. Sensitivity is calculated as the proportion of teenagers who said they smoked *and* who had high concentrations of cotinine, divided by all real smokers according to the urine test. Put another way, it is the true positives divided by all positives. In this example, smoking was underreported, so the sensitivity of the self-report was .75. Specificity is the proportion of teenagers who accurately reported they did not smoke: the true negatives divided by all negatives. In our example, specificity is .92. There was less overreporting of smoking ("faking bad") than underreporting ("faking good"). We would conclude that the sensitivity of the self-reports was moderate, but the specificity was good.

Other related indicators often are calculated with such data. **Predictive values** are posterior probabilities—the probability of an outcome after the results are known. A **positive predictive value** (or PPV) is the proportion of people with a positive result who have the target outcome. In our example, the PPV is the proportion of teens who said they smoke who actually *do* smoke, according to the cotinine test results. Thirty out of thirty-five

of those who reported smoking had high concentrations of cotinine, and so PPV = .86. A **negative predictive value** (NPV) is the proportion of people who have a negative "score" on the focal measure who also have a negative result on the gold standard. As shown in Table 15.2, 55 out of the 65 teenagers who reported not smoking actually were nonsmokers, and so NPV in our example is .85.

Reporting **likelihood ratios** has come into favor because they summarize the relationship between specificity and sensitivity in a single number. The *positive likelihood ratio* (LR+) is the ratio of true positives to false positives. The formula for LR+ is sensitivity, divided by 1 minus specificity. For the data in Table 15.2, LR+ is 9.04: we are nine times more likely to find that a self-report of smoking really *is* for a true smoker than it is for a nonsmoker. The *negative likelihood ratio* (LR−) is the ratio of false-negative results to true-negative results. For the data in Table 15.2, the LR− is 0.27, indicating that we are substantially less likely to find that a self-report of nonsmoking is false than we are to find that it reflects a true nonsmoker.

These criterion validity indicators are often used when a *cutpoint* on a continuous focal measure is used to classify patients into two categories, which we discuss next.

> **TIP** In Chapter 1, we discussed categories of evidence-based practice (EBP)-related questions, such as Therapy, Prognosis, and so on. One category concerns the accuracy of diagnostic or screening tests. The methods discussed in this section on criterion validity are especially important for providing evidence for this type of EBP question.

Criterion Validity With a Continuous Measure and a Dichotomous Criterion

When the measure being assessed is continuous and the criterion is dichotomous, criterion validation often uses an approach that involves plotting each score on the index measure against its specificity and sensitivity for correct classification based on the dichotomous criterion.

The indicators we calculated for the data in Table 15.2 are contingent upon the value that we established for cotinine concentration (200 ng/mL). Sensitivity and specificity would be different if we used 100 ng/mL as indicative of smoking status. There is almost invariably a tradeoff between the sensitivity and specificity of a measure. When sensitivity is increased to include more true positives, the proportion of true negatives declines. Therefore, a common task in developing new measures for which there is a continuous gold standard is to find an appropriate **cutoff point** (or *cutpoint*)—that is, a score to distinguish cases and noncases.

Researchers use a **receiver operating characteristic curve** (**ROC curve**) to identify the best cutoff point. In an ROC curve, the sensitivity of an instrument (i.e., the rate of correctly identifying a case vis-à-vis an established criterion) is plotted against the false-positive rate (i.e., the rate of incorrectly classifying someone as a case, which is the inverse of its specificity) over a range of different scores on the focal measure. The score (cutoff point) that yields the best balance between sensitivity and specificity can then be determined. The optimum cutoff is at or near the shoulder of the ROC curve.

Figure 15.2 presents an ROC curve from a study to assess the criterion validity of a brief cognitive screening instrument (the Montreal Cognitive Assessment, MoCA) for adolescents with congenital heart disease (Pike et al., 2017). The criterion was a longer, widely accepted measure of cognition for this population—the General Memory Index (GMI). Scores on the GMI were dichotomized for "caseness" at 85. In this figure, sensitivity and 1 minus specificity are plotted for each MoCA score. The upper left corner represents sensitivity at its highest possible value (1.0) and false positives at its lowest possible value (.00).

In ROC analyses, the **area under the curve** (**AUC**) can be used as a validity parameter. Desirable AUC values (close to 1.00) are found when the curve hugs close to the upper left corner. When the curve is close to the diagonal, the AUC value is .50, indicating that the measure cannot differentiate between those who are positive and negative on the criterion. Values of .70 are usually considered evidence of adequate validity. The AUC for the data portrayed in Figure 15.2 is .84. The cutoff score for the MoCA in this example was set at 26. At this cutoff value, sensitivity was .94 and specificity was .80; the PPV was .70 and NPV was .96.

> **Example of Sensitivity, Specificity, Predictive Values, and Likelihood Ratio**
> Curley and an interprofessional team (2018) developed and tested the Braden QD scale for predicting pressure injury risk in pediatric patients. Using data from a sample of 625 patients in eight medical centers, the sensitivity and specificity at a cutoff score of 13 on the Braden QD were .86 and .59, respectively. The PPV was .15 and the NPV was .98. The positive likelihood ratio was 2.09.

Construct Validity

For many abstract attributes (constructs), no gold standard criterion exists, so other validation avenues must be pursued. The third component within the validity domain of our measurement taxonomy (Figure 15.1) is construct validity. The construct validity question is this: What attribute is *really* being measured? Borrowing from

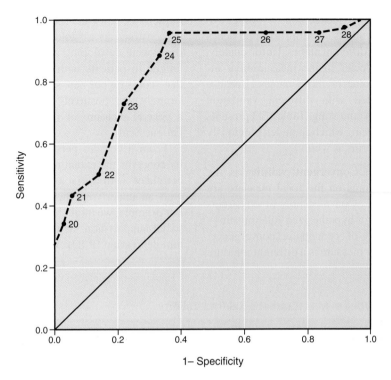

FIGURE 15.2 Receiver operating characteristic (ROC) curve for Montreal Cognitive Assessment Screener for Adolescents and Young Adults with Congenital Heart Disease. (Adapted with permission from Pike, N., Poulsen, M., & Woo, M. (2017). Validity of the Montreal Cognitive Assessment Screener for adolescents and young adults with and without congenital heart disease. *Nursing Research, 66*, 222–230.)

esteemed methodologists Shadish, Cook, and Campbell (2002), we define **construct validity** as the degree to which evidence about a measure's scores in relation to other scores supports the inference that the construct has been appropriately represented.

Evidence for construct validity comes from tests of hypotheses about the nature of the construct and scores on the focal measure. The researcher must speculate: If my instrument is, in fact, really measuring construct X, then how would I expect the scores to perform? In a construct validation, the instrument developer must have a firm conceptualization not only of the construct itself (as in a content validity effort), but also a conceptualization of how the construct is related to other constructs. In other words, there needs to be an overarching conceptual model of processes and traits of relevance to the construct.

Construct validity encompasses three aspects: hypothesis-testing construct validity, structural validity, and cross-cultural validity.

Hypothesis-Testing Construct Validity

Hypothesis-testing validity involves testing to corroborate hypotheses about the focal measure. In hypothesis-testing construct validations, hypotheses are developed about relationships between scores on the focal measure and scores on measures of other constructs; data are collected to test the hypotheses with a sample from a specified population; and validity conclusions are reached based on results of the hypothesis tests. A successful construct validation effort requires ingenuity. Researchers must challenge themselves to develop diverse and complementary ways of testing whether their measure is, indeed, measuring the construct of interest.

Different types of evidence can be brought to bear on construct validity, leading to approaches that have been given different names. Unfortunately, there are inconsistencies in the measurement literature regarding some of those names. Because the terms associated with different validation approaches are often confusing, Table 15.3 presents a quick summary chart, which includes previously discussed validity terms as well.

Convergent Validity. Convergent validity is the degree to which scores on the focal measure are correlated with scores on measures of constructs with which there is a hypothesized relationship—that is, the degree of conceptual convergence. Sometimes the other measure is a different measure of the same construct (but not a measure that could be construed as a "gold standard"). For example, if we were developing a new, specific measure of fatigue in patients with cancer, we might predict that scores on our new scale would correlate fairly strongly and positively with patients' scores on a general measure of fatigue, such as the Piper Fatigue Scale.

From a broader perspective, convergent validity concerns the extent to which the focal measure correlates with variables in a manner consistent with an underlying theory or conceptual model. For example, we might hypothesize that inadequate social support is a factor contributing to postpartum depression (PPD). We could test the construct

TABLE 15.3 • Types of Measurement-Related Validity

TYPE OF VALIDITY	EXPLANATION
Content and face validity	
Face validity	Concerns whether a measure "looks" as though it is measuring the relevant construct
Content validity	Concerns the adequacy of content for multicomponent measures
Criterion validity	
Concurrent validity	Tests whether a measure is consistent with a criterion (a gold standard), measured at the same time
Predictive validity	Tests whether a measure is consistent with a criterion (a gold standard), measured at a future point in time
Construct validity: Hypothesis testing	
Convergent validity	In the absence of a gold standard, tests the correlation between the focal measure and a measure of a construct with which conceptual convergence is expected
Known-groups (discriminative) validity	Tests the degree to which a measure can discriminate between groups known to differ with regard to the focal construct
Divergent (discriminant) validity	Tests that the focal measure is not a measure of a different construct other than the one intended
Construct validity: Other	
Structural validity	Tests whether a measure captures the hypothesized dimensionality of a construct
Cross-cultural validity	Concerns the extent to which a translated or adapted measure is equivalent to the original

validity of a PPD scale by examining the correlation between scores on this scale with those on a measure of social support. In essence, researchers reason as follows:

- According to theory or prior evidence, construct X is positively related to construct Y.
- Instrument A is a measure of construct X; instrument B is a valid measure of construct Y.
- Scores on A and B are correlated positively, as predicted.
- Therefore, it is inferred that A is a valid measure of X.

This logical analysis does not offer proof of construct validity but yields supportive evidence. Construct validation is an ongoing evidence-building enterprise. With convergent validity, the validity parameter is typically the correlation coefficient between two measures—most often Pearson's *r*.

Example of Convergent Validity

Ciupitu-Plath and colleagues (2018) assessed the psychometric properties of the German version of the Weight Bias Internalization Scale (WBIS-Y) with 191 overweight adolescents. In their construct validation efforts, they hypothesized that the youth's scores on the WBIS would correlate positively with their body mass index and negatively with self-esteem, self-efficacy, and health-related quality of life. Their hypotheses were supported.

Known-Groups Validity. Known-groups validity, which has also been called *discriminative validity,* tests hypotheses about a measure's ability to discriminate between two or more groups known (or expected) to differ on the construct of interest. For example, we might hypothesize that women who had planned their pregnancy would have more favorable scores on a postpartum depression scale than women whose pregnancy was unwanted. If the scores on the PPD measure do not differ for the two groups, one might question the scale's validity, given the existing evidence that women whose pregnancies are wanted are less susceptible than other women to PPD. We would not necessarily expect large differences; some women in both groups would likely suffer from PPD. We would, however, hypothesize differences in

average group scores. The known-groups approach is one of the most widely used methods of assessing construct validity.

A key difference between convergent validity and known-groups validity concerns how the validation variable is measured. Continuous scores on a comparator construct can be used to create "known" groups by dividing the sample into subgroups for known-groups validity, or the continuous scores can be used to test a correlation for convergent validity. It is best to divide sample members into subgroups for a known-groups validation when there is a well-established cutpoint for "caseness."

Example of the Known-Groups Technique

Martin, Martin, and Redshaw (2017) developed and tested a short birth satisfaction scale, using items from the Birth Satisfaction Scale-Revised (BSS-R). Consistent with their hypothesis, birth satisfaction scores using the new short scale were significantly higher for mothers with a normal vaginal delivery compared to mothers who had an interventional delivery (e.g., with forceps or by caesarean birth).

Divergent Validity. Divergent validity (which is often called *discriminant validity*) concerns evidence that a measure is *not* a measure of a different construct. We use the term *divergent* because it is a good contrast with *con*vergent validity and also because of possible confusion between the terms discriminant and discriminative (known-groups) validity.

In a divergent validation, researchers typically measure both the focal attribute and a similar—but distinct—attribute as a means of ensuring that the two are not really measures of the same construct but with different labels. Thus, in a divergent validation, the hypothesis is that the two measures are only weakly correlated.

Sometimes hypotheses for construct validations are stated in relative rather than absolute terms, especially when there are both convergent and divergent hypotheses. For example, an absolute hypothesis for a new PPD scale might predict that scores would correlate only modestly with scores on a measure of anxiety about maternal role performance, to distinguish the PPD construct from maternal anxiety. For a relative hypothesis, we might predict that scores on a PPD scale would correlate more strongly with scores on a general measure of depression (convergent validity) than with scores on the maternal anxiety scale (divergent validity).

The primary approach to divergent validation is to compute correlation coefficients. Researchers should stipulate in advance how "weak" a correlation would need to be as evidence of divergent validity, either in absolute or relative terms.

> **Example of Convergent and Divergent Validity**
> Jurgens and colleagues (2017) undertook a psychometric assessment of the Heart Failure Somatic Perception Scale (HFSPS) as a measure of patient symptom perception. The researchers assessed convergent validity by testing a hypothesized relationship between scores on the HFSPS and on a physical limitation subscale. Divergent validity was tested by correlating scores on the HFSPF with scores on a self-care management scale.

> **TIP** An approach known as the **multitrait–multimethod matrix method** (MTMM) is a significant construct validation tool that involves tests of both convergent and divergent validity (Campbell & Fiske, 1959). Few nurse researchers have used an MTMM in its full form. The MTMM is explained more fully in Polit and Yang (2016).

Construct Validity Evidence. Most researchers identify multiple hypotheses for their construct validity work and include several different types of validation approaches in a single study. As a result, drawing conclusions about a measure's construct validity is typically more complex than interpreting results for other measurement properties, such as reliability. For many measurement parameters, only a single number needs to be interpreted. For example, when an ICC is computed with test–retest data, that value *is* the estimated reliability. However, there is seldom a single "validity coefficient" in construct validation, because typically several hypotheses are tested. Indeed, the more supporting evidence there is, the greater the confidence one can have about the measure's validity. An instrument does not possess or lack validity; it is a question of degree. An instrument's validity is not proved, established, or demonstrated but rather is supported to a greater or lesser extent by evidence. However, when there are multiple hypotheses, results may be "mixed"—some hypotheses are supported and others are not. This fact means that it is wise for researchers to establish a priori standards for how much confirmatory evidence is considered sufficient.

Structural Validity

Another aspect of construct validity is called structural validity. **Structural validity** refers to the extent to which the structure of a multi-item scale adequately reflects the hypothesized dimensionality of the construct being measured. Structural validity concerns which dimensions of a broader construct are captured by the instrument and whether the dimensions are consistent with theory. For example, we might conceptualize pain as having two dimensions: pain severity and pain interference. After developing a scale based on this conceptualization, we would want to test whether we were successful in capturing and distinguishing the two dimensions. Content validity work ideally paves the way for a good conceptualization of a construct's multiple dimensions.

Assessments of structural validity rely on a statistical procedure called factor analysis, which is computationally complex, but it is conceptually fairly simple. **Factor analysis** is a method for identifying clusters of related items—that is, dimensions underlying a broad construct. Each dimension, or **factor**, represents a relatively unitary attribute. The procedure is used to identify and group together different items measuring an underlying attribute. In effect, factor analysis constitutes another means of testing hypotheses about the interrelationships among variables and of formulating evidence of convergence and divergence at the item level.

As we discuss in the next chapter, there are two broad classes of factor analysis—exploratory and confirmatory. *Exploratory factor analysis* is an important tool in the development of multi-item scales. *Confirmatory factor analysis*, however, is the preferred method for testing structural validity hypotheses about the dimensionality of a scale.

It is important to note that information about a measure's structural validity does not constitute sufficient evidence of a measure's construct validity. Factor analysis can confirm a hypothesis that a complex construct has, for example, three underlying dimensions, but such an analysis does not in and of itself address the central construct validity question: Does this instrument really measure the construct it purports to measure?

Example of Structural Validation

Riegel and colleagues (2019) tested the psychometric properties of the revised Self-Care of Heart Failure Index (SCHFI). Data were collected from 626 patients in five sites. Structural validity was assessed using confirmatory factor analysis (CFA). The sample was randomly split into two subsamples and the CFA results from one subsample were confirmed in a CFA of the second subsample.

TIP Structural validity is only relevant for multi-item reflective scales and not formative indexes. Factor analysis relies on items with strong intercorrelations.

Cross-Cultural Validity

A third type of construct validity is cross-cultural validity, which is relevant for measures that have been translated or adapted for use with a different cultural group than that for the original instrument. We define **cross-cultural validity** as the degree to which the components (e.g., items) of a translated or culturally adapted measure perform adequately and equivalently, individually and collectively, relative to their performance on the original instrument.

Developing a high-quality and cross-culturally valid instrument requires even more time and effort than starting from scratch with a new instrument. Yet, without such efforts, it would be impossible to understand health outcomes globally. If, for example, we want to learn whether health-related quality of life differs across countries, comparisons cannot be made with disparate instruments. Several coordinated multinational efforts have been undertaken to adapt widely used English-language health scales, such as the Mini-Mental State Examination and a quality-of-life scale called the SF-36. Also, many item banks of health outcomes have been translated for use in CAT as part of the PROMIS® initiative.

The methods used in cross-cultural validation are complex and multifaceted, and many of them require high levels of statistical sophistication. An overview of some of these methods, together with some guidance on undertaking a translation or adaptation of an instrument, is presented in the Supplement to this chapter on thePoint. **S** More detailed information is offered in Polit and Yang (2016).

RELIABILITY OF CHANGE SCORES

Two domains in our measurement taxonomy relate to measurements over time. Both of these domains concern change scores, so we briefly discuss the issue of measuring change.

Measuring Change

How does one measure whether a change in a construct has occurred? For some attributes, there is only one option: measuring it on two occasions and comparing the values—in other words, subtracting one value from the other to calculate a **change score** that represents the amount of change between two scores. If we want to learn, for example, whether a patient's blood pressure has decreased, we need to know what it was initially and what it is now and calculate the difference. For patient-reported outcomes, there are two other alternatives: asking patients directly whether a change has occurred and asking them to report retrospectively what their status was previously and then comparing it to their current status. Unfortunately, all three methods have potential problems.

In clinical trials, statisticians have argued against using change scores as the dependent variables in the analysis of treatment effects. When patients are randomized to groups, it is recommended that scores at the posttest be used as the outcome variables, rather than change scores. A major emphasis in randomized trials is on *difference scores* (the average difference between the randomized groups at posttest), rather than on *change scores.*

Yet, it is of inherent substantive interest to understand how much patients in all arms of a trial have changed. Some nonexperimental studies seek to describe outcomes over the course of an illness, which requires a direct examination of how scores have evolved. And, at the level of an individual patient, assessments of improvement, deterioration, or stability over time as measured by change scores may be the focus of clinical assessment and decision-making.

Change scores can be affected by several factors that can threaten their accuracy and validity. A major concern with change scores is the inevitability of measurement error. Change scores—the difference between an imperfectly reliable score at time 1 and another imperfectly reliable score at time 2—potentially can magnify a small change or mask a large one. The greater the degree of unreliability, the greater the risk that a change score will be misleading.

The reliability of change domain focuses on this issue: how do we know when a change score is "real" and not merely a random fluctuation? Except for measures created within an item response theory framework, reliable change has most often been assessed by computing one of two indexes: the smallest detectable change (SDC) or the reliable change index (RCI).

The Smallest Detectable Change

The usual approach to assessing the reliability of group-level change is to test the statistical significance of a group's change in scores from one point in time to another, using tests we describe in Chapter 18. From a measurement perspective, however, statistical significance may not be an informative way to understand change—and significance tells us nothing about whether a change was reliable for individuals.

Reliable change for continuous data often is estimated using an index called the **smallest**

detectable change (SDC) or the *minimal detectable change (MDC).*[4] An SDC can be defined as a change in scores that is beyond measurement error—a change of sufficient magnitude that the probability is low that it resulted from random error.

Operationally, the SDC is a change score that falls outside the limits of agreement on a Bland–Altman plot. As noted earlier, the LOA can be estimated using test–retest data from a stable population. The limits of agreement are an estimate of the probable range of score differences between a test and a retest, for a stable population over a specified interval. If a change score falls outside the LOA, there can be greater confidence that the change is reliable. High measurement error makes it more difficult to detect true change—underscoring the importance of using measures with high reliability.

Earlier we noted that the LOA for the self-esteem scores in Table 15.1 was about 7.0 (actually, 7.1). Suppose that we evaluated an intervention designed to improve the self-esteem and mental health of adolescents. The scores in Table 15.1 are from a test–retest administration of the scale but suppose that the time 2 scores were baseline values for a test of the intervention. Three months after the intervention, we would readminister the self-esteem scale (time 3). Based on the LOA, any improvement in self-esteem scores of 7 points or greater in a participant's score would be considered indicative of real (reliable) improvement in self-esteem.

Example of the Smallest Detectable Change
Lee and colleagues (2016) assessed the Heart Quality of Life (HeartQoL) measure with 105 patients who had ischemic heart disease. The 95% limits of agreement were .07 + .67 for the physical subscale and .04 + .70 for the emotional subscale. The SDC was .67 and .70 for these two subscales, respectively.

---

[4]The term "minimal detectable change" is often used in the medical literature. We use "smallest detectable change" to be consistent with COSMIN. The SDC has also been called the "smallest detectable *difference*" or "minimal detectable *difference*," but, like the COSMIN group, we prefer "smallest detectable *change*" to emphasize the focus on *change* scores.

The Reliable Change Index

The SDC is similar to another index that is widely used in the field of psychotherapy. The **reliable change index (RCI)** was proposed by Jacobson and colleagues (1984, 1991) as an element of a two-part process for assessing the clinical significance of patients' improvement as a result of psychotherapy. Jacobson argued that, to be clinically meaningful, a change score on psychotherapy outcomes must pass the test of being "real"—that is, a change beyond measurement error.

The RCI is calculated by using a formula that includes the amount of measurement error for the scale, as estimated by the standard error of measurement.[5] The cutoff values for reliable change are similar (but not identical) for the RCI and the SDC. In our example of the self-esteem scores in Figure 15.1, the SDC is 7.10 and the RCI is. 7.33. The RCI is discussed in greater detail in the Supplement to Chapter 21 **Ⓢ**.

> **Example of the Reliable Change Index**
> Bond and an interdisciplinary team (2016) studied neurocognitive changes in patients with head and neck cancer. Study participants underwent neurocognitive testing at baseline and then 3 months after chemoradiation treatment. Patients' changes in performance were assessed using the reliable change index.

RESPONSIVENESS

The final domain in our measurement taxonomy also concerns measurements over time. We define the measurement property of **responsiveness** as the ability of a measure to detect change over time in a construct that has changed, commensurate with the amount of change that has occurred. Just as reliability can be extended to apply to change scores, responsiveness represents the extension of validity over time. Validity concerns whether a measure is truly capturing the intended construct, and responsiveness concerns whether a change score is truly capturing a real change in the construct.

> **TIP** Before COSMIN, there was no consensus about what responsiveness is or how to know when it has been achieved. Terwee and colleagues (2003), in a systematic review of the quality-of-life literature, found 25 definitions of responsiveness. The COSMIN group brought together health measurement experts who reached agreement in defining responsiveness as the validity of change scores.

Validity and responsiveness share many features, the main difference being the timeframe. The methods used to assess responsiveness overlap with methods used to assess validity. Validity and responsiveness are also both challenging to assess. Assessments require researchers to be creative in developing useful hypotheses. Furthermore, both responsiveness and validity rely on ongoing evidence building. The more evidence that can be brought to bear on a measure's responsiveness, the greater the confidence one has in the measure's capacity to capture true change in a construct. This evidence-building feature of both cross-sectional and longitudinal validity (responsiveness) means that there is no single number to quantify its value.

Psychometricians have not traditionally considered responsiveness as a measurement property. We agree with the COSMIN group, however, that responsiveness merits consideration. Change is critically important to healthcare professionals who hope to achieve improvements with clients.

Two broad approaches have been used in assessing responsiveness, similar to approaches used in validity testing: a criterion approach and a construct approach.

The Criterion Approach to Responsiveness

Like criterion validation, the criterion approach to responsiveness requires a gold standard—a well-established and reliable criterion that indicates that a change in the target construct has occurred. This approach to responsiveness assessment has also been called an **anchor-based approach**, with the criterion serving as the anchor.

A criterion-based assessment of responsiveness sometimes involves an examination of the relationship between changes on the target measure

---

[5]For 95% confidence, the formula for the RCI is 1.96 times $\sqrt{2 \times \text{SEM}^2}$.

and changes on the criterion, which corresponds directly to a longitudinal assessment of criterion validity. For example, earlier in the chapter, we used a study by Bowen and colleagues (2017) to illustrate criterion validity. These researchers correlated scores on a new measure of physical and cognitive performance for residents in assisted living facilities (the PCPT ALF) with scores on two gold standard performance measures. To assess the responsiveness of the PCPT ALF, they could compute the correlation between *changes* on this scale and *changes* on the gold standard scales. The implicit hypothesis in such a responsiveness assessment is that change scores on the focal measure are consistent with change scores on the criterion. When formal testing supports such a hypothesis, then the evidence supports the focal measure's responsiveness (longitudinal validity).

Another strategy for testing criterion-based responsiveness involves the use of a single-item **global rating scale** or **GRS** (also known as a **health transition rating**) as the criterion (DeVet et al., 2011). A GRS involves asking patients to rate directly the degree to which their status on the focal construct has changed over a time interval in which change is presumed to have occurred. Figure 15.3

provides an example of a 7-point GRS, which asks patients to rate changes in their ability to perform activities of daily living. Such a GRS would be relevant for assessing the responsiveness of a physical function or activities of daily living (ADL) scale—for example, for measuring improvements in patients' physical function 3 months after a health-promotion intervention.

Let us suppose we were assessing the responsiveness of a physical function scale, such as the Barthel Index (BI). We might administer the BI just prior to the intervention and then 3 months later. At the 3-month point, patients would also be asked to complete the GRS shown in Figure 15.3. Several statistical approaches could be used to test the BI's responsiveness. For example, the average BI change scores could be statistically compared for patients who said they had any improvement on the GRS (response options 1, 2, or 3) and patients who did not report improvements (options 4-7). Alternatively, change scores on the BI could be plotted on an ROC curve against the sensitivity and specificity for predicting the GRS criterion: improved versus did not improve. The AUC would provide the estimate of responsiveness.

The Construct Approach to Responsiveness

The construct approach to evaluating a measure's responsiveness is analogous to a hypothesis-testing construct validation. Researchers develop and test hypotheses about changes on the focal measure in relation to other phenomena. Sometimes, the hypotheses concern an expected change on the construct resulting from a treatment of well-established efficacy (e.g., changes in quality of life after hip replacement). Alternatively, the hypotheses may concern the nature and magnitude of relationship between changes on the focal measure on the one hand and changes on measures of constructs that are theoretically linked to the focal construct on the other.

When hypotheses are developed about how changes in a focal measure are related to changes in other measures, a full array of strategies and analytic methods can be used, analogous to those

---

Please rate the changes you have experienced in the past three months with regard to *your ability to perform regular activities of daily living*, such as standing up from a sitting position or taking a bath or shower:

1. Very much better
2. Much better
3. A little better
4. No change
5. A little worse
6. Much worse
7. Very much worse

Shaded response options show one possible cut point on the criterion: Responses 1–3 (any improvement) versus 4–7 (no improvement)

FIGURE 15.3 Example of a global rating scale for a criterion-related assessment of responsiveness for an activities of daily living (ADL) scale.

described for hypothesis-testing construct validity. For example, some hypotheses are designed to support what might be called *convergent responsiveness*—the degree to which change scores on the focal measure are correlated with change scores on a measure of a construct with which a relationship is hypothesized. Similarly, it would be possible to hypothesize that changes on the focal construct, as captured in change scores on the focal measure, are *not* associated (or only weakly associated) with changes on another, unrelated measure (*divergent responsiveness*). Another option is *known-groups responsiveness,* the longitudinal extension of known-groups validity. In this approach, researchers test the hypothesis that changes on the focal measure are different for groups known (or hypothesized) to have different amounts of change.

Conceptually, construct-focused responsiveness assessment is an extension of construct validation, but procedurally there has been greater complexity in evaluating responsiveness. Polit and Yang (2016) provide more details about so-called responsiveness indexes and about **distribution-based approaches** to assessing responsiveness, which were given this label because they are based on change score distributions.

Example of Responsiveness Assessment
Wong and coresearchers (2017) tested the psychometric properties of the International Prostate Symptom Score (IPSS) in a sample of Chinese patients with benign prostatic hyperplasia. Using distribution-based methods, the researchers found evidence of responsiveness for the IPSS and three of its four subscales.

TIP When you select an instrument to use in a study, you should seek evidence of its psychometric soundness by examining the instrument developers' report. The report ideally would provide evidence regarding all the measurement properties discussed in this chapter—but information about reliability of change scores and responsiveness may be absent. You should also consider evidence about the quality of the measure from others who have used it. Each time the scale "performs" as hypothesized, this constitutes supplementary evidence for its validity and possibly its responsiveness.

CRITICAL APPRAISAL OF DATA QUALITY IN QUANTITATIVE STUDIES

If data are seriously flawed, a study cannot contribute useful evidence. Therefore, in drawing conclusions about a study's evidence, you should consider whether researchers have taken appropriate steps to ensure high-quality measurements of key constructs. Research consumers need to ask: Can I trust the data in this study? Are the measurements of key constructs reliable and valid, and are change scores reliable and responsive?

Information about data quality should be provided in every quantitative research report. Reliability estimates are usually reported because they are easy to communicate. Ideally, for composite scales, the report should provide internal consistency reliability coefficients based on data from the study itself, not just from previous research. Interrater or interobserver reliability is especially crucial for coming to conclusions about data quality in observational studies. The values of the reliability coefficients should be sufficiently high to support confidence in the findings. In studies with nonsignificant findings, pay special attention to reliability information because the unreliability of measures can undermine statistical conclusion validity.

Validity is more difficult to document in a report than reliability. At a minimum, researchers should defend their choice of existing measures based on validity information from the developers, and they should cite the relevant publication. If a study involves the use of a screening or diagnostic measure, information should also be provided about its sensitivity and specificity.

Box 15.1 provides some guidelines for critically appraising aspects of the data quality of quantitative measures. The guidelines are available in the Toolkit of the accompanying *Resource Manual* for your use and adaptation. Francis and colleagues (2016) have also developed a checklist for evaluating patient-reported outcome measures.

BOX 15.1 Guidelines for Critically Appraising Measurement and Data Quality in Quantitative Studies

1. Was there congruence between the research variables as conceptualized (i.e., as discussed in the introduction of the report) and as operationalized (i.e., as described in the method section)?
2. If operational definitions (or scoring procedures) were specified, did they clearly indicate the rules of measurement? Do the rules seem sensible? Were data collected in such a way that measurement errors were minimized (e.g., training of data collectors)?
3. Did the report describe the measurement properties of the instruments used to measure key study constructs? Was the rationale for using the chosen instruments based on data quality issues (e.g., better measurement properties than alternative measures of the same construct)?
4. Did the report offer evidence of the reliability of the measures used in the study? Did the evidence come from the research sample itself, or was it based on other studies? If the latter, is it reasonable to conclude that data quality would be similar for the research sample as for the reliability sample (e.g., are sample characteristics similar)?
5. If reliability was reported, which estimation method was used? Was this method appropriate? Should an alternative or additional method of reliability appraisal have been used? Was the appropriate reliability coefficient computed (e.g., an ICC for test–retest reliability)? Is the reliability sufficiently high? Was measurement error reported?
6. Did the report offer evidence of the validity of the measures? Assuming validity evidence came from other studies, is it reasonable to believe that data quality would be similar for the research sample as for the validity sample (e.g., are the sample characteristics similar)?
7. If validity information was reported, which validity approach was used? Was this method appropriate? Does the validity of the instruments appear to be adequate?
8. If the study involved computing change scores, was information provided about the reliability of change scores? Was evidence about the responsiveness of change scores provided?
9. If there was information about the measurement properties of key instruments used in the study, what conclusion can you reach about the quality of the data in the study?
10. Were the research hypotheses supported? If not, might data quality have played a role in the failure to confirm the hypotheses?

RESEARCH EXAMPLE

In this section, we describe a study that used a wide variety of types of data and strategies to enhance data quality.

Study: Associations between hormonal biomarkers and cognitive, motor, and language development status in very low-birthweight (VLBW) infants (Cho et al., 2017)

Statement of purpose: The purpose of this study was to examine relationships between testosterone and cortisol with measures of infants' cognitive, motor and language development in VLBW infants.

Design: A total of 62 mother–infant pairs participated in the study. Data were collected through record review,

maternal self-report, biomarkers, and observation. Mother–infant interactions were observed at 3 and 6 months corrected age (CA), and infant development was assessed at 6 months CA.

Instruments and data quality: *Records data:* Information about infant demographics and neonatal history was extracted from medical records. *Maternal self-reports.* Maternal reports were used to collect data on infant health history after discharge from the neonatal intensive care unit (NICU). The researchers indicated that they asked about the presence or absence of health problems rather than about frequency of occurrence, to reduce the risk of recall bias. *Biomarker data:* Samples of saliva for measuring cortisol and testosterone levels were collected 1 hour before or after a feeding to avoid contamination. Three saliva samples were obtained within a 2-hour period, and the values were averaged to enhance reliability. The lab technician who determined the testosterone and cortisol levels was blinded to infant characteristics, to minimize the risk of any bias. *Observational measures:* The infant's developmental status was assessed using a widely used measure, the Bayley Scales of Infant Development-III (BSID-III). Cho et al. provided information about the scale's strong reliability and validity as assessed in instrument development studies. For example, the reliability of the BSID-III for preterm infants was reported as .89 to .96 (the type of reliability was not indicated). Evidence of the BSID-III's convergent validity was also reported. Mother–infant interactions were videotaped for 15 minutes on two occasions. Mothers were asked to interact with their infants as they usually do. Two coders used a validated coding scheme to code 5 maternal behaviors and 5 infant behaviors. The behaviors were combined into global interactive behaviors "to reduce multiplicity during data analysis" (p. 353). For mothers, the two behaviors were attention and restrictiveness and for infants they were social behaviors and negativism. Interrater reliabilities were computed using Cohen's kappa and, on average, were .82 for maternal behaviors and .90 for infant behaviors. Although the researchers did look at changes in mother–infant interactions between the 3-month and 6-month observations, no information was provided regarding the reliability of change or responsiveness. As noted earlier, nurse researchers are only beginning to consider longitudinal measurement issues.

Key findings: The researchers found that, after statistically controlling for mother–infant interactions and other variables, high testosterone levels were positively related to language development in male infants. High cortisol levels were negatively associated with the motor development of female infants.

SUMMARY POINTS

- **Measurement** involves assigning numbers to objects to represent the amount of an attribute, according to rules. When researchers invent rules to capture a construct, they create a **measure** of the construct.

- **Psychometrics** is the branch of psychology concerned with the theory and methods of psychological measurement, and psychometrics have influenced health measurement. **Classical test theory (CTT)** is one major psychometric theory of measurement and **item response theory (ITT)** is another.

- Within CTT, **obtained scores** from a measure are conceptualized as having a **true score** component (the value that would be obtained for a hypothetical perfect measure of the attribute) and an error component, or **error of measurement**, that represents measurement inaccuracies. Sources of measurement error include situational contaminants, response set biases, and transient personal factors, such as fatigue.

- Measures can vary in several ways, including whether they are *generic* (broadly applicable) or *specific* to certain types of people, such as disease-specific measures. Measures can be **static** (the same instrument for everyone) or **adaptive**, with different questions from an *item bank* being administered to different people, usually using **computerized adaptive testing**.

- For multi-item measures, another distinction is important. In **reflective scales**, the items are viewed as being *caused by* the construct—responses are reflections of the underlying attribute. In a **formative index**, the items are viewed as defining the construct.

- A panel of health measurement experts defined key **measurement properties** in the **COSMIN** initiative. The taxonomy presented in this book modified the COSMIN taxonomy to include two cross-sectional measurement properties (reliability and validity) and two longitudinal measurement properties (reliability of change scores and responsiveness).

- Many measurement properties can be assessed by computing a statistic that estimates a **measurement parameter**. Several parameter estimates involve computing a **correlation coefficient** that indicates the magnitude and direction of a relationship between two variables. Correlation coefficients can range from −1.00 (a **perfect negative relationship**) through .00 to +1.00 (a **perfect positive relationship**).

- **Reliability** is the extent to which scores for people *who have not changed* are the same for repeated measurements, under several situations, including repetition on different occasions (test–retest and intrarater reliability), by different persons (interrater reliability), on different versions of a measure (parallel test reliability), or with different items on a multi-item instrument (internal consistency).
- Assessments of **test–retest reliability** involve administering a measure twice to assess the stability of scores. When scores are continuous, the preferred index of test–retest reliability is the **intraclass correlation coefficient (ICC)**. Reliability coefficients such as the ICC range from .00 to 1.00, with higher values reflecting greater reliability.
- **Interrater reliability** involves assessing the congruence of ratings or classifications of two or more independent observers. When observers make classifications, interrater agreement is usually assessed using the **kappa** statistic, which is an index of chance-adjusted **proportion of agreement**.
- **Internal consistency**, a component in the reliability domain, concerns the extent to which all the instrument's items are measuring the same attribute; it is usually assessed by **Cronbach alpha**. Internal consistency is not relevant for formative indexes.
- A third component in the reliability domain is measurement error, for which there are two indexes that indicate the precision of a score. The **standard error of measurement (SEM)**, which quantifies "typical error" on a measure, is in the units of measurement of the measure itself. Another index is called the **limits of agreement (LOA)** on a *Bland–Altman plot*. The LOA can be used to identify how much differences in scores in a retest study are reasonable if the attribute has in fact not changed.
- **Validity,** a second domain the measurement taxonomy, is the degree to which an instrument measures what it purports to measure. Validity has multiple components.
- **Face validity** refers to whether the instrument appears, on the face of it, to be measuring the appropriate construct.

- **Content validity** is the extent to which an instrument's content (its items) adequately captures the construct being measured. Expert ratings on the relevance of items can be used to compute **content validity index (CVI)** information. An **item CVI (I-CVI)** represents the proportion of experts rating an item as relevant. A **scale CVI (S-CVI)** using the averaging method is the average of all I-CVI values for the set of items on the scale.
- **Criterion-related validity** (which includes both **predictive validity** and **concurrent validity**) is the extent to which scores on an instrument are an adequate reflection of a "gold standard" criterion. When both the focal measure and the criterion are continuous measures, correlation coefficients are used to estimate criterion validity.
- When both the focal measure and the criterion are dichotomous, criterion-related validity is assessed with indexes of **diagnostic accuracy**, namely sensitivity and specificity. **Sensitivity** is the instrument's ability to identify a case correctly (i.e., its rate of yielding true positives). **Specificity** is the instrument's ability to identify noncases correctly (i.e., its rate of yielding true negatives).
- Sensitivity is sometimes plotted against specificity in a **receiver operating characteristic curve (ROC curve)** to determine the optimum **cutoff point** for caseness with continuous measures. An ROC yields an index called the **area under the curve (AUC)** that can be used as an index of criterion validity.
- **Construct validity,** a third component in the validity domain, concerns what abstract construct an instrument is actually measuring. One aspect is **hypothesis-testing construct validity**: the extent to which hypotheses about what the instrument is measuring can be supported. Key approaches include **convergent validity**, the degree to which there is conceptual convergence between scores on the focal measure and another measure; **known-groups validity**, the extent to which hypotheses about groups expected to differ on a measure are supported; and **divergent validity**, the extent to which hypotheses about what an instrument does *not* measure are supported.

- Another aspect of construct validity is **structural validity**, which concerns the extent to which evidence supports hypotheses about the dimensionality of a complex construct. A statistical tool called **factor analysis** is used to assess structural validity.
- **Cross-cultural validity,** another aspect of construct validity, concerns the degree to which the items on a translated or culturally adapted scale perform adequately and equivalently in relation to their performance on the original instrument.
- Change is often measured by computing a **change score** that is the difference in value between two measurements. A major issue with change scores is that they tend to amplify measurement error, and hence a third domain in the taxonomy concerns the **reliability of a change score**.
- Two indexes summarize whether a change in a person's score over time is reliable or merely reflects random fluctuations. One is the **smallest detectable change (SDC)**, which is a value that is outside the limits of agreement. The **reliable change index (RCI)** is a similar index that is based on a formula using the standard error of measurement.
- The final domain in the measurement taxonomy is **responsiveness**, which refers to the ability of a measure to detect change over time in a construct that has changed. Responsiveness, the longitudinal analog of validity, can be assessed by testing hypotheses about how changes in the focal measure are consistent with changes in other measures.
- Assessments of responsiveness, like validity, can involve a criterion approach or a construct approach. Some researchers used **health transition ratings** (also called **global rating scales**) as the criterion for change.

STUDY ACTIVITIES

Study activities are available to instructors on thePoint

REFERENCES CITED IN CHAPTER 15

Ambrosio, L., Portillo, M., Rodriguez-Blazquez, C., Martinez-Castillo, J., Rodriguez-Violante, M., Serrano-Duenas, M., … Martinez-Martin, P. (2016). Satisfaction with Life Scale (SLS-6): First validation study in Parkinson's disease population. *Parkinsonism & Related Disorder, 25,* 52–57.

*Bikker, A., Fitzpatrick, B., Murphy, D., Foster, L., & Mercer, S. (2017). Assessing the consultation and relational empathy (CARE) measure in sexual nurses' consultations. *BMC Nursing, 16,* 71.

Bland, J. M. & Altman, D. G. (1986). Statistical methods for assessing agreement between two methods of clinical measurement. *Lancet, 327,* 307–310.

Bond, S., Dietrich, M., Gilbert, J., Ely, E., Jackson, J., & Murphy, B. (2016). Neurocognitive function in patients with head and neck cancer undergoing primary or adjuvant chemoradiation treatment. *Supportive Care in Cancer, 24,* 4433–4442.

Bowen, M., Rowe, M., Wesek, M., Ibrahim, S., & Shea, J. (2017). The Physical and Cognitive Performance Test for residents in assisted living facilities. *Journal of the American Geriatric Society, 65,* 1543–1548.

Brod, M., Tesler, L., & Christensen, T. (2009). Qualitative research and content validity: Developing best practices based on science and experience. *Quality of Life Research, 18,* 1263–1278.

*Campbell, D. T., & Fiske, D. W. (1959). Convergent and discriminant validation by the multitrait-multimethod matrix. *Psychological Bulletin, 56,* 81–105.

Cella, D., Gershon, R., Lai, J., & Choi, S. (2007). The future of outcome measurement: Item banking, tailored short forms, and computerized adaptive testing. *Quality of Life Research, 16*(Suppl. 1), 133–141.

**Cho, J., Holditch-Davis, D., Su, X., Phillips, V., Biasini, F., & Carlo, W. (2017). Associations between hormonal biomarkers and cognitive, motor, and language developmental status in very low birth weight infants. *Nursing Research, 66,* 350–358.

Ciupitu-Plath, C., Wiegand, S., & Babitsch, B. (2018). The Weight Bias Internalization Scale for Youth: Validation of a specific tool for assessing internalized weight bias among treatment-seeking German adolescents with overweight. *Journal of Pediatric Psychology, 43,* 40–51.

Coleman, S., Smith, I., McGinnis, E., Keen, J., Muir, D., Wilson, L., … Nixon, J. (2018). Clinical evaluation of a new pressure ulcer risk assessment instrument, the Pressure Ulcer Risk Primary or Secondary Evaluation Tool (PURPOSE T). *Journal of Advanced Nursing, 74,* 407–424.

Curley, M., Hasbani, N., Quigley, S., Stellar, J., Pasek, T., Shelley, S., … Wypij, D. (2018). Predicting pressure injury risk in pediatric patients: The Braden QD scale. *The Journal of Pediatrics, 192,* 189–195.

DeVellis, R. F. (2017). *Scale development: Theory and application* (4th ed.). Thousand Oaks, CA: Sage Publications.

DeVet, H. C. W., Terwee, C., Mokkink, L. B., & Knol, D. L. (2011). *Measurement in medicine: A practical guide.* Cambridge: Cambridge University Press.

Egger-Rainer, A. (2018). Determination of content validity of the Epilepsy Monitoring Unit Comfort Questionnaire using the content validity index. *Journal of Nursing Measurement, 26*, 398–410.

Folstein, M., Folstein, S., White, T., & Messer, M. (2010). *MMSE-2: User's manual.* Lutz, FL: PAR.

*Francis, D. O., McPheeters, M., Noud, M., Penson, D., & Feurer, I. (2016). Checklist to operationalize measurement characteristics of patient-reported outcome measures. *Systematic Reviews, 5*, 129.

Holmes, T. H., & Rahe, R. (1967). The Social Readjustment Rating Scale. *Journal of Psychosomatic Research, 11*, 213–218.

Jacobson, N. S., Follette, W. C., & Revenstorf, D. (1984). Psychotherapy outcome research: Methods for reporting variability and evaluating clinical significance. *Behavior Therapy, 15*, 336–352.

Jacobson, N. S., & Truax, P. (1991). Clinical significance: A statistical approach to defining meaningful change in psychotherapy research. *Journal of Consulting and Clinical Psychology, 59*, 12–19.

*Jurgens, C., Lee, C., & Riegel, B. (2017). Psychometric analysis of the Heart Failure Somatic Perception Scale as a measure of patient symptom perception. *Journal of Cardiovascular Nursing, 32*, 140–147.

Lee, L., Chinna, K., Bulgiba, A., Abdullah, K., Abidin, I., & Hofer, S. (2016). Test-retest reliability of HeartQOL and its comparability to the MacNew heart disease health-related quality of life questionnaire. *Quality of Life Research, 25*, 351–357.

*Martin, C., Martin, C., & Redshaw, M. (2017). The Birth Satisfaction Scale-Revised Indicator (BSS-RI). *BMC Pregnancy & Childbirth, 17*, 277.

Mokkink, L. B., Terwee, C., Patrick, D., Alonso, J., Stratford, P., Knol, D. L., ... DeVet, H. C. W. (2010a). The COSMIN study reached international consensus on taxonomy, terminology, and definitions of measurement properties for health-related patient-reported outcomes. *Journal of Clinical Epidemiology, 63*, 737–745.

*Mokkink, L. B., Terwee, C., Patrick, D., Alonso, J., Stratford, P., Knol, D. L., ... DeVet, H. C. W. (2010b). The COSMIN checklist for assessing the methodological quality of studies on measurement properties of health status instruments: An international Delphi study. *Quality of Life Research, 19*, 539–549.

Nunnally, J., & Bernstein, I. H. (1994). *Psychometric theory* (3rd ed.). New York: McGraw-Hill.

Olsen, L., Ishikawa, T., Masse, L., Chan, G., & Brussoni, M. (2018). Risk Engagement and Protection Survey (REPS): Developing a validating a survey tool on fathers' attitudes towards child injury protection and risk engagement. *Injury Protection, 24*, 106–112.

Pike, N., Poulsen, M., & Woo, M. (2017). Validity of the Montreal Cognitive Assessment screener for adolescents and young adults with and without congenital heart disease. *Nursing Research, 66*, 222–230.

Polit, D. F. (2014). Getting serious about test-retest reliability: A critique of retest research and some recommendations. *Quality of Life Research, 23*, 1713–1720.

Polit, D. F., & Beck, C. T. (2006). The content validity index: Are you sure you know what is being reported? *Research in Nursing & Health, 29*, 489–497.

Polit, D. F., Beck, C. T., & Owen, S. V. (2007). Is the CVI an acceptable indicator of content validity? Appraisal and recommendations. *Research in Nursing & Health, 30*, 459–467.

Polit, D. F. & Yang, F. M. (2016). *Measurement and the measurement of change: A primer for health professionals.* Philadelphia: Lippincott.

Radloff, L.S. (1977). The CES-D scale: A self -report depression scale for research in the general population. *Applied Psychological Measurement, 1*, 385–401.

Radwin, L., Cabral, H., Seibert, M., Stolzmann, K., Meterko, M., Evans, L., ... Bokhour, B. (2019). Patient-centered care in primary care scale: Pilot development and psychometric assessment. *Journal of Nursing Care Quality, 34*, 34–39.

Riegel, B., Barbaranelli, C., Carlson, B., Sethares, K., Daus, M., Moser, D., ... Vellone, E. (2019). Psychometric testing of the Revised Self-Care of Heart Failure Index. *Journal of Cardiovascular Nursing, 34*(2), 183–192.

Shadish, W. R., Cook, T. D., & Campbell, D. T. (2002). *Experimental and quasi-experimental designs for generalized causal inference.* Boston, MA: Houghton Mifflin Co.

Streiner, D. L. (2003). Being inconsistent about consistency: When coefficient alpha does and doesn't matter. *Journal of Personality Assessment, 80*, 217–222.

Terwee, C. B., Dekker, F., Wiersinga, W., Prummel, M., & Bossuyt, P. (2003). On assessing responsiveness of health-related quality of life instruments: Guidelines for instrument evaluation. *Quality of Life Research, 12*, 349–362.

*Terwee, C. B., Mokkink, L. B., Knol, D. L., Ostelo, R., Bouter, L. M., & DeVet, H. C. W. (2012). Rating the methodological quality in systematic reviews of studies on measurement properties: A scoring system for the COSMIN checklist. *Quality of Life Research, 21*, 651–657.

Thoyre, S., Pados, B., Park, J., Estrem, H., McComish, C., & Hodges, E. (2018). The Pediatric Eating Assessment Tool: Factor structure and psychometric properties. *Journal of Pediatric Gastroenterology and Nutrition, 66*, 299–305.

Wong, C., Choi, E., Chan, S., Tsu, J., Fan, C., Chu, P., ... Lam, C. (2017). Use of the International Prostate Symptom Score (IPSS) in Chinese male patients with benign prostatic hyperplasia. *The Aging Male, 20*, 241–249.

A link to this open-access article is provided in the Toolkit for Chapter 15 in the **Resource Manual.** ✖

**This journal article is available on the Point *for this chapter.*

16 | Developing and Testing Self-Report Scales

Researchers sometimes are unable to find a suitable instrument to operationalize a construct. This may occur when the construct is new but often results from limitations of existing instruments. This chapter provides an overview of the steps involved in developing high-quality self-report scales. The scope of this chapter is fairly narrow. Specifically, we focus on multi-item reflective scales and, primarily, scales rooted in classical test theory.

> **TIP** The development of high-quality scales is a lengthy, labor-intensive process that requires some statistical sophistication. We urge you to think carefully before embarking on a scale development endeavor and to consider involving a psychometric consultant if you proceed.

BEGINNING STEPS: CONCEPTUALIZATION AND ITEM GENERATION

Conceptualizing the Construct

A sound, insightful conceptualization of the construct to be measured is essential. You will not be able to quantify an attribute adequately if you do not thoroughly understand the **latent trait** (the underlying construct) you wish to capture. For reflective scales, the latent trait is the *cause* of people's responses to questions, which drives their scores on the measure. You cannot develop items to produce the right score if you are unclear about the construct. Thus, the first step in scale development is to become an *expert* on the construct.

Complex constructs have a number of different *dimensions*, and it is important to identify and understand each one. This is partly a content validity consideration: for the scale to be content valid, there must be items representing all facets of the construct. All scales—or subscales of a broader scale—need to be *unidimensional* (measuring a single construct or facet of a construct) and internally consistent.

During the early conceptualization, you also need to think about related constructs that should be differentiated from the target construct. If you are measuring, say, self-esteem, you have to be sure you can differentiate it from similar but distinct constructs, such as self-confidence. In thinking about the dimensions of the target construct, you should be certain that they are truly facets of the construct and not a different construct altogether.

You should also have an explicit conceptualization of the population for whom the scale is intended. For example, a general anxiety scale may not be suitable for measuring childbearing anxiety in pregnant women. There are arguments for developing patient-specific scales, particularly with respect to item relevance and face validity. On the other hand, a highly focused scale reduces the ability to make comparisons across populations. The point is that you should have a clear view of how and with whom the scale will be used. Without a good grasp of the population, it will be difficult to consider such issues as reading levels and cultural appropriateness in wording the items.

Deciding on the Type of Scale

Before items can be generated, you need to decide on the type of scale you wish to create, because item characteristics vary by scale type. Our focus is restricted to multi-item reflective scales, which are also featured in several books on scale development that can be consulted for more detail (DeVellis, 2017; Polit & Yang, 2016; Streiner et al., 2015). Two broad categories of scales fall into this category: traditional summated rating scales and latent trait scales.

Traditional summated rating scales (Chapter 14) are based in classical test theory (CTT). In CTT, items are presumed to be roughly comparable indicators of the underlying construct. The items gain strength in approximating a hypothetical true score through their aggregation. Traditional scales rely on items that are deliberately redundant, in the hope that multiple indicators of the construct will converge on the true score and balance out error.

Item response theory (IRT) is an alternative to CTT that is growing in popularity for scale development. IRT methods are complex and require statistical sophistication. We note a few characteristics of IRT here and provide further information in the Supplement to this chapter on thePoint. 🅢

In CTT, traits are modeled at the level of the observed scale score, whereas in IRT, the models are at the level of observed item responses. The goal of IRT is to allow researchers to gain understanding of the characteristics of items independent of the people who complete them. *Latent trait scales* based on IRT models can use items like the ones used in CTT, such as items in a Likert-type format. In fact, a person completing a scale would likely not know whether it had been developed within the CTT or IRT framework. But a person *developing* a scale must decide which measurement theory is being used. Items on a CTT scale are designed to be similar to each other to tap the underlying construct in a comparable

manner, but items on a latent trait IRT scale tap different levels of the attribute being measured.

As an example, suppose we were developing a scale to measure risk-taking behavior in adolescents. In a CTT scale, the items might include statements about risk-taking of similar intensity, to which respondents would respond with graded responses corresponding to frequency or strength of endorsement. The aggregate of responses would array respondents along a continuum indicating the propensity to take risks. In an IRT scale, the items themselves would be chosen to reflect different levels of risk-taking (e.g., not eating vegetables, smoking cigarettes, having unprotected sex, texting while driving). Each item could be described as having a different *difficulty*. It is "easier" to agree with or admit to lower-risk items than higher-risk items. Measurements based on an IRT model result in information about the *location* of both items and people on a trait continuum. If a pool of unidimensional items can readily be ordered into a hierarchy of difficulty, then a good IRT model fit is plausible.

Generating an Item Pool: Getting Started

An early step in scale construction is to develop a pool of possible items. Items—which collectively constitute the operational definition of the construct—need to be carefully crafted to reflect the latent variable they are designed to measure. This is often easier to do as a team, because different people articulate an idea in diverse ways. Here are some possible sources for generating an **item pool**:

1. *Existing instruments.* Sometimes it is possible to adapt an existing scale rather than starting from scratch. Adaptations may involve adding, deleting, or rewording items—for example, to simplify wording for a population with low reading skills. Permission from the author of the original scale should be sought because published scales are copyright-protected.
2. *The literature.* Ideas for item content often come from a thorough understanding of prior research.
3. *Concept analysis.* A related source of ideas is a concept analysis. Walker and Avant (2019) offer concept analysis strategies that could be used to develop items for a scale.

4. *In-depth qualitative research.* In-depth inquiry relating to the key construct is a rich source of items. A qualitative study can help you to understand the dimensions of a phenomenon and can give you actual phrases for items. If you are unable to undertake an in-depth study, pay attention to the verbatim quotes in published qualitative reports about your construct.

5. *Clinical observations.* Patients in clinical settings may be an excellent source of items. Ideas for items may come from direct observation of patients' behaviors in relevant situations or from listening to their comments.

Example of Sources of Items

Wu and colleagues (2018) developed bone health scales for adolescents with cancer in Mandarin. The items were developed based on a prior qualitative study, theoretical considerations using Social Cognitive Theory, the clinical expertise of the lead researcher, and a review of the literature.

DeVellis (2017) urged scale developers to start writing scale items without a lot of critical review in the early stages. Perhaps a good way to begin if you are struggling is to develop a simple statement with the key construct mentioned in it. For example, if the construct is test anxiety, you might start with, "I get anxious when I take a test." This could be followed by similar statements worded differently (e.g., "Taking tests makes me nervous.").

Making Decisions About Item Features

In preparing to write items, you need to make decisions about such issues as the number of items to develop, the form of the response options, whether to include positively and negatively worded items, and how to deal with time.

Number of Items

In the CTT framework, a **domain sampling model** is assumed, which involves the random sampling of a homogeneous set of items from a hypothetical universe of items on the construct. Of course, sampling from a *universe* of all possible items does not happen in reality. The idea is to generate a fairly exhaustive set of item possibilities, given the construct's theoretical demands. For a traditional scale, redundancy (except for trivial word substitutions) is a good thing. The goal is to measure the construct with a set of items that capture its essence in slightly different ways so that irrelevant aspects of individual items cancel each other out.

There is no magic formula for how many items should be developed, but our advice is to generate a large pool of items. As you proceed, many items will be discarded. Longer scales tend to be more internally consistent, so starting with a large number of items promotes the likelihood of developing an internally consistent scale. DeVellis (2017) recommends starting with 3 to 4 times as many items as you will have in your final scale (e.g., 30-40 items for a 10-item scale), but the minimum should be 50% more (e.g., 15 items for a 10-item scale).

Response Options

Scale items involve both a *stem* (often a declarative statement) and *response options*. Traditional Likert scales involve response options on a continuum of agreement, but other continua are possible, such as frequency (never/always), importance (very important/unimportant), quality (excellent/very poor), and likelihood (definitely/definitely not).

How many response options should there be? There is no simple answer, but keep in mind the goal is to array people on a continuum, and so variability is essential. Variability can be enhanced by including a lot of items, numerous response options, or both. However, there is no merit in creating the illusion of precision when it does not exist. With 15 response options, for example, the difference between a score of 12 and 13 might not be meaningful. Moreover, too many options can be confusing.

Most scales have items with five to seven options, with verbal descriptors attached to each option and, often, numbers placed under the descriptors to further help respondents find an appropriate place on the continuum. An odd number of items give respondents an opportunity to be neutral or ambivalent (i.e., to choose a midpoint). Some scale developers prefer an even number (e.g., 4 or 6) to force even slight tendencies and to avoid equivocation. However, some respondents may actually *be* neutral or ambivalent, so a midpoint option allows them to express it. The midpoint can be labeled with such phrases as "neither agree nor disagree," "undecided," "agree and disagree equally," or simply "?".

> **TIP** Here are some frequently used words for response options, with midpoint terms not listed:
> - Strongly disagree, disagree, agree, strongly agree
> - Never, almost never (or rarely), sometimes (or occasionally), often (or frequently), almost always (or always)
> - Very important, important, somewhat important, of little importance, unimportant
> - Definitely not, probably not, possibly, probably, very probably, definitely
> - With no trouble, with a little trouble, with some trouble, with a lot of trouble, not able to do

Positive and Negative Stems

A generation ago, psychometricians advised scale developers to deliberately include both positively and negatively worded statements and to reverse-score negative items. As an example, consider these two items for a scale of depression: "I frequently feel blue," and "I rarely feel sad." The objective was to include items that would minimize the possibility of an acquiescence response set—the tendency to agree with statements regardless of their content.

Many experts currently advise against including negative and positive items on a scale. Some respondents are confused by reversing polarities. Responding to item with negative stems appears to be an especially difficult cognitive task for younger respondents. Some research suggests that acquiescence can be minimized by putting the most positive response options (e.g., strongly agree) at the end of the list rather than at the beginning.

Item Intensity

In a traditional summated rating scale, the intensity of the statements (stems) should be similar and fairly strongly worded. If items are worded such that almost anyone would agree with them, the scale will not be able to discriminate between people with different amounts of the underlying

trait. For example, an item such as "Good health is important" would generate almost universal agreement. On the other hand, statements should not be so extremely worded as to result in universal rejection. For a latent trait scale, scale developers seek a range of item intensities. Yet, even on an IRT-based scale, there is no point in including items with which almost everyone would either agree or disagree.

Item Time Frames

Some items make an explicit reference to time (e.g., "In the past week I have had trouble falling asleep"), but others do not (e.g., "I have trouble falling asleep"). Sometimes instructions to a scale can designate a temporal frame of reference (e.g., "In answering the following questions, please indicate how you have felt in the past week"). And yet other scales ask respondents to respond in terms of a time frame: "In the past week, I have had trouble falling asleep: Every day, 5-6 days…Never."

A time frame should not emerge as a consequence of item development. You should decide in advance, based on your conceptual understanding of the construct and the needs for which the scale is being constructed, how to deal with time.

> **Example of Handling Time in a Scale**
> The Postpartum Depression Screening Scale asks respondents to indicate their emotional state in the previous 2 weeks—for example, over the last 2 weeks I: "…had trouble sleeping even when my baby was asleep" and "…felt like a failure as a mother" (Beck & Gable, 2000, 2001). The 2-week period was chosen because it parallels the duration of symptoms required for a diagnosis of major depressive episode according to the DSM-V criteria.

Wording the Items

In addition to the suggestions on question wording, we provided in Chapter 14, some additional tips specific to scale items are as follows:

1. *Clarity.* Scale developers should strive for clear, unambiguous items. Words should be chosen with the educational and reading level of the target population in mind. In most cases, this

means developing a scale at about the seventh grade reading level. You should use words that everyone understands and strive to have everyone reach the same conclusion about what the words mean.

2. *Length.* Avoid long sentences or phrases and eliminate unnecessary words. For example, "It is fair to say that in the scheme of things I do not get enough sleep," could more simply be worded, "I do not get enough sleep."

3. *Double negatives.* It is preferable to word things affirmatively ("I am usually happy" than negatively ("I am not usually sad"), but double negatives should always be avoided ("I am *not* usually *un*happy").

4. *Double-barreled items.* Avoid putting two or more ideas in a single item. For example, "I am afraid of insects and snakes" is a bad item because a person who is afraid of insects but not snakes (or vice versa) would not know how to respond.

> **TIP** Here are some tips for scale developers who anticipate a translation into another language: (1) avoid metaphors, idioms, and colloquialisms; (2) use specific words rather than ones open to interpretation (e.g., "daily" rather than "frequently"); (3) avoid pronouns—repeat nouns to avoid ambiguity; (4) write in the present tense and avoid the subjunctive mode; and (5) use words with a Latin root if translation into a Romance language is expected (Hilton & Skrutkowski, 2002).

PRELIMINARY EVALUATION OF ITEMS

Internal Review

Once a large item pool has been generated, it is time for critical appraisal. Care should be devoted to such issues as whether individual items capture the construct, are grammatical, and are well-worded. The initial review should also consider whether the items taken together adequately embrace the nuances of the construct.

It is imperative to assess the scale's **readability**, unless the scale is intended for a highly educated

population. There are different approaches for assessing the reading level of written documents, but many methods require several hundreds of words of text and thus are not suited to evaluating scale items.

Many word processing programs provide some information about readability. In Microsoft Word, for example, you could type your items on a list and then get readability statistics for the items as a whole or for individual items, as described in Chapter 7. For example, take the following two sets of items for measuring fatigue:

Set A	Set B
I am frequently exhausted.	I am often tired.
I invariably get insufficient sleep.	I don't get enough sleep.

The Word software tells us that the items in set A have a *Flesch–Kincaid grade level* of 12.0 and a *Flesch reading ease score* of 4.8. (Reading ease scores rate text on a 100-point scale, with higher values associated with greater ease.) Set B, by contrast, has a grade level of 1.8 and a reading ease score of 89.4. Streiner et al. (2015) warn that word processing–based readability scores should be interpreted cautiously, but it is clear from the foregoing analysis that the second set of items would be superior for a population that includes people with limited education. A general principle is to avoid long sentences and words with four or more syllables.

> **Example of Assessing Readability**
> Moser and colleagues (2017) carefully developed a measure of diabetic peripheral neuropathy symptoms for youth aged 8 to 17 years. Items were assessed for readability using the Flesch–Kincaid reading level test. On average, items were written at a third-grade level. The researchers presented a table that showed the reading level of all 25 items.

Input From the Target Population

In the next step, the initial pool of items is pretested. In a conventional pretest, a small sample (20-40 people) representing the target population is invited to complete the items. Researchers then look for items with high rates of nonresponse, items with limited variability, items with numerous midpoint responses (fence-sitting), or items with the majority of responses at either extreme (*floor effects* or *ceiling effects*). Such items are candidates for deletion or revision.

Developments in cognitive science over the past 25 years have paved the way for a different approach to pretesting, often as a supplement to standard pretests. In **cognitive questioning**, people are asked to reflect upon their interpretation of the items and their answers so that the underlying process of response selection is better understood.

There are two basic approaches to cognitive interviewing. One is called the **think-aloud method**, wherein respondents are asked to explain step-by-step how they processed the question and arrived at an answer. A second approach is to conduct an interview in which the interviewer uses a series of targeted **probes** that encourage reflection about underlying cognitive processes. The Toolkit offers suggestions for cognitive questioning. ❇

> **Example of Cognitive Questioning**
> Gibbs and an interprofessional team (2017) used cognitive questioning with 12 patients with a chronic disease to guide revisions to the Nutrition Literacy Assessment instrument for use in primary care. The researchers presented a table that summarized themes that emerged during the interviews and the revision decisions that resulted. In all, 17 items were modified and 5 items were deleted.

TIP When questioning pretest respondents about the clarity or meaning of the items, avoid using the word "item," which is research jargon (e.g., do not say, "Did any *items* confuse you?").

As an alternative or supplement to pretests, *focus groups* can also be used at this stage in scale development. Two or three groups can be convened to discuss whether, from the respondents' perspective, the items are understandable, linguistically and culturally appropriate, inoffensive, and relevant to the construct.

External Review by Experts

External review of the revised items by a panel of experts should be undertaken to assess the scale's **content validity**. It is advisable to undertake two rounds of review, if feasible—the first to refine or remove faulty items or to add new items and the second to formally assess the content validity of the items and scale. We discuss some procedures for such a two-step strategy.

Selecting and Recruiting the Experts

The panel of experts should include people with strong credentials regarding the construct being measured and the target population. In the first round, it is also desirable to include experts on scale construction.

In the initial phase of a two-part review, we advise having an expert panel of 8 to 12 members, with a good mix in terms of roles (e.g., clinicians, researchers) and disciplines. For example, for a scale designed to measure fear of dying in the elderly, the experts might include nurses, gerontologists, and psychiatrists. If the scale is intended for broad use, it might be advantageous to recruit experts from various regions because of possible regional variations in language. The second panel for formally assessing the content validity of a more refined set of items should consist of three to five experts in the content area.

> **Example of an Expert Panel**
> Sanchez and colleagues (2019) developed a scale to measure barriers to seeking frequent dental care among patients with cardiovascular disease. An expert panel of clinicians, educators, and academics in the fields of dentistry, cardiology, and allied health reviewed the scale for content validity.

Experts are typically sent materials that include a cover letter, background information about the construct and target population, reviewer instructions, and a questionnaire soliciting their opinion. A critical component of the packet is a careful explanation of the construct's conceptualization, including an explication of the construct's dimensions that would be captured in subscales.

TIP The Toolkit section of the *Resource Manual* includes a sample cover letter and other material relating to expert review.

Preliminary Expert Review: Content Validation of Items

The experts' job is to evaluate individual items and the overall scale (and any subscales), using guidelines established by the scale developer. The first panel of experts is usually invited to rate each item along several dimensions, such as clarity of wording, relevance of the item to the construct, and appropriateness for the target population (e.g., developmental or cultural appropriateness). Experts can be asked to make judgments dichotomously (e.g., ambiguous/clear) or along a continuum. As noted in the previous chapter, relevance is most often rated as follows: 1 = *not relevant*, 2 = *somewhat relevant*, 3 = *quite relevant*, and

4 = *highly relevant*. Table 16.1 shows a possible format for a content validation assessment of relevance.

The questionnaire usually asks for detailed comments about items judged to be unclear, not relevant, or not appropriate, such as how wording might be improved, or why the item is deemed not to be relevant. In a first phase, experts are sometimes asked for overall recommendations—for example, retain the item exactly as worded, make major revisions to the item, make minor revisions to the item, and drop the item entirely.

In addition to evaluating each item, the initial expert panel should be asked whether the items taken together adequately cover the construct domain. Experts should be asked for specific guidance on items or subdomains that should be added. For scales constructed within an IRT framework, experts can also be asked whether the items span a continuum of difficulty.

TABLE 16.1 • Example of a Content Validation Form

The scale items shown below have been developed to measure one dimension of the construct of safe sexual behaviors among adolescents, namely **assertiveness.** Please read each item and score it for its relevance in representing this concept.

Assertiveness is defined as the use of verbal and interpersonal skills to negotiate protection during sexual activities.

Item	Not Relevant	Somewhat Relevant	Quite Relevant	Highly Relevant
1. I ask my partner about his/her sexual history before having intercourse.	1	2	3	4
2. I don't have sex without asking the person if he/she has been tested for HIV/AIDS.	1	2	3	4
3. When I am having sex with someone for the first time, I insist that we use a condom.	1	2	3	4
4. I don't let my partner talk me into having sex without knowing something about how risky it would be.	1	2	3	4

Please comment on any of these items, including possible revisions or substitutions, or your thoughts about why an item is not relevant to the concept of assertiveness. Please suggest any additional items you feel would improve the measurement of assertiveness relating to adolescents' safe sexual behaviors.

The standard method for computing an item-level **content validity index** (I-CVI) is the number giving a rating of 3 or 4 on the 4-point relevance scale, divided by the number of experts. For example, if five experts rated an item as 3 and one rated the item as 2, the I-CVI would be .83. Because of the risk of chance agreement, we recommend I-CVIs of .78 or higher (Polit et al., 2007). This means that when there are four or fewer experts, there must be 100% agreement. When there are five to eight experts, one rating of "not relevant" can be tolerated.

Items with lower-than-desired I-CVIs need careful scrutiny. If there are disagreements among the experts on individual items (or if there is agreement about lack of relevance), the items should be revised or dropped.

Content Validation of the Scale

In the second round of content validation, a smaller group of experts (3-5) can be used to evaluate the relevance of the revised set of items and to compute the scale content validity (S-CVI). Although it is possible to use a new group of experts, we recommend using a subset from the first panel—information from the first round can be used to select the most qualified judges. With information from round 1, for example, you can perhaps identify experts who did not understand the task, who were not as familiar with the construct as you thought, or who seemed biased. In other words, data from the first round can be analyzed with a view toward evaluating the performance of the experts, not just the items.

Here are a few considerations when selecting experts based on their ratings in the first round. First, experts who rated every item as "highly relevant" (or "not relevant") may not be sufficiently discriminating. Second, consider omitting an expert who gave high ratings to items that were judged by most others to not be relevant. Third, the proportion of items judged relevant should be computed for all judges. For example, if an expert rated 8 out of 10 items as relevant, the proportion for that judge would be .80. The pattern across experts can be examined for "outliers." If the average proportion

across raters is, for example, .80, you might consider not inviting back experts whose average proportion was either very low (e.g., .50) or very high (e.g., 1.00). Useful qualitative feedback from an expert in round 1 might indicate both content capability and a commitment to the project. Finally, items known *not* to be relevant can be included in the first round to identify judges who wrongly say the items are relevant and so may not really be experts.

After ratings of relevance are obtained for a revised set of items, the S-CVI can be computed. There is more than one way to compute an S-CVI. We recommend the approach that averages across I-CVIs. On a 10-item scale, for example, if the I-CVIs for 5 items were .80 and the I-CVIs for the remaining 5 items were 1.00, then the S-CVI/Ave would be .90. An S-CVI/Ave of .90 or higher is desirable.

In summary, a scale can be judged to have excellent content validity if all its items have I-CVIs of .78 or higher and the scale has an S-CVI (using the averaging approach) of .90 or higher. This requires strong items, skillful experts, and clear instructions to the experts regarding the underlying constructs and the rating task.

> **TIP** When you describe content validation in a report, be specific about your criteria for accepting items (i.e., the cutoff value for your I-CVIs and the S-CVI). The report should indicate the range of obtained I-CVI values, and the method used to compute the S-CVI.

FIELD TESTING THE INSTRUMENT

At this point, you will have whittled down and refined your items based on your own and others' careful scrutiny. The next step is to undertake a quantitative assessment of the items, which requires that they be administered to a fairly large assessment sample. Testing a new instrument is a full study in and of itself, and care must be taken to design the study to yield useful evidence about the scale's worth. Important steps include the development of a sampling plan and data collection strategy.

Developing a Sampling Plan

The sample for testing the scale should be representative of the population for whom the scale is intended and should be large enough to support complex analyses. If it is not possible to administer the items to a random sample (as is typical), it is advantageous to recruit a sample from multiple sites to enhance representativeness and to assess geographic variation in responding to items. Other strategies to enhance representativeness should be sought, as well—for example, making sure that the sample includes older and younger respondents, men and women, people with varying educational and ethnic backgrounds, and so on, if these characteristics are relevant. You may also need to take steps to ensure that the sample includes the right subgroups of people for a "known-groups" validation.

How large is a "large" sample? There is neither consensus among experts nor hard-and-fast rules. Some suggest that 300 is an adequate number to support a factor analysis (Nunnally & Bernstein, 1994), whereas others offer guidance in terms of a ratio of items to respondents. Ten people per item are often recommended. That means that if you have 20 items, your sample should be at least 200. Having a sufficiently large sample is essential to ensure stability in estimating inter-item relationships. For assessments of test–retest reliability, a smaller subsample of participants (e.g., 50-100) is usually sufficient.

You should make efforts to recruit a sample that is heterogeneous on the target attribute. Reliability and internal consistency estimates are dampened when the scores are not sufficiently diverse.

Developing a Data Collection Plan

A decision has to be made concerning how to administer the instrument (e.g., by mail, over the Internet). You should choose an approach that best approximates how the scale typically would be administered after it is finalized.

The instrument should include the scale items and basic demographic information. If the intent is to estimate test–retest reliability, then contact information needs to be obtained for scheduling the second administration—and the same is true if the reliability of change scores and responsiveness are being assessed.

Thought also needs to be given to including other measures for validity assessments, if validation efforts are carried out with the development sample. Measures of constructs hypothesized to be correlated with the target construct usually should be included. If the data confirm a relationship predicted by theory or prior research, this would lend evidence to the new scale's validity.

> **TIP** In deciding on what other measures to administer, keep in mind that respondents' willingness to cooperate may decline as the instrument gets longer.

Preparing for Data Collection

As with all data collection efforts, care should be taken to make the instrument attractive, professional-looking, and easy to understand. Instructions for completing the instrument should be clear and a readability assessment should be undertaken. Guidance in understanding the endpoints of response options might be needed if points along the continuum are not explicitly labeled. The instructions should encourage candor. Sometimes social desirability can be minimized by stating that there are no right or wrong answers.

One other consideration is how to sequence the items in the instrument. At issue is something that is called a *proximity effect*, the tendency to be influenced in responding to an item by the response given to the previous item. This effect would tend to artificially inflate estimates of internal consistency. One approach to deal with this is the random ordering of items. An alternative, for scales designed to measure several related dimensions, is to systematically alternate items that are expected to be scored into different subscales.

ANALYSIS OF SCALE DEVELOPMENT DATA

The analysis of data from multi-item scales is a topic about which entire books have been written. We provide only an overview. We assume that readers of this section have basic familiarity with statistics. Those who need a refresher should consult Chapters 17-19.

Basic Item Analysis

Each item on the preliminary scale needs to be evaluated empirically in an **item analysis**. Within classical test theory, what is desired is an item that has a high correlation with the true score of the underlying construct. We cannot assess this directly, but if each item is a measure of that construct, then the items should correlate with one another.

The degree of **inter-item correlation** can be assessed by inspecting the *correlation matrix* of all the items. If there are items with substantial negative intercorrelations, some should perhaps be *reverse-scored*. Unless intentional, however, negative correlations are likely to reflect problems and may signal the need to remove items. For items on the same subscale, inter-item correlations between .30 and .70 are recommended, with correlations lower than .30 suggesting little congruence with the underlying construct and ones higher than .70 suggesting over-redundancy. However, the evaluation depends on the number of items in the scale. An average inter-item correlation of .57 is needed to achieve a coefficient alpha of .80 on a 3-item scale, but an average of only .29 is needed for a 10-item scale (DeVellis, 2017).

A next step is to compute preliminary total scale or subscale scores and then calculate correlations between items and total scores on the subscales they are intended to represent. If item scores do not correlate well with scale scores, the item is probably measuring something else and will lower the reliability of the scale. There are two types of **item-scale correlations**, one in which the total score includes the item under consideration (*uncorrected*) and another in which the item is removed in calculating the total scale score. The latter (*corrected*) approach is preferable because the inclusion of the item on the scale inflates the correlation coefficients. The standard advice is to eliminate items whose item-scale correlation is less than .30.

Descriptive information for each item should also be examined. Items should have good variability—without it, they will not correlate with the total scale and will dampen internal consistency. Means for the items that are close to the center of the range of possible scores are also desirable (e.g., a mean near 4 on a 7-point scale). Items with means near one extreme or the other tend not to discriminate well among respondents; also, such items may perform poorly if a goal is to assess changes because there may be no room for further improvement or deterioration (i.e., *floor* or *ceiling effects*).

Example of an Item Analysis

Burchill and colleagues (2018) performed an item analysis in their field testing of the Personal Workplace Safety Instrument for Emergency Nurses (PWSI-EN). Their sample consisted of 305 emergency nurses from 16 hospitals. They eliminated two items whose item-total correlations were low (both <.15).

Exploratory Factor Analysis

A set of items is not necessarily a scale—the items form a scale only if they have a common underlying construct. **Factor analysis** disentangles complex interrelationships among items and identifies items that "go together" as unified concepts. This section deals with a type of factor analysis known as **exploratory factor analysis (EFA)**, which essentially assumes no a priori hypotheses about the dimensionality of a set of items.

Suppose we developed 50 items measuring women's attitudes toward menopause. We could form a scale by adding together scores from several individual items, but which items should be combined? Would it be reasonable to combine all 50 items? Probably not, because the 50 items are not all tapping the same thing—there are various *dimensions* to women's attitude toward menopause. One dimension may relate to aging and another to loss of reproductive ability. Other items may involve sexuality. These multiple dimensions to women's attitudes toward menopause should be measured on separate subscales. Women's attitude on one dimension may be independent of their attitude on another. Dimensions of a construct are usually identified during initial conceptualization and content validation. Preconceptions about dimensions, however, do not always "pan out" when tested against actual responses. Factor analysis offers an objective method of clarifying the underlying dimensionality of a set of items. Underlying dimensions in the analysis are called **factors**, which are weighted combinations of items.

> **TIP** Before undertaking an EFA, you should evaluate the *factorability* of your set of items. Procedures for a factorability assessment are described in Polit (2010) and Polit and Yang (2016).

Factor Extraction

EFA involves two phases. The first phase (**factor extraction**) condenses items into a smaller number of factors and is used to identify the number of underlying dimensions. The goal is to extract clusters of highly interrelated items from a correlation matrix. There are various methods of performing the first step, each of which uses different criteria for assigning weights to items. A widely used factor extraction method is **principal components analysis (PCA)** and another is **principal axis factor analysis**. Our discussion focuses mostly on PCA, although the two methods often lead to the same conclusion about dimensionality.

Factor extraction yields an *unrotated factor matrix*, which contains coefficients or *weights* for all original items on each extracted factor. Each extracted factor is a weighted linear combination of all the original items. For example, with three items, a factor would be item 1 (times a weight) + item 2 (times a weight) + item 3 (times a weight). In the PCA method, weights for the first factor are computed such that the average squared weight is maximized—this permits a maximum amount of variance to be extracted by that factor. The second factor, or linear weighted combination, is formed so that the highest possible amount of variance is extracted from what *remains* after the first factor. The factors thus represent independent sources of variation in the data matrix.

Factoring should continue until no further meaningful variance is left—a criterion must be applied to decide when to stop extraction. Several criteria can be described by illustrating information from a factor analysis. Table 16.2 presents fictitious values for eigenvalues, percentages of variance accounted for, and cumulative percentages of variance accounted

TABLE 16.2 • Summary of Factor Extraction results

FACTOR	EIGENVALUE	PERCENTAGE OF VARIANCE EXPLAINED	CUMULATIVE PERCENTAGE OF VARIANCE EXPLAINED
1	12.32	29.2	29.2
2	8.57	23.3	52.5
3	6.91	15.6	68.1
4	2.02	8.4	76.5
5	1.09	6.2	82.7
6	0.98	5.8	88.5
7	0.80	4.5	93.0
8	0.62	3.1	96.1
9	0.47	2.2	98.3
10	0.25	1.7	100.0

for, for 10 factors. **Eigenvalues** are equal to the sum of the squared item weights for the factor. Many researchers establish as their cutoff point for extraction eigenvalues of 1.0 or greater. In our example, the first five factors meet this criterion. Another cutoff benchmark, called the *scree test,* is based on discontinuities: A sharp drop in the percentage of explained variance indicates a possible termination point. In Table 16.2, we might argue that there is considerable discontinuity between the third and fourth factors—that is, that three factors should be extracted. Another guideline concerns the amount of variance explained by the factors. Some advocate that the factors extracted should account for at least 60% of the total variance, and that for any factor to be meaningful it must account for at least 5% of the variance. In our table, the first three factors account for 68.1% of the total variance. Six factors contribute 5% or more to the total variance.

So, should we extract three, five, or six factors? One approach is to see whether there is any convergence among the criteria. In our example, two criteria (the scree test and total variance test) suggest three factors. Another approach is to see whether any of the rules yields a number consistent with our original conceptualization. In our example, if we had designed the items to represent three theoretically meaningful subscales, we might consider three factors to be the right number because the data provide sufficient support for that conclusion.

> **TIP** Polit (2010) provides a "walk-through" demonstration of how decisions are made in undertaking an exploratory factor analysis.

Factor Rotation

The second phase of factor analysis—**factor rotation**—is performed on factors that have met extraction criteria, to make the factors more interpretable. The concept of rotation can be best explained graphically. Figure 16.1 shows two coordinate systems, marked by axes A1 and A2 and B1 and B2. The primary axes (A1 and A2) represent factors I and II, respectively, as defined *before* rotation. Points 1 through 6 represent six

items. The weights for each item can be determined in reference to these axes. For instance, before rotation, item 1 has a weight of .80 on factor I and .85 on factor II, and item 6 has a weight of −.45 on factor I and .90 on factor II. Unrotated axes account for a maximum amount of variance, but interpretability is enhanced by rotating the axes so that clusters of items are distinctly associated with a factor. In the figure, B1 and B2 represent rotated factors. After rotation, items 1, 2, and 3 have large weights on factor I and small weights on factor II, and the opposite is true for items 4, 5, and 6.

Researchers choose from two types of rotation. Figure 16.1 illustrates **orthogonal rotation**, in which factors are kept at right angles to one another. Orthogonal rotations maintain the independence of factors—that is, orthogonal factors are uncorrelated with one another. **Oblique rotations** permit rotated axes to depart from a 90-degree angle. In our figure, an oblique rotation would have put axis B1 between items 2 and 3

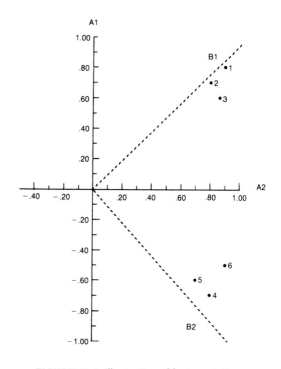

FIGURE 16.1 Illustration of factor rotation.

and axis B2 between items 5 and 6. This placement strengthens the clustering of items around an associated factor but results in correlated factors. Some writers argue that orthogonal rotation leads to greater theoretical clarity; others claim it is unrealistic. Advocates of oblique rotation point out that if the concepts *are* correlated, then the analysis should reflect this fact. In developing a scale with multiple dimensions, we likely would expect the dimensions to be correlated, and so oblique rotation might well be more meaningful. This can be assessed empirically: if an oblique rotation is specified, the correlation between factors is computed. If the correlations are low (e.g., less than .15 or .20), an orthogonal rotation may be preferred because it yields a simpler model.

Researchers work with a **rotated factor matrix** in interpreting the factor analysis. As an example, Table 16.3 shows factor analysis information for the final 12 items on the Uncivil Behavior in Clinical Nursing Education (UBCNE) scale (Anthony et al., 2014). The entries under each factor are the weights or **factor loadings**. For orthogonally rotated factors, factor loadings can range from -1.00 to $+1.00$ and can be interpreted like correlation coefficients—they express the correlation between items and factors. In this example, item 1 is highly correlated with factor 1, .83. By examining factor loadings, we can find which items "belong" to a factor. In this example, items 1, 2, 4, 7, 8, 11, and 12 had sizable loadings on factor 1. Loadings with an absolute value of .40 or higher often are used as cutoff values, but somewhat smaller values may be acceptable if it makes theoretical sense to do so. The underlying dimensionality of the items can then be interpreted. By inspecting the content of these seven items, we can search for a common theme that makes them "go together." The developers of the UBCNE called this first factor *Hostile/Mean/Dismissive.* Items 3, 5, 6, 9, and 10 had high loadings on factor 2, which they named *Exclusionary Behavior.* The naming of factors is a process of identifying underlying constructs—this naming often would have occurred during the conceptualization phase.

The results of the factor analysis can be used not only to identify the dimensionality of the construct but also to make decisions about item retention and deletion. If items have low loadings on all factors, they likely are good candidates for deletion (or revision, if you can detect wording problems that may have caused different respondents to infer different

TABLE 16.3 • Factor Loadings: Uncivil Behavior in Clinical Nursing Education

HOW OFTEN HAVE YOU HAD A SITUATION WHERE A NURSE:	FACTOR 1	FACTOR 2
1. Embarrassed you …	**.83**[a]	.18
2. Rolled their eyes at you	**.73**	.30
3. Gave you an incomplete report	.02	**.70**
4. Used an inappropriate tone …	**.77**	.19
5. Avoided taking a report from you	.24	**.75**
6. Avoided giving you a report	.21	**.82**
7. Made snide remarks …	**.58**	.30
8. Raised their voice …	**.76**	.23
9. Did not involve you in a patient care decision …	.23	**.70**
10. Did not pass on patient information …	.18	**.78**
11. Told you that you were incompetent	**.82**	$-.07$
12. Refused to help you	**.77**	.18

Adapted from Table 6 and Appendix B of Anthony, M., Yastik, J., MacDonald, D., & Marshall, K. (2014). Development and validation of a tool to measure incivility in clinical nursing education. *Journal of Professional Nursing, 30*, 48–55.

[a]High loadings are bolded; these are the ones used to name and interpret the factors. Factor 1 was named *Hostile/Mean/Dismissive* and factor 2 was named *Exclusionary Behavior.*

meanings). Items with high loadings on multiple factors may also be candidates for deletion. In the development of the UBCNE, the researchers deleted six items that had high loadings on more than one factor (e.g., "Told you to go ask your instructor"). Items with marginal loadings (e.g., .35) but that had good content validity could be retained for the internal consistency analysis.

> **TIP** If you have a very large sample, consider dividing the sample in half at random, running the factor analysis and internal consistency analysis with one subsample, and then rerunning them with the second one as a cross-validation.

> **Example of an Exploratory Factor Analysis**
> Shin and colleagues (2018) developed a scale to measure menstrual health in adolescent girls in Korea and tested it with a sample of 230 students. After eliminating 10 items through item analysis, the researchers did an EFA on the remaining 29 items. Five theoretically meaningful factors were extracted.

Internal Consistency Analysis

After a final set of items is selected based on the item and factor analysis results, an analysis should be undertaken to calculate coefficient alpha. Alpha, it may be recalled, provides an estimate of a key measurement property of multi-item scales: internal consistency reliability.

Most general-purpose statistical programs calculate the value of coefficient alpha for the full scale—and for a hypothetical scale when each individual item is removed. If the overall alpha is extremely high, it may be prudent to eliminate redundancy by deleting items that do not make a large contribution to alpha. (Sometimes removal of a faulty item actually *increases* alpha.) A modest reduction in reliability is sometimes worth the benefit of lowering respondent burden. Scale developers must consider the best trade-off between brevity and internal consistency.

Internal consistency estimates tend to capitalize on chance factors in a sample of respondents and may be lower in a new sample. Thus, you should aim for alphas that are a bit higher in the development sample than ones you would consider minimally acceptable so that if the alphas decay they will still be adequate. This is especially true if the development sample is small.

Test–Retest Reliability Analysis

Although test–retest reliability analysis has not been a standard feature of psychometric assessment in nursing research, we urge developers of new scales to gather information about both internal consistency and test–retest reliability. The COSMIN group considers test–retest reliability a particularly important indicator of a scale's quality.

An issue of importance in a retest study is the timing of the retest relative to the initial administration. Timing decisions must balance the risks for different potential sources of error. When the time interval is too brief, carryover effects (the memory of answers on the previous measurement and the desire to be consistent) can lead to artificially high estimates of reliability. But other factors—including true change—could depress reliability coefficients. Some experts advise that the time interval between measurements should be in the vicinity of 1 to 2 weeks. Polit (2014) has offered several suggestions for strategies to improve decision-making about the retest interval and for basing decisions on evidence or theory about an attribute's stability, rather than assumptions. She also provides guidance on using test–retest results to identify items that may benefit from revision.

SCALE REFINEMENT AND VALIDATION

In some scale development efforts, the bulk of work is over at this point. For example, if you developed a scale as part of a larger substantive project because you were unable to identify a good measure of a key construct, you may be ready to pursue your substantive analyses. If, however, you are developing a scale for others to use, a few more steps are needed.

Revising the Scale

The analyses undertaken in the development study often suggest the need to revise or add items. For example, if subscale alpha coefficients are lower than .80 or so, consideration should be given to adding items for subsequent testing. In thinking about new items, a good strategy is to examine items that had high factor loadings because they may offer clues for good new items.

Before deciding that your scale is finalized, it is prudent to examine the content of the items in the scale. Sometimes alphas are inflated by items that have similar wording, so decisions about retaining or removing items are best made by also considering content validity information. It may be worthwhile to reexamine the I-CVIs of each item in making final decisions.

Scoring the Scale

Scoring a composite summated rating scale is easy: item scores are typically just added together (with reverse scoring of items, if appropriate) to form subscale scores. Subscale scores are sometimes added together to form total scale scores—although this is not always justifiable. Some scale developers create a total score that is the *average* across items so that the total score is on the same scale as the items. In either case, all items are weighted equally. Such scoring involves an implicit assumption that each item is equally important as a measure of the target construct.

> **TIP** It may sometimes be attractive to have differential weighting of items to reflect differences in the items' contribution to the measure—although weighting usually has been found to have little effect on a scale's measurement properties (Streiner et al., 2015). Thus, unitary weighting of items is typical for most composite scales.

Conducting a Validation Study

Scales designed for use by others require validity assessments. Scale developers who are not able to do a separate validation study should strive to undertake many of the activities described in this section with data from the original development sample. Designing a validation study entails much of the same issues (and advice) as designing a development study, in terms of sample composition, sample size, and data collection strategies. The exception is that if efforts will be made to assess longitudinal measurement properties, a longitudinal design is needed.

Confirmatory Factor Analysis

Confirmatory factor analysis (CFA) is playing an increasingly important role in validation studies. CFA is preferable to EFA as an approach to construct (structural) validity because CFA is a hypothesis-testing approach—testing the hypothesis that the items belong to specific factors, rather than having the dimensionality of a set of items emerge empirically, as in EFA.

CFA is a subset of an advanced class of statistical techniques known as **structural equation modeling** (SEM). CFA differs from EFA in a number of respects, many of which are technical. One concerns the estimation procedure. Many statistical procedures used by nurse researchers employ what is called *least-squares estimation*. In SEM, the estimation procedure is *maximum likelihood estimation*. Least-squares procedures have several stringent assumptions that are generally untenable—for example, the assumption that variables are measured without error. SEM can accommodate measurement error and avoid other restrictions.

CFA involves testing a **measurement model**, which specifies the hypothesized relationships among underlying constructs and the *manifest variables*—that is, the items. Loadings on the factors (the *latent variables*) provide a method for evaluating relationships between observed variables (the items) and unobserved variables (the construct's factors).

We illustrate with an example of a scale designed to measure two aspects of fatigue: physical fatigue and mental fatigue. In the example shown in Figure 16.2, both types of fatigue are captured by five items: items I1 to I5 for physical fatigue and

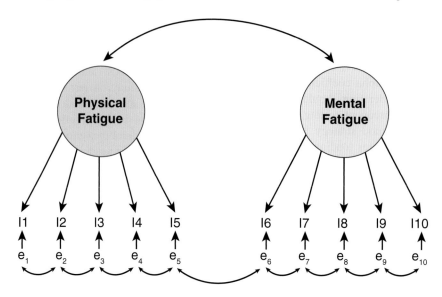

FIGURE 16.2 Example of a measurement model.

items I6 to I10 for mental fatigue. According to the model, item responses are caused by respondents' level of physical and mental fatigue (the straight arrows indicate hypothesized causal paths) and are also affected by error (e_1 through e_{10}). It is expected that error terms are correlated, as indicated by the curved lines connecting the errors. Correlated measurement errors on items might arise from a person's desire to "look good"—a factor that would systematically affect all item scores. The two fatigue constructs also are hypothesized to be correlated.

The hypothesized measurement model would be tested against actual data. The analysis would yield loadings of observed variables on the latent variables, the correlation between the two latent variables, and correlations among the error terms. The analysis would also indicate whether the overall model fit is good, based on several *goodness-of-fit statistics*.

CFA is a complex topic, and we have described only basic characteristics. Further reading on the topic is imperative for those wishing to pursue it (e.g., Brown, 2015; Kline, 2016).

Example of Confirmatory Factor Analysis

Oh and colleagues (2018) assessed the validity of the Arthritis Self-Management Assessment Tool (ASMAT). They used confirmatory factor analysis with a sample of 150 Korean patients to test hypotheses about three domains of self-management. The CFA indicated that the 32-item scale corresponded with the three conceptual constructs of arthritis self-management.

TIP Bott and colleagues (2018) have written an article about free and accessible software (CBID) for performing confirmatory factor analyses and combining patient data with expert data from content validity assessments. A link to the software is provided in the Toolkit.

Other Validation Activities

A validation effort would be incomplete without undertaking additional activities, such as ones described in Chapter 15. The assessment of criterion or construct validity primarily relies on correlational evidence. In criterion-related validity, scores on the new scale are correlated with an external gold standard criterion. In construct validity, scores on the scale can, for example, be correlated with measures of constructs hypothesized to be related to the target construct; or supplementary measures of the same construct (convergent validity); or measures of a closely related but distinguishable construct (divergent validity). Validation using a known-groups approach requires selecting people with membership in groups expected to be different, on average, on the scale. It is desirable to produce as much validity evidence as possible.

> **TIP** If a CFA is not possible, it is still advisable to undertake a "confirmatory" factor analysis using EFA with the validation sample. Comparisons between the original and new factor analyses can be made with respect to factor structure, loadings, variance explained, and so on. In the new analysis, the number of factors to be extracted and rotated can be prespecified, as this is now the working hypothesis about the underlying dimensionality of the construct.

Longitudinal Measurement Properties

In both clinical work and research, measurements of health outcomes are often made on two or more occasions to assess whether a change occurred. Scale developers who anticipate that their scales will be used to measure change should assess the reliability of change scores on the measure and its responsiveness (longitudinal construct validity).

Such assessments inherently require a longitudinal design so that measurements can be made twice. The study should be designed using a population in which change is expected to occur over a specified interval. This may be a population in which deterioration is anticipated (e.g., patients with a progressive disease) or a population receiving a treatment known to be effective. In terms of the time interval between measurements, enough time should have elapsed that one could reasonably expect change on the focal construct for a sizable subset of the sample. However, lengthy time periods may create several problems, including attrition.

Using our definition of responsiveness as longitudinal validity (Chapter 15), it follows that much of the advice we offered with regard to construct validation is relevant here. As with assessments of construct validity, multiple hypothesis tests are desirable for examining a measure's responsiveness—which typically means correlating change scores on the focal measure with change scores on other measures with which a relationship is expected. When a known-groups approach to responsiveness assessment is adopted, comparison groups whose change trajectories are expected to differ are needed. Further advice on testing responsiveness is offered in Polit and Yang (2016).

INTERPRETABILITY OF SCALE SCORES

In addition to the four measurement properties identified in our taxonomy (Figure 15.1), another important aspect of measurement concerns interpretability—that is, understanding what a score *means*. The COSMIN group defined **interpretability** as "the degree to which one can assign qualitative meaning—that is, clinical or commonly understood connotations—to an instrument's quantitative scores or change in scores" (Mokkink et al., 2010, p. 743).

A raw score on a scale is seldom directly interpretable. What does a score of 16 on the Center for Epidemiologic Studies Depression (CES-D) depression scale mean, for example? We briefly discuss some ways to enhance the interpretability of scale scores.

> **TIP** Ideally, if you expect the scale to be used by others, you should create a manual for its use. Guidelines for preparing manuals are published in *Standards for Educational and Psychological Testing* (AERA, APA, & NCME Joint Committee, 2014). Scale developers should consider registering a copyright, even if they do not plan to publish the scale commercially.

Percentiles

Raw score values from a scale can be made more interpretable by converting them to percentiles. A **percentile** indicates the percentage of people who score below a particular score. Percentiles provide information about how a person performs relative to others and are easily interpreted by most people. Percentiles can range from the 0th to the 99th percentile, and the 50th percentile corresponds to the median. Percentile values are most useful when they are determined with a large, representative sample.

Standard Scores

Standard scores transform raw scores into values that have been stripped of the original measurement metric. The transformation makes it possible to compare people on a measure along an easily interpretable scale, without needing to understand the raw score value. Standard scores also make it possible to compare a person's performance on multiple measures with different metrics (e.g., a 10-item fatigue scale and a 5-item pain scale).

Standard scores are expressed in terms of their relative distance from the mean, in standard deviation (*SD*) units. A standard score of .00 corresponds to a raw score at the scale's mean—regardless of what that mean is. A standard score of 1.0 corresponds to a score 1 *SD* above the mean, and a standard score of −1.0 corresponds to a score 1 *SD* below the mean. Standard scores can be readily calculated from raw scores once the mean and *SD* have been calculated (see Chapter 19).

It is often easier to work with score values that do not have negative values and decimal points. Standard scores can be transformed to have any desired mean and *SD*, and certain transformations are particularly common. In particular, standard scores with a mean of 50 and an *SD* of 10 are widely used and are called **T scores.** With T scores, a score of, say, 60, is immediately interpretable, even without knowing much about the scale—it is a score one standard deviation above the mean.

Norms

In some cases, it might be desirable to standardize a new scale and establish norms. This typically occurs if it is expected that the scale will be widely used—and used by people who will rely on comparative information to help them evaluate scores. Norms are often established for key demographic subgroups.

A good sampling plan is critical in a norming effort. The sample should be geographically dispersed and representative of the population for whom the scale is intended. A large standardization sample is required so that subgroup values are stable.

Norms are often expressed in terms of percentiles. For example, an adult male with a score of 72 on the scale might be at the 80th percentile, but a female with the same score might be at the 85th percentile. Nunnally and Bernstein (1994) offer guidelines for norming instruments.

Cutoff Points

Interpretation of scores can often be facilitated if the instrument developer establishes *cutpoints* for classification purposes. Cutpoints are typically used as the basis for making decisions about needed treatments or further assessments. Sometimes cutpoints are defined in terms of percentiles. For example, for children's weights, those below the 5th percentile are considered underweight (or, in infants, "failure to thrive"), whereas those above the 95th percentile are considered overweight. In other cases, the cutpoints are designated with standard scores. For example, the World Health Organization defines osteoporosis as a standard score on a bone mineral density test at or below −2.5, which is 2½ *SD*s below the mean for women in their 30s. Cutpoints that are linked to the measure's distribution are considered *norm-referenced.*

Various methods—both empirical and subjective—have been developed for establishing cutoff points for raw scale scores. As described in Chapter 15, a frequently used method is the construction of receiver operating characteristic (ROC) curves to identify the cutpoint that maximizes and balances sensitivity and specificity. Scale developers who intend to develop ROC curves need to select highly reliable criteria for dividing people into groups (e.g., those with and those without the condition being screened), and the criteria must be independent of participants' responses on the scale.

> **TIP** It may be important to develop guidelines for interpreting *change scores*. If you are developing a scale that will be used to capture change (for example, as an outcome measure in an intervention study), then you should make an effort to establish the value of a *minimal important change* (Chapter 21) and the *smallest detectable change* (Chapter 15) for your scale.

CRITICAL APPRAISAL OF SCALE DEVELOPMENT STUDIES

Articles about scale development appear regularly in nursing journals. If you are planning to use a scale in a substantive study, carefully review the methods used to construct the scale and to evaluate its psychometric adequacy. Remember that you run the risk of undermining the statistical conclusion validity of your study (that is, of having insufficient power for testing your hypotheses) if you use a scale with weak reliability. And you can run the risk of poor construct validity in your study if your measures are not strong proxies for key constructs.

Box 16.1 (also found in the Toolkit) provides broad guidelines for evaluating a research report on the development and validation of a scale.

BOX 16.1 Guidelines for Critically Appraising Scale Development and Assessment Reports

1. Did the report offer a clear definition of the construct being measured? Did it provide sufficient context for the study through a summary of the literature and discussion of relevant theory? Is the population for whom the scale intended adequately described?
2. Did the report indicate how items were generated? Do the procedures seem sound? Was information provided about the reading level of scale items?
3. Did the report describe content validation efforts, and was the description thorough? Is there evidence of good content validity?
4. Were appropriate efforts made to refine the scale (e.g., through pretests, cognitive questioning, item analysis)?
5. Was the development/validation sample of participants appropriate in terms of representativeness, size, and diversity?
6. Was factor analysis used to evaluate or validate the scale's dimensionality? If yes, did the report offer evidence to support the factor structure and the naming of factors?
7. Were appropriate methods used to assess the scale's internal consistency and reliability? Were estimates of reliability and internal consistency sufficiently high?
8. Were appropriate methods used to assess the scale's criterion or construct validity? Is the evidence about the scale's validity persuasive? What other validation methods would have strengthened inferences about the scale's worthiness?
9. Were efforts made to assess the reliability of change scores and the responsiveness of the new measure?
10. Did the report provide information for scoring the scale and interpreting scale scores—for example, means and standard deviations, cutoff scores, norms?

Additionally, many important evaluative questions with regard to reporting and study design for measurement studies have been incorporated into a series of checklists prepared by the COSMIN group (Terwee et al., 2012).

RESEARCH EXAMPLE

In this section we describe the development and testing of a widely used scale that was carefully created by one of this book's authors.

Studies: Postpartum Depression Screening Scale: Development and psychometric testing (Beck & Gable, 2000); Further validation of the Postpartum Depression Screening Scale (Beck & Gable, 2001); Postpartum Depression Screening Scale: Spanish version (Beck & Gable, 2003).

Background: Beck studied postpartum depression (PPD) in a series of qualitative studies, using both phenomenologic and grounded theory approaches. Based on her in-depth understanding of PPD, she sought to develop a scale that could be used to screen for PPD, the Postpartum Depression Screening Scale (PDSS). Beck and an expert psychometrician undertook methodologic studies to develop, refine, and validate the PDSS to screen women for PPD and to translate the scale into Spanish.

Scale development: The PDSS is a summated rating scale designed to tap seven dimensions, such as sleep disturbances, eating disturbances, and mental confusion. A 56-item pilot form of the PDSS was initially developed with 8 items per dimension, using a 5-point response option scale. Themes from Beck's qualitative research were used to craft the items for the seven dimensions. The reading level of the final PDSS was assessed to be at the third-grade level and the Flesch reading ease score was 92.7.

Content validity: Content validity was enhanced by using direct quotes from the qualitative studies as items on the scale (e.g., "I felt like I was losing my mind"). The pilot form was subjected to two content validations with a panel of five content experts. Feedback from these procedures led to some item revisions.

Construct validity: The PDSS was administered to a sample of 525 new mothers in six states (Beck & Gable, 2000). Preliminary item analyses resulted in the deletion of several items, based on item-total correlations. The PDSS was finalized as a 35-item scale with seven subscales, each with 5 items. This version of the PDSS was subjected to confirmatory factor analyses, which involved a validation of Beck's hypotheses about how individual items mapped onto underlying constructs, such as *mental confusion.* Item response theory analysis was also used and provided supporting evidence of the scale's construct validity. In a subsequent study, Beck and Gable (2001) administered the PDSS and two other depression scales to 150 new mothers and tested hypotheses about how scores on the PDSS would correlate with scores on other scales. The results indicated good convergent validity.

Internal consistency: In both studies, Beck and Gable evaluated the internal consistency of the PDSS and its subscales. Subscale alphas were high, ranging from .83 to .94 in the first study and from .80 to .91 in the second study. Figure 16.3 shows an internal consistency analysis printout (from the Statistical Package for the Social Sciences, or SPSS, Version 17.0) for the five items on the Mental Confusion subscale from the first study. In panel A, we see that Cronbach alpha for the 5-item subscale is high, .912. The first column of panel B (Item Statistics) identifies subscale items by number: Item 11, item 18, and so on. Item 11, for example, is the item "I felt like I was losing my mind." The item means and standard deviations for the 522 cases suggest adequate variability on each item. Panel C shows intercorrelations among the five items. The correlations are fairly high, ranging from .601 for item 25 with 53 to .814 for item 11 with 25. Panel D (Summary Item Statistics) presents descriptive item statistics. In panel E, the fourth column ("Corrected Item-Total Correlation") presents correlation coefficients for the relationship between women's score on an item and their score on the subscale, after removing the item from the scale. Item 11 has a corrected item-total correlation of .799, which is very high; all five items have excellent correlations with the total subscale score. The final column shows what the internal consistency would be if an item were deleted. If Item 11 were removed from the subscale and only 4 items remained, the reliability coefficient would be .888—less than the reliability for all 5 items

A   **Reliability Statistics**

Cronbach's Alpha	Cronbach's Alpha Based on Standardized Items	N of Items
.912	.912	5

B   **Item Statistics**

	Mean	Std. Deviation	N
Item 11	2.36	1.424	522
Item 18	2.21	1.270	522
Item 25	2.21	1.374	522
Item 39	2.40	1.351	522
Item 53	2.28	1.349	522

C   **Inter-Item Correlation Matrix**

	Item 11	Item 18	Item 25	Item 39	Item 53
Item 11	1.000	.654	.814	.646	.649
Item 18	.654	1.000	.603	.659	.751
Item 25	.814	.603	1.000	.652	.601
Item 39	.646	.659	.652	1.000	.724
Item 53	.649	.751	.601	.724	1.000

D   **Summary Item Statistics**

	Mean	Minimum	Maximum	Range	Maximum / Minimum	Variance	N of Items
Item Means	2.292	2.205	2.399	.194	1.088	.008	5
Item Variances	1.835	1.612	2.029	.416	1.258	.023	5
Inter-Item Correlations	.675	.601	.814	.213	1.354	.006	5

E   **Item-Total Statistics**

	Scale Mean if Item Deleted	Scale Variance if Item Deleted	Corrected Item-Total Correlation	Squared Multiple Correlation	Cronbach's Alpha if Item Deleted
Item 11	9.09	21.371	.799	.715	.888
Item 18	9.24	23.006	.770	.623	.895
Item 25	9.25	22.097	.769	.691	.894
Item 39	9.06	22.290	.869	.610	.894
Item 53	9.18	22.176	.781	.666	.891

FIGURE 16.3 Statistical Package for the Social Sciences (SPSS) internal consistency analysis for the Mental Confusion subscale of the Postpartum Depression Screening Scale.

(.912). Deleting any of the items on the subscale would reduce its internal consistency but only by a rather small amount.

Criterion-related validity: In the second study, Beck and Gable correlated scores on the PDSS with an expert clinician's diagnosis of PPD for each woman (the criterion). The coefficient was .70, which was higher than the correlations between the clinical diagnosis and scores on other depression scales, indicating its superiority as a screening instrument. Additionally,

ROC curves were constructed to examine the sensitivity and specificity of the PDSS at different cutoff points, using the expert diagnosis to establish PPD caseness. In this sample, 46 of the 150 mothers had a diagnosis of major or minor depression. To illustrate the trade-offs the researchers made, the ROC curve (Figure 16.4) revealed that with a cutoff score of 95 on the PDSS, the sensitivity would be only .41, meaning that only 41% of the women actually diagnosed with PPD would be identified. A score of 95 has a

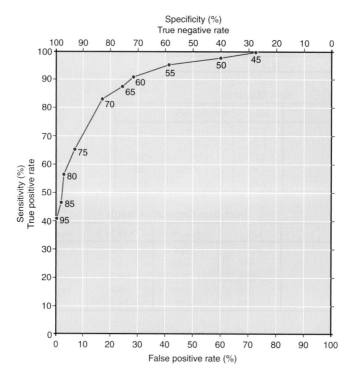

FIGURE 16.4 Receiver operating characteristic (ROC) curve for Postpartum Depression Screening Scale.

specificity of 1.00, meaning that all cases *without* an actual PPD diagnosis would be accurately screened out. At the other extreme, a cutoff score of 45 would have 1.00 sensitivity but only .28 specificity (i.e., 72% false positive), an unacceptable rate of overdiagnosis. Beck and Gable recommended a cutoff score of 60, which would accurately screen in 91% of true PPD cases and would mistakenly screen in 28% who do not have PPD. Beck and Gable found that this cutoff point correctly classified 85% of their sample. In their ROC analysis, the area under the curve was excellent, .91.

Spanish translation: Beck collaborated with translation experts to develop a Spanish version of the PDSS. Eight bilingual translators from four backgrounds (Mexican, Puerto Rican, Cuban, and South American) translated and back-translated the items. The translators met as a committee to review each others' wordings and to arrive at a consensus. Both the English and Spanish versions were then administered, in random order, to a bilingual sample. Scores on the two

versions correlated highly (e.g., .98 on the "Sleeping/ Eating Disturbances" subscale). Coefficient alpha was .95 for the total scale and ranged from .76 to .90 for subscales. CFA yielded information that was judged to indicate an adequate fit with the hypothesized measurement model, and screening performance was found to be good (Beck & Gable, 2005). Another psychometric assessment of the Spanish version was undertaken by Lara and colleagues (2013) in Mexico, who found comparably good measurement properties.

Other translations: The PDSS has been translated into several other languages (e.g., Chinese, Portuguese, Turkish, Hungarian, Thai), and psychometric assessments in all cases suggest that the instrument has strong measurement properties. In the Turkish version of the PDSS, the 15-day test–retest reliability, which was not reported in other papers, was high, r = .86 (Karaçam, & Kitiş, 2008). In the Hungarian version, the parallel forms reliability for the English and Hungarian versions was .97 (Hegedus & Beck, 2012).

Responsiveness: Responsiveness of the PDSS was not assessed by the scale developers. There is, however, evidence that PPD as measured by the PDSS is sensitive to interventions and to changes over time, suggesting good responsiveness of the scale. For example, in a study of the effects of kangaroo mother care in Brazil, scores on the PDSS dropped during the time the infants were in the NICU, consistent with the researchers' hypotheses (de Alencar et al., 2009). In an analysis of the effects of a psychoeducation intervention for pregnant women with abuse-related posttraumatic stress, Rowe et al. (2014) reported a significant decrease in PDSS scores. Zhao et al. (2018) examined how women's perinatal depression scores as measured on the PDSS changed across the perinatal period.

SUMMARY POINTS

- Scale development begins with a sound conceptualization of the construct (the **latent trait**) to be measured, including its *dimensionality*.
- An early step in scale construction is the generation of items. Common sources for items include existing instruments, the research literature, concept analyses, qualitative studies, and clinical observations.
- In classical test theory, a **domain sampling model** is assumed; the basic notion is to sample a homogeneous set of items from a hypothetical universe of items.
- In generating items, a number of decisions must be made, including how many items to generate (typically a large number initially), what continuum to use for the response options, how many response options there should be, whether to include positive and negative item stems, how intensely worded the items will be, and what to do about references to time.
- Items should be inspected for clarity, length, and avoidance of jargon and double negatives; the scale's **readability** should also be assessed.
- External review of the preliminary pool of items should be undertaken, including review by members of the target population (e.g., via a small pretest that could include **cognitive questioning**).
- **Content validity** should be built into the scale through careful efforts to conceptualize the construct and through content validation by a panel of experts—including the calculation of a quantitative index such as the CVI to summarize the experts' judgments of the relevance of scale items.
- Once content validity has been established at a satisfactory level, the scale must be administered to a development sample—typically 300 or more respondents who are representative of the target population.
- Data collected from the development sample are then analyzed using a number of techniques, including **item analysis** (e.g., a scrutiny of **inter-item correlations** and **item-scale correlations**), **exploratory factor analysis (EFA)**, internal consistency analysis, and test–retest reliability analysis.
- EFA is used to reduce a large set of variables into a smaller set of underlying dimensions, called **factors.** Mathematically, each factor is a linear combination of variables in a data matrix.
- The first phase of EFA **(factor extraction)** identifies clusters of items that are strongly intercorrelated and helps to define the number of underlying dimensions in the items. A widely used factor extraction method is **principal components analysis (PCA)**; another is **principal axis factor analysis.**
- The second phase of factor analysis involves **factor rotation**, which enhances the interpretability of the factors by aligning items more distinctly with a particular factor. Rotation can be either **orthogonal** (which maintains the independence of the factors) or **oblique** (which allows correlated factors). **Factor loadings** of the items on the rotated factor matrix are used to interpret and name the factors.
- After the scale is finalized based on the preliminary analyses, steps are taken to validate the scale, using a variety of validation techniques; one widely used approach to assess structural validity is **confirmatory factor analysis (CFA)**.

- CFA involves tests of a **measurement model**, which stipulates the hypothesized relationship between latent traits and *manifest variables* (items). CFA is a subset of sophisticated statistical techniques called **structural equation modeling**.
- The **interpretability** of scale scores can be enhanced using such approaches as computing **percentiles**, converting raw scores to **standard scores** and developing **norms** and meaningful **cutoff points**.

STUDY ACTIVITIES

Study activities are available to instructors on thePoint.

REFERENCES CITED IN CHAPTER 16

AERA, APA, & NCME Joint Committee. (2014). *Standards for educational and psychological testing* (5th rev.). Washington: American Psychological Association.

Anthony, M., Yastik, J., MacDonald, D., & Marshall, K. (2014). Development and validation of a tool to measure incivility in clinical nursing education. *Journal of Professional Nursing, 30*, 48–55.

Beck, C. T., & Gable, R. K. (2000). Postpartum Depression Screening Scale: Development and psychometric testing. *Nursing Research, 49*, 272–282.

Beck, C. T., & Gable, R. K. (2001). Further validation of the Postpartum Depression Screening Scale. *Nursing Research, 50*, 155–164.

Beck, C. T., & Gable, R. K. (2003). Postpartum Depression Screening Scale: Spanish version. *Nursing Research, 52*, 296–306.

Beck, C. T., & Gable, R. K. (2005). Screening performance of the Postpartum Depression Screening Scale—Spanish version. *Journal of Transcultural Nursing, 16*, 331–338.

Bott, M., Karanevich, A., Garrard, L., Price, L., Mudaranthakam, D., & Gajewski, B. (2018). Confirmatory factor analysis alternative: Free, accessible CBID software. *Western Journal of Nursing Research, 40*, 257–269.

Brown, T. (2015). *Confirmatory factor analysis for applied research* (2nd ed.). New York: Guilford Press.

Burchill, C., Bena, J., & Polomano, R. (2018). Psychometric testing of the Personal Workplace Safety Instrument for Emergency Nurses. *Worldviews on Evidence Based Nursing, 15*, 97–103.

De Alencar, A., Arraes, L., de Albuquerque, E., & Alves, J. (2009). Effect of kangaroo mother care on postpartum depression. *Journal of Tropical Pediatrics, 55*, 36–38.

DeVellis, R. F. (2017). *Scale development: Theory and application* (4th ed.). Thousand Oaks, CA: Sage Publications.

*Gibbs, H., Harvey, S., Owens, S., Boyle, D., & Sullivan, D. (2017). Engaging experts and patients to refine the Nutrition Literacy Assessment Instrument. *BMC Nutrition, 3*, 7.

Hegedus, K. S., & Beck, C. T. (2012). Development and psychometric testing of the Postpartum Depression Screening Scale: Hungarian version. *International Journal for Human Caring, 16*, 54–58.

Hilton, A., & Skrutkowski, M. (2002). Translating instruments into other language: Development and testing processes. *Cancer Nursing, 25*, 1–7.

Karaçam, Z., & Kitiş, Y. (2008). The Postpartum Depression Screening Scale: Its reliability and validity for the Turkish population. *Türk Psikiyatri Dergesi, 19*, 187–196.

Kline, R. B. (2016). *Principles and practice of structural equation modeling* (4th ed.). New York: The Guilford Press.

Lara, M., Navarette, L., Navarro, C., & Le, H. (2013). Evaluation of the psychometric measures for the Postpartum Depression Screening Scale – Spanish version for Mexican women. *Journal of Transcultural Nursing, 24*, 378–386.

Mokkink, L. B., Terwee, C., Patrick, D., Alonso, J., Stratford, P., Knol, D. L., … DeVet, H. (2010). The COSMIN study reached international consensus on taxonomy, terminology, and definitions of measurement properties for health-related patient-reported outcomes. *Journal of Clinical Epidemiology, 63*, 737–745.

*Moser, J., Lipman, T., Langdon, D., & Bevans, K. (2017). Development of a youth-report measure of DPN symptoms: Conceptualization and content validation. *Journal of Clinical and Translational Endocrinology, 9*, 55–60.

Nunnally, J., & Bernstein, I. H. (1994). *Psychometric theory* (3rd ed.). New York: McGraw-Hill.

Oh, H., Han, S., Kim, S., & Seo, W. (2018). Development and validity testing of an arthritis self-management assessment tool. *Orthopaedic Nursing, 37*, 24–35.

Polit, D. F. (2010). *Statistics and data analysis for nursing research* (2nd ed.). Upper Saddle River, NJ: Pearson.

Polit, D. F. (2014). Getting serious about test-retest reliability: A critique of retest research and some recommendations. *Quality of Life Research, 23*, 1713–1720.

Polit, D., Beck, C., & Owen, S. (2007). Is the CVI an acceptable indicator of content validity? Appraisal and recommendations. *Research in Nursing & Health, 30*, 459–467.

Polit, D. F., & Yang, F. M. (2016). *Measurement and the measurement of change: A primer for health professionals.* Philadelphia: Lippincott.

Rowe, H., Sperlich, M., Cameron, H., & Seng, J. (2014). A quasi-experimental outcomes analysis of a psychoeducation intervention for pregnant women with abuse-related posttraumatic stress. *Journal of Obstetric, Gynecologic, and Neonatal Nursing, 43*, 282–293.

**Sanchez, P., Salamonson, Y., Everett, B., & George, A. (2019). Barriers and predictors associated with accessing oral healthcare among patients with cardiovascular disease in Australia. *Journal of Cardiovascular Nursing, 34*, 208–214.

Shin, H., Park, Y., & Cho, I. (2018). Development and psychometric validation of the Menstrual Health Instrument (MHI) for adolescents in Korea. *Health Care for Women International, 9*, 1–20.

Streiner, D. L., Norman, G. R., & Cairney, J. (2015). *Health measurement scales: A practical guide to their development and use* (5th ed.). Oxford: Oxford University Press.

*Terwee, C. B., Mokkink, L. B., Knol, D. L., Ostelo, R., Bouter, L. M., & DeVet, H. C. W. (2012). Rating the methodological quality in systematic reviews of studies on measurement properties: A scoring system for the COSMIN checklist. *Quality of Life Research, 21*, 651–657.

Walker, L. O., & Avant, K. C. (2019). *Strategies for theory construction in nursing* (6th ed.). Upper Saddle River, NJ: Prentice Hall.

Wu, W., Liu, C., Jou, S., Hung, G., & Liang, S. (2018). Development of feasibility of Mandarin-language bone health scales for adolescents with cancer in Taiwan. *Nursing & Health Sciences, 20*, 197–205.

Zhao, Y., Munro-Kramer, M. L., Shi, S., Wang, J., & Luo, J. (2018). A longitudinal study of perinatal depression among Chinese high-risk pregnant women. *Women and Birth, 31*, e395–e402.

A link to this open-access article is provided in the Toolkit for Chapter 16 in the Resource Manual.

**This journal article is available on thePoint for this chapter.*

17 | Descriptive Statistics

Statistical analysis enables researchers to organize and communicate numeric information. Mathematic skill is not required to grasp basic statistics—only logical thinking ability is needed. In this book, we focus on explaining which statistics to use in different situations, and on how to understand what statistical results mean.

Statistics can be descriptive or inferential. **Descriptive statistics** are used to describe and synthesize data—for example, percentages are descriptive statistics. When a descriptive index is calculated from population data, it is a **parameter**. A descriptive index from a sample is a **statistic**. Research questions are about parameters, but researchers calculate statistics to estimate them and use **inferential statistics** to make inferences about the population. This chapter discusses descriptive statistics, and Chapter 18 focuses on inferential statistics. We first discuss levels of measurement because analytic options depend on how variables are measured.

LEVELS OF MEASUREMENT

Scientists have developed a system for classifying measures. The four **levels of measurement** are nominal, ordinal, interval, and ratio.

Nominal Measurement

The lowest level of measurement is **nominal measurement**, which involves assigning numbers to classify characteristics into categories. Examples of variables amenable to nominal measurement include gender, blood type, and marital status.

The numbers used in nominal measurement have no quantitative meaning. If we code married people as 1 and not married people as 2, the number 2 does not mean "more than" 1. The numbers are only symbols representing different values of marital status. We easily could use 1 for not married, 2 for married. Nominal measurement provides no information about an attribute except equivalence. If we were to "measure" the gender of Nate, Alan, Cathy, and Diane by assigning them the codes 1, 1, 2, and 2, respectively, this means Nate and Alan are equivalent on the gender attribute but are not equivalent to Cathy and Diane.

Nominal measures must have categories that are mutually exclusive and collectively exhaustive. For example, if we were measuring blood type, we might use these codes: 1 = A, 2 = B, and 3 = O. The requirement for collective exhaustiveness would not be met if there were people in a sample whose blood type was AB. Numbers in nominal measurement cannot be treated mathematically. It is not meaningful to calculate the average marital status of a sample, but we can compute percentages. In a sample of 50 patients with 30 not married and 20 married, we could say that 60% were not married and 40% were married.

Ordinal Measurement

Ordinal measurement involves sorting people based on their relative ranking on an attribute. This measurement level goes beyond categorization: Attributes are *ordered* according to some criterion. Ordinal measurement captures not only equivalence but also relative rank.

Consider this ordinal scheme for measuring ability to perform activities of daily living: (1) completely dependent, (2) needs another person's assistance, (3) needs mechanical assistance, and (4) completely independent. The numbers signify incremental ability to perform activities of daily living. People coded 4 are equivalent to each other with regard to functional ability *and*, relative to those in the other categories, have more of the attribute.

Ordinal measurement does not, however, tell us anything about how much greater one level is than another. We do not know if being completely independent is twice as good as needing mechanical assistance. Nor do we know if the difference between needing another person's assistance and needing mechanical assistance is the same as that between needing mechanical assistance and being completely independent. Ordinal measurement tells us only the relative ranking of the attribute's levels.

As with nominal measures, mathematic operations with ordinal-level data are restricted—for example, averages are usually meaningless. Frequency counts, percentages, and several other statistics to be discussed later are appropriate for ordinal-level data.

Interval Measurement

Interval measurement occurs when researchers can assume equivalent distance between rank-ordering on an attribute. The Fahrenheit temperature scale is an example: a temperature of 60°F is 10°F warmer than 50°F. A 10°F difference similarly separates 40°F and 30°F, and the two differences in temperature are equivalent. Interval-level measures are more informative than ordinal ones, but interval measures do not

communicate absolute magnitude. For example, we cannot say that 60°F is twice as hot as 30°F. The Fahrenheit scale uses an arbitrary zero point: zero degrees does not signify an absence of heat. Most psychosocial scales are assumed to yield interval-level data.

Interval scales expand analytic possibilities—in particular, interval-level data can be averaged meaningfully. It is reasonable, for example, to compute an average daily body temperature for hospital patients.

Ratio Measurement

Ratio measurement provides information about ordering on the critical attribute, the intervals between objects, *and* the absolute magnitude of the attribute because there is a rational, meaningful zero. Many physical measures provide ratio-level data. A person's weight, for example, is measured on a ratio scale. We can say that someone who weighs 200 pounds is twice as heavy as someone who weighs 100 pounds.

Because ratio measures have an absolute zero, all arithmetic operations are permissible. Statistical procedures suitable for interval-level data are also appropriate for ratio-level data.

Example of Different Measurement Levels

Zenk and colleagues (2018) examined the impact of community food environment on the weight loss effects of a weight management program for veterans. The presence versus absence of 10 chronic health conditions (e.g., diabetes, hypertension) were dichotomous nominal-level variables. Measures of the community food environment, such as number of fast food restaurants within a mile of the veterans' house, were captured as ordinal variables (e.g., 0, 1-4, 5-11, or 12+). The body mass index was a ratio-level variable.

TIP Nominal-level measures are often called *categorical*. Variables measured on an interval- or ratio-level scale are often called *continuous* variables.

Comparison of the Levels

The four levels of measurement form a hierarchy, with ratio scales at the top and nominal measurement at the base. Moving from a higher to a lower level of measurement results in an information loss. For example, if we measured a woman's weight in pounds, this would be a ratio measure. If we categorized the weights into three groups (e.g., under 125, 125-175, and 176+), this would be an ordinal measure. With this scheme, we would not be able to differentiate a woman who weighed 125 from one who weighed 175 pounds—we have much less information with ordinal information. This example illustrates another point: With information at one level, it is possible to convert data to a lower level, but the converse is not true. If we were given only the ordinal measurements, we could not reconstruct actual weights.

It is not always easy to identify a variable's level of measurement. Nominal and ratio measures usually are discernible, but the distinction between ordinal and interval measures is more problematic. Some methodologists argue that most psychological measures that are treated as interval measures are really ordinal measures. Although instruments such as Likert scales produce data that are, strictly speaking, ordinal, many analysts believe that treating them as interval measures results in too few errors to warrant using less powerful statistical procedures.

TIP In operationalizing variables, it is best to use the highest measurement level possible because they are more powerful and precise. Sometimes, however, group membership is more informative than continuous scores, especially for clinicians who need "cutpoints" for making decisions. For example, for some purposes, it may be more relevant to designate infants as being of low versus normal birth weight (nominal level) than to use actual birth weight values (ratio level). But it is best to *measure* at the higher level and then convert to a lower level if appropriate.

FREQUENCY DISTRIBUTIONS

When quantitative data are unanalyzed, it is difficult to discern even general trends. Consider the 60 numbers in Table 17.1, which are fictitious scores of 60 patients on a six-item anxiety scale—scores that we will consider as interval level. Inspection of the numbers does not help us understand patients' anxiety. A set of data can be described in terms of three characteristics: the shape of the distribution of values, central tendency, and variability. In this section, we focus on a distribution's shape.

Constructing Frequency Distributions

Frequency distributions are used to organize numeric data. A **frequency distribution** is a

TABLE 17.1 • Patients' Anxiety Scores

22	27	25	19	24	25	23	29	24	20
26	16	20	26	17	22	24	18	26	28
15	24	23	22	21	24	20	25	18	27
24	23	16	25	30	29	27	21	23	24
26	18	30	21	17	25	22	24	29	28
20	25	26	24	23	19	27	28	25	26

TABLE 17.2 • Frequency Distribution of Patients' Anxiety Scores

SCORE (X)	FREQUENCY (f)	PERCENTAGE (%)
15	1	1.7
16	2	3.3
17	2	3.3
18	3	5.0
19	2	3.3
20	4	6.7
21	3	5.0
22	4	6.7
23	5	8.3
24	9	15.0
25	7	11.7
26	6	10.0
27	4	6.7
28	3	5.0
29	3	5.0
30	2	3.3
	$N = 60 = \Sigma f$	$\Sigma\% = 100.0\%$

systematic arrangement of values from lowest to highest, together with a count of the number of times each value was obtained. Our 60 anxiety scores are shown in a frequency distribution in Table 17.2. We can readily see the highest and lowest scores, the most common score, where the bulk of scores clustered, and how many patients were in the sample (total sample size is typically depicted as *N*). None of this was apparent before we organized the data.

Frequency distributions consist of two parts: observed score values (the *X*s) and the frequency of cases at each value (the *f*s). Scores are listed in order in one column, and corresponding frequencies are listed in another. The sum of numbers in the frequency column must equal the sample size. In less verbal terms, $\Sigma f = N$, which means the sum of (signified by Greek sigma, Σ) the frequencies (*f*) equals the sample size (*N*).

It is useful to display percentages for each value, as shown in column 3 of Table 17.2. Just as the sum of all frequencies should equal *N*, the sum of all percentages should equal 100.

Frequency data can be displayed graphically. Graphs for displaying interval- and ratio-level data include **histograms** and **frequency polygons**, which are constructed in a similar fashion. First, score values are arrayed on a horizontal (X) axis, with the lowest value on the left, ascending to the highest value on the right. Frequencies or percentages are displayed vertically. A histogram is constructed by drawing bars above the score classes to the height corresponding to the frequency for that score. Figure 17.1 shows a histogram for the anxiety score data. Frequency polygons are similar, but dots corresponding to the frequencies are placed above each score (Figure 17.2). The dots are connected by straight lines and show the distribution's shape.

Shapes of Distributions

A distribution is **symmetric** if, when folded over, the two halves are superimposed. All the distributions in Figure 17.3 are symmetric. With real data sets, distributions are rarely perfectly symmetric,

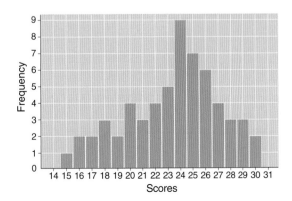

FIGURE 17.1 Histogram of patients' anxiety scores.

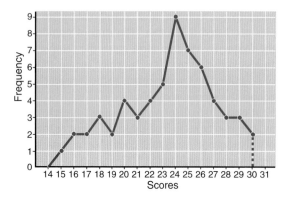

FIGURE 17.2 Frequency polygon of patients' anxiety scores.

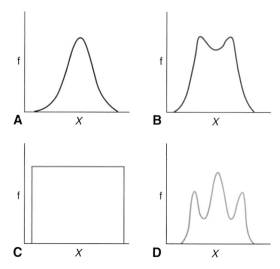

FIGURE 17.3 Examples of symmetric distributions.

but minor discrepancies are ignored in characterizing a distribution's shape.

In **skewed** (asymmetric) distributions, the peak is off center and one tail is longer than the other. When the longer tail points to the right, the distribution is **positively skewed** (Figure 17.4A). Personal income, for example, is positively skewed. Most people have low to moderate incomes, with relatively few high-income people in the tail. If the tail points to the left, the distribution is **negatively skewed** (Figure 17.4B). Age at death is negatively skewed: most people are at the upper end of the distribution, with relatively few dying at an early age. Patients' anxiety scores (Figure 17.2) were negatively skewed—high scores were more common than low ones.

Modality is a second aspect of a distribution's shape. A **unimodal distribution** has only one peak

(i.e., a value with high frequency), whereas a **multimodal distribution** has two or more peaks. A distribution with two peaks is **bimodal**. Figure 17.3A is unimodal, and Figure 17.3B and D illustrate multimodal distributions. Symmetry and modality are independent: skewness is unrelated to how many peaks a distribution has.

Some distributions have special names. Of particular importance is the **normal distribution** (sometimes called a *Gaussian distribution* or *bell-shaped curve*). A normal distribution is symmetric, unimodal, and not too peaked (Figure 17.3A). Many human attributes (e.g., height, intelligence) approximate a normal distribution.

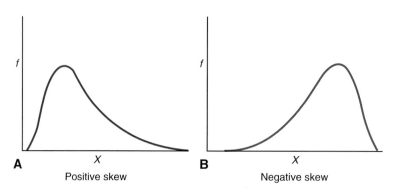

FIGURE 17.4 Examples of skewed distributions.

CENTRAL TENDENCY

Frequency distributions are a good way to clarify data patterns, but often a pattern is of less interest than an overall summary. Researchers ask such questions as, "What is the average body temperature of infants during bathing?" or "What is the average weight loss of patients with cancer?" Such questions seek a single number to best represent a distribution. Because an index of typicalness is more likely to come from the center of a distribution than from an extreme, such indexes are called measures of **central tendency**. Lay people use the term *average* to designate central tendency. Researchers avoid this term because there are three indexes of central tendency: the mode, the median, and the mean.

The Mode

The **mode** is the most frequently occurring score value in a distribution. In the following distribution, the mode is 53:

50 51 51 52 53 53 53 53 54 55 56

The score of 53 occurred four times, a higher frequency than for any other score. The mode of patients' anxiety scores (Table 17.2) is 24. In multimodal distributions, there is more than one score value with high frequencies. Modes are a quick way to determine a "popular" score, but they are rather unstable. By *unstable*, we mean that modes tend to fluctuate from sample to sample drawn from the same population.

The Median

The **median** is the point in a distribution above and below which 50% of cases fall. As an example, consider the following set of values:

2 2 3 3 4 5 6 7 8 9

The value that divides the cases exactly in half is 4.5, the median for this set of numbers. The point that has 50% of the cases above and below it is halfway between 4 and 5. For the patient anxiety scores, the median is 24. An important characteristic of the median is that it does not take into account the quantitative values of scores—it is an index of average *position* in a distribution and is thus insensitive to extremes. In the above set of numbers, if the value of 9 were changed to 99, the median would remain 4.5. Because of this property, the median is often a preferred index of central tendency with skewed distributions. In research reports, the median may be abbreviated as **Md** or **Mdn**.

The Mean

The **mean,** often symbolized as M or $\overline{X}$, is the sum of all scores divided by the number of scores. The mean is what people usually refer to as the *average*. The mean of the patients' anxiety scores is 23.4 ($1405 \div 60$). Let us compute the mean weight of eight people with the following weights: 85, 109, 120, 135, 158, 177, 181, and 195:

$$\overline{X} = \frac{85 + 109 + 120 + 135 + 158 + 177 + 181 + 195}{8} = 145$$

Unlike the median, the mean is affected by every score. If we were to exchange the 195-pound person in this example for one weighing 275 pounds, the mean would increase from 145 to 155. Such a substitution would leave the median unchanged.

The mean is the most widely used measure of central tendency. When researchers work with interval-level or ratio-level measurements, the mean, rather than the median or mode, is usually the statistic reported.

Comparison of the Mode, Median, and Mean

The mean is the most stable index of central tendency. If repeated samples were drawn from a population, means would fluctuate less than modes or medians. Sometimes, however, the primary interest is to understand what is typical, in which case a median might be preferred. If we wanted to know about the economic well-being of U.S. citizens, for example, we would get a distorted impression by considering mean income, which would be inflated by the wealth of a minority. The median would better reflect how a typical person fares financially.

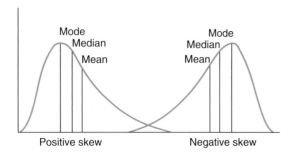

FIGURE 17.5 Relationships of central tendency indexes in skewed distributions.

FIGURE 17.6 Two distributions of different variability.

When a distribution is symmetric and unimodal, the three indexes of central tendency coincide. In skewed distributions, the values of the mode, median, and mean differ. The mean is always pulled in the direction of the long tail, as shown in Figure 17.5. A variable's level of measurement plays a role in determining the appropriate index of central tendency to use. In general, the mode is most suitable for nominal measures, the mode or median is appropriate for ordinal measures, and the mean is appropriate for interval and ratio measures.

VARIABILITY

Two distributions with identical means could differ in **variability**—how spread out or dispersed the data are. Consider the two distributions in Figure 17.6, which represent fictitious scores for students from two schools on an IQ test. Both distributions have a mean of 100, but the score patterns differ. School A has a wide range of scores, from below 70 to above 130. In school B, by contrast, there are few low scores and few high scores. School A is more **heterogeneous** (i.e., more variable) than school B, and school B is more **homogeneous** than school A.

Researchers compute an index of variability to express the extent to which scores in a distribution differ from one another. Two common indexes are the range and standard deviation.

The Range

The **range** is simply the highest score minus the lowest score in a distribution. In the example of

patients' anxiety scores, the range is 15 (30 − 15). In the examples shown in Figure 17.6, the range for school A is about 80 (140 − 60), and the range for school B is about 50 (125 − 75).

The chief virtue of the range is computational ease, but, being based on only two scores, the range is unstable. From sample to sample from a population, the range tends to fluctuate widely. Another limitation is that the range ignores variations in scores between the two extremes. In school B of Figure 17.6, suppose one student obtained a score of 60 and another obtained a score of 140. The range of both schools would then be 80, despite clear differences in heterogeneity. For these reasons, the range is used mainly as a crude descriptive index.

> **TIP** Another index of variability is called the *interquartile range (IQR)*, which is calculated based on *quartiles*. The IQR indicates the range of scores within which the middle 50% of score values lie. IQRs are infrequently reported but play a role in detecting extreme values (*outliers*). For more detailed information, see the Supplement to Chapter 20 on thePoint.

The Standard Deviation

The most widely used measure of variability is the standard deviation. The **standard deviation** indicates the *average amount* of deviation of values from the mean and is calculated using every score. In research reports, the standard deviation is often abbreviated as **SD**.

A variability index needs to capture the degree to which scores deviate from one another. This concept of deviation is represented in the range by the minus sign, which produces an index of deviation, or difference, between two score points. The standard deviation is also based on score differences. In fact, the first step in calculating a standard deviation is to compute deviation scores for each score. A **deviation score** (symbolized as x) is the difference between an individual score and the mean, i.e., $x = X - \overline{X}$. If a person weighed 150 pounds and the sample mean were 140, then the person's deviation score would be +10.

Because we want an *average* deviation, you might think that a good variability index could be computed by summing all deviation scores and then dividing by the number of cases. The problem is that the sum of a set of deviation scores is always zero. Table 17.3 presents deviation scores for nine numbers. As shown in the second column, the sum of the xs is zero. Deviations above the mean always balance exactly deviations below the mean.

The standard deviation overcomes this problem by having each deviation score squared before summing. After dividing by the number of cases (minus 1), the square root is taken to bring the index back to the original unit of measurement. The formula for the standard deviation is:

$$SD = \sqrt{\frac{\sum x^2}{N-1}}$$

> **TIP** For calculating the *SD* of a *population*, the formula has *N* rather than *N* − 1 in the denominator. Differences in the results from the two formulas are negligible unless the sample size is small. Statistical programs use *N* − 1 to compute *SD*s.

A standard deviation has been worked out for the data in Table 17.3. First, a deviation score is calculated for each of the nine raw scores by subtracting the mean ($\overline{X} = 7$) from them. Each deviation score is squared (column 3), converting all values to positive numbers. The squared deviation scores are summed ($\Sigma x^2 = 28$), divided by 8 (N − 1), and a square root taken to yield an *SD* of 1.87.

TABLE 17.3 • Computation of a Standard Deviation

X	$x = X - \overline{X}$	$x^2 = (X - \overline{X})^2$
4	−3	9
5	−2	4
6	−1	1
7	0	0
7	0	0
7	0	0
8	1	1
9	2	4
10	3	9
$\Sigma X = 63$	$\Sigma x = 0$	$\Sigma x^2 = 28$
$\overline{X} = 7$		

$$SD = \sqrt{\frac{28}{8}} = \sqrt{3.50} = 1.87$$

> **TIP** The standard deviation often is shown in relation to the mean without a formal label. For example, patients' anxiety scores might be shown as $M = 23.4 \ (3.7)$ or $M = 23.4 \pm 3.7$, where 23.4 is the mean and 3.7 is the standard deviation.

A related variability index is the **variance**, which is the value of the standard deviation before taking the square root. In other words, variance = SD^2. In our example, the variance is 1.87^2 or 3.50. The variance is rarely reported because it is not in the same unit of measurement as the original data, but it is important in statistical tests we discuss in Chapter 18.

A standard deviation is more difficult to interpret than other statistics, such as the mean. In our example, we calculated $SD = 1.87$. One might ask, 1.87 *what?* What does the number mean? First, the standard deviation is a variability index for a set of scores. If two distributions had a mean of 25.0, but one had an *SD* of 7.0 and the other had an *SD* of 3.0, we would know that the first sample was more heterogeneous.

Second, think of a standard deviation as an average of deviations from the mean. The mean tells us the single best value for summarizing a distribution; a standard deviation tells us how much, on average, scores deviate from that mean. A standard deviation can thus be interpreted as our degree of error when we use a mean to describe the entire sample.

The standard deviation can also be used to interpret individual scores in a distribution. Suppose we had weight data from a sample whose mean weight was 150 pounds with *SD* = 10. The *SD* provides a *standard* of variability. Weights greater than 1 *SD* away from the mean (i.e., greater than 160 or less than 140 pounds) are at a greater than the average "distance" from the mean.

In normal distributions, there are roughly 3 *SD*s above and 3 *SD*s below the mean. To illustrate, suppose we had normally distributed scores with a mean of 50 and an *SD* of 10 (Figure 17.7). In a normal distribution, a fixed percentage of cases falls within certain distances from the mean. Sixty-eight percent of cases fall within 1 *SD* of the mean (34%

above and 34% below the mean). In our example, nearly 7 out of 10 scores fall between 40 and 60. Ninety-five percent of scores in a normal distribution fall within 2 *SD*s from the mean. Only a handful of cases—about 2% at each extreme—lie more than 2 *SD*s from the mean. In the figure, we can see that a person with a score of 70 had a higher score than about 98% of the sample.

In summary, the *SD* is a useful variability index for describing a distribution and interpreting individual scores. Like the mean, the standard deviation is a stable estimate of a parameter and is the preferred index of a distribution's variability.

TIP Descriptive statistics (e.g., percentages, means, standard deviations) are most often used to summarize sample characteristics, describe key research variables, and document methodologic features (e.g., response rates), rather than to answer research questions; inferential statistics (Chapter 18) are used for this purpose. The Toolkit section of the accompanying *Resource Manual* includes some table templates for displaying descriptive information that can be "filled in" with descriptive results.

Example of Descriptive Statistics
Lucas-de la Cruz and colleagues (2018) studied the influence of sleep characteristics on metabolic syndrome (MetS) in Spanish children. Sophisticated statistical analyses were performed, but the researchers also presented descriptive information about the characteristics of the 210 children in their sample. For example, their mean age was 9.2 (*SD* = .74), their mean BMI was 18.7 (*SD* = 3.81), and their average sleep efficiency was 92.8% (*SD* = 3.12). Girls comprised 54.8% of the sample.

BIVARIATE DESCRIPTIVE STATISTICS

The mean, mode, and standard deviation are **univariate** (one-variable) **descriptive statistics** that describe one variable at a time. Most research is about relationships between variables, and **bivariate** (two-variable) **descriptive statistics** describe such relationships, often through crosstabs tables and correlation indexes.

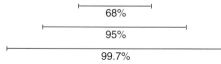

FIGURE 17.7 Standard deviations (SDs) in a normal distribution.

Crosstabs Tables

A **crosstabs table** (or *contingency table*) is a two-dimensional frequency distribution in which the frequencies of two variables are crosstabulated. Suppose we had data on patients' gender (male–female) and whether they were nonsmokers, light smokers (<1 pack of cigarettes a day), or heavy smokers (≥1 pack a day). The question is whether there is a tendency for men to smoke more heavily than women or vice versa (i.e., whether there is a relationship between smoking and gender). Fictitious data on these two variables are shown in Table 17.4. Six **cells** are created by placing one variable (gender) on one dimension and the other variable (smoking status) on the other. Each sample member is allocated to a cell based on their status on the two variables. For example, a woman who does not smoke would be counted in the upper left of the six cells. After all participants are allocated to the appropriate cells, percentages are computed. The crosstab allows us to see that, in this sample, women were more likely than men to be nonsmokers (45.4% versus 27.3%) and less likely to be heavy smokers (18.2% versus 36.4%). Crosstabs tables are used with nominal data or ordinal data with few ranks. In the present example, gender is nominal, and smoking status, as defined, is ordinal.

Crosstabs tables are easy to construct by hand or by commands to a computer. A key issue is which variable to put in the rows and which in the columns. Crosstabs tables are often set up such that the percentages in a column add to 100%, as in Table 17.4. However, cell percentages can be computed based on either row totals or column totals. In Table 17.4, the number 10 in the first cell (nonsmoking women) was divided by the *column* total (i.e., total number of women—22) to arrive at the percentage of women who were nonsmokers (45.4%). This cell *could* have shown 62.5%—the percentage of non-smokers who were women (10 ÷ 16). Thus, care must be taken in reading crosstabs tables.

Example of Crosstabulations

Luz and colleagues (2019) studied characteristics that differentiate formal from informal nurse champions who spread innovations in healthcare organizations. A table in the report showed whether 93 nurse champions were formal (performing in a formal organizational role) or informal in relation to such characteristics as gender, type of project, and professional tenure. For example, 67% of the formal champions had a tenure of less than 15 years, compared to 42% of the informal champions.

Correlation

Relationships between two variables are usually described through **correlation** procedures. Correlation coefficients, briefly described in Chapter 15, can be computed with two variables measured on the ordinal, interval, or ratio scale. The correlation question is: To what extent are two variables related to each other? For example, to

---

TABLE 17.4 • Contingency Table for Gender and Smoking Status Relationship

| SMOKING STATUS | GENDER | | | | | |
| | WOMEN | | MEN | | TOTAL | |
	n	%	*n*	%	*n*	%
Nonsmoker	10	45.4	6	27.3	16	36.4
Light smoker	8	36.4	8	36.4	16	36.4
Heavy smoker	4	18.2	8	36.4	12	27.3
TOTAL	22	100.0	22	100.0	44	100.0

what degree are anxiety scores and blood pressure readings correlated?

Correlations between two variables can be graphed on a **scatter plot** (*scatter diagram*) using a coordinate graph. Values for one variable (X) are scaled on the horizontal axis, and values for the other variable (Y) are scaled vertically (Figure 17.8). This graph presents data for 10 people (a–j). For person a, the values for X and Y are 2 and 1, respectively. To graph person a's position, we go two units to the right along the X axis and one unit up on the Y axis. The letters on the plot are shown to help identify individuals, but normally only dots appear.

In a scatter plot, the direction of the slope of points indicates the direction of the correlation. A positive correlation occurs when high values on one variable are associated with high values on a second variable. If the slope of points begins at the lower left corner and extends to the upper right corner, the relationship is positive. In the current example, X and Y are positively related. People with high scores on variable X tended to have high scores on variable Y, and low scorers on X tended to score low on Y.

A negative relationship is one in which high values on one variable are related to low values on the other. Negative relationships on a scatter plot are depicted by points that slope from the upper left corner to the lower right corner, as in Figure 17.9A and D.

When relationships are *perfect*, it is possible to predict perfectly the value of one variable by knowing the value of the second. For instance, if all people who were 6 feet 2 inches tall weighed 180 pounds, all people who were 6 feet 1 inch tall weighed 175 pounds, and so on, then weight and height would be perfectly, positively related. In such a situation, we would only need to know a person's height to know his or her weight. On a scatter plot, a perfect relationship is represented by a sloped straight line (Figure 17.9C). When a relationship is not perfect, as is usually the case, one can interpret the *degree* of correlation by seeing how closely the points cluster around a straight line. The closer the points are around a diagonal slope, the stronger the correlation. When the points are scattered all over the graph, the relationship is low or nonexistent. Various degrees and directions of relationships are shown in Figure 17.9.

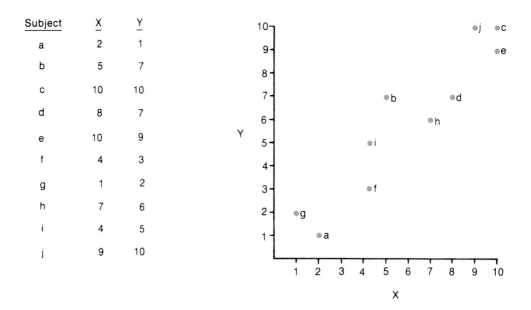

FIGURE 17.8 Construction of a scatter plot.

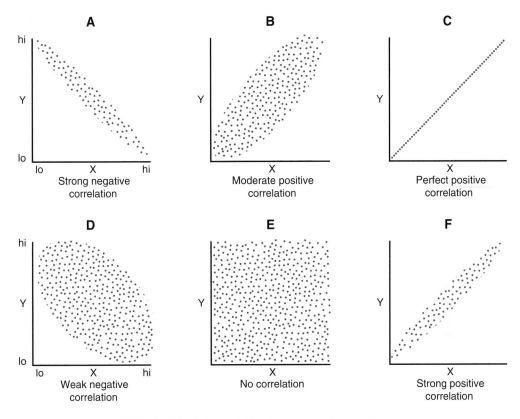

FIGURE 17.9 Various relationships graphed on scatter plots.

 The Supplement to this chapter illustrates printouts for a variety of descriptive statistics using widely used statistical software called the *Statistical Package for the Social Sciences* (SPSS).

It is more efficient to express relationships by computing a correlation coefficient, an index with values ranging from −1.00 for a perfect negative correlation, through zero for no relationship, to +1.00 for a perfect positive correlation. The higher the absolute value of the coefficient (i.e., the value disregarding the sign), the stronger the relationship. A correlation of −.30, for instance, is stronger than a correlation of +.20.

The most widely used correlation index is the **product-moment correlation coefficient**, also called **Pearson's** *r*. This coefficient is computed with variables measured on an interval or ratio scale. **Spearman's rho (ρ)** is a correlation index for ordinal-level data. The calculation of these correlation statistics is laborious and seldom performed by hand. (Computational formulas are available in statistics textbooks, such as that by Polit, 2010.)

It is difficult to offer guidelines on what to interpret as strong or weak relationships because it depends on the variables. If we measured patients' body temperatures orally and rectally, a correlation (*r*) of .70 between the two values would be low. For most psychosocial variables (e.g., stress and illness severity), an *r* of .70 is high; correlations between such variables are typically in the .30 to .40 range.

Correlation coefficients are sometimes displayed in a two-dimensional **correlation matrix**, in which every variable is displayed in both a row and a column and coefficients are displayed at the intersections. An example of a correlation matrix is presented at the end of this chapter.

RISK INDEXES

Several descriptive statistical indexes can be used to facilitate clinical decision-making. These indexes reflect the realization that risk and risk reduction must be interpreted within a context. If an intervention reduces the risk of an adverse event three times over, but the initial risk is miniscule, the intervention may be too costly to be practical. Both absolute and relative differences in risks are important in clinical decision-making.

TIP The indexes described in this section are often not reported in nursing journal articles but often can be calculated by readers. Further information about the use and interpretation of these indexes can be found in Guyatt et al. (2015) and Polit (2010).

We focus in this section on describing risk for dichotomous outcomes (e.g., alive/dead, had a fall/did not have a fall) in relation to exposure versus nonexposure to a potentially beneficial treatment. This situation results in a 2 × 2 crosstabs table with four cells, as depicted in Table 17.5, which shows labels for the four cells so that computations can be explained. *Cell a* is the number with an undesirable outcome (e.g.,

TABLE 17.5 • Indexes of Risk and Association in a 2 × 2 Table

EXPOSURE	OUTCOME		TOTAL
	UNDESIRABLE OUTCOME	**DESIRABLE OUTCOME**	
Yes, exposed (E) to intervention—experimentals (or, NOT exposed to a risk factor)	a	b	$a+b$
No, not exposed (NE) to intervention—controls (or, exposed to a risk factor)	c	d	$c+d$
Total	$a+c$	$b+d$	$a+b+c+d$

Absolute risk, exposed group (AR_E) $\quad = \quad a/(a+b)$

Absolute risk, nonexposed group (AR_{NE}) $\quad = \quad c/(c+d)$

Absolute risk reduction (ARR) $\quad = \quad AR_{NE} - AR_E$

Relative risk (RR) $\quad = \quad \dfrac{AR_E}{AR_{NE}}$

Relative risk reduction (RRR) $\quad = \quad \dfrac{ARR}{AR_{NE}}$

Odds, exposed group ($Odds_E$) $\quad = \quad a/b$

Odds, nonexposed group ($Odds_{NE}$) $\quad = \quad c/d$

Odds ratio (OR) $\quad = \quad \dfrac{Odds_E}{Odds_{NE}}$

Number needed to treat (NNT) $\quad = \quad \dfrac{1}{ARR}$

death) in an intervention group; *cell b* is the number with a desirable outcome (e.g., survival) in an intervention group; and *cells c* and *d* are the two outcome possibilities for a nonexposed (control) group. We can now explain the meaning and calculation of several indexes of interest to clinicians.

Absolute Risk

Absolute risk can be computed for those exposed to an intervention (or risk factor) and for those not exposed. **Absolute risk (AR)** is the proportion of people who experienced an undesirable outcome in each group. We illustrate this and other indexes with fictitious data from an intervention study in which 200 smokers were randomly assigned to a smoking cessation intervention or to a control group (Table 17.6). Smoking status 3 months after the intervention is the outcome variable. In this example, the absolute risk of continued smoking was .50 in the intervention group and .80 in the control group. The risk of an undesirable outcome for a treatment group is sometimes called the *experimental event rate (EER),* and the risk of an adverse outcome for untreated people is sometimes called the *baseline risk rate* or the *control event rate (CER).* In the absence of the intervention, 20% of those in the experimental group might have stopped smoking anyway, but the intervention boosted the rate to 50%.

> **TIP** The computations shown in Table 17.5 specifically reflect risk indexes that assume that the intervention exposure will be beneficial, and that information for the *undesirable* outcome will be in cells a and c. If good outcomes rather than bad ones are put in cells a and c, formulas would have to be modified. For example, AR_E would then be b/(a + b), and so on. Similarly, if the research question involved the association between an adverse outcome and a hypothesized risk factor (e.g., the risk that smoking is associated with a cardiovascular accident), the group exposed to the risk factor (e.g., those who smoke) should be in the *bottom* row (cells c and d) and not the top row—or, again, the formulas would need to be adapted. As a general rule, to use the formulas shown in Table 17.6, the cell in the lower left corner (cell c) should be predicted to reflect the highest percentage of undesirable outcomes.

Absolute Risk Reduction

The **absolute risk reduction (ARR)**, sometimes called the *risk difference* or *RD*, represents a comparison of the two risks. It is computed by subtracting the absolute risk for the exposed group from the absolute risk for the untreated group. This index indicates the estimated proportion of people who would be spared the undesirable outcome through exposure to the intervention. In our example, the value of ARR is .30: 30% of the control group participants would presumably have stopped smoking if they had received the intervention, over and above the 20% who stopped without it.

Relative Risk

Relative risk (RR), or the *risk ratio*, represents the estimated proportion of the original risk of an adverse outcome (in our example, continued smoking) that persists when people are exposed to the intervention. To compute an RR, the absolute risk for exposed people is divided by the absolute risk for nonexposed people. In our fictitious example, the RR is .625. This means that the risk of continued smoking after the smoking cessation intervention is estimated to be 62.5% of what it would have been in its absence.

Relative Risk Reduction

Relative risk reduction (RRR) is another useful index for evaluating the effectiveness of an intervention. RRR is the estimated proportion of untreated risk that is reduced through exposure to the intervention. This index is computed by dividing the ARR by the absolute risk for the control group. In our example, RRR = .375. This means that the smoking cessation intervention decreased the relative risk of continued smoking by 37.5%, compared to not having had the intervention.

Odds Ratio

The **odds ratio (OR)** is a widely reported index, even though it is less intuitively meaningful than RR as an index of risk. The **odds**, in this context, is

TABLE 17.6 • Hypothetical Data for Smoking Cessation Example Illustrating Risk Index Calculation

EXPOSURE TO SMOKING CESSATION INTERVENTION	OUTCOME		TOTAL
	CONTINUED SMOKING	STOPPED SMOKING	
Yes, exposed: E (experimental group)	50 (*a*)	50 (*b*)	100
No, not exposed: NE (control group)	80 (*c*)	20 (*d*)	100
TOTAL	130	70	200

Absolute risk, exposed group (AR_E)   =   50 / 100   =   .50
Absolute risk, nonexposed group (AR_{NE})   =   80 / 100   =   .80
Absolute risk reduction (ARR)   =   .80 − .50   =   .30
Relative risk (RR)   =   .50 / .80   =   .625
Relative risk reduction (RRR)   =   .30 / .80   =   .375

Odds ratio (OR) $= \dfrac{(50 / 50)}{(80 / 20)} = .25$

Number needed to treat   =   1 / .30   =   3.33

the proportion of people *with* the adverse outcome relative to those *without* it. In our example, the odds of continued smoking for the experimental group is 50 (the number who continued smoking) divided by 50 (the number who stopped), or 1. The odds for the control group is 80 divided by 20, or 4. The **odds ratio** is the ratio of these two odds, or .25 in our example. The estimated odds of continuing to smoke are one-fourth as high among those in the intervention group as among those in the control group. Turned around, we could say that the estimated odds of continued smoking is four times higher among smokers who did not get the intervention as among those who did.

TIP Odds ratios can be computed when the independent variable is not dichotomous, using a statistical procedure described in Chapter 19. For example, we could estimate the odds ratio for obesity among adults in four different income groups, using one of the groups as a reference.

Number Needed to Treat

A final index of interest is the **number needed to treat (NNT),** which represents an estimate of how many people would need to receive a treatment or intervention to prevent one undesirable outcome. NNT is computed by dividing 1 by the value of the absolute risk reduction. In our example, ARR = .30, and so NNT is 3.33. About three smokers would need to be exposed to the intervention to avoid one person's continued smoking. The NNT is inversely related to the RRR. An intervention that is twice as effective with regard to relative risk reduction will cut the number needed to treat in half. The NNT is especially valuable for decision-makers because it can be integrated with monetary information to determine if an intervention is cost-effective.

Example of Relative Risk and Number Needed to Treat
Forni and colleagues (2018) tested the effectiveness of a new polyurethane foam multilayer dressing in the sacral area to prevent pressure ulcers in the elderly with hip fractures. Pressure ulcers occurred in 4.5% of the patients in the intervention group and 15.4% of those in the control group. The relative risk was .29 with an NNT of 9.

BOX 17.1 Guidelines for Critically Appraising Descriptive Statistics

1. Did the report include descriptive statistics? Do these statistics sufficiently describe major characteristics of the sample?
2. Were descriptive statistics used appropriately—for example, were descriptive statistics used to describe sample characteristics, key variables, and methodologic features of the study, such as response rate or attrition rate? Were they used to answer research questions when inferential statistics would have been more appropriate?
3. Were the correct descriptive statistics used—for example, was a mean presented when percentages would have been more informative? If the median was used rather than the mean, was this appropriate?
4. Was the descriptive information presented in a useful format—for example, were tables used effectively? Is information in the text and the tables redundant? Is information in the text and tables consistent with each other? Were the tables clear, with a good title, carefully labeled headings, and good table notes?
5. Were any risk indexes computed? If not, would they have been useful?

TIP Various tools on the Internet facilitate the calculation of risk indexes. Links to these and other useful websites are available in the Toolkit for you to "click" on directly.

CRITICAL APPRAISAL OF DESCRIPTIVE STATISTICS

Descriptive statistics help to set the stage for understanding quantitative evidence. Descriptive statistics are useful for communicating information about the study sample. Readers of reports cannot draw inferences about the study's applicability without understanding who the participants were with regard to key demographic characteristics and health-related attributes.

In addition to describing sample characteristics, descriptive statistics are useful in communicating information about the baseline values of key outcome variables in longitudinal or intervention studies, or correlations between a set of independent variables. Methodologic information about study quality also typically relies on descriptive statistics—for example, response rates and attrition rates are typically shown as percentages, and means are used to characterize such things as time elapsed between two interviews.

Descriptive statistics are sometimes used to directly address research questions in studies that are primarily descriptive. However, when only descriptive statistics are presented, readers should think about whether the inclusion of inferential statistics would have been preferable. If a research question is about a *population*, and not just about the particular people who participated in the research, inferential statistics are needed.

In critically appraising the researcher's use of descriptive statistics, readers can consider whether the information was adequate, whether the correct statistical indexes were used, and whether it was presented in a clear and efficient manner. Box 17.1 (which is also found in the Toolkit) presents some guiding questions for a critical appraisal of the descriptive statistics presented in a research report.

RESEARCH EXAMPLE

We conclude this chapter with an example of a study that presented several of the descriptive statistics mentioned in this chapter.

Study: Physical activity among female adolescents in Jeddah, Saudi Arabia (Bajamal et al., 2017).

Statement of purpose: The overall purpose of this study was to examine relationships among self-reported physical activity and cognitive and affective variables among female Saudi adolescents 13 to 18 years of age.

Methods: The sample of female Saudis was recruited from 10 randomly selected intermediate and high schools in Jeddah, a large city in Saudi Arabia. Those who met the eligibility criteria completed surveys and were measured for height and weight. The survey included demographic questions and scales to measure physical activity (PA), perceived barriers to physical activity, and other PA-related variables. The final sample included 383 adolescents.

Analysis and findings: The researchers undertook numerous complex analyses that are not described here. In terms of descriptive statistics, they presented information about the participants' background characteristics. Table 17.7 summarizes a few variables that were measured on the ordinal scale. This table shows, for example, that the adolescents were about equally divided across grade groupings, and that about half came from families where both the mother and father had college degrees. About one out of four of these adolescents was either overweight or obese.

Findings about interrelationships among variables were presented in a correlation matrix. An adapted version of this matrix, with selected variables, is presented in Table 17.8.[a] This table lists, on the left, six variables: participants' scores on (1) the physical activity scale, (2) perceived barriers to PA scale, (3) PA self-efficacy scale, (4) PA enjoyment scale, (5) commitment to PA scale, and (6) age. The numbers in the top row correspond to the six variables: 1 is physical activity scores, and so on. The correlation matrix shows, in the first column, the correlation coefficients (*r*) between PA scores with all six variables. At the intersection of row 1 and column 1, we find the value 1.00, which simply indicates that PA scores are perfectly correlated with themselves. The next entry in the first column is the correlation between PA scores and perceived barriers to PA. The value of −.20 indicates a modest negative relationship: those who have higher levels of physical activity had somewhat lower perceived barriers to physical activity. The next entry (.29) indicates a modest positive relationship between PA and PA self-efficacy: those who engaged in more

---

[a]Although we present only descriptive information in Table 17.8, Bajamal et al. also presented inferential statistical information in their correlation matrix—that is, they identified correlations that were statistically significant.

TABLE 17.7 • Selected Demographic Characteristics of Female Saudi Adolescents in the Study Sample (*N* = 338)

SAMPLE CHARACTERISTIC	FREQUENCY (*n*)	PERCENT (%)
Grade		
7th or 8th	126	32.9
9th or 10th	118	30.8
11th or 12th	139	36.3
Mother's education level		
Intermediate school or lower	86	22.4
High school	116	30.3
Undergraduate degree or higher	181	47.3
Father's education level		
Intermediate school or lower	53	13.8
High school	119	31.1
Undergraduate degree or higher	211	55.1
BMI category		
Thin	70	18.3
Normal weight	216	56.4
Overweight	67	17.5
Obese	30	7.8

Adapted from Table 1 of Bajamal, E., Robbins, L., Ling, J., Smith, B., Pfeiffer, K., & Sharma, D. (2017). Physical activity among female adolescents in Jeddah, Saudi Arabia: A health promotion model-based path analysis. *Nursing Research, 66,* 473–482.

physical activity had somewhat higher scores on the self-efficacy for PA scale. Age was unrelated to most of the outcomes, except PA: there was a tendency for older girls to engage in less physical activity. The two right-hand columns of this table show the means and *SD*s for all six variables. For example, the girls were,

TABLE 17.8 • Correlation Matrix for Selected Study Variables Relating to Physical Activity in Female Saudi Adolescents

VARIABLE	1	2	3	4	5	6	MEAN	SD
1. Physical activity (PA) score	1.00						2.1	0.7
2. Perceived barriers to PA score	−.20	1.00					1.4	0.4
3. PA self-efficacy score	.29	−.18	1.00				1.8	0.6
4. PA enjoyment score	.27	−.31	.35	1.00			2.4	0.5
5. Commitment to PA scores	.32	−.18	.48	.44	1.00		1.9	0.6
6. Age	−.21	.00	−.05	.00	−.01	1.00	15.4	1.7

Adapted from Table 2 of Bajamal, E., Robbins, L., Ling, J., Smith, B., Pfeiffer, K., & Sharma, D. (2017). Physical activity among female adolescents in Jeddah, Saudi Arabia: A health promotion model-based path analysis. *Nursing Research, 66*, 473–482.

on average, 15.4 years old ($SD = 1.7$). Mean scores on the PA scale ($M = 2.1$) indicated fairly low levels of physical activity in this sample.

SUMMARY POINTS

- There are four **levels of measurement**: (1) **nominal measurement**—the classification of characteristics into mutually exclusive categories, (2) **ordinal measurement**—the ranking of objects based on their relative standing on an attribute, (3) **interval measurement**—indicating not only the ranking of objects but the amount of distance between them, and (4) **ratio measurement**—distinguished from interval measurement by having a rational zero point.
- **Descriptive statistics** enable researchers to summarize and describe quantitative data.
- **Frequency distributions** impose order on raw data. Numeric values are ordered from lowest to highest, accompanied by a count of the number (or percentage) of times each value was obtained.
- **Histograms** and **frequency polygons** are methods of displaying frequency information graphically.
- Data for a variable can be described in terms of the shape of the distribution, central tendency, and variability.

- A distribution is **symmetric** if its two halves are mirror images of each other. A **skewed** distribution is asymmetric, with one tail longer than the other.
- In **positively skewed distributions,** the long tail points to the right (e.g., personal income); in **negatively skewed distributions,** the tail points to the left (e.g., age at death).
- The **modality** of a distribution refers to the number of peaks: A **unimodal distribution** has one peak, and a **multimodal distribution** has more than one peak.
- A **normal distribution** (*bell-shaped curve*) is symmetric, unimodal, and not too peaked.
- Measures of **central tendency** are indexes that represent the average or typical value of a set of scores. The **mode** is the value that occurs most frequently in a distribution. The **median** is the point above which and below which 50% of the cases fall. The **mean** is the arithmetic average of all scores. The mean is a preferred index of central tendency because of its *stability* from sample to sample drawn from a population.
- Measures of **variability**—how spread out the data are—include the range and standard deviation. The **range** is the distance between the highest and lowest scores. The **standard deviation** (*SD*) indicates how much, on average, scores deviate from the mean.

- The *SD* is calculated by first computing **deviation scores**, which indicate the degree to which a person's score deviates from the mean. The **variance** is equal to the *SD* squared. In a normal distribution, 95% of scores fall within 2 *SD*s above and below the mean.
- **Bivariate descriptive statistics** describe relationships between two variables.
- A **crosstabs table** is a two-dimensional frequency distribution in which the frequencies of two nominal- or ordinal-level variables are crosstabulated.
- **Correlation coefficients** describe the direction and magnitude of a relationship between two variables. Researchers most often compute the **product-moment correlation coefficient** (**Pearson's *r***), used with interval- or ratio-level variables. The **Spearman rho coefficient** is used to correlate ordinal-level variables.
- Graphically, the relationship between two continuous variables can be displayed on a **scatter plot.**
- Several risk indexes describe outcomes in relation to exposures (to interventions or risk factors) for a two-group (e.g., experimental versus control) situation with dichotomous outcomes (e.g., alive/dead). These indexes are useful in clinical decision-making.
- **Absolute risk reduction (ARR)** expresses the estimated proportion of people who would be spared an adverse outcome through exposure to an intervention (or lack of exposure to a risk). **Relative risk (RR)** is the estimated proportion of the original risk of an adverse outcome that persists among people exposed to an intervention. **Relative risk reduction (RRR)** is the estimated proportion of untreated risk that is reduced through exposure to the intervention. The **odds ratio (OR)** is the ratio of the odds for the treated versus untreated group, with **odds** reflecting the proportion of people with the adverse outcome relative to those without it. The **number needed to treat (NNT)** is an estimate of how many people would need to receive the intervention to prevent one adverse outcome.

STUDY ACTIVITIES

Study activities are available to instructors on thePoint.

REFERENCES CITED IN CHAPTER 17

**Bajamal, E., Robbins, L., Ling, J., Smith, B., Pfeiffer, K., & Sharma, D. (2017). Physical activity among female adolescents in Jeddah, Saudi Arabia: A health promotion model-based path analysis. *Nursing Research, 66*, 473–482.

Forni, C., D'Allessandro, F., Gallerani, P., Genco, R., Bolzon, A., Bombino, C., … Taddia, P. (2018). Effectiveness of using a new polyurethane foam multi-layer dressing in the sacral area to prevent the onset of pressure ulcer in the elderly with hip fractures: A pragmatic randomised controlled trial. *International Wound Journal, 15*, 383–390.

Guyatt, G., Rennie, D., Meade, M., & Cook, D. (2015). *Users' guide to the medical literature: A manual for evidence-based clinical practice* (3rd ed.). New York: McGraw Hill.

*Lucas-de la Cruz, L., Martín-Espinosa, N., Cavero-Redondo, I., González-Garcia, A., Díez-Fernández, A., Martínez-Vizcaíno, V., & Notario-Pacheco, B. (2018). Sleep patterns and cardiometabolic risk in schoolchildren from Cuenca, Spain. *PLoS One, 13*, e0191637.

Luz, S., Shadmi, E., Admi, H., Peterfreund, I., & Drach-Zahavy, A. (2019). Characteristics and behaviours of formal versus informal nurse champions and their relationship to innovation success. *Journal of Advanced Nursing, 75*, 85–95.

Polit, D. F. (2010). *Statistics and data analysis for nursing research* (2nd ed.). Upper Saddle River, NJ: Pearson.

*Zenk, S., Tarlov, E., Wing, C., Matthews, S., Tong, H., Jones, K., & Powell, L. (2018). Long-term weight loss effects of a behavioral weight management program: Does the community food environment matter? *International Journal of Environmental Research and Public Health, 15*(2).

A link to this open-access article is provided in the Toolkit for Chapter 17 in the Resource Manual. ✖

****This journal article is available on** thePoint *for this chapter.*

18 | Inferential Statistics

Inferential statistics, based on the **laws of probability**, allow researchers to draw conclusions about a population, given data from a sample. Inferential statistics would help us with such questions as, "What can I infer about 1-minute Apgar scores of premature babies (the population) after calculating a mean Apgar score of 6.9 in a sample of 500 premature babies?" Inferential statistics provide a framework for making objective judgments about the reliability of sample statistics as estimates of population parameters. Different researchers applying inferential statistics to the same data are likely to draw the same conclusions.

SAMPLING DISTRIBUTIONS

To estimate population parameters, representative samples should be used, and probability sampling is the best way to get representative samples (Chapter 13). Inferential statistics assume random sampling from populations, an assumption that is widely violated. The validity of statistical calculations does depend, however, on the extent to which results from the sample are similar to what you would have obtained had you randomly selected people from the population.

Even when random sampling *is* used, sample characteristics are seldom identical to population characteristics. Suppose we had a population of 50,000 nursing school applicants whose mean score on a standardized entrance exam was 500.0 with a standard deviation (*SD*) of 100.0. Suppose we wanted to estimate the population mean from the scores of a random sample of 25 students. Would we expect a mean of *exactly* 500.0 for the sample? Obtaining the exact population value is unlikely. Let us say the sample mean is 505.1. If a new random sample were drawn, we might obtain a mean of, say, 497.8. The tendency for statistics to fluctuate from one sample to another reflects **sampling error**. The challenge is to decide whether sample values are good estimates of population parameters.

Researchers compute statistics with only *one* sample, but to understand inferential statistics we must perform a mental exercise. Consider drawing a sample of 25 students from the population of 50,000, calculating a mean, replacing the students, and drawing a new sample. Each mean is one datum. If we drew 100,000 such samples, we would have 100,000 means (data points) that could be used to construct a frequency polygon (Figure 18.1). This distribution is a **sampling distribution of the mean**. A sampling distribution is theoretical—in practice no one draws consecutive samples from a population and plots their means. Sampling distributions are the basis of inferential statistics.

Characteristics of Sampling Distributions

When an infinite number of samples are randomly drawn from a population, the sampling distribution of the mean has certain characteristics.

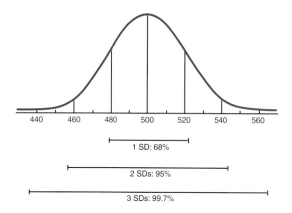

FIGURE 18.1 A sampling distribution of the mean.

(Our example of 100,000 samples is large enough to approximate these characteristics.) Sampling distributions of means are normally distributed, and the mean always equals the population mean. In the example shown in Figure 18.1, the mean of the sampling distribution is 500.0, the same as the population mean.

Remember that when data are normally distributed, 68% of values fall between ±1 *SD* from the mean. Because a sampling distribution of means is normally distributed, we can say that the probability is 68 out of 100 that any randomly drawn sample mean lies between +1 *SD* and −1 *SD* of the population mean. Thus, if we knew the standard deviation of the sampling distribution, we could interpret the accuracy of a sample mean.

Standard Error of the Mean

The standard deviation of a sampling distribution of the mean is called the **standard error of the mean (*SEM*)**. The word *error* signifies that the various means in the sampling distribution have some error as estimates of the population mean. The smaller the *SEM*—that is, the less variable the sample means—the more accurate is a single mean as an estimate of the population value.

No one actually constructs a sampling distribution, so how can its standard deviation be computed? Fortunately, there is a formula for estimating the *SEM* from a single sample, using two pieces of information: the sample's standard deviation and sample size. The equation for the SEM is: $SD/\sqrt{N}$.

In our example, if we use this formula to calculate the *SEM* for an *SD* of 100.0 with a sample of 25 students, we obtain:

$$SEM = \frac{100.0}{\sqrt{25}} = 20.0$$

The standard deviation of the sampling distribution in our example is 20.0, as shown in Figure 18.1. This *SEM* is an estimate of how much sampling error there is from one sample mean to another when samples of 25 are randomly drawn and the *SD* is 100.0.

Given that a sampling distribution of means follows a normal curve, we can estimate the probability of drawing a sample with a certain mean. With a sample size of 25 and a population mean of 500.0, the chances are about 95 out of 100 that any sample mean will fall between 460 and 540 (i.e., 2 *SD*s above and below the mean). Only 5 times out of 100 would the mean of a randomly selected sample exceed 540 or be less than 460. Only 5 times out of 100 would we get a sample whose mean deviated from the population mean by more than 40 points.

Because the *SEM* is partly a function of sample size, we need only increase sample size to increase the accuracy of our estimate. If we used a sample of 100 applicants, rather than 25, the SEM would be 10 (i.e., $100/\sqrt{100} = 10.0$). In this situation, the chances are about 95 out of 100 that a sample mean will be between 480 and 520. The chances of drawing a sample with a mean very different from the population mean are reduced as sample size increases because large numbers promote the likelihood that extreme values will cancel each other out.

ESTIMATION OF PARAMETERS

Statistical inference consists of two techniques: (1) estimation of parameters and (2) hypothesis testing. Parameter estimates have not traditionally been presented in nursing research reports, but that situation is changing. The push for evidence-based practice (EBP) has heightened interest among practitioners in learning not only whether a hypothesis was supported (via hypothesis testing) but also the estimated value of a population parameter and the degree of accuracy of the estimate (via parameter estimation). Many medical research journals *require* that estimation information be reported because it is useful to clinicians (Braitman, 1991). In this section we present general concepts relating to parameter estimation and offer some examples based on one-variable descriptive statistics.

Confidence Intervals

Parameter estimation is used to estimate a parameter—for example, a mean, a proportion, or a mean difference between two groups (e.g., experimental and control group members). Estimation can take two forms: point estimation or interval estimation. **Point estimation** involves calculating a single statistic to estimate the population parameter. To continue with the earlier example, if we calculated the mean entrance exam score for a sample of 25 applicants and found that it was 510.0, then this would be the point estimate of the population mean.

Interval estimation is useful because it indicates a range of values within which the parameter has a specified probability of lying. With interval estimation, researchers construct a **confidence interval** (**CI**) around the estimate; the upper and lower limits are **confidence limits**. Constructing a confidence interval around a sample mean establishes a range of values for the population value as well as the probability of being right—the estimate is made with a certain degree of confidence. By convention, researchers usually use either a 95% or a 99% confidence interval.

Confidence Intervals Around a Mean

Calculating confidence limits around a mean involves using the *SEM*. In a normal distribution, 95% of the scores lie within about 2 *SD*s (more precisely, 1.96 *SD*s) from the mean. In our example, suppose the point estimate for mean entrance exam scores is 510.0, and the *SD* is 100.0. The *SEM* for a sample of 25 would be 20.0. We can build a 95% confidence interval with the following formula:

$$\text{CI } 95\% = (\bar{X} \pm 1.96 \times SEM)$$

That is, confidence is 95% that the population mean lies between the values equal to 1.96 times

the *SEM*, above and below the sample mean. In the example at hand, we would obtain the following:

$$\text{CI } 95\% = \left(510.0 \pm \left(1.96 \times 20.0\right)\right)$$
$$\text{CI } 95\% = \left(510.0 \pm \left(39.2\right)\right)$$
$$\text{CI } 95\% = \left(470.8 \leq \mu \leq 549.2\right)$$

The final statement may be read as follows: confidence is 95% that the population mean (symbolized by the Greek letter mu [μ] by convention) is between 470.8 and 549.2. This would be stated in a research report as 95% CI = 470.8 to 549.2, or 95% CI (470.8, 549.2).

Confidence intervals reflect the researchers' risk of being wrong. With a 95% CI, researchers accept the probability that they will be wrong five times out of 100. A 99% CI sets the risk at only 1% by allowing a wider range of possible values. The formula is as follows:

$$\text{CI } 99\% (\bar{X} \pm 2.58 \times SEM)$$

The 2.58 reflects the fact that 99% of all cases in a normal distribution lie within ±2.58 *SD* units from the mean. In the example, the 99% confidence interval would be:

$$\text{CI } 99\% = \left(510.0 \pm \left(2.58 \times 20.0\right)\right)$$
$$\text{CI } 99\% = \left(510.0 \pm \left(51.6\right)\right)$$
$$\text{CI } 99\% = \left(458.4 \leq \mu \leq 561.6\right)$$

The price of having a reduced risk of being wrong is reduced *precision*. With 95% confidence, the range of the CI was about 80 points; with 99% confidence, the range is more than 100 points. The acceptable risk of error depends on the nature of the problem. In research with implications for the health of individual patients, a stringent 99% confidence interval might be used; for most studies, a 95% confidence interval usually is sufficient.

Confidence Intervals Around Proportions and Risk Indexes

Calculating confidence intervals around a proportion or percentage is important, especially with regard to risk estimates. Consider, for example, this question: "What proportion of people exposed to a certain hazard will contract a disease?" This question calls for an estimated proportion (an absolute risk index, as described in Chapter 17) that is more useful if it is reported within a 95% confidence interval.

For proportions based on dichotomous variables, as in the above question (positive/negative for a disease), the theoretical distribution is a **binomial distribution**. A binomial distribution is the probability distribution of the number of "successes" (e.g., heads) in a sequence of independent yes/no trials (e.g., a coin toss), each of which yields "success" with a specified probability.

Building confidence intervals around a proportion is computationally complex, and so we do not provide formulas here, but certain features of confidence intervals around proportions are worth noting. First, the CI is rarely symmetric around a sample proportion. For example, if 3 out of 30 sample members were positive for an outcome (e.g., hospital readmission), the estimated population proportion would be .10 and the 95% CI would be from .021 to .265. Second, the width of the CI depends on both the sample size and the value of the proportion. The smaller the sample, the wider the CI. And, the closer the sample proportion is to .50, the wider the CI. For example, with a sample size of 30, the range for a 95% CI for a proportion of .50 is .374 (.313, .687), while the range for a proportion of .10 is only .188 (.021, .265). Finally, the CI for a proportion never extends below 0 or above 1.0, but a CI can be constructed around an *obtained* proportion of 0 or 1.0. For example, if 0 out of our 30 participants were readmitted to the hospital, the estimated proportion would be .00 and the 95% CI would be from .00 to .116.

It is advisable to construct confidence intervals around all the risk indexes described in the previous chapter, such as the ARR, RRR, OR, and NNT. The computed value of these indexes from study data represents a "best estimate" and confidence intervals indicate the estimate's precision. Clearly, clinical inference is enhanced when information about a plausible range of values for risk indexes is presented. An easy method for constructing 95% CIs around major risk indexes is to use an online calculator, such as the one in the Evidence-Based Medicine Toolbox (https://ebm-tools.knowledgetranslation.net/calculator/prospective/).

Example of CIs Around Odds Ratios

Gray and Giuliano (2018) studied the relationship between characteristics of incontinent patients in acute care facilities and the risk of facility-acquired sacral pressure injury. They found, for example, that the odds ratio for such an injury for those who were immobile versus those who were mobile was 3.30 (95% CI = 2.38-4.59).

HYPOTHESIS TESTING

Statistical **hypothesis testing** provides objective criteria for deciding whether hypotheses are supported by data. Suppose we hypothesized that participation in a stress management program would reduce anxiety levels among patients with cancer. The sample is 25 control group patients who do not participate in the program and 25 patients who do. The mean posttreatment anxiety score for the intervention group is 15.8 and that for controls is 17.9. Should we conclude that the hypothesis is correct? Group differences are in the predicted direction, but the results might represent sampling error. With a new sample, group means might be nearly identical. Statistical hypothesis testing allows researchers to make objective decisions about whether study results likely reflect chance sample differences or true population differences.

The Null Hypothesis

Hypothesis testing is based on negative inference. In our example, patients participating in the intervention had lower mean anxiety scores than control group patients. There are two possible explanations: (1) the intervention was successful in reducing anxiety; or (2) the differences resulted from chance factors. The first explanation is our research hypothesis, and the second is the null hypothesis. The **null hypothesis**, it may be recalled, states that there is no relationship between variables. Statistical hypothesis testing is basically a process of rejection. It cannot be demonstrated directly that the research hypothesis is correct but, using theoretical sampling distributions, it can be shown that the null hypothesis has a high probability of being wrong. Researchers seek to reject the null hypothesis through various **statistical tests**.

The null hypothesis in our example can be stated formally as follows:

$$H_0 : \mu_E = \mu_C$$

The null hypothesis (H_0) is that the mean population anxiety score for experimental group patients (μ_E) is the same as that for controls (μ_C). The **alternative**, or research, **hypothesis** (H_A) is that the means are *not* the same:

$$H_A : \mu_E \neq \mu_C$$

Null hypotheses are accepted or rejected based on sample data, but hypothesis testing is used to make inferences about the population.

Type I and Type II Errors

Researchers decide whether to accept or reject a null hypothesis by determining how *probable* it is that observed results are due to chance. Researchers cannot know with certainty whether a null hypothesis is or is not true based on data from a sample. They can only conclude that hypotheses are *probably* true or *probably* false, and there is always a risk of error.

Researchers can make two types of statistical error: rejecting a true null hypothesis or accepting a false null hypothesis. Figure 18.2 summarizes possible outcomes of researchers' decisions. Researchers make a **Type I error** by rejecting a null hypothesis that is, in fact, true. For instance, if we concluded that a drug was more effective than a placebo in reducing cholesterol, when in fact the observed differences in cholesterol levels resulted from sampling fluctuations, this would be a Type I error—a false positive conclusion. Conversely, if we concluded that group differences in cholesterol resulted by chance, when in fact the drug *did* reduce cholesterol, this would be a **Type II error**—a false negative conclusion. In the context of drug testing, a good way to think about statistical error can be expressed as follows: A Type I error might allow an ineffective drug to come onto the market, but a Type II error might *prevent* an effective drug from coming onto the market.

Level of Significance

Researchers never know when they have made an error in statistical decision making. The validity of a null hypothesis could be known only by collecting data from the population. Researchers control the *risk* of a Type I error by selecting a **level of significance**, which signifies the probability of incorrectly rejecting a true null hypothesis.

The two most frequently used significance levels (referred to as **alpha** or α) are .05 and .01. With a .05 significance level, we accept the risk that out of 100 samples drawn from a population, a true null hypothesis would be rejected 5 times. With a .01 significance level, the risk of a Type I error is *lower*: in only 1 sample out of 100 would we erroneously reject the null hypothesis. The minimum acceptable level for α usually is .05. A stricter level (e.g., .01 or .001) may be needed when the decision has important consequences.

The actual situation is that the null hypothesis is:

		True	False
The researcher calculates a test statistic and decides that the null hypothesis is:	True (Null accepted)	Correct decision	Type II error (False negative)
	False (Null rejected)	Type I error (False positive)	Correct decision

FIGURE 18.2 Outcomes of statistical decision making.

> **TIP** A group of prominent researchers and statisticians have made a controversial proposal to "redefine statistical significance" by using a threshold of .005 rather than .05 for inferences of statistical significance (Benjamin et al., 2017). Their argument is based, in part, on the fact that many significant findings cannot be replicated. It remains to be seen if their viewpoint will predominate in the years ahead.

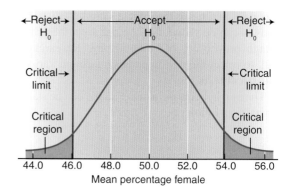

FIGURE 18.3 Critical regions in the sampling distribution for a two-tailed test: Gender bias example.

Naturally, researchers want to reduce the risk of committing both types of error, but unfortunately lowering the risk of a Type I error increases the risk of a Type II error. The stricter the criterion for rejecting a null hypothesis, the greater the probability of accepting a false null hypothesis. Researchers must deal with tradeoffs in establishing criteria for statistical decision making, but the simplest way of reducing the risk of a Type II error is to increase sample size. Type II errors are discussed later in this chapter.

Critical Regions

By selecting a significance level, researchers establish a decision rule. That rule is to reject the null hypothesis if the test statistic falls at or beyond the limits that establish a **critical region** on an applicable theoretical distribution, and to accept the null hypothesis otherwise. The critical region indicates whether the null hypothesis is *improbable*, given the results.

An example from our study of gender bias in nursing research (Polit & Beck, 2013) illustrates the statistical decision-making process. We examined whether males and females are equally represented as study participants in nursing studies—that is, whether the average percentage of females across studies in four leading nursing research journals was 50.0 as one would expect if there was no bias. The null hypothesis is H_0: $\mu = 50.0$, and the alternate hypothesis is H_A: $\mu \neq 50.0$. We found, using a consecutive sample of 300 studies published over a 2-year period, that the mean percentage of female study participants was 74.1. Using statistical procedures, we tested the hypothesis that the mean of 74.1 was not merely a chance fluctuation from a population mean of 50.0.

In hypothesis testing, researchers assume the null hypothesis is true and then gather evidence to disprove it. Assuming a mean percentage of 50.0 for the population of nursing studies, a theoretical sampling distribution can be constructed. The standard error of the mean in this example is about 2.0, as shown in Figure 18.3.

Based on normal distribution characteristics,[1] we can determine *probable* and *improbable* values of sample means from the population of nursing studies. If, as is assumed in the null hypothesis, the population mean is 50.0, then 95% of all sample means would fall between 46.0 and 54.0, i.e., within 2 *SD*s above and below the mean of 50.0. The obtained sample mean of 74.1 is in the critical region considered *improbable* if the null hypothesis were true—in fact, any value greater than 54.0% female would be improbable with alpha = .05. In our study, the probability of obtaining an average of 74.1% female by chance alone was less than 1 in 10,000. We rejected the null hypothesis that the mean percentage of females in nursing studies was 50.0. We would not be justified in saying that we had *proved* our hypothesis because the possibility of having made a Type I error remains—but the possibility is, in this case, remote. We can *accept* the alternative hypothesis

---

[1]Strictly speaking, the appropriate theoretical distribution in this example is the *t* distribution, but with a large *N*, the *t* and normal distributions are highly similar.

that the population mean is not 50.0—i.e., that males and females are not equally represented as participants in nursing studies.

> **TIP** Levels of significance are analogous to the CI values described earlier—an alpha of .05 is analogous to the 95% CI, and an alpha of .01 is analogous to the 99% CI. In our example of gender bias, the 95% CI around the mean percentage female of 74.1 was 71.1 to 77.1.

Statistical Tests

Researchers test hypotheses by computing **test statistics** with their data. For every test statistic, there is a related theoretical distribution. The value of the computed test statistic is compared to values of the critical limits for the relevant distribution.

When researchers calculate a test statistic that is beyond the critical limit, the results are said to be **statistically significant**. The word *significant* does not mean *important* or *clinically meaningful*. In statistics, *significant* means that obtained results are not likely to have been the result of chance, at a specified level of probability. A **nonsignificant result** means that an observed result could reflect chance fluctuations.

> **TIP** When the null hypothesis is retained (i.e., when results are nonsignificant), this is sometimes referred to as a *negative result*. Negative results are often disappointing to researchers and may lead to rejection of a manuscript by journal editors. Research reports with negative results are not rejected because editors are prejudiced against certain types of outcomes; they are rejected because negative results are inconclusive and difficult to interpret. A nonsignificant result indicates that the result *could* have occurred as a result of chance and provides no evidence that the research hypothesis is or is not correct.

One-Tailed and Two-Tailed Tests

In most hypothesis-testing situations, researchers use **two-tailed tests**. This means that both tails

of the sampling distribution are used to determine improbable values. In Figure 18.3, for example, the critical region that contains 5% of the sampling distribution's area involves 2½% in one tail of the distribution and 2½% in the other. If the significance level were .01, the critical regions would involve ½% in each tail.

When researchers have a strong basis for a directional hypothesis, they sometimes use a **one-tailed test**. For example, if we did an RCT to test a program to improve prenatal practices among rural women, we would expect birth outcomes for the two groups not to just be *different*; we would expect program participants to *benefit*. It could be argued that it does not make sense to use the tail of the distribution signifying *worse* outcomes in the intervention group.

In one-tailed tests, the critical region of improbable values is in only one tail of the distribution—the tail corresponding to the direction of the hypothesis, as illustrated in Figure 18.4. Using our earlier gender bias example, the research hypothesis being tested might be that the population mean is *greater than* 50.0—i.e., that, on average, females are overrepresented in nursing studies. When a one-tailed test is used, the critical 5% area of "improbability" covers a bigger area of the specified tail, so one-tailed tests are less conservative. Thus, it is easier to reject the null hypothesis with a one-tailed test than with a two-tailed test. In our gender bias example, with an alpha of .05, a sample mean of

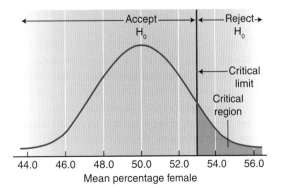

FIGURE 18.4 Critical region in the sampling distribution for a one-tailed test: Gender bias example.

53.0 or greater would result in rejecting the null hypothesis for a one-tailed test, rather than 54.0 for a two-tailed test.

One-tailed tests are controversial. Most researchers use a two-tailed test even if they have a directional hypothesis. In reading research reports, one can assume that two-tailed tests were used unless one-tailed tests are specifically mentioned. When there is a strong theoretical reason for a directional hypothesis and for assuming that findings in the opposite direction are virtually impossible, however, a one-tailed test might be warranted. In the remainder of this chapter, the examples are for two-tailed tests.

TIP You should choose a one-tailed test only if you state a directional hypothesis in advance of statistical testing. And, you must be prepared to attribute any observed group differences in the "wrong" direction to chance, even if the group differences are large.

Parametric and Nonparametric Tests

There are two broad classes of statistical tests, parametric and nonparametric. **Parametric tests** involve estimation of a parameter, require measurements on at least an interval scale, and involve several assumptions, such as the assumption that the variables are normally distributed in the population. **Nonparametric tests**, by contrast, do not estimate parameters. They involve less restrictive assumptions about the shape of the variables' distribution than do parametric tests.

Parametric tests are more powerful than nonparametric tests and are usually preferred, but there is some disagreement. Purists insist that if the requirements of parametric tests are not met, they are inappropriate. Statistical studies have shown, however, that statistical decision making is not affected when the assumptions for parametric tests are violated if sample sizes are large. Nonparametric tests are most useful when data cannot in any manner be construed as interval-level, when the distribution is markedly nonnormal, or when the sample size is very small.

TIP Some statisticians advise that when N is 50 or greater, it may not be necessary to use nonparametric statistics, unless the population has a markedly unusual distribution. Such advice invokes the **central limit theorem**, which, briefly, concerns the fact that when samples are large, the theoretical distribution of sample *means* tends to follow a normal distribution— *even if* the variable itself is not normally distributed in the population. With small Ns, you cannot rely on the central limit theorem, so probability values could be wrong if a parametric test is used.

Between-Subjects Tests and Within-Subjects Tests

Another distinction in statistical tests concerns the nature of the comparisons. When comparisons involve different people (e.g., men versus women), the study uses a between-subjects design, and the statistical test is a **test for independent groups**. Other designs involve a single group of people—for example, with a crossover design, participants are exposed to two or more treatments. In within-subjects designs, comparisons are not independent because the same people are used in all conditions, and the appropriate statistical tests are **tests for dependent groups**.

Overview of Hypothesis-Testing Procedures

This chapter describes several bivariate statistical tests. We have emphasized applications rather than computations, but urge you to consult other references (e.g., Dancey et al., 2012; Gravetter et al., 2018; Polit, 2010) for fuller explanations. In this research methods textbook, our goal is to provide an overview of the use and interpretation of some common statistical tests.

Each statistical test has a particular application, but the process of testing hypotheses is basically the same. The steps are as follows:

1. *Select an appropriate test statistic.* Figure 18.5 provides a quick reference guide for selecting many widely used bivariate statistical tests. (Multivariate tests are discussed in Chapter 19.) Researchers must consider such factors as which measurement levels were used, whether a

Level of Measurement of Dependent Variable	Group Comparisons: Number of Groups (the Independent Variable)				Correlational Analyses (to Examine Relationship Strength)
	2 Groups		3+ Groups		
	Independent Groups Tests	Dependent Groups Tests	Independent Groups Tests	Dependent Groups Tests	
Nominal (categorical)	χ^2 (or Fisher's exact test)	McNemar's test	χ^2	Cochran's Q	Phi coefficient (dichotomous) or Cramér's V (not restricted to dichotomous)
Ordinal (rank)	Mann–Whitney U test**	Wilcoxon signed-rank test	Kruskal– Wallis H test	Friedman test	Spearman's rho (or Kendall's tau)
Interval or ratio (continuous)*	Independent group t-test	Paired t-test	ANOVA	RM- ANOVA	Pearson's r
	Multifactor ANOVA for 2+ independent variables				
	RM-ANOVA for 2+ groups x 2+ measurements over time				

*For distributions that are markedly nonnormal or samples that are small, the nonparametric tests in the row above may be needed.
**The Mann–Whitney U test is also known as the Wilcoxon rank-sum test.

FIGURE 18.5 Quick guide to bivariate statistical tests.

parametric test is justified, whether a dependent groups test is appropriate, and whether the focus is correlations or group comparisons—and how many groups are being compared.

2. *Establish the level of significance.* Researchers establish the criterion for accepting or rejecting the null hypothesis. An α of .05 has been considered acceptable in most circumstances.

3. *Select a one-tailed or two-tailed test.* In most cases, a two-tailed test should be used.

4. *Compute a test statistic.* Using collected data, researchers calculate a test statistic.

5. *Determine the degrees of freedom* (symbolized as *df*). **Degrees of freedom** refers to the number of observations free to vary about a parameter. The concept is too complex for full elaboration, but *df* is easy to compute.

6. *Compare the test statistic with a tabled value.* Theoretical distributions for test statistics enable researchers to determine whether the test statistic (Step 4) is beyond the range of what is *probable* if the null hypothesis were true. Computed test statistic values are compared to values in a table. If the absolute value of the test statistic

is larger than the tabled value, the results are statistically significant. If the computed value is smaller, the results are nonsignificant.

When analyses are done by a computer, as is usually the case, researchers follow only the first three steps and then give commands to the computer. The computer calculates the test statistic, degrees of freedom, and the *actual* probability that the null hypothesis is true. For example, the computer may show that the two-tailed probability (*p*) of an intervention group being different from a control group by chance alone is .025. This means that only 25 times out of 1,000 would a group difference as large as the one obtained reflect chance differences rather than true intervention effects. The computed probability can then be compared with the desired significance level (alpha). If the significance criterion were .05, then the results would be significant because .025 is more stringent than .05. By convention, any computed probability greater than .05 (e.g., .20) indicates nonsignificance (sometimes abbreviated *NS*)—that is, a result that could have occurred by chance in more than 5 out of 100 samples.

TIP The reference guide in Figure 18.5 does not include every test you may need, but it does include bivariate tests most often used by nurse researchers. Many resources are available online to help you select an appropriate test, including interactive decision-tree tools. Links to useful websites are included in the Toolkit of the *Resource Manual* for you to click on directly.

In the sections that follow, several common bivariate statistical tests are described. It is important to note that our introduction to inferential statistics is simplified and neglects important issues such as specific assumptions underlying various tests. We urge readers to grasp statistical principles before undertaking quantitative analyses.

TESTING DIFFERENCES BETWEEN TWO GROUP MEANS

A common research situation involves comparing two groups of participants on a continuous outcome variable. For instance, we might compare an experimental and control group of patients with regard to their mean blood pressure. Or, we might contrast men and women with regard to mean depression scores.

The parametric test for differences in two means is the *t*-test. A *t*-test can be used when there are two independent groups (e.g., experimental versus control), and when the sample is dependent (e.g., mean pretreatment and posttreatment scores for the same people).

TIP A one-sample *t*-test can be used to compare mean values of a single group to a hypothesized value. One-sample *t*-tests were used in Polit and Beck's (2013) study of gender bias in nursing studies, which tested obtained mean values against a hypothesized value of 50.0, as previously described.

t-Tests for Independent Groups

Suppose we wanted to test the effect of early discharge of maternity patients on perceived maternal competence. We administer a scale of perceived maternal competence at discharge to 20 primiparas who had a vaginal birth: 10 who remained in the hospital 25 to 48 hours (regular discharge group) and 10 who were discharged within 24 hours of giving birth (early discharge group). In Table 18.1 we see that mean scores for these two groups are 25.0 and 19.0, respectively. Are these differences *reliable* (i.e., would they be found in the population of early-discharge and later-discharge mothers?), or do group differences reflect chance factors?

Note that the 20 scores in Table 18.1—10 per group—vary from one person to another. Some variability reflects individual differences in perceived maternal competence. Some variability might be due to measurement error (e.g., the scale's imperfect reliability), some could result from participants' moods on a particular day, and so forth. The research question is: Can a portion of the

TABLE 18.1 • Fictitious Data for *t*-Test Example: Scores on a Perceived Maternal Competence Scale for Regular-Discharge and Early-Discharge Mothers

REGULAR-DISCHARGE MOTHERS	EARLY-DISCHARGE MOTHERS
30	23
27	17
25	22
20	18
24	20
32	26
17	16
18	13
28	21
29	14
Mean = 25.0	Mean = 19.0
$t = 2.86$; $df = 18$; $p = .011$	

variability reliably be attributed to the independent variable—time of discharge from the hospital? The t-test allows us to answer this question objectively. The hypotheses are:

$$H_0 : \mu_A = \mu_B \qquad H_A : \mu_A \neq \mu_B$$

To test these hypotheses, we would compute a t-statistic. The formula for the t statistic uses group means, variability, and sample size to calculate a value for t. When the data from Table 18.1 are used in the formula, the value of t is 2.86. Next, degrees of freedom are calculated. In this situation, degrees of freedom equal the total sample size minus 2 ($df = 20 - 2 = 18$). A table of critical t values is shown in Table A-1, Appendix A. Degrees of freedom are listed in the left column, and different alpha values are shown in the top rows. The shaded column shows values for $\alpha = .05$ for a two-tailed test. We find in this column that for $df = 18$, the tabled value of t is 2.10. *This value establishes an upper limit to what is probable if the null hypothesis is true.* Thus, the calculated t of 2.86, which is larger than the tabled value of the statistic,[2] is improbable (i.e., statistically significant). We can now say that the primiparas discharged early had significantly lower perceptions of maternal competence than those who were not discharged early. The group difference in perceived maternal competence is sufficiently large that it is unlikely to reflect merely chance fluctuations. If a computer were used to analyze the data, the output would show the *exact* probability, which is .011. This means that in only 11 out of 1,000 samples would we expect a group difference in means of 6.0 points by chance alone.

> **Example of Independent *t*-Tests**
> Chiu and colleagues (2018) studied the effects of resistance training on body composition and functional capacity among sarcopenic obese residents in long-term care facilities. They found, for example, that the mean postintervention grip strength among those in the intervention group was 29.8 kg, compared to 20.4 kg in the comparison group; according to the t-test, this difference was statistically significant, $p < .001$.

---

[2]The tabled t values should be compared to the absolute value of the calculated t. Thus, if the calculated t were -2.86, then the results would still be significant.

When multiple tests are run with the same data—that is, when there are multiple outcomes—the risk of a Type I error increases. One t-test with an $\alpha = .05$ has a 5% probability of a Type I error. Two t-tests with the same data set, however, have a probability of 9.75% of one spurious significant result, and with three tests the risk goes up to 14.3%. Researchers sometimes apply a **Bonferroni correction** when they run multiple tests, to establish a more conservative alpha level. For example, if the desired α is .05, and there are three separate tests, the corrected alpha needed to reject the null hypothesis for *all* tests would be .017, not .05. The correction is computed by dividing the desired α by the number of tests—e.g., $.05/3 = .017$. If we concluded that mean group differences were significant for three tests at or below $p = .017$, there would be only a 5% probability of wrongly rejecting the null across all three comparisons. The Bonferroni correction can, however, be problematic in that it tends to increase the risk of a Type II error—incorrectly concluding there is no statistical association when in fact there is one.

Confidence Intervals for Mean Differences

Confidence intervals can be constructed around the difference between two means, and the results provide information about both statistical significance (i.e., whether the null hypothesis should be rejected) and precision of the estimated difference. Because CI information is more useful in clinical applications than p values, it is sometimes preferred—although nursing journals have not required it, as many medical journals have.

In the example in Table 18.1, the mean maternal competence scores were 25.0 in the regular discharge group and 19.0 in the early discharge group. Using a formula to compute the *standard error of the difference*, CIs can be constructed around the mean difference of 6.0. For a 95% CI, the confidence limits in our example are 1.6 and 10.4. This means that we can be 95% confident that the true difference in population means on the scores for early- and regular-discharge mothers lies somewhere between these limits.

In the *t*-test analysis, we obtained an estimate of mean group differences (6.0) and learned that the group differences were probably not spurious ($p = .011$). The CI information tells us the range within which the mean difference probably lies. We can see from the CI that the mean difference is significant at the .05 level *because the range does not include 0.* Given that there is a 95% probability that the mean difference is not lower than 1.6, this means that there is less than a 5% probability that there is no difference at all—thus, the null hypothesis can be rejected.

Because the CI does not give exact probabilities about the plausibility of the null hypothesis, it is often useful to present both parameter estimation and hypothesis testing information. In the current example, the results could be reported as follows: "Mothers who were discharged early had significantly lower maternal competence scores (19.0) than mothers with a regular discharge (26.0) ($t = 2.86$, $df = 18$, $p = .011$). The mean difference of 6.0 had a 95% CI of 1.6 to 10.4." Such information is more conveniently displayed in tables when there are multiple outcomes.

TIP The Toolkit section of the accompanying *Resource Manual* includes table templates that may be useful for presenting findings from analyses described in this chapter.

Paired *t*-Tests

Researchers sometimes obtain two measurements from the same people, or from paired sets of participants (e.g., siblings). When means for two sets of scores are not independent, researchers should use a **paired *t*-test**—a *t*-test for dependent groups.

Suppose we were studying the effect of a special diet on the cholesterol level of elderly men. A sample of 50 men is selected, and their cholesterol levels are measured at baseline and then after 2 months on the special diet. The hypotheses being tested are

$$H_0 : \mu_{X1} = \mu_{X2} \qquad H_A : \mu_{X1} \neq \mu_{X2}$$

where X_1 = pretreatment cholesterol levels

X_2 = posttreatment cholesterol levels

A *t*-statistic then would be computed from pretest and posttest data, using a different formula than for the independent groups *t*-test. The obtained *t* would be compared with tabled *t*-values. For this type of *t*-test, degrees of freedom equal the number of paired observations minus one ($df = N - 1$). Confidence intervals can be constructed around mean differences for paired as well as independent means.

Example of Paired *t*-Tests
In a pilot study of a holistic meditation intervention for patients with heart failure, psychosocial distress was measured before and after the 12-week program (Heo et al., 2018). In the paired *t*-test analyses, health-related quality of life improved significantly and severity of depressive symptoms decreased significantly (both $p < .001$).

Nonparametric Two-Group Tests

In certain two-group situations, a nonparametric test may be needed—for example, if the outcome variable is on an ordinal scale, or if the distribution is markedly nonnormal. The **Mann–Whitney *U* test**, the nonparametric analogue of an independent groups *t*-test, involves assigning ranks to the two groups of scores. The sum of the ranks for the two groups can be compared by calculating the *U* statistic. (This test is sometimes referred to as the *Wilcoxon rank-sum test*.) When ordinal-level data are paired (dependent), the Wilcoxon signed-rank test can be used. The **Wilcoxon signed-rank test** involves taking the difference between paired scores and ranking the absolute difference.

TESTING MEAN DIFFERENCES WITH THREE OR MORE GROUPS

Analysis of variance (**ANOVA**) is the parametric procedure for testing differences between means when there are three or more groups. The statistic computed in ANOVA is the ***F*-ratio**. ANOVA decomposes total variability in an outcome variable into two parts: (1) variability attributable to the independent variable; and (2) all other variability, such as individual differences, measurement error, and so on. Variation *between* groups is contrasted to variation *within* groups to get an *F*-ratio. When differences between groups are large relative to variation within groups, the probability is high that the independent variable is related to, or has caused, group differences.

One-Way ANOVA

Suppose we were comparing the effectiveness of alternative interventions to help people stop smoking. One group of smokers receives nurse counseling (group A); a second group receives peer counseling—i.e., from a former smoker (group B); and a third control group receives no special treatment (group C). The outcome variable is 1-day cigarette consumption measured 1 month after the intervention. Thirty smokers who wish to quit smoking are randomly assigned to one of the three conditions. **One-way ANOVA** tests the following hypotheses:

$$H_0 : \mu_A = \mu_B = \mu_C \qquad H_A : \mu_A \neq \mu_B \neq \mu_C$$

The null hypothesis is that the population means for posttreatment cigarette smoking are the same for all three groups, and the alternative

(research) hypothesis is inequality of means. Table 18.2 presents fictitious data for 30 participants. The mean numbers of posttreatment cigarettes smoked in 1 day are 16.6, 19.2, and 34.0 for groups A, B, and C, respectively. These means are different, but are they significantly different—or do differences reflect random fluctuations?

In calculating an *F*-statistic, total variability in the data is broken down into two sources. The portion of the variance due to group status (i.e., exposure to different treatments, the independent variable) is reflected in the **sum of squares between groups**, or SS$_B$. The SS$_B$ is the sum of squared deviations of individual group means from the overall **grand mean** for all participants.

The second component is the **sum of squares within groups**, or SS$_W$. This index is the sum of the squared deviations of each individual score from its *own* group mean. SS$_W$ indicates variability attributable to individual differences, measurement error, and so on.

Recall from Chapter 17 that the formula for calculating a sample variance is $\Sigma x^2 \div N - 1$. The two sums of squares are like the numerator of this variance equation: both SS$_B$ and SS$_W$ are sums of squared deviations from means. So, to compute variance within and variance between groups, we

TABLE 18.2 • Fictitious Data for a One-Way ANOVA: Number of Cigarettes Smoked in 1 Day, 1 month Postintervention in Three Treatment Groups

GROUP A NURSE COUNSELING		GROUP B PEER COUNSELING		GROUP C UNTREATED CONTROL	
28	19	0	27	33	35
0	24	31	0	54	0
17	0	26	3	19	43
20	21	30	24	40	39
35	2	24	27	41	36
$\bar{X}_A = 16.6$		$\bar{X}_B = 19.2$		$\bar{X}_C = 34.0$	
$F = 4.98, df = 2, 27, p = .01$					

must divide the sums of squares by something similar to $N - 1$, namely degrees of freedom for each sum of squares. For between groups, $df_B = G - 1$ (number of groups minus 1). For within groups, df_W is the number of participants less 1, for each group.

In an ANOVA context, the variance is referred to as the **mean square** (MS). The formulas for the mean square between groups and the mean square within groups are

$$MS_B = \frac{SS_B}{df_B} \qquad MS_W = \frac{SS_W}{df_W}$$

The F-ratio statistic is the ratio of these mean squares, or

$$F = \frac{MS_B}{MS_W}$$

The ANOVA summary table (Table 18.3) shows that the calculated F-statistic in our example is 4.98. For $df = 2$ and 27 and $\alpha = .05$, the tabled F value is 3.35 (see Table A-2 in Appendix A for values from the theoretical F distribution). Because our obtained F-value of 4.98 exceeds 3.35, we reject the null hypothesis that the population means are equal. The *actual* probability, calculated by computer, is .014. Mean group differences in the number of posttreatment cigarettes smoked in 1 day are beyond chance expectations. In only 14 samples out of 1,000 would differences this great be obtained by chance alone.

The data support the research hypothesis that different treatments were associated with different cigarette smoking, but we cannot tell from the test

whether treatment A was significantly more effective than treatment B. Statistical analyses known as **multiple comparison procedures** (or **post hoc tests**) are needed. Their function is to isolate the differences between group means that are responsible for rejecting the overall ANOVA null hypothesis. Note that it is *not* appropriate to use a series of t-tests (group A versus B, A versus C, and B versus C) because this would increase the risk of a Type I error. Multiple comparison methods are described in most intermediate statistical textbooks, such as that by Polit (2010).

> **Example of a One-Way ANOVA**
> Bonsaksen and an interprofessional team (2019) studied differences in general self-efficacy across several sociodemographic groups in the Norwegian population. Using ANOVA with data from 1,787 Norwegians, they found, for example, that there was a significant difference in perceived self-efficacy among employment status groups (e.g., working, retired, etc.) ($F = 15.8$, $p < .001$).

Two-Way ANOVA

One-way ANOVA is used to test mean group differences for a single independent variable, such as participants in three different interventions. Data from studies with multiple factors, as in a factorial design, can be analyzed by *multifactor ANOVA*. In this section, we describe principles for **two-way ANOVA**.

Suppose we wanted to compare the effectiveness of two alternative smoking cessation modalities (in-person and by telephone) led by nurse counselors versus peer counselors (ex-smokers). We randomly assign a sample of 40 smokers to one

TABLE 18.3 • ANOVA Summary Table for Example of Posttreatment Smoking After Intervention

SOURCE OF VARIANCE	SS	df	MEAN SQUARE	F	p
Between groups	1,761.9	2	880.9	4.98	.014
Within groups	4,772.0	27	176.7		
Total	6,533.9	29			

of the four treatment conditions. One month after the intervention, participants report the number of cigarettes they smoked the previous day. Fictitious data for this example are shown in Table 18.4.

With two independent variables, three hypotheses are tested. First, we are testing the effectiveness, for both modalities, of nurse counseling versus peer counseling. Second, we are testing whether postintervention smoking differs for in-person counseling versus telephone counseling, regardless of who does the counseling. These are tests for **main effects**. Third, we are testing **interaction effects** (i.e., differential effects for the two counselor types in the two modalities). Interaction concerns whether the effect of one independent variable is consistent for all levels of a second independent variable.

...A reveal that participants ...group smoked less, on those ... Peer Counseling group exposed ...icipants who got in- ...than those who got got peer co... us 23.0); and that in-person cou... smoked less when ANOVA on these ... but those who effects were statistica...hen exposed to

Multifactor ANOVA...g a two-way way analyses. In theory, ...whether the pendent variables is possibl...ed to two- studies with more than two fa...of inde- ...practice ...rare.

TABLE 18.4 • Fictitious Data for a Two-Way (2 × 2) ANOVA: Number of Cigarettes Smoked in One day, 1 month Postintervention for Type of Counselors and Counseling Modality Groups

FACTOR B—MODALITY	FACTOR A—TYPE OF COUNSELORS				TOTAL
	NURSES (1)		PEERS (2)		
In-Person (1)	24	25	27	23	In-Person $\bar{X}_{B1} = 21.0$
	28	38	0	18	
	2	21	45	20	
	19	0	29	12	
	27	36	22	4	
	$\bar{X}_{A1B1} = 22.0$		$\bar{X}_{A2B1} = 20.0$		
Telephone (2)	10	16	36	27	Telephone $\bar{X}_{B2} = 23.0$
	21	18	41	0	
	17	3	28	49	
	0	25	37	35	
	33	17	5	42	
	$\bar{X}_{A1B2} = 16.0$		$\bar{X}_{A2B2} = 30.0$		
Total	Nurse Counselors: $\bar{X}_{A1} = 19.0$		Peer Counselors: $\bar{X}_{A2} = 25.0$		$\bar{X}_T = 22.0$

re used
les, as we

Other statis
with three
discuss in

Repeated **(RM-ANOVA)** is
Repeated one of which is when
used in asures of the same out-
there ar articipant. For instance, in
come v gic measures such as blood
some s e might be collected before,
pressu l medical procedure. In this sit-
durin y RM-ANOVA is an extension of
uatio. It can be used with a single group
a p tudinally, or in a crossover design with
stud ore different conditions. (In Chapter 19
thr ss RM-ANOVA for mixed designs.)
we
an example, suppose we wanted to compare
thr interventions for preterm infants, with regard
to effects on infants' feeding rates: (1) nonnutritive
sucking; (2) nonnutritive sucking plus music; or (3)
music alone. Using an experimental repeated measures crossover design, infants participating in the
study are randomly assigned to different orderings
of the three treatments. Bottle feeding rate, the outcome, is measured after the treatments. The null
hypothesis for this study is that type of intervention
is unrelated to feeding rate (i.e., $\mu_1 = \mu_2 = \mu_3$). The
alternative hypothesis is that feeding rate and type
of intervention are related (i.e., that the three population means are not equal).

We would find in such a study that there was
riability in feeding rates both across infants
hin each condition, and across the three treat-
t conditions within infants. As was true with
ANOVA situations, total variability in the
me is represented by the total sum of squares,
can be partitioned into contributing compo-
n RM-ANOVA, three sources of variation
te to total variability:

$$SS_{total} = SS_{treatments} + SS_{subjects} + SS_{error}$$

nally, *sum of squares-treatments* is
sum of squares-between in regular
epresents the effect of the indepen-
(When measurements are taken at

multiple points without an intervention, it may be
called *sum of squares-time*.) The *sum of squares-
error* is similar to the sum of squares-within in regular ANOVA: both represent variations associated
with random fluctuations. The third component,
sum of squares-subjects, has no counterpart in a
simple ANOVA, because those being compared in
regular ANOVA are different people. The $SS_{subjects}$
term captures individual differences, the effects
of which are consistent across conditions. That is,
some infants tend to have high feeding rates and
others tend to have low feeding rates, regardless of
treatment. Because individual differences can be
statistically isolated from the error term (random
fluctuation), RM-ANOVA yields a more sensitive
test of the relationship between the independent
and dependent variables than between-subjects
ANOVA. By statistical isolation, we mean that
variability attributable to individual differences is
removed from the denominator in computing the F
statistic.

Example of RM-ANOVA

Yates and colleagues (2018) studied changes over
time in caregiving demand and caregiving difficulty
among spousal caregivers of CABG patients. Scores
on the Caregiving Burden Scale were obtained at
early hospital discharge and 3 and 6 months later.
The data were analyzed for within-group changes.
The results indicated a significant decline over time
in caregiving demands ($p < .001$) and caregiving difficulties ($p = .02$).

Nonparametric "Analysis of Variance"

Nonparametric tests do not actually analyze variance, but there are nonparametric analogues to
ANOVA when a parametric test is not appropriate.
The **Kruskal–Wallis test** is a generalized version
of the Mann-Whitney U test, based on assigning
ranks to the scores of various groups. This test is
used when the number of groups is greater than
two and a one-way test for independent samples is
desired. When multiple measures are obtained from
the same subjects, the **Friedman test** for "analysis of variance" by ranks can be used. Both tests
are described in Polit (2010) and other statistics
textbooks.

TESTING DIFFERENCES IN PROPORTIONS

Tests discussed thus far involve continuous dependent variables, when group means are being compared. In this section, we examine tests of group differences when the outcome is on a nominal scale.

The Chi-Square Test

The **chi-square** (χ^2) **test** is used to test hypotheses about group differences in proportions, as when a crosstabs table has been created. Suppose we were studying the effect of nursing instruction on patients' compliance with a self-medication regimen. Nurses implement a new instructional strategy with 100 randomly assigned experimental patients, while 100 control group patients get the usual instruction. The research hypothesis is that a higher proportion of people in the intervention group than in the control group will be compliant.

The chi-square statistic is computed by comparing **observed frequencies** (i.e., values observed in the data) and expected frequencies. Observed frequencies for our example are shown in Table 18.5. As this table shows, 60 experimental participants (60%), but only 40 controls (40%), reported self-medication compliance after the intervention. The chi-square test enables us to decide whether a difference in proportions of this magnitude is likely to reflect a real treatment effect or only chance fluctuations. **Expected frequencies** are the cell frequencies that would be found if there were

no relationship between the two variables. In this example, if there were no relationship between the two groups, the expected frequency would be 50 people per cell because, overall, exactly half the participants (100 out of 200) complied.

The chi-square statistic is computed by summarizing differences between observed and expected frequencies for each cell. Formulas and computations are not shown here, but in our example, $\chi^2 = 8.00$. For chi-square tests, *df* equals the number of rows minus 1 times number of columns minus 1. In the current case, $df = 1 \times 1 = 1$. With 1 *df*, the tabled value (Table A-3 of Appendix A) from a theoretical chi-square distribution that must be exceeded to establish significance at the .05 level is 3.84. The obtained value of 8.00 is much larger than would be expected by chance (actual $p = .005$). We can conclude that a significantly larger proportion of experimental patients than control patients were compliant.

Example of Chi-Square Test
Using chi-square analysis, Snyder and colleagues (2018) analyzed differences in women's reports of workplace support for breastfeeding in various employment sectors (e.g., health care, education, management/professional, service). For example, in the women's response to a question about whether the employer supported their breastfeeding goals, group differences were significant ($p = .03$), with the management/professional group having the highest percentage saying "yes" (81.9%) and the service sector having the lowest (66.1%).

TABLE 18.5 • Observed Frequencies for Chi-Square Example: Patient Compliance in Two Treatment Groups

PATIENT COMPLIANCE	GROUP		TOTAL
	CONTROL	EXPERIMENTAL	
Compliant	40	60	100
Noncompliant	60	40	100
Total	100	100	200
$X^2 = 8.00$, $df = 1$, $p = .005$			

Confidence Intervals for Differences in Proportion

As with means, it is possible to construct confidence intervals around the difference between two proportions. To do this, we would need to calculate the *standard error of the difference of proportions*. In the example used to explain the chi square statistic (Table 18.5), the difference in proportions was .20 ($p < .01$), and the *SE* of the difference is .069. The 95% CI in this example is .06 to .34. We can be 95% confident that the true population difference in compliance rates between those exposed to the intervention and those not exposed is between 6% and 34%. This interval does not include 0%, indicating that we can be 95% confident that group differences are "real."

Other Tests of Proportions

Sometimes a chi-square test is not appropriate. When the total sample size is small (total N of 30 or fewer) or when there are cells with small frequencies (5 or fewer), **Fisher's exact test** should be used to test the significance of differences in proportions. When the proportions being compared are from two paired groups (e.g., when a pretest–posttest design is used to compare changes in proportions on a dichotomous variable), the appropriate test is **McNemar's test**.

TESTING CORRELATIONS

The statistical tests discussed thus far are used to test *group* differences—they involve situations in which the independent variable is a nominal-level variable. In this section, we consider statistical tests used when both the independent variable and the outcome variable are ordinal, interval, or ratio.

Pearson's *r*

Pearson's *r*, the correlation coefficient calculated when two variables are measured on at least the interval scale, is both descriptive and inferential. Descriptively, the correlation coefficient summarizes the magnitude and direction of a relationship between two variables. As an inferential statistic, *r* is used to test hypotheses about population correlations, which are symbolized as ρ, the Greek letter rho. The null hypothesis is that there is no relationship between two variables; the alternate hypothesis is that a relationship exists in the population:

$$H_0 : \rho = 0 \qquad H_A : \rho \neq 0$$

For instance, suppose we studied the relationship between patients' self-reported level of stress and the pH level of their saliva. In a sample of 50 people, we find that $r = -.29$, indicating a modest tendency for people with high stress scores to have low pH levels. But does the coefficient of $-.29$ reflect a random fluctuation, observable only for the people in our sample, or is the relationship likely to be true in the population? We can compare our computed r to a tabled value from a theoretical distribution for r. Degrees of freedom for r equal the number of participants minus 2, or $(N - 2)$. With $df = 48$, the tabled value for r for a two-tailed test with $\alpha = .05$ (Table A-4 in Appendix A) is .2803. Because the absolute value of the calculated r is .29, the null hypothesis can be rejected. We accept the research hypothesis that the correlation between stress and saliva acidity in the population is not zero.

Pearson's *r* can be used in both within-group and between-group situations. The example about the relationship between stress scores and the pH levels is a between-group situation: The question is whether people with high stress scores tend to have significantly lower pH levels than *different* people with low stress scores. If stress scores were obtained from the same people (e.g., before and after surgery), the correlation between the two scores would be a within-group situation.

Example of Pearson's *r*
Wijdenes and colleagues (2019) studied factors that correlated with nurses' compassion fatigue. The researchers found, for example, that nurses' levels of burnout were significantly negatively correlated with compassion fatigue ($r = -.69, p < .001$).

Other Tests of Bivariate Relationships

Pearson's *r* is a parametric statistic. When the assumptions for a parametric test are violated, or when the data are ordinal-level, then the appropriate coefficient of correlation is either **Spearman's rho** (r_S) or **Kendall's tau**. The values of these statistics range from -1.00 to $+1.00$, and their interpretation is similar to that of Pearson's *r*. Another correlation statistic that is used to correlate a dichotomous variable with a continuous one is called a **point-biserial correlation coefficient**. Interpretation of this statistic requires knowing how the dichotomous variable was coded (usually, it is 1 versus 0).

Measures of the magnitude of relationships can also be computed with nominal-level data. For example, the **phi coefficient** (Φ) is an index describing the relationship between two dichotomous variables. **Cramér's V** is an index of relationship applied to crosstabs tables larger than 2×2. Both statistics are based on the chi-square statistic and yield values that range between .00 and 1.00, with higher values indicating a stronger association between variables.

 Inferential statistics are almost invariably calculated using statistical software. The Supplement to this chapter illustrates how the *Statistical Package for the Social Sciences* (SPSS) can be used to test hypotheses.

POWER ANALYSIS AND EFFECT SIZE

Many published nursing studies (and even more *un*published ones) have nonsignificant findings, and many of these could reflect Type II errors. As indicated earlier, researchers set the probability of committing a Type I error (a false positive) as the significance level, alpha (α). The probability of a Type II error (a false negative) is **beta** (β). The complement of beta ($1 - \beta$) is the *probability of detecting a true relationship or group difference* and is the **power** of a statistical test. Polit and Sherman (1990) found that many published nursing studies have insufficient power, placing them at risk

for Type II errors—although a more recent study has found that, on average, power has improved in nursing studies, perhaps because of heightened awareness (Gaskin & Happell, 2014). Nevertheless, even in the more recent analysis, many studies were found to be **underpowered**.

Power analysis is used to reduce the risk of Type II errors and strengthen statistical conclusion validity by estimating in advance how big a sample is needed. There are four components in a power analysis, three of which must be known or estimated:

1. *The significance criterion, α.* Other things being equal, the more stringent this criterion, the lower the power.
2. *The sample size, N.* As sample size increases, power increases.
3. *The effect size* (ES). ES is an estimate of how wrong the null hypothesis is—that is, how strong the relationship between the independent variable and the outcome is in the population.
4. *Power, or $1 - \beta$.* This is the probability of rejecting a false null hypothesis.

Researchers typically use power analysis at the outset of a study to estimate the sample size needed to avoid a Type II error. To estimate needed sample size (N), researchers must specify α, ES, and $1 - \beta$. Researchers usually establish the risk of a Type I error (α) as .05. The conventional standard for $1 - \beta$ is .80. With power equal to .80, there is a 20% risk of committing a Type II error. Although this risk may seem high, a stricter criterion requires sample sizes larger than many researchers could afford.

With α and $1 - \beta$ specified, the information needed to solve for N is ES, the estimated population effect size. The **effect size** is the magnitude of the relationship between the research variables. When relationships (effects) are strong, they can be detected at significant levels even with small samples. With modest relationships, large sample sizes are needed to avoid Type II errors.

In using power analysis to estimate sample size needs, the population effect size is not *known*; if it were known, there would be no need for the new study. Effect size must be estimated using available evidence and theory. In essence, the effect size estimate represents the researcher's *hypothesis* about how strong relationships are. Researchers sometimes use findings from a pilot study as a basis for the estimate—although we explain in Chapter 29 why this is risky. More often an effect size is calculated based on findings from earlier studies on a similar problem. When there are *no* relevant earlier findings and when theory offers only broad guidance, researchers use conventions based on expectations of a *small*, *medium*, or *large* effect. Most nursing studies have modest (small-to-medium) effects.

> **TIP** Researchers can usually find several studies from which the effect size can be estimated. In such a case, the estimate should be based on the one with the most reliable results. Researchers can also estimate effect size by combining information from multiple high-quality studies through averaging or weighted averaging.

Procedures for estimating effects and sample size needs vary from one statistical situation to another. We focus mainly on two-group mean-difference situations.

Sample Size Estimates for Testing Differences Between Two Means

Suppose we were testing the hypothesis that cranberry juice reduces the urinary pH of diet-controlled patients. We plan to assign some patients randomly to a control condition (no cranberry juice) and others to an experimental condition in which they will be given 300 mL of cranberry juice for 5 days. How large a sample is needed for this study, given a desired α of .05 and power of .80?

To answer this, we must first estimate ES. In a two-group situation in which mean differences are of interest, ES is usually designated as **Cohen's *d***, the formula for which is.

$$d = \frac{\mu_1 - \mu_2}{\sigma}$$

The effect size (*d*) is the difference between the two population means, divided by the population

standard deviation (σ). These population values are never known but are estimated. For example, suppose we found an earlier nonexperimental study that compared the urinary pH of people who had or had not ingested cranberry juice in the previous 24 hours. The earlier study is a reasonable starting point. Suppose the results were as follows:

$$\overline{X}_1 \text{ (no cranberry juice)} = 5.70$$
$$\overline{X}_2 \text{ (cranberry juice)} = 5.50$$
$$SD = .50$$

The estimated value of *d* would be .40:

$$d = \frac{5.70 - 5.50}{.50} = .40$$

Table 18.6 presents approximate sample size requirements for various effect sizes and powers, for $\alpha = .05$ (for two-tailed tests), in a two-group mean-difference situation. We find in this table that the estimated *n* (number *per group*) to detect an effect size of .40 with power equal to .80 is 99 people. Assuming that the earlier study provided a good estimate of the population effect size, the total number of people needed in the new study would be about 200, with half assigned to the control group (no cranberry juice) and the other half assigned to the experimental group. With a sample size smaller than 200, there would be a greater than 20% chance of a false negative conclusion, i.e., a Type II error. For example, a sample size of 128 (64 per group) would result in an estimated 40% chance of incorrect nonsignificant results.

If there is no prior research, researchers can, as a last resort, estimate whether the expected effect is small, medium, or large. By convention (Cohen, 1988), the value of *ES* in a two-group test of mean differences is estimated at .20 for small effects, .50 for medium effects, and .80 for large effects. With an α value of .05 and power of .80, the *n* (number of participants per group) for studies with expected small, medium, and large effects would be 394, 64, and 25, respectively. Most nursing studies cannot expect effect sizes in excess of .50; those in the range of .20 to .40 are most common. In Polit and Sherman's (1990) analysis of effect sizes for

TABLE 18.6 • Approximate Sample Sizes[a] per Group Needed to Achieve Selected Levels of Power as a Function of Estimated Effect Size for Test of Difference of Two Means, for $\alpha = .05$

POWER	ESTIMATED EFFECT SIZE (d)[b]										
	.10	.15	.20	.25	.30	.35	.40	.50	.60	.70	.80
.60	979	435	245	157	109	80	62	40	28	20	16
.70	1,233	548	309	198	137	101	78	50	35	26	20
.80	1,576	701	394	253	176	129	99	64	44	33	25
.90	2,103	935	526	337	234	172	132	85	59	43	33
.95	2,594	1,154	649	416	289	213	163	105	73	53	41

[a]Sample size requirements for each group; total sample size would be twice the number shown.
[b]Estimated effect size (d) is the estimated population mean group difference divided by the estimated population standard deviation or $(\mu_1 - \mu_2)/s$.

studies published in two nursing research journals, the average effect size for *t*-test situations was .35. A medium effect should be estimated only when the effect is so substantial that it can be detected by the naked eye (i.e., without formal research procedures).

> **TIP** Performing a power analysis based on estimates of an effect size is an *evidence-based* approach to designing a new study—that is, the new study uses evidence from earlier studies to estimate how many sample members will be needed to achieve an effect that seems plausible in light of what is already known. A useful supplementary approach is to ask, How big an effect would be needed to be clinically relevant? If effect-size estimates are both evidence-based and clinically meaningful, the study will be stronger.

Sample Size Estimates for Other Bivariate Tests

Power analysis can be undertaken for the other statistical tests described in this chapter. It is relatively easy to do a power analysis online (we suggest several relevant websites in the Toolkit with the *Resource Manual* 🌐). Here we discuss only a few basic features for situations in which ANOVA, Pearson's *r*, or a chi-square situation would be the basis for doing the power analysis.

There are alternative approaches to doing a power analysis in an ANOVA context. The simplest approach is to estimate **eta-squared** (η^2), which is an ES index indicating the proportion of variance explained in ANOVA. Eta-squared equals the sum of squares between (SS_B) divided by the total sum of squares (SS_T) and can be used directly as the estimate of effect size if sum of squares information is available. When eta-squared cannot be estimated, researchers can estimate whether effects are likely to be small, medium, or large. For ANOVA situations, the conventional estimates for small, medium, and large effects would be values of η^2 equal to .01, .06, and .14, respectively. Assuming $\alpha = .05$ and power $= .80$, this corresponds to sample size requirements of about 319, 53, or 22 subjects *per group* in a three-group study, and about 272, 44, and 19 *per group* in a four-group study,[3] (for the data in Table 18.2 and shown in an ANOVA summary table in Table 18.3, $\eta^2 = .27$, a large effect).

---

[3]Power tables are not provided here for ANOVA and chi-square situations.

TABLE 18.7 • Approximate Sample Sizes Necessary to Achieve Selected Levels of Power as a Function of Estimated Population Correlation, With $\alpha = .05$

	ESTIMATED POPULATION CORRELATION COEFFICIENT (ρ)[a]										
POWER	.10	.15	.20	.25	.30	.35	.40	.50	.60	.70	.80
.60	489	217	122	78	54	39	30	19	13	9	7
.70	614	272	152	97	67	49	37	23	16	11	8
.80	785	347	194	123	85	62	47	29	19	13	10
.90	1,047	463	258	164	112	81	61	37	25	17	12
.95	1,296	575	322	204	141	101	80	50	32	22	18

[a]Estimated effect size (r) is the estimated population correlation coefficient (ρ).

For Pearson correlations, the ES index is an estimate of ρ, the population correlation coefficient. Thus, the value of the correlation coefficient (r) from a relevant earlier study can be used directly as the estimated effect size. Table 18.7 shows sample size requirements for various effect sizes and powers when $\alpha = .05$ and the test statistic is Pearson's r. For example, if our estimated population correlation was .25, we would need a sample size of 123 for power = .80. With a sample this size, we can expect that we would wrongly reject a true null hypothesis 5 times out of 100 and wrongly retain a false null hypothesis 20 times out of 100. When prior estimates of effect size are unavailable, the conventional values of small, medium, and large effect sizes in a bivariate correlation situation are .10, .30, and .50, respectively (i.e., samples of 785, 85, and 29 for a power of .80 and a significance level of .05). In Polit and Sherman's (1990) study, the average correlation in nursing studies was found to be around .20.

Estimating sample size requirements for testing group differences in proportions is complex. The effect size for crosstabs tables is influenced not only by expected differences in proportions (e.g., 60% in one group versus 40% in another, a 20-percentage point difference), but also by the absolute values of the proportions. Effect sizes are *larger* (and thus sample size needs are *smaller*) at the extremes than near the midpoint. A 20-percentage point difference is easier to detect if the percentages are 10% and 30% than if they are near the middle, such as 60% and 40%. Because of this fact, it is difficult to offer information on values for small, medium, and large effects. We can, however, give *examples* of differences in proportions that conform to the conventions in a 2 × 2 situation:

Small: .05 versus .10, .20 versus .29, .40 versus .50, .60 versus .70, .80 versus .87
Medium: .05 versus .21, .20 versus .43, .40 versus .65, .60 versus .82, .80 versus .96
Large: .05 versus .34, .20 versus .58, .40 versus .78, .60 versus .92, .80 versus .96

For example, if the expected proportion for a control group were .40, the researcher would need about 385, 70, and 24 per group if values higher than .40 were expected for the experimental group and the effect was expected to be small, medium, and large, respectively. As in other situations, researchers are encouraged to avoid using the conventions in favor of more precise estimates based on existing evidence. If the conventions cannot be avoided, conservative estimates should be used to minimize the risk of obtaining nonsignificant results.

Example of a Power Analysis

Miyamoto and colleagues (2018) described a protocol for a randomized trial of a mobile health–enabled nurse coaching intervention designed to improve self-efficacy among adults with type 2 diabetes. A goal of recruiting 300 participants (150 for each arm) was established, based on a power analysis that took into account an expected rate of 16% attrition. Power was set to .80.

TIP Although power analysis is frequently used to estimate sample size needs, an alternative is to use *precision estimation*, which uses a confidence interval framework to estimate an appropriate sample size (Corty & Corty, 2011). Another approach is to consider benchmarks for *clinical significance* (Chapter 21) when estimating sample size needs.

Effect Size Calculations in Completed Studies

Power analysis concepts are sometimes used after analyses are completed to calculate estimated population effects based on *actual N*s. In this situation, power, alpha, and *N* are known, and so the task is to solve for ES. Effect sizes provide readers and clinicians with estimates about the magnitude of effects—an important issue in EBP. Effect size information can be crucial because, with large samples, even tiny effects can be statistically significant. *p* values tell you whether results are likely to be *real*, but effect sizes can suggest whether they are important. Effect size estimates are needed in doing meta-analyses (see Chapter 30), and so when these values are presented in a report, they are helpful to meta-analysts.

Example of Calculated Effect Size

Cheung and colleagues (2019) did a pilot trial to test the preliminary efficacy of a cognitive stimulating play intervention for older people with early to moderate dementia. Those in the intervention group had significantly higher scores than those in the control group on tests of memory storage ($p = .006$) and retrieval functions ($p = .018$), and the effect sizes were moderate ($\eta^2 = .19 - .25$).

CRITICAL APPRAISAL OF INFERENTIAL STATISTICAL ANALYSES

It is difficult to critically appraise researchers' data analysis decisions without good training in statistics. Nevertheless, there are certain things you can do to evaluate statistical analyses even if your background in statistics is modest.

You can begin by asking whether the report presents the results of statistical tests for all study hypotheses, and whether the researchers undertook analyses to address questions about the study's internal validity. For example, in a case-control study, was the comparability of the groups assessed (i.e., were analyses undertaken to test for selection biases)? Did groups differ with regard to attrition? As noted in Chapter 10, both analytic and design decisions can affect statistical conclusion validity. When sample size is small, when participation in an intervention is low, or when a weak statistical procedure is used in lieu of a more powerful one, then the risk of drawing the wrong conclusion about the research hypotheses is heightened. Threats to statistical conclusion validity should be considered when research hypotheses are not supported.

Other issues important in a thorough appraisal are whether the researcher used the right statistical tests, whether the statistical information reported is adequate to meet readers' information needs, and whether the results were presented in a clear and thoughtful manner, with a judicious combination of information reported in the text and in well laid-out tables. Box 18.1 (which is also found in the Toolkit) presents some guiding questions for critically appraising bivariate inferential statistics in a research report. ✖

TIP You may find it helpful to consult the glossary of statistical symbols in the inside back cover if you find a symbol in a report that you do not recognize. Some symbols included in this glossary are not explained in this book; it may be necessary to refer to a statistics textbook for further information.

BOX 18.1 Guidelines for Critically Appraising Bivariate[a] Inferential Analyses

1. Did the report include any bivariate inferential statistics? Was a statistical test performed for each hypothesis or research question? If inferential statistics were not used, should they have been?

2. Were statistical tests used to strengthen inferences about the study's internal validity (e.g., to test for selection bias or attrition bias)? If not, should they have been?

3. Were the selected statistical tests appropriate, given the level of measurement of the variables and the nature of the hypotheses?

4. Were parametric tests used? Does it appear that the use of parametric tests was appropriate? If nonparametric tests were used, was a rationale provided, and does the rationale seem sound?

5. Was information provided about both hypothesis testing and estimation of parameters? Were effect sizes reported?

6. In general, did the report provide a rationale for the use of the selected statistical tests? Did the report contain sufficient information for you to judge whether appropriate statistics were used?

7. Were the results of any statistical tests significant? What do the tests tell you about the plausibility of the research hypotheses? Were effects sizable?

8. Were the results of any statistical tests nonsignificant? Is it plausible that these reflect Type II errors? What factors might have undermined the study's statistical conclusion validity?

9. Was an appropriate amount of statistical information reported? Are the findings clearly and logically organized?

10. Were tables or figures used judiciously to summarize large amounts of statistical information? Are the tables clearly presented, with good titles and carefully labeled column headings? Is the information in the text consistent with the information presented in the tables? Is the information totally redundant?

───

[a]Most of these questions are equally appropriate for critically appraising the multivariate statistics described in Chapter 19.

RESEARCH EXAMPLE

We conclude this chapter with an example of a study that used some of the statistical tests described in this chapter.

Study: The effect of interactive text message follow-up on health-promoting lifestyle of patients with acute coronary syndrome (Moradi et al., 2017).

Statement of purpose: The purpose of this study was to test the effectiveness of interactive text message follow-up aimed at enhancing health-promoting lifestyles among patients with acute coronary syndrome (ACS).

Methods: A sample of 100 patients suffering from ACS was randomly assigned to an intervention or a control group. The researchers did a power analysis that indicated they needed 43 per group, but they

recruited 50 per group in case of attrition. Six text messages that promoted healthy lifestyle choices were sent to the intervention group members each week for 12 weeks, and participants could respond to the text and ask questions. Control group members were sent one health-related (but not health promoting) message each week, but they could not text back to the researchers. The Walker Health Promoting Lifestyle (WHPL) questionnaire was administered to all participants at baseline and 3 and 4 months later. The researchers hypothesized that participating in the intervention would result in improved scores on the scale.

Analysis and Findings: The researchers used numerous bivariate statistical tests to analyze their data. First, baseline characteristics of the two groups were compared. For example, using an independent groups *t*-test, the mean age for the experimental and control group participants was 54.3 and 56.1, respectively (*NS*). Chi-squared tests were used to compare the groups on nominal-level characteristics, such as gender and marital status. The groups did not differ significantly on background traits.

Using independent group *t*-tests, the researchers tested differences in the groups' scores at 3 and 4 months post baseline, and at both time periods group differences were highly significant ($p < .001$). For example, at 4 months after beginning the intervention, the experimental group had a significantly higher total mean score on the WHPL scale: 163.1, compared to 120.0 for the controls; baseline scores, by contrast, were not significantly different (119.3 and 115.6, respectively).

Finally, the researchers used one-way repeated measures ANOVAs to examine changes in WHPL scores from baseline to the 3- and 4-month follow-ups. For the total scores and scores on all six subscales, the improvements over time were highly significant for the intervention group ($p < .001$), but also were modestly improved and significant in the control group ($p = .04$).

SUMMARY POINTS

- **Inferential statistics**, which are based on **laws of probability**, allow researchers to make inferences about a population based on data from a sample; it offers a framework for deciding whether **sampling error** resulting from sampling fluctuations is too high to provide reliable population estimates.
- The **sampling distribution of the mean** is a theoretical distribution of the means of an infinite number of samples drawn from a population. The sampling distribution of means is normally distributed, so the probability that a given sample value will be obtained can be ascertained.
- The **standard error of the mean** (*SEM*)—the standard deviation of this theoretical distribution—indicates the degree of average error of a sample mean; the smaller the *SEM*, the more accurate are the sample estimates of the population mean.

- Statistical inference consists of parameter estimation and hypothesis testing. **Parameter estimation** is used to estimate a population parameter from a sample statistic.
- **Point estimation** is a descriptive value of the population estimate (e.g., a mean or odds ratio). **Interval estimation** provides the upper and lower limits of a range of values—the **confidence interval (CI)**—between which the population value is expected to fall, at a specified probability. A 95% CI indicates a 95% probability that the true population value lies between the upper and lower **confidence limits**.
- **Hypothesis testing** through statistical procedures enables researchers to make objective decisions about the validity of their hypotheses.
- The **null hypothesis** states that there is no relationship between research variables, and that any observed relationship is due to chance. Rejection of the null hypothesis lends support to the research hypothesis.
- A **Type I error** occurs when a null hypothesis is incorrectly rejected (a false positive). A **Type II error** occurs when a null hypothesis is wrongly accepted (a false negative).
- Researchers control the risk of a Type I error by establishing a **level of significance** (or **alpha** [α] level), which is the probability that such an error will occur. The .05 level means that in only 5 out of 100 samples would the null hypothesis be rejected when it should have been accepted.
- In testing hypotheses, researchers compute a **test statistic** and then determine whether the statistic falls at or beyond the **critical region** on a relevant theoretical distribution. If the value of the test statistic indicates that the null hypothesis is "improbable," the result is **statistically significant** (i.e., obtained results are not likely to have occurred by chance, at the specified level of probability).
- Most hypothesis testing involves **two-tailed tests**, in which both ends of the sampling distribution are used to define the region of improbable values; a **one-tailed test** may be appropriate if there is a strong rationale for an a priori directional hypothesis.

- **Parametric tests** involve the estimation of at least one parameter, the use of interval- or ratio-level data, and the assumption of normally distributed variables; **nonparametric tests** are used when the data are nominal or ordinal or when a normal distribution cannot be assumed—especially when samples are small.
- **Tests for independent groups** compare different groups of people (between-subjects design), and **tests for dependent groups** compare the same group of people over time or conditions (within-subjects designs).
- Two common statistical tests are the *t*-test and **analysis of variance** (**ANOVA**), both of which are used to test the significance of the difference between group means; ANOVA is used when there are three or more groups (**one-way ANOVA**) or when there is more than one independent variable (e.g. **two-way ANOVA**). **Repeated measures ANOVA (RM-ANOVA)** is used when there are multiple means being compared over time.
- The **chi-square test** (χ^2) is used to test hypotheses about differences in proportions. For small samples or small cell sizes, **Fisher's exact test** should be used.
- Statistical tests to measure the magnitude of bivariate relationships and to test whether the relationship is significantly different from zero include **Pearson's *r*** for interval-level data, **Spearman's rho** and **Kendall's tau** for ordinal-level data, and the **phi coefficient** and **Cramér's V** for nominal-level data. A **point-biserial correlation coefficient** can be computed when one variable is dichotomous and the other is continuous.
- Confidence intervals can be constructed around almost any computed statistic, including differences between means, differences between proportions, and correlation coefficients. CI information is valuable to clinical decision-makers, who need to know more than whether differences are probably real.
- **Power analysis** is a method of estimating either the likelihood of committing a Type II error or sample size requirements. Power analysis involves four components: desired significance level (α), **power** ($1 - \beta$), sample size (N), and estimated **effect size** (ES). Effect size estimates convey important information about the magnitude of effects in a study and are a useful supplement to *p* values and CI values. **Cohen's *d*** is a widely used effect size index summarizing mean-difference effects between two groups.

STUDY ACTIVITIES

Study activities are available to instructors on thePoint.

REFERENCES CITED IN CHAPTER 18

*Benjamin, D. J., Berger, J., Johannesson, M., Nosek, B., Wagenmakers, E., Berk, R., Johnson, V…. (2017). *Redefine statistical significance.* Paper downloaded December 14, 2018 from https://scholar.harvard.edu/files/dtingley/files/sig-naturehumanbehaviour.pdf.

Bonsaksen, T., Lerdal, A., Heir, T., Ekeberg, O., Skogstad, L., Grimholt, T., & Schou-Bredal, I. (2019). General self-efficacy in the Norwegian population: Differences and similarities between sociodemographic groups. *Scandinavian Journal of Public Health.* doi:10.1177/1403494818756701.

Braitman, L. (1991). Confidence intervals assess both clinical significance and statistical significance. *Annals of Internal Medicine, 114,* 515–517.

Cheung, D., Li, B., Lai, D., Leung, A., Yu, C., & Tsang, K. (2019). Cognitive stimulating play intervention for dementia: A feasibility randomized controlled trial. *American Journal of Alzheimer's Disease and Other Dementias, 34*(1), 63–71.

*Chiu, S., Yang, R., Yang, R., & Chang, S. (2018). Effects of resistance training on body composition and functional capacity among sarcopenic obese residents in long-term care facilities: A preliminary study. *BMC Geriatrics, 18,* 21.

Cohen, J. (1988). *Statistical power analysis for the behavioral sciences* (2nd ed.). Hillsdale, NJ: Lawrence Erlbaum Associates.

Corty, E. W., & Corty, R. (2011). Setting sample size to ensure narrow confidence intervals for precise estimation of population values. *Nursing Research, 60,* 148–154.

Dancey, C., Reidy, J., & Rowe, R. (2012). *Statistics for the health sciences: A non-mathematical introduction.* Thousand Oaks, CA: Sage Publications.

Gaskin, C., & Happell, B. (2014). Power, effects, confidence, and significance: An investigation of statistical practices in nursing research. *International Journal of Nursing Studies, 51,* 795–806.

Gravetter, F., Wallnau, L., & Forzano, L. (2018). *Essentials of statistics for the behavioral sciences* (9th ed.). Belmont, CA: Wadsworth Publishing.

*Gray, M., & Giuliano, K. (2018). Incontinence-associated dermatitis, characteristics and relationship to pressure injury: A multisite epidemiologic analysis. *Journal of Wound, Ostomy & Continence Nursing, 45*, 63–67.

Heo, S., McSweeney, J., Ounpraseuth, S., Shaw-Devine, A., Fier, A., & Moser, D. (2018). Testing a holistic meditation intervention to address psychosocial distress in patients with heart failure: A pilot study. *Journal of Cardiovascular Nursing, 33*, 126–134.

*Miyamoto, S., Dharma, M., Fazio, S., Tang-Feldman, Y., & Young, H. (2018). mHealth technology and nurse health coaching to improve health in diabetes: Protocol for a randomized controlled trial. *JMIR Research Protocols, 7*, e45.

*Moradi, A., Moeini, M., & Sanei, H. (2017). The effect of interactive text message follow-up on health promoting lifestyle of patients with acute coronary syndrome. *Iranian Journal of Nursing and Midwifery Research, 22*, 287–293.

Polit, D. F. (2010). *Statistics and data analysis for nursing research* (2nd ed.). Upper Saddle River, NJ: Pearson.

Polit, D. F., & Beck, C. T. (2013). Is there still gender bias in nursing research? An update. *Research in Nursing & Health, 36*, 75–83.

Polit, D. F., & Sherman, R. (1990). Statistical power in nursing research. *Nursing Research, 39*, 365–369.

Snyder, K., Hansen, K., Brown, S., Portratz, A., White, K., & Dinkel, D. (2018). Workplace breastfeeding support varies by employment type: The service workplace disadvantage. *Breastfeeding Medicine, 13*, 23–27.

**Wijdenes, K., Badger, T., & Sheppard, K. (2019). Assessing compassion fatigue risk among nurses in a large urban trauma center. *Journal of Nursing Administration, 49*, 19–23.

Yates, B., Park, E., Hug, A., Kupzyk, K., & Skradski, S. (2018). Changes over time in caregiving demand and difficulty in spousal caregivers of coronary artery bypass graft surgery patients. *Applied Nursing Research, 39*, 1–3.

*A link to this open-access article is provided in the Toolkit to Chapter 18 in the **Resource Manual.** ✪

**This journal article is available on the⬤Point for this chapter.

19 | Multivariate Statistics

Scientists, in their efforts to explain or predict phenomena, have recognized that two-variable studies are often inadequate. The classic approach to data analysis, which involved studying the effect of a single independent variable on an outcome, is being replaced by sophisticated **multivariate**[a] **statistics**.

Multivariate statistics are computationally formidable. Our purpose is to provide a general understanding of how, when, and why multivariate statistics are used, without working out computations. Nevertheless, we must present more formulas than we did in the previous two chapters because, to read and create tables with results from multivariate procedures, you must understand underlying components. This chapter introduces a few frequently used multivariate techniques—although we acknowledge that many of the sophisticated analytic procedures that are coming increasingly into use—such as *generalized estimating equations (GEE)*—are not covered in this overview. Those needing more comprehensive coverage of multivariate statistics should consult books such as those by Tabachnick and Fidell (2018), Pituch and Stevens (2016), or Hair et al. (2019).

---

[a]We use the term *multivariate* in this chapter to refer to analyses with at least three variables.

TIP Multivariate statistics are never computed manually. We present examples of output from several multivariate analyses using the *Statistical Package for the Social Sciences* (SPSS) in the Supplement to this chapter. 🅢

One widely used multivariate procedure is multiple regression analysis, which is used to analyze the relationship between two or more independent variables and a continuous dependent variable. The terms **multiple correlation** and **multiple regression** will be used almost interchangeably, consistent with the strong bond between correlation and regression. To comprehend this bond, we first explain simple (i.e., bivariate) regression.

SIMPLE LINEAR REGRESSION

Regression analysis is used to predict outcomes. In simple regression, one independent variable (X) is used to predict a dependent variable (Y). For instance, we could use simple regression to predict stress scores from noise levels. The higher the correlation between two variables, the more accurate the prediction. If the correlation between diastolic and systolic blood pressure were perfect (i.e., if $r = 1.00$), we would need to measure only one to know the value of the other. Few variables are perfectly correlated, and so predictions made through regression analysis usually are imperfect.

The basic linear regression equation is

$$Y' = a + bX$$

where Y' = predicted value of dependent variable Y
a = intercept constant
b = regression coefficient
X = actual value of independent variable X

Regression analysis solves for a and b, and so a prediction about Y can be made for any value of X. You may remember from high school algebra that the preceding equation is the algebraic equation for a straight line. **Linear regression** is used to determine a straight-line fit to the data that minimizes deviations from the line.

As an illustration, consider the data in Table 19.1 for five people on two strongly correlated variables, X and Y ($r = .90$). If we used the five pairs of X and Y values to solve for a and b in a regression equation, we would be able to predict Y values for *any* person for whom we have information on variable X.

We do not show the formulas for computing the values of a and b here but suffice it to say they are straightforward calculations involving deviation scores from X and Y values. As shown at the bottom of Table 19.1, the solution to the regression

equation is $Y' = 1.5 + .9X$. Now suppose that the X values in column 1 are the only data we have, and we want to predict values for Y. For the first person, $X = 1$; we would predict that $Y = 1.5 + (.9)(1)$, or 2.4. Column 3 shows Y' values for each X. These numbers show that Y' does not equal Y, the *actual* values obtained (column 2). Most **errors of prediction** (*e*) are small, as shown in column 4. Errors of prediction occur because the correlation between X and Y is not perfect. Only when $r = 1.00$ or -1.00 does $Y' = Y$. The regression equation solves for a and b in a way that minimizes such errors. More precisely, the solution minimizes the sums of squares of prediction errors—standard regression analysis is said to use **least-squares estimation**, which is why it is sometimes called *ordinary least squares*, or *OLS*, *regression*. In column 5 of Table 19.1, the error terms—called **residuals**—have been squared and summed to yield a value of 7.60. Any values of a and b other than 1.5 and .9 would yield a larger sum of squared residuals.

Figure 19.1 shows the solution to this regression analysis graphically. Actual X and Y values are plotted with circles. The line running through these points represents the regression solution. The intercept (a) is the point at which the line crosses the Y axis, which is 1.5. The slope (b) is the angle of the line. With $b = .90$, the line slopes so that for every 4 units on the X axis, we must go up 3.6 units ($.9 \times 4$)

TABLE 19.1 • Example of Simple Linear Regression

(1) X	(2) Y	(3) Y'	(4) e	(5) e²
1	2	2.4	−0.4	0.16
3	6	4.2	1.8	3.24
5	4	6.0	−2.0	4.00
7	8	7.8	0.2	0.04
9	10	9.6	0.4	0.16
$\overline{X} = 5.0$	$\overline{Y} = 6.0$		0.0	$\sum e^2 = 7.60$

$r = .90$
$Y' = a + bX = 1.5 + .9X$

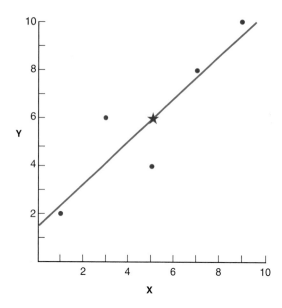

FIGURE 19.1 Example of simple linear regression.

on the *Y* axis. The line thus embodies the regression equation. To predict a value for *Y*, we would go to the point on the *X* axis for an obtained *X* value, go up to vertically to the point on the regression line directly above the *X* score, and then read the predicted *Y'* value horizontally on the *Y* axis. For example, for an *X* value of 5, we would predict a *Y'* of 6, indicated by the star.

Correlation coefficients express how variation in one variable is associated with variation in another. The square of r (r^2) tells us the proportion of variance in *Y* that is accounted for by *X*. In our example, $r = .90$, so $r^2 = .81$. This means that 81% of the variability in *Y* values can be understood in terms of variability in *X* values. The remaining 19% is variability due to other factors. Thus, the stronger the correlation, the better the prediction; the stronger the correlation, the greater the percentage of variance explained.

MULTIPLE LINEAR REGRESSION

The correlation between two variables is rarely perfect, and so researchers often try to improve predictions of *Y* by including multiple independent variables—which are called **predictor variables** in a multiple regression context.

Basic Concepts for Multiple Regression

Suppose we wanted to predict graduate nursing students' grade-point averages (GPAs). Not all applicants can be accepted, so we want to select those with the greatest likelihood of success. Suppose we had previously found that students with high scores on the verbal portion of an entrance exam (EE-V) tended to get better grades than those with lower EE-V scores. The correlation between EE-V and graduate GPAs is .50. With only 25% ($.50^2$) of the variance of graduate GPA accounted for, there will be many errors of prediction: Many admitted students will not perform as well as expected, and many rejected applicants would have made good students. It may be possible, by adding information, to make more accurate predictions through multiple regression. The basic multiple regression equation is

$$Y' = a + b_1 X_1 + b_2 X_2 + \ldots b_k X_k$$

where Y' = predicted value for dependent variable *Y*
    a = intercept constant
    k = number of predictor (independent) variables
b_1 to b_k = regression coefficients for the *k* variables
X_1 to X_k = scores or values on the *k* independent variables

In our example of predicting graduate nursing students' GPAs, suppose we hypothesized that undergraduate GPA (GPA-U) and scores on the quantitative portion of the entrance exam (EE-Q) would improve the prediction of graduate GPA. Suppose the resulting equation were

$$Y' = .4 + .05(\text{GPA-U}) + .003(\text{EE-Q}) + .002(\text{EE-V})$$

For instance, suppose an applicant had an EE-V score of 600, an EE-Q score of 550, and a GPA-U of 3.2. The predicted graduate GPA would be

$$Y' = .4 + .05(3.2) + .003(550) + .002(600) = 3.41$$

We can assess the degree to which adding two predictor variables improved our ability to predict graduate school performance through the multiple correlation coefficient. In bivariate correlation, the index is Pearson's r. With two or more independent variables, the index is the **multiple correlation coefficient**, or R. Unlike r, R does not have negative values. R varies from .00 to 1.00, showing the *strength* of relationship between several independent variables and a dependent variable but not *direction*. R, when squared (R^2), indicates the proportion of variance in Y accounted for by the combined, simultaneous influence of the predictor variables.

R^2 provides a way to evaluate the accuracy of a prediction equation. Suppose that with the three predictors in the current example, the value of $R = .71$. This means that 50% ($.71^2$) of the variation in graduate GPA can be explained by the two EE scores and undergraduate grades. Adding two predictors doubled the variance accounted for by EE-V alone, from .25 to .50.

The multiple correlation coefficient is never less than the highest bivariate correlation between a predictor and the outcome variable. Table 19.2 presents a correlation matrix with the rs for all pairs of variables in this example. The predictor most strongly correlated with graduate grades is GPA-U, $r = .60$. The value of R could not be less than .60.

R is more readily increased when predictors have low correlations among themselves. In the current case, the correlations range from .40 (between EE-Q and GPA-U) to .70 (EE-Q and EE-V). All correlations are fairly substantial, which helps to explain why R is not much higher than the r between the GPA-GRAD and GPA-U alone (.71 compared with .60). This somewhat puzzling phenomenon reflects redundancy of information among predictors. When correlations among independent variables are high, they add little predictive power to each other. With low correlations among predictors, each can contribute something unique to predicting an outcome. In our example, GPA-U predicts 36% of Y's variance ($.60^2$). The remaining two independent variables do not contribute as much as we would expect by considering their bivariate correlation with graduate GPA. Their *combined* added contribution is only 14% ($.50 - .36 = .14$), which is small because the two test scores have redundant information with undergraduate grades.

As more predictors are added to the equation, increments to R tend to decline. It is rare to find predictor variables that correlate well with an outcome but negligibly with one another. Redundancy is difficult to avoid as more and more variables are added. The inclusion of predictor variables beyond the first three or four typically does little to improve the proportion of variance accounted for or the accuracy of prediction.

> **TIP** When predictors are too highly correlated, a problem called **multicollinearity** can occur, which can lead to unstable results. Most researchers assess the risk of multicollinearity before finalizing their regression model. The Supplement for this chapter shows how multicollinearity can be evaluated. **Ⓢ**

Dependent variables in multiple regression analysis, as in ANOVA, should be measured on an interval or ratio scale. Predictor variables, on the

TABLE 19.2 • Correlation Matrix for Graduate Nursing Student Grade Example

	GPA-GRAD	GPA-U	EE-Q	EE-V
GPA-GRAD	1.00			
GPA-U	.60	1.00		
EE-Q	.55	.40	1.00	
EE-V	.50	.50	.70	1.00

EE, entrance examination; EE-Q, entrance examination quantitative score; EE-V, entrance examination verbal score; GPA, grade-point average; GPA-GRAD, graduate GPA; GPA-U, undergraduate GPA.

other hand, can either be interval- or ratio-level variables *or* categorical variables. Categorical variables usually are coded as dichotomous **dummy variables**, with the code of 1 designating the presence of an attribute and 0 designating its absence. For example, if females were coded 1 and males were coded 0, the code of 1 would represent "femaleness." A text such as that by Polit (2010) can be consulted for information on how to use and interpret dichotomous dummy variables.

Tests of Significance

Multiple regression analysis is not used solely (or even primarily) to develop prediction equations. Researchers typically test hypotheses about relationships among variables in the analysis. Several tests address different questions.

Tests of the Overall Equation and *R*

The basic null hypothesis in multiple regression is that the population multiple correlation coefficient equals zero. The test for the significance of *R* is based on principles analogous to those for ANOVA. With ANOVA, the *F*-ratio statistic is the ratio of the mean squares between, divided by mean squares within. In multiple regression, the form is similar:

$$F = \frac{SS_{\text{due to regression}} / df_{\text{regression}}}{SS_{\text{of residuals}} / df_{\text{residuals}}}$$
$$= \frac{\text{Mean Square}_{\text{due to regression}}}{\text{Mean Square}_{\text{of residuals}}}$$

As in ANOVA, variance from the independent variables is contrasted with variance attributable to other factors, or error. In our example of predicting graduate GPAs, suppose a multiple correlation coefficient of .71 ($R^2 = .50$) was calculated for a sample of 100 graduate students. The computed value of the *F*-statistic in this example is 32.05. The tabled value of *F* (with *df* = 3 and 96) for a significance level of .01 is about 4.00; thus, the probability that *R* = .71 resulted from chance fluctuations is considerably less than .01.

Example of Multiple Regression
Takei and colleagues (2019) used multiple regression to study factors associated with vegetable intake (VI) in pregnant Japanese women. In their sample of 273 pregnant women, the median energy-adjusted VI was 140 g/1,000 kcal. Several factors were predictive of VI, both negatively (e.g., pregnancy-associated nausea, $p = .006$) and positively (e.g., exercise habits, $p = .001$). The R^2 for all predictors was .27.

Tests for Adding Predictors

Another question researchers may want to answer is: Does *adding* X_k to the regression significantly improve the prediction of *Y* over that achieved with X_{k-1}? For example, does a third predictor increase our ability to predict *Y* after two predictors have been used? An *F*-statistic can be computed to answer this question.

In the current example, let us say that X_1 = GPA-U; X_2 = EE-Q; and X_3 = EE-V. We can then symbolize various correlation coefficients as follows:

$R_{y.1}$ = the correlation of *Y* with GPA-U = .60
$R_{y.12}$ = the correlation of *Y* with GPA-U *and* EE-Q = .71
$R_{y.123}$ = the correlation of *Y* with all three predictors = .71

We can see that EE-V scores made no independent contribution to the multiple correlation coefficient. The value of $R_{y.12}$ is identical to the value of $R_{y.123}$. We cannot tell at a glance, however, whether adding X_2 to X_1 *significantly* increased the prediction of *Y*. What we want to know is whether X_2 would improve predictions in the population, or if its added predictive power in this sample resulted from chance. In the current example, the value of the *F*-statistic for testing whether adding EE-Q scores significantly improves our prediction of *Y* is 27.16. If we consulted a table for the theoretical distribution of *F* with *df* = 1 and 97 and a significance level of .01, we would find that the critical value is about 6.90. Therefore, adding EE-Q to the regression equation with GPA-U significantly improved the accuracy of predicting graduate GPA, beyond the .01 level.

Tests of the Regression Coefficients

When a regression coefficient (b) is divided by its standard error, the result is a value for the t statistic, which can be used to assess the significance of individual predictors. A significant t indicates that the regression coefficient (b) is significantly different from zero.

In simple regression, the value of b indicates the amount of change in predicted values of Y for a specified rate of change in X. In multiple regression, the coefficients represent the number of units the dependent variable is predicted to change for each unit change in a predictor variable *when the effects of other predictors are held constant.* "Holding constant" other predictors means that they are statistically controlled, a feature that can enhance a study's internal validity. If a regression coefficient is significant when confounding variables are included in the regression equation, it means that the predictor associated with the coefficient contributed significantly to the regression, even after confounding variables are taken into account.

Strategies for Handling Predictors in Multiple Regression

Three alternative strategies for entering predictor variables into regression equations are simultaneous, hierarchical, and stepwise regressions.

Simultaneous Multiple Regression

The most basic strategy, **simultaneous multiple regression**, enters all predictor variables into the regression equation at the same time. One regression equation is developed, and statistical tests indicate the significance of R and of individual regression coefficients. This strategy is most appropriate when there is no basis for considering any particular predictor as causally prior to another, and when the predictors are of comparable importance to the research question.

Hierarchical Multiple Regression

Many researchers use **hierarchical multiple regression**, which involves entering predictors into the equation in a series of steps. Researchers control the order of entry, with the order typically based on theoretical considerations. For example, some predictors may be thought of as causally or temporally prior to others, in which case they could be entered in an early step. Another important reason for using hierarchical regression is to examine the effect of a key independent variable after first removing (controlling) the effect of confounding variables.

> **Example of Hierarchical Multiple Regression**
> Staneva and colleagues (2018) explored psychological factors associated with adverse birth outcomes. They used hierarchical regression to enter predictors in two steps. Medical complications (e.g., infections, excessive bleeding, preeclampsia, placenta complications) were entered in the first step; measures of psychological distress (e.g., anxiety, low social support) were entered in the second block.

With hierarchical regression, researchers determine the number of steps and the number of predictors included in each step. When several variables are added as a block, as in the Staneva example, the analysis is a simultaneous regression for those variables at that stage. Thus, hierarchical regression can be considered a controlled sequence of simultaneous regressions.

Stepwise Multiple Regression

Stepwise multiple regression involves *empirically* selecting the combination of independent variables with the most predictive power. In stepwise multiple regression, predictors enter the regression equation in the order that produces the greatest increments to R^2. The first step selects the single best predictor of the outcome variable, i.e., the independent variable with the highest bivariate correlation with Y. The second variable to enter the equation is the one that produces the largest increase to R^2 when used simultaneously with the predictor selected in the first step. The procedure continues until no additional predictor significantly increases the value of R^2.

Figure 19.2 illustrates stepwise multiple regression. Suppose that the first variable (X_1), has a correlation of .60 with Y ($r^2 = .36$). Variable X_1 accounts for the portion of the variability of Y represented by the hatched area in step 1 of the figure.

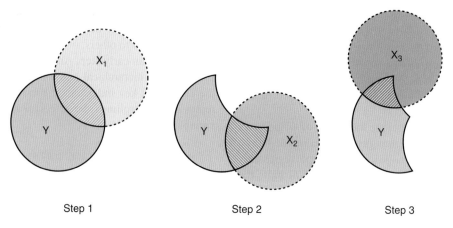

FIGURE 19.2 Visual representation of stepwise multiple regression analysis.

This hatched area is, in effect, removed from further consideration, because this portion of Y's variability is explained. The variable chosen in step 2 is not always the X variable with the second largest correlation with Y. The selected predictor is the one that explains the largest portion of what *remains* of Y's variability after X_1 has been taken into account. Variable X_2, in turn, removes a second part of Y so that the independent variable selected in step 3 is the one that accounts for the most variability in Y after *both* X_1 and X_2 are removed.

Example of Stepwise Multiple Regression

Barbe and colleagues (2018) used stepwise multiple regression to study the relationship between psychosocial factors and aspects of work function among nurses who provide direct patient care. For example, in predicting scores on a work function subscale measuring nurses' lack of energy and motivation, the only predictor stepped into the regression equation was perceived stress. Depression, sleep disturbances, and subjective cognitive complaints (e.g., poor memory) were not significant with stress controlled. The final R^2 was .15, $p < .01$.

TIP Stepwise regression is controversial because variables are entered into the regression equation based on statistical rather than theoretical criteria. If stepwise regression is used, cross-validation is recommended (e.g., by dividing the sample in half and running two independent series of regressions).

Relative Contribution of Predictors

Scientists want not only to predict phenomena, but to explain them. Predictions can be made in the absence of understanding. For instance, in our graduate school example, we could predict performance moderately well without explaining *why* the factors contributed to students' success. For practical applications, it may be sufficient to make accurate predictions, but researchers typically want to understand phenomena.

In multiple regression, one approach to understanding a phenomenon is to explore the relative importance of predictor variables. Unfortunately, determining the relative contributions of independent variables in predicting an outcome is a thorny issue. When predictor variables are correlated, as they usually are, there is no ideal way to disentangle the effects of variables in the equation.

It may appear that the solution is to compare the contributions of the Xs to R^2. In our graduate school example, GPA-U accounted for 36% of Y's variance; EE-Q explained an additional 14%. Should we conclude that undergraduate grades are more than twice as important as EE-Q scores in explaining graduate school grades? This conclusion would be inaccurate because the order of entry of variables in a regression equation affects their apparent contribution. If these two predictor variables were entered in reverse order (i.e., EE-Q first), R^2 would remain unchanged at .50; however, EE-Q's contribution would be .30 (.55²), and GPA-U's contribution would be .20 (.50 − .30). This is because whatever variance the independent variables have in common is attributed to the first variable entered in the analysis.

Another approach to assessing the relative importance of the predictors is to compare regression coefficients. Earlier, we presented an equation for multiple regression that included *a* (the constant), and *b*s (regression coefficients) for each predictor. The *b* values cannot be directly compared because they are in the units of original scores, which differ from one *X* to another. X_1 might be in milliliters, X_2 in degrees Fahrenheit, and so forth. The use of **standard scores** (or *z* **scores**) eliminates this problem by transforming all variables to scores with a mean of 0.0 and a standard deviation (*SD*) of 1.00 (Chapter 16). Transforming regular scores to *z* scores is easy—they are the difference between a score and the mean of that score divided by the standard deviation, or:

$$z_x = \frac{X - \overline{X}}{SD_x}$$

In standard score form, the regression equation uses standard scores (*z*s) instead of raw scores (*X*s), and the regression coefficients for each *z* are *standardized regression coefficients*, called **beta** (*β*) **weights**. With all the *β*s in the same measurement units, can their relative size shed light on the relative importance of predictors? Many researchers have interpreted beta weights in this fashion, but there are problems in doing so. These regression coefficients will be the same no matter what the order of entry of the variables. The difficulty, however, is that regression weights are unstable. Values of *β* tend to fluctuate from sample to sample. Moreover, when a variable is added to or subtracted from the equation, beta weights change. Because values of the regression coefficients fluctuate, it is difficult to attach theoretical importance to them.

One of the best solutions is to compare the **squared semipartial correlation coefficients** (*sr²*) of the predictors. It is beyond the scope of this book to explain this index in detail, but we note that the *sr²* is useful because it indicates a predictor's unique contribution to variability in the dependent variable—that is, the contribution after other predictors are controlled.

Regression Results

There are no standard table formats for presenting regression results, and different formats are relevant depending on whether standard, hierarchical, or stepwise regression has been performed. The most frequently reported elements are *β*, R^2, and *p* values. We illustrate a table of regression results using a study of predictors of moral distress in a sample of critical care nurses in the United States (Hiler et al., 2018). The researchers hypothesized that nurses' moral distress could be predicted by perceptions of their practice environments. They used a two-step hierarchical regression in which they first entered scores on five self-reported measures of the nurses' perceptions of workplace plus an objective indicator—whether the ICU in which they worked had been recognized by a Beacon Award. In the second step, the researchers' entered predictors corresponding to participants' characteristics—their age and job satisfaction. Table 19.3 shows results for the final model in which all predictors were in the equation.

The first column shows the order of entry (in blocks) of the eight predictors, which are listed in the second column. The next column shows values for the standardized beta coefficients. The last column shows whether each predictor was statistically significant. For example, the nurses' perception of collegial nurse–physician relations (NPR) was a highly significant predictor of the nurses' degree of moral distress. The negative coefficient for beta (−.18) indicates that higher scores on the NPR scale were associated with lower scores on the moral distress scale. This is significant (*p* = .001): the probability is 1 in 1,000 that the relationship between NPR scores and moral distress scores is spurious. Also, older nurses have lower moral distress scores than younger ones (*p* = .001). The results suggest that certain aspects of the nurses' practice environment are significantly associated with moral distress even after controlling for the nurses' age and job satisfaction. Other factors

TABLE 19.3 • Multiple Regression Analysis Results: Predictors of Moral Distress in U.S. Critical Care Nurses ($N = 328$)

STEP[a]	PREDICTOR	BETA	p
1	Nurses' participation in hospital affairs	−.04	ns
1	Perceptions of nursing foundations for quality of care (patient safety)	−.12	ns
1	Nurse managers' ability, leadership, and support of nurses	−.00	ns
1	Staffing and resource adequacy	−.19	.003
1	Collegial nurse–physician relations (NPR scale)	−.18	.001
1	Beacon Award designation (1 = yes, 0 = no)	−.03	ns
2	Age	−.14	.001
2	Job satisfaction	−.22	<.001

For Step 1 regression: $R^2 = .25$, $F = 17.65$, $p < .001$.

For final regression: $R^2 = .30$, $F = 17.07$, $p < .001$.

Change in R^2 from Step 1 to Step 2: $F = 11.77$, $p < .001$.

[a]In this hierarchical regression, variables were entered in two steps, as designated. Parameter estimates for beta are shown for the step 2 results only.

Adapted from Table 3, Hiler, C., Hickman, R., Reimer, A., & Wilson, K. (2018). Predictors of moral distress in a U.S. sample of critical care nurses. *American Journal of Critical Care, 27,* 59–65.

(e.g., perceptions of nurse managers' leadership ability, Beacon award designation) were not significant independent predictors of moral distress.

At the bottom of the table, we see that the value of R^2 for the final model was .30, which is significant at $p < .001$. Adding age and job satisfaction in step 2 significantly increased the value of R^2, from .25 to .30 ($p < .001$). The remaining 70% of variation in levels of moral distress is explained by factors not included in the regression model.

TIP Some table templates for presenting multivariate results are included in the Toolkit of the accompanying *Resource Manual.*

Power Analysis for Multiple Regression

Small samples are especially problematic in multiple regression and other multivariate procedures. Inadequate sample size can lead to Type II errors and erratic regression coefficients.

One approach to estimating sample size needs concerns the ratio of predictor variables to total number of cases. Tabachnick and Fidell (2018) suggest this guideline: N should be greater than 50, plus 8 times the number of predictors. So, with 5 predictors, the sample size should be greater than 90 (50 + [8 × 5]). Some experts recommend a ratio of 20 to 1 for simultaneous and hierarchical regression and a ratio of 40 to 1 for stepwise. More cases are needed for stepwise regression because this procedure capitalizes on the idiosyncrasies of a specific data set.

Another way to estimate sample size needs is to perform a power analysis. The number of participants needed to reject the null hypothesis that R equals zero is estimated based on effect size, number of predictors, desired power, and the significance criterion. In multiple regression, the estimated effect size is a function of the value of R^2. Researchers must either predict the value of R^2 on the basis of earlier research or use the convention that effect size will be small ($R^2 = .02$), moderate ($R^2 = .13$), or large ($R^2 = .30$).

Table 19.4 presents sample size estimates for 2 to 10 predictors and various values of R^2, for power = .80 and alpha = .05. As an example, suppose we were planning a study to predict functional ability in nursing home residents using five predictor variables. We estimate a moderate effect size ($R^2 = .13$) and want to achieve a power of .80 and $\alpha = .05$. A sample of about 92 nursing home residents is needed to detect a population R^2 of .13 with five predictors, with a 5% chance of a Type I error and a 20% chance of a Type II error.

> **TIP** Several websites (many of which are in the Toolkit for you to click on) do instantaneous power calculations and sample size estimates for many multivariate procedures.

ANALYSIS OF COVARIANCE

Analysis of covariance (ANCOVA) has much in common with multiple regression, but it also has features of ANOVA. Like ANOVA, ANCOVA is used to compare the means of two or more groups, and the central question is the same: Are mean group differences likely to be *real* or spurious? Like multiple regression, ANCOVA allows researchers to control confounding variables statistically.

Uses of Analysis of Covariance

ANCOVA is especially useful in certain situations. For example, if a nonequivalent control group design is used to test an intervention, researchers must consider whether obtained results are influenced by preexisting group differences. When control through randomization is lacking, ANCOVA offers post hoc statistical control. Even in true experiments, ANCOVA can result in more precise estimates of group differences because, even with randomization, there are typically slight differences between groups. ANCOVA adjusts for initial differences so that the results more precisely illuminate the effect of an intervention.

Strictly speaking, ANCOVA should not be used with existing groups because randomization is an underlying assumption of ANCOVA. This assumption is often violated, however; when randomization is not feasible, ANCOVA can sometimes improve a study's internal validity.

TABLE 19.4 • Power Analysis Table for Multiple Regression: Sample Size Estimates to Test the Null Hypothesis that $R^2 = .00$, for Power = .80, and $\alpha = .05$ with 2-10 Predictor Variables

NO. OF PREDICTORS	ESTIMATED POPULATION R^2										
	.02	.04	.06	.08	.10	.13	.15	.20	.25	.30	.40
2	478	230	152	113	89	67	58	42	32	26	18
3	543	261	173	128	102	77	66	48	37	30	21
4	597	287	190	141	112	85	73	53	41	33	24
5	643	309	205	153	121	92	79	57	45	36	26
6	684	329	218	163	129	98	84	61	48	39	28
7	721	347	231	172	136	104	89	65	51	41	30
8	755	375	242	180	143	109	94	69	54	44	32
9	788	380	252	188	150	114	98	72	56	46	33
10	818	395	262	196	156	119	102	75	59	48	35

Shaded columns indicate conventions for small, medium, and large effect sizes.

ANCOVA Procedures

Suppose we were testing the effectiveness of bio-feedback therapy on patients' anxiety. A group in one hospital is exposed to the treatment, and a comparison group in another hospital is not. Patients' anxiety levels are measured both before and after the intervention; thus, pretest anxiety scores can be statistically controlled through ANCOVA. In this situation, the outcome variable is the posttest anxiety scores, the independent variable is experimental/comparison group status, and the **covariate** is pretest anxiety scores. Covariates are usually continuous variables (e.g., anxiety scores), but can be dichotomous variables (male/female); the independent variable is a nominal-level variable.

ANCOVA tests the significance of differences between group means after adjusting scores on the outcome variable to remove the effect of covariates. In essence, the first step in ANCOVA is the same as the first step in hierarchical multiple regression. Variability in the outcome that can be explained by the covariate is removed from further consideration. ANOVA is performed on what remains of Y's variability to see whether, once the covariate is controlled, differences between group means are statistically significant.

Let us consider another example to explore further aspects of ANCOVA. Suppose we were testing the effectiveness of weight-loss diets, and we randomly assigned 30 people to 1 of 3 groups. ANCOVA, using pretreatment weight as the covariate, permits a more sensitive analysis of weight change than simple ANOVA. Some hypothetical data for such a study

are shown in Table 19.5. Two aspects of the weight values in this table are discernible. First, despite random assignment to treatment groups, group means at baseline are different. Participants in diet B differ from those in diet C by an average of 10 pounds (175 versus 185 pounds). This difference reflects chance fluctuations and is not significant ($F = 0.45$, $p = .64$). Second, posttreatment means are also different by a maximum of only 10 pounds (160-170). However, the mean number of pounds *lost* ranged from 10 pounds for diets A and B to 25 pounds for diet C.

When we perform an ordinary ANOVA testing group differences in posttreatment weights, we get an F of 0.55, indicating nonsignificant mean group differences ($p = .58$). Based on ANOVA, we would conclude that all three diets had comparable effects on weight loss.

Now let us use ANCOVA to analyze the data. The first step breaks total variability in posttreatment weights into two components: (1) variability explained by the covariate (pretreatment weights) and (2) residual variability. The covariate accounts for a significant amount of variance, which is not surprising because there is a strong relationship between pretreatment and posttreatment weights: people who started out especially heavy tended to stay that way, relative to others in the sample. In the second step, residual variance is broken down to reflect between-group and within-group contributions. The resulting F of 17.54 ($df = 2, 26$) is significant beyond the .001 level. We can conclude that, after controlling for initial weight, there is a significant difference in weight loss in the different diet groups.

TABLE 19.5 • Fictitious Data for ANCOVA Example: Comparison of Pre- and Posttreatment Weights for Three Diet Interventions

	DIET A	DIET B	DIET C	TOTAL
Pretreatment weight, mean (*SD*)	180.0 (23.5)	175.0 (22.5)	185.0 (24.6)	180.0 (23.1)
Posttreatment weight, mean (*SD*)	170.0 (21.7)	165.0 (22.0)	160.0 (20.3)	165.0 (20.0)
ANOVA $F(2, 27)$ for mean group differences in posttreatment weight = 0.55, $p = .58$				
ANCOVA $F(1, 26)$ for covariate (pretreatment weight) = 309.88, $p < .001$				
ANCOVA $F(2, 26)$ for mean group differences in posttreatment weight = 17.54, $p < .001$				

This fictitious example was contrived so that an ANOVA result of "no difference" would be altered by adding a covariate. Most actual results are less dramatic. Nonetheless, ANCOVA yields a more sensitive statistical test than ANOVA because the covariate reduces the error term (within-group variability), against which treatment effects are compared.

Theoretically, it is possible to use any number of covariates. It is seldom advisable, however, to use more than two or three. For one thing, a large number of covariates is often unnecessary because of the typically high degree of redundancy beyond the first few. Moreover, each covariate uses up a degree of freedom; fewer degrees of freedom means that a higher F is required for significance. For instance, with 2 and 26 df, an F of 5.53 is required for significance at the .01 level, but with 2 and 23 df (i.e., adding three covariates), an F of 5.66 is needed.

Selection of Covariates

Useful covariates are almost always available. Background characteristics, such as age and gender, are often good candidates. Background characteristics are especially important to control if they are predictors of the outcome and there are differences between the groups being compared. The literature is a good source of information about factors correlated with outcomes.

A baseline measure of the outcome is an excellent covariate, invariably strongly correlated with the final outcome. However, RM-ANOVA is an alternative to ANCOVA when analyzing data from studies with pretest–posttest designs. *Propensity scores*, discussed briefly in Chapter 9, can be powerful covariates. Propensity scores capture group differences on a broad range of attributes because they represent an attempt to model group differences using available data. The use of propensity scores as covariates is described by Qin et al. (2008) and Schroeder et al. (2016).

In general, it is important to select covariates that have strong reliability. Measurement errors can lead to overadjustments or underadjustments of the mean and can contribute to Type I or Type II errors.

Adjusted Means

In our example of the three diets, the significant ANCOVA F test indicates that at least one of the three groups had a posttreatment weight that is significantly different from the overall grand mean, after adjusting for pretreatment weights. It sometimes is useful to examine **adjusted means**, that is, group means on the outcome variable after adjusting for (i.e., removing the effect of) covariates. In our example of posttreatment weights for participants in three diet interventions, the adjusted means for diets A, B, and C were 170.0, 169.4, and 155.6, respectively—values that clearly indicate differences among those exposed to the different diets.

When ANCOVA results in a significant group F test, researchers can reject the null hypothesis that the adjusted group means are equal. As with ANOVA, further analysis is needed to assess which pairs of adjusted group means are significantly different from one another. In our example, post hoc tests revealed that the mean weight for diet C is significantly different from that for both diets A and B, but diets A and B are not significantly different from each other.

> **TIP** For ANCOVA, an eta squared statistic can be computed to summarize the magnitude of the *adjusted* effect of the independent variable on the dependent variable. Estimates of eta squared can be used in a power analysis to estimate sample size needs when planning a study. In general, when ANCOVA is used with carefully selected covariates, the analysis of group differences is more powerful than with ANOVA because error variance is reduced. In our example of the three diets, the value of adjusted eta squared is .57.

Example of ANCOVA

Looman and colleagues (2018) tested the effects of a telehealth care coordination intervention on health-related quality-of-life outcomes of children with medical complexity. Children, randomized into two intervention groups or a usual-care control group, were compared on such outcomes as functional status and health-related quality of life 24 months after the start of the interventions. ANCOVA was used to test postintervention group differences, controlling for baseline scores on the outcomes.

OTHER LEAST-SQUARES MULTIVARIATE TECHNIQUES

Many multivariate statistics discussed thus far are related. For example, ANOVA and multiple regression are similar. Both techniques analyze total variability in a continuous dependent measure, and contrast variability due to independent variables with that attributable to error. By tradition, experimental data typically are analyzed by ANOVA, and correlational data are analyzed by regression.

A broad class of statistical techniques are subsumed under the **general linear model (GLM)**, which include techniques that fit data to straight-line (linear) solutions. The GLM is the foundation for such procedures as the *t*-test, ANOVA, and multiple regression. The GLM is an important model because of its generality and applicability to numerous research situations, but a thorough understanding of the GLM requires advanced statistical training. In this section, other GLM methods are briefly introduced.

Repeated-Measures ANOVA for Mixed Designs

In Chapter 18 we discussed one-way repeated-measures ANOVA (RM-ANOVA), which is appropriate when one group of people is measured at multiple points. Many RCTs involve randomly assigning participants to different treatment groups, and then collecting postintervention data several times. When there are only two data collection points (e.g., a pretest and a posttest), ANCOVA is often used to test the null hypothesis that group means are equal, after removing the effect of pretest (baseline) scores. When data are collected three or more times, a **repeated-measures ANOVA for mixed designs** is often used.

As an example, suppose we collected heart rate data at 2 hours (T1), 4 hours (T2), and 6 hours (T3) postsurgery for people in an intervention and control group. Structurally, the ANOVA for analyzing these data would look similar to a 2 × 3 multifactor ANOVA, but calculations would differ in this mixed design—mixed because it involves both a within-subject factor and a between-subject factor. An *F*-statistic would be computed to test for a *between-subjects effect* (i.e., differences between experimentals and controls). This statistic would indicate whether, across all time periods, mean heart rate differed in the two groups. Another *F*-statistic would be computed to test for a *within-subjects effect* or time factor (i.e., differences at T1, T2, and T3). This statistic would indicate whether, for both groups, mean heart rates differed over time. Finally, an **interaction effect** would be tested to assess whether group differences varied across time. In mixed design RM-ANOVA, the interaction effect usually is of primary importance. When people are randomized to treatment groups, we would expect their mean values at baseline to be equivalent—but if there are treatment effects, group means would differ at subsequent points of data collection, thus resulting in a time × treatment interaction.

Tests within the GLM have several basic assumptions, all of which are fully described in statistics textbooks. Assumptions such as normality of the distributions and the equality of variances apply to most GLM procedures, but ANOVA and most of its variants are fairly **robust** to violation of assumptions (i.e., violations tend not to affect the accuracy of statistical decision-making). However, RM-ANOVA has some unique assumptions—the assumption of *sphericity* and the related assumption of *compound symmetry*, both of which are too complex to elaborate here. RM-ANOVA is not, unfortunately, robust to violations of these assumptions. Furthermore, there are different opinions about how to detect and address violations. Thus, RM-ANOVA tends to be more complex than many procedures discussed thus far. Polit (2010) and advanced statistical texts offer suggestions on using RM-ANOVA.

> **Example of a Mixed Design RM-ANOVA**
> Yang and Chen (2018) used a mixed design to test whether an aerobic exercise intervention for postnatal women affected their stress, fatigue, and sleep quality. Data for these outcomes were collected at baseline and 4 and 12 weeks later for women randomized to either the intervention group or the control group. RM-ANOVA revealed significant improvements for those in the intervention group.

Multivariate Analysis of Variance

Multivariate analysis of variance (MANOVA) is the extension of ANOVA to more than one outcome. MANOVA is used to test the significance of differences in group means for multiple dependent variables, considered simultaneously. For instance, if we wanted to test the effect of two methods of exercise on diastolic *and* systolic blood pressure, MANOVA would be appropriate. Researchers often analyze such data by performing two separate ANOVAs. Strictly speaking, this practice is not appropriate. Separate ANOVAs imply that the outcomes were independent when, in fact, they were obtained from the same people and are correlated. MANOVA takes the intercorrelations of outcomes into account. ANOVA is, however, a more widely understood procedure than MANOVA, and thus its results may be more easily communicated to a broad audience.

MANOVA can be extended in ways analogous to ANOVA. For example, it is possible to perform **multivariate analysis of covariance (MANCOVA)**, which allows for the control of confounding variables (covariates) when there are two or more outcome variables.

TIP If you opt to use simpler analyses to enhance the accessibility of the evidence to clinical audiences (e.g., three separate ANOVAs rather than a MANOVA), you should run the analyses both ways. Then, you could present bivariate results (e.g., from ANOVAs) in the report and state whether the more complex analysis (e.g., MANOVA) yielded comparable results.

Example of MANOVA
Thorlton and Collins (2018) studied the beliefs of college students regarding the consumption of energy beverages. One analysis involved a MANOVA to analyze gender differences in student's perceptions, intents, attitudes, and behavior regarding energy drink consumption. Gender differences were statistically significant, with men more positive toward energy beverages than women: $F(8, 264) = 4.26$, $p < .001$.

LOGISTIC REGRESSION

Logistic regression is a widely used multivariate technique. Like multiple regression, logistic regression analyzes the relationship between multiple independent variables and a dependent variable and yields a predictive equation. Logistic regression, however, relies on an estimation procedure that has less restrictive assumptions than multivariate procedures within the GLM and is used to predict categorical outcomes.

TIP A least-squares procedure for predicting categorical outcomes is called *discriminant analysis.* Although popular two decades ago, discriminant analysis is infrequently used and has been superseded by logistic regression.

Basic Concepts for Logistic Regression

Logistic regression uses **maximum likelihood estimation (MLE)**. Maximum likelihood estimators are ones that estimate the parameters most likely to have generated the observed data. Confirmatory factor analysis, discussed in Chapter 16, also uses MLE.

Logistic regression has few assumptions about the underlying distribution of variables. Logistic regression is well suited to many clinical questions because it models the probability of an outcome. For example, we might be interested in modeling the probability of engaging in breast self-examination, or the probability of a patient fall.

Logistic regression transforms the probability of an event occurring (e.g., that a patient will fall) into its odds. As discussed in Chapter 17, **odds** reflect the ratio of two probabilities: the probability of an event occurring, to the probability that it will not occur. For example, if 10% of patients fall, the odds would be .10 divided by .90, or .111.

Probabilities, which range between zero and one, are then transformed into continuous variables that range between zero and infinity. Because this range is still restricted, a further transformation is performed, namely calculating the logarithm of the odds. The range of this new variable (the **logit**, short for *log*istic probability un*it*) is from minus to plus infinity. Using the continuous logit as the outcome variable, a maximum likelihood procedure estimates the coefficients of the independent variables.

The solution yields an equation that predicts the logit from a weighted combination of independent variables, plus a constant, much like a multiple regression equation. The interpretation, however, is different because the equation does not predict *actual* values of the dependent variable. In logistic regression, a regression coefficient (*b*) can be interpreted as the change in the log odds associated with a one-unit change in the associated predictor variable.

The Odds Ratio

A logistic regression equation is hard to interpret because we do not think in terms of log odds. The equation can, however, be transformed back to yield information in terms of odds rather than log odds. The factor by which the odds change is the *odds ratio* (*OR*), the risk index we discussed in Chapter 17.

For example, suppose that we used logistic regression to predict the probability of performing breast self-examination. One of the predictors might be whether the woman has a family member (e.g., a sister) who had breast cancer. A logistic regression analysis might indicate that the *OR* was 12.1, with all other predictors in the equation held constant. (This is often called an *adjusted odds ratio*.) The odds ratio provides an estimate (around which confidence intervals can be built) of relative risk—the risk of an event occurring given one condition, versus the risk of it occurring given a different condition. In our example, we would estimate that the "risk" of performing breast self-examination is about 12 times greater if a woman has a family history of breast cancer than if she does not, with other factors controlled.

TIP Just as there is simple regression with least-squares estimation—i.e., the prediction of an outcome variable based on a single independent variable—*bivariate logistic regression* is also possible. This is often done to produce estimates of *unadjusted* (or *crude*) odds ratios—i.e., odds ratios without controlling other variables.

Variables in Logistic Regression

The outcome variable in logistic regression is a dichotomous variable. The outcome is typically coded 1 to represent an event or a characteristic (e.g., had a fall, is obese), and 0 to represent the absence of the event or characteristic (no fall, not obese). Predictor variables can be continuous variables, categorical variables, or interaction terms. Although there are no strict limits to the number of predictors that can be included, it is best to achieve a parsimonious model with strong predictive power using a small set of good predictors.

When continuous variables are the predictors, the odds ratio is interpreted somewhat differently than with categorical variables. For example, suppose we were predicting whether a nursing home resident would have a fall, and one predictor variable was age. Suppose we found, for example, that the *OR* associated with age was 1.10. This means that for every additional year of age, the odds of falling increased by 10%, with everything else in the model held constant.

Dummy-coded variables are a common method of representing dichotomous predictors, such as smokes cigarettes (1) versus does not smoke cigarettes (0). For variables with more than two categories, a series of dummy variables is needed. For example, if marital status were a predictor variable in a logistic regression for predicting breast self-examination, a bivariate logistic analysis could provide estimates of the relative risk of different marital statuses (e.g., never married, currently married, formerly married) on breast self-examination. In such an analysis, one group would be the **reference group**, with an *OR* of 1.0, and the other two groups would have *OR*s in relation to the reference group. As a hypothetical example, if the *OR* for a never-married reference group was 1.0 and the *OR* for currently married was 1.23, this means that married women were 23% more likely to perform breast self-examination than never-married women.

As with multiple regression, predictors in multiple regression can be entered into the equation if different ways. The options include simultaneous, hierarchical, and stepwise entry.

Significance Tests in Logistic Regression

Researchers usually want to assess the overall reliability of the model, i.e., whether the set of predictors, taken as a whole, is significantly better than chance in predicting the probability of the outcome. Unfortunately, assessing the goodness of fit of a logistic regression model can be confusing because there are several different tests, and different authors use different names for the tests. Another potential source of confusion is that some tests indicate goodness of fit by a significant result, and others indicate goodness of fit by a *non*significant result. We briefly describe two approaches but recommend further reading in advanced textbooks such as Tabachnick and Fidell (2018) or Hosmer et al. (2013).

One statistic in logistic regression is the **likelihood index**, which is the probability of the observed results, given parameters estimated in the analysis. If the overall model fits the data perfectly, the likelihood index is 1.0. Because the likelihood index is typically a small decimal, it is usually transformed by multiplying it by -2 times the log of the likelihood. The transformed index ($-2LL$) is a small number when the fit is good; in a perfect fit, the value is zero. The chi-square statistic is then used to test the null hypothesis that all of the b regression coefficients are zero, in a **likelihood ratio test**. A **goodness-of-fit statistic**, which has a chi-squared distribution, is the analogue of the overall F test in multiple regression. This statistic is based on the residuals for all cases in the analysis—which is the difference between the observed probability of an event and the predicted probability. This statistic is thus a mechanism for evaluating the fit of the predictive model. The likelihood ratio test also can be used to evaluate the significance of *improvement* to $-2LL$ with successive entry of predictors, when hierarchical or stepwise regression is performed.

An alternative approach to testing the overall model is the **Hosmer–Lemeshow test**, which compares the prediction model to a hypothetically "perfect" model. In brief, the perfect model is one that contains the exact set of predictors needed to duplicate the observed frequencies in the outcome. The full model can be tested against the perfect model by computing differences between observed frequencies and expected frequencies—i.e., those expected in the perfect model. With this test, a *nonsignificant* chi-square is desired. A nonsignificant result indicates that the model being tested is not reliably different from the perfect model. In other words, nonsignificance supports the inference that the model adequately duplicates the observed frequencies of the outcome.

> **TIP** There is no consensus on which approach for an overall model test is better, but logistic regression software programs can perform both tests, and some researchers present both results.

It is also possible to test the significance of individual predictors in the model—just as the t statistic is used in multiple regression. A frequently used statistic for this purpose is the **Wald statistic**, which is distributed as a chi-square. Significance can also be assessed by examining the confidence intervals around the odds ratios. If the 95% CI includes the value of 1.0, this indicates that the OR was not statistically significant at the .05 level.

Effect Size in Logistic Regression

Statisticians have worked on developing an effect size index for logistic regression that is analogous to R^2 in multiple regression. The main problem, however, is that R^2 in multiple regression can be interpreted as the percentage of variance in the outcome explained by the predictors, but this is more complex with a dichotomous outcome. Despite difficulties in achieving a good analog to least squares–based R^2, several **pseudo R^2** measures have been proposed for logistic regression. These indexes should be reported as approximations to an R^2 rather than as the percentage of variance explained. A statistic called the **Nagelkerke R^2** is the most frequently reported pseudo R^2 index.

> **Example of Logistic Regression**
> Siegmund and colleagues (2018) sought to identify factors predictive of hospital readmission among patients with metabolic syndrome who received cardiac rehabilitation. In their logistic regression analysis, they found that white race (OR = .50) and high functional capacity (OR = .80) were protective against readmission within the first 90 days.

SURVIVAL AND EVENT HISTORY ANALYSIS

Some outcomes are time-related. **Survival analysis** is widely used by epidemiologists when the dependent variable is a time interval between an initial event (e.g., onset of a disease) and a terminal event (e.g., death). Survival analysis calculates a survival score, which compares survival time for one participant with that for others. When researchers are interested in group comparisons—for example, comparing the survival function of people in an intervention group versus a control group—a statistic can be computed to test the null hypothesis that the groups are sampled from the same survival distribution.

Survival analysis can be applied to many situations unrelated to mortality. For example, survival analysis could be used to analyze such time-related phenomena as length of time in labor, length of stay in hospital, or length of time breastfeeding. Survival analysis can be used when time-related data are **censored**, that is, the observation period does not cover all possible events. As an example, if the outcome were hospital readmission and data are collected 2 years after release, the data are censored because there will be readmissions beyond the 2-year period. Further information about survival analysis can be found in Hosmer et al. (2008).

Extensions of survival analysis have been developed that allow researchers to examine determinants of survival-type transitions in a multivariate framework. In these analyses, independent variables are used to model the risk (or hazard) of experiencing an event at a given point in time, given that one has not experienced the event before that time. The most common specification of the hazard is known as the *Cox proportional hazards model*. Further information about **Cox regression** may be found in O'Quigley (2008).

Example of Cox Regression
Kim and an interprofessional team (2018) used Cox regression to study the association between low levels of high-density lipoprotein cholesterol (HDL-C) and the onset of a mood disorder. In their sample of over 400,000 Koreans, they found that females (but not males) with low levels of HDL-C had an increased risk of mood disorder onset.

CAUSAL MODELING

Causal modeling involves testing a hypothesized causal explanation of a phenomenon, typically with data from nonexperimental (observational) studies. In a causal model, researchers posit causal linkages among three or more variables, and then test whether hypothesized pathways from the causes to the effect are consistent with the data. Casual modeling is not a method for discovering causes; rather, it is a method applied to a prespecified model formulated based on prior knowledge and theory.

> **TIP** Although causal modeling is most often performed with data from nonexperimental studies, it can also be used to test hypotheses about paths of mediation in randomized controlled trials.

Casual modeling is often referred to as **path analysis**. Until recently, nurse researchers performed path analysis primarily using ordinary least squares estimation. In fact, it is possible to conduct a path analysis with a series of multiple regression analyses. We begin our explanation of path analysis within an OLS framework.

Path analytic results are usually displayed in a **path diagram**, and we use such a diagram (Figure 19.3) to illustrate key concepts. This model postulates that the outcome variable, patients' functional ability (V4), is influenced by patients' capacity for self-care (V3); this, in turn, is affected by nursing actions (V1) and the severity of their illness (V2). The model in Figure 19.3 is a **recursive model**, which means that the causal flow is unidirectional. It is hypothesized that V2 is a cause of V3, but not that V3 is a cause of V2.

Path analysis distinguishes exogenous and endogenous variables. Determinants of an **exogenous variable** lie outside the model. In Figure 19.3, nursing actions (V1) and illness severity (V2) are exogenous; no attempt is made in the model to elucidate what causes different nursing actions or different degrees of illness. An

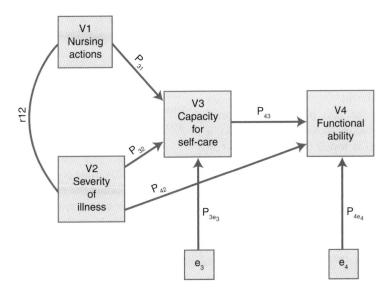

FIGURE 19.3 Example of a path diagram.

endogenous variable, by contrast, is one whose variation is hypothesized to be affected by other variables in the model. In our example, self-care capacity (V3) and functional ability (V4) are endogenous.

Causal linkages are shown on a path diagram by arrows drawn from presumed causes to presumed effects. In our illustration, severity of illness is hypothesized to affect functional ability both directly (path p_{42}) and indirectly through the *mediating variable* self-care capacity (paths p_{32} and p_{43}). Correlated exogenous variables are indicated by curved lines, as shown by the curved line between nursing actions and illness severity.

Ideally, the model would totally explain the outcome, but this almost never happens because there are other determinants, which are **residual variables**. The two boxes labeled e in Figure 19.3 denote a composite of all determinants of self-care capacity (e_3) and functional ability (e_4) that are not in the model. If we could identify and measure additional causes and incorporate them into the theory, the model could be strengthened.

Path analysis solves for **path coefficients**, which are the weights representing the effect of one variable on another. In Figure 19.3, causal paths indicate that one variable (e.g., V3) is caused by another (e.g., V2), yielding a path labeled p_{32}. In research reports, path symbols would be replaced by actual path coefficients. Path coefficients are standardized partial regression slopes. For example, path p_{32} is equal to $\beta_{32.1}$—the beta weight between variables 2 and 3, holding variable 1 constant. Because path coefficients are in standard form, they indicate the proportion of a standard deviation difference in the caused variable that is directly attributable to a 1 *SD* difference in the specified causal variable. Thus, path coefficients provide an indication about the relative importance of various determinants.

Structural equations modeling (SEM) using maximum likelihood estimation is a more powerful approach to path analysis that avoids several problems in OLS estimation, notably difficulties in meeting assumptions. Unlike an OLS approach, SEM can accommodate measurement errors, correlated residuals, and **nonrecursive models** that allow for reciprocal causation. Another attractive feature of SEM is that it can be used to analyze causal models involving one or more *latent* *variables*—a variable representing a construct that is not measured directly (Chapter 16). In SEM, latent variables are captured by two or more measured (manifest) variables that are indicators of the construct.

When there are latent variables, SEM proceeds in two phases. In the first phase, which corresponds to a confirmatory factor analysis (CFA), a measurement model is tested (Chapter 16). When there is evidence of an adequate fit of the data to the hypothesized measurement model, the theoretical causal model is tested by structural equation modeling.

SEM yields information about the hypothesized causal parameters—i.e., path coefficients that are presented as beta weights. The coefficients indicate the expected amount of change in the (latent) endogenous variable that is caused by a change in the (latent) causal variable. SEM programs yield information on the significance of individual paths. The overall fit of the model to the data can be tested by means of several statistics, such as the **goodness-of-fit index (GFI)** and **adjusted goodness-of-fit index (AGFI)**. For both indexes, a value of .90 or greater indicates a good fit.

Path analysis using SEM has gained popularity among nurse researchers but is a complex procedure. Readers interested in further information can consult Loehlin and Beaujean (2017).

Example of a Path Analysis

Xu and colleagues (2018) tested a causal model (using SEM) to explain quality of life (QOL) scores for patients with type 2 diabetes. The model predicted that overactive bladder severity affected QOL both directly and indirectly—through the patients' help-seeking behavior and their perceptions of their bladder condition's bother.

CRITICAL APPRAISAL OF MULTIVARIATE STATISTICS

As noted in the previous chapter, it is difficult to critically appraise researchers' statistical analysis without statistical skills. This caution is even more relevant when it comes to multivariate analyses.

As with bivariate statistics, one issue is whether the researcher selected the right tests. The selection of a multivariate procedure depends on several factors, including the nature of the research question and the measurement level of the variables. (It also depends on whether the data conformed to various assumptions underlying the tests—an issue we did not address in this brief chapter.) Table 19.6, which summarizes some of the major features of multivariate statistics discussed in this chapter, may help you assess the appropriateness of an analytic approach. It might also be noted that studies in which multivariate statistics were *not* used might well be critiqued in terms of whether they *should* have been used. As we illustrated, results from a bivariate test can sometimes be altered by controlling confounding variables. Conversely, some researchers apply multivariate statistics when their sample size is too small to justify their use.

No specific appraisal guidelines for multivariate statistics are presented in this chapter, but most of the questions presented in Box 18.1 are also relevant for researchers' use of complex statistics.

TIP The statistical analyses described in this chapter concern the analysis of data from individuals. Methods for analyzing dyadic/family data have been developed, some within a framework called the Actor-Partner Interdependence Model (Fitzpatrick et al., 2016; Kenny & Ledermann, 2010).

TABLE 19.6 • Guide to Selected Multivariate Analyses

		MEASUREMENT LEVEL[a] OF VARIABLES[b]			NUMBER OF VARIABLES[b]		
TEST NAME	PURPOSE	IV	DV	CV	IVs	DVs	CV
Multiple regression/correlation	To test the relationship between 2+ IVs and 1 DV; to predict a DV from 2+ IVs	Nominal, continuous	Continuous	—	2+	1	—
Analysis of covariance (ANCOVA)	To test the difference between the means of 2+ groups while controlling for 1+ covariate	Nominal	Continuous	Nominal, continuous	1+	1	1+
Mixed design RM-ANOVA	To test mean differences for 2+ groups for outcomes measured multiple times	Nominal	Continuous	Nominal, continuous	1+	1	1+
Multivariate analysis of variance (MANOVA)	To test the difference between the means of 2+ groups for 2+ DVs simultaneously	Nominal	Continuous	—	1+	2+	—
Multivariate analysis of covariance (MANCOVA)	To test the difference between the means of 2+ groups for 2+ DVs simultaneously, while controlling for 1+ covariate	Nominal	Continuous	Nominal, continuous	1+	2+	1+
Logistic regression	To test the relationship between 2+ IVs and 1 DV; to predict the probability of an event; to estimate relative risk	Nominal, continuous	Nominal	—	2+	1	—

[a]Measurement levels: Continuous = interval-level or ratio-level.

[b]Variables: IV, independent variables; DV, dependent variable; CV, covariate.

RESEARCH EXAMPLE

We conclude with a summary of a study that used multivariate procedures.

Study: The influence of comorbidities, risk factors, and medications on sexual activity in individuals aged 40 to 59 years with and without cardiac conditions (Steinke et al., 2018).

Statement of purpose: The purpose of this study was to explore factors predictive of sexual activity among middle-aged people with and without cardiac problems such as heart failure, coronary heart disease, angina, and myocardial infarction.

Methods: The study was a secondary analysis of data from the National Health and Nutrition Examination Survey (NHANES), which involves a nationally representative sample of noninstitutionalized adults in the United States. The researchers selected respondents between the ages of 40 and 59 years who had completed relevant questions about cardiovascular disease, comorbidities, medication use, and sexual activity. The sample size for the analyses was 1,741 (889 men and 852 women). Data on a broad range of demographic characteristics were available for the study sample. The outcome variable was a dichotomous variable that characterized participants as sexually inactive (no or only one episode of sexual activity in the past year) or sexually active (more than one episode). The main analysis involved logistic regression.

Analysis and findings: Overall, 94% of the sample was sexually active. The researchers first looked at bivariate relationships between cardiac conditions and sexual activity. They found that individuals with coronary heart disease, angina, or myocardial infarction were significantly less likely to have had sexual activity than those without these conditions. The use of certain medications (e.g., statins) was also associated with less sexual activity. Smoking and a perceived weight problem were also related to diminished sexual activity. The researchers then tested five predictors of sexual activity, using logistic regression: gender, smoking status, chest pain when walking uphill, a weight problem, and one or more cardiac condition. The Hosmer–Lemeshow test suggested that the model fit the data adequately, and all variables except gender were significant predictors of sexual activity. For example, the value of the Wald statistic for the variable "chest pain when walking uphill" was 33.02, $p < .0004$. Although the overall model was statistically significant, the value of the Nagelkerke R^2 was only .07, suggesting that although cardiac conditions, smoking and weight problems significantly affect sexual activity, many other factors also influence the sexual activity of people in the 40 to 59 year age range.

SUMMARY POINTS

- **Multivariate statistics** are increasingly being used in nursing research to untangle complex relationships among three or more variables.
- Simple **linear regression** is used to predict the values of one variable based on values of

a second variable. **Multiple regression** is a method of predicting a continuous dependent variable based on two or more independent (**predictor**) variables.

- **Multiple correlation coefficients** (R) can be squared (R^2) to estimate the proportion of variability in the outcome variable accounted for by the predictors. The F-statistic is used to test the overall regression model and changes to R^2 as new predictors are introduced.
- The regression equation yields **regression coefficients** (**bs**) for each predictor that, when raw scores are converted to **standard scores**, are called **beta weights** (βs).
- **Simultaneous multiple regression** enters all predictor variables into the regression equation at the same time. **Hierarchical multiple regression** enters predictors into the equation in a series of steps controlled by researchers. **Stepwise multiple regression** enters predictors in steps using a statistical criterion for order of entry.
- **Analysis of covariance (ANCOVA)**, an extension of ANOVA, removes the effect of confounding variables (**covariates**) before testing whether mean group differences on the outcome variable are statistically significant.
- **Mixed design RM-ANOVA** is used to test mean differences between groups (between-subjects factor) over time (within-subjects factor). In mixed design RM-ANOVAs, the interaction term (time × group) usually is of primary interest.
- **Multivariate analysis of variance (MANOVA)** is the extension of ANOVA to situations in which there is more than one outcome variable.
- The **general linear model (GLM)** encompasses a broad class of frequently used statistical techniques that fit data to straight-line (linear) solutions, including t-tests, ANOVA, ANCOVA, and multiple regression.
- **Least-squares estimation** used within GLM minimizes the square of **errors of prediction** (the **residuals**). An alternative is **maximum likelihood estimation** (**MLE**), which estimates the parameters most likely to have generated observed data.

- **Logistic regression**, which is based on MLE, is used to predict categorical outcomes. Logistic regression yields an **odds ratio** that is an index of relative risk for each predictor, that is, the risk of an outcome occurring given one condition, versus the risk of it occurring given a different condition, while controlling other predictors.

- The overall logistic regression model can be tested with a **likelihood ratio test** that uses a **goodness-of-fit chi-square** statistic. An alternative is the **Hosmer–Lemeshow** test that tests how close the model is to a perfect model. Individual predictors can be tested with the **Wald statistic**. Several **pseudo** R^2 indexes can be used to summarize overall effect size for logistic regression; the most widely reported is the **Nagelkerke** R^2.

- **Survival analysis** and other related event history methods, such as **Cox regression**, are used when the dependent variable of interest is a time interval (e.g., length of time in hospital).

- **Causal modeling** involves the development and testing of a hypothesized causal explanation of a phenomenon.

- **Path analysis**, a method for testing causal models, involves the preparation of a **path diagram** that stipulates hypothesized causal links among variables. Path analysis can be performed using least-squares estimation, but currently is more likely to involve **structural equations modeling** (**SEM**), an MLE approach to causal modeling.

STUDY ACTIVITIES

Study activities are available to instructors on thePoint.

REFERENCES CITED IN CHAPTER 19

Barbe, T., Kimble, L., & Rubenstein, C. (2018). Subjective cognitive complaints, psychosocial factors and nursing work function in nurses providing direct patient care. *Journal of Advanced Nursing, 74*, 914–925.

*Fitzpatrick, J., Gareau, A., Lafontaine, M., & Gaudreau, P. (2016). How to use the Actor-Partner Interdependence Model (APIM) to estimate different dyadic patterns in MPLUS: A step-by-step tutorial. *Quantitative Methods for Psychology, 12*, 74–86.

Hair, J. F., Black, W., Babin, B., & Anderson, R. (2019). *Multivariate data analysis* (8th ed.). Upper Saddle River, NJ: Prentice-Hall.

*Hiler, C., Hickman, R., Reimer, A., & Wilson, K. (2018). Predictors of moral distress in a US sample of critical care nurses. *American Journal of Critical Care, 27*, 59–65.

Hosmer, D., Lemeshow, S., & May, S. (2008). *Applied survival analysis: Regression modeling of time to event data* (2nd ed.). New York: John Wiley.

Hosmer, D., Lemeshow, S., & Sturdivant, R. (2013). *Applied logistic regression* (3rd ed.). New York: John Wiley & Sons.

Kenny, D. A., & Ledermann, T. (2010). Detecting, measuring, and testing dyadic patterns in the Actor-Partner Interdependence Model. *Journal of Family Psychology, 24*, 359–366.

Kim, S., Han, K., Jang, S., & Park, E. (2018). The association between low level of high-density lipoprotein cholesterol and mood disorder using time-dependent analysis. *Journal of Affective Disorders, 225*, 317–325.

Loehlin, J. C., & Beaujean, A. (2017). *Latent variable models: An introduction to factor, path, and structural equation analysis* (5th ed.). New York: Routledge.

Looman, W., Hullsiek, R., Pryor, L., Mathiason, M., & Finkelstein, S. (2018). Health-related quality of life outcomes of a telehealth care coordination intervention for children with medical complexity: A randomized controlled trial. *Journal of Pediatric Health Care, 32*, 63–75.

O'Quigley, J. (2008). *Proportional hazards regression.* New York: Springer.

Pituch, K., & Stevens, J. (2016). *Applied multivariate statistics for the social sciences* (6th ed.). New York: Routledge.

Polit, D. F. (2010). *Statistics and data analysis for nursing research* (2nd ed.). Upper Saddle River, NJ: Pearson.

*Qin, R., Titler, M., Shever, L., & Kim, T. (2008). Estimating effects of nursing intervention via propensity score analysis. *Nursing Research, 57*, 444–452.

*Schroeder, K., Jia, H., & Smaldone, A. (2016). Which propensity score method best reduces confounder imbalance? An example from a retrospective evaluation of a childhood obesity intervention. *Nursing Research, 65*, 465–474.

Siegmund, L., Albert, N., McClelland, M., Bena, J., & Morrison, S. (2018). Functional capacity but not early uptake of cardiac rehabilitation predicts readmission in patients with metabolic syndrome. *Journal of Cardiovascular Nursing, 33*, 306–312.

Staneva, A., Morawska, A., Bogossian, F., & Wittkowski, A. (2018). Maternal psychological distress during pregnancy does not increase the risk for adverse birth outcomes. *Women & Health, 58*, 92–111.

**Steinke, E., Mosack, V., & Hill, T. (2018). The influence of comorbidities, risk factors, and medications on sexual activity in individuals aged 40 to 59 years with and without cardiac conditions: US National Health and Nutrition Examination Survey, 2011 to 2012. *Journal of Cardiovascular Nursing, 33*, 118–125.

Tabachnick, B. G., & Fidell, L. S. (2018). *Using multivariate statistics* (7th ed.). Upper Saddle River, NJ: Pearson Education.

Takei, H., Shiraishi, M., Matsuzaki, M., & Haruna, M. (2019). Factors related to vegetable intake among pregnant Japanese women: A cross-sectional study. *Appetite, 132,* 175–181.

Thorlton, J., & Collins, W. (2018). Underlying beliefs associated with college student consumption of energy beverages. *Western Journal of Nursing Research, 40,* 5–19.

*Xu, D., Zhao, M., Huang, L., & Wang, K. (2018). Overactive bladder symptom severity, bother, help-seeking behavior, and quality of life in patients with type 2 diabetes: A path analysis. *Health and Quality of Life Outcomes, 16,* 1.

Yang, C., & Chen, C. (2018). Effectiveness of aerobic gymnastic exercise on stress, fatigue, and sleep quality during postpartum: A pilot randomized controlled trial. *International Journal of Nursing Studies, 77,* 1–7.

A link to this open-access article is provided in the Toolkit for Chapter 19 in the **Resource Manual.**

This journal article is available on thePoint *for this chapter.*

20 | Processes of Quantitative Data Analysis

In this chapter, we offer an overview of the steps often taken to prepare for the analysis of quantitative data. Most of these activities would be undertaken *before* performing the statistical analyses described in the last few chapters, but we have positioned this chapter here because some of the material requires some familiarity with statistics.

Figure 20.1 shows what the flow of tasks in a quantitative analysis might look like, organized in phases. Progress in analyzing quantitative data is seldom as linear as this figure suggests, but it provides a framework for discussing key steps in the analytic process.

PREANALYSIS PHASE

The first phase of a quantitative analysis involves various clerical and administrative tasks, such as logging in forms, reviewing data for completeness and legibility, retrieving pieces of missing information, and assigning identification (ID) numbers. Another task involves selecting statistical software for doing the data analyses. Two widely used statistical software packages are the Statistical Package for the Social Sciences (SPSS) and the Statistical Analysis System (SAS), but there are many others. Next, researchers must code the data and enter them onto computer files to create a **dataset** (the total collection of data for all sample members).

Coding Quantitative Data

Coding is the process of transforming data into symbols—usually numbers. Certain variables are inherently quantitative (e.g., age, body temperature) and do not require coding, unless the data are gathered in categories (e.g., younger than 50 years of age versus 50 or older). Even with "naturally" quantitative data, researchers need to inspect their data. All responses should be of the same form and precision. For example, for the variable *height* in the nonmetric system, researchers need to decide whether to record feet and inches as two separate "variables" or to convert the information entirely to inches. Whichever method is adopted, it must be used consistently for all participants. There must also be consistency in handling information reported by sample members with different degrees of precision (e.g., a decision about how to code a response such as 5 feet 2½ inches).

Most data from structured instruments can be precoded, with codes designated before data are collected. For example, questions with fixed response alternatives can be preassigned a numeric code and is sometimes printed on the data collection form, such as: under age 50 = 1 and 50 and older = 2. Codes are often arbitrary, as in the case of the variable gender. Whether a female participant is coded 1 or 2 has no analytic importance so long as females are consistently assigned one code and males another code.

435

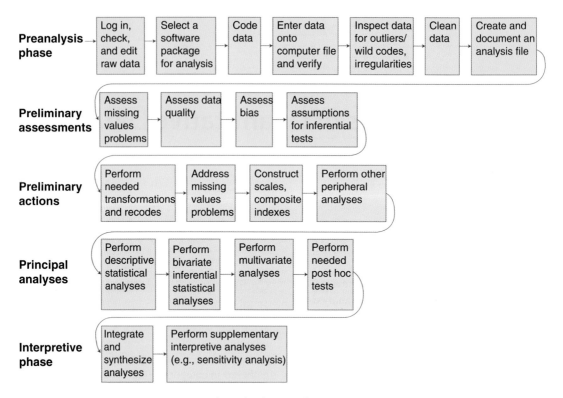

FIGURE 20.1 Flow of tasks in analyzing quantitative data.

Respondents sometimes can check off more than one response to a question, as in the following question that might be used in a study about irritable bowel syndrome:

Which of the following symptoms have you experienced in the past week? (Check all that apply).
Abdominal pain
Bloating
Constipation
Diarrhea
Flatulence

With questions of this type, responses must be coded as though there were five separate questions: "Did you experience abdominal pain?" "Did you experience bloating?" and so on. Each check is treated as a "yes." The question yields five variables, with one code (e.g., 1) signifying "yes" and another code (e.g., 0) signifying "no."

If data from open-ended questions are going to be used in quantitative analysis, they must be coded. Sometimes researchers can develop codes ahead of time, but unstructured data often are collected because responses cannot be anticipated. In such situations, researchers typically review a sizable portion of the data to understand content and then develop a coding scheme.

A code is needed for each variable for every sample member, even if there is no response. **Missing values** can be of various types. A person answering a question may be undecided, refuse to answer, or say, "Don't know." When skip patterns are used, there is missing information for questions that are irrelevant to some respondents. A single missing values code may suffice, but it may be important to distinguish different types of missing data using different codes (e.g., distinguishing refusals and *don't know*s).

The choice of what code to use for missing data is often arbitrary, but missing values codes must be ones that have not been used for actual pieces of information. Some researchers use blanks, periods, or negative values for missing information. Some use 9 as the missing code because this value is out of the range of real codes for many variables.

Precise coding instructions should be documented in a coding manual. Coders, like observers and interviewers, must be properly trained, and intercoder (or intracoder) reliability checks are recommended.

Entering, Verifying, and Cleaning Data

Coded data typically are transferred onto a data file via keyboard entry, but other options (e.g., scanning of forms, importing electronic health records information) are also available. Various programs can be used for data entry, including spreadsheets or databases. Major software packages for statistical analysis have data editors that make data entry fairly easy.

> **TIP** Sometimes sample members enter their own data directly onto a computer file—for example, when they complete an online questionnaire. This is clearly advantageous in terms of efficiency and costs.

Figure 20.2 shows a screenshot of a data file for the Statistical Package for the Social Sciences (SPSS). These are the data used to illustrate various analyses in the Supplements 🅂 to Chapters 17–19, and this screenshot appears in all three Supplements. This data file is very small: a 30 × 7 matrix, with 30 rows (1 for each participant) and 7 columns for the variables—i.e., one variable per column.

Each variable in a dataset has to be named. Usually the variable name is abbreviated—for example, in Figure 20.2, we can see that the variable names are all short (GROUP, BWEIGHT, etc.). The software allows users to enter a more detailed description of each variable. For example, for the variable BWEIGHT, the extended label is "Infant birthweight in ounces." This full name would appear on all output, rather than BWEIGHT. The Supplement to this chapter on thePoint shows a screenshot with extended variable information.🅂

Each participant's unique ID should be entered in the file along with her or his actual data, because this would allow you to go back to original sources if something needed to be verified. The ID number normally is entered as the first variable of the record, as in Figure 20.2.

The variables BWEIGHT, AGE, and PRIORS in this dataset are ones that are "naturally" quantitative (number of ounces, years, and prior pregnancies). Other variables had to be coded. GROUP, for example, uses a coding scheme of 1 for intervention group members and 2 for control group members. SMOKE is coded 1 for those who smoke and 0 for those who do not. We use a 1-2 code for GROUP because this coding would ensure that in output with statistical results the intervention group information would be first, which is the convention in research reports. We used a dummy 0-1 code for SMOKE to make regression results easier to interpret.

Data entry is prone to error, so it is essential to verify entries and correct mistakes. One method is to compare visually the numbers on a printout of the data file with codes on the original source, and another is to double-enter data. There are also special verifying programs designed to perform comparisons during direct data entry.

Even verified data need to be cleaned. **Data cleaning** involves two types of checks. The first is a check for outliers and wild codes. **Outliers** are values that lie outside the normal range. Outliers can be found by inspecting frequency distributions, paying special attention to the lowest and highest values. (Most researchers begin data analysis by constructing frequency distributions for all variables in their dataset.) Some outliers are true, legitimate values (e.g., an annual income of $1 million in a distribution where the mean is $50,000), but sometimes they result from data entry errors.

Another problem is **wild codes**—that is, codes that are not possible. For example, the variable gender might have these codes: 1 = female, 2 = male, 3 = other, and "blank" = missing. If someone were coded 5 for gender, there is an error. The computer could show the ID number of the faulty record, and the correct code could then be tracked down.

File Edit View Data Transform Analyze Direct Marketing Graphs Utilities Add-ons

	ID	GROUP	AGE	PRIORS	SMOKE	BWEIGHT	REPEAT
1	1	1	17	1	1	107	1
2	2	1	14	0	0	101	0
3	3	1	21	3	0	119	0
4	4	1	20	2	0	128	1
5	5	1	15	1	1	89	0
6	6	1	19	0	1	99	0
7	7	1	19	1	0	111	0
8	8	1	18	1	1	117	1
9	9	1	17	0	0	102	1
10	10	1	20	0	0	120	0
11	11	1	13	0	1	76	0
12	12	1	18	0	1	116	0
13	13	1	16	0	0	100	1
14	14	1	18	0	0	115	0
15	15	1	21	2	1	113	0
16	16	2	19	0	0	111	1
17	17	2	21	1	0	108	0
18	18	2	19	2	1	95	0
19	19	2	17	0	1	99	0
20	20	2	19	0	0	103	1
21	21	2	15	0	1	94	0
22	22	2	17	1	0	101	1
23	23	2	21	2	0	114	0
24	24	2	20	1	0	97	0
25	25	2	18	0	1	99	1
26	26	2	18	0	1	113	0
27	27	2	19	1	0	89	0
28	28	2	20	0	0	98	0
29	29	2	17	0	0	102	0
30	30	2	19	1	1	105	0

Notes:

GROUP:	Group status,	1 = Experimental group	2 = Control group
AGE:	Mother's age in years		
PRIORS:	Number of prior pregnancies		
SMOKE:	Mother's smoking status,	1 = Smokes	0 = Does not smoke
BWEIGHT:	Infant's birthweight, in ounces		
REPEAT:	Had repeat pregnancy within 18 months,	1 = Yes	0 = No

FIGURE 20.2 Fictitious dataset for intervention study with low-income pregnant adolescents (screenshot of an SPSS data file).

TIP Such checks will never reveal all errors. If a male were incorrectly coded 1 for gender in the coding scheme just mentioned, the mistake might not be detected. Errors can have a big effect on the analysis and interpretation of data, so it is important to code, enter, verify, and clean data with care.

A second data-cleaning procedure involves **consistency checks**, which focus on internal data consistency. In this task, researchers check for errors by testing compatibility of data within a case. For example, one question in a survey might ask current marital status, and another might ask number of marriages. If the data were internally consistent, respondents who answered "Single, never married" to the first question should have a zero (or a missing values code) for the second. Researchers should search for opportunities to check the consistency of entered data.

Osborne (2013) has devoted an entire book to a discussion of data cleaning. Another very useful resource is a brief open-access paper on this topic by Van den Broeck and colleagues (2005). Dziadkowiec and colleagues (2016) offer advice on cleaning data extracted from electronic health records.

Example of Data Verification and Cleaning

Minnick and colleagues (2017) studied the recruitment of junior nursing research faculty and views about the junior nursing research faculty pool in a survey of administrators in U.S. programs offering research doctorates. Here is how the researchers described preparing their dataset for analysis: "After entry into an SPSS data file, all data were subjected to tests for outliers. We conducted >25 random checks of surveys returned by mail for data entry errors" (p. 20).

Creating and Documenting the Analysis Files

The decisions that researchers make about coding and variable naming should be fully documented. Memory should not be trusted; several weeks after coding, researchers may no longer remember if males were coded 1 and female were coded 2, or vice versa. Moreover, colleagues may wish to borrow the data for a secondary analysis. Documentation should always be sufficiently thorough that someone unfamiliar with the original study could use the data.

Documentation usually involves preparing a codebook. A **codebook** is a listing of each variable together with information about placement in the file, codes associated with the values of the variable, and other basic information. Codebooks can be generated by statistical or data entry programs.

PRELIMINARY ASSESSMENTS AND ACTIONS

Researchers typically undertake several preanalytic activities before they test their hypotheses. Several preparatory activities are discussed next.

Assessing and Handling Missing Values Problems

Researchers strive to have data values for all participants on all key variables but usually find that their datasets have some **missing values**. An appropriate solution to a missing values problem depends on such factors as the extent of missing data, the importance of the variables with missing data, and the pattern of missingness.

There are three missing values patterns. The first, and most desirable, is **missing completely at random (MCAR)**, which occurs when cases with missing values are just a random subset of all cases. When data are MCAR, analyses remain unbiased—but missing values are seldom MCAR.

Data are considered **missing at random (MAR)** if missingness is related to variables in the dataset (e.g., gender)—but *not* related to the value of the variable that has the missing values. For example, if missing values for depression occur more frequently for men than for women—but not for people who are most or least depressed—the pattern of missingness may be MAR.

The third pattern is **missing not at random (MNAR)**, a pattern in which the value of the variable that is missing *is* related to its missingness (e.g., those declining to report their income tend to be rich). Missing values that are MAR or MNAR can result in biased results. Solutions are most readily accomplished when missing data are MAR and not MNAR—though it is difficult to know which of these two patterns applies.

A first step in analyzing missing data is to assess the extent of the problem by examining frequency distributions on a variable-by-variable basis. Another step is to examine the cumulative extent of missing values (e.g., what percentage of cases had no variables missing, one variable missing, and so on). Another task is to evaluate the randomness of missing values. A simple procedure is to divide the sample into two groups—those with and without missing data on a specified variable. The two groups can then be compared in terms of their characteristics to assess whether the two groups are comparable in terms of key demographic or clinical variables (e.g., Were men more likely than women to leave certain questions blank? Was the mean age of those with missing values different from that of people without missing values?).

Until recently, examining patterns of missingness was a tedious process, which may explain why some researchers simply ignore the problem of missing data (and therefore remain susceptible to the risk of bias that can be introduced). Now, however, programs in widely used statistical software have greatly simplified this important task. For example, the Missing Values Analysis (MVA) module within SPSS offers powerful means of detecting and handling missing values.

Once researchers have assessed the extent and patterning of missing values, they must address the problem. There are three basic types of solutions: deletions, imputations, and mixed modeling within longitudinal datasets. We discuss the first two here; information about sophisticated modeling solutions are discussed in Son et al. (2012).

Missing Data and Deletions
Listwise deletion (also called *complete case analysis*) is simply the analysis of those cases for which there are no missing data. Listwise deletion is based on an implicit assumption of MCAR. Researchers who use this method typically have not made a formal assessment of the extent to which MCAR is probable, but rather are simply disregarding the problem of missing data.

Perhaps the most widely used (but not the best) approach is to delete cases selectively, on a variable-by-variable basis by means of **pairwise deletion** (also called *available case analysis*). For example, in a test of an intervention to reduce patient anxiety, the outcomes might be blood pressure and self-reported anxiety. If 10 people from the sample 100 failed to complete the anxiety scale, we might base the analyses of anxiety data on the 90 people who completed the scale but use the full sample of 100 in the blood pressure analysis. If the number of cases fluctuates widely across outcomes, the results are difficult to interpret because the sample is essentially a "moving target."

TIP Computer programs like SPSS use either listwise or pairwise deletion as the **default** (i.e., the option that will be used in the analysis unless there are specific instructions to the contrary).

Researchers sometimes use pairwise deletion in analyses involving a correlation matrix. From one pair of variables in the matrix to another, the number of cases can vary considerably. Although such correlation matrixes may provide useful descriptive information, it is not wise to use pairwise deletion for correlation-based multivariate analyses such as multiple regression or factor analysis because the correlations are calculated on nonidentical subsets of people.

Another option is to delete a variable entirely. This option may be suitable when there are a lot of missing values for a variable that is not central to the analysis. Recommendations for how much missing data should drive this decision range from 15% to 40% of cases (Fox-Wasylyshyn & El-Masri, 2005).

Missing Data and Imputations
Preferred methods for addressing missing values involve **imputation**—that is, "filling in" missing data with values believed to be good estimates of what the values would have been, had they not been missing. An attractive feature of imputation is that it allows researchers to maintain full sample size, and thus statistical power is not compromised. The risk is that the imputations will be poor estimates of real values, leading to biases of unknown magnitude and direction.

The simplest procedure is **mean substitution** or *median substitution*, which involves using "typical" sample values to replace missing data that are continuous. For example, if a person's age were missing and if the average age of sample members were 45.2 years, we could substitute the value 45.2 in place of the missing values code. Mean substitution is, like listwise deletion, popular because of its simplicity. Yet, even though mean substitution increases sample size and leaves variable means unchanged, it is rarely the best approach. Regardless of what the underlying pattern of missingness is, mean imputation leads to underestimations of variance, and variance is what most statistical analyses are all about.

A refinement on mean substitution is to use the mean value for a relevant subgroup—called a **subgroup** (or *conditional*) **mean substitution**. The assumption is that a better estimate of the missing value can be obtained by making the substitution conditional on participants' characteristics. For example, rather than replacing a missing age value with 45.2, we could replace a man's missing value with men's mean age, and a woman's mean value with women's mean age. This is a better option than mean substitution because the substituted values are presumably closer to the real values and because variance is not reduced as much. Nevertheless, conditional (subgroup) mean substitution is not a preferred approach, except when overall missingness is low.

> **TIP** When data are missing for items on a multi-item scale, it may be appropriate to replace a missing value with the mean of other similar items from the person with the missing value, an approach that assumes that people are "internally consistent" across similar questions. Such **case mean substitution**, which uses person-specific information to inform the estimate, has the advantage of not throwing out data altogether (listwise deletion) and not assuming that a person is similar to all others in a sample or subgroup (mean substitution). Case mean substitution has been found to be an acceptable method of imputation at the item level, even compared to more sophisticated methods. An example showing how to do case mean substitution is provided in the Toolkit.

Researchers are increasingly using imputation methods that make more extensive use of data in the dataset. One method uses regression analysis to "predict" the correct value of missing data. Suppose we found that participants' age was correlated with gender, education, and health status. Based on data from those with complete data, age could be regressed on these three variables to predict age for people with missing age data but whose values for the three other variables were not missing. Regression-based imputation is more accurate than previously discussed strategies, although variability remains underestimated.

Even more sophisticated solutions have been developed. Maximum likelihood estimation is useful because it uses all data points in a dataset to construct estimated replacement values. **Expectation maximization (EM)** involves using an iterative procedure with a maximum-likelihood–based algorithm to produce the best parameter estimates.

An approach called **multiple imputation (MI)** is currently considered the best method for addressing missing values problems. MI addresses a fundamental issue—the uncertainty of any given estimate—by imputing several (m) estimates of the missing data, and each estimate has an element of randomness introduced. Results from analyses across the m imputations are later pooled. MI has not often been used because of its complexity and the limited availability of appropriate software, but recent versions of the SPSS MVA module (version 17.0 and higher) do offer multiple imputation. Patrician (2002) has described multiple imputation in some detail.

Example of Handling Missing Values

Okura and an interprofessional team (2018) studied the health beliefs and health checkup behavior of nearly 5,000 community-dwelling older adults in Japan. Multiple imputation was used to address problems with missing data.

It might be noted that the issue of missingness has been given a lot of attention in the analysis of data from randomized controlled trials (RCTs) because attrition in trials is common. The "gold standard" for analyzing data from RCTs is to use an **intention-to-treat (ITT) analysis**, which involves analyzing outcome data from all participants who were randomized, regardless of whether they dropped out of the study. A true ITT analysis is achieved only if there are no missing outcome data or if missing values are accounted for in the analysis, such as through imputation. A resource for advice on how to achieve ITT is offered in Polit and Gillespie (2010). Polit and Gillespie (2009) found, in their analysis of 124 nursing trials, that 75% of the RCTs had missing outcome data, and one out of four had 20% or more missing values. Only about 10% of the studies used imputation or mixed effects modeling in their ITT analyses. The approach most often used to impute values for missing outcome variables in these RCTs was a procedure called **last observation carried forward (LOCF)**, which imputes the missing outcome using the previous measurement of that same outcome. For example, if data were collected 1 month and 3 months after the intervention, but data for the 3-month outcome were missing for some participants, the 1-month value would replace the missing value. LOCF is no longer considered the best approach.

Procedures for dealing with missing data are discussed at greater length in McKnight and colleagues (2007), Enders (2010), and Molenberghs et al. (2015). Also, links to some open-access articles relating to the handling of missing values are available in the Toolkit. ⊗

Assessing Data Quality

Assessing data quality is another preanalytic task. For example, when a composite scale is used, researchers should assess its internal consistency (Chapter 15). The distribution of data values for key variables also should be examined to assess any anomalies, such as limited variability, extreme skewness, or the presence of ceiling or floor effects. A **ceiling effect** occurs when values for a variable are restricted at the upper end of a continuum, and a **floor effect** occurs when values are restricted at the lower end. For example, a vocabulary test for 10-year-olds likely would yield a clustering of high scores in a sample of 11-year-olds, creating a ceiling effect that would reduce correlations between test scores and other characteristics of the children. Conversely, there likely would be a clustering of low scores on the same test with a sample of 9-year-olds, resulting in a floor effect with similar consequences. Floor and ceiling effects

are of special concern when the goal is to measure change: if a measure has floor or ceiling effect, improvement (or deterioration) will not be adequately captured.

Earlier we discussed outliers in connection with efforts to clean a dataset to ensure data accuracy. Legitimate outliers—extreme scores that are true values—are a data quality issue. Outliers can distort study results and cause errors in statistical decision-making, and so outliers should be scrutinized. By convention, a value is considered an **extreme outlier** if it is greater than three times the *interquartile range (IQR)* above the third quartile or below the first quartile. The IQR, as noted briefly in Chapter 17, is an index of variability. Methods for detecting and addressing outlier problems are discussed in Polit (2010).

> **Example of Extreme Outliers**
> Kovach and Ke (2016) wrote about an experience that Kovach had in using an existing dataset to predict future health problems of nursing home residents. She found in a preliminary multiple regression analysis that the predictors accounted for 42% of the variance in her outcome ($R^2 = .42$). In a more formal analysis, she removed one extreme outlier and found that the R^2 dropped by 20 points, to .22. The authors offered some advice about the management of outliers.

> **TIP** For those using the Statistical Package for the Social Sciences (SPSS), the EXPLORE routine is invaluable in making assessments of data quality. We illustrate this in the Supplement to this chapter on thePoint. ⓢ

Assessing Bias

Researchers often undertake preliminary analyses to assess biases, including the following:

- *Nonresponse (volunteer) bias.* If possible, researchers should assess whether a biased subset of people participated in a study. If there is information about the characteristics of all people who were asked to participate (e.g., demographic information from hospital records), researchers should compare the characteristics of those who did and did not agree to participate to assess the nature of any biases.

- *Selection bias.* When nonrandomized comparison groups are used (e.g., in quasi-experimental studies), researchers should check for selection biases by comparing the groups' baseline characteristics. Detected differences should, if possible, be controlled—for example, through analysis of covariance—especially if a characteristic is a strong predictor of the dependent variable.
- *Attrition bias.* In studies with multiple points of data collection, it is important to check for attrition biases by comparing people who did and did not continue to participate in later waves of data collection, based on baseline characteristics.

In performing any of these analyses, significant group differences are often an indication of bias, and such bias must be taken into consideration in interpreting and discussing the results. To the extent possible, biases should be controlled in testing the principal hypotheses.

TIP It is not considered appropriate to test the significance of group differences on baseline variables in randomized controlled trials—even though this practice is adopted widely, and results are often reported in tables (Pocock et al., 2002). If randomization and allocation were done properly and the sample size is adequate, one would expect 5% of the group differences to be significant, when $\alpha = .05$—and this does not signify a bias. Experts advise that it is preferable to control for significant predictors of the outcome, even if group differences are not significant, than to control for a baseline variable with significant group differences but weakly related to the outcome.

Example of Assessing Bias

In their case–control study, Munday and colleagues (2018) studied the incidence of perioperative hypothermia in women undergoing spinal anesthesia for cesarean birth with versus without intrathecal morphine. To assess selection bias, the two groups of women were compared in terms of demographic variables (e.g., age, BMI) and numerous clinical variables. Two significant differences were found out of dozens of variables examined.

Testing Assumptions for Statistical Tests

Most statistical tests are based on several **assumptions**—conditions that are presumed to be true and, when violated, can lead to erroneous conclusions. For example, parametric tests assume that variables are distributed normally. Frequency distributions, scatter plots, and other assessment procedures provide researchers with information about whether underlying assumptions for statistical tests have been upheld.

Statistical indexes of skewness or peakedness are available to test whether the shape of the distribution is significantly skewed or peaked or flat. Many software programs include the *Kolmogorov–Smirnov test*, which tests that a distribution does not deviate significantly from a normal distribution.

Example of Testing Assumptions

Azarmnejad and colleagues (2017) tested the effectiveness of a familiar auditory stimulus (recorded maternal voices) on hospitalized neonates' physiologic responses to procedural pain. The Kolgmogorov–Smirnov test was used to test outcomes for departures from normality. For outcomes whose distribution was nonnormal, nonparametric statistical analyses were used.

Performing Data Transformations

Raw data often need to be modified or transformed before hypotheses can be tested. Various **data transformations** can easily be handled through commands to the computer. For example, the scoring direction of some items on multi-item scales might need to be reversed before item scores can be summed. Guidance on *item reversals* was presented in Chapter 16.

Sometimes researchers want to create a variable that is a cumulative **count** of variables in the dataset. For example, suppose we asked people to indicate which types of illegal drug they had used in the past month, from a list of 10 options. Use of each drug would be answered independently as a yes (e.g., coded 1) or no (e.g., coded 0). We could create a new variable of number of different drugs used, representing a count of all the "1" codes for the 10 drug items. Other transformations involve **recodes** of original values. Recoding is often used to create *dummy variables* for multivariate analyses.

Transformations also can be undertaken to render data appropriate for statistical tests. For example, if a distribution is nonnormal, a transformation can sometimes help to make parametric procedures appropriate. A logarithmic transformation, for example, tends to normalize positively skewed distributions.

TIP The Toolkit in the accompanying *Resource Manual* includes a table with data transformations that may help to correct skewed distributions. The table also identifies the SPSS functions that would be used for the transformations.

When you do transformations, it is important to check that they were done correctly by examining a sample of values for the original and transformed variables. This can be done by instructing the computer to list, for a sample of cases, the values of the newly created variables and the original variables used to create them.

Example of Transforming Variables
Kobayashi and an interprofessional team (2017) studied morning-to-afternoon changes in the distribution characteristics of salivary cortisol and immunoglobulin A concentrations in a sample of 113 healthy young males. The researchers used a logarithmic transformation of afternoon cortisol values to make the distribution almost normal, but the transformation did not improve the distribution of morning values.

Performing Additional Peripheral Analyses

Depending on the study, additional peripheral analyses may be needed before proceeding to substantive analyses. It is impossible to catalog all such analyses, but we offer a few examples to alert readers to the kinds of issues that need some thought.

Data Pooling

Researchers sometimes obtain data from more than one source—for example, when researchers recruit participants from multiple sites or when data are obtained from multiple cohorts. The risk is that participants from different sites/cohorts may not really be drawn from the same population, and so it is wise

to evaluate whether **pooling** of data is warranted (Knapp & Brown, 2014). This type of evaluation involves comparing participants from the different sites or cohorts in terms of key research variables or comparing the extent to which correlations between key variables are similar across sites/cohorts.

Example of Testing for Pooling
Hung and colleagues (2015) studied gender differences in the association between adolescent drinking and perceived parental attitudes toward underage drinking. Data were obtained from two cohorts of adolescents, with about 2,000 in each cohort. The researchers found no evidence of a cohort effect, and so the two cohorts were pooled.

Testing Ordering (Carryover) Effects

When a crossover design is used (i.e., people are randomly assigned to different orderings of treatments), researchers should assess whether outcomes are different for people in the different treatment-order groups. That is, did getting A before B yield different outcomes than getting B before A? In essence, such tests offer evidence that it is legitimate to pool the data from alternative orderings.

Example of Testing for Ordering Effects
Abdeyazdan and coresearchers (2016) used a crossover design to assess the effects of nesting and swaddling on the sleep duration of premature infants in the NICU. Half the infants were randomized to a nest-swaddle condition and the other half were in the swaddle-nest condition. In both cases, there was a 2-minute washout period. The researchers did an analysis to examine whether the sequencing itself had an effect on infant sleeping and found that it did not.

PRINCIPAL ANALYSES

At this point in the analysis process, researchers have a cleaned dataset, with missing data problems resolved and transformations completed; they also have some understanding of data quality and biases. They can now proceed with more substantive data analyses.

Planning the Substantive Data Analysis

In many studies, researchers collect data on dozens of variables. They cannot analyze every variable in relation to all others, and so a plan to guide data analysis must be developed. One approach is to prepare a list of the analyses to be undertaken, specifying both the variables and the statistical test to be used. Another approach is to develop table shells. **Table shells** are layouts of how researchers envision presenting their findings, without numbers filled in. Once a table shell is prepared, researchers can do the analyses needed to complete the table. (The table templates in the Toolkit of the accompanying *Resource Manual,* for Chapters 17-19, can be used as a basis for table shells ⊗). Researchers do not need to adhere rigidly to table shells, but they provide a good mechanism for organizing the analysis of large amounts of data.

Substantive Analyses

Substantive analyses typically begin with descriptive analyses. Researchers usually develop a profile of the sample and may look descriptively at correlations among variables. These initial analyses may suggest further analyses or further data transformations that were not originally envisioned. They also give researchers an opportunity to become familiar with their data.

TIP When you explore your data, resist the temptation of going on a "fishing expedition," that is, hunting for *any* significant relationships. The facility with which computers can generate statistics makes it easy to run analyses indiscriminately. The risk is that you will serendipitously find significant correlations between variables as a function of chance. For example, in a correlation matrix with 10 variables—which results in 45 nonredundant correlations—there are likely to be two to three *spurious* significant correlations when alpha = .05 (i.e., .05 × 45 = 2.25).

Researchers then perform statistical analyses to test their hypotheses. Researchers whose data analysis plan calls for multivariate analyses (e.g.,

MANOVA) often begin with bivariate analyses (e.g., a series of ANOVAs). The primary statistical analyses are complete when all research questions are addressed and when table shells have the applicable numbers in them.

Sensitivity Analyses

Sometimes supplementary analyses can facilitate interpretation of the results or strengthen conclusions. An important example is the use of **sensitivity analyses**, which are analyses that test research hypotheses using different assumptions or different strategies. One example is testing alternative strategies to address missing values problems. Some strategies are appropriate under varying conditions, so sensitivity analyses to understand how different strategies affect substantive results are valuable. Another example is running analyses with and without legitimate outliers to see if the results change. Thabane and colleagues (2013) offer a tutorial on sensitivity analyses.

Example of Sensitivity Analysis
Pickham and colleagues (2018) studied the clinical effectiveness of a wearable patient sensor to improve compliance with turning protocols and thus prevent pressure ulcers in acutely ill patients in ICUs. The intervention group had significantly fewer hospital-acquired pressure injuries (HAPIs) than the control group. Sensitivity analysis was performed to compare results for intention-to-treat and per-protocol analyses, and similar results were obtained.

RESEARCH EXAMPLE

We conclude this chapter by describing a study that provided considerable detail about data management and analyses. Even though this study is not recent, it provides a useful overview of the steps the researchers took in their analyses—steps that are infrequently reported. The study described here was a feasibility study for a larger and more recent study (Kintner et al., 2015a, 2015b), but the more recent reports have less information about topics covered in this chapter.

Study: Randomized clinical trial of a school-based academic and counseling program for older school-age students (Kinter & Sikorskii, 2009).

Statement of purpose: The purpose of this feasibility study was to gather preliminary evidence about the efficacy of an academic and counseling program for older elementary students with asthma, in terms of cognitive, behavioral, psychosocial, and quality-of-life outcomes.

Method: The researchers used a two-group cluster randomized design with a sample of fourth- to sixth-grade students aged 9 to 12 years. Three schools were randomly assigned: One received the SHARP (Staying Healthy—Asthma Responsible and Prepared) program, and two schools were assigned to a control group. A total of 66 students were included in the sample. Students in the SHARP program met weekly for 10 weeks to discuss asthma management. There was also a community component for family members, friends, and others. Data were collected at baseline and after the intervention for such outcomes as knowledge of asthma, asthma health behaviors, acceptance of asthma, participation in life activities, and illness severity.

Analyses: The researchers collected and managed their data using laptop computers: "The system included quality-control methods to restrict field ranges and values, to provide internal consistency checks, to prevent entry of erroneous data, and to track missing data" (p. 326). Virtually no missing data were found in completed surveys. There were, however, four dropouts (all in the intervention group) before the Time 2 data collection, and data for one control group member could not be used. Reasons for all participant loss were reported. The researchers noted that "an intention-to-treat approach was adopted for analysis" (p. 326). The researchers looked at distributions for all variables to assess data quality and evaluate whether assumptions for statistical tests had been met. Internal consistency estimates were computed for all scales. The baseline characteristics of students in the two groups were compared to assess selection biases. Because the groups differed on some baseline measures, baseline values were statistically controlled to estimate program effects. The researchers also compared the characteristics of those who completed the study and those who did not and found no significant differences. Postintervention outcomes for the two groups were assessed using complex hierarchical models. The researchers computed adjusted mean scores, as well as effect size indexes, for all outcomes.

Results: Compared with students in the control group, students in the SHARP program had statistically significant improvements in asthma knowledge, use of risk reduction behaviors, and other outcomes, with sizeable effect sizes of d greater than .70. Moderate (but not statistically significant) effects (d between .30 and .50) were observed for two other outcomes.

SUMMARY POINTS

- Researchers who collect quantitative data typically progress through a series of steps in the analysis and interpretation of their data. Careful researchers lay out a data analysis plan in advance to guide that progress.
- Quantitative data typically must be **coded** into numerical values; codes need to be developed for legitimate data and for **missing values.** Decisions about coding and variable naming are documented in a **codebook.**
- **Data entry** is an error-prone process that requires verification and **data cleaning.** Cleaning involves checks for **outliers** (values that lie outside the normal range of values) and **wild codes** (codes that are not legitimate), as well as **consistency checks** (checks for internally consistent information).
- Decisions on handling missing values must be based on the amount of missing data and how missing data are patterned (i.e., the extent to which missingness is random). Addressing missing data is important for undertaking **intention-to-treat analyses.**
- The three missing values patterns are: (1) **missing completely at random (MCAR)**, which occurs when cases with missing values are just a random subsample of all cases in the sample; (2) **missing at random (MAR)**, which occurs if missingness is related to other variables but is *not* related to the variable that has the missing values; and (3)

missing not at random (MNAR), a pattern in which the value of the variable that is missing is related to its missingness.

- Two basic missing values strategies involve **deletion** or **imputation**. Deletion strategies include deleting cases with missing values (i.e., **listwise deletion**), selective **pairwise deletion** of cases, or deleting variables with missing values. Imputation strategies include **mean substitution**, regression-based estimation of missing values, **expectation maximization (EM) imputation,** and **multiple imputation (MI)**, which is considered the best approach.

- Raw data often need to be transformed for analysis. Examples of **data transformations** include reversing the coding of items, recoding the values of a variable (e.g., for creating dummy variables), and transforming data to meet statistical assumptions (e.g., through logarithmic transformations to achieve normality).

- Researchers usually undertake additional steps to assess data quality, such as evaluating the internal consistency of scales, examining distributions for **extreme outliers** that are legitimate values and analyzing the magnitude and direction of any biases, such as nonresponse bias, selection bias, and attrition bias.

- Another assessment may involve a scrutiny for possible **ceiling effects** (which occurs when values for a variable are restricted at the upper end of a continuum) or **floor effects** (which occurs when values are restricted at the lower end).

- Sometimes peripheral analyses involve tests to determine whether **pooling** of participants is warranted in tests for **site/cohort effects** or **ordering effects.**

- Once the data are fully prepared for substantive analysis, researchers should develop a formal analysis plan, to reduce the temptation to go on a "fishing expedition." One approach is to develop **table shells**, i.e., fully laid-out tables without numbers in them.

- Supplementary statistical analyses can sometimes facilitate interpretation (e.g., doing **sensitivity analyses** that test whether results hold true under different assumptions or with different statistical procedures).

STUDY ACTIVITIES

Study activities are available to instructors on thePoint.

REFERENCES CITED IN CHAPTER 20

*Abdeyazdan, A., Mohammadian-Ghahfarokhi, M., Ghazavi, Z., & Mohammadizadeh, M. (2016). Effects of nesting and swaddling on the sleep duration of premature infants hospitalized in neonatal intensive care units. *Iranian Journal of Nursing and Midwifery Research, 21*, 552–556.

Azarmnejad, E., Sarhangi, F., Javadi, M., Rejeh, N., Amirsalari, S., & Tadrisi, A. (2017). The effectiveness of familiar auditory stimulus on hospitalized neonates' physiologic responses to procedural pain. *International Journal of Nursing Practice, 23*(3), 1–7.

*Dziadkowiec, O., Callahan, T., Ozkaynak, M., Reeder, B., & Welton, J. (2016). Using a data quality framework to clean data extracted from the electronic health record: A case study. *eGEMS, 4*, 1–15.

Enders, C. K. (2010). *Applied missing data analysis*. New York: The Guilford Press.

Fox-Wasylyshyn, S., & El-Masri, M. (2005). Handling missing data in self-report measures. *Research in Nursing & Health, 28*, 488–495.

*Hung, C., Chang, H., Luh, D., Wu, C., & Yen, L. (2015). Do parents play different roles in drinking behaviours of male and female adolescents? A longitudinal follow-up study. *BMJ Open, 5*(4), e007179.

*Kintner, E., Cook, G., Marti, N., Allen, A., Stoddard, D., Harmon, P, … Van Egeren, L. (2015b). Effectiveness of a school- and community-based academic asthma health education program on use of effective asthma self-care behaviors in older school-age students. *Journal for Specialists in Pediatric Nursing, 20*, 62–75.

Kintner, E., Cook, G., Marti, N., Stoddard, D., Gomes, M., Harmon, P., & Van Egeren, L. (2015a). Comparative effectiveness on cognitive asthma outcomes of the SHARP academic asthma health education and counseling program and a non-academic program. *Research in Nursing & Health, 38*, 423–435.

*∗**Kintner, E., & Sikorskii, A. (2009). Randomized clinical trial of a school-based academic and counseling program for older school-age students. *Nursing Research, 58*, 321–331.

Knapp, T. R., & Brown, J. (2014). Ten statistics commandments that almost never should be broken. *Research in Nursing & Health, 37*, 347–351.

*Kobayashi, H., Song, C., Ikei, H., Park, B., Kagawa, T., & Miyazaki, Y. (2017). Diurnal changes in distribution characteristics of salivary cortisol and immunoglobulin A concentrations. *International Journal of Environmental Research & Public Health, 14*(9).

Kovach, C., & Ke, W. (2016). Handling those pesky statistical outliers. *Research in Gerontological Nursing, 9*, 206–207.

McKnight, P., McKnight, K., Sidani, S., & Figueredo, A. (2007). *Missing data: A gentle introduction*. New York: The Guilford Press.

Minnick, A. F., Norman, L., & Donaghey, B. (2017). Junior research track faculty in U.S. schools of nursing: Resources and expectations. *Nursing Outlook, 65*, 18–26.

Molenberghs, G., Fitzmaurice, G., Kenward, M., Tsiatis, A., & Verbeke, G. (2015). *Handbook of missing data methodology*. Boca Raton, FL: Taylor & Francis.

Munday, J., Osborne, S., & Yates, P. (2018). Intrathecal morphine-related perioperative hypothermia in women undergoing cesarean delivery: A retrospective case-control study. *Journal of Perianesthesia Nursing, 33*, 3–12.

Okura, M., Ogita, M., Yamamoto, M., Nakai, T., Numata, T., & Arai, H. (2018). Health checkup behavior and individual health beliefs in older adults. *Geriatrics & Gerontology International, 18*, 338–351.

Osborne, J. E. (2013). *Best practices in data cleaning: A complete guide to everything you need to do before and after collecting your data*. Thousand Oaks, CA: Sage Publications.

Patrician, P. A. (2002). Multiple imputation for missing data. *Research in Nursing & Health, 25*, 76–84.

*Pickham, D., Berte, N., Pihulic, M., Valdez, A., Mayer, B., & Desai, M. (2018). Effect of a wearable patient sensor on care delivery for preventing pressure injuries in acutely ill adults: A pragmatic randomized clinical trial (LS-HAPI study). *International Journal of Nursing Studies, 80*, 12–19.

Pocock, S. J., Assmann, S., Enos, L., & Kasten, L. (2002). Subgroup analysis, covariate adjustment and baseline comparisons in clinical trial reporting: Current practice and problems. *Statistics in Medicine, 21*, 2917–2930.

Polit, D. F. (2010). *Statistics and data analysis for nursing research* (2nd ed.). Upper Saddle River, NJ: Pearson.

Polit, D. F., & Gillespie, B. (2009). The use of the intention-to-treat principle in nursing clinical trials. *Nursing Research, 58*, 391–399.

Polit, D. F., & Gillespie, B. (2010). Intention-to-treat in randomized controlled trials: Recommendations for a total trial strategy. *Research in Nursing & Health, 33*, 355–368.

Son, H., Friedman, E., & Thomas, S. A. (2012). Application of pattern mixture models to address missing data in longitudinal data analysis using SPSS. *Nursing Research, 61*, 195–203.

*Thabane, L., Mbuagbaw, L., Zhang, S., Samaan, Z., Marcucci, M., Ye, C., … Goldsmith, C. (2013). A tutorial on sensitivity analyses in clinical trials: The what, why, when, and how. *BMC Research Methodology, 13*, 92.

*Van den Broeck, J., Cunningham, S., Eeckles, R., & Herbst, K. (2005). Data cleaning: Detecting, diagnosing, and editing data abnormalities. *PLoS Medicine, 2*, 10.

A link to this open-access article is provided in the Toolkit for Chapter 20 in the Resource Manual. ✪

**This journal article is available on thePoint for this chapter.*

21

Clinical Significance and Interpretation of Quantitative Results

In this chapter, we discuss the issue of interpreting statistical results. We begin with some general interpretive guidelines and then discuss an important emerging topic in health research: clinical significance.

INTERPRETATION OF QUANTITATIVE RESULTS

The analysis of research data provides the **results** of the study. These results need to be evaluated and interpreted, giving thought to the study's theoretical basis, existing research evidence, and limitations of the research methods used. Interpretation of statistical results forms the basis for the Discussion section of quantitative research reports.

Issues in Interpretation

The interpretive task is complex, requiring methodologic and substantive skills. Interpretation is difficult to teach, but we offer advice about ways of making sound inferences from study results.

The Interpretive Mindset
Evidence-based practice (EBP) encourages clinicians to make decisions based on a careful assessment of "best evidence." Thinking critically and demanding evidence are also part of a research interpreter's job. Just as clinicians must ask, "What *evidence* is there

that this intervention or strategy will be beneficial?" so should research interpreters ask, "What *evidence* is there that the results are real, true, and important?" This is precisely why nurses need to develop skills in understanding research methods and appraising research reports. To be a good interpreter of your research results, it is appropriate to adopt a skeptical attitude, challenging the results until you are confident that the results are real and important.

> **TIP** You should ask such questions as: Is it *plausible* that my results were affected by selection biases? Is it *plausible* that if I had used a different instrument, or had gotten a larger sample, or had less attrition, my results would change? You hope that the answers to such questions are "no," but you should start with the working assumption that the answer is "maybe" until you have satisfied yourself that this is not true (*Plausibility assessments* in the context of quasi-experimental research were discussed in Supplement B to Chapter 10).

Aspects of Interpretation
Interpreting the results of a study involves attending to different but overlapping considerations:

- The credibility and accuracy of the results
- The precision of the estimate of effects
- The magnitude of effects and importance of the results

- The meaning of the results, especially regarding causality
- The generalizability and applicability of the results
- The implications of the results for practice, theory development, or further research

Credibility of Quantitative Results

One of the most important interpretive tasks is to assess whether the results are *correct*. This corresponds to the first EBP question we posed in Chapter 2 with regard to appraising research evidence: To what extent is the evidence valid? If the results are not credible, the remaining interpretive issues (meaning, magnitude, and so on) are not likely to matter.

Research findings are meant to reflect "truth in the real world." The findings are intended to be proxies for the true state of affairs in actual community or healthcare settings. Inference is the vehicle for linking results to the real world. Inferences about what is true in the real world are valid, however, to the extent that the researchers have made rigorous methodologic decisions. To come to a conclusion about whether the results closely approximate "truth in the real world," each aspect of the study—its design, procedures, sampling plan, measurements, and analytic approach—must be subjected to critical scrutiny.

There are various ways to assess credibility, including the use of the critical appraisal guidelines we have offered throughout this book. Here we share additional perspectives.

Proxies and Credibility

Researchers begin with abstract constructs and then devise ways to operationalize them. Constructs are linked to reality in a series of approximations, each of which affects interpretation because at each step there is potential for misrepresentation. The better the proxies, the more credible the results are likely to be. In this section, we illustrate successive proxies using sampling concepts, to highlight the potential for inferential challenges.

When researchers formulate research questions or hypotheses, the population is typically broad and abstract. Population specifications are delineated later, when eligibility criteria are defined. For example, suppose we wanted to test the effectiveness of an intervention to increase physical activity in low-income women. Figure 21.1 shows the series of steps between the abstract population construct (low-income women) and the *actual* women who participated in the study. Using data from the actual sample on the far right, the researcher would like to make inferences about the effectiveness of the intervention for a broader group, but each proxy along the way represents a potential problem for achieving the desired inference. In interpreting a study, readers must consider how *plausible* it is that the actual sample reflects the recruited sample, the accessible population, the target population, and then the population construct.

Table 21.1 presents a description of a hypothetical scenario in which the researchers moved from a population construct of low-income women to an actual sample of 161 women who participated in the study. The table shows some questions that a person trying to make inferences about the study results might ask—these represent inferential challenges. Answers to these questions would affect the interpretation of whether the intervention *really* is effective with low-income women—or only with motivated, cooperative welfare recipients from two neighborhoods of Los Angeles who recently got approved for public assistance.

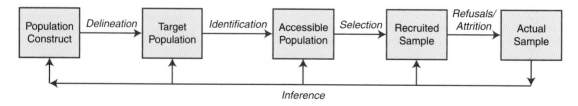

FIGURE 21.1 Inferences about populations: From the analysis sample to the population construct.

TABLE 21.1 • Successive Proxies in Sampling Example: From the Population Construct to the Analysis Sample

ELEMENT	DESCRIPTION	POSSIBLE INFERENTIAL CHALLENGES
Population construct	Low-income women	
Target population	All women who receive public assistance (cash welfare) in California	• Why only welfare recipients—why not the working poor? • Why California?
Accessible population	All women who receive public assistance in Los Angeles and who speak English or Spanish	• Why Los Angeles? • What about non-English/non-Spanish speakers?
Recruited sample	A consecutive sample of 300 female welfare recipients (English or Spanish speaking) who applied for benefits in January 2020 at two randomly selected welfare offices in Los Angeles	• Why only new applicants—what about women with long-term receipt? • Why only two offices? Are these representative? • Is January a typical month?
Actual sample	161 women from the recruited sample who fully participated in the study	• Who refused to participate (or was too ill, and so on) and why? • Who dropped out of the study, and why?

As Figure 21.1 suggests, researchers in our example made a series of methodologic decisions that affect inferences, and these decisions must be scrutinized in assessing study credibility. However, participant behavior and external circumstances also affect the results and need to be considered in the interpretation. In our example in Table 21.1, 300 women were recruited but only 161 provided usable data for analysis. The final sample of 161 almost surely would differ in important ways from the 139 who were not in the study, and these differences affect inferences about the value of the study evidence.

We illustrated how successive proxies in a study, from the abstract to the concrete, can affect inferences with regard to sampling, but we could focus on other aspects of the study. For example, Figure 21.2 considers successive proxies for an intervention for these women. As with our previous illustration, researchers move from an abstraction on the left (here, a theory about why an intervention might have beneficial outcomes), through the design of protocols that purport to operationalize the theory, to the actual implementation and use of the intervention on the right. Researchers want the right side

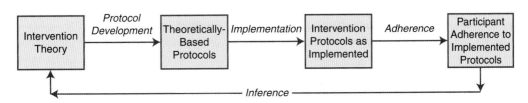

FIGURE 21.2 Inferences about interventions: From actual program operations to the intervention theory.

to be a good proxy for the left side—and, in interpreting their results, they must assess the plausibility that they were successful in the transformation.

Credibility and Validity

Studies inherently involve making inferences. We *infer* that scores on a depression scale are, in fact, capturing the depression construct. We *infer* that a sample can tell us something about a population. We use inferential statistics to make inferences about parameters. Inference and validity are inextricably linked. Indeed, research experts Shadish and colleagues (2002) defined validity as "the approximate truth of an inference" (p. 34). To be careful interpreters, researchers must seek evidence within their study that desired inferences are, in fact, valid.

In Chapter 10, we discussed four types of validity that play a key role in assessing the credibility of quantitative results: statistical conclusion validity, internal validity, external validity, and construct validity. Let us use our sampling example (Figure 21.1 and Table 21.1) to demonstrate the relevance of methodologic decisions to all four types of validity—and hence to inferences about study results.

First, let us consider construct validity—a term that has relevance for many aspects of a study. In our example, the population construct was *low-income women,* which was the basis of the eligibility criteria stipulating public assistance recipients. There are, however, alternative operationalizations of the population construct—for example, women with incomes below the official poverty level. Construct validity, it may be recalled, involves inferences from the particulars of the study to higher-order constructs. So it is fair to ask, Do the specified eligibility criteria adequately capture the population construct, low-income women?

Statistical conclusion validity—the extent to which correct inferences can be made about whether relationships between key variables are "real"—is also affected by sampling decisions. Ideally, researchers would do a power analysis to estimate how large a sample is needed. In our example, let us say we estimated (based on previous research) a small-to-moderate effect size for the intervention,

$d = .40$. For a power of .80, with risk of a Type I error set at .05, we would need a sample of about 200 participants. The actual sample of 161 yields a nearly 30% risk of a Type II error, i.e., falsely concluding that the intervention was not successful.

External validity—the generalizability of the results—is also affected by sampling decisions. To whom would it be safe to generalize the results in this example—to the population construct of low-income women? to all welfare recipients in California? to all new welfare recipients in Los Angeles who speak English or Spanish? Inferences about the extent to which the study results correspond to "truth in the real world" must take sampling decisions and sampling problems (e.g., recruitment and retention difficulties) into account.

Finally, internal validity (the extent to which a causal connection between variables can be inferred) is also affected by sample composition. In particular (in this example), differential attrition would be a concern. Were those in the intervention group more likely (or less likely) than those in the control group to drop out of the study? If so, any observed differences in physical activity outcomes could be caused by individual differences in the two groups (for example, differences in motivation), rather than by the intervention itself.

Methodologic decisions and the careful implementation of those decisions—whether they be about sampling, intervention design, measurement, research design, or analysis—inevitably affect study validity and the interpretation of results.

Credibility and Bias

Part of a researcher's job in doing a study is to translate abstract constructs into plausible and meaningful proxies. Another job is to eliminate or reduce biases—or, as a last resort, to detect and understand them. In interpreting results, the risk for various biases should be assessed and taken into account when drawing conclusions.

Biases are factors that create distortions and undermine researchers' efforts to capture and reveal "truth in the real world." Biases are pervasive. It is not so much a question of whether there *are* biases in a study, so much as what types of bias are present, and how extensive and systematic the biases are. We have discussed many types of bias—some reflect design inadequacies (e.g., selection bias), others reflect recruitment or sampling problems (nonresponse bias), others are related to measurement (social desirability bias). To our knowledge, there is no comprehensive listing of biases that might arise in a study, but Table 21.2 presents a list of some of the biases and errors mentioned in this book. This list is not all-inclusive but is meant to serve as a reminder of potential problems to consider in interpreting study results.

TIP The Toolkit of the accompanying *Resource Manual* includes a longer list of biases, with definitions and notes. Different disciplines use different names for the same or similar biases, but the names are not especially important—what is important is to understand how different forces can distort the results and affect inferences.

Credibility and Corroboration

Yet another strategy for assessing credibility is to seek corroboration for results. Corroboration can come from both internal and external sources, and the concept of *replication* is an important one in both cases. Interpretations are aided by considering prior research on the topic, for example. Interpreters can examine whether the study results replicate (are congruent with) those of other studies. Consistency across studies supports the credibility of the findings.

Researchers can pursue opportunities for replication themselves. For example, in multisite studies, if results are similar across sites, this suggests that something "real" is occurring with some regularity. Triangulation can be another form of replication and sometimes can help to corroborate results. For example, if results are similar across different measures of an outcome, then there can be greater confidence that the results are "real" and do not reflect some peculiarity of an instrument. When mixed results occur, interpreters must dig deeper to uncover the reason.

Finally, we are strong advocates of mixed methods studies, a special type of triangulation (Chapter 27). When findings from the analysis of qualitative data are consistent with the results of statistical analyses, internal corroboration can be especially powerful and persuasive.

TABLE 21.2 • Selected List of Major Potential Biases or Errors in Quantitative Studies

RESEARCH DESIGN	SAMPLING	MEASUREMENT	ANALYSIS
Expectation bias	Sampling error	Social desirability bias	Type I error
Hawthorne effect	Volunteer bias	Acquiescence bias	Type II error
Performance bias	Nonresponse bias	Naysayers bias	
Detection bias		Extreme response set bias	
Contamination of treatments		Recall/memory bias	
Carryover (ordering) effects		Ceiling effects	
Noncompliance bias		Floor effects	
Selection bias/threat		Reactivity	
Attrition bias/threat		Observer biases	
History bias/threat			

Precision of the Results

The results of statistical hypothesis testing indicate whether an observed relationship or group difference is probably real and replicable. A p value in hypothesis testing indicates how unlikely it is that the null hypothesis is true—it is not an estimate of a numeric value of direct relevance to clinicians. A p value offers information that is important, but incomplete.

Confidence intervals (CIs), by contrast, communicate how precise the study results are—that is, they indicate not only the estimate of an effect but also the range within which the actual effect probably lies. Dr. David Sackett, a founding father of the EBP movement, had this to say about confidence intervals: "*P* values on their own are…not informative…By contrast, CIs indicate the strength of evidence about quantities of direct interest, such as treatment benefit. They are thus of particular relevance to practitioners of evidence-based medicine" (2000, p. 232). It is hoped nurse researchers will increasingly report CIs because of their value for interpreting study results and assessing their potential utility for nursing practice.

Magnitude of Effects and Importance

In quantitative studies, results that support the researcher's hypotheses are described as *significant*. A careful analysis of study results involves evaluating whether, in addition to being statistically significant, the effects are large and clinically important.

Attaining statistical significance does not necessarily mean that the results are meaningful to nurses and clients. Statistical significance indicates that the results are unlikely to be due to chance—not that they are necessarily valuable. With large samples, even modest relationships are statistically significant. For instance, with a sample of 500, a correlation coefficient of .10 is significant at the .05 level, but a relationship this weak may have little practical value. Estimating the magnitude and importance of effects is relevant to the issue of clinical significance, a topic we discus later in this chapter.

Meaning of the Results

In quantitative studies, standard statistical results are in the form of p values, effect sizes, and confidence intervals, to which researchers must attach meaning once they have concluded that these results are credible. Many questions about the meaning of statistical results reflect a desire to interpret causal connections.

Interpreting what results mean usually is not challenging in descriptive studies. For example, suppose we found that, among patients undergoing electroconvulsive therapy (ECT), the percentage who experience an ECT-induced headache is 59.4% (95% CI = 56.3, 63.1). This result is directly meaningful and interpretable. But if we found that headache prevalence is significantly lower for patients in a cryotherapy intervention group than for patients given acetaminophen, we would need to interpret what the results mean. In particular, we need to interpret whether it is plausible that cryotherapy *caused* reductions in headaches. Even if the results are deemed to be "real," i.e., statistically significant, interpretation involves coming to conclusions about internal validity when a causal inference is sought.

In this section, we discuss the interpretation of various research outcomes within a hypothesis-testing context, with an emphasis on causal interpretations. In thinking about causal interpretations, we encourage you to review the criteria for causal relationships (Chapter 9).

Interpreting Hypothesized Results

Interpreting statistical results is easiest when hypotheses are supported, i.e., when there are *positive results*. In this situation, interpretations have been partly achieved beforehand because researchers have brought together prior findings, theory, and logic in developing hypotheses. This groundwork forms the context within which specific interpretations are made.

It is important to avoid the temptation of going beyond the data to explain what results mean, however. As an example, suppose we hypothesized that pregnant women's anxiety level about labor and delivery is correlated with the number of children they have borne. The data reveal a significant negative relationship between anxiety levels and parity ($r = -.30$). We interpret this to mean that increased experience with childbirth results in decreased anxiety. Is this conclusion supported by the data? The conclusion seems logical, but in fact, there is nothing in the data that leads to this interpretation. An important, indeed critical, research precept is: *correlation does not prove causation*. The finding that two variables are related offers no evidence suggesting which of the two variables—if either—caused the other. In our example, perhaps causality runs in the opposite direction, i.e., a woman's anxiety level influences how many children she bears. Or perhaps a third variable, such as the woman's relationship with her husband, influences both anxiety and number of children. Inferring causality is especially difficult in studies with a nonexperimental design.

> **TIP** Froman and Owen (2014) have written a helpful paper about avoiding inappropriate causal language in research reports. They point out that researchers often use misleading "loaded words" that suggest a casual link even when the study design does not support a causal inference—words like *impact, effect*, and *determinant*.

Alternative explanations for the findings should always be considered. Researchers sometimes can test rival hypotheses directly. If competing interpretations can be ruled out, so much the better, but every angle should be examined to see if one's own explanation has been given adequate competition.

Empirical evidence supporting research hypotheses never constitutes *proof* of their veracity. Hypothesis testing is probabilistic. There is always a possibility that observed relationships resulted from chance—that is, that a Type I error occurred. Researchers must be tentative about their results and about interpretations of them. Even when the results are in line with expectations, researchers should draw conclusions with restraint and should give due consideration to limitations identified in assessing the credibility of the results.

> **Example of Corroboration of a Hypothesis**
> Wargo-Sugleris and colleagues (2018) tested hypotheses about the relationship between acute care nurses' job satisfaction, successful aging, and delaying retirement. Consistent with hypotheses, successful aging (a construct that incorporated good health, self-assessments of work ability, and use of sick leave) was associated with job satisfaction and intention to delay retirement. The researchers concluded that "environment and successful aging are important areas that have an impact on job satisfaction and delay of retirement in older nurses" (p. 911).

This study is an example of the challenges of interpreting findings in correlational studies. The researchers' interpretation was that successful aging had an *impact* on job satisfaction—a word that implies a causal interpretation. This is a conclusion supported by earlier research and consistent with theory. Yet nothing in the data rules out the possibility that nurses' job satisfaction affects nurses' successful aging, or that a third factor might cause both job dissatisfaction and health issues captured in the successful aging measure. The researchers' interpretation is plausible, but their cross-sectional design makes it difficult to rule out other explanations. A major threat to the internal validity of the inference in this study is temporal ambiguity—that is, whether job dissatisfaction preceded indicators of successful aging.

> **TIP** A mistake that many researchers make is to qualitatively interpret the *p* values in statistical tests. A *p* value of .0001 is not "more significant" than a *p* value of .05. The outcome of a significance test is dichotomous: the result either is or is not significant. Similarly, a *p* value of .08 is not "marginally significant;" if one has established alpha = .05, the result is not significant (Hayat, 2010). Mechanisms other than *p* values are needed to interpret magnitude and importance, as we discuss later in this chapter.

Interpreting Nonsignificant Results

Nonsignificant results pose interpretative problems because statistical tests are geared toward disconfirmation of the null hypothesis. Failure to reject a null hypothesis can occur for many reasons, and the real reason is usually difficult to discern. The null hypothesis *could* actually be true, for example: a nonsignificant result could accurately reflect the absence of a relationship among research variables. On the other hand, the null hypothesis could be false, in which case a Type II error has been committed. Nonsignificant results are inconclusive.

Retention of a false null hypothesis can result from several methodologic problems, such as poor internal validity, an anomalous sample, a weak statistical procedure, or unreliable measures. In particular, failure to reject null hypotheses is often a consequence of insufficient power resulting from too small a sample.

In any event, a retained null hypothesis should not be considered as proof of the *absence* of relationships among variables. *Nonsignificant results provide no evidence of the truth or the falsity of the hypothesis.* Interpreting nonsignificant results can, however, be aided by considering such factors as sample size and effect size estimates.

> **Example of Nonsignificant Results**
> Griffin, Polit, and Byrnes (2007) hypothesized that nurses' stereotypes of patients (based on patients' gender, race, and attractiveness) would influence the nurses' pain treatment recommendations for children in pain. The hypotheses were not supported: there was no evidence of stereotyping. The conclusion that stereotyping probably did not occur was bolstered by the fact that the sample was fairly large (*N* = 334) and the effect sizes were extremely low.

Because statistical tests support the rejection of null hypotheses, they are not well-suited for testing *actual* research hypotheses about the absence of relationships or about group equivalence. Yet sometimes this is exactly what researchers want to do—and this is especially true in clinical situations in which the goal is to assess if one practice is as effective as another (an *equivalence trial*) or not less effective than another (a *noninferiority trial*). When the actual research hypothesis is null (i.e., a prediction of no group difference or no relationship),

additional strategies must be used to provide supporting evidence. In particular, it is important to compute effect sizes and confidence intervals to show that the risk of a Type II error was small. There may also be clinical standards that can be used to corroborate that nonsignificant—but predicted—results are plausible. In noninferiority and equivalence trials, clinical parameters must be stipulated for undertaking a power analysis (Tunes da Silva et al., 2009).

> **Example of Support for a Hypothesized Nonsignificant Result**
> Potts and an interprofessional team (2019) conducted a randomized noninferiority trial to test whether a vibrating cold device is not inferior to the standard of care (4% topical lidocaine cream) in reducing children's pain when they require IV insertion in the emergency department. In their sample of 224 children, the two treatments were equally effective in reducing pain and distress.

Interpreting Unhypothesized Significant Results

Unhypothesized significant results can occur in two situations. The first involves exploring relationships that were not anticipated during the design of the study. For example, in examining correlations among variables in the dataset, a researcher might notice that two variables that were not central to the research questions were nevertheless significantly correlated—and interesting. To interpret serendipitous findings, it is wise to consult the literature to see if similar relationships had been previously observed—and to recommend a replication.

> **Example of a Serendipitous Significant Finding**
> In a secondary analysis of data from a national survey, Must and colleagues (2017) studied the effect of age on the prevalence of obesity among U.S. youth with and without autism spectrum disorder (ASD). They found, consistent with expectations, that the odds of obesity among children with ASD, but not among those without ASD, increased from ages 10 to 17. Unexpectedly, they found that while white children with ASD experienced increases in obesity, minority children with ASD experienced declines.

The second situation is more perplexing, and it does not happen often: obtaining results *opposite* to those hypothesized. For instance, a researcher might hypothesize that individualized teaching about AIDS risks is more effective than group instruction, but the results might indicate that group instruction was significantly better. Some researchers view such situations as awkward, but research should not be undertaken primarily to corroborate researchers' predictions but rather to arrive at truthful evidence. The interpretation of such findings should involve comparisons with other research, a consideration of alternative theories, and—if possible—in-depth interviews with a subsample of study participants.

Example of Significant Results Contrary to Hypotheses

Griggs and Crawford (2017) studied the relationship between hope, emotional well-being, and health-risk behaviors in a sample of nearly 500 university freshmen. Contrary to the researchers' hypothesis, higher levels of hope were associated with more—not less—sexual risk-taking behaviors and alcohol use.

Interpreting Mixed Results

Interpretation is often complicated by *mixed results*: some hypotheses are supported by the data, but others are not. Or a hypothesis may be accepted with one measure of the outcome but rejected with a different measure. When only some results run counter to a prediction, the research methods are the first aspect of the study deserving scrutiny. Differences in the validity and reliability of the various measures may account for such discrepancies, for example. Or, the sample size might be sufficiently large when effects are large but insufficient for more modest effects. On the other hand, mixed results may suggest that a theory needs to be qualified or that certain constructs within the theory need to be reconceptualized. Mixed results sometimes present opportunities for conceptual advances because efforts to make sense of disparate pieces of evidence may lead to a breakthrough.

In summary, interpreting the meaning of research results is a demanding task but offers the possibility of intellectual rewards. Interpreters must play the role of scientific detectives, trying to make pieces of the puzzle fit together so that a coherent picture emerges.

> **TIP** A major strength of mixed methods research is that it can prove invaluable in interpreting results, especially if the results are not consistent with expectations.

Generalizability and Applicability of the Results

Researchers are rarely interested in discovering relationships among variables for a specific sample of people at a specific point in time. If a new nursing intervention is found to be successful, others may want to adopt it. Thus, an important interpretive question is whether the intervention will "work" or whether relationships will "hold" in other settings, with other people. Part of the interpretive process involves asking, "To what groups, environments, and conditions can the results of the study reasonably be applied?" In interpreting the study results with regard to the generalizability, it is useful to consider our earlier discussion about proxies. For which higher-order constructs, which populations, which settings, or which versions of an intervention were the study operations good "stand-ins"? We discuss the issue of generalizability and applicability of research evidence at greater length in Chapter 31.

Implications of the Results

Once you have reached conclusions about the credibility, precision, importance, meaning, and generalizability of your results, you are ready to think about their implications. You might consider the implications with respect to future research (What should other researchers working in this area do? What is the right "next step"?) or theory development (What are the implications for nursing theory?). A key issue, though, is the implications of the evidence for nursing practice. Specific suggestions for implementing the results of the study in real nursing contexts are valuable.

TIP In interpreting your data, remember that others will be reviewing your interpretation with a critical and perhaps even a skeptical eye. The job of consumers is to make decisions about the credibility and utility of the evidence, which is likely to be affected by how much support you offer for the validity and meaning of your results.

CLINICAL SIGNIFICANCE

Attaining statistical significance does not indicate whether a finding is clinically meaningful or relevant. With a large enough sample, a trivial relationship can be statistically significant. Broadly speaking, we define **clinical significance** as the practical importance of research results in terms of whether they have genuine, palpable effects on the daily lives of patients or on the healthcare decisions made on their behalf.

More than 20 years ago, LeFort (1993) wrote, in a prominent nursing journal, about the "recent interest" in clinical significance—but that interest has had a bigger impact on fields other than nursing. Relatively few nurse researchers comment on the clinical significance of their findings when discussing their results. When nurse researchers mention clinical significance, they often use the phrase loosely and ambiguously, or sometimes they establish a criterion for clinical significance without offering a rationale (Bruner et al., 2012; Polit, 2017).

In fields other than nursing, notably in medicine and psychotherapy, a lot of attention has recently been paid to two key challenges relating to clinical significance: developing a conceptual definition of what it means and developing a way to operationalize it. Consensus has not been reached on either front, but a few conceptual and statistical solutions are used with considerable regularity. In this section we briefly describe recent advances in defining and operationalizing clinical significance. Further information is available in Polit and Yang (2016).

In statistical hypothesis testing, a fair degree of consensus was reached decades ago that a *p* value of .05 would be the standard for statistical significance—although this criterion continues to be

debated. It is unlikely that a uniform standard will ever be adopted with regard to clinical significance, however, in part because it is a more complex concept than statistical significance. For example, in some cases *no change* over time could be clinically significant if it means that a group with a progressive disease has not experienced deterioration. In other cases, clinical significance is associated with improvements. Another issue concerns whose *perspective* on clinical significance is considered. Sometimes clinicians' perspective is paramount because of implications for health management (e.g., regarding blood pressure values), whereas for other outcomes the patient's view is what matters (e.g., about pain or quality of life). Two other issues concern whether clinical significance is for group-level findings or for individual patients and whether clinical significance is attached to point-in-time outcomes or to change scores. Most of the work that has been done to date, and therefore most of our discussion here, is about the clinical significance of *change scores* for individual patients. We begin, however, with a brief discussion of group-level clinical significance.

Clinical Significance at the Group Level

Many studies concern group-level comparisons. For example, one-group pretest–posttest designs involve comparing a group at two (or more) points in time, to test whether, on average, a change in outcomes has occurred. In randomized controlled trials (RCTs) and case–control studies, the comparisons are about average differences in outcomes for different groups of people. These comparisons are subjected to hypothesis-testing procedures, and statistical tests lead to decisions about rejecting the null hypothesis.

Group-level clinical significance (which is sometimes called *practical significance*) typically involves using statistical information other than *p* values to draw conclusions about the importance of the results. The most widely used statistics for this purpose are effect size (ES) indexes, confidence intervals (CIs), and number needed to treat (NNT). Many medical journals insist that information about CIs and effect sizes be reported. Yet, it has been found that only a minority of articles in top nursing research journal report on CIs or effect sizes (Gaskin & Happell, 2014; Polit, 2017).

Effect size indexes summarize the magnitude of a relationship or change score and thus provide insights into how a group, *on average*, might benefit from a treatment (or be spared a harm). A clinically significant finding at the group level means that the effect size is sufficiently large to have relevance for the "average" patient.

Confidence intervals are espoused by several writers as useful tools for understanding clinical significance (e.g., Fethney, 2010). CIs provide the most plausible range of values, at a given level of confidence, for the unknown population parameter, such as means on an outcome after treatment. Fethney provided an example that illustrated how CIs were used in a study evaluating an intervention for premature infants. A weight gain value was established a priori as clinically significant by a panel of experts, and then a CI around the obtained mean weight gain was calculated to see if the CI encompassed the designated value.

NNTs are sometimes promoted as useful indicators of clinical significance in clinical trials because the information is in a format that is relatively easy to understand. For example, if the NNT for an important outcome is found to be 2.0, only two patients have to receive a treatment in order for one patient to benefit. If the NNT is 10.0, however, 9 patients out of 10 receiving the treatment would get no benefit.

When using any of the group-level indexes mentioned, researchers should designate in advance what would constitute clinical significance—just as they would establish an alpha value for statistical significance. For example, would an ES of .20 (for the *d* index described in Chapter 18) be considered clinically significant? A *d* of .20 was described by Cohen (1988) as a "small" effect, but sometimes small improvements can have clinical relevance. Claims about attainment of clinical significance for groups should be based on reasonable criteria. Table 21.3 presents some traditional guidelines for interpreting the strength of relationships for *d*, *r*, and the NNT, based on the work of Kraemer and colleagues (2003).

> **TIP** In Chapter 18, we discussed using a power analysis to estimate sample size needs during the planning stage of the study based on a goal of detecting statistical significance. A compelling approach is to estimate sample size needs that will support goals for both clinical and statistical significance.

Clinical Significance at the Individual Level

Clinicians usually are not interested in what happens in a *group* of people—they are concerned with individual patients. A key goal in evidence-based practice (EBP) is to personalize "best evidence" into decisions for a specific patient's needs, within

TABLE 21.3 • Traditional Guidelines for Interpreting Relationship Strength

SIZE OF THE EFFECT	EFFECT SIZE (*d*)	EFFECT SIZE (*r*)	NNT
Small	.20	.10	8.9
Moderate	.50	.30	3.6
Large	.80	.50	2.3
Very large	≥ 1.00	$\geq .70$	≤ 1.9

NNT, number needed to treat

Adapted from Kraemer, H., Morgan, G., Leech, N., Gliner, J., Vaske, J., & Harmon, R. (2003). Measures of clinical significance. *Journal of the American Academy of Child and Adolescent Psychiatry, 42,* 1524–1529, Table 1.

a particular clinical context. Efforts to draw conclusions about clinical significance at the individual level can thus be directly linked to EBP goals.

Dozens of approaches to defining and operationalizing clinical significance at the individual level have been developed, but they share one thing in common: they involve establishing a **benchmark** (or *threshold*) that designates the value on a measure or a change score that would be considered clinically meaningful. When there is a benchmark for clinical significance, *each person in a study can be classified as to whether their score or change score is clinically significant.* Before looking at how the benchmarks have been established, we consider alternative definitions of clinical significance.

> **TIP** The operationalization of clinical significance is linked to measurement interpretability, which is one of the elements in our measurement property taxonomy (Figure 15.1).

Conceptual Definitions of Clinical Significance

Dozens of definitions of clinical significance can be found in the health literature; most definitions concern changes in measures of patient outcomes. The various definitions fall mainly into one of four categories.

One definitional category is linked to statistical issues discussed in Chapter 15—whether a change score is statistically reliable. Some have reasoned that if a patient's improved score on an outcome is more than random error, the improvement has clinical significance.

> **Example of Defining Reliable Change as Clinical Significance**
> Bond and colleagues (2016) studied change in neurocognitive performance of patients with head and neck cancer undergoing chemoradiation treatment. They used the reliable change index to assess clinically meaningful declines in performance.

Reliable change also figures into a definition of clinical significance that appeared in the psychotherapy literature in the early 1990s. Jacobson and Truax (1991) proposed that a clinically significant change for patients undergoing a psychotherapeutic intervention would involve a reliable improvement *and* a

return to "normal" functioning. They proposed several ways of deciding whether individual patients in a study had changed sufficiently to meet this criterion of normalcy. Their approach, sometimes referred to as the *J-T approach*, has been used for outcomes other than those used in psychotherapy research, such as in studies using measures of physical function as key outcomes (e.g., Mann et al., 2012). The J-T approach is described more fully in the Supplement to this chapter on the book's website. **S**

> **Example of Using the J-T Approach**
> Da Mata and colleagues (2018) presented a fully worked-out example of applying the J-T approach in a trial, testing the clinical effectiveness of a home care program after prostatectomy. The researchers first assessed whether scores on a knowledge measure had changed reliably, using the reliable change index. They then used an approach suggested by Jacobson and Truax for establishing a benchmark of clinical significance.

> **TIP** "Normalcy" sometimes can be defined as improvements that represent a return to a desirable value—especially for biophysiologic outcomes such as blood pressure or cholesterol levels. Thresholds for these outcomes are available in clinical guidelines.

A third way to conceptualize clinical significance is not linked to change scores explicitly. Tubach and colleagues (2006, 2007) argued that patients are more interested in "feeling good" than in simply "feeling better." In their view, a clinically significant state occurs when patients achieve an outcome that they perceive as important and meaningful. Tubach et al. called their benchmark the **patient acceptable symptom state (PASS).** The PASS approach is discussed in greater detail in Polit and Yang (2016).

The fourth way of conceptualizing clinical significance dominates in medicine. In a paper cited hundreds of times in the medical literature, Jaeschke and colleagues (1989) offered the following definition: "The minimal clinically important difference (MCID) can be defined as the smallest difference in score in the domain of interest which patients perceive as beneficial and which would mandate, in the absence of troublesome side effects and excessive cost, a change in the patient's management" (p. 408). Although these researchers, and many after them, have referred to the threshold for clinical significance as a *minimal important difference* (MID) or *minimal clinically important difference* (MCID), we follow the COSMIN group in using the term **minimal important change (MIC)** (DeVet et al., 2011) because the focus is on individual *change* scores (not group *differences*). We focus on methods of operationalizing this benchmark.

Operationalizing Clinical Significance: Establishing the MIC Benchmark

To our knowledge, the definition of the MIC offered by Jaeschke and colleagues (1989) has never been fully operationalized. For example, side effects and costs are not typically taken into consideration in the thresholds, and input on how much change would trigger a change in patient management is seldom sought. Thus, although the Jaeschke et al. definition regarding change score benchmarks has been cited extensively, researchers have gone in many different directions in translating and quantifying it. Nevertheless, the focus on *patient input* to establish the MIC has had a profound effect on establishing benchmarks for patient-reported outcomes (PROs).

Benchmarks for clinically important change are usually the number of change score points on a PRO that an individual patient must achieve, but benchmarks sometimes are a percentage change. Two MICs are established for some measures: one MIC denoting the threshold for clinically significant improvement and a second MIC as the threshold for clinically significant deterioration.

Dozens of methods have been used to derive MICs for widely used healthcare measures—and the developers of many new multi-item scales now make efforts to estimate the MIC as part of the psychometric assessment of their instrument. Methods of establishing the MIC benchmark mainly fall into three categories.

A traditional approach to setting a benchmark for health outcomes is to obtain input from a panel of healthcare experts—often called a *consensus panel*. For example, the Initiative on Methods, Measurement, and Pain Assessment in Clinical Trials (IMMPACT) convened a special panel on clinical significance, and one recommendation of the consensus review was that a 30% improvement in self-reported pain intensity (e.g., on a visual analog scale) be considered the benchmark for moderately important clinical change and that a 50% decrease in pain be the benchmark for substantial change (Dworkin et al., 2008).

The COSMIN group has advocated a different approach. They defined the MIC as "the smallest change in score in the construct to be measured which patients perceive as important" (De Vet et al., 2011, p. 245). Even this definition has led to different interpretations: some researchers have emphasized the "smallest" aspect in looking at a change score, and others have emphasized the "important" aspect. This divergence can be best explained with an illustration.

A widely used method of establishing the MIC value is called an **anchor-based approach**. This approach requires administering the focal measure on two occasions to a sample of people in which change is expected, so that change scores can be computed. At the second administration, information about an "anchor" is also obtained. The anchor is a criterion for establishing the MIC benchmark on the focal scale. The anchor often is a single-item **global rating scale** (GRS), as we described in Chapter 15 in our discussion of the criterion approach to responsiveness.

Indeed, we can use the same example as the one shown in Figure 15.3, which illustrated a 7-point GRS for assessing the responsiveness of a physical function (PF) scale. Figure 21.3 shows the mean scores on our physical function scale for each response category on the GRS. If we wanted to operationalize the MIC for the PF scale in a manner that emphasized the *smallest* noticeable improvement in score ("a little better"), we might conclude that the MIC for the PF scale was 2.17. In this case, any change in a person's score of 3 or better would be interpreted as clinically significant. Other researchers, however, have argued that "minimal change" is an insufficient criterion. They would opt for using the GRS rating of "much better" as their anchor for establishing the MIC for the PF scale. In that case, the MIC in this example would be 3.89; a person's change would be deemed clinically significant only if their change score on the scale was 4

Please rate the changes you have experienced in the past three months with regard to *your ability to perform regular activities of daily living*, such as standing up from a sitting position or taking a bath or shower:

GRS Rating	Mean Change Score on Focal Physical Function Scale (Posttest – Baseline)
1. Very much better	5.50
2. Much better	**3.89**
3. A little better	**2.17**
4. No change	0.75
5. A little worse	-1.89
6. Much worse	-4.03
7. Very much worse	-5.98

Highlighted categories indicate possible MIC thresholds.

FIGURE 21.3 Example of a global rating scale anchor used to establish a minimal important change (MIC) for improvement on a physical function scale.

points or higher. Other statistical approaches can be used to establish an MIC using anchor-based methods, notably the use of a receiver operating characteristic (ROC) curve analysis.

Note that despite the widespread endorsement of using patients' input in defining clinical significance for PROs, it is almost always the researcher, not the patient, who defines what is "minimally important." When reading about the MIC or when using a previously obtained MIC value in a study to assess clinical significance, it is crucial to understand how the researcher defined "minimally important."

TIP The anchor used as the criterion for the MIC need not be based on patients' self-reported change on a GRS. For example, the anchor for a physical functioning scale could be based on performance tests.

Calculating an MIC using an anchor-based approach requires a lot of work, and it also requires a careful research design with a large sample of people whose changes over time are expected to vary. Using an anchor-based approach, an MIC must be established for every new scale; moreover, the MIC value is population-specific. The MIC on a measure of pain intensity might be different for a population experiencing chronic pain than for

a population recovering from surgery—and in a group with chronic pain, a separate threshold might be needed for both improvement and deterioration.

These complexities have led to a third approach to defining the MIC—one that uses the distributional characteristics of a measure. **Distribution-based methods** rely on the statistical characteristics of a sample, and they express the MIC as a standardized metric. The most frequently used metric is based on Cohen's (1988) effect size index, operationalized at the individual level as a fraction of the standard deviation (SD). Most often, the MIC using this approach is set to a threshold of 0.5—i.e., one half a standard deviation based on the distribution of baseline scores (Norman et al., 2003, 2004). Norman and colleagues found that there was "remarkable" consistency supporting a threshold equivalent to an SD of 0.5. They argued that this consistency was unlikely to be a coincidence and could be tied to theory and evidence on the psychology of human discrimination. They concluded that a change of 0.5 SD in baseline scores is a defensible benchmark for interpreting an individual's change score as important.

An MIC threshold value in change score units using this distribution approach can be easily computed. For example, if the baseline SD for a scale were 6.0, then the MIC using the 0.5 SD criterion would be 3.0. This value, like any MIC, can be used as the benchmark to classify individual patients as having or not having experienced clinically meaningful change.

An alternative distribution-based method is to establish the value of the MIC based on measurement error (see Chapter 15). A number of researchers have suggested using the standard error of measurement (SEM) to establish the threshold. Norman and colleagues (2003) pointed out that for measures with a test–retest reliability of .75, the 0.5 *SD* threshold is exactly equivalent to 1 SEM.

There is no consensus on which approach to calculating the MIC yields the most helpful benchmark of clinical significance, but many people agree that none is ideal. The anchor-based approach is preferred by the COSMIN group, but it adds more work to the burdensome effort of constructing and evaluating new scales. It has also been argued that a single GRS is a poor choice for the anchor, because a single item is unreliable and subject to recall bias.

MICs based on distribution approaches are appealing because they are easy to compute, but it is often difficult to communicate what such an MIC represents. A persistent criticism of distribution methods is that they yield values that are not linked to any clinical yardstick—they do not embody any notion of "meaningfulness" or "importance." Another problem with MICs based on *SD*s is that the value is dependent on the heterogeneity of the population under study. Those who have suggested distribution-based MICs often emphasize that they are a reasonable starting point or "an approximate rule of thumb in the absence of more specific information" (Norman et al., 2003, p. 590).

Triangulation of Methods for the MIC

Because there is no "gold standard" approach to setting the MIC, some experts argue that it is advantageous to triangulate information from more than one approach (e.g., Revicki et al., 2008). Many approaches to triangulation have been adopted. For example, some researchers have combined information from multiple anchors, including anchors reflecting both patients' and clinicians' perspectives. Most efforts at triangulation involve using both a distribution method, such as 1 SEM, plus an anchor-based method. This particular type of triangulation has the merit of enhancing the likelihood that a change score value is not only clinically meaningful but also reliable.

An example of triangulation comes from the field of respiratory medicine. Patel and colleagues (2013) sought to establish the MIC for King's Brief Interstitial Lung Disease Questionnaire (K-BILD). These researchers used two distribution methods (1 SEM and .3 *SD*), a clinical anchor (a forced vital capacity change of at least 7% from baseline) and patients' responses on four GRSs. Integrating all information, the researchers established the MIC on the K-BILD at 8 points.

Example of Estimating MICs

Chen and an interprofessional team (2018) triangulated anchor-based and distribution-based methods to estimate the minimum important change for four fixed-length PROMIS® pain interference scales. For example, for patients in pain, MIC estimates ranged from 2 to 3 points in T-score points (i.e., scores with a mean of 50 and *SD* of 10).

Procedures for Clinical Significance Inquiries

Nurse researchers who wish to assess the clinical significance of their results for individual participants, using some of the procedures described in this chapter, should begin by coming to conclusions about how they wish to conceptualize clinical significance. This is most easily illustrated in the context of intervention research. Clinical significance can have many meanings, and so the researcher must be clear at the outset about treatment goals. Is the goal to have patients achieve *real change*? Return to *normal functioning*? Achieve a *favorable state*? Or experience change at a level that is *minimally important*?

If researchers decide in advance how they want to approach clinical significance, they will be in a better position to operationalize it when they plan their studies. For example, if "return to normal functioning" is the treatment goal, the researchers should investigate whether there are measures of key outcomes for which normative information is readily available. If depression, for instance, is an outcome, then a researcher interested in assessing clinically significant changes in depression should select a depression scale with published norms or recommended cutpoints. If, on the other hand, the treatment goal is for patients to achieve meaningful improvements, then researchers should search the literature for MIC values for their outcome measures. MIC values have been reported for many health scales. MIC values are population-specific, so it is important to identify MIC thresholds that are appropriate for study participants. By looking for MIC information before the study is underway, researchers may be able to select between alternative measures of a construct.

Example of Using MIC Values From Previous Research

Garvin and colleagues (2017) studied how much weight reduction was needed to achieve minimal clinically important improvements in health-related quality of life (HRQOL) scores among African Americans. The researchers used a value of the MIC for a measure of HRQOL that was established in a previous study.

Triangulation is sometimes adopted by those who wish to *use* existing benchmarks of clinical significance. For example, Fleet and colleagues (2014) studied the effect of a subcutaneous administration of fentanyl in childbirth on changes in the women's pain scores, as measured on a 100 cm visual analog scale (VAS) for pain. MIC values for the VAS in four earlier studies ranged from 0.9 to 1.3 cm. Fleet and colleagues used 1.2 cm as their benchmark for clinically meaningful improvement and concluded that 78% of the women in their sample had a clinically significant reduction in pain.

TIP The Toolkit in the *Resource Manual* provides a few examples of MIC values that have been proposed for several health measures. We emphasize that these MICs are illustrative, as a means of showing that MIC information can be located in the literature. We found these examples by searching in PubMed, using as search terms the name of a construct (e.g., depression) or a scale (e.g., Beck Depression Inventory), combined with the terms "minimal important" OR "minimum important" OR "minimum clinically important."

Many measures that are widely used by nurse researchers have not, however, been subjected to analysis for establishing an MIC—which suggests avenues for new research. When no MIC benchmark has been established for an outcome of interest, nurse researchers may have to adopt a distribution-based approach to estimating it.

Responder Analysis

A number of researchers (including nurse researchers) have used MIC values to interpret group-level findings. The MIC is, however, an index that concerns *individual* changes, not group differences. Experts have warned that it is not appropriate to interpret mean differences in relation to the MIC (Guyatt et al., 2002; Wyrwich et al., 2013). For example, if the MIC on an important outcome has been reported as 4.0 points, this value should not be used to interpret mean group differences for clinical significance. If the mean group difference were found to be 3.0, for instance, it would be inappropriate to conclude that the results were not clinically significant. A mean difference of 3.0 almost certainly implies that a sizable percentage of the participants achieved a meaningful benefit—i.e., an improvement of 4 points or more.

MIC thresholds can, however, be used to create new outcomes that facilitate the interpretation of group differences. Once the MIC is established, researchers can classify all people in the study in terms of their having attained or not attained the threshold. Study participants can be classified as *responders* or *nonresponders* (e.g., to an intervention) based on an established threshold of meaningful change. Then, researchers can undertake a **responder analysis** that compares the percentage of responders in the study groups (e.g., those in the intervention and those in the control group). A distinct advantage of a responder analysis is that it is easy to understand and can facilitate comparisons across trials or across different outcomes in a trial.

Example of a Responder Analysis

Horrocks and colleagues (2015) tested the effectiveness of percutaneous tibial nerve stimulation versus sham stimulation in the treatment of fecal incontinence. Their primary outcome was number of weekly fecal incontinence episodes (FIEs), and they established as their benchmark for clinical improvement a 50% reduction in FIEs. The percentage of responders who met this threshold was compared for the two groups.

TIP By classifying people as responders and nonresponders, researchers can go on to examine who did and did not respond at clinically significant levels and explore their characteristics and treatment experiences.

CRITICAL APPRAISAL OF INTERPRETATIONS

Researchers offer their interpretation of the findings and discuss what the findings might imply for nursing in the Discussion section of research reports. When critically appraising a study, your own interpretation and inferences can be contrasted against those of the researchers.

As a reviewer, you should be wary if a discussion section fails to point out any limitations. Researchers are in the best position to detect and assess the impact of sampling deficiencies, practical constraints, data quality problems, and so on, and it is a professional responsibility to alert readers to these difficulties. Moreover, when researchers note methodologic shortcomings, readers have some confidence that these limitations were considered in interpreting the results. Of course, researchers are unlikely to note all relevant shortcomings of their own work. The task of reviewer is to independently assess limitations and to challenge conclusions that do not appear to be warranted.

In addition to comparing your interpretation with that of the researchers, your appraisal should also draw conclusions about the stated implications of the study. Some researchers make grandiose claims or offer unfounded recommendations based on modest results.

We have discussed the issue of clinical significance at some length in this chapter. The conceptualization and operationalization of clinical significance have not received much attention in nursing (Polit, 2017). We hope that nurse researchers will pay more attention to this issue in the years ahead.

Some guidelines for evaluating researchers' interpretation and implications are offered in Box 21.1.

BOX 21.1   Guidelines for Critically Appraising Interpretations in Discussion Sections of Quantitative Research Reports

INTERPRETATION OF THE FINDINGS

1. Are all important results discussed?
2. Did the researchers discuss the limitations of the study and their possible effects on the credibility of the research evidence? In discussing limitations, were key threats to the study's validity and possible biases noted?
3. What types of evidence were offered in support of the researchers' interpretation, and was that evidence persuasive? If results were "mixed," were possible explanations offered? Were results interpreted in light of findings from other studies?
4. Did the researchers make any unwarranted causal inferences? Were alternative explanations for the findings considered? Were the rationales for rejecting these alternatives convincing?
5. Did the interpretation take into account the precision of the results and/or the magnitude of effects?
6. Did the researchers discuss the generalizability of the findings? Did they draw any unwarranted conclusions about generalizability?

IMPLICATIONS OF THE FINDINGS AND RECOMMENDATIONS

1. Did the researchers discuss the study's implications for clinical practice, nursing theory, or future nursing research? Did they make specific recommendations?
2. If yes, are the stated implications appropriate, given the study's limitations and the magnitude of the effects—as well as evidence from other studies? Are there important implications that the report neglected to include?

CLINICAL SIGNIFICANCE

1. Did the researchers mention clinical significance? Did they make a distinction between statistical and clinical significance? Did they identify explicit criteria for clinical significance?
2. If yes, was clinical significance interpreted in terms of group-level information (e.g., effect sizes) or individual-level results? If the latter, how was clinical significance operationalized?

RESEARCH EXAMPLE

We conclude this chapter with an example of a study that examined clinical significance.

Study: Effectiveness of a community-based nurse–pharmacist managed pain clinic (Hadi et al., 2016).

Statement of purpose: The purpose of this study was to evaluate the effectiveness of a community-based pain clinic jointly managed by a nurse and pharmacist.

Method: The researchers evaluated a community-based pain clinic that involved having a pharmacist come to the clinic 1 day per week to conduct a medication review. The nursing intervention focused on educating patients about pain and encouraging them to develop self-management skills. The researchers undertook a mixed methods study with in-depth qualitative interviews embedded in a quasi-experimental pretest–posttest design. A total sample of 79 patients completed baseline questionnaires that included measures of pain intensity (the primary outcome), physical functioning, anxiety, depression, and chronic pain grade. Only 36 patients completed follow-up questionnaires at discharge from the pain management service because the service was unexpectedly decommissioned.

Analyses: Within-subjects tests (paired t-tests, Wilcoxon signed-ranks test) were used to test the statistical significance of changes in participants' outcomes from baseline to follow-up. Using benchmarks recommended by the IMMPACT consensus panel for interventions targeting pain, the researchers assessed the number of patients who demonstrated clinically important change.

Results: At discharge, there was a statistically significant reduction for median "worst pain" and "average pain" intensity (both $p = .02$). Using recommended values for the MIC from IMMPACT, the researchers found that 37% of the patients achieved minimum clinically important improvements in pain intensity (10%-20% reduction), 6% achieved moderate improvement (>30%), and 6% achieved substantial improvement (>50%). Pain interference with physical activity was significantly improved for the group ($p = .02$), and 40% of the patients achieved a minimum clinically important change. Changes from baseline to follow-up for other outcomes were not statistically significant.

Discussion: The researchers devoted some of their discussion to linking their qualitative findings to their quantitative findings. In particular, they talked about the link between chronic pain and anxiety and depression. They noted that the joint pain clinic appeared not to have had an effect on the patients' emotional functioning and speculated that this could be the result of the small sample size or the use of insensitive measures. They advised that "These issues require further exploration" (p. 226). The researchers pointed out that their analysis with the MIC helped to "improve clinical interpretation of the results" (p. 226) and concluded that, based on the service's apparent positive effect on pain intensity, "interdisciplinary community-based pain clinics run by nurses and pharmacists have the potential to improve chronic pain management in the community" (p. 226). Although the Discussion did not link the findings to other evidence, it was noted earlier in the report (in the introduction) that a similar previous study also found a significant reduction in pain intensity. The researchers urged that the findings be interpreted with care because of the small sample size—although they did not mention potential threats to internal validity resulting from the use of a fairly weak research design. They pointed out, however, that the quantitative results suggesting significant improvements in pain intensity were corroborated during the qualitative interviews with patients, who provided positive feedback about the value of the pain clinic.

SUMMARY POINTS

- The interpretation of quantitative research **results** (the outcomes of the statistical analyses) typically involves consideration of the (1) credibility of the results; (2) precision of estimates of effects; (3) magnitude of effects; (4) underlying meaning of the results; (5) generalizability of results; and (6) implications for future research, theory development, and nursing practice.
- Inference is central to interpretation. Researchers' methodologic decisions affect the inferences that can be made about the correspondence between study results and "truth in

the real world." A cautious outlook is appropriate in drawing conclusions about the credibility and meaning of study results.

- An assessment of a study's credibility can involve various approaches, one of which involves evaluating the degree of congruence between abstract constructs or idealized methods on the one hand and the proxies actually used on the other. Credibility assessments can also involve an analysis of validity threats and biases that could undermine the accuracy of the results. Corroboration (replication) of results is another approach in a credibility assessment.

- Broadly speaking, **clinical significance** refers to the practical importance of research results—i.e., whether the effects are genuine and palpable in the daily lives of patients or in the management of their health. Clinical significance has not received sufficient attention in nursing research.

- Clinical significance for group-level results is often inferred based on such statistics as effect size indexes, confidence intervals, and number needed to treat. However, clinical significance is most often discussed in terms of effects for individual patients—especially, whether they have achieved a clinically meaningful change in outcomes.

- Definitions and operationalizations of clinical significance for individuals typically involve using a **benchmark** or threshold that designates the amount of change on an outcome that is meaningful. At the conceptual level, clinical significance has been defined in terms of whether a change in the attribute is real (reliable), whether a patient in a dysfunctional state returns to normal functioning, whether a patient has achieved a symptom state that is acceptable to them, and whether the amount of change in an attribute can be considered minimally important.

- The efforts to operationalize clinical significance in medical fields have mostly focused on the last definition. The goal of such efforts is to establish a benchmark (change score value) on a health measure that can be considered a **minimal important change (MIC)**, also called a *minimal important difference (MID)* and *minimal clinically important difference* (MCID).

- The MIC benchmark is a value for the number of change score points that an individual patient must achieve to be counted as having a clinically important change.

- The primary methods of establishing the MIC for a measure are (1) through a consensus panel, (2) using an **anchor-based approach** that often involves linking changes on the focal measure to a criterion for meaningful change, and (3) using a **distribution-based method** that bases the MIC on the distributional characteristics of the sample (e.g., 0.5 *SD* of a baseline distribution or 1 standard error of measurement). Triangulation of approaches is increasingly common.

- MICs cannot legitimately be used to interpret group means or differences in means. However, the MIC can be used to ascertain whether each person in a sample has or has not achieved a change greater than the MIC, and then a **responder analysis** can be undertaken to compare the percentage of responders in different study groups.

STUDY ACTIVITIES

Study activities are available to instructors on thePoint.

REFERENCES CITED IN CHAPTER 21

Bond, S., Dietrich, M., Gilbert, J., Ely, E., Jackson, J., & Murphy, B. (2016). Neurocognitive function in patients with head and neck cancer undergoing primary or adjuvant chemoradiation treatment. *Supportive Care in Cancer, 24*, 4433–4442.

Bruner, S., Corbett, C., Dupler, A., & Gates, B. (2012). Clinical significance as it relates to evidence-based practice. *International Journal of Nursing Knowledge, 23*, 62–74.

**Chen, C., Kroenke, K., Stump, T., Kean, J., Carpenter, J., Krebs, E., … Monahan, P. (2018). Estimating minimally important differences for the PROMIS pain interference scales: Results from 3 randomized clinical trials. *Pain, 159*, 775–782.

Cohen, J. (1988). *Statistical power analysis for the behavioral sciences* (2nd ed.). Hillsdale, NJ: Lawrence Erlbaum Associates.

*Da Mata, L., Bernardes, M., Azevedo, C., Chianca, T., Pereira, M., & de Carvalho, E. (2018). Jacobson and Truax method: Evaluation of the clinical effectiveness of a home care program after prostatectomy. *Revista Latino-Americana de Enfermagem, 26*, e3003.

DeVet, H., Terwee, C., Mokkink, L., & Knol, D. (2011). *Measurement in medicine: A practical guide*. Cambridge: Cambridge University Press.

Dworkin, R., Turk, D., Wyrwich, K., Beaton, D., Cleland, C., Farrar, J., ... Zavisic, S. (2008). Interpreting the clinical importance of treatment outcomes in chronic pain clinical trials: IMMPACT recommendations. *Journal of Pain, 9*, 105–121.

Fethney, J. (2010). Statistical and clinical significance, and how to use confidence intervals to help interpret both. *Australian Critical Care, 23*, 93–97.

Fleet, J., Jones, M., & Belan, I. (2014). Subcutaneous administration of fentanyl in childbirth: An observational study on the clinical effectiveness of fentanyl for mother and neonate. *Midwifery, 30*, 36–42.

Froman, R. D., & Owen, S. (2014). Why you want to avoid being a causist. *Research in Nursing & Health, 37*, 171–173.

Garvin, J., Williams, L., Joshua, T., Looney, S., & Marion, L. (2017). Percent weight reduction required to achieve minimal clinically important improvements in health-related quality of life among African Americans: A secondary analysis of the fit body and soul study. *Applied Nursing Research, 36*, 100–105.

Gaskin, C., & Happell, B. (2014). Power, effects, confidence, and significance: An investigation of statistical practices in nursing research. *International Journal of Nursing Studies, 51*, 795–806.

Griffin, R., Polit, D., & Byrnes, M. (2007). Stereotyping and nurses' treatment of children's pain. *Research in Nursing & Health, 30*,655–666.

Griggs, S., & Crawford, S. (2017). Hope, core self-evaluations, emotional well-being, health-risk behaviors, and academic performance in university freshmen. *Journal of Psychosocial Nursing and Mental Health Services, 55*, 33–42.

Guyatt, G. H., Osoba, D., Wu, A., Wyrwich, K., Norman, G. R., & the Clinical Significance Consensus Meeting Group. (2002). Methods to explain the clinical significance of health status measures. *Mayo Clinic Proceedings, 77*, 371–383.

Hadi, M., Alldred, D., Briggs, M., Marczewski, K., & Closs, S. (2016). Effectiveness of a community-based nurse-pharmacist managed pain clinic: A mixed methods study. *International Journal of Nursing Studies, 53*, 219–227.

Hayat, M. J. (2010). Understanding statistical significance. *Nursing Research, 59*, 219–223.

*Horrocks, E., Bremner, S., Stevens, N., Norton, C., Gilbert, D., O'Connell, P, ... Knowles, C. (2015). Double-blind randomised controlled trial of percutaneous tibial nerve stimulation versus sham electrical stimulation in the treatment of fecal incontinence. *Health Technology Assessments, 19*, 1–164.

*Jacobson, N. S., & Truax, P. (1991). Clinical significance: A statistical approach to defining meaningful change in psychotherapy research. *Journal of Consulting and Clinical Psychology, 59*, 12–19.

Jaeschke, R., Singer, J., & Guyatt, G. H. (1989). Measurement of health status: Ascertaining the minimal clinically important difference. *Controlled Clinical Trials, 10*, 407–415.

Kraemer, H., Morgan, G., Leech, N., Gliner, J., Vaske, J., & Harmon, R. (2003). Measures of clinical significance. *Journal of the American Academy of Child and Adolescent Psychiatry, 42*, 1524–1529.

LeFort, S. M. (1993). The statistical versus clinical significance debate. *Image: The Journal of Nursing Scholarship, 25*, 57–62.

Mann, B. J., Gosens, T., & Lyman, S. (2012). Quantifying clinically significant change: A brief review of methods and presentation of a hybrid approach. *The American Journal of Sports Medicine, 40*, 2385–2393.

Must, A., Eliasziw, M., Phillips, S., Curtin, C., Kral, T., Segal, M., ... Bandinit, L. (2017). The effect of age on the prevalence of obesity among US youth with autism spectrum disorder. *Childhood Obesity, 13*, 25–35.

Norman, G. R., Sloan, J., & Wyrwich, K. W. (2003). Interpretation of changes in health-related quality of life: The remarkable universality of half a standard deviation. *Medical Care, 41*, 582–592.

Norman, G. R., Sloan, J., & Wyrwich, K. W. (2004). The truly remarkable universality of half a standard deviation: Confirmation through another look. *Expert Review of Pharmacoeconomics & Outcomes Research, 4*, 581–586.

Patel, A., Siegert, R., Keir, G., Bajwah, S., Barker, R., Maher, T., ... Birring, S. (2013). The minimal important difference of the King's Brief Interstitial Lung Disease Questionnaire (K-BILD) and forced vital capacity in interstitial lung disease. *Respiratory Medicine, 107*, 1438–1443.

Polit, D. F. (2017). Clinical significance in nursing research: A discussion and descriptive analysis. *International Journal of Nursing Studies, 52*, 1746–1753.

Polit, D. F. & Yang, F. M. (2016). *Measurement and the measurement of change: A primer for health professionals*. Philadelphia: Lippincott.

Potts, D., Davis, K., Elci, O., & Fein, J. (2019). A vibrating cold device to reduce pain in the pediatric emergency department: A randomized clinical trial. *Pediatric Emergency Care, 35*(6), 419–425.

Revicki, D., Hays, R., Cella, D., & Sloan, J. (2008). Recommended methods for determining responsiveness and minimally important differences for patient-reported outcomes. *Journal of Clinical Epidemiology, 61*, 102–109.

Sackett, D., Straus, S., Richardson, W., Rosenberg, W., & Haynes, R. (2000). *Evidence-based medicine*. (2nd ed.). Edinburgh: Churchill Livingston.

Shadish, W. R., Cook, T. D., & Campbell, D. T. (2002). *Experimental and quasi-experimental designs for generalized causal inference*. Boston: Houghton Mifflin.

Tubach, F., Dougados, M., Falissard, B., Baron, G., Logeart, I., & Ravaud, P. (2006). Feeling good rather than feeling better matters more to patients. *Arthritis & Rheumatism, 55*, 526–530.

*Tubach, F., Ravaud, P., Beaton, D., Boers, M., Bombardier, C., Felson, D., … Dougados, M. (2007). Minimal clinically important improvement and patient acceptable symptom state for subjective outcome measures in rheumatic disorders. *Journal of Rheumatology, 34*, 1139–1193.

*Tunes da Silva, G. T., Logan, B., & Klein, J. (2009). Methods for equivalence and noninferiority testing. *Biology of Blood and Marrow Transplantation, 15*, 120–127.

Wargo-Sugleris, M., Robbins, W., Lane, C., & Phillips, L. (2018). Job satisfaction, work environment and successful aging: Determinants of delaying retirement among acute care nurses. *Journal of Advanced Nursing, 74*, 900–913.

Wyrwich, K. W., Norquist, J., Lenderking, W., Acaster, S., & the Industry Advisory Committee of ISOQOL. (2013). Methods for interpreting change over time in patient-reported outcome measures. *Quality of Life Research, 22*, 475–483.

***A link to this open-access article is included in the Toolkit for Chapter 21 in the* Resource Manual.** ✴

****This journal article is available on** thePoint *for this chapter.*

Part 4

DESIGNING AND CONDUCTING QUALITATIVE STUDIES TO GENERATE EVIDENCE FOR NURSING

22 | Qualitative Research Design and Approaches

THE DESIGN OF QUALITATIVE STUDIES

Quantitative researchers specify a research design before collecting their data and rarely depart from that design once the study is underway. In qualitative research, by contrast, the design typically evolves over the course of the study. Qualitative researchers use an **emergent design** that takes shape as they make ongoing decisions reflecting what they have already learned. An emergent design is a reflection of the researchers' desire to have the inquiry based on participants' realities and viewpoints, which are unknown at the outset (Lincoln & Guba, 1985).

Characteristics of Qualitative Research Design

Qualitative inquiry has been used in different disciplines, and each has developed methods for addressing particular types of questions. However, some characteristics of qualitative research design cut across disciplinary boundaries. In general, qualitative design:

- Is flexible, capable of adjusting to new information during data collection;
- Tends to be holistic, aimed at understanding the whole;

- Often involves merging various data collection strategies;
- Requires researchers to become intensely involved; and
- Relies on ongoing analysis of the data to formulate subsequent strategies and to determine when to stop collecting data.

Qualitative researchers often put together a complex array of data, derived from a variety of sources and using a variety of methods. This process has sometimes been described as **bricolage** and the qualitative researcher has been referred to as a *bricoleur*—a person who "is adept at performing diverse tasks, ranging from interviewing to intensive reflection and introspection" (Denzin & Lincoln, 2011, p. 5).

Qualitative Design and Planning

Although design decisions are not prespecified, qualitative researchers typically do advance planning to support an emergent design. Planning is especially useful with regard to the following:

- Selecting a broad inquiry framework or tradition (described in the next section) to guide design decisions
- Determining the maximum amount of time available for the study, given costs and other constraints

- Developing a broad data collection strategy and identifying opportunities for enhancing trustworthiness (e.g., through triangulation)
- Collecting relevant site materials (e.g., maps, organizational charts, resource directories)
- Identifying the types of equipment needed for collecting data (e.g., audio recording equipment, computer tablets)
- Identifying personal biases, views, and presuppositions vis-à-vis the phenomenon, as well as ideological stances (reflexivity)

Thus, qualitative researchers need to plan for a variety of circumstances, but decisions about how to deal with them must be resolved when the social context is better understood. By allowing for and anticipating an evolution of strategies, qualitative researchers seek to make their research design responsive to the situation and to the phenomenon under study.

Qualitative Design Features

In Chapter 8, we discussed various features of research design, three of which are relevant to qualitative research—comparisons, settings, and timeframes. Here we briefly review these aspects of qualitative design.

Qualitative researchers seldom explicitly plan a comparative study (e.g., comparing children who have or do not have cancer). Nevertheless, patterns emerging in the data often suggest that certain comparisons are relevant and illuminating. Indeed, as Morse (2004) noted in an editorial in *Qualitative Health Research*, "All description requires comparisons" (p. 1323). Inevitably in categorizing qualitative information and evaluating whether categories are saturated, there is a need to compare "this" to "that." Morse pointed out that qualitative comparisons are often not dichotomous: "life is usually on a continuum" (p. 1324). Of course, comparisons sometimes *are* planned in qualitative studies (e.g., a comparison of nurses' and patients' perspectives about a phenomenon). Moreover, qualitative researchers can sometimes plan for the *possibility* of comparisons by selecting richly diverse people as participants.

Example of Comparisons in a Qualitative Study
Lin and colleagues (2018) conducted in-depth interviews in four hospitals and compared the views of patients with advanced cancer and their oncologists regarding family involvement in conversations about goals of care. Four themes were common to patients and oncologists (e.g., patient–family disagreements), but two additional themes emerged in the patients' data—the effects of cancer on the entire family and the relationship between the oncologist and family members.

In terms of research settings, qualitative researchers usually collect their data in real-world, naturalistic settings. And, whereas quantitative researchers usually strive to collect data in one type of setting to maintain constancy in environmental conditions (e.g., conducting all interviews in participants' homes), qualitative researchers may deliberately strive to study phenomena in a variety of natural contexts.

Regarding timeframes, qualitative research can be either cross-sectional, with one data collection point, or longitudinal, with multiple data collection points over an extended time period, to observe the evolution of some phenomenon. Sometimes qualitative researchers plan for a longitudinal design, but sometimes a decision to study a phenomenon longitudinally may be made after preliminary analysis of the data.

Example of a Longitudinal Qualitative Study
Armuand and an interprofessional team (2018) conducted an in-depth longitudinal study to explore how men and women experience the threat of infertility resulting from cancer treatment. Nine women and seven men were interviewed after initiation of treatment and then 2 years later.

Causality and Qualitative Research

The issue of causality, which has been controversial throughout the history of science, is especially contentious in qualitative research. Some qualitative researchers think that causality is not an appropriate construct within the constructivist paradigm.

Lincoln and Guba (1985) devoted a chapter of their book to a critique of causality and argued that it should be replaced with a concept they called *mutual shaping*. According to their view of mutual and simultaneous shaping, "Everything influences everything else, in the here and now. Many elements are implicated in any given action, and each element interacts with all of the others in ways that change them all while simultaneously resulting in something that we…label as outcomes or effects" (p. 151).

Others, however, believe that causal explanation is not only a legitimate pursuit in qualitative research, but also that qualitative methods are especially well-suited to understanding causal relationships. For example, Maxwell (2012) argued that qualitative research is important for causal explanations, noting that they "depend on the in-depth understanding of meanings, contexts, and processes that qualitative research can provide" (p. 655).

In attempting to not only describe but to explain phenomena, qualitative researchers who undertake in-depth studies will inevitably reveal patterns and processes suggesting causal interpretations. These interpretations can be subjected to more systematic testing using more controlled methods of inquiry.

Overview of Qualitative Research Traditions

Despite some features common to many qualitative designs, a variety of approaches can be taken— but there is no agreed-upon classification system for these approaches. One system is to categorize qualitative research according to disciplinary traditions. These traditions (or *inquiry frameworks*) vary in their conceptualization of the types of questions that are important and the methods considered appropriate for answering them.

The research traditions and frameworks that have provided a theoretical underpinning for qualitative studies in healthcare fields come from such disciplines as anthropology, psychology, and sociology. As shown in Table 22.1, each discipline has focused on one or two broad domains of inquiry. Researchers in each tradition have developed

methodologic strategies for the design and conduct of relevant studies. Thus, once a researcher has identified what aspect of the human experience is of greatest interest, there is typically a wealth of advice available about methods likely to be productive in designing and undertaking the study.

In this chapter, we focus particular attention on the traditions that have inspired many nurse researchers—ethnography, phenomenology, and grounded theory. The Supplement to this chapter on thePoint provides brief descriptions of other traditions and discusses secondary analyses of qualitative datasets. 🅢

TIP Sometimes a research report identifies more than one tradition as the framework for a qualitative inquiry (e.g., a phenomenologic study using grounded theory methods). Such "method slurring" (Baker et al., 1992) has been criticized because each research tradition has different intellectual assumptions and methodologic guidelines. However, as noted by Nepal (2010), echoing some of the sentiments expressed in an editorial by Janice Morse (2009), mixed qualitative methods may be viable when "the researcher has ascertained, from the beginning…, that the research questions cannot be answered in their entirety unless and until there are two different qualitative methods used" (p. 281).

ETHNOGRAPHY

Ethnography, the research tradition of anthropologists, involves the description and interpretation of cultural behavior. Ethnographies are a blend of a process and a product—fieldwork and written text. Fieldwork is how the ethnographer comes to understand a culture, and the ethnographic text is how that culture is communicated and portrayed. Because *culture* is not visible or tangible, it must be constructed through ethnographic writing. Culture is inferred from the words, actions, and products of members of a group.

Ethnographic research is sometimes concerned with broadly defined cultures (e.g., a Nigerian village culture) in a **macroethnography.** Ethnographies often focus on more narrowly defined cultures in a **microethnography** or **focused ethnography** (Cruz

TABLE 22.1 • Overview of Qualitative Research Traditions

DISCIPLINE	DOMAIN	RESEARCH TRADITION/INQUIRY FRAMEWORK	AREA OF INQUIRY
Anthropology	Culture	Ethnography	Holistic view of culture
		Ethnoscience (cognitive anthropology)[a]	Mapping of the cognitive world of a culture; a culture's shared meanings, semantic rules
Psychology/ philosophy	Lived experience	Phenomenology	Experiences of individuals within their lifeworld
		Hermeneutics	Interpretations and meanings of individuals' experiences
		Phenomenography	Differences in the ways in which people experience or think about a phenomenon
Psychology	Behavior	Ethology[a]	Behavior observed over time in natural context
		Ecological psychology[a]	Behavior as influenced by the environment
Sociology	Social settings and interactions	Grounded theory	Social structural processes within a social setting
		Ethnomethodology[a]	Manner by which shared agreement is achieved in social settings
		Semiotics[a]	Manner by which people make sense of social interactions
Sociolinguistics	Human communication	Discourse analysis[a]	Forms and rules of conversation
History	Past behavior, events, and conditions	Historical research[a]	Description and interpretation of historical events

[a]Brief descriptions of these frameworks are included in the Supplement to this chapter on thePoint. **S**

& Higginbottom, 2013). Microethnographies are fine-grained studies of either small units in a group or culture (e.g., the culture of homeless shelters), or of specific activities in an organizational unit (e.g., how nurses communicate with children in an emergency department). An underlying assumption of the ethnographer is that every human group eventually evolves a culture that guides the members' view of the world and the way they structure their experiences.

Example of a Focused Ethnography

Wright and colleagues (2018) conducted a focused ethnography to explore how midwives in antenatal clinics in South Australia organize their antenatal care consultations with pregnant women.

Ethnographers seek to learn from members of a cultural group—to understand their world view. Ethnographic researchers sometimes refer to "emic" and "etic" perspectives (terms from linguistics—phon*emic* versus phon*etic*). An **emic perspective** is the way members of a culture envision their world—the insiders' view. The emic is the local language, concepts, or means of expression used by members of the group under study to characterize their experiences. The **etic perspective** is the outsiders' interpretation of the experiences of that culture; it is the language used by those doing the research to refer to the same phenomena. Ethnographers strive to acquire an emic perspective of a culture. Moreover, they strive to reveal **tacit knowledge** about the culture that is so deeply embedded in cultural experiences that members do not talk about it or may not even be consciously aware of it.

Ethnographic research typically is labor-intensive, requiring long periods (months or even years) in the field. The study of a culture requires a certain level of intimacy with members of the cultural group, and such intimacy can only be developed over time. The concept of *researcher as instrument* is frequently used by anthropologists to describe the significant role ethnographers play in analyzing and interpreting a culture.

Three types of information usually are sought by ethnographers: cultural behavior (what members of the culture do), cultural artifacts (what people make and use), and cultural speech (what people say). This implies that ethnographers rely on a variety of data sources, including observations, in-depth interviews, records, and physical evidence such as photographs and diaries. Ethnographers often use a **participant observation** strategy in which they make observations of the culture while participating in its activities. Ethnographers observe people day after day in their natural environments to observe behavior in an array of circumstances. Ethnographers also enlist the help of **key informants** to help them understand and interpret the activities being observed.

Some ethnographers undertake an **egocentric network analysis**, which focuses on patterns of relationships and networks of individuals. Each person has his or her own network of relationships that are presumed to contribute to the person's behaviors and attitudes. In studying these networks, researchers develop lists of a person's network members (called *alters*) and seek to understand the scope and nature of interrelationships. Network data from such efforts are often quantified and analyzed statistically. Egocentric network analysis is used to understand features of personal networks and has been used to explain such phenomena as longevity, coping with crisis, and risk taking.

Example of an Egocentric Network Analysis
Using an egocentric network analysis, Crotty and colleagues (2015) studied the service and social support networks of people with mental illness and type 2 diabetes. Participants identified small social networks with few friendship ties.

The product of ethnographic research usually is a rich, holistic description and interpretation of the culture. Among healthcare researchers, ethnography provides access to the health beliefs and practices of a culture. Ethnographic inquiry can thus help to facilitate understanding of behaviors affecting health and illness.

In addition to written reports, ethnographers have recently used their research as the basis for performance ethnographies. **A performance ethnography** has been described as a scripted and staged reenactment of ethnographically derived notes that reflect an interpretation of the culture. Smith and Gallo (2007) have described how applications of performance ethnography can be used in nursing.

A rich array of ethnographic methods has been developed and cannot be fully described in this general textbook. More information may be found in Fetterman (2010) and LeCompte and Schensul (2010). Three variants of ethnographic research (ethnonursing research, institutional ethnography, and autoethnography) are described here, and a fourth (critical ethnography) is described later in this chapter.

Ethnonursing Research

Many nurse researchers have undertaken ethnographies. Leininger coined the phrase **ethnonursing research**, which she defined as "the study and analysis of the local or indigenous people's viewpoints, beliefs, and practices about nursing care behavior and processes of designated cultures" (1985, p. 38). In conducting an ethnonursing study, investigators use a broad theoretical framework to guide the research, such as Leininger's Theory of Culture Care Diversity and Universality (Leininger and McFarland, 2006; McFarland & Wehbe-Alamah, 2015).

McFarland and Wehbe-Alamah (2015) described several enablers to support researchers' efforts in conducting ethnonursing research. *Enablers* are ways to discover complex phenomena like human care. Two of the enablers are the Stranger-Friend Model and the Observation-Participation-Reflection Model. The stranger–friend enabler guides researchers in mapping their progress and becoming aware of their feelings, behaviors, and responses as they transition from a stranger to trusted friend. The phases of Leininger's observation-participation-reflection enabler go from (1) primary observation and active listening, (2) primary observation with limited participation, (3) primary participation with continuing observations, to (4) primary reflection and reconfirmation of results with informants.

Example of an Ethnonursing Study
Pennafort and colleagues (2016) conducted an eth-nonursing study to explore the influence of network and social support in caring for children with type 1 diabetes in Brazil. The researchers used Leininger's observation-participation-reflection model to collect and analyze their data.

Institutional Ethnography

An ethnographic approach called **institutional ethnography** was pioneered by Dorothy Smith, a Canadian sociologist (1999). Institutional ethnography has been used in such fields as nursing, social work, and community health to study the organization of professional services, examined from the perspective of clients or frontline workers. Institutional ethnography seeks to understand the social determinants of people's everyday experiences in institutional settings. The focus is on social organization and institutional processes, and so research findings can play a role in organizational change.

In institutional ethnography, a person's actions in the social world are labeled as "social relations."

Relations of *ruling* occur when social relations involve powerful coordination in people's lives and day-to-day activities. Where individuals are situated in the social location within an institution dictates relations of ruling.

Institutional ethnographers study the complexities of social and ruling relations. Rankin (2013) emphasized that an important step in an institutional ethnography is to decide on a standpoint within the organization of social relations. It is from that standpoint that the researcher studies how activities are socially organized. The research question focuses on "how does it happen?"

Example of Institutional Ethnography
MacKinnon and colleagues (2018) conducted an institutional ethnography to study the work experiences and interrelationships of nurses and LPNs working on redesigned care delivery teams in Canada.

TIP A relatively new approach, called **video-reflexive ethnography** (VRE), is gaining in popularity in healthcare settings. VRE is a collaborative visual method used by healthcare professionals to understand and interpret healthcare professionals' work practices and patient experiences (Carroll & Mesman, 2018).

Autoethnography

Ethnographers are often "outsiders" to the culture under study. A type of ethnography that involves self-scrutiny (including the study of groups or cultures to which researchers belong) is **autoethnography** (sometimes called *insider research* or *peer research*). Autoethnography offers numerous advantages, the most obvious being ease of access and recruitment and the ability to obtain candid, in-depth data based on preestablished trust and rapport. Another potential advantage is the researcher's ability to detect subtle nuances that an outsider might miss or take months to uncover. A potential limitation, however, is the researcher's inability to be objective about group (or self) processes, which can result in unsuspected myopia about important but sensitive issues. Autoethnography requires researchers to maintain consciousness of their role and monitor their internal state and their interactions with others during the study.

Chang (2016) noted that successful autoethnographies need to provide not only a rich description of personal experiences but also a "sociocultural interpretation of such experiences" (p. 443). Chang recommends that autoethnographers ask themselves five evaluative questions, such as whether the autoethnography uses authentic data. (A list of Chang's five questions is presented in the Toolkit for this chapter in the *Resource Manual* ⊗.) Ellis and Bochner (2000) suggest methodologic strategies for autoethnographic work. Peterson (2015) has argued for greater use of autoethnography in nursing research.

Example of an Autoethnography
Eileen and colleagues (2017) described an autoethnography that explored the experience of nurses working in a medical school in New Zealand—which they characterized as "crossing professional cultures."

PHENOMENOLOGY

Phenomenology, rooted in a philosophical tradition developed by Husserl and Heidegger, is an approach to understanding people's everyday life experiences. Phenomenologic researchers ask: What is the *essence* of this phenomenon as experienced by these people and what does it *mean?* Phenomenologists assume there is an *essence*—an essential invariant structure—that can be understood, in much the same way that ethnographers assume that cultures exist. Essence is what makes a phenomenon what it is, and without which it would not be what it is. Phenomenologists investigate subjective phenomena in the belief that critical truths about reality are grounded in people's lived experiences. The phenomenologic approach is especially useful when a phenomenon has been poorly defined.

Phenomenologists believe that lived experience gives meaning to each person's perception of a phenomenon. The goal of phenomenologic inquiry is to understand lived experience and the perceptions to which it gives rise. Four aspects of lived experience of interest to phenomenologists are *lived space*, or spatiality; *lived body*, or corporeality; *lived time*, or temporality; and *lived human relation*, or relationality.

Phenomenologists view human existence as meaningful and interesting because of people's consciousness of that existence. The phrase **being-in-the-world** (or *embodiment*) is a concept that acknowledges people's physical ties to their world—they think, see, hear, feel, and are conscious through their bodies' interaction with the world.

In phenomenologic studies, in-depth conversations are the main data source, with researchers and informants as coparticipants. Through in-depth conversations, researchers strive to gain entrance into the informants' world, to have full access to their experiences as lived. Multiple interviews or conversations are sometimes needed. Typically, phenomenologic studies involve a small number of study participants—often fewer than 15. For some phenomenologic researchers, the inquiry includes not only gathering information from informants but also efforts to experience the phenomenon through participation, observation, and introspective reflection.

TIP The notion that "insider research" can be a useful strategy in phenomenologic inquiries has emerged recently. Johnston and colleagues (2017) have described methodologic considerations relating to nurse researchers using their own experience of a phenomenon within a phenomenologic study.

Phenomenologists share their insights in rich, vivid reports. A phenomenologic text describing study results should help readers "see" something in a way that enriches their understanding of an experience. van Manen (1997) warned that if a phenomenologic text is flat and boring, it "loses power to break through the taken-for-granted dimensions of everyday life" (p. 346). A wealth of resources on phenomenologic methods is available, including such classic sources as Giorgi (2009), Colaizzi (1973), or van Manen (1990, 2014).

There are several variants and methodologic interpretations of phenomenology. The two main schools of thought are descriptive phenomenology and interpretive phenomenology (hermeneutics). Lopez and Willis (2004) and Matua and Van Der Wal (2015) provide useful discussions about the need to differentiate the two in nursing.

Descriptive Phenomenology

Descriptive phenomenology was developed by Husserl (1962), who was primarily interested in the question: What do we know as persons? His philosophy emphasized descriptions of human experience. Descriptive phenomenologists insist on the careful description of ordinary conscious experience of everyday life—a description of "things" as people experience them. These "things" include hearing, seeing, believing, feeling, remembering, deciding, evaluating, and acting. Two acts are key to Husserl's philosophical approach: bracketing (also called *epoché*) and reduction. **Bracketing** is the process of identifying and holding in abeyance preconceived beliefs and opinions about the phenomenon under study. Bracketing helps to remove influences that can block access to the meaning of a phenomenon. Phenomenologic **reduction** is a meditative and liberating practice wherein the phenomenologist attains a more attentive openness by constantly questioning the meaning of an experience.

Descriptive phenomenologic studies often involve the following four general steps: bracketing, intuiting, analyzing, and describing. Bracketing can never be achieved totally, but researchers strive to bracket out the world and any presuppositions in an effort to confront the data in pure form. Bracketing is an iterative process that involves preparing, evaluating, and providing systematic ongoing feedback about the effectiveness of the bracketing. Phenomenologic researchers (as well as other qualitative researchers) often maintain a **reflexive journal** in their efforts to bracket. Ahern (1999) provided 10 tips to help qualitative researchers with bracketing through notes in a reflexive journal:

1. Make note of interests that, as a researcher, you may take for granted.
2. Clarify your personal values and identify areas in which you know you are biased.
3. Identify areas of possible role conflict.

4. Recognize gatekeepers' interest and make note of the degree to which they are favorably or unfavorably disposed toward your research.
5. Identify any feelings you have that may indicate a lack of neutrality.
6. Describe new or surprising findings in collecting and analyzing data.
7. Reflect on and profit from methodologic problems that occur during your research.
8. Even after data analysis is complete, reflect on how you write up your findings.
9. Reflect on whether the literature review is truly supporting your findings, or whether it is expressing the similar cultural background that you have.
10. Consider whether you can address any bias in your data collection or analysis by interviewing a participant a second time or reanalyzing the transcript in question.

Intuiting, the second step in descriptive phenomenology, occurs when researchers remain open to the meanings attributed to the phenomenon by those who have experienced it. Phenomenologic researchers then proceed to the analysis phase (i.e., extracting significant statements, categorizing, and making sense of the essential meanings of the phenomenon), as we describe in Chapter 25. Finally, the descriptive phase occurs when researchers come to understand and define the phenomenon.

> **TIP** Descriptive phenomenology is often called the *Duquesne School* of phenomenology, named for three psychology professors who developed descriptive phenomenologic methods at Duquesne University—Colaizzi, Giorgi, and van Kaam.

Example of a Descriptive Phenomenologic Study
Leyva-Moral and colleagues (2019) used a descriptive phenomenologic approach to study the experience of growing old while living with HIV in Spain.

Interpretive Phenomenology and Hermeneutics

Nurse researchers have also used methods that can be described as interpretive phenomenology, which encompasses several approaches to inquiry.

Heideggerian Hermeneutics

Heidegger, a student of Husserl, moved away from his professor's philosophy into **interpretive phenomenology (hermeneutics)**. To Heidegger (1962), the critical question is: What is *being*? He stressed interpreting and understanding—not just describing—human experience. His premise is that the lived experience is inherently an interpretive process. Heidegger argued that hermeneutics is a basic characteristic of human existence. Indeed, the term hermeneutics refers to the art and philosophy of interpreting the meaning of an object (such as a *text*, work of art, and so on). The goals of interpretive phenomenologic research are to enter another's world and to discover the practical wisdom, possibilities, and understandings found there.

Gadamer (1976), another influential phenomenologist, described the interpretive process as a circular relationship known as the **hermeneutic circle** where one understands the whole of a text (for example, a transcribed interview) in terms of its parts and the parts in terms of the whole. In his view, researchers enter into a dialogue with the text and continually question its meaning.

Interpretive phenomenologists, like descriptive phenomenologists, rely primarily on in-depth interviews with individuals who have experienced the phenomenon of interest, but they may go beyond a traditional approach to gathering and analyzing data. For example, interpretive phenomenologists sometimes augment their understandings of the phenomenon through an analysis of supplementary texts, such as novels, poetry, or other artistic expressions—or they use such materials in their conversations with study participants.

In an interpretive phenomenologic study, bracketing does not necessarily occur. For Heidegger, it was impossible to bracket one's being-in-the-world. Hermeneutics presupposes prior understanding on the part of the researcher. Gearing (2004) described *reflexive bracketing*—in which researchers attempt to identify internal suppositions to facilitate greater transparency, but without bracketing them out—as a tool for hermeneutical inquiry. Interpretive phenomenologists ideally approach each interview text with openness—they must be open to hearing what the text is saying. As Heidegger (1971) stated, "We

never come to thoughts. They come to us" (p. 6). Guidance in undertaking a hermeneutic phenomenologic nursing study is offered by Cohen and colleagues (2000); analytic methods for hermeneutic inquiry that were developed by nurse researchers (Benner, 1994; Dieckelmann et al., 1989) are described in Chapter 25.

> **Example of a Hermeneutic Study**
> Harris and colleagues (2018) used a hermeneutic approach in their study that explored the meaning of living with uncertainty for people diagnosed with motor neurone disease (MND). An interpretive analysis of in-depth interviews with four people with MND revealed an illness trajectory that was tied to uncertainty.

The Utrecht School of Phenomenology

Another approach comes from the *Utrecht School* in the Netherlands. The Utrecht School incorporates components of both descriptive and interpretive phenomenology. Influenced by the Utrecht school, van Manen (1990) noted that "Hermeneutic phenomenology tries to be attentive to both terms of its methodology: it is a descriptive (phenomenologic) methodology because it wants to be attentive to how things appear, it wants to let things speak for themselves; it is an interpretive (hermeneutic) methodology because (of) its claim that there are no such things as uninterpreted phenomena" (p. 180). For van Manen (2017), phenomenology is a science of examples: examples are reflected on to discover exemplary aspects of the meaning of a phenomenon. We discuss van Manen's methods in greater detail in Chapter 25.

Interpretive Phenomenologic Analysis (IPA)

In some recent studies, nurse researchers have cited the work of a group of psychological phenomenologists, who have described an approach called **interpretive phenomenologic analysis** or **IPA** (Smith, Flowers, & Larkin, 2009). The focus of IPA is on the subjective experiences of persons—their *lifeworld*. Studying individuals' experiences requires interpretation on the part of the researcher and the participant because it is not possible to directly access a person's lifeworld. There are three key principles to IPA: (1) it investigates the phenomenon of experience of a person, (2) it requires intense interpretation and engagement with the data obtained from the person, and (3) it is examined in detail.

Example of Interpretive Phenomenologic Analysis

Liu and Chiang (2017) used IPA to explore how end-of-life nurses in Taiwan interpret their care experience and how they transform their experience and mindset.

Reflective Lifeworld Research (RLR)

A nurse researcher and colleagues in Sweden (Dahlberg et al., 2008) have created another approach that combines descriptive and interpretive phenomenology, called **reflective lifeworld research** (RLR). Lifeworlds can be reached through an open attitude, which requires sensitivity toward the things being studied. Dahlberg and colleagues use the term *bridling* rather than *bracketing* to describe having an open and respectful attitude that permits the phenomenon being studied to present itself. Their view is that *bracketing* points backwards, as the researcher's energy is focused on restraining preunderstanding. A goal of RLR is to enable a reflection on taken-for-granted assumptions so that the phenomenon being studied can show itself more fully. "The understanding process is…slowed down in order to let new and surprising meanings arise that otherwise might have been clouded by the researcher's own preunderstandings or established meanings of the phenomenon" (Dahlberg et al., 2016, pp. 3–4).

Example of Reflective Lifeworld Research

In their study of the lived experiences of hospital stays for patients undergoing urgent ostomy services, Herlufsen and Brødgaard (2017) were guided by the reflective lifeworld research approach.

The Parse Phenomenologic-Hermeneutic Research Method

Some nurse researchers use approaches that have been formulated by Rosemarie Rizzo Parse (2014) based on her Humanbecoming Paradigm. Parse's

methods have been evolving. Most recently, she has proposed two modes of inquiry under this paradigm: humanbecoming hermeneutic sciencing (Parse 2016a) and Parsesciencing (2016b).

In **humanbecoming hermeneutic sciencing**, the researcher's aim is to uncover emergent meanings of universal living experiences that are expressed in published texts and artforms. It consists of three phases: discoursing with penetrating engaging, interpreting with quiescent beholding, and understanding with inspiring envisaging. Parse acknowledges that "yet there remains a knowing that the vessel of inquiry can never be filled. There is always the veil of mystery, the barely seen" (Parse, 2016a, p. 129).

Parse's (2016b) second mode of inquiry is **Parsesciencing**, which she describes as "coming to know the meanings of universal humanuniverse living experiences" (p. 271). Parsesciencing consists of dialoging-engaging, distilling-fusing, and heuristic interpreting. Using these three phases, the researcher's purpose is to discover universal humanuniverse living experiences through descriptions from "historians"—the individuals who agree to describe their experiences. Data are gathered in the first phase through dialoging-engaging, which are not interviews per se, but rather unique dialogues in which the researcher is a true presence with participants who are asked to talk about the experience being studied. In the next phases, the researcher dwells with the descriptions and strives to attain higher levels of abstraction.

Example of Parse's Phenomenologic Method

Doucet (2018) used Parse's method to investigate the living experience of feeling peaceful. Through engagement with 12 participants living in a community, the researcher identified the structure: feeling peaceful is contentedness amid tribulation.

Phenomenography

Phenomenography is another approach to studying how phenomena are conceived and understood. An important assumption in phenomenography is that people differ in terms of how they experience the world, but differences can be described and understood by others. Phenomenographers distinguish between first-order perspectives—what the essence of something really is, that is, the actual phenomenon—and second-order perspectives—how a phenomenon is perceived and conceptualized. The second-order perspective is the focus of phenomenography. In a phenomenographic study, researchers strive to understand the qualitatively different ways in which people experience a phenomenon or think about it. In analyzing their data, phenomenographers sort perceptions emerging from the data into categories of description. The categories, which are logically related to one another, become the phenomenographic essence of the phenomenon. A good resource for learning more about phenomenography is the book by Marton and Booth (1997).

Example of a Phenomenographic Study
Svensson and Wåhlin (2018) undertook a phenomenographic study of patients' perceptions of what it is like to be cared for by a specialized palliative care team in home-based palliative care. The researchers interviewed 14 patients receiving such care and identified four categories of description (e.g., "It is safe to receive care at home").

GROUNDED THEORY

Grounded theory has contributed to the development of many middle-range nursing theories. Grounded theory was formulated in the 1960s as a systematic method of qualitative inquiry by two sociologists, Glaser and Strauss (1967).

Grounded theory tries to account for actions in a substantive area from the perspective of those involved. Grounded theory researchers seek to understand actions by focusing on the main concern or problem that the individuals' behavior is designed to address (Glaser, 1998). The manner in which people resolve this main concern is called the **core variable**. One type of core variable is called a **basic social process (BSP)**. The goal of grounded theory is to discover this main concern and the basic social process that explains how people continually resolve it. The main concern must be discovered from the data.

Conceptualization is a key aspect of grounded theory (Glaser, 2003). Grounded theory researchers generate conceptual categories and their properties and integrate them into a substantive theory grounded in the data. Through this conceptual process, the generated grounded theory represents an abstraction based on participants' actions and their meanings. The grounded theorist uncovers and names latent patterns (categories) from the participants' accounts. Glaser emphasized that concepts transcend time, place, and person. "In grounded theory, behavior is a pattern that a person engages in; it is not the person. People are not categorized, behavior is" (p. 53).

Grounded theory methods constitute an entire approach to the conduct of field research. For example, a study that follows Glaser and Strauss's method does not begin with a focused research problem; the problem emerges from the data. In a grounded theory study, both the problem and the process used to resolve it are discovered.

A fundamental feature of grounded theory research is that data collection, data analysis, and sampling of participants occur simultaneously. The grounded theory process is recursive: researchers collect data, categorize them, describe the emerging central phenomenon, and then recycle earlier steps. In-depth interviews and observation are the most common data sources in grounded theory studies, but other data sources such as documents may also be used.

A procedure called **constant comparison** is used to develop and refine theoretically relevant categories. Categories elicited from the data are constantly compared with data obtained earlier so that commonalities and variations can be determined. As data collection proceeds, the inquiry becomes increasingly focused on emerging theoretical concerns.

Example of a Grounded Theory Study
Uengwongsapat and colleagues (2018) used Glaser's approach to grounded theory to explore the process of Thai adolescents becoming first-time fathers with an unplanned pregnancy. "Growing into teen fatherhood" emerged as the basic social process by which the fathers transitioned into the fatherhood role through many conflicts and challenges.

Like most theories, a grounded theory is modifiable as the researcher (or other researchers) collects new data. Modification is an ongoing process and is the method by which theoretical completeness is enhanced (Glaser, 2001). As more data are found and more qualitative studies are published in the substantive area, the grounded theory can be modified to accommodate new or different dimensions.

Example of a Modification of a Grounded Theory Study

Beck (2012) modified her 1993 grounded theory study, "Teetering on the Edge," which was a substantive theory of postpartum depression. After Beck's original study had been conducted, 27 additional qualitative studies of postpartum depression in women from other cultures had been published. The results from these 27 transcultural studies were compared with the findings from the original grounded theory. Maximizing differences among comparative groups is a powerful method for enhancing theoretical properties and extending the theory.

TIP Glaser and Strauss (1967) distinguished two types of grounded theory: substantive and formal. **Substantive theory** is grounded in data on a specific substantive area, such as postpartum depression. It can serve as a springboard for **formal grounded theory**, which is at a higher level of conceptualization and is abstract of time, place, and persons. The goal of formal grounded theory is not to discover a new core variable but to develop a theory that goes beyond the substantive grounded theory and extends the general implications of the core variable.

Alternate Views of Grounded Theory: Strauss and Corbin

In 1990, Strauss and Corbin published what was to become a controversial book, *Basics of Qualitative Research: Grounded Theory Procedures and Techniques*. The authors stated that the book's purpose was to provide beginning grounded theory researchers with basic procedures involved for building theory at the substantive level.

Glaser, however, disagreed with some of the procedures advocated by Strauss (his original coauthor) and Corbin (a nurse researcher). Glaser published a rebuttal in 1992, *Emergence versus Forcing: Basics of Grounded Theory Analysis.* Glaser believed that Strauss and Corbin developed a method that is not grounded theory but rather what he called "full conceptual description." According to Glaser, the purpose of grounded theory is to generate concepts and theories about their relationships that explain, account for, and interpret variation in behavior in the substantive area under study. *Conceptual description*, in contrast, is aimed at describing the full range of behavior of what is occurring in the substantive area, "irrespective of relevance and accounting for variation in behavior" (Glaser, 1992, p. 19). In their latest edition, Corbin and Strauss (2015) stated that their method reflects Strauss' approach to doing grounded theory which is based on the philosophies of pragmatism and interactionism.

Nurse researchers have conducted grounded theory studies using both the original Glaser and Strauss and the Strauss and Corbin approaches. Heath and Cowley (2004) provide a comparison of the two approaches. We describe analytic differences in Chapter 25.

Example of Strauss and Corbin's Grounded Theory Methods

Milhomme and colleagues (2018) used Corbin and Strauss' grounded theory approach in their effort to explain the surveillance process that expert nurses employ in critical care.

Constructivist Grounded Theory: Charmaz

Strauss and Glaser had different training and backgrounds. Strauss, trained at the University of Chicago, had a background in symbolic interaction and pragmatist philosophy. Glaser, by contrast, came from a tradition of positivism and quantitative methods at Columbia University. In one of Glaser's (2005) later publications, in which he discussed the takeover of grounded theory by symbolic interaction, he argued that "grounded theory is a general inductive method possessed by no discipline or theoretical perspective or data type" (p. 141).

In recent years, an approach called **constructivist grounded theory** has emerged. A leading advocate is sociologist Kathy Charmaz, who has sought to bring the Chicago School antecedents of grounded theory into the forefront again. She has called for returning to the pragmatist foundation which "assumes that interaction is inherently dynamic and interpretive and addresses how people create, enact, and change meanings and actions" (Charmaz, 2014, p. 9). Charmaz views Glaser and Strauss' (and Strauss and Corbin's) versions of grounded theory as being based in the positivist tradition. Her position is that what is missing from their objective grounded theory method is the researcher's influence on the data collected and analyzed, and interactions between the researcher and participants.

Charmaz uses the term, constructivist, "to acknowledge subjectivity and the researcher's involvement in the construction and interpretation of data" (2014, p.14). In her approach, the developed grounded theory is seen as an interpretation. The analyzed data are acknowledged to be constructed from shared experiences and relationships between the researcher and the participants. Charmaz's view is that "we start with the assumption that social reality is multiple, processual, and constructed, then we must take the researcher's position, privileges, perspective, and interactions into account as an inherent part of the research reality (p. 13). Reflexivity of both the researcher's own interpretations and the interpretations of the participants is important. Higginbottom and Lauridsen (2014) have described how Charmaz's approach is similar to and different from original grounded theory.

Example of a Constructivist Grounded Theory

Butler and colleagues (2019) used constructivist grounded theory methods to explore the influence on the pediatric intensive care environment on parent–healthcare provider relationship when a child dies in the PICU. The researchers found that the PICU environment either welcomes parents of dying children into the care team or demotes them to the status of a "watcher."

> **TIP** Beginning qualitative researchers should be aware that a grounded theory study is a lengthier and more complex process than a phenomenologic study. This may be important to consider if there are constraints in the amount of time you can devote to a study.

OTHER TYPES OF QUALITATIVE RESEARCH

Qualitative studies often can be characterized in terms of the disciplinary research traditions discussed in the previous section. However, several other important types of qualitative research also deserve mention. This section discusses qualitative research that is not associated with any particular discipline.

Case Studies

Case studies are in-depth investigations of a single entity (or small number of entities), which could be an individual, family, institution, community, or other social unit. In a case study, researchers obtain a wealth of descriptive information and may examine relationships among different phenomena or may examine trends over time. Case study researchers attempt to analyze and understand issues that are important to the history, development, or circumstances of the entity under study.

One way to think of a case study is to consider what is at center stage. In most studies, whether qualitative or quantitative, a certain phenomenon or variable (or set of variables) is the core of the inquiry. In a case study, the *case* itself is central. As befits an intensive analysis, the focus of case studies is typically on understanding *why* a person thinks, behaves, or develops in a particular manner rather than on *what* his or her status, progress, or actions are. It is not unusual for probing research of this type to require detailed study over a considerable period. Data are often collected that relate not only to the person's present state but also to past experiences and situational factors relevant to the problem being examined.

Yin (2018) has described several designs for case studies. A **single case study** is an appropriate design when (1) it is a critical case in testing a well-formulated theory, (2) it represents an extreme or unique case, (3) it is a representative or typical case, (4) it is a revelatory case, or (5) it is a longitudinal case. A **multiple case design** is a study that involves more than one case. Single and multiple case studies can be either holistic or embedded. In a **holistic design**, the global nature of a case—be it an individual, community, or organization—is examined. An **embedded design** involves multiple units of analysis. A wide variety of data can be used in case studies, including data from interviews, observations, documents, and artifacts.

A distinction is sometimes drawn between an intrinsic and instrumental case study. In an *intrinsic case study*, researchers do not have to select the case. For instance, a process evaluation of implementing an innovation is often a case study of a particular program or institution; the "case" is a given. In an *instrumental case study*, researchers begin with a research question or problem and seek a case that offers illumination. The aim is to use the case to understand a phenomenon of interest. In such a situation, a case is usually selected not because it is typical but rather because it can maximize what can be learned about the phenomenon.

Although understanding a particular case is the central concern of case studies, they are sometimes a useful way to explore phenomena that have not been rigorously researched. The information obtained in case studies can be used to develop hypotheses to be tested more rigorously in subsequent research. The intensive probing that characterizes case studies often leads to insights concerning previously unsuspected relationships. Furthermore, case studies may serve the important role of clarifying concepts or of elucidating ways to capture them.

TIP Case study research is not a distinct methodology (Sandelowski, 2011). Many ethnographies focus on a specific "case," as do many historical studies. Although case studies typically involve the collection of in-depth qualitative information, some case studies are quantitative and use statistical methods to analyze data. And some case studies used mixed methods (i.e., both qualitative and quantitative approaches).

The greatest strength of case studies is the depth that is possible when a limited number of individuals, institutions, or groups are being investigated. Case studies provide researchers with opportunities of having an intimate knowledge of a person's condition, thoughts, actions (past and present), intentions, and environment. On the other hand, this same strength is a potential weakness because researchers' familiarity with the person or group may make objectivity difficult. Perhaps the biggest concern about case studies is generalizability: If researchers discover important relationships, it is difficult to know whether the same relationships would occur with others. However, case studies can play a role in challenging generalizations based on other types of research.

It is important to recognize that case study *research* is not simply anecdotal descriptions of a particular incident or patient, such as a case report. Case study research is a disciplined process and typically requires a long period of data collection. The writings of Yin (2018) and Baxter and Jack (2008) are good resources for learning more about case study research.

Example of a Case Study
Goicolea and colleagues (2019) used a multiple embedded case study of four primary healthcare teams in Spain to learn how team-level conditions influence the healthcare professionals' responses to intimate partner violence.

Narrative Analyses

Narrative analysis focuses on *story* as the object of inquiry, to examine how individuals make sense of events in their lives. Narratives are viewed as a type of "cultural envelope" into which people pour their experiences (Riessman, 1991). What distinguishes narrative analysis from other types of qualitative research designs is its focus on the broad contours of a narrative; stories are not fractured and dissected. The broad underlying premise of narrative research is that people most effectively make sense of their world—and communicate these meanings—by constructing, reconstructing, and narrating stories. Individuals construct stories when they wish to understand specific events and situations that require linking an inner world of desire and motive to an external world of observable actions. Narrative analysts explore *form* as well as content, asking "Why was the story told that way?" (Riessman, 2008).

A number of approaches can be used to examine stories. One approach is Burke's (1969) **pentadic dramatism**. For Burke, there are five key elements of a story: act, scene, agent, agency, and purpose. Analysis of a story "will offer some kind of answers to these five questions: what was done (act), when or where it was done (scene), who did it (agent), how he did it (agency), and why (purpose)" (p. xv). The five terms of Burke's pentad are meant to be understood paired together as ratios such as, act: agent, act: scene, agent: agency, and purpose: agent. The analysis focuses on the internal relationships and tensions of these five terms to each other. Each pairing in the pentad provides a different way of directing the researcher's attention. What drives the narrative analysis is not just the interaction of the pentadic terms but an imbalance between two or more terms. Bruner (1991) modified Burke's pentad with the addition of a sixth term that he called Trouble. Bruner included this sixth element to provide more focus in narrative analysis on Burke's imbalance between the terms in his pentad.

Example of a Narrative Analysis, Burke's Approach

Tobin, Murphy-Lawless, and Beck (an author of this textbook) (2014) conducted a narrative analysis of asylum-seeking women's experience of childbirth in Ireland. Twenty-two mothers participated in unstructured interviews lasting from 40 minutes to 1½ hours. Burke's pentad of terms was used to analyze these narratives and revealed numerous accounts of scene: agent and act: agency imbalances in the women's experiences. Highlighted in their narratives was the lack of communication, connection, and culturally competent care.

Another approach is that of Riessman (1993, 2008), whose method of thematic narrative analysis involves protecting each story as a whole and not fragmenting them. Each story is analyzed

separately for themes. Then all the stories are compared to identify common themes for a *mega story*. Specific stories can be chosen by the researcher to illustrate common themes. The narrative analyst remains focused on the content of the stories rather than how or why the stories are told. Riessman (1993) described five levels of experience in the research process for narrative analysts:

1. Attending: participants create personal meaning by actively thinking about reality in new ways. Participants reflect and remember their experiences; they compose their own realities.
2. Telling: participants "re-present" the events of an experience. They share the event by recounting characters, significant events, and their interpretation of the experience. The interviewer takes part in the narrative by listening to the story and asking questions (to clarify/further understand the story). As participants tell their story, they are also creating a vision of themselves.
3. Transcribing: participants' stories are typically captured through video or audio recording. The analyst then creates a written narrative representing the conversation.
4. Analyzing: the researcher analyzes each individual transcript. Similarities are noted and a "mega story" is created by defining critical moments within narratives and making meaning out of each story. The analyst also makes decisions about form, order, and style of presentation of the narratives.
5. Reading: the final level of experience in the research process is reading. Drafts are commonly shared with colleagues. The researcher frequently incorporates this editorial feedback into a final report that reflects the researcher's interpretation of the narrative.

Example of a Narrative Analysis Using Riessman's Approach

Hall, Hutson, and West (2018) used Riessman's method of narrative analysis in their study of end-of-life needs of people with HIV or AIDS in rural Appalachia. The study involved the analysis of the stories told by eight men and women, whose narratives were fraught with tensions, contradictions, and paradoxes.

Descriptive Qualitative Studies

Many qualitative studies have a link to one of the research traditions discussed in this chapter. Many other qualitative studies, however, claim no particular disciplinary or methodologic roots. The researchers may simply indicate that they have conducted a qualitative study or a naturalistic inquiry, or they may say that they have done a *content analysis* or a *thematic analysis* of their qualitative data (i.e., an analysis of themes and patterns that emerge in the narrative content). We refer to the many qualitative studies that do not have a formal name as **descriptive qualitative studies**, although they are sometimes called *generic qualitative inquiries* (Patton, 2015).

Sandelowski (2000), in a widely read article, noted that in doing descriptive qualitative studies, researchers tend not to penetrate their data in any interpretive depth. These studies present comprehensive summaries of a phenomenon or of events. Qualitative descriptive designs tend to be eclectic, and they often borrow or adapt methodologic techniques from other qualitative traditions, such as constant comparison.

In a more recent article, Sandelowski (2010) warned researchers not to call their studies *qualitative description* "after the fact to give a name to poorly conceived and conducted studies" (p. 80). She noted that qualitative descriptive studies produce findings closer to the data ("data-near") than studies within such traditions as phenomenology or grounded theory, but that good qualitative descriptions are still interpretive products. She recognized that her 2000 article had provided justification for studies that primarily reproduce raw data and stated that she "never intended to communicate…that qualitative description removes the researcher's obligation to do any analyzing or interpreting at all" (p. 79). Rather than being a distinct methodologic classification, qualitative description is perhaps viewed as a "distributed residual category" (p. 82) that signals a "confederacy" of diverse groups of qualitative researchers.

Example of a Descriptive Qualitative Study
O'Brien and colleagues (2019) undertook a descriptive qualitative study to explore the perceptions of nurses and other healthcare professionals regarding spiritual care and the impact of spiritual care training on their clinical roles.

Sally Thorne (2008) expanded qualitative description into a realm she called **interpretive description**. Her book outlined an approach that extends "beyond mere description and into the domain of the 'so what' that drives all applied disciplines" (p. 33) such as nursing. While acknowledging that her approach is neither novel nor distinctive, Thorne emphasizes the importance of having a disciplinary conceptual frame (such as nursing): "Interpretive description becomes a conceptual maneuver whereby a solid and substantive logic derived from the disciplinary orientation justifies the application of specific techniques and procedures outside of their conventional context" (p. 35). An important thrust of her approach is that it requires integrity of purpose from an actual practice goal and seeks to generate new insights that can help shape applications of qualitative evidence to practice.

Thorne (2013) has acknowledged that she developed interpretive description to free qualitative nurse researchers from the constraints of qualitative methodologies. She noted that "the nursing disciplinary mind never truly accepts standardization; it always seeks to ensure that there is room for necessary variation" (p. 296). Interpretive description holds no attachment to any one qualitative method, but rather it uses the wealth of research techniques available. Thorne offered examples of typical research questions for interpretive description, such as, "What are the common ways in which patients' experience …?" (p. 298).

Example of an Interpretive Descriptive Study
Doull and colleagues (2018) used interpretive description in a study that explored why lesbian and bisexual girls aged 14 to 18 years choose not to use barriers to prevent sexually transmitted infection during female-to-female sex.

RESEARCH WITH IDEOLOGICAL PERSPECTIVES

Some qualitative researchers conduct inquiries within an ideological framework, to focus attention on the problems or needs of certain groups and to effect change. These approaches, which are sometimes described as being within a **transformative paradigm** (Mertens, 2007), are briefly described in this section.

Critical Theory

Critical theory originated with a group of Marxist-oriented German scholars in the 1920s, referred to as the Frankfurt School. A critical researcher is concerned with a critique of society and with envisioning new possibilities.

Critical social science is typically action-oriented. Its broad aim is to integrate theory and practice such that people become aware of disparities and become inspired to change them. Critical researchers reject the idea of an objective, disinterested inquirer and pursue a transformation process. An important feature of critical theory is that it calls for inquiries that foster enlightened self-knowledge and sociopolitical action. Critical theory also involves a self-reflective aspect. To prevent a critical theory of society from becoming yet another self-serving ideology, critical theorists must account for their own transformative effects.

A critical inquiry often begins with a thorough analysis of aspects of a problem. For example, critical researchers might analyze and critique taken-for-granted assumptions that underlie the problem, the language used to depict the situation, or the biases of prior researchers studying the problem. Critical researchers often triangulate multiple methodologies and emphasize multiple perspectives (e.g., alternative racial or social class perspectives) on problems. They typically interact with study participants in ways that emphasize participants' expertise. Some of the features that distinguish more traditional qualitative research and critical research are summarized in Table 22.2.

Critical theory has played an especially important role in ethnography. **Critical ethnography** focuses on raising consciousness and aiding emancipatory goals in the hope of effecting social change. Critical ethnographers address the historical, social, political, and economic dimensions of cultures and their value-laden agendas. An assumption in critical ethnographic research is that actions and thoughts are mediated by power relationships. Critical ethnographers attempt to increase the political dimensions of cultural research and undermine oppressive systems—there is an explicit

TABLE 22.2 • Comparison of Traditional Qualitative Research and Critical Research

ISSUE	TRADITIONAL QUALITATIVE RESEARCH	CRITICAL RESEARCH
Research aims	Understanding; reconstruction of multiple constructions	Critique; transformation; consciousness-raising; advocacy
View of knowledge	Transactional/subjective; knowledge is created in interaction between investigator and participants	Transactional/subjective; value-mediated and value-dependent; importance of historical insights
Methods	Dialectic: truth is arrived at logically through conversations	Dialectic and didactic: dialogue designed to transform naivety and misinformation
Evaluative criteria for inquiry quality	Authenticity; trustworthiness	Historical situatedness of the inquiry; erosion of ignorance; stimulus for change
Researcher's role	Facilitator of multivoice reconstruction	Transformative agent; advocate; activist

political purpose. Cook (2005) has argued that critical ethnography is especially well-suited to health promotion research because both are concerned with enabling people to take control of their own situation.

Carspecken (1996) developed a five-stage approach to critical ethnography that has been found useful in nursing studies (e.g., Bidabadi et al., 2019) and in health promotion research. Madison (2012) also provides guidance about critical theory methods.

Example of a Critical Ethnography
Laging and colleagues (2018) conducted a critical ethnography in two Australian nursing homes. Their study, which involved observations and in-depth interviews, focused on how nurses and personal-care assistants manage a deteriorating nursing home resident. They found that limited organizational support for nurses contributed to potentially avoidable hospital transfers.

Feminist Research

In **feminist research,** the focus is on gender domination and discrimination within patriarchal societies. Like critical researchers, feminist researchers seek to establish collaborative and nonexploitative relationships with their informants, to avoid objectification, and to conduct research that is transformative.

Gender is the organizing construct in feminist research, and investigators seek to understand how gender and a gendered social order have shaped women's lives and their consciousness. The aim is to ameliorate the "invisibility and distortion of female experience in ways relevant to ending women's unequal social position" (Lather, 1991, p. 71).

Although feminist researchers agree on the importance of focusing on women's diverse situations and the relationships that frame those situations, there are many variants of feminist inquiry. Three broad models (within each of which there is diversity) have been identified: (1) *feminist empiricism*, whose adherents usually work within fairly standard norms of qualitative inquiry but who seek to portray more accurate pictures of the social realities of women's lives; (2) *feminist standpoint*

research, which holds that inquiry ought to begin in and be tested against the lived everyday sociopolitical experiences of women, and that women's views are particular and privileged; and (3) *feminist postmodernism*, which stresses that "truth" is a destructive illusion and views the world as endless stories, texts, and narratives. In nursing and health care, feminist empiricism and feminist standpoint research have been most prevalent.

TIP An emerging construct is *intersectionality,* a term used to designate overlapping or intersecting social identities (e.g., gender and race) and related systems of oppression or discrimination. Intersectionality emphasizes that multiple social identities intersect to create a whole that differs from its components. Caiola and colleagues (2017), for example, studied how African American mothers with HIV describe their situation at the intersection of gender, race, and social inequality.

The scope of feminist research ranges from studies of the subjective views of individual women to studies of social movements, structures, and broad policies that affect (and often exclude) women. Feminist research methods typically include in-depth, interactive, and collaborative individual or group interviews that offer the possibility of reciprocally educational encounters. Feminists usually seek to negotiate the meanings of the results with those participating in the study and to be self-reflective about what they themselves are experiencing and learning.

Feminist research, like other research that has an ideological perspective, has raised the bar for the conduct of ethical research. With the emphasis on trust, empathy, and nonexploitative relationships, proponents of these newer modes of inquiry view any type of deception or manipulation as abhorrent. Those interested in feminist methodologies may wish to consult the writings of Hesse-Biber (2014) or Brisolara et al. (2014).

Example of Feminist Research
Clarke, Barnes and Ross (2018) used feminist theory and methods in their study of women who underwent electroconvulsive therapy and whose narratives revealed concerns about the informed consent process.

Participatory Action Research

A type of research known as participatory action research is closely allied to both critical research and feminist research. **Participatory action research (PAR)**, one of several types of *action research* that originated in the 1940s with social psychologist Kurt Lewin, is based on a recognition that the production of knowledge can be political and can be used to exert power. Action researchers typically work with groups or communities that are vulnerable to the control or oppression of a dominant group or culture.

In participatory action research, researchers and study participants collaborate in defining the problem, selecting research methods, analyzing the data, and deciding on the use to which findings are put. The aim of PAR is to produce not only knowledge but also action and consciousness-raising. Researchers seek to empower people through the process of constructing and using knowledge. The PAR tradition has as its starting point a concern for the powerlessness of the group under study. Thus, a key objective is to produce an impetus that is directly used to make improvements through education and sociopolitical action.

In PAR, research methods take second place to processes of collaboration that can motivate, increase self-esteem, and generate community solidarity. "Data-gathering" strategies are not only the traditional methods of interview and observation (including both qualitative and quantitative approaches) but may include storytelling, sociodrama, drawing and painting, plays and skits, and other activities designed to encourage people to find creative ways to explore their lives, tell their stories, and recognize their own strengths. Koch and Kralik (2006) offer a useful resource for learning more about PAR for health care, and Balbale and colleagues (2016) have described how participatory methods can be used in quality improvement projects.

Example of PAR

Caswell and an interprofessional team (2019) conducted a PAR project to learn about how best to support family carers in home-based end-of-life care. The project involved the development of a training program to enhance the knowledge and skills of volunteers and support workers who coordinate care with bereaved family carers.

CRITICAL APPRAISAL OF QUALITATIVE DESIGNS

Evaluating a qualitative design is often difficult. Qualitative researchers do not always document design decisions and seldom describe the process by which such decisions were made. Researchers often do, however, indicate whether the study was conducted within a specific qualitative tradition, and this information can be used to come to some conclusions. For example, if a report indicated that the researcher conducted 2 months of fieldwork for an ethnographic study, there would be reason to suspect that insufficient time had been spent in the field to obtain an emic perspective of the culture under study. Ethnographic studies may also be suspect if their only source of information was from interviews, rather than from a broader range of data sources, particularly observations.

In a grounded theory study, look for evidence about when the data were collected and analyzed. If all the data were collected before analysis, you might question whether constant comparison was used correctly. Glaser and Strauss (1967) offered four properties on which a grounded theory should be evaluated: fitness, understanding, generality, and control. The theory should fit the substantive area for which the data were collected. A grounded theory should increase the understanding of persons working in that substantive area. Also, the categories in the grounded theory should be abstract enough to allow the theory to be a general guide to changing situations—but not so abstract to decrease their sensitizing features. Lastly, the substantive theory must be sufficiently flexible that people who want to apply the grounded theory in practice can modify and control it if necessary.

In appraising a phenomenologic study, you should first determine if the study is descriptive or interpretive. This will help you to assess how closely the researcher kept to the basic tenets of that qualitative research tradition. For example, in a descriptive phenomenologic study, did the researcher bracket? When critically appraising phenomenologic studies, in addition to evaluating the methods, you should look at their power to demonstrate the meaning of the phenomena being studied.

BOX 22.1   Guidelines for Critically Appraising Qualitative Designs

1. Was a research tradition for the qualitative study identified? If none was identified, can one be inferred? If more than one was identified, is this justifiable or does it suggest "method slurring"?
2. Is the research question congruent with a qualitative approach and with the specific research tradition (i.e., is the domain of inquiry for the study congruent with the domain encompassed by the tradition)? Are the data sources, research methods, and analytic approach congruent with the research tradition?
3. How well is the research design described? Are design decisions explained and justified? Does it appear that the researcher made all design decisions up-front, or did the design emerge during data collection, allowing researchers to capitalize on early information?
4. Is the design appropriate, given the research question? Does the design lend itself to a thorough, in-depth, intensive examination of the phenomenon of interest? What design elements, if any, might have strengthened the study (e.g., a longitudinal perspective rather than a cross-sectional one)?
5. Did the researcher spend a sufficient amount of time doing fieldwork or collecting the research data?
6. Was there evidence of reflexivity in the design?
7. Was the study undertaken with an ideological perspective? If so, is there evidence that ideological methods and goals were achieved? (e.g., was there evidence of full collaboration between researchers and participants? Did the research have the power to be transformative, or is there evidence that a transformative process occurred?)

van Manen (1997) called for phenomenologic researchers to address five textual features in their reports: lived thoroughness (placing the phenomenon concretely in the lifeworld), evocation (vividly bringing the phenomenon into presence), intensification (giving key phrases their full value), tone (letting the text speak to the reader), and epiphany (suddenly grasping the meaning).

The guidelines in Box 22.1 are designed to assist you in critically appraising the designs of qualitative studies.

RESEARCH EXAMPLES

Nurse researchers have conducted studies in all of the qualitative research traditions described in this chapter, and several actual examples have been cited. In the following sections, we present more detailed descriptions of three qualitative nursing studies.

Research Example of an Ethnographic Study

Study: Health care experiences of Korean women divers (Jeju haenyeos) (Kim & Kim, 2018).

Statement of Purpose: Jeju haenyeos are female divers who collect seafood while holding their breath, without equipment. They work in groups and have developed a unique culture. The study sought to explore the health beliefs and experiences of the Jeju haenyeos and how they manage and maintain their health in their daily work lives.

Setting: The research was conducted in the eastern part of Jeju in South Korea.

Method: An ethnographic approach was used, with fieldwork conducted over a 4-month period. The researchers received permission from the Jeju haeyeos' association chairperson to observe the participants at work. A 73-year-old diver who had started working at the age of 5 years served as a key informant. She provided rich information about the divers' health management and access to other divers. She allowed the researcher to stay in her home for 3 days so she could observe the divers' daily lives and interactions. Observations were also made in the fitting rooms before dives and at a seawall where the diving occurred. The researchers conducted individual face-to-face interviews with 14 other divers. On average, the divers in the study had been working for 55 years.

Key findings: The main theme of the divers' health management approach was "a life of listening to the body and mind, controlling greed, and adjusting work for safe diving." (p. 756). The study revealed that the divers led communal lives centered on their work and promoted safety by working collectively. The researchers found, however, that the Jeju haenyeos used a range of preventive drugs before work to relieve their minds and bodies. They also used other drugs and lacked understanding of how the diverse drugs potentially interact.

Research Example of a Phenomenologic Study

Study: Keeping it together and falling apart: Women's dynamic experience of birth (Hall, Foster, & Young, 2018).

Statement of purpose: The purpose of this phenomenologic study was to explore the complexity of women's birth experience in the context in which they occur.

Sample: Study participants were eight healthy women aged 23 to 38 who had an uncomplicated vaginal birth at term and who had given birth to a healthy infant. One birth was a home birth and seven were hospital births.

Method: In-depth interviews were conducted at two points in time. The first interview was completed 2 to 10 weeks postpartum, and the second was completed 6 to 16 weeks postpartum. Interviews, which lasted between 25 and 90 minutes, were conducted in a private place of the women's choosing—most often, their own homes. The women were asked to tell their birth story in as much detail as possible and were probed for more detail about their emotions, physical sensations, and experiences of time and space. The interviews were audio-recorded and professionally transcribed for analysis. The data were analyzed using van Manen's phenomenologic method.

Key findings: The analysis revealed that the phenomenon of childbirth involved a dynamic that fluctuated between "keeping it together" and "falling apart." The changes in the women's emotions were created by a sensitive feedback loop between the women and their environments, the physical space, and interactions with other people who were present. During their labor, the women wanted an authentic human connection.

Research Example of a Grounded Theory Study

Study: Student veterans' construction and enactment of resilience: A constructivist grounded theory study (Reyes et al., 2018).

Statement of purpose: Military veterans transitioning to civilian life—and to college—face many challenges. The purpose of the study was to understand how college student veterans construct and enact resilience within their academic and personal (nonacademic) lives.

Method: The researchers used a constructivist grounded theory approach to explore the resilience of student veterans. Face-to-face interviews were conducted with 20 university student veterans (16 men and 4 women) in the state of Nevada, all of whom had been deployed or served in combat in a branch of the U.S. military. The in-depth interviews, which lasted 1.5 to 2 hours, were recorded. Two key questions were, "Would you please share some of your experiences of stress and difficulties as a university student since your return from military service?" and "How were you able to manage the issues around your stress and difficulties?" (p. 39). An iterative process of data collection and analysis was used: After each interview, the researchers analyzed the data and developed initial concepts, which were further explored in subsequent interviews. Constant comparison was applied. After 20 interviews, theoretical saturation was achieved and data collection stopped.

Key findings: The researchers identified the core category as the process of *integrating*, which represents student veterans' construction and enactment of resilience. Their resilience is a result of integrating and resolving challenges in their academic and personal lives. Resilience entailed a complex process of transitioning from military to civilian life and an iterative journey between positive adaptation and transient difficulties.

SUMMARY POINTS

- Qualitative research involves an **emergent design**—a design that emerges in the field as the study unfolds. Although qualitative design is flexible, qualitative researchers plan for broad contingencies that pose decision opportunities for study design in the field.

- As *bricoleurs*, qualitative researchers tend to be creative and intuitive, putting together an array of data drawn from many sources to develop a holistic understanding of a phenomenon.
- Qualitative research traditions have their roots in anthropology (e.g., ethnography and *ethnoscience*); philosophy (phenomenology, hermeneutics, and phenomenography); psychology (*ethology* and *ecological psychology*); sociology (grounded theory, *ethnomethodology*, and *semiotics*); sociolinguistics (*discourse analysis*); and history (*historical research*).
- **Ethnography** focuses on the culture of a group of people and relies on extensive fieldwork that usually includes **participant observation** and in-depth interviews with **key informants.** Ethnographers strive to acquire an **emic** (insider's) perspective of a culture rather than an **etic** (outsider's) perspective.
- Ethnographers use the concept of *researcher as instrument* to describe the researcher's significant role in analyzing and interpreting a culture. The product of ethnographic research is typically a holistic description of the culture, but sometimes the products are **performance ethnographies** (interpretive scripts that can be performed).
- Nurses sometimes refer to their ethnographic studies as **ethnonursing research.** Other types of ethnographic work include **institutional ethnographies** (which focus on the organization of professional services from the perspective of the frontline workers or clients) and **autoethnographies** or *insider research* (which focuses on the group or culture to which the researcher belongs).
- **Phenomenology** seeks to discover the *essence* and *meaning* of a phenomenon as it is experienced by people, mainly through in-depth interviews with people who have had the relevant experience.
- In **descriptive phenomenology**, which seeks to describe lived experiences, researchers strive to **bracket** out preconceived views and to **intuit** the essence of the phenomenon by remaining open to meanings attributed to it by those who have experienced it. **Interpretive phenomenology (hermeneutics)** focuses on interpreting the meaning of experiences, rather than just describing them. Various approaches to interpretive phenomenology have been developed, including **interpretive phenomenologic analysis (IPA)**, **reflective lifeworld research (RLR)**, and Parse's research methods (**humanbecoming hermeneutic sciencing** and **Parsesciencing**).
- **Phenomenography** involves gaining an understanding of the different ways in which people experience or think about a phenomenon.
- **Grounded theory** aims to discover theoretical precepts grounded in the data. Grounded theory researchers try to account for people's actions by focusing on the main concern that the behavior is designed to resolve. The manner in which people resolve this main concern is the **core variable.** The goal of grounded theory is to discover this main concern and the **basic social process (BSP)** that explains how people resolve it.
- Grounded theory uses **constant comparison**: categories elicited from the data are constantly compared with data obtained earlier.
- A controversy among grounded theory researchers concerns whether to follow the original Glaser and Strauss procedures or to use the adapted procedures of Strauss and Corbin; Glaser argued that the latter approach does not result in *grounded theories* but rather in *conceptual descriptions.*
- More recently, Charmaz's **constructivist grounded theory** has emerged as a method to emphasize interpretive aspects in which the grounded theory is constructed from shared experiences and relationships between the researcher and study participants.
- **Case studies** are intensive investigations of a single entity or a small number of entities, such as individuals, groups, organizations, or communities; such studies usually involve collecting data over an extended period. Case study designs can be **single** or **multiple**, and **holistic** or **embedded.**
- **Narrative analysis** focuses on *story* in studies in which the purpose is to explore how people make sense of events in their lives. Several different structural approaches can be used to analyze narrative data, including, for example, Burke's **pentadic dramatism.**

- **Descriptive qualitative studies** are "generic" qualitative inquiries that do not fit into any disciplinary tradition but that aim at rich description of a phenomenon. Qualitative description has been expanded into a realm called **interpretive description,** which emphasizes the importance of having a disciplinary conceptual frame, such as nursing.
- Research is sometimes conducted within an ideological perspective, and such research tends to rely primarily on qualitative research.
- **Critical theory** entails a critique of existing social structures; critical researchers strive to conduct inquiries that involve collaboration with participants and foster enlightened self-knowledge and transformation. **Critical ethnography** applies the principles of critical theory to the study of cultures.
- **Feminist research**, like critical research, is designed to be transformative; the focus is on how gender domination and discrimination shape women's lives and their consciousness.
- **Participatory action research (PAR)** produces knowledge through close collaboration with groups or communities that are vulnerable to control or oppression by a dominant social group; in PAR research, methods take second place to emergent processes that can motivate people and generate community solidarity.

STUDY ACTIVITIES

Study activities are available to instructors on thePoint.

REFERENCES CITED IN CHAPTER 22

Ahern, K. J. (1999). Ten tips for reflexive bracketing. *Qualitative Health Research, 9*, 407–411.

Armuand, G., Wettergren, L., Nilsson, J., Rodriguez-Wallberg, K., & Lampic, C. (2018). Threatened fertility: A longitudinal study exploring experiences of fertility and having children after cancer treatment. *European Journal of Cancer Care, 27*, e12798.

Baker, C., Wuest, J., & Stern, P. N. (1992). Method slurring: The grounded theory/phenomenology example. *Journal of Advanced Nursing, 17*, 1355–1360.

Balbale, S., Locatelli, S., & LaVela, S. (2016). Through their eyes: Lessons learned using participatory methods in health care quality improvement projects. *Qualitative Health Research, 26*, 1382–1392.

*Baxter, P., & Jack, S. (2008). Qualitative case study methodology: Study design and implementation for novice researchers. *The Qualitative Report, 13*, 544–559.

Beck, C. T. (2012). Exemplar: Teetering on the edge. A continually emerging substantive theory of postpartum depression. In Munhall, P. (Ed.). *Nursing Research: A qualitative perspective* (5th ed., pp. 225–256). Sudbury, MA: Jones & Bartlett Publishers.

Benner, P. (1994). The tradition and skill of interpretive phenomenology in studying health, illness, and caring practices. In Benner, P. (Ed.). *Interpretive phenomenology* (pp. 99–127). Thousand Oaks, CA: Sage.

Bidabadi, F., Yazdannik, A., & Zargham-Boroujeni, A. (2019). Patient's dignity in intensive care unit: A critical ethnography. *Nursing Ethics, 26*, 738–752.

Brisolara, S., Seigart, S., & SenGupta, S. (Eds.). (2014). *Feminist evaluation and research: Theory and practice*. New York: Guilford Press.

Bruner, J. (1991). *Acts of meaning*. Cambridge, MA: Harvard University Press.

Burke, K. (1969). *A grammar of motives*. Berkley, CA: University of California Press.

Butler, A., Copnell, B., & Hall, H. (2019). The impact of the social and physical environments on parent-healthcare provider relationships when a child dies in PICU: Findings from a grounded theory study. *Intensive & Critical Care Nursing, 50*, 28–35.

Caiola, C., Barroso, J., & Docherty, S. (2017). Capturing the social location of African American mothers living with HIV: An inquiry into how social determinants of health are framed. *Nursing Research, 66*, 209–221.

Carroll, K., & Mesman, J. (2018). Multiple researcher roles in video-reflexive ethnography. *Qualitative Health Research, 28*, 1145–1156.

Carspecken, P. F. (1996). *Critical ethnography in educational research*. New York: Routledge.

*Caswell, G., Hardy, B., Ewing, G., Kennedy, S., & Seymour, J. (2019). Supporting family carers in home-based end-of-life care: Using participatory action research to develop a training programme for support workers and volunteers. *BMJ Supportive & Palliative Care, 9*, e4.

Chang, H. (2016). Autoethnography in health research: Growing pains? *Qualitative Health Research, 26*, 443–451.

Charmaz, K. (2014). *Constructing grounded theory: A practical guide through qualitative analysis* (2nd ed.). Thousand Oaks, CA: Sage Publications.

Clarke, K., Barnes, M., & Ross, D. (2018). I had no other option: Women, electroconvulsive therapy, and informed consent. *International Journal of Mental Health Nursing, 27*, 1077–1085.

Cohen, M.Z., Kahn, D., & Steeves, R. (2000). *Hermeneutic phenomenological research: A practical guide for nurse researchers*. Thousand Oaks, CA: Sage.

Colaizzi, P. F. (1973). *Reflection and research in psychology*. Dubuque, Iowa: Kendall/Hunt Publishing Co.

Cook, K. E. (2005). Using critical ethnography to explore issues in health promotion. *Qualitative Health Research, 15*, 129–138.

Corbin, J., & Strauss, A. (2015). *Basics of qualitative research: Techniques and procedures for developing grounded theory* (4th ed.). Thousand Oaks, CA: Sage Publications.

*Crotty, M., Henderson, J., Ward, P., Fuller, J., Rogers, A., Kralik, D., & Gregory, S. (2015). Analysis of social networks supporting the self-management of type 2 diabetes for people with mental illness. *BMC Health Services Research, 15*, 257.

Cruz, E. V., & Higginbottom, G. (2013). The use of focused ethnography in nursing research. *Nurse Researcher, 20*, 36–43.

Dahlberg, K., Dahlberg, H., & Nyström, M. (2008). *Reflective lifeworld research*. Lund, Sweden: Studentlitteratur.

*Dahlberg, H., Ranheim, A., & Dahlberg, K. (2016). Ecological caring: Revisiting the original ideas of caring science. *International Journal of Qualitative Studies on Health and Well-being, 11*, 33344.

Denzin, N. K., & Lincoln, Y. S. (Eds.). (2011). *Handbook of qualitative research* (4th ed.). Thousand Oaks, CA: Sage.

Diekelmann, N. L., Allen, D., & Tanner, C. (1989). *The NLN criteria for appraisal of baccalaureate programs: A critical hermeneutic analysis*. New York: NLN Press.

Doucet, T. (2018). Feeling peaceful: A universal living experience. *Nursing Science Quarterly, 31*, 55–65.

Doull, M., Wolowic, J., Saewyc, E., Rosario, M., Prescott, R., & Ybarra, M. (2018). Why girls choose not to use barriers to prevent sexually transmitted infection during female-to-female sex. *Journal of Adolescent Health, 62*, 411–416.

Eileen, M., Peter, G., Bernadette, J., Lindsay, M., & Christine, B. (2017). Crossing professional cultures: A qualitative study of nurses working in a medical school. *Contemporary Nurse, 14*, 1–14.

Ellis, C., & Bochner, A. P. (2000). Autoethnography, personal narrative, reflexivity. In Denzin, N. K. & Lincoln, Y. S. (Eds.), *Handbook of qualitative research* (2nd ed., pp. 733–768). Thousand Oaks, CA: Sage.

Fetterman, D. M. (2010). *Ethnography: Step by step* (3rd ed.). Thousand Oaks, CA: Sage.

Gadamer, H. G. (1976). *Philosophical hermeneutics* (D. E. Linge, Ed. & Trans.). Berkeley: University of California Press.

Gearing, R. E. (2004). Bracketing in research: A typology. *Qualitative Health Research, 14*, 1429–1452.

Giorgi, A. (2009). *The descriptive phenomenological method in psychology: A modified Husserlian approach*. Pittsburgh: Duquesne University Press.

Glaser, B. (1992). *Emergence versus forcing: Basics of grounded theory analysis*. Mill Valley, CA: Sociology Press.

Glaser, B. (1998). *Doing grounded theory: Issues and discussions*. Mill Valley, CA: Sociology Press.

Glaser, B. (2001). *The grounded theory perspective: Conceptualization contrasted with description*. Mill Valley, CA: Sociology Press.

Glaser, B. (2003). *The grounded theory perspective II: Description's remodeling of grounded theory methodology*. Mill Valley, CA: Sociology Press.

Glaser, B. (2005). *The grounded theory perspective III: Theoretical coding*. Mill Valley, CA: Sociology Press.

Glaser, B. G., & Strauss, A. (1967). *The discovery of grounded theory: Strategies for qualitative research*. New York: Aldine de Gruyter.

*Goicolea, I., Marchal, B., Hurtig, A., Vives-Cases, C., Briones-Vozmediano, E., & San Sebastian, M. (2019). Why do certain primary health care teams respond better to intimate partner violence than others? A multiple case study. *Gaceta Sanitaria, 33*, 169–176.

Hall, P., Foster, J., Yount, K., & Jennings, B. (2018). Keeping it together and falling apart: Women's dynamic experience of birth. *Midwifery, 58*, 130–136.

Hall, J., Hutson, S., & West, F. (2018). Anticipating needs at end of life in narratives related by people living with HIV/AIDS in Appalachia. *American Journal of Hospice & Palliative Care, 35*, 985–992.

Harris, D., Jack, K., & Wibberley, C. (2018). The meaning of living with uncertainty for people with motor neurone disease. *Journal of Clinical Nursing, 27*, 2062–2071.

Heath, H., & Cowley, S. (2004). Developing a grounded theory approach: A comparison of Glaser and Strauss. *International Journal of Nursing Studies, 41*, 141–150.

Heidegger, M. (1962). *Being and time*. New York: Harper & Row.

Heidegger, M. (1971). *Poetry, language, thought*. New York: Harper & Row.

Herlufsen, P., & Brødgaard, A. (2017). The lived experiences of persons hospitalized for construction of an urgent fecal ostomy. *Journal of Wound, Ostomy, & Continence Nursing, 44*, 557–561.

Hesse-Biber, S. (Ed.). (2014). *Feminist research practice: A primer* (2nd ed.). Thousand Oaks, CA: Sage Publications.

Higginbottom, G., & Lauridsen, E. (2014). The roots and development of constructivist grounded theory. *Nurse Researcher, 21*, 8–13.

Husserl, E. (1962). *Ideas: General introduction to pure phenomenology*. New York: Macmillan.

Johnston, C., Wallis, M., Oprescu, F., & Gray, M. (2017). Methodological considerations related to nurse researchers using their own experience of a phenomenon within phenomenology. *Journal of Advanced Nursing, 73*, 574–584.

Kim, J. I., & Kim, M. (2018). Health care experiences of Korean women divers (Jeju Haenyeos). *Qualitative Health Research, 28*, 756–765.

Koch, T., & Kralik, D. (2006). *Participatory action research in healthcare*. Chichester, UK: Wiley.

Laging, B., Kenny, A., Bauer, M., & Nay, R. (2018). Recognition and assessment of residents' deterioration in the nursing home setting: A critical ethnography. *Journal of Clinical Nursing, 27*, 1452–1463.

Lather, P. (1991). *Getting smart: Feminist research and pedagogy with/in the postmodern*. New York: Routledge.

LeCompte, M., & Schensul, J. (2010). *Designing and conducting ethnographic research: An introduction* (2nd ed.). Plymouth, UK: AltaMira Press.

Leininger, M. M. (Ed.). (1985). *Qualitative research methods in nursing*. New York: Grune and Stratton.

Leininger, M. M., & McFarland, M. (2006). *Culture care diversity and universality: A worldwide nursing theory* (2nd ed.). Sudbury, MA: Jones & Bartlett.

**Leyva-Moral, J., Martínez-Batlle, F., Vásquez-Naveira, M., Hernández-Fernández, K., & Villar-Salqueiro, M. (2019). The experience of growing old while living with HIV in Spain: A phenomenological study. *Journal of the Association of Nurses in AIDS Care, 30*, 111–118.

Lincoln, Y. S., & Guba, E. G. (1985). *Naturalistic inquiry*. Newbury Park, CA: Sage.

Lin, J., Smith, C., Feder, S., Bickell, N., & Schulman-Green, D. (2018). Patients' and oncologists' views on family involvement in goals of care conversations. *Psychooncology, 27*, 1035–1041.

Liu, Y., & Chiang, H. (2017). From vulnerability to passion in the end-of-life care: The lived experience of nurses. *European Journal of Oncology Nursing, 31*, 30–36.

Lopez, K. A., & Willis, D. G. (2004). Descriptive versus interpretive phenomenology: Their contributions to nursing knowledge. *Qualitative Health Research, 14*, 726–735.

*MacKinnon, K., Butcher, D., & Bruce, A. (2018). Working to full scope: The reorganization of nursing work in two Canadian community hospitals. *Global Qualitative Nursing Research, 5*.

Madison, D. S. (2012). *Critical ethnography: Methods, ethics, and performance* (2nd ed.). Thousand Oaks, CA: Sage.

Marton, F., & Booth, S. (1997). *Learning and awareness*. Mahwah, NJ: Erlbaum.

Matua, G., & Van der Wal, D. (2015). Differentiating between descriptive and interpretive phenomenological research approaches. *Nurse Researcher, 22*, 22–27.

Maxwell, J. (2012). The importance of qualitative research for causal explanation in education. *Qualitative Inquiry, 18*, 655–661.

McFarland, M. R., & Wehbe-Alamah, H. B. (2015). *Leininger's culture care and diversity and universality: A worldwide nursing theory*. Burlington, MA: Jones & Bartlett Learning.

Mertens, D. M. (2007). Transformative paradigm: Mixed methods and social justice. *Journal of Mixed Methods Research, 1*, 212–225.

Milhomme, D., Gagnon, J., & Lachasseur, K. (2018). The clinical surveillance process as carried out by expert nurses in a critical care context: A theoretical explanation. *Intensive & Critical Care Nursing, 44*, 24–30.

Morse, J. M. (2004). Qualitative comparison: Appropriateness, equivalence, and fit. *Qualitative Health Research, 14*, 1323–1325.

Morse, J. M. (2009). Mixing qualitative methods. *Qualitative Health Research, 19*, 1523.

Nepal, V. (2010). On mixing qualitative methods. *Qualitative Health Research, 20*, 281.

O'Brien, M., Kinloch, K., Groves, K., & Jack, B. (2019). Meeting patients' spiritual needs during end-of-life care: A qualitative study of nurses' and healthcare professionals' perceptions of spiritual care training. *Journal of Clinical Nursing, 28*, 182–189.

Parse, R. R. (2014). *The Humanbecoming Paradigm: A transformational worldview*. Pittsburgh, PA: Discovery International Publication.

Parse, R. R. (2016a). Humanbecoming hermeneutic sciencing: Reverence, awe, betrayal, and shame in the lives of others. *Nursing Science Quarterly, 29*, 128–135.

Parse, R. R. (2016b). Parsesciencing: A basic science model of inquiry. *Nursing Science Quarterly, 29*, 271-274.

Patton, M. Q. (2015). *Qualitative research & evaluation methods* (4th ed.). Thousand Oaks, CA: Sage.

*Pennafort, V., Queroz, M., Nascimento, L., & Guedes, M. (2016). Network and social support in family care of children with diabetes. *Revista Brasileira de Enfermagem, 69*, 912–919.

Peterson, A. L. (2015). A case for the use of autoethnography in nursing research. *Journal of Advanced Nursing, 71*, 226–233.

Rankin, J. M. (2013). Institutional ethnography. In Beck, C.T. (Ed.). *Routledge international handbook of qualitative nursing research* (pp. 242–255). New York: Routledge.

Reyes, A., Kearney, C., Isla, K., & Bryant, R. (2018). Student veterans' construction and enactment of resilience: A constructivist grounded theory study. *Journal of Psychiatric and Mental Health Nursing, 25*, 37–48.

Riessman, C. K. (1991). Beyond reductionism: Narrative genres in divorce accounts. *Journal of Narrative and Life History, 1*, 41–68.

Riessman, C. K. (1993). *Narrative analysis*. Newbury Park, CA: Sage Publications.

Riessman, C. K. (2008). *Narrative methods for the human sciences*. Thousand Oaks, CA: Sage.

*Sandelowski, M. (2000). Whatever happened to qualitative description? *Research in Nursing & Health, 23*, 334–340.

Sandelowski, M. (2010). What's in a name? Qualitative description revisited. *Research in Nursing & Health, 33*, 77–84.

Sandelowski, M. (2011). "Casing" the research case study. *Research in Nursing & Health, 34*, 153–159.

Smith, D. E. (1999). *Writing the social: Critique, theory, and investigation*. Toronto: University of Toronto Press.

Smith, J. A., Flowers, P., & Larkin, M. (2009). *Interpretive phenomenological analysis: Theory, method and research*. Los Angeles: Sage Publications.

Smith, C. A., & Gallo, A. (2007). Applications of performance ethnography in nursing. *Qualitative Health Research, 17*, 521–528.

Strauss, A., & Corbin, J. (1990). *Basics of qualitative research: Grounded theory procedures and techniques*. Newbury Park, CA: Sage Publications.

Svensson, G., & Wåhlin, I. (2018). Patient perceptions of specialised hospital-based palliative home care: A qualitative study using a phenomenographical approach. *International Journal of Palliative Nursing, 24*, 22–32.

Thorne, S. (2008). *Interpretive description.* Walnut Creek, CA: Left Coast Press.

Thorne, S. (2013). Interpretive description. In Beck, C. T. (Ed.). *Routledge international handbook of qualitative nursing research* (pp. 295–306). New York: Routledge.

Tobin, C., Murphy-Lawless, J., & Beck, C. T. (2014). Childbirth in exile: Asylum seeking women's experience of childbirth in Ireland. *Midwifery, 30*, 831–838.

Uengwongsapat, C., Kantaruska, K., Klunklin, A., & Sansiriphun, N. (2018). Growing into teen fatherhood: A grounded theory study. *International Nursing Review, 65*, 244–253.

Van Manen, M. (1990). *Researching lived experience.* New York: SUNY Press.

Van Manen, M. (1997). From meaning to method. *Qualitative Health Research, 7*, 345–369.

Van Manen, M. (2014). *Phenomenology of practice: Meaning-giving methods in phenomenological research and writing.* Walnut Creek, CA: Left Coast Press.

Van Manen, M. (2017). Phenomenology in its original sense. *Qualitative Health Research, 27*, 810–825.

Wright, D., Pincombe, J., & McKellar, L. (2018). Exploring routine hospital antenatal care consultations: An ethnographic study. *Women and Birth, 31*, e162–e169.

Yin, R. (2018). *Case study research: Design and methods* (6th ed.). Thousand Oaks, CA: Sage.

A link to this open-access article is provided in the Toolkit for Chapter 22 in the **Resource Manual.** ✪

**This journal article is available on thePoint for this chapter.*

23 | Sampling in Qualitative Research

In Chapter 13, we presented concepts relating to sampling in quantitative research. Sampling in qualitative studies is quite different. Qualitative studies almost always use small, nonrandom samples. This does not mean that qualitative researchers are unconcerned with the quality of their samples, but rather that they use different considerations in selecting participants who will strengthen their findings. Indeed, as Patton (2015) has noted in his widely read book on qualitative methods, "What you sample is what you have something to say about in the end" (p. 244). This chapter describes sampling approaches used by qualitative researchers.

THE LOGIC OF QUALITATIVE SAMPLING

Quantitative researchers measure attributes and study relationships in a population. A representative sample is desired in quantitative studies to enhance the likelihood that the measurements accurately reflect and can be generalized to the population. The aim of most qualitative studies, by contrast, is to discover *meaning* and to uncover multiple realities, not to generalize to a population.

Qualitative researchers begin with the following types of sampling question in mind: Who would be an information-rich data source for my study?

Whom should I talk to or observe to maximize my understanding of the phenomenon? A critical first step in qualitative sampling is selecting settings with potential for information richness. As the study progresses, new sampling questions emerge, such as: Who can confirm my understandings? Challenge my understandings? Enrich my understandings? Thus, as with the overall design in qualitative studies, sampling often is emergent and capitalizes on early findings to guide subsequent direction.

> **TIP** Individuals are not always the *unit of analysis* in qualitative studies. Glaser and Strauss (1967) have noted that "incidents" or experiences are sometimes the basis for analysis. An information-rich informant may contribute dozens of incidents (e.g., stressful life events), and so even a small number of informants can generate a large sample for analysis.

Qualitative researchers do not articulate an explicit population to whom results are intended to be generalized, but they do establish the kinds of people who are eligible to participate in their research. A prime criterion is whether a person has experienced the phenomenon, culture, or process that is under study. Practical issues, such as costs, accessibility, and health constraints also affect who can be included in the sample.

Example of Eligibility Criteria in a Qualitative Study

In their interpretive phenomenologic study, Lamb and colleagues (2019) explored the meaning of conscience for nurses in the context of conscientious objection (CO) in clinical practice. To be included, nurses had to speak English, be employed as an RN in a healthcare setting in Ontario, and had to have made a CO in clinical practice.

TYPES OF QUALITATIVE SAMPLING

Several different approaches to sampling in qualitative research are reviewed in this section. Despite differences, however, a few key features that characterize most sampling strategies have been distilled from an analysis of the qualitative literature (Curtis et al., 2000).

- Participants are not selected randomly. A random sample is not considered the best method of selecting people who will make good informants, that is, people who are knowledgeable, articulate, reflective, and willing to talk at length with researchers.
- Samples tend to be small and studied intensively, with each participant provided a wealth of data. Typically, qualitative studies involve fewer (and sometimes much fewer) than 50 participants.
- Sample members are not prespecified; their selection is emergent.
- Sample selection is driven largely by conceptual requirements rather than by a desire for representativeness.

Convenience Sampling

Qualitative researchers often begin with a convenience sample, which is sometimes called a *volunteer sample*. Volunteer samples are especially likely to be used when researchers need to have participants come forward and identify themselves. For example, if we wanted to study the experiences of people with frequent nightmares, we might recruit sample members by placing a notice on a bulletin board or on Internet sites, requesting people with frequent nightmares to contact us. In this situation, we would be less interested in obtaining a representative sample of people with nightmares, than in obtaining a diverse group representing various experiences with nightmares.

Sampling by convenience is easy, but it is not a preferred sampling approach, even in qualitative studies. The goal in qualitative studies is to extract the greatest possible information from the few cases in the sample, and a convenience sample may not provide the most information-rich sources. However, a convenience sample may be an economical way to begin the sampling process, relying on other strategies later.

Convenience sampling may also work well with participants who need to be recruited from a particular clinical setting or from a specific organization. Thorne (2008), however, has advised that in such situations the researcher should carefully reflect on and understand any peculiarities of the study context. In essence, researchers must consider whether participants' narrations reflect the experience of the healthcare or organizational setting to a greater extent than the experience of the phenomenon under study.

Example of a Convenience Sample

Durante and coresearchers (2019) undertook a qualitative study to describe caregiver contributions to self-care management and maintenance for patients with heart failure. A convenience sample of 40 caregivers was recruited from outpatient cardiovascular clinics in three Italian hospitals.

Snowball Sampling

Qualitative researchers, like quantitative researchers, sometimes use snowball (or *chain*) sampling, asking early informants to refer other study participants. Snowball sampling has advantages over convenience sampling from a broad population. The first is that it may be more cost-efficient. Researchers may spend less time screening people to determine if they are appropriate for the study, for example. Furthermore, with an introduction from the referring person, researchers may have an easier time establishing a trusting relationship with new participants. Finally, researchers can more readily specify the characteristics that they want new participants to have. For example, in the study of people with nightmares, we could ask early respondents if they knew anyone else who had the same problem *and* who was verbally expressive. We could also ask for referrals to people who would add new dimensions to the sample, such as people who vary in age, race, socioeconomic status, and so on.

A weakness of this approach is that the eventual sample might be restricted to a rather small network of acquaintances. Moreover, the quality of the referrals may be affected by whether the referring sample members trusted the researcher and truly wanted to cooperate.

> **TIP** Researchers should be careful about protecting the rights of the individuals who are referred. It is wise to suggest that early informants first check with the potential referrals to make sure they are interested in participating before their names are shared with the researcher. This is especially true if the study focuses on sensitive issues (e.g., suicide attempts).

Example of Snowball Sampling

Lauder and colleagues (2018) conducted a qualitative descriptive study of mothers' experiences of caring for a child with early-onset scoliosis. Snowball sampling assisted in the recruitment of parents.

Purposive Sampling

Qualitative sampling may begin with volunteer informants and may be supplemented with new participants through snowballing, but many qualitative studies eventually evolve to a purposive (or *purposeful*) sampling strategy—that is, selecting specific cases that will most benefit the study.

More than a dozen purposive sampling strategies have been identified (Patton, 2015). We briefly describe several strategies to illustrate the diverse approaches qualitative researchers have used to meet their conceptual and substantive needs—although researchers themselves do not necessarily use these labels for their sampling plans. As an organizing structure, we have adapted the typology of purposive sampling proposed by Teddlie and Tashakkori (2009).

> **TIP** Some qualitative researchers appear to call their sample *purposive* simply because they "purposely" selected people who have experienced the phenomenon of interest. However, exposure to the phenomenon is an eligibility criterion—the group of interest comprises people with that exposure. If the researcher then recruits *any* person with the desired experience, the sample is selected by convenience, not purposively. Purposive sampling implies an intent to choose *particular* exemplars or *types* of people who can best enhance the researcher's understanding of the phenomenon.

Sampling for Representativeness or Comparative Value

The first broad category of purposive sampling involves two general goals: (1) sampling to find examples that are typical or representative of a broader group on a dimension of interest or (2) sampling to set up the possibility of comparisons across different types of cases on a dimension of interest.

Maximum variation sampling is the most widely used method of purposive sampling. It involves purposefully selecting persons (or settings) with variation on dimensions of interest. By selecting participants with diverse backgrounds, researchers invite enrichments of and challenges to emerging conceptualizations. Maximum variation sampling might involve ensuring that people with diverse backgrounds are represented in the sample (ensuring that there are men and women, poor and affluent people, and so on). It might also involve deliberate attempts to include people with different viewpoints about the phenomenon under study. For example, researchers might use snowballing to ask early participants for referrals to people who hold different points of view. One major advantage of maximum variation sampling is that any common patterns emerging despite the diversity of the sample are likely to be capturing core experiences.

Maximum variation sampling is often an emergent approach: Information from initial participants helps to guide the subsequent selection of a diverse group of participants. However, there may be an advantage to having some upfront insights into the dimensions of variation that will likely prove productive. The factors that affect the health or wellness experience under scrutiny can often be anticipated or identified in advance, and having a mental list of such factors can be useful in ensuring sufficient diversity in the sample.

Example of Maximum Variation Sampling

Stormorken and colleagues (2017) studied factors that affect the illness trajectory of patients with postinfectious fatigue syndrome. A sample of 26 adults was selected from patients who fell ill with gastrointestinal infection that resulted from a contaminated water supply in Bergen, Norway. Using maximum variation sampling, the researchers selected patients who varied with regard to age, gender, education, income, marital status, and functional disability.

Although maximum variation sampling is one of the most popular approaches to sampling in qualitative research, other types of purposive sampling include the following:

- **Homogeneous sampling** deliberately reduces variation and permits a more focused inquiry; researchers may use this approach if they wish to understand a particular group of people especially well.
- **Typical case sampling** involves selecting cases that illustrate or highlight what is typical, average, normal, or representative. Identifying typical cases can help the researcher understand key aspects of a phenomenon as they are manifested under ordinary circumstances.
- **Stratified purposive sampling** involves selecting participants in distinct subgroups along a single dimension (e.g., pain levels above average, average, or below average). In this approach, each "stratum" would comprise a fairly homogeneous sample.
- **Extreme (deviant) case sampling** (also called *outlier sampling*) provides opportunities for learning from the most unusual and extreme informants—cases that at least on the surface

seem like "exceptions to the rule" (e.g., outstanding successes and notable failures). Most often, this approach is a supplement to other sampling strategies—extreme cases are sought to develop a richer or more nuanced understanding of the phenomenon under study.

- **Intensity sampling** is similar to extreme case sampling but with less emphasis on the extremes. Intensity samples involve information-rich cases that manifest the phenomenon of interest intensely but not as extreme or potentially distorting manifestations. The goal in intensity sampling is to select rich cases that offer *strong* examples of the phenomenon.
- **Reputational case sampling** involves selecting cases based on a recommendation of an expert or key informant. This approach, most often used in ethnographies, is useful when researchers have little information about how best to proceed with sampling and must rely on recommendations from others.

Many of these sampling strategies require that researchers have some knowledge about the study context. For example, to choose extreme cases, typical cases, or homogenous cases, researchers must have information about the range of variation of the phenomenon and how it manifests itself. Early participants may be helpful in pursuing these sampling strategies.

Sampling Special or Unique Cases

The second broad category of purposive sampling involves selecting special or unique cases. In these approaches, individual cases or a specific group of cases are the focus of the investigation. Several of these approaches are especially likely to be used in case study research.

Criterion sampling involves selecting cases that meet a predetermined criterion of importance. For example, in studying patient satisfaction with nursing care, researchers might sample only those patients whose responses to questions upon discharge expressed a complaint about nursing care. Criterion sampling has the potential for identifying and understanding cases that are fertile with experiential information on the phenomenon of interest.

> **Example of Criterion Sampling**
> Hamilton and colleagues (2018) explored the use of spirituality to make sense of the end-of-life and bereavement experiences of African American families. Criterion sampling guided their selection of 19 African Americans who lost a family member to cancer.

Yin (2014), whose work on case study research is widely cited, described **revelatory case sampling.** This approach involves identifying and gaining access to a single case representing a phenomenon that was previously inaccessible to research scrutiny.

> **Example of Revelatory Case Sampling**
> Mamier and Winslow (2014) used revelatory case sampling to describe the contrasting perspectives between a family caregiver (a wife) and a professional provider regarding placement decision-making for the husband, who was diagnosed with Alzheimer's disease.

A final type of special-case sampling is **sampling of politically important cases.** This approach is used to select or search for politically sensitive cases (or sites) for analysis. Sometimes, politically salient cases or sites can enhance the visibility of a study or increase the likelihood that it has an impact. The approach sometimes is used to select *out* politically sensitive locales or individuals, to avoid attracting unwanted attention.

Sampling Sequentially

Several of the purposive strategies already described can be combined in a single study. For example, extreme case sampling could occur after an initial strategy such as maximum variation sampling. The strategies in this third broad category of purposive sampling involve a gradual, and often planned, sequence of sampling. One such strategy, theory-based or theoretical sampling, is discussed separately in the next section.

Opportunistic sampling (or *emergent sampling*) involves adding new cases to a sample based on changes in research circumstances as data are being collected or in response to new leads and opportunities that may develop in the field. As the researcher gains greater knowledge of a setting or a phenomenon, on-the-spot sampling decisions can take advantage of unfolding events. This approach, although seldom labeled as opportunistic sampling, is used often in qualitative research because of its flexible and emergent nature.

Sampling confirming and disconfirming cases tends to be used toward the end of data collection. This approach involves testing ideas and assessing the viability of emergent findings and conceptualizations with new data. **Confirming cases** are additional cases that fit researchers' conceptualizations and offer enhanced credibility, richness, and depth to the analysis and conclusions. **Disconfirming cases** (or **negative cases**) are examples that do not fit and serve to challenge researchers' interpretations. These negative cases may simply be "exceptions that prove the rule," but they may be exceptions that disconfirm earlier insights and suggest rival explanations about the phenomenon. These cases can bring to light how the original conceptualization needs to be revised or expanded.

> **Example of Sampling Negative Cases**
> Matthew-Maich and colleagues (2013) explored the processes and strategies used by frontline leaders to support the uptake of best practice breastfeeding guidelines by nurses in maternity care practice settings. They used several approaches to sampling 58 health professionals and 54 clients. They noted that they undertook negative case interviewing "whenever gaps or inconsistencies were noted in the data codes or categories" (p. 1761).

Theoretical Sampling

Although Patton (2015) categorized theoretical sampling as a type of purposive sampling, we devote a separate section to this sampling strategy because of its importance in grounded theory. Glaser (1978) defined theoretical sampling as "the process of data collection for generating theory whereby the analyst jointly collects, codes, and analyzes his data and decides what data to collect next and where to find them, in order to develop his theory as it emerges" (p. 36). The process of sampling theoretically is guided by the developing grounded theory. Theoretical sampling is not envisioned as a single, unidirectional line. This complex sampling technique requires researchers to be involved with multiple lines and directions as they go back and forth between data and categories in the emerging theory. Theoretical sampling supports the constant comparative method that is a key feature of grounded theory research.

In Glaser's view, theoretical sampling is not the same as purposive sampling. The purpose of theoretical sampling is to discover categories and their properties and to offer interrelationships that occur in the substantive theory. "The basic question in theoretical sampling is: what groups or subgroups does one turn to next in data collection?" (Glaser, 1978, p. 36). These groups are not chosen before the research begins but only as they are needed for their theoretical relevance for developing emerging categories.

Most reports on grounded theory studies state that theoretical sampling was used. However, as noted by McCrae and Purssell (2016), many grounded theory studies do not demonstrate the use of theoretical sampling. The following example by one of this book's authors provides insights into an effective theoretical sampling strategy.

Example of a Theoretical Sampling

Beck (2002) used theoretical sampling in her grounded theory study of mothering twins during the first year of life. A specific example of theoretical sampling concerned what the mothers kept referring to as the "blur period"—the first few months of caring for the twins. Initially, Beck interviewed mothers whose twins were around 1 year of age. Her rationale was that these mothers would be able to reflect over the entire first year of mothering the multiples. When these mothers referred to the "blur period," Beck asked them to describe this period more fully. The mothers said they could not provide many details about this period because "it was such a blur!" Beck then chose to interview mothers whose twins were 3 months of age or younger, to ensure that mothers still immersed in the "blur period" would be able to provide rich detail about what this phase of mothering twins was like.

TIP No matter what type of qualitative sampling you use, you should keep a journal or notebook to jot down ideas and reminders regarding the sampling. Memos to yourself will help you remember valuable ideas about your sample.

SAMPLE SIZE IN QUALITATIVE RESEARCH

In qualitative studies, sample size should be based on informational needs. One guiding principle that is often used is **data saturation**—that is, sampling to the point at which no new information is obtained and redundancy is achieved. The goal is to generate enough in-depth data to illuminate the patterns, categories, and dimensions of the phenomenon under study. Redundancy, and hence sample size, can be affected by the type of sampling strategy used. For example, a larger sample is likely to be needed with maximum variation sampling than with typical case sampling.

Morse (2000) noted that the number of participants needed to reach saturation depends on several factors. One factor concerns the scope of the research question: the broader the scope, the more participants likely will be needed. A broader scope may mean not only more interviews with people who have experienced the phenomenon but also a search for supplementary data sources.

Data quality can also affect sample size. If participants are good informants who can reflect on their experiences and communicate effectively, saturation can be achieved with a relatively small sample. For this reason, convenience sampling may require more cases to achieve saturation than purposive or theoretical sampling.

TIP Malterud and colleagues (2016) have argued that sample size in qualitative studies should be guided by *information power* rather than saturation: the more *information* a sample holds, the fewer participants are needed. In their view, information power depends on such factors as the study aim, the use of established theory, and the quality of the data.

Another issue that can affect sample size is the sensitivity of the phenomenon being studied. If the topic is one that is deeply personal, participants may be more reluctant to fully share their thoughts. Thus, to obtain sufficient data for a deep understanding of sensitive or controversial phenomena, more participants may be needed.

Greater amounts of data can be created by increasing the sample size, but sometimes depth and richness in the data can be achieved by longer, more intense interviews (or observations) or by going back to the same participants more than once. Multiple interviews often have the advantage of not only generating more data but also yielding better-quality data if participants are more forthcoming in later sessions because of increased trust.

Morse (2000) noted that sample size can be affected by the availability of what she called *shadowed data*. These are data from participants who are able to discuss not only their own experiences but also the experiences of others. Morse noted that shadowed data can provide researchers "with some idea of the range of experiences and the domain of the phenomenon beyond the single participant's personal experience" (p. 4). Shadowed data can help inform decisions relevant to purposive and theoretical sampling.

The skills and experience of the researcher also can affect sample size. Researchers with strong interviewing or observational skills often require fewer participants because they are more successful in putting participants at ease, encouraging candor, and soliciting important revelations. Thus, students who are just starting out on a qualitative project are likely to require a larger sample size to achieve data saturation than their more experienced mentors.

One final suggestion that may be especially important for beginning researchers is to "test" whether data saturation has been achieved. Essentially, this involves adding one or two cases after achieving informational redundancy to ensure that no new information emerges.

> **Example of Data Saturation**
> Shamaskin-Garroway and colleagues (2018) studied the inpatient hospitalization experience of American women veterans. Data were collected from 25 women who had been hospitalized in a Veterans Administration hospital. The sample size "was determined once thematic saturation was achieved when no new information concepts emerged from additional interviews" (p. 602).

> **TIP** Sample size estimation can create practical dilemmas if you are seeking approval or funding for a project. Patton (2015) recommended that, in a proposal, researchers should specify *minimum* samples that would reasonably be adequate for understanding the phenomenon. Additional cases can then be added, as necessary, to achieve saturation.

SAMPLING IN THE THREE MAIN QUALITATIVE TRADITIONS

There are similarities among the various qualitative traditions with regard to sampling: samples are small, probability sampling is not used, and final sampling decisions usually take place during data collection. However, there are some differences as well.

Sampling in Ethnography

Ethnographers may begin by adopting a "big net" approach—that is, mingling with and having conversations with as many members of the culture under study as possible. Although they may converse with many people, they often rely heavily on a smaller number of key informants. **Key informants** (or *cultural consultants*) are individuals who are highly knowledgeable about the culture or organization and who develop ongoing relationships with the researcher. These key informants are often the researcher's main link to the "inside."

Key informants are chosen purposively, guided by the ethnographer's informed judgments. Developing a pool of potential key informants often depends on ethnographers' prior knowledge to construct a relevant framework. For example, an ethnographer might make decisions about different types of key informants to seek out based on roles (e.g., physicians, nurse practitioners) or on some other substantively meaningful distinction. Once a pool of potential key informants is developed, the primary considerations for final selection are the informants' level of knowledge about the culture and their willingness to collaborate with the ethnographer in revealing and interpreting the culture.

> **TIP** It is prudent not to choose key informants too quickly. The first participants who volunteer to be key informants may be atypical members of the culture being studied. If ethnographers align themselves with marginal members of the culture, this may prevent gaining access to other valuable informants (Bernard, 2018).

Sampling in ethnography typically involves more than selecting informants because observation and other means of data collection play an important role in helping researchers understand a culture. Ethnographers have to decide not only *whom* to sample but *what* to sample as well. For example, ethnographers need to make decisions about observing *events* and *activities*, about examining *records* and *artifacts*, and about exploring *places* that provide clues about the culture. Key informants can play an important role in helping ethnographers decide what to sample.

Sampling in Phenomenologic Studies

Phenomenologists tend to rely on very small samples—typically 10 to 15 participants. One key principle guides sample selection for a phenomenologic study: all participants must have experienced the phenomenon and must be able to articulate what it is like to have lived that experience. Although phenomenologic researchers seek participants who have had the targeted experiences, they also want to explore diversity of individual experiences. Thus, they may specifically look for people with demographic or other differences who have shared a common experience.

> **Example of a Sample in a Phenomenologic Study**
> Ramsayer and colleagues (2019) used a hermeneutic approach to study maternal emotions during the first 3 postnatal months. The researchers stated that "purposeful sampling was used to explore multiple perspectives of individuals using a wide range of participants" (p. 3). For example, the sample of 15 mothers included ones who gave birth for the first time and ones with previous birth experiences.

Sampling in Grounded Theory Studies

Grounded theory research is typically done with samples of about 20 to 30 people, using theoretical

sampling. The goal in a grounded theory study is to select informants who can best contribute to the evolving theory. Sampling, data collection, data analysis, and theory construction occur concurrently. Study participants are selected serially and contingently (i.e., contingent on the emerging conceptualization). Sampling might evolve as follows:

1. The researcher begins with a general notion of where and with whom to start. The first few cases may be solicited purposively, by convenience, or through snowballing.
2. In the early part of the study, a strategy such as maximum variation sampling might be used, to gain insights into the range and complexity of the phenomenon under study.
3. The sample is adjusted in an ongoing fashion. Emerging conceptualizations help to inform the theoretical sampling process.
4. Sampling continues until saturation is achieved.
5. Final sampling may include a search for confirming and disconfirming cases to test, refine, and strengthen the theory.

Draucker and colleagues (2007) have provided particularly useful guidance regarding the actual implementation of theoretical sampling, based on strategies used in their study of responses to sexual violence. Their article included a model for a "theoretical sampling guide."

> **Example of a Sample in a Grounded Theory Study**
> Akbar and colleagues (2017) studied the coping process of Iranian nurses dealing with job stress using a grounded theory approach. The study participants were 15 nurses, 3 head nurses, and 1 nursing supervisor from academic general hospitals. The researchers began with purposive sampling, making efforts to select a diverse group in terms of gender and shifts. The last 12 participants were selected based on theoretical demands, and sampling continued until all categories and concepts were saturated.

TRANSFERABILITY

Qualitative researchers seldom worry explicitly about generalizability. The goal of most qualitative studies is to provide a contextualized understanding of human experience through the intensive study of a few cases. Sampling decisions are not guided by a desire to generalize to a target population.

Yet, in our evidence-based practice environment, the issue of applying research findings beyond the particular people who took part in a study is important. Indeed, Groleau and colleagues (2009), in discussing generalizability, have argued that an important goal of qualitative studies is to shape the opinion of decision-makers whose actions affect people's health and well-being. They noted that "it is not qualitative data itself that must have a direct impact on decision makers but the insights they foster in relation to the problem under investigation" (p. 418). Many who have written about generalizability in qualitative research attempt to find a balance between the generalizable and the particular through *reasonable extrapolation*.

Firestone (1993) developed a useful typology depicting three models of generalizability. The first model is extrapolating from a sample to a population, the model on which sampling in quantitative research is based, as discussed in Chapter 13. The second model is analytic or conceptual generalization, and the third is case-to-case translation, which is more often referred to as transferability—both of which have relevance for qualitative research. In **analytic generalization**, the goal is to generalize from the particulars to a broader theory. Case-to-case translation (**transferability**) involves judgments about whether findings from an inquiry can be extrapolated to a different setting or group of people. **Thick description**—richly thorough depictions of research settings and the sample of study participants (or events)—is needed in qualitative reports to support transferability. Analytic generalization and transferability are described more fully in the Supplement to this chapter on thePoint. Ⓢ

CRITICAL APPRAISAL OF QUALITATIVE SAMPLING PLANS

Qualitative researchers do not always fully describe their method of identifying, recruiting, and selecting participants. Yet, readers will have difficulty drawing conclusions about the study findings without understanding researchers' sampling strategies. Indeed, there have been increased demands for making sampling decisions and processes in qualitative research more "public" (Onwuegbuzie & Leech, 2007). To facilitate transferability, qualitative reports should ideally describe the following:

- The type of sampling approach used (e.g., snowball, purposive, theoretical), together with an indication of how variation was dealt with (for example, in maximum variation sampling, the dimensions chosen for diversification);
- Eligibility criteria for inclusion in the study;
- The nature of the setting or community;
- The time period during which data were collected;
- The number of participants, and a rationale for the sample size, such as an explicit statement that data saturation was achieved; and
- The main characteristics of participants (e.g., age, gender, length of illness, and so forth).

Inadequate description of the sampling strategy can undermine assessments of the strategy's success. Moreover, if the description is vague, it will be difficult for readers to reach conclusions about whether the evidence can be applied in their clinical practice. In appraising a report you should evaluate whether the researcher provided an adequately rich description of the sample and the context in which the study was carried out so that someone interested in transferring the findings could make an informed decision.

Various writers have proposed criteria for evaluating sampling in qualitative studies. Morse (1991), for example, advocated two criteria: adequacy and appropriateness. *Adequacy* refers to the sufficiency and quality of the data the sample yielded. An adequate sample provides data without "thin" spots. When the researcher has truly obtained data saturation, the resulting description or theory is richly textured and complete.

Appropriateness concerns the methods used to select a sample. An appropriate sample is one resulting from the identification and use of participants who can best supply information according to the

> **BOX 23.1** Guidelines for Critically Appraising Qualitative Sampling Designs
>
> 1. Is the setting or context adequately described? Is the setting appropriate for the research question? Is there an explanation of why the setting was chosen?
> 2. Are the sample selection procedures clearly delineated? What type of sampling strategy was used?
> 3. Were the eligibility criteria for the study specified? How were participants recruited into the study? Did the recruitment strategy yield information-rich participants?
> 4. Given the information needs of the study—and, if applicable, its qualitative tradition—was the sampling approach appropriate? Are dimensions of the phenomenon under study adequately represented?
> 5. Is the sample size adequate and appropriate for the qualitative tradition of the study? Did the researcher indicate that saturation had been achieved?
> 6. Do the findings suggest a richly textured and comprehensive set of data without any apparent "holes" or thin areas? Did the sample contribute sufficiently to analytic generalization?
> 7. Are key characteristics of the sample described (e.g., age, gender)? Is a rich description of participants and context provided, allowing for an assessment of the transferability of the findings?

conceptual requirements of the study. Researchers should use a strategy that yields the fullest possible understanding of the phenomenon of interest. A sampling approach that excludes negative cases or that fails to include participants with unusual experiences may not meet the information needs of the study.

Curtis and colleagues (2000) proposed six criteria for evaluating qualitative sampling strategies. These criteria are as relevant for a self-evaluation by qualitative researchers as for an appraisal by readers. First, the sampling strategy should be relevant to the tradition, conceptual framework, and research question addressed by the research. Second, the sample should yield rich information on the phenomenon under study. Third, the sample should enhance the analytic generalizability of the findings. Fourth, the sample should produce believable descriptions, in the sense of being true to real life. Fifth, the strategy should be ethical. Finally, the sampling plan should be feasible in terms of resources, time, and researcher's skills—and the researcher's or participants' ability to cope with the data collection process.

Some specific questions that can be used to critically appraise sampling in a qualitative study are presented in Box 23.1.

RESEARCH EXAMPLE

Examples of various approaches to sampling in qualitative research have been presented throughout this chapter. In this section, we describe more fully the sampling plan used in an ethnographic study.

Study: "Meal realities"—An ethnographic exploration of hospital mealtime environment and practice (Ottrey et al., 2018).

Purpose: The researchers sought to understand patterns of mealtime culture, environment, and social practice in hospital wards from the perspective of hospital staff, volunteers, and visitors.

Method: The researchers used an ethnographic approach to obtain a comprehensive understanding of mealtime environment and practice. A major goal was to identify the challenges experienced by staff, volunteers, and visitors at mealtimes. Data were collected by means of observations at mealtimes and in-depth personal interviews that were audio-recorded.

Sampling strategy: The study settings were wards from two sites in a publicly funded healthcare network in Melbourne, Australia. The two wards were selected purposively to be similar. Both had a subacute focus and were similar in size, staffing, organizational structure, and food service systems. Study participants were staff, volunteers, and visitors who were present on the study wards at mealtimes—everyone meeting these criteria was eligible to be observed and interviewed. A purposive sample of leaders from key professions involved in nutritional care was also invited to be interviewed, but there was no single key informant in this study. The lead investigator conducted 67 hours of fieldwork. Observations were conducted at breakfast, lunch, and dinner across 7 days of the week. Observations began about 40 minutes before meal service and lasted until meal trays were collected. More than 150 staff, volunteers, and visitors were observed during 35 observation periods. Interviews were conducted with participants who were either identified through observation or by nomination from other participants. Interviews lasted, on average, about 45 minutes. In all, 61 participants were interviewed.

Key findings: The report provided thick description about mealtime experiences in the hospital wards. The researchers found that staff, volunteers, and visitors strive for patient-centeredness at mealtimes, but the routine and structured nature of the meal and care systems was in constant tension with efforts to provide patients the care they needed.

SUMMARY POINTS

- Qualitative researchers use the conceptual demands of the study to select articulate and reflective informants with certain types of experience in an emergent way, typically capitalizing on early learning to guide subsequent sampling decisions. Qualitative samples tend to be small, nonrandom, and intensively studied.
- Sampling in qualitative inquiry may begin with a convenience (or *volunteer*) sample. Snowball (*chain*) sampling may also be used.
- Qualitative researchers often use **purposive sampling** to select data sources that enhance information richness. Various purposive sampling strategies have been used by qualitative researchers and can be loosely categorized as (1) sampling for representativeness or comparative value; (2) sampling special or unique cases; or (3) sampling sequentially.

- An important purposive strategy in the first category is **maximum variation sampling,** which entails purposely selecting cases with a range of variation. Other strategies used for comparative purposes include **homogeneous sampling** (deliberately reducing variation), **typical case sampling** (selecting cases that illustrate what is typical), **extreme case sampling** (selecting the most unusual or extreme cases), **intensity sampling** (selecting cases that are intense but not extreme), **stratified purposeful sampling** (selecting cases within defined strata), and **reputational case sampling** (selecting cases based on a recommendation of an expert or key informant).
- Purposive sampling in the "special cases" category includes **criterion sampling** (studying cases that meet a predetermined criterion of importance), **revelatory case sampling** (identifying and gaining access to a case representing a phenomenon that was previously inaccessible to research scrutiny), and **sampling politically important cases** (searching for and selecting or deselecting politically sensitive cases or sites).
- Although many qualitative sampling strategies unfold while in the field, purposive sampling in the "sequential" category involves deliberative emergent efforts and includes **theoretical sampling** (selecting cases based on their contribution to important constructs) and **opportunistic sampling** (adding new cases based on changes in research circumstances or in response to new leads that develop in the field). Another important sequential strategy is **sampling confirming and disconfirming cases**—that is, selecting cases that enrich or challenge the researchers' conceptualizations.
- A guiding sample size principle is **data saturation**—sampling to the point at which no new information is obtained and redundancy is achieved. Factors affecting sample size include data quality, researcher skills and experience, and scope and sensitivity of the problem.
- Ethnographers make numerous sampling decisions, including not only *whom* to sample but *what* to sample (e.g., activities, events, documents, artifacts); **key informants,** who serve

as guides and interpreters of the culture, often assist with sampling decisions.

- Phenomenologists typically work with a small sample of people (15 or fewer) who meet the criterion of having lived the experience under study.

- Grounded theory researchers typically use *theoretical sampling* in which sampling decisions are guided in an ongoing manner by the emerging theory. Samples of about 20 to 30 people are typical in grounded theory studies.

- Two models of generalizability have relevance for qualitative research. In **analytic generalization**, researchers strive to generalize from particulars to broader conceptualizations and theories. **Transferability** involves judgments about whether findings from an inquiry can be extrapolated to a different setting or group of people. **Thick description**—richly thorough depictions of research settings and participants—is needed in qualitative reports to support transferability.

STUDY ACTIVITIES

Study activities are available to instructors on thePoint.

REFERENCES CITED IN CHAPTER 23

*Akbar, R., Elahi, N., Mohammadi, E., & Khoshknab, F. (2017). How do the nurses cope with job stress? A study with grounded theory approach. *Journal of Caring Sciences, 6*, 199–211.

Beck, C. T. (2002). Releasing the pause button: Mothering twins during the first year of life. *Qualitative Health Research, 12*, 593–608.

Bernard, H. R. (2018). *Research methods in anthropology: Qualitative and quantitative approaches* (6th ed.). Lanham, MD: AltaMira Press.

Curtis, S., Gesler, W., Smith, G., & Washburn, S. (2000). Approaches to sampling and case selection in qualitative research: Examples in the geography of health. *Social Science & Medicine, 50*, 1001–1014.

Draucker, C., Martsoff, D., Ross, R., & Rusk, T. (2007). Theoretical sampling and category development in grounded theory. *Qualitative Health Research, 17*, 1137–1148.

**Durante, A., Paturzo, M., Mottola, A., Alvaro, R., Dickson, V., & Vellone, E. (2019). Caregiver contribution to self-care in patients with heart failure: A qualitative descriptive study. *Journal of Cardiovascular Nursing, 34*, E28–E35.

*Firestone, W. A. (1993). Alternative arguments for generalizing from data as applied to qualitative research. *Educational Researcher, 22*, 16–23.

Glaser, B. (1978). *Theoretical sensitivity*. Mill Valley, CA: The Sociology Press.

Glaser, B. G., & Strauss, A. (1967). *The discovery of grounded theory: Strategies for qualitative research*. New York: Aldine de Gruyter.

Groleau, D., Zelkowitz, P., & Cabral, I. (2009). Enhancing generalizability: Moving from an intimate to a political voice. *Qualitative Health Research, 19*, 416–426.

Hamilton, J., Best, N., Wells, J., & Worthy, V. (2018). Making sense of loss through spirituality: Perspectives of African American family members who have experienced the death of a close family member to cancer. *Palliative & Supportive Care, 16*, 662–668.

Lamb, C., Evans, M., Babenko-Mould, Y., Wong, C., & Kirkwood, K. (2019). Nurses' use of conscientious objection and the implications for conscience. *Journal of Advanced Nursing, 75*, 594–602.

Lauder, B., Sinclair, P., & Maguire, J. (2018). Mothers' experience of caring for a child with early onset scoliosis: A qualitative descriptive study. *Journal of Clinical Nursing, 27*, e1549–e1560.

Malterud, K., Siersma, V., & Guassora, A. (2016). Sample size in qualitative interview studies: Guided by information power. *Qualitative Health Research, 26*, 1753–1760.

Mamier, I., & Winslow, B. (2014). Divergent views of placement decision-making: A qualitative case study. *Issues in Mental Health Nursing, 35*, 13–20.

Matthew-Maich, N., Ploeg, J., Jack, S., & Dobbins, M. (2013). Leading on the frontlines with passion and persistence: A necessary condition for breastfeeding best practice guideline uptake. *Journal of Clinical Nursing, 22*, 1759–1770.

McCrae, N., & Pursell, E. (2016). Is it really theoretical? A review of sampling in grounded theory studies in nursing journals. *Journal of Advanced Nursing, 72*, 2284–2293.

Morse, J. M. (1991). Strategies for sampling. In Morse, J. M. (Ed.), *Qualitative nursing research: A contemporary dialogue*. Newbury Park, CA: Sage.

Morse, J. M. (2000). Determining sample size. *Qualitative Health Research, 10*, 3–5.

*Onwuegbuzie, A., & Leech, N. (2007). Sampling designs in qualitative research: Making the sampling process more public. *The Qualitative Report, 12*, 238–254.

Ottrey, E., Porter, J., Huggins, C., & Palermo, C. (2018). "Meal realities"—An ethnographic exploration of hospital mealtime environment and practice. *Journal of Advanced Nursing, 74*, 603–613.

Patton, M. Q. (2015). *Qualitative research and evaluation methods* (4th ed.). Thousand Oaks, CA: Sage.

Ramsayer, B., Fleming, V., Robb, Y., Deery, R., & Cattell, T. (2019). Maternal emotions during the first three postnatal months: Gaining an hermeneutic understanding. *Women and Birth.* doi:10.1016/j.wombi.2018.11.002.

Shamaskin-Garroway, A., Knobf, M., Adams, L., & Haskell, S. (2018). "I think it's pretty much the same, as it should be": Perspectives of inpatient care among women veterans. *Qualitative Health Research, 28,* 600–609.

*Stormorken, E., Jason, L., & Kirkevolv, M. (2017). Factors impacting the illness trajectory of post-infectious fatigue syndrome: A qualitative study of adults' experiences. *BMC Public Health, 17,* 952.

Teddlie, C., & Tashkkori, A. (2009). *Foundations of mixed methods research.* Thousand Oaks, CA: Sage Publications.

Thorne, S. (2008). *Interpretive description.* Walnut Creek, CA: Left Coast Press.

Yin, R. (2014). *Case study research: Design and methods* (5th ed.). Thousand Oaks, CA: Sage.

*A link to this open-access article is provided in the Toolkit for Chapter 23 in the **Resource Manual.** ⊗

**This journal article is available on the Point *for this chapter.*

24 | Data Collection in Qualitative Research

This chapter provides an overview of data collection approaches used in qualitative research, with a focus on self-reports and observations.

DATA COLLECTION ISSUES IN QUALITATIVE STUDIES

In qualitative studies, data collection usually is more fluid than in quantitative research; decisions about types of information to collect evolve in the field. For example, as researchers gather and digest their data, they may realize that it would be fruitful to pursue a new line of questioning. Even while allowing for and profiting from this flexibility, however, qualitative researchers make several up-front decisions about data collection, and need to be prepared for problematic situations that may arise in the field.

Types of Data for Qualitative Studies

Qualitative researchers typically begin a study knowing the most likely sources of data, while not ruling out other possible sources that might come to light as data collection progresses. The primary method of collecting qualitative data is by interviewing study participants. Observation is used in many qualitative studies as well. Physiologic data are rarely collected in a constructivist inquiry,

except perhaps to describe participants' characteristics or to ascertain eligibility for the study.

Table 24.1 compares the types of data used by researchers in the three main qualitative traditions, as well as other aspects of the data collection process for each tradition. Ethnographers typically collect a wide array of data, with observation and interviews being the primary methods. Ethnographers also examine products of the culture under study, such as documents, artifacts, photographs, and so on. Phenomenologists and grounded theory researchers rely primarily on in-depth interviews, although observation and documents may also play a role in grounded theory studies.

Field Issues in Qualitative Studies

Collecting qualitative data often gives rise to several important concerns, which are particularly salient in ethnographies. Ethnographic researchers must deal with such issues as gaining entrée, negotiating for space and privacy for interviewing and recording data, deciding on an appropriate role (i.e., the extent to which they will participate in the culture's activities), and taking care not to exit from the field prematurely. Ethnographers also need to be able to cope with culture shock and should have a high tolerance for uncertainty and ambiguity. Other field issues apply to most qualitative research.

TABLE 24.1 • Comparison of Data Collection Issues in Three Qualitative Traditions

ISSUE	ETHNOGRAPHY	PHENOMENOLOGY	GROUNDED THEORY
Types of data	Primarily observation and interviews, plus artifacts, documents, photographs, genealogies, maps, social network diagrams	Primarily in-depth interviews, sometimes diaries, other written materials	Primarily individual interviews, sometimes group interviews, observation, participant journals, documents
Unit of data collection	Cultural systems	Individuals	Individuals
Data collection points	Mainly longitudinal	Mainly cross-sectional	Cross-sectional or longitudinal
Length of time for data collection	Typically long, many months or years	Typically moderate	Typically moderate
Data recording	Field notes, logs, interview notes/recordings	Interview notes/recordings	Interview notes/recordings, memoing, observational notes
Salient field issues	Gaining entrée, reactivity, determining a role, learning how to participate, encouraging candor and other interview logistics, loss of objectivity, premature exit, reflexivity	Bracketing one's views, building rapport, encouraging candor, listening while preparing what to ask next, keeping "on track," handling emotionality	Building rapport, encouraging candor, listening while preparing what to ask next, keeping "on track," handling emotionality

Gaining Trust

Qualitative researchers must gain and maintain a high level of trust with participants and strive to achieve *empathic neutrality*. This may be a delicate balancing act: researchers must try to "be like" the people being studied while at the same time keeping a certain distance. "Being like" participants means that researchers should be sensitive to such issues as styles of dress, modes of speech, and customs. In ethnographic research, it is important not to take sides on any controversial issue and not to appear strongly affiliated with a particular subgroup of the culture—especially with leaders or prominent members of the culture. It is often impossible to gain the trust of the larger group if researchers appear close to those in power.

Preparing for the Intensity of Data Collection

In qualitative studies, data collection can be an intense and exhausting experience, especially if the phenomenon being studied is an illness experience or other stressful life event (e.g., domestic violence). Petty (2017) has written about "emotion work" in qualitative inquiry, referring to qualitative researchers' emotional responses in exploring difficult experiences. Collecting high-grade qualitative data requires deep concentration and energy. The process can be an emotional strain for which researchers need to prepare—Petty refers to this as cultivating "emotional intelligence." One way to deal with this is to collect data at a pace that minimizes stress (e.g., one interview a day) and to engage in emotionally releasing activities (e.g., exercising) between interviews. It may also be helpful to debrief about any feelings of distress with a coresearcher, colleague, or advisor.

Emotional Involvement With Participants

Qualitative researchers need to guard against getting too emotionally involved with participants, a pitfall that has been called "**going native**." Researchers who get too close to participants run several risks, including compromising their ability to collect meaningful and trustworthy data, and becoming overwhelmed with participants' suffering. It is important, of course, to be supportive and to listen carefully to people's concerns, but it usually is not advisable to try to solve participants' problems or to share personal problems with them. If participants need help, it is better to give advice about where they can get it than to give it directly.

Reflexivity

As noted in Chapter 8, reflexivity is an important concept in qualitative data collection. Reflexivity refers to researchers' awareness of themselves as part of the data they are collecting. Researchers need to be conscious of the part they play in their own study and reflect on how their own experiences can affect the data they obtain. McNair and colleagues (2008) have discussed how reflexivity can be used to enhance in-depth interviewing skills.

Example of Reflexivity
Nilson (2017) wrote a thoughtful paper highlighting her personal journey of "reflective development" that she, as a non-Aboriginal white researcher, underwent to be fully positioned in everyday lives in a rural Australian Aboriginal community. She used reflexivity to examine and contextualize her judgments and preconceptions, which promoted openness to differing viewpoints and alternative perspectives.

Recording and Storing Qualitative Data

In addition to thinking about the types of data to be gathered, qualitative researchers need to plan for how data will be recorded and stored. To ensure that interview data are participants' actual verbatim responses, qualitative interviews should

be recorded and subsequently transcribed rather than relying on interviewer notes. Notes tend to be incomplete and may be affected by the interviewer's personal views or by memory lapses. Moreover, note-taking can distract interviewers, whose main job is to listen intently and direct the flow of questioning based on what has already been said.

TIP In addition to traditional audio-recording equipment, new technologies are emerging to facilitate recording in the field. For example, digital voice recorders with transcription capabilities allow researchers to record and transfer voice data to a personal computer using a USB interface. Some digital voice recorders come bundled with voice recognition software. A recent innovation is the *smartpen*—a ballpoint pen with an embedded computer and digital audio recorder—that can record up to 200 hours of audio. When used with *digital paper*, the smartpen records written material for uploading to a computer and synchronizes the notes with any material that was audio-recorded.

Environmental distractions are a common pitfall in recording interviews. A quiet setting without disruptions is ideal but is not always possible. The second author of this book (Beck) has conducted many challenging interviews. As an example, a mother of three children was interviewed in her home about her experience with postpartum depression. The interview was scheduled during the toddlers' normal naptime, but when Beck arrived, the toddlers had already taken their nap. The television was on to occupy the toddlers, but they kept trying to play with the audio recorder. The 6-week-old baby was fussy, crying through most of the interview. The background noise level on the recording made accurate transcription difficult.

TIP Some researchers use their smartphones to record interviews, which requires special precautions to ensure the security of the interviews. There are special cell phone apps that can encrypt the interview data. Without special encryption, the interviews should be transferred from a cell phone to a secure device as soon as possible and deleted from the cell phone.

When observations are made, detailed observational notes must be maintained, unless it is possible to video-record. Observational notes should be made shortly after an observational session, usually onto a computer file. Whatever method is used to record observations, researchers need to go into the field with the equipment or supplies needed to record their data and to be sure that the equipment is functioning properly.

Grounded theory (and other) researchers write **analytic memos** that document researchers' ideas about their analyses (e.g., how some categories are interrelated). These memos can vary in length from a sentence to multiple pages. Charmaz (2014) offers guidance on preparing grounded theory notes and memos.

If assistants are used to conduct interviews, qualitative researchers need to hire appropriate staff and train them to elicit rich and vivid descriptions. Qualitative interviewers need to be good listeners; they need to hear all that is being said, rather than trying to anticipate what is coming next. A good data collector must be self-aware and attentive to participants (e.g., paying attention to nonverbal behavior). Qualitative data collectors must be able to create an atmosphere that safely allows for the sharing of experiences and feelings. Respect and authentic caring for participants are critical.

> **TIP** In qualitative studies, data are sometimes collected by a single researcher working alone. In such cases, self-training and self-preparation are important. When a team of researchers works together on a qualitative study, attention needs to be paid to team issues related to fieldwork and to group decision-making (Hall et al., 2005).

QUALITATIVE SELF-REPORT TECHNIQUES

Unstructured or loosely structured self-report methods provide narrative data for qualitative analysis. Most qualitative self-report data are collected through interviews rather than by self-administered questionnaires.

Types of Qualitative Self-Reports

Researchers use various approaches in collecting qualitative self-report data. The main methods are described here.

Unstructured Interviews

Researchers who do not have preconceived views of the content or flow of information to be gathered may conduct completely **unstructured interviews**. Unstructured interviews are conversational and are the mode of choice when researchers do not have a clear idea of what it is they do not know. Researchers using unstructured interviews do not have a set of prepared questions because they do not yet know what to ask or even where to begin—they let participants tell their stories, with little interruption. Phenomenologic, grounded theory, and ethnographic studies may involve unstructured interviews, especially at the outset.

Researchers using a completely unstructured approach often begin by informally asking a broad question (a **grand tour question**) relating to the research topic, such as, "What happened when you first learned you had AIDS?" Subsequent questions are more focused, guided by responses to the broad question. Some respondents may request direction after the initial question is posed, perhaps asking, "Where should I begin?" Respondents should be encouraged to begin wherever they wish.

Van Manen (1990) provided suggestions for guiding a phenomenologic interview in a manner likely to produce rich descriptions of the experience under study:

- "Describe the experience from the inside, as it were; almost like a state of mind: the feelings, the mood, the emotions, etc.
- Focus on a particular example or incident of the object of experience: describe specific events, an adventure, a happening, a particular experience.
- Try to focus on an example of the experience which stands out for its vividness, or as it was the first time.
- Attend to how the body feels, how things smell(ed), how they sound(ed), etc." (pp. 64–65).

Kahn (2000), discussing unstructured interviews in hermeneutic studies, recommended interviews that resemble conversations. If the experience under study is an ongoing one, Kahn suggested obtaining as much detail as possible about the participant's daily life. For example, a question that can be used is, "Pick a normal day for you and tell me what happened" (p. 62). If the experience being studied is primarily in the past, then Kahn advocated beginning with a general question such as, "What does this experience mean to you?" (p. 63) and then probing for more detail until the experience is thoroughly described.

Example of Unstructured Interviews

Ho and colleagues (2018) examined the experiences of foreign domestic helpers (FDHs) working with community-dwelling older people in Hong Kong. The study addressed the helpers' transition from a task-oriented relationship to caring companion. Unstructured interviews were conducted with 11 female FDHs. The researchers began with, "Let's start by introducing ourselves" and then asking, "What comes to your mind when you think about caring for an older person who is a member of your employer's family?" (p. 3).

In grounded theory, questioning changes as the theory is developed. At the outset, interviews are similar to open-ended conversations using unstructured interviews. Glaser and Strauss (1967) suggested researchers initially should just sit back and listen to participants' stories. Later, as the theory emerges, researchers ask more direct questions related to categories in the grounded theory. The more direct questions can be answered rather quickly, and so the interviews tend to get shorter as the grounded theory develops.

Ethnographic interviews are also unstructured. Spradley (1979) describes three types of questions used to guide interviews: descriptive, structural, and contrast questions. *Descriptive questions* ask participants to describe their experiences in their own language and are the backbone of ethnographic interviews. *Structural questions* are more focused and help to develop the range of terms in a category

or domain. Last are *contrast questions*, which are asked to distinguish differences in the meaning of terms and symbols.

Example of Ethnographic Interviewing

Mirhaghi and an interprofessional team (2016) conducted an ethnographic study to gain an understanding of emergency department nursing and the triage of nonemergent patients. The interview questions consisted of a sequence of descriptive, structural, and then contrast questions according to Spradley's method.

Semistructured Interviews

Researchers sometimes want to be sure that a specific set of topics is covered in their qualitative interviews. They know what they want to ask but cannot predict what the answers will be. Their role in the process is somewhat structured, whereas the participants' is not. In such **focused** or **semistructured interviews**, researchers prepare a written **topic guide**, which is a list of areas or questions to be covered with each participant. The interviewer's job is to encourage participants to talk freely about all the topics on the guide and to tell stories in their own words. This technique ensures that researchers will obtain all the information required and yet gives people the freedom to provide as many illustrations and explanations as they wish.

In preparing a topic guide, questions should be ordered in a logical sequence—perhaps chronologically or perhaps from the general to the specific. Interviewers need to be attentive, however, because respondents often volunteer information about questions that are later on the list. The topic guide might include suggestions for *probes* designed to elicit more detailed information. Examples of such probes include, "What happened next?" and "When that happened, how did you feel?" Questions that require one- or two-word responses, such as "yes" or "no," should be avoided. Questions should give people an opportunity to provide rich, detailed information about the phenomenon under study. McIntosh and Morse (2015) have described different types of semistructured interviews.

Example of Semistructured Interviews

Skilbeck and colleagues (2018) conducted an ethnographic study to understand how older people with health problems experience frailty in their daily lives. The topic guide used to interview 10 older people in their own homes covered four areas. One area, for example, was the participants' understanding of frailty and included such questions as "What do you understand by the term 'frail'?" and "In considering this description would you consider yourself to be frail?" (p. 5).

Focus Group Interviews

Focus group interviews have become popular in the study of health problems. In a focus group interview, a group of people (usually five or more) is assembled for a discussion, although some focus group discussions are conducted online. The interviewer (or **moderator**) guides the discussion according to a written set of questions or topics to be covered, as in a semistructured interview. Focus group sessions are carefully planned discussions that take advantage of group dynamics and synergies for accessing rich information in an economical manner.

Typically, the people selected are fairly homogeneous, to promote a comfortable group dynamic. People usually feel more at ease expressing their views when they share a similar background with other group members. Thus, if the overall sample is diverse, it is best to organize focus groups for people with similar characteristics (e.g., in terms of age or gender). Several writers have suggested that the optimal group size for focus groups is 6 to 12 people, but some have advised even smaller groups when the topic is emotionally charged or sensitive.

TIP In recruiting group members, it is usually wise to recruit one or two more people than is considered optimal, because of the risk of no-shows. Monetary incentives can help reduce this risk. It is also important to call recruits the night before the session to confirm attendance.

Moderators play a critical role in the success of focus group interviews. At the start of a session, moderators establish some ground rules with the participants. For example, they might advise participants to please speak one at a time, to be respectful of each other, and to maintain the confidentiality of what is said in the group. Moderators must take care to solicit input from all group members and not let a few vocal people dominate the discussion. Researchers other than the moderator should be present to take detailed observational notes about each session.

A major advantage of a group format is that it is efficient—researchers obtain the viewpoints of many people in a short time. Moreover, focus groups capitalize on the fact that members react to what is being said by others, thereby potentially leading to deeper expressions of opinion. Focus group interviews are also usually stimulating to respondents, but one problem is that some people are uncomfortable about communicating their views in front of a group. Another concern is that the dynamics of the session may foster a group culture that could inhibit individual expression as "group think" takes hold. Studies of focus groups suggest that they are similar to individual interviews in terms of number and quality of ideas generated (Kidd & Parshall, 2000), but some critics have worried about whether data from focus groups are as "natural" as data obtained from individual interviews (Morgan, 2001).

The researcher's *questioning route*—the series of questions used to guide the interview—is key to effective focus group sessions. A typical 2-hour focus group session should include about 12 questions. Krueger and Casey (2015) provided these guidelines for developing a good questioning route:

1. Brainstorm.
2. Sequence the questioning. Arrange general questions first and then more specific questions. Ask positive questions before negative ones.
3. Phrase the questions. Use open-ended questions. Ask participants to think back and reflect on their personal experiences. Avoid asking "why" questions. Keep questions simple and make your questions sound conversational. Be careful about giving examples.
4. Estimate the time for each question. Consider the following when estimating time: the complexity of the questions, the category of questions, level of participant's expertise, the size of the focus group, and the amount of discussion you want related to the question.

5. Obtain feedback from others.
6. Revise the questions.
7. Test the questions.

Rothwell and colleagues (2016) have proposed a *deliberative discussion* approach to certain types of focus group studies. In such studies, researchers develop methods of educating and informing participants about the focal topic prior to the group interview. They argue that this approach can "promote more quality data from informed opinions" (p. 734).

Focus groups have been used by researchers in many qualitative research traditions and can play a role in feminist, critical theory, and participatory action research. Nurse researchers have offered excellent guidance on studies with focus groups (e.g., Carey, 2016; Côté-Arsenault, 2013), and books on how to do focus group research are available (e.g., Carey & Asbury, 2012; Krueger & Casey, 2015). The Toolkit in the accompanying *Resource Manual* also has additional resources on focus groups. ✪

Example of Focus Group Interviews
Schenck and co-researchers (2019) studied different perspectives on patient and family engagement with reduction in harm in hospitals. Focus group interviews were conducted in two acute care facilities in different states in the United States, with four groups in both sites: (1) recently hospitalized patients and family members; (2) nurses; (3) physician hospitalists; and (4) physical therapists and pharmacists. Questions in the 90-minute sessions relied on topic guides.

Joint Interviews

Nurse researchers are sometimes interested in phenomena that involve interpersonal relationships. For example, the phenomenon might be the grief that mothers *and* fathers experience on losing a child, or the experiences of patients with AIDS *and* their caretakers. In such cases, it can be productive to conduct **joint (dyadic) interviews** in which two or more people are simultaneously questioned, using either an unstructured or semistructured format. Unlike focus group interviews, which typically involve group members who do not know each other, joint interviews involve respondents who are intimately related.

Joint interviews usually supplement rather than replace individual interviews, because there are things that cannot readily be discussed in front of the other party (e.g., criticisms of the other person's behavior). Joint interviews can be especially helpful, however, when researchers want to *observe* the dynamics between two key actors. Voltelen and colleagues (2018) and Zarhin (2018) have described ethical issues to consider when conducting joint interviews with couples or close relatives.

Example of Joint Interviews
Ye and colleagues (2017) conducted 20 joint interviews with couples (20 patients and their partners) to identify factors that are facilitators of and barriers to successful treatment of obstructive sleep apnea.

Diaries and Journals

Personal **diaries** have long been used as a source of data in historical research. It is also possible to generate new data for a study by asking study participants to maintain a diary or journal over a specified period—or by asking them to share a diary they wrote. Diaries can be useful in providing an intimate and detailed description of a person's everyday life.

The diaries may be completely unstructured; for example, individuals who have undergone organ transplantation could be asked to spend 10 to 15 minutes a day jotting down their thoughts and feelings. Frequently, however, participants are requested to make entries into a diary regarding a specific aspect of their experience, sometimes in a semistructured format (e.g., about their appetite or sleeping). Nurse researchers have used health diaries to collect information about how people prevent illness, maintain health, experience morbidity, and treat health problems.

Although diaries are a useful means of learning about ongoing experiences, one limitation is that they can be used only by people with adequate literacy skills, although there are examples of studies in which diary entries were audio-recorded rather than written out. Diaries also require a high level of participant cooperation.

Example of Diaries
Ten Hoeve and colleagues (2018) studied the clinical experiences of novice nurses during their first 2 years after graduation. A sample of 19 novice nurses maintained weekly diaries. The nurses were asked to address the following questions in their diary entries: "Please describe a personal or work-related experience from the past week that really was important to you. What was the experience? In what situation? How did you reflect on this experience and how did it affect your work?" (p. e1615).

Photo Elicitation and Photovoice

Photo elicitation involves an interview stimulated and guided by photographic images. This procedure, most often used in ethnographies, is a method that can break down barriers between researchers and study participants and promote a collaborative discussion (Frith & Harcourt, 2007). The photographs sometimes are ones that researchers have made of the participants' world, through which researchers can gain insights into the new culture. Participants may need to be continually reassured that their taken-for-granted explanations of the photos are providing useful information. Photo elicitation can also be used with photos that participants have in their homes, although in such case, researchers have less time to frame useful questions and no opportunity to select the photos that will be the stimulus for discussion.

Researchers are also using an increasingly popular technique of asking participants to take photographs themselves and then interpret them, a method called **photovoice**. Photovoice can be used as a strategy to promote empowerment and give voice to participants in addressing social and political change and thus is often used in participatory action research (Liebenberg, 2018). Oliffe and colleagues (2008) offered useful suggestions for a four-part strategy of analyzing participant-produced photographs, and Jaiswal and colleagues (2016) offered 12 tips to facilitate a photovoice project. Photovoice can be an empowering data collection strategy, but ethical challenges may emerge because people not involved in the research are often photographed (Caiola et al., 2018; Creighton et al., 2018).

Example of a Study With Photovoice
Chew and Lopez (2018) explored self-care in Singaporean patients with heart failure. The 16 participants were asked to take photographs that represented their promotion of self-care, and the photos were then discussed in subsequent in-depth interviews.

Video-Stimulated Recall Interviews

A related technique is called a **stimulated recall interview**, which is used to explore how people approach social interactions. The researcher video-records study participants engaging in various activities in social situations. Then, in follow-up interviews, the researcher discusses aspects of the participants' behavior with them. For example, the interviewer might probe how the person chose from various options in deciding how to react to the behavior and actions of others. Stimulated recall interviews are considered a valuable tool for investigating cognitive processes in connection with specific events. Stimulated recall has most often been used in ethnographic research (Dempsey, 2010).

Example of Stimulated Recall Interviews
Burden and colleagues (2018) studied how nurse mentors form judgments and reach conclusions about student nurses' competence. The researchers video-recorded mentors conducting assessments and providing feedback to students. The stimulated recall interviews were undertaken with a purposive sample of 17 final placement mentors.

TIP **Digital storytelling** is an emergent method for collecting short first-person accounts in an electronic format. Digital stories are usually 3 to 5 minutes long and can include a person's photographs or drawings, video segments, and audio recording in the person's own voice. It is being used in community-based participatory research to address health inequities in vulnerable, underrepresented populations. Briant and colleagues (2016) have described the power of digital storytelling as a culturally relevant tool in health promotion projects.

Self-Report Narratives on the Internet

In addition to the possibility of soliciting narrative data on the Internet through structured or semi-structured "interview" methods (as we describe in the next section), a potentially rich data source for qualitative researchers involves narrative self-reports available directly on the Internet. For example, researchers can enter into long conversations with other users in a chat room.

Some data that can be analyzed qualitatively are simply "out there," as when a researcher enters a chat room, blog site, or online forum and analyzes the content of existing, unsolicited messages. As pointed out by Keim-Malpass et al. (2014), the Internet is a rich source of interactive and socially mediated data, giving rise to "*Internet ethnography*." Interest has focused, in particular, on illness blogs as a means of studying illness experiences.

Using the Internet to access narrative data has obvious advantages. This approach is economical and allows researchers to obtain information from geographically dispersed and perhaps remote Internet users. However, a number of ethical concerns have been raised, and authenticity and other methodologic challenges need to be considered (Corti & Fielding, 2016; Smith et al., 2017). Germain and three other Ph.D. students (2018) have discussed the benefits and challenges of doing online research for their doctoral dissertations.

> **Example of an Analysis of Facebook Posts**
> Gage-Bouchard and co-researchers (2017) examined how caregivers of patients with cancer use personal Facebook pages for cancer-related communication. The researchers examined themes in cancer-related exchanges in 12 months of data from 18 Facebook pages hosted by parents of children with leukemia.

Other Unstructured Self-Reports

We have described the primary means of collecting in-depth self-report, but other forms of unstructured self-reports have been developed. Examples include:

- **Life history interviews**, which are individual interviews directed at documenting a person's life story or an aspect of it that has developed over the life course;

- **Oral histories**, a method often used by historical researchers to gather personal recollections about events or issues;
- The **critical incidents technique**, a method of gathering in-depth information about specific incidents experienced by participants; and
- The **think-aloud method**, which involves obtaining real-time narrative data about how a person solves a problem or makes a decision.

These methods are briefly described, and some examples are provided, in the Supplement to this chapter on thePoint. **S**

Gathering Qualitative Self-Report Data Through Interviews

The purpose of gathering narrative self-report data is to enable researchers to construct reality in a way that is consistent with the constructions of the people being studied. This goal requires researchers to take steps to overcome communication barriers and to enhance the flow of meaning. Asking good questions and eliciting good narrative data are more difficult than you might think. This section offers some suggestions about gathering qualitative self-report data through in-depth interviews. Further advice is offered by Rubin and Rubin (2012) and Brinkman and Kvale (2015).

Locating the Interview

Researchers must decide where the interviews will take place. For one-on-one interviews, in-home interviews are often preferred because interviewers can then observe the participants' world and take observational notes. When in-home interviews are not desired by participants (e.g., if they prefer more privacy), it is wise to identify alternatives, such as an office, coffee shop, and so on. The important thing is to select places that offer privacy, that protect against interruptions insofar as possible, and that are suitable for recording purposes. It is sometimes useful to let participants select the setting, but the setting may be dictated by circumstances, as when interviews take place while participants are hospitalized.

Settings for focus group sessions should be selected carefully and, ideally, should be neutral.

Churches, hospitals, or other settings that are strongly identified with particular values or expected behaviors may not be suitable, depending on the topic. The location should be comfortable, accessible, easy to find, and acoustically amenable to audio recording.

Most qualitative interviews are conducted in person, but new technologies have opened up other options. For example, videoconferencing makes it possible to conduct face-to-face interviews with participants remotely (Irani, 2019). Videoconferencing is advantageous from the perspective of having both a visual and auditory record of the interview.

Example of Videoconferencing Interviews
Lee and colleagues (2015) conducted a qualitative study of the sexual needs and concerns of men who have sex with men following treatment for prostate cancer. Sixteen men were interviewed, some in face-to-face interviews and others via videoconferencing.

Another option is to conduct interviews using Skype, Facebook, or other synchronous online services, which have become widely available. Janghorban and colleagues (2014) have noted that such services can be used for both individual interviews and small focus group interviews. Such technologies are especially useful for gathering data from geographically dispersed participants or from people living in rural areas. Virtual focus groups open the door for including people who are unable or unwilling to participate in traditional focus groups that meet physically in a room.

Liamputtong (2011) has described the advantages of virtual focus groups. For example, in addition to being relatively inexpensive, participants' inhibitions are often lessened, anonymity can be enhanced, and pressures to conform can be reduced. The potential disadvantages of online focus groups include limits to group interaction, comments that are short and direct, and limited opportunity for the moderator to drive in-depth conversations (Carey, 2016). However, Woodyatt and colleagues (2016), in their comparison of data from in-person and online focus groups on a sensitive topic, found less sharing of in-depth stories in the in-person groups, but noted that "the content of the data generated is remarkably similar" (p. 741).

Study participants can also be "interviewed" asynchronously (not in real time) via emails or on social media platforms. A distinct advantage of online interviewing is that participants' narratives are already typed, thus avoiding the expense of transcribing recorded interviews. James and Busher (2012) and Fritz and Vandermause (2018) have offered advice about Internet interviewing. Asynchronous methods have also been used with focus groups (e.g., Biedermann, 2018).

Example of Internet Interviewing
Beck and Watson (2016) conducted a phenomenologic study via the Internet about women's experiences of posttraumatic growth following a traumatic childbirth. A recruitment notice was posted on the website of Trauma and Birth Stress, a charitable trust in New Zealand, dedicated to supporting women who have experienced birth trauma. Women who were interested in participating e-contacted Beck. Each woman was asked to respond to the following statement: "Please describe for us in as much detail as you can remember your experiences of any positive changes in your beliefs or life as a result of your traumatic childbirth. Any specific examples you can share about your posttraumatic growth will be extremely valuable in helping to educate clinicians so that they can provide better care to mothers who have experienced a traumatic childbirth."

TIP In an Internet environment, researchers need to devote time and effort to crafting individual email responses to make sure all participants feel valued and understand that their narratives made important contributions to the study.

In-depth telephone interviews are also possible but are relatively rare, perhaps reflecting a bias (Novick, 2008). The argument against telephone interviews concerns the absence of visual cues—although that is also true in asynchronous Internet interviews. Mealer and Jones (2014) have described methodologic and ethical issues relating to telephone interviewing on sensitive topics.

Preparing for In-Depth Interviews
Although qualitative interviews are conversational, this does not mean that they are entered into casually. The conversations are purposeful and require advance preparation. For example, careful thought

should be given to the wording of questions. To the extent possible, the wording should make sense to respondents and reflect their world view. Researchers and respondents should, for example, have a common vocabulary. If the researcher is studying a culture or a group that uses distinctive terms or slang, efforts should be made before data collection begins to understand those terms and their nuances.

Researchers usually prepare for the interview by developing, mentally or in writing, the broad questions to be asked (or the initial questions, in unstructured interviews). Sometimes it is useful to do a practice interview with a stand-in respondent. It is a good idea to ask any sensitive questions late in the interview after rapport has been established.

> **TIP** Memorize key questions if you have written them out, so that you will be able to maintain eye contact with participants.

It is important to decide in advance how to present yourself—as a researcher, a nurse, an ordinary person like participants, a humble "learner," and so on. An advantage of assuming the nurse role is that people often trust nurses. Yet, people may be overly deferent if nurses are perceived as better educated or more knowledgeable than they are. Moreover, participants may use the interview as an opportunity to ask health questions or to solicit opinions about health practitioners. Jack (2008) provided some guidelines to support nurse researchers in their reflections on role conflicts in qualitative interviewing.

For interviews done in the field, researchers must anticipate needs for equipment and supplies. Preparing a checklist of all such items is helpful. The checklist typically would include recording equipment, laptop computers or tablets, batteries or chargers, consent and demographic forms, notepads, and pens. Other possibilities include incentive payments, cookies or donuts to help break the ice, and distracting toys or books if children will be home. It may be necessary to bring proper identification to assure participants of the legitimacy of the visit. And, if the topic under study is likely to elicit emotional narratives, tissues should be readily at hand.

Conducting the Interview

Qualitative interviews are typically long, sometimes lasting hours. Researchers often find that the respondents' construction of their experience begins to emerge after lengthy, in-depth dialogues. Interviewers must prepare respondents for the interview by putting them at ease. Part of this process involves sharing pertinent information about the study (e.g., about confidentiality), and another part is using the first few minutes for ice-breaking exchanges of conversation before actual questioning begins. Up-front "small talk" can help to overcome stage fright, which can occur for both interviewers and respondents. Participants may be particularly nervous when interviews are being recorded. They typically forget about the recorder after the interview is underway, so the first few minutes should be used to help both parties "settle in."

Participants will not share much information with interviewers they do not trust. Close rapport with respondents provides access to richer information and to intimate details of their stories. Interviewer personality plays a role in developing rapport: Good interviewers are usually congenial people who are able to see the situation from the respondent's perspective. Nonverbal communication can be critical in conveying concern and interest. Facial expressions, nods, and so on help to set the tone for the interview. Gaglio and colleagues (2006) have offered some insights about developing rapport in primary care settings.

A critical skill for in-depth interviewers is being a good listener. It is especially important not to interrupt respondents, to "lead" them, to offer advice or opinions, or to counsel them. The interviewer's job is to listen intently to the respondents' stories. Only by attending carefully to what respondents are saying can interviewers develop appropriate follow-up questions. Even when a topic guide is used, interviewers must not let the flow of dialogue be bound by those questions.

> **TIP** In-depth interviewers must be comfortable with pauses and silences and should let participants set the pace. Interviewers can encourage respondents with nonspecific prompts, such as "Mmhm."

Interviewers need to be prepared for strong emotions, such as anger, fear, or grief, to surface. Narrative disclosures can "bring it all back" for respondents, which can be a cathartic or therapeutic experience if interviewers create an atmosphere of concern and caring—but it can also be stressful.

Interviewers may need to manage potential crises during the interviews (MacDonald & Greggans, 2008). One problem is a flawed recording of the interview. Thus, even when interviews are recorded, notes should be taken immediately after the interview to ensure the highest possible reliability of data and to prevent total information loss. Interruptions (usually the telephone) and other distractions are other common problems when interviewing in participants' homes. If respondents are willing, telephones can be controlled by unplugging them or turning them off. Interruptions by personal intrusions of friends or family members may be more difficult to manage. In some cases, the interview may need to be terminated and rescheduled—for example, when a woman is discussing domestic violence and the perpetrator enters and stays in the room.

Interviewers should strive for positive closure to interviews. The last questions in in-depth interviews should usually be along these lines: "Is there anything else you would like to tell me?" or "Are there any other questions that you think I should have asked you?" Such probes can often elicit a wealth of important information. In closing, interviewers normally ask respondents whether they would mind being contacted again, in the event that additional questions come to mind after reflecting on the information, or in case interpretations of the information need to be verified.

> **TIP** It is usually unwise to schedule back-to-back interviews. You should not cut short the first interview to be on time for a next one, and you may be too emotionally drained for another interview. It is also important to have an opportunity to write out notes, impressions, and analytic ideas, and it is best to do this when an interview is fresh in your mind.

Postinterview Procedures

Recorded interviews should be listened to and checked for audibility and completeness soon after

the interview is over. If there have been problems with the recording, the interview should be reconstructed in as much detail as possible. Listening to the interview may also suggest possible follow-up questions that could be asked if respondents are recontacted. Morse and Field (1995) recommend that interviewers listen to the recordings objectively and critique their own interviewing style, so that improvements can be made in subsequent interviews.

Steps also need to be taken to ensure that interview transcriptions are done with rigor (see the Supplement to Chapter 25 for more information about transcriptions) 🅢. Transcriptionists, like interviewers, can be affected by hearing heart-wrenching interviews. Researchers may need to warn transcriptionists about upcoming interviews that are particularly stressful and allow transcribers the opportunity to talk about their reaction to interviews (Lalor et al., 2006).

> **TIP** Transcriptions can be the most expensive part of a study. It generally takes about 4 to 5 hours of transcription time for every hour of interviewing. New and improved voice recognition computer software may help with transcribing interviews.

Evaluation of Qualitative Self-Report Approaches

In-depth interviews are a flexible approach to gathering data and offer distinct advantages. In clinical situations, for example, it is often appropriate to let people talk freely about their problems and concerns, allowing them to take much of the initiative in directing the flow of information. Unstructured self-reports may allow investigators to ascertain what the basic issues or problems are, how sensitive or controversial the topic is, how individuals conceptualize and talk about the problems, and what range of opinions or behaviors exists relevant to the topic. In-depth interviews may also help elucidate the underlying meaning of a pattern or relationship repeatedly observed in more structured research. On the other hand, qualitative self-reports are extremely time-consuming and demand strong skills for gathering high-quality data.

UNSTRUCTURED OBSERVATION

Qualitative researchers sometimes collect loosely structured observational data, often as a supplement to self-report data. The aim is to understand the behaviors and experiences of people as they actually occur in naturalistic settings.

Unstructured observational data are most often gathered in field settings through **participant observation**. Participant observers participate in the functioning of the social group under investigation and strive to observe, ask questions, and record information within the contexts and structures that are relevant to group members. Participant observation is characterized by prolonged periods of social interaction between researchers and participants, in the participants' sociopolitical and cultural milieu.

Example of Participant Observation

In their ethnographic study, Van Meurs and colleagues (2018) sought to understand the extent to which nurses explored spiritual issues with hospitalized cancer patients during daily caregiving. Participant observation was used to collect data during four shifts at the medical oncology department of an academic hospital. The researcher, who was a chaplain wearing the same uniform as the nurses, observed nurses, participated in their actions, and interviewed them after the shift.

Not all qualitative observational research is *participant* observation (i.e., with observations occurring from *within* the group under study). Some unstructured observations involve watching and recording behaviors without participating in activities.

Example of Unstructured Nonparticipant Observation

O'Brien and colleagues (2018) conducted a grounded theory study focused on how nurses minimize risk within perioperative settings. In addition to interviews with 37 nurses working in 11 different perioperative settings, the researchers undertook 33 hours of nonparticipant observation.

Nevertheless, if a key research objective is to learn how group interactions and activities give meaning to human behaviors and experiences, then participant observation is an appropriate method. The members of any group or culture are influenced by assumptions they take for granted, and observers can, through active participation as members, hope to gain access to these assumptions. Participant observation is most often used by ethnographers but also by grounded theory researchers and researchers with ideological perspectives.

The Observer—Participant Role in Participant Observation

The role that observers play in the groups under study is important because the observers' social position determines what they are likely to see. That is, the behaviors that are likely to be available for observation depend on observers' position in a network of relations.

McFarland and Wehbe-Alamah (2015), in describing Leininger's methods, depicted a participant observer's role as evolving through a four-phase sequence:

1. Primarily observation and active listening
2. Primarily observation with limited participation
3. Primarily participation with continued observation
4. Primary reflection and reconfirmation of findings with informants

In the initial phase, researchers observe and listen to those under study to obtain a broad view of the situation. This phase allows both observers and the observed to "size up" each other, to become acquainted, and to become comfortable interacting. In the next phase, observation is enhanced by a modest degree of participation. By participating in the group's activities, researchers can study people's behaviors as well as people's reactions. In phase 3, researchers become more active participants, learning by the actual experience of doing rather than just by watching and listening. In phase 4, researchers reflect on what transpired and how people interacted with and reacted to them.

Junker (1960) described a somewhat different continuum that does not assume an evolving process: complete participant, participant as observer, observer as participant, and complete observer. Complete participants conceal their identity as researchers, entering the group ostensibly as regular members. For example, a nurse researcher might accept a job as a clinical nurse with the express intent of studying, in a concealed fashion, some aspect of the clinical environment. At the other extreme, complete observers do not attempt participation in the group's activities, but rather make observations as outsiders. At both extremes, observers may have difficulty asking probing questions: complete participants may arouse suspicion if they make inquiries not congruent with a participant role, and complete observers may not have personal access to, or the trust of, those being observed. Most observational fieldwork lies in between these two extremes.

Example of Participant-Observer Roles

In their focused ethnography, Aagaard and colleagues (2017) explored the professional identity of registered nurse anesthetists (RNAs) in Denmark. Participant observations were conducted with patients scheduled for surgery and with the nurse anesthetists in charge of the patients during the surgical procedures. "The first author became familiar with the different groups of patients, clinical activities of nurses working in the surgical wards, and RNAs working in the two units of the Department of Anesthesiology. These participant observations provided knowledge of patients' hospitalization plan." (p. 621).

TIP Being a fully participating member of a group does not *necessarily* offer the best perspective for studying a phenomenon—just as being an actor in a play does not offer the most advantageous view of the performance.

Getting Started

Observers must overcome two initial hurdles: gaining entrée into the social group or culture under study and establishing rapport and developing trust within the social group. Without gaining entrée, the study cannot proceed; but without the group's trust, researchers could be restricted to "front-stage" knowledge (Leininger, 1985), that is, information distorted by the group's protective facades. The observer's goal is to "get back stage"—to learn about the realities of the group's experiences and

behaviors. This section discusses some practical and interpersonal aspects of getting started in the field.

Gaining an Overview

In the earliest stage of observational fieldwork, it is often useful to gather some written or pictorial descriptive material that provides an overview of the site. In an institutional setting, for example, it is helpful to obtain a floor plan, an organizational chart, an annual report, and so on. Then, a preliminary personal tour should be undertaken to gain familiarity with its ambiance and to note major activities, social groupings, and transactions.

In community studies, ethnographers sometimes conduct a **windshield survey** (or *windshield tour*), which involves an intensive exploration (sometimes in an automobile, and hence the name) to "map" important features of the community. Such community mapping can document community resources (e.g., churches, businesses, public transportation, community centers), community liabilities (e.g., vacant lots, empty stores, dilapidated buildings), and social and environmental characteristics (e.g., condition of streets and buildings, traffic patterns, types of signs, children playing in public places). A protocol for a windshield survey is included in the Toolkit of the accompanying *Resource Manual.*

Example of a Windshield Survey

Ballantyne-Rice and colleagues (2016) undertook a community assessment that explored factors affecting the health and wellness of older adults living in an assisted living facility. The researchers did a windshield survey to better understand The Lodge community and surrounding suburban areas.

Establishing Rapport

After gaining entrée into a setting and obtaining permissions and suggestions from gatekeepers, the next step is to enter the field. It may be possible just to "blend in" or ease into a social group, but often researchers walk into a "head-turning" situation in which they stand out as strangers. Participant observers often find that, for their own comfort level and for that of participants, it is best to have a brief, simple explanation about their presence. Except in rare cases, deception is neither necessary nor recommended, but vagueness has many advantages. People rarely want to know *exactly* what researchers are studying, they simply want an introduction and enough information to satisfy their curiosity and erase suspicions about the researchers' ulterior motives.

After initial introductions with members of the group, it is usually best to keep a low profile. At the beginning, researchers are not yet familiar with the customs, language, and norms of the group, and it is critical to learn these things. Politeness and friendliness are essential, but ardent socializing is not appropriate at the early stages of fieldwork. As rapport is developed and trust is established, researchers can play a more active participatory role and collect observational data in earnest.

> **TIP** Your initial job is to listen intently and learn what it takes to fit into the group, that is, what you need to do to become accepted as a member. To the extent possible, you should downplay any expertise you might have. Your goal is to gain people's trust and to move relationships to a deeper level.

Gathering Unstructured Observational Data

Participant observers typically place few restrictions on the nature of the data collected, in keeping with the goal of minimizing observer-imposed meanings and structure. Nevertheless, participant observers often have a broad plan for the types of information to be gathered. Among aspects likely to be considered relevant are the following:

1. *The physical setting.* What are key features of the setting? What is the context within which human behavior unfolds? What behaviors are promoted (or constrained) by the physical environment?
2. *The participants.* What are the characteristics of the people being observed? How many people are there? What are their roles? Who is given free access to the setting—who "belongs"? What brings these people together?
3. *Activities and interactions.* What are people doing and saying? Is there a discernible progression of activities? How do people interact with

one another? How—and how often—do they communicate? What type of emotions do they show during their interactions? How are participants interconnected to one another or to activities underway?
4. *Frequency and duration.* When did the activity or event begin, and when is it scheduled to end? How much time has elapsed? Is the activity a recurring one, and if so, how regularly does it recur? How typical of such activities is the one that is under observation?
5. *Precipitating factors.* Why is the event or interaction happening? What contributes to how the event or interaction unfolds?
6. *Organization.* How is the event or interaction organized? How are relationships structured? What norms or rules are in operation?
7. *Intangible factors.* What did *not* happen (especially if it ought to have happened)? Are participants saying one thing verbally but communicating different messages nonverbally? What types of things were disruptive to the activity or situation?

Clearly, this is far more information than can be absorbed in a single session (and not all categories may be relevant to the research question). However, this framework provides a starting point for thinking about observational possibilities while in the field. (This list of features amenable to in-depth observation is included in the Toolkit ⊗.)

> **TIP** When we enter a social setting in our everyday lives, we unconsciously process many of the questions on this list. Usually, however, we do not consciously *attend* to our observations and impressions in any systematic way and are not careful about making note of the details that contribute to our impressions. This is precisely what participant observers must learn to do.

Spradley (1980) distinguished three levels of observation that typically occur during fieldwork. The first level, **descriptive observation**, tends to be broad and helps observers figure out what is going on. During descriptive observations, researchers attempt to observe as much as possible. Later in the inquiry, observers do **focused** observations of carefully selected events and interactions. Based on the research aims and on what has been learned from descriptive observations, participant observers begin to focus more sharply on key aspects of the setting. From these focused observations, they may develop a system for organizing observations, such as a taxonomy or category system. **Selective observations** are the most highly focused and are undertaken to facilitate comparisons between categories or activities. Spradley describes these levels as analogous to a funnel, with an increasingly narrow and more systematic focus.

While in the field, participant observers need to decide how to sample observations and select observational locations. **Single positioning** means staying in a single location for a period to observe behaviors and transactions in that location. **Multiple positioning** involves moving around the site to observe behaviors from different locations. **Mobile positioning** involves following a person throughout a given activity or period. It is usually useful to use a combination of positioning approaches.

Because participant observers cannot spend a lifetime in one site and cannot be in more than one place at a time, observation is almost always supplemented with information from unstructured interviews or conversations. For example, key informants may be asked to describe what went on in a meeting that the observer was unable to attend or to describe events that occurred before the observer entered the field. In such a case, the informant functions as the observer's observer.

Recording Observations

Participant observers may be tempted to put more emphasis on the *participation* and *observation* parts of their research than on the recording of those activities. Without systematic recording of observational data, however, the project can flounder. Observational information cannot be trusted to memory; it must be diligently recorded as soon after the observations as possible.

Types of Observational Records
The most common forms of record-keeping in participant observation are logs and field notes,

but photographs and video recordings may also be used. A **log** (or **field diary**) is a daily record of events and conversations in the field. A log is a chronological listing of how researchers have spent their time and can be used for planning, for keeping track of expenses, and for reviewing what work has already been completed. Box 24.1 presents an example of a log entry from Beck's (2002) grounded theory study of mothers of twins.

Field notes are broader, more analytic, and more interpretive than a simple listing of occurrences. Field notes represent the observer's efforts to record information and to synthesize and understand the data. Phillippi and Lauderdale (2018) have written an excellent guide to preparing field notes in qualitative research.

TIP Field notes are valuable in many types of qualitative studies, not just in studies involving participant observation. Field notes are an important means of documenting contextual information and should be maintained even when the only data source is from interviews.

The Content of Field Notes
Participant observers' field notes contain a narrative account of what is happening in the field; they serve as the data for analysis. Most "field" notes are not written while observers are literally in the field but rather are written after an observational session in the field has been completed.

Field notes are usually lengthy and time-consuming to prepare. Observers need to discipline themselves to provide a wealth of detail, the meaning and importance of which may not emerge for weeks. Descriptions of what has transpired must include enough contextual information about time, place, and actors to portray the situation fully. *Thick description* is the goal for participation observers' field notes (as it is in describing a completed qualitative study).

TIP Especially in the early stages of fieldwork, a general rule of thumb is this: When in doubt, write it down.

BOX 24.1 Example of a Log Entry: Mothering Multiples Grounded Theory Study

Log entry for Mothers of Multiples Support Group Meeting
July 15, 1999 10–11:30 AM

This is my fourth meeting that I have attended. Nine mothers came this morning with their twins. One other woman attended. She was pregnant with twins. She came to the support group for advice from the other mothers regarding such issues as what type of stroller to buy, etc. All the moms sat on the floor with their infants placed on blankets on the floor next to them. Toddlers and older children played together off to the side with a box of toys. I sat next to a mom new to the group with her twin 4-month-old girls. I helped her hold and feed one of the twins. On my other side was a mom who had signed up at the last meeting to participate in my study. I hadn't called her yet to set up an appointment. She asked how my research was going. We then set up an appointment for next Thursday at 10 AM at her home for me to interview her. The new mother that I sat next to also was eager to participate in the study. In fact, she said we could do the interview right after the meeting ends today, but I couldn't due to another meeting. We scheduled an interview appointment for next Thursday at 1 PM. I also set up a third appointment for an interview for next week with I.K. for Monday at 1 PM. She had participated in an earlier study of mine. She came right over to me this morning at the support group meeting.

From the author's records for the study reported in the following paper: Beck, C. T. (2002). Releasing the pause button: Mothering twins during the first year of life. *Qualitative Health Research, 12*, 593–608.

Field notes are both descriptive and reflective. **Descriptive notes** (or **observational notes**) are objective descriptions of observed events and conversations. Information about actions, dialogue, and context is recorded as completely and objectively as possible. Sometimes descriptive notes are recorded on loosely structured forms analogous to topic guides to ensure that key information is captured. ✳

Reflective notes, which document the researcher's personal experiences, reflections, and progress while in the field, can serve several purposes:

- **Methodologic notes** are reflections about observational strategies. Sometimes observers do things that do not "work," and methodologic notes document thoughts about new approaches or about why a strategy was especially effective. Methodologic notes also can provide instructions or reminders about how subsequent observations will be made.
- **Analytic notes** (or **theoretical notes**) document researchers' thoughts about how to make sense of what is going on. These notes serve as a starting point for subsequent analysis.

- **Personal notes** are comments about researchers' own feelings in the field. Almost inevitably, field experiences give rise to emotions and challenge researchers' assumptions. It is essential to reflect on such feelings, because there is no other way to know whether they are influencing what is being observed. Personal notes can also contain reflections relating to ethical dilemmas.

Box 24.2 presents examples of various types of field notes from Beck's (2002) study of mothering twins.

Reflective notes are typically not integrated into the descriptive notes but are kept separate as parallel notes; they may be maintained in a journal or a series of self-memos. Strauss and Corbin (1990) argue that reflective memos help researchers to achieve analytic distance from the actual data and play a critical role in the project's success.

TIP Personal notes should begin even before entering the field. By recording your feelings and expectations, you will have a baseline against which to compare feelings and experiences that emerge in the field.

BOX 24.2 Example of Field Notes: Mothering Multiples Grounded Theory Study

Observational notes: O.L. attended the mothers of multiples support group again this month but she looked worn out today. She was not as bubbly as she had been at the March meeting. She explained why she was not doing as well this month. She and her husband had just found out that their house has lead-based paint in it. Both twins do have increased lead levels. She and her husband are in the process of buying a new home.

Analytic notes: So far, all the mothers have stressed the need for routine in order to survive the first year of caring for twins. Mothers, however, have varying definitions of routine. I.R. had the firmest routine with her twins. B.L. is more flexible with her routine, i.e., the twins are always fed at the same time but are not put down for naps or bed at night at the same time. Whenever one of the twins wants to go to sleep is fine with her. B.L. does have a daily routine in regards to housework. For example, when the twins are down in the morning for a nap, she makes their bottles up for the day (14 bottles total).

Methodologic notes: The first sign-up sheet I passed around at the Mothers of Multiples Support Group for women to sign up to participate in interviews for my grounded theory study only consisted of two columns: one for the mother's name and one for her telephone number. I need to revise this sign-up sheet to include extra columns for the age of the multiples, the town where the mother lives, and older siblings and their ages. My plan is to start interviewing mothers with multiples around 1 year of age so that the moms can reflect back over the process of mothering their infants for the first 12 months of their lives.

Right now, I have no idea of the ages of the infants of the mothers who signed up to be interviewed. I will need to call the nurse in charge of this support group to find out the ages.

Personal notes: Today was an especially challenging interview. The mom had picked the early afternoon for me to come to her home to interview her because that is the time her 2-year-old son would be napping. When I arrived at her house, her 2-year-old ran up to me and said hi. The mom explained that he had taken an earlier nap that day and that he would be up during the interview. So in the living room with us during our interview were her two twin daughters (3 months old) swinging in the swings and her 2-year-old son. One of the twins was quite cranky for the first half hour of the interview. During the interview, the 2-year-old sat on my lap and looked at the two books I had brought as a little present. If I did not keep him occupied with the books, he would keep trying to reach for the microphone of the tape recorder.

From the author's records for the study reported in the following paper: Beck, C. T. (2002). Releasing the pause button: Mothering twins during the first year of life. *Qualitative Health Research, 12,* 593–608.

The Process of Writing Field Notes

The success of participant observation depends on the quality of the field notes, and timing is important to quality. Field notes should be written as soon as possible after an observation is made. The longer the interval between an observation and field note preparation, the greater the risk of forgetting or distorting the data. With long delays, details will be forgotten and memory of what was observed may be biased by things that happened subsequently.

TIP Be sure not to talk to anyone about your observation before you have had a chance to write up the observational notes. Such discussions could color what you record.

Participant observers cannot usually write their field notes while they are in the field, in part because this would distract them from their job of being keen observers, and because it would undermine their role as ordinary members.

Researchers must develop the skill of making detailed mental notes that can later be committed to a permanent record. Observers often try to jot down unobtrusively a phrase or sentence that will later serve as a reminder of an event, conversation, or impression. Many experienced field-workers use the tactic of frequent trips to the bathroom to record these **jottings**, either in a small notebook or onto a recording device. With the widespread use of cell phones, researchers can also excuse themselves to make a call, and "phone in" their jottings. Observers use jottings to develop more extensive field notes.

> **TIP** It is important to schedule enough time to record field notes after an observation. An hour of observation can take 3 to 4 hours to record. Try to find a quiet place for writing up field notes, preferably a location where you can work undisturbed for several hours.

Observational field notes should be as detailed as possible. This means that hundreds of pages of field notes typically will be created, and so systems need to be developed for managing them. For example, each entry should have the date and time the observation was made, the location, and the name of the observer (if several are working as a team). It is useful to give observational sessions a name that will trigger a memory (e.g., "Emotional Outburst by a Patient with Ovarian Cancer").

Thought also needs to be given to how to record participants' dialogue. The goal is to record conversations as accurately as possible, but it is not always possible to make verbatim recordings if researchers are trying to maintain a stance as regular group members. Procedures are needed to distinguish different levels of accuracy in recording dialogue (e.g., by using quotation marks and italics for true verbatim recordings, and a different designation for paraphrasings).

> **TIP** Observation, participation, and record-keeping are exhausting, labor-intensive activities. It is important to establish the proper pace of these activities to ensure the highest possible quality notes for analysis.

Evaluation of Participant Observation

Participant observation can provide a deeper and richer understanding of human behaviors and social situations than is possible with structured observation. Participant observation is particularly valuable for its ability to "get inside" a situation and provide understanding of its complexities. Furthermore, this approach is inherently flexible and gives observers the freedom to reconceptualize problems after becoming more familiar with the situation. Participant observation is a good method for answering questions about phenomena that are difficult for insiders to explain because these phenomena are taken for granted.

Like all research methods, however, participant observation faces potential problems. Observer bias and observer influence are prominent risks. Observers may lose objectivity in viewing and recording observations; they may also inappropriately sample events and situations to be observed. Once researchers begin to participate in a group's activities, the possibility of emotional involvement becomes a salient concern. Researchers in their member role may fail to attend to research-relevant aspects of the situation or may develop a myopic view on issues of importance to the group. Participant observation may thus be unsuitable when the risk of identification is strong. Another important issue concerns the ethical dilemmas that often emerge in participant observation studies. Finally, the success of participant observation depends on the observer's observational and interpersonal skills—skills that may be difficult to cultivate.

On the whole, participant observation and other unstructured observational methods are extremely profitable for in-depth research in which researchers wish to develop a comprehensive description and conceptualization of phenomena within a social setting or culture.

> **TIP** Although this chapter emphasized the two most frequently used methods of collecting unstructured data (self-reports and observation), we encourage you to think about other data sources, such as documents. Miller and Alvarado (2005) offer useful suggestions for incorporating documents into qualitative nursing research.

CRITICAL APPRAISAL OF DATA COLLECTION IN QUALITATIVE RESEARCH

It is usually not easy to appraise the decisions that researchers have made in collecting qualitative data because details about those decisions are seldom spelled out in research reports. In particular, there is often scant information about participant observation. It is not uncommon for a report to simply say that the researcher undertook participant observation, without descriptions of how much time was spent in the field, what exactly was observed, how observations were recorded, and what level of participation was involved. In fact, we suspect that many projects described as having used a participant observation approach were unstructured observations with little actual participation. Thus, an appraisal may focus on how much information

the research report provided about the data collection methods used. Even though space constraints in journals make it impossible for researchers to fully elaborate their methods, researchers have a responsibility to communicate basic information about their approach so that readers can assess the quality of evidence that the study yields. Researchers should provide examples of questions asked and types of observations made.

As we discuss in Chapter 26, *triangulation* of multiple data collection methods provides opportunities for qualitative researchers to enhance the quality of their data. Thus, an important issue to consider in evaluating unstructured data is whether the types and amount of data collected are sufficiently rich to support an in-depth, holistic understanding of the phenomena under study. Box 24.3 provides guidelines for critically appraising the collection of unstructured data.

BOX 24.3 Guidelines for Critically Appraising Unstructured Data Collection Methods

1. Was the collection of unstructured data appropriate to the study aims?
2. Given the research question and the characteristics of study participants, did the researcher use the best method of capturing study phenomena (i.e., self-reports, observation)? Should supplementary data collection methods have been used to enrich the data available for analysis?
3. If self-report methods were used, did the researcher make good decisions about the specific method used to solicit information (e.g., focus group interviews, semistructured interviews, and so on)? Was the modality of obtaining the data appropriate (e.g., in-person interviews, telephone interviews, Internet questioning, etc.)?
4. If a topic guide was used, did the report present examples of specific questions? Were the questions appropriate and thorough? Did the wording encourage full and rich responses?
5. Were interviews recorded and transcribed? If interviews were not recorded, what steps were taken to ensure the accuracy of the data?
6. Were self-report data gathered in a manner that promoted high-quality responses (e.g., in terms of privacy, efforts to put respondents at ease, etc.)? Who collected the data, and were they adequately prepared for the task?
7. If observational methods were used, did the report adequately describe what the observations entailed? What did the researcher actually observe, in what types of settings did the observations occur, and how often and over how long a period were observations made? Were decisions about positioning described?
8. What role did the researcher assume in terms of being an observer and a participant? Was this role appropriate?
9. How were observational data recorded? Did the recording method maximize data quality?

RESEARCH EXAMPLE

This section provides an example of a qualitative study that collected a rich variety of unstructured data.

Study: Healthy Canadian adolescents' perspectives of cancer using metaphors: A qualitative study (Woodgate & Busolo, 2017).

Statement of purpose: The purpose of this study was to extend knowledge about Canadian adolescents' perspectives of cancer and cancer prevention, including how they conceptualize and understand cancer risk.

Design: The researchers used an ethnographic approach that involved the use of multiple data collection methods. A purposive sample of 75 adolescents was recruited, with efforts made to achieve variation in age, gender, ethnicity, cancer experience, and urban-rural residence. Data collection took place over a 3-year period.

Data collection: Two face-to-face interviews were planned for each adolescent, with the second one scheduled 4 to 5 weeks after the first. Each interview, lasting between 60 and 90 minutes, was digitally recorded and transcribed. For the first interview, the topic guide (which had been thoroughly pretested) included open-ended questions about cancer risk and prevention (e.g., "How do people get cancer? When you hear the word 'cancer,' what does it make you think of?"). Photovoice methods were also introduced. The participants were given cameras and were asked to take pictures of what they felt depicted cancer, cancer risks, and cancer prevention over a period of a month. Then, in the second interview, 53 adolescents shared 557 photos with the research team. Participants were asked to describe every picture, what was happening, and what the pictures meant to them. They were guided by such questions as, "How does this [picture] relate to cancer?". Finally, 14 participants took part in four focus group interviews, each with 3 to 4 adolescents. The focus group interviews were used to supplement and confirm emerging themes on cancer and cancer prevention. Field notes were maintained to describe verbal and nonverbal behaviors of participants after individual and focus group interviews.

Key findings: The researchers used the data to identify cancer-related metaphors that the adolescents used. Four metaphors emerged from the data: Loss (cancer as the sick patient and death itself); Military (cancer as a battle); Living thing (haywire cells); and Faith (cancer as God's will).

SUMMARY POINTS

- Qualitative researchers typically adopt flexible data collection plans that evolve as the study progresses. Self-reports are the most frequently used type of data in qualitative studies, followed by observation. Ethnographers are likely to combine these two data sources with other sources such as the products of the culture (e.g., photographs, documents, artifacts).

- Qualitative researchers often confront such fieldwork issues as gaining participants' trust, pacing data collection to avoid being overwhelmed by the intensity of data, avoiding emotional involvement with participants ("**going native**"), and maintaining reflexivity (awareness of the part they play in the study and possible effects on their data).

- Qualitative researchers need to plan for how their data will be recorded and stored. If technical equipment is used (e.g., audio recorders, video recorders), care must be taken to select equipment that functions properly in the field.

- Unstructured and loosely structured self-reports, which offer respondents and interviewers latitude in their questions and answers, yield rich narrative data for qualitative analysis.

- Methods of collecting qualitative self-report data include: (1) **unstructured interviews**, which are conversational discussions on the topic of interest; (2) **semistructured** (or **focused**) **interviews**, in which interviewers are guided by a **topic guide** listing broad questions to be asked; (3) **focus group interviews**, which involve discussions with small, homogeneous groups; (4) **joint interviews**, which involve simultaneously talking with members of a dyad; (5) **diaries** and journals, in which participants maintain ongoing records about some aspects of their lives; (6) **photo elicitation interviews**, which are stimulated and guided by photographic images and **photovoice**, which involves having participants take photos themselves; (7) **stimulated recall interviews** that involve video recordings of participants in social interactions, followed by interviews; and (8) narrative materials available on the Internet. Additional methods include **life histories, oral histories, critical incident interviews,** and **think-aloud methods.**

- In preparing for in-depth interviews, researchers learn about the language and customs of participants, formulate broad questions, make decisions about how to present themselves, develop ideas about interview settings, and take stock of equipment needs.

- Most qualitative interviews take place in face-to-face situations, but technological advances are making remote synchronous interviewing possible (e.g., via Skype).

- Conducting good in-depth interviews requires considerable skill in putting people at ease, developing trust, listening intently, and managing possible crises in the field.

- Ethnographers (and other qualitative researchers) also collect unstructured observational data, often through **participant observation.** Participant observers obtain information about the dynamics of social groups or cultures within members' own frame of reference.

- In the initial phase of participant observation studies, researchers are primarily observers gaining an understanding of the site, sometimes including *windshield surveys* to get a "lay of the land." Researchers later become more active participants.

- Observations tend to become more focused over time, ranging from **descriptive observation** (broad observations) to **focused observation** of more carefully selected events or interactions, and then to **selective observations** designed to facilitate comparisons.

- Participant observers usually select events to be observed through a combination of **single positioning** (observing from a fixed location),

multiple positioning (moving around the site to observe in different locations), and **mobile positioning** (following a person around a site).

- **Logs** of daily events and **field notes** are the major methods of recording unstructured observational data. Field notes are both descriptive and reflective.

- Descriptive notes (or **observational notes**) are detailed, objective accounts of what transpired in an observational session. Observers strive for detailed, thick description.

- **Reflective notes** include **methodologic notes** that document observers' thoughts about their strategies; **analytic notes** (or **theoretical notes**) that represent ongoing efforts to make sense of the data; and **personal notes** that document observers' feelings and experiences.

- In-depth unstructured data collection methods tend to yield data of considerable richness and are useful in gaining an understanding about little-researched phenomena, but they are time-consuming and yield a volume of data that are challenging to analyze.

STUDY ACTIVITIES

Study activities are available to instructors on thePoint.

REFERENCES CITED IN CHAPTER 24

Aagaard, K., Sørensen, E. E., Rasmussen, B. S., & Laursen, B. S. (2017). Identifying nurse anesthetists' professional identity. *Journal of Perianesthesia Nursing, 32*, 619–630.

Ballantyne-Rice, M., Chopp, K., Evans, L., Ho, V., Hsiung, W., Simon, M., … Donnelly, T. (2016). A client-centered community engagement project: Improving the health and wellness of older adults in an assisted living facility. *Journal of Gerontological Nursing, 42*, 44–51.

Beck, C. T. (2002). Releasing the pause button: Mothering twins during the first year of life. *Qualitative Health Research, 12*, 593–608.

Beck, C. T., & Watson, S. (2016). Posttraumatic growth following birth trauma: "I was broken. Now I am unbreakable". *MCN: American Journal of Maternal Child Nursing, 41*, 264–271.

Biedermann, N. (2018). The use of Facebook for virtual asynchronous focus groups in qualitative research. *Contemporary Nurse, 54,* 26–34.

*Briant, K., Halter, A., Marchello, N., Escareno, M., & Thomson, B. (2016). The power of digital storytelling as a culturally relevant health promotion tool. *Health Promotion & Practice, 17,* 793–801.

Brinkman, S., & Kvale, S. (2015). *InterViews: Learning the craft of qualitative research interviewing* (3rd ed.). Thousand Oaks, CA: Sage.

Burden, S., Topping, A., & O'Halloran, C. (2018). Mentor judgements and decision-making in the assessment of student nurse competence in practice. *Journal of Advanced Nursing, 74,* 1078–1089.

Caiola, C., Barroso, J., & Docherty, S. (2018). Black mothers living with HIV picture the social determinants of health. *Journal of the Association of Nurses in AIDS Care, 29,* 204–219.

Carey, M. A. (2016). Focus groups—what is the same, what is new, what is next? *Qualitative Health Research, 26,* 731–733.

Carey, M. A., & Asbury, J. (2012). *Focus group research.* Walnut Creek, CA: Left Coast Press.

Charmaz, K. (2014). *Constructing grounded theory.* Thousand Oaks, CA: Sage.

Chew, H., & Lopez, V. (2018). Empowered to self-care: A photovoice study in patients with heart failure. *Journal of Transcultural Nursing, 29,* 410–419.

*Corti, L., & Fielding, N. (2016). Opportunities from the digital revolution: Implications for researching, publishing, and consuming qualitative research. *Sage Open,* 1–16.

Côté-Arsenault, D. (2013). Focus groups. In Beck, C. T. (Ed.), *Routledge handbook of qualitative nursing research* (pp. 307–318). New York: Routledge.

Creighton, G., Oliffe, J., Ferlatte, O., Bottorff, J., Broom, A., & Jenkins, E. (2018). Photovoice ethics: Critical reflections from men's mental health research. *Qualitative Health Research, 28,* 446–455.

Dempsey, N. (2010). Stimulated recall interviews in ethnography. *Qualitative Sociology, 33,* 349–367.

Frith, H., & Harcourt, D. (2007). Using photographs to capture women's experiences with chemotherapy: Reflecting on the method. *Qualitative Health Research, 17,* 1340–1350.

Fritz, R., & Vandermause, R. (2018). Data collection via in-depth email interviewing: Lessons from the field. *Qualitative Health Research, 28,* 1640–1649.

Gage-Bouchard, E., LaValley, S., Mollica, M., & Beaupin, L. (2017). Cancer communication on social media: Examining how cancer caregivers use Facebook for cancer-related communication. *Cancer Nursing, 40,* 332–338.

Gaglio, B., Nelson, C., & King, D. (2006). The role of rapport: Lessons learned from conducting research in a primary care setting. *Qualitative Health Research, 16,* 723–734.

Germain, J., Harris, J., Mackay, S., & Maxwell, C. (2018). Why should we use online research methods? Four doctoral health student perspectives. *Qualitative Health Research, 28,* 1650–1657.

Glaser, B. G., & Strauss, A. (1967). *The discovery of grounded theory: Strategies for qualitative research.* New York: Aldine de Gruyter.

Hall, W. A., Long, B., Bermbach, N., Jordan, S., & Patterson, K. (2005). Qualitative teamwork issues and strategies: Coordination through mutual adjustment. *Qualitative Health Research, 15,* 394–410.

*Ho, K., Chiang, V., Leung, D., & Ku, B. (2018). When foreign domestic helpers care for and about older people in their homes: I am maid or a friend. *Global Qualitative Nursing Research, 5,* 1–10.

Irani, E. (2019). The use of videoconferencing for qualitative interviewing: Opportunities, challenges, and considerations. *Clinical Nursing Research, 28,* 3–8.

*Jack, S. (2008). Guidelines to support nurse-researchers reflect on role conflict in qualitative interviewing. *The Open Nursing Journal, 2,* 58–62.

Jaiswal, D., To, M. J., Hunter, H., Lane, C., States, C., Cameron, B., … MacLeod, A. (2016). Twelve tips for medical students to facilitate a photovoice project. *Medical Teacher, 38,* 981–986.

James, N., & Busher, H. (2012). Internet interviewing. In Gubrium, J. F., & Holstein, J. A. (Eds.), *Handbook of interview research: The complexity of the craft* (2nd ed., pp. 177–192). Thousand Oaks, CA: Sage.

*Janghorban, R., Latifinejad Roudsair, R., & Taghipour, A. (2014). Skype interviewing: The new generation of online synchronous interview in qualitative research. *International Journal of Qualitative Studies on Health and Well-Being, 9,* 24152.

Junker, B. H. (1960). *Field work: An introduction to the social sciences.* Chicago: University of Chicago Press.

Kahn, D. L. (2000). How to conduct research. In Cohen, M. Z., Kahn, D. L., & Steeves, R. H. (Eds.), *Hermeneutic phenomenological research* (pp. 57–70). Thousand Oaks, CA: Sage.

Keim-Malpass, J., Steeves, R., & Kennedy, C. (2014). Internet ethnography: A review of methodological considerations for studying online illness blogs. *International Journal of Nursing Studies, 51,* 1686–1692.

Kidd, P. S., & Parshall, M. B. (2000). Getting the focus and the group: Enhancing analytic rigor in focus group research. *Qualitative Health Research, 10,* 293–308.

Krueger, R., & Casey, M. (2015) *Focus groups: A practical guide for applied research* (5th ed.). Thousand Oaks, CA: Sage.

Lalor, J.G., Begley, C., & Devane, D. (2006). Exploring painful experiences: Impact of emotional narratives on members of a qualitative research team. *Journal of Advanced Nursing, 56,* 607–616.

Lee, T., Handy, A., Kwan, W., Oliffe, J., Brotto, L., Wassersug, R., & Dowsett, G. (2015). Impact of prostate cancer treatment on the sexual quality of life for men-who-have-sex-with-men, *The Journal of Sexual Medicine, 12,* 2378–2386.

Leininger, M,. (Ed.). (1985). *Qualitative research methods in nursing.* New York: Grune and Stratton.

Liamputtong, P. (2011). *Focus group methodology: Principles and practice.* Los Angeles, CA: Sage Publications.

Liebenberg, L. (2018). Thinking critically about photovoice: Achieving empowerment and social change. *International Journal of Qualitative Methods, 17*, 1–9.

MacDonald, K., & Greggans, A. (2008). Dealing with chaos and complexity: The reality of interviewing children and families in their own homes. *Journal of Clinical Nursing, 17*, 3123–3130.

McFarland, M. R., & Wehbe-Alamah, H. B. (2015). *Leininger's culture care diversity and universality: A worldwide nursing theory*. Burlington, MA: Jones & Bartlett Learning.

*McIntosh, M., & Morse, J. M. (2015). Situating and constructing diversity in semi-structured interviews. *Global Qualitative Nursing Research, 2*, 1–12.

*McNair, R., Taft, A., & Hegarty, K. (2008). Using reflexivity to enhance in-depth interviewing skills for the clinical researcher. *BMC Medical Research Methodology, 8*, 73.

Mealer, M., & Jones, R. (2014). Methodological and ethical issues related to qualitative telephone interviews on sensitive topics. *Nurse Researcher, 21*, 32–37.

Miller, F., & Alvarado, K. (2005). Incorporating documents into qualitative nursing research. *Journal of Nursing Scholarship, 37*, 348–353.

*Mirhaghi, A., Heydari, A., Ebrahimi, M., & Bahmani, M. (2016). Nonemergent patients in the emergency department: An ethnographic study. *Trauma Monthly, 21*, e23260.

Morgan, D. L. (2001). Focus group interviewing. In Gubrium, J. F., & Holstein, J. A. (Eds.), *Handbook of interview research: Context and method* (2nd ed., pp. 141–159). Thousand Oaks, CA: Sage.

Morse, J. M., & Field, P. A. (1995). *Qualitative research methods for health professionals* (2nd ed.). Thousand Oaks, CA: Sage.

Nilson, C. (2017). A journey toward cultural competence: The role of researcher reflexivity in indigenous research. *Journal of Transcultural Nursing, 28*, 119–127.

*Novick, G. (2008). Is there a bias against telephone interviews in qualitative research? *Research in Nursing & Health, 31*, 391–398.

Oliffe, J., Bottorff, J., Kelly, M., & Halpin, M. (2008). Analyzing participant-produced photographs from an ethnographic study of fatherhood and smoking. *Research in Nursing & Health, 31*, 529–539.

O'Brien, B., Andrews, T., & Savage, E. (2018). Anticipatory vigilance: A grounded theory study of minimising risk within the perioperative setting. *Journal of Clinical Nursing, 27*, 247–256.

Petty, J. (2017). Emotion work in qualitative research: Interviewing parents about neonatal care. *Nurse Researcher, 25*, 26–30.

Phillippi, J., & Lauderdale, J. (2018). A guide to field notes for qualitative research. *Qualitative Health Research, 28*, 381–388.

Rothwell, E., Anderson, R., & Botkin, J. (2016). Deliberative discussion focus groups. *Qualitative Health Research, 26*, 734–740.

Rubin, H., & Rubin, I. S. (2012). *Qualitative interviewing: The art of hearing data* (3rd ed.). Thousand Oaks, CA: Sage.

Schenck, E., Bryant, R., Van Son, C., & Odom-Maryon, T. (2019). Perspectives on patient and family engagement with reduction in harm. *Journal of Nursing Care Quality, 34*, 73–79.

*Skilbeck, J., Arthur, A., & Seymour, J. (2018). Making sense of frailty: An ethnographic study of the experience of older people living with complex health problems. *International Journal of Older People Nursing, 13*(1).

*Smith, H., Bulbul, A., & Jones, C. (2017). Can online discussion sites generate quality data for research purposes? *Frontiers in Public Health, 5*, 156.

Spradley, J. (1979). *The ethnographic interview*. New York: Holt Rinehart & Winston.

Spradley, J. P. (1980). *Participant observation*. New York: Holt, Rinehart & Wilson.

Strauss, A., & Corbin, J. (1990). *Basics of qualitative research: Grounded theory procedures and techniques*. Newbury Park, CA: Sage.

Ten Hoeve, Y., Kunnen, S., Brouwer, J., & Roodbol, P. (2018). The voice of nurses: Novice nurses' first experiences in a clinical setting. *Journal of Clinical Nursing, 27*, e1612–e1626.

Van Manen, M. (1990). *Researching lived experience: Human science for an action sensitive pedagogy*. London, Ontario: Althouse Press.

**Van Meurs, J., Smeets, W., Vissers, K., Groot, M., & Engels, Y. (2018). Nurses exploring the spirituality of their patients with cancer. *Cancer Nursing, 41*, E39–E45.

Voltelen, B., Konradsen, H., Ostergaard, B. (2018). Ethical considerations when conducting joint interviews with close relatives or family. *Scandinavian Journal of Caring Sciences, 32*(2), 515–526.

*Woodgate, R. L., & Busolo, D. (2017). Healthy Canadian adolescents' perspectives of cancer using metaphors: A qualitative study. *BMJ Open, 7*, e013958.

Woodyatt, C., Finneran, C., & Stephenson, R. (2016). In-person versus online focus group discussions: A comparative analysis of data quality. *Qualitative Health Research, 26*, 741–749.

Ye, L., Antonelli, M., Willis, D., Kayser, K., Malhotra, A., & Patel, S. (2017). Couples' experiences with continuous positive airway pressure treatment: A dyadic perspective. *Sleep Health, 3*, 362–367.

Zarhin, D. (2018). Conducting joint interviews with couples: Ethical and methodological challenges. *Qualitative Health Research, 28*, 844–854.

***A link to this open-access article is provided in the Toolkit for Chapter 24 in the* Resource Manual. ✖

****This journal article is available on* thePoint *for this chapter.*

25 | Qualitative Data Analysis

Qualitative data come from a variety of sources, such as verbatim interview transcripts, observational field notes, and diaries kept by study participants. This chapter describes methods for analyzing such narrative data.

INTRODUCTION TO QUALITATIVE ANALYSIS

The purpose of data analysis is to organize, provide structure to, and elicit meaning from data. In qualitative studies, data collection and data analysis often occur concurrently, rather than after all data are collected. When the person collecting the data is the person who analyzes the data, the search for important concepts and patterns begins as data collection is underway.

Qualitative analysis is a labor-intensive activity that requires creativity, conceptual sensitivity, and sheer hard work. We begin by discussing some general issues.

Qualitative Analysis Challenges

Qualitative data analysis is very challenging. There are no universal rules for analyzing qualitative data, and the absence of standard procedures makes it hard to explain how to do such analyses. It is also difficult for researchers to describe their analytic process at length in a report and to present findings in a way that their validity is apparent.

A second challenge of qualitative analysis is the enormous amount of work required. In most studies, hundreds of pages (and sometimes thousands of pages) of transcribed interviews and field notes have to be read, reread, coded and recoded, analyzed, and interpreted.

Another challenge comes in reducing data for reporting purposes. Quantitative results can often be summarized in a few tables. Qualitative researchers, by contrast, must balance the need to be concise with the need to maintain the richness and evidentiary value of their data.

TIP Students often view qualitative analyses as mystifying and daunting. In this edition, we have included numerous explicit examples of and supports for qualitative analysis in the Toolkit in the accompanying *Resource Manual*. We designate the availability of a relevant resource with the Toolkit icon.

Decisions in Qualitative Analysis

Qualitative researchers make numerous decisions that affect the analytic process. Not all decisions are independent—that is, one decision may affect another decision. In this section, we discuss some key decisions for qualitative analysts.

Who Will Do the Analysis?

Many qualitative studies are undertaken by a single researcher who designs the study, selects participants, collects the data, and then analyzes the data. In some studies, however, two to three researchers work collaboratively on analytic tasks. Increasingly, qualitative analysis is being undertaken by interprofessional teams that include both clinicians and researchers from different disciplines—and may even include lay people. Some approaches to qualitative analysis are specifically geared to teamwork. Having multiple analysts may sometimes enhance the trustworthiness of a qualitative study but can be time-consuming because teams typically meet regularly to arrive at a consensus.

Who Will Do the Transcriptions?

Audio-recorded interviews and field notes are major data sources in qualitative studies. Verbatim transcription of the recordings is a critical step in preparing for data analysis. Without accurate transcriptions, the data available for analysis could be flawed. Some have argued that the person who leads the analysis should do the transcriptions, as a way to get immersed in the data. As noted by Braun and Clarke (2006), "The process of transcription, while it may seem time-consuming, frustrating, and at times boring, can be an excellent way to start familiarizing yourself with the data" (p. 87). Others, however, urge transcriptions by professionals as a means of enhancing consistency and accuracy. The Supplement to this chapter on the book's website offers guidance on qualitative data transcription. **S**

Will Coding and Analysis Be Inductive or Deductive?

An early step in most qualitative analyses is the coding and indexing of data so that relevant segments can be retrieved for analysis. In most cases, the codes will be inductive—that is, driven by the data themselves. With an *inductive* (or "bottoms-up") *approach*, analysts identify meaningful concepts that appear with some regularity in the data. In a so-called *deductive*

(or "top-down") *approach*, researchers begin with an a priori framework that typically is based on an existing theory, prior research, or personal conceptualization. In such an approach, the researcher codes the data into a preexisting coding frame (sometimes called a *template*), although modifications may be necessary to accommodate the data. Critics worry that researchers who use an existing coding frame risk premature analytic closure, but a deductive approach can be productive when the inquiry is guided by an existing theory.

> **Example of Using an Existing Framework**
> Grigsby (2018) conducted a qualitative study of African American mothers talking about sexual health with their preadolescent daughters. They used the Theory of Planned Behavior as the organizing framework for their coding and analysis.

> **TIP** Sometimes a so-called *abductive approach* is used, which combines induction and deduction. Graneheim and colleagues (2017), for example, described a study that began with inductive coding, and the initial codes called to mind the construct of human territoriality. A theory of human territoriality was then used deductively to identify themes in the data. Caoila and colleagues (2017) started with an a priori coding scheme (see the Toolkit) and then moved to a more inductive strategy.

How Much of the Data Should Be Coded?

Some qualitative researchers have argued that only the salient portions of a qualitative dataset need to be coded and analyzed. With nonrelevant parts of a record left uncoded, the primary segments can be subjected to more intensive analysis. Others believe that everything should be subjected to preliminary coding—even if some segments are coded "Other" or "Not applicable." Saldaña (2016) advises beginning researchers to code everything.

Will the Focus of the Analysis Be Description or Interpretation?

Some qualitative researchers have as a central aim a rich and thorough description of a phenomenon. Others seek to describe *and* to interpret the meaning of the phenomenon. A distinction is sometimes made between an analysis of the manifest content versus the latent content of the narrative material. The *manifest content* is the actual words and actions of study participants; analyses of manifest content are primarily descriptive in nature, with modest interpretation. Analyses of *latent content* involve a search for underlying ideas and conceptualizations. Efforts are made to understand the broader meanings that underpin what is articulated in the data. Description may be an important and worthwhile goal in some studies, but cultivating the full potential of the data requires efforts to interpret what the data mean. Graneheim and colleagues (2017) have noted that description and interpretation are not dichotomous but lie on a continuum.

What Will Be the Final Product?

Relatedly, researchers should have a sense of what their final product will be. If the focus of the research is primarily description, the final product may take the form of a list of categories or a *taxonomy*—i.e., an orderly system of classification. Morgan (2018) has noted that most qualitative results are reported as theories, models, or themes—with themes being the most typical format. *Themes* are meaningful patterns in the data and can be descriptive or interpretive. Morgan describes *models* as "low-level theories" that connect themes and are often presented in graphic form. *Theories* specify links between a set of themes *and* they explain why they are related in a specified manner. Grounded theory research is explicitly geared toward theory development. Researchers should decide upfront whether they will pursue a theory-building analysis.

Will Computer Software Be Used in the Analysis?

Software to facilitate the management and analysis of qualitative data is used with growing regularity. Some experts have advised beginning researchers—or those whose dataset is small—to use primarily manual (paper-and-pencil) methods. The rationale for this advice is that manual methods allow researchers to get closer to their data, and that

the time spent learning the software may reduce the time available for actual analysis. Qualitative software does, however, offer many advantages.

Will the Analysis Involve Counting?

Most qualitative analyses involve a search for important themes or core constructs. Sometimes, especially with a strategy called *content analysis,* there is a literal count of the number of times a theme (or even a word) appears in the data. Such frequency counts are extremely easy when software is used. Most qualitative researchers do not undertake a formal analysis of thematic prevalence, and yet they *do* often characterize their findings using such statements as, "Most participants described…" or "Many respondents experienced…" Both "many" and "most" suggest at least a loose accounting.

Sandelowski (2001) expressed her belief that numbers are underutilized in qualitative research because of two myths: first, that real qualitative researchers *do not* count, and second, that qualitative researchers *cannot* count. Numbers can be helpful in highlighting the complexity of qualitative data. Numbers may also be useful in testing interpretations and conclusions and in describing events and experiences (although Sandelowski warned of the pitfalls of overcounting). We discuss this issue further in the chapter on mixed methods research (Chapter 27).

Will the Analysis Follow a Formal Guideline?

Although there are no universal rules for analyzing qualitative data, numerous guidelines have been developed. In traditions such as phenomenology, ethnography, and grounded theory, *multiple* guides have been proposed by different experts, and researchers must choose the one that appears most relevant, appealing, or feasible. We briefly describe major analytic systems within these three disciplinary traditions later in this chapter.

Many qualitative studies are not done within one of these research traditions, however. Qualitative analysis has been criticized for being "opaque" or "mysterious," and most beginning researchers struggle with the analysis task. To address these problems, several broad guidelines have been developed to make the task more understandable, transparent, and manageable, and researchers can decide which one (if any) to follow.

The Qualitative Analysis Process

The analysis of qualitative data is a complex and creative process that is fundamentally iterative and nonlinear. This means that analysts move forward and backward between various analytic tasks in their effort to discern the meaning of the data.

Broad processes of qualitative data analysis are shown in Figure 25.1, but there are some caveats. Some qualitative analyses do not involve all activities in this figure. For example, *coding* is commonly used as a preliminary data management and analysis step in many—but not all—studies. Relatively few qualitative studies involve the development of a theory. Also, Figure 25.1 suggests a more linear set of activities than is ever the case. Nevertheless, the figure offers a broad overview of common sequences in the analysis of qualitative data and illustrates that qualitative researchers move from a massive amount of particulars (the data) to smaller, more general units of understanding.

One activity in the figure is, however, universal. First and foremost, analysts must totally immerse themselves in their data. A good analysis requires researchers to scrutinize their data carefully and deliberatively, reading transcriptions over and over (and relistening to recordings) in search of understanding. Insights cannot occur until researchers "live" their data. Relatedly, conscientious analysts get into the habit of writing down their thoughts and observations in the margins of the transcripts and in **analytic memos** as they read through the data and reflect upon their meaning and importance.

Analysis and interpretation often rely on the development of a coding system that allows the researchers to index and retrieve segments for closer scrutiny. **Precoding** typically occurs during data collection, as researchers read interview transcripts or field notes to help them hone their questioning and select new participants. Precoding typically involves circling, underlining, or highlighting passages or concepts that strike the analyst as significant or noteworthy. Without precoding (at least mentally if not in writing), researchers would not be able to discern when their data are saturated.

When data collection is complete, analysts usually develop a more formal coding scheme and then apply the codes to segments of the data—and then refine the codes as they seek to "dig deeper" or to verify the coding. Coding is an important mechanism for organizing the data and is also a process that stimulates insights.

The actual analysis of the data may involve multiple iterations of reading the entire dataset, developing new higher-order codes, looking for patterns, grouping codes into categories, identifying relationships among the categories, forming and reforming

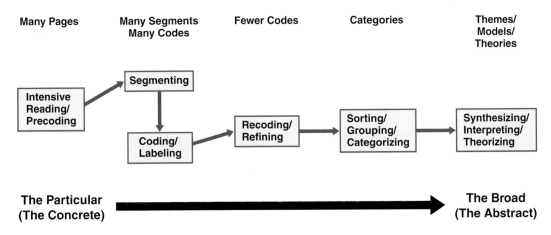

FIGURE 25.1 Broad overview of qualitative analysis processes.

conceptualizations, exploring the properties and dimensions of categories and themes, and continually testing the formulations against the data. Morse and Field (1995) noted that qualitative analysis is a "process of fitting data together, of making the invisible obvious, of linking and attributing consequences to antecedents. It is a process of conjecture and verification, of correction and modification, of suggestion and defense" (p. 126).

> **TIP** Given the nonprescriptive nature of most qualitative analysis, it might be said that it is a process best learned by *doing* it.

CODING AND QUALITATIVE DATA MANAGEMENT

Qualitative analysis often begins with efforts to organize and manage the mass of narrative data, while at the same time developing ideas about what is going on in the data. In the next few sections, we discuss the widely used strategy of *coding* the data, but we acknowledge that not all qualitative researchers agree on the benefits of coding (e.g., St. Pierre & Jackson, 2014).

Developing a Coding Scheme

In qualitative analysis, a **code** is used to identify (in a data segment, such as a phrase, sentence, or paragraph) an interesting, salient, evocative, or essential feature of the data in relation to the phenomenon under investigation. Most coding schemes in qualitative analyses are data-driven and developed through induction as analysts read and reread their data.

> **TIP** Many qualitative researchers move from initial codes to higher-order analytic procedures, such as grouping codes into categories or clustering categories into themes. However, in some research traditions, notably grounded theory, there are *multiple* cycles of coding. Our discussion in this section focuses on initial coding.

Developing a high-quality inductive coding scheme requires a careful reading of the data, with

an eye to identifying underlying concepts. Even if computer software will be used to *apply* codes to the data, most coding schemes are *developed* using paper-and-pencil methods—that is, by using printed copies of transcripts or field notes and writing preliminary codes next to the relevant segment. Typically, this process involves formatting the pages with two columns—one for the data and the other for the codes.

Codes can take many forms. Saldaña (2016) recommends that the codes be entire words or phrases, such as those shown in the right column of Table 25.1, which shows an excerpt from Beck and Gable's (2012) study about secondary traumatic stress experienced by nurses during traumatic births. Depending on the nature of the coding, the codes can be nouns ("immobility," "fatigue"), adjectives ("powerless," "fearful"), verb phrases ("gained a lot of weight"), gerund-based phrases ("losing hope"), or even questions ("What went wrong?").

> **TIP** In lieu of words, some qualitative researchers use abbreviations (e.g., DEPR for depression) or alpha-numerics (A1, B2) (see the Toolkit) that correspond to verbal codes.

In developing preliminary codes, it is useful to select a mix of cases, to maximize opportunities for diverse content. One strategy is to deliberately select materials that vary along key dimensions, such as participant characteristics (e.g., men versus women), role (patient versus caretaker), or time-related factors (e.g., patients with different time elapsed since a diagnosis). A substantial sample of the data should be read before the scheme is applied to the dataset.

> **TIP** Saldaña (2016) has identified several skills and characteristics that promote excellence in coding. These include good organizational skills, flexibility, creativity, perseverance, and the capacity to deal with ambiguity. He also noted that having an extensive vocabulary is a desirable attribute, because word choices matter. He recommended using tools such as a thesaurus and dictionary while coding.

TABLE 25.1 • Example of a Coded Excerpt

DATA EXTRACT	CODES
"One of the most traumatic birth experiences happened a few years ago but I still remember it as though it were yesterday. A grand multipara came to labor and delivery in labor. This was her 9th pregnancy. The doctor, who I don't really get along with, treated her like a piece of dirt. He delivered the baby with no complications. He immediately put the baby in the warmer without letting the mom see or hold her baby. He then proceeded to put his hand inside of her practically halfway up his arm to start pulling her placenta out! She was yelling 'something's not right—it's never hurt like this before!' I walked away from the bed but went back to be with her because she was still screaming. I felt like I was watching a rape! **I felt so helpless**. He's one of those doctors that for whatever reason seems to get away with anything. I talked to my case manager about it and how upset I was. Nothing was ever done. I felt **so powerless**. I really **feel that I failed my patient**. She was counting on me to keep her safe. **I let her down**. To this day I **still think about it and what I could have done differently. I should have protected my patient and advocated for her, but I didn't**."	*Felt helpless* *Felt powerless—person in authority was causing unnecessary trauma* *Feel like I failed my patient* *What could have been done differently?* *I let my patient down*

From the author's (unpublished) coding scheme for the study reported in the following paper: Beck, C., & Gable, R. (2012). A mixed methods study of secondary traumatic stress in labor and delivery nurses. *Journal of Obstetric, Gynecologic, & Neonatal Nursing, 41*, 747–760.

There are no straightforward or easy guidelines for the task of developing codes—and no magic number for how many codes are needed. Sometimes researchers develop 100 or more codes in a study, although "code proliferation" can complicate subsequent analytic work. Some methodologists advocate "lean coding" using a small number of codes (e.g., Creswell, 2013). Typically, researchers create a set of 20 to 40 initial codes. The number of codes depends on the nature of the research question, the focus of the coding (e.g., coding manifest versus latent content), and the level of detail desired. When the analytic segments being coded are phrases or sentences, many codes are needed to capture the detailed information. Fewer codes are needed if the "chunks" being coded are entire paragraphs. Table 25.1 shows an example of fairly detailed coding.

Saldaña (2016) has identified 27 different types of "first-cycle" coding approaches that vary along several dimensions, such as amount of detail and level of abstraction. Here are some examples, with coded excerpts from a study of hunger and food insecurity in low-income families (Polit et al., 2000):

- **Descriptive coding** uses mainly nouns as codes and is often the method of choice of beginning qualitative researchers; it does not, however, provide much insight into meaning.
  - *Excerpt:* "The other day, we ran out of everything and we had to go to a church and get food"
  - *Code:* Food pantry use
- **Process coding** often involves using gerunds as codes to connote action and observable activity (including conceptual action) in the data.
  - *Excerpt:* "The other day, we ran out of everything and we had to go to a church and get food"
  - *Code:* Running out of food (or, Using community resources)

- **Concept coding** involves using a word or phrase to represent symbolically a broad meaning beyond observable facts or behaviors; the codes are usually nouns or gerunds.
  - *Excerpt:* "The other day, we ran out of everything and we had to go to a church and get food"
  - *Code:* Coping with the risk of hunger
- **In vivo coding** (also called "literal" or "verbatim" coding) involves using participant-generated words and phrases; it is used as initial coding in many grounded theory studies but is also applied in other types of qualitative research.
  - *Excerpt:* "The other day, we <u>ran out of everything</u> and we <u>had to go to a church and get food</u>"
  - *Codes:* Ran out of everything; Had to go to a church and get food
- **Holistic coding** involves using codes to grasp broad ideas in large "chunks" of data, rather than coding smaller segments.
  - *Excerpt:* "I buy on deals. I learned how to, you know, what to buy and what not to buy. Where to shop, where to look for sales. I'll go to all the stores. And I clip coupons from the paper and stuff. But sometimes that's not enough. The other day, we ran out of everything and we had to go to a church and get food."
  - *Code:* Food management strategies

TIP Saldaña (2016) acknowledges that some researchers, especially those doing phenomenologic research, label and analyze portions of the data with an extended thematic statement rather than a shorter code. He refers to this type of "coding" as theming the data. An example, based on a phenomenologic study by Beck and Watson (2016), is included in the Toolkit.

As these examples show, the same excerpt can be coded in various ways—there is no single "right" way to code data, and two people are unlikely to develop identical codes for the same data. Sometimes researchers explore alternative ways of coding their data until they achieve a desirable solution. When working in teams, the team should reach a decision about the type of coding to use; team members should independently develop codes and then collaboratively work toward achieving a consensus.

The nature of the research question and the desired end product are likely to influence the type of codes that are created. For example, if the research question were "What is it like for poor families to experience food insecurity?", descriptive coding is unlikely to be productive. It might be suitable if the research question were, "What strategies do poor families use to manage food insecurity?" Descriptive qualitative studies are especially likely to use descriptive or process coding.

Example of a Descriptive Coding Scheme

Dykeman and colleagues (2018) used individual and focus group interviews to explore the views of community service providers regarding the implementation of older adult fall prevention interventions. The data were coded into categories of barriers to such interventions and suggested strategies.

Studies designed to be interpretive are likely to involve abstract, conceptual codes for the latent content (e.g., "Coping with the risk of hunger"). In creating conceptual codes, researchers closely examine segments of the data and compare them to other segments for similarities and dissimilarities to figure out the meaning of those phenomena. This is part of the *constant comparison* process which, although developed within the context of grounded theory research, is widely advocated for other types of qualitative inquiry. The researcher asks questions such as the following about discrete events, incidents, or statements:

What is this?
What is going on?
What does it stand for?
What else is like this?
What is this distinct from?

Important concepts that emerge from close examination of the data are then given a label. These labels are necessarily abstractions, but they should be sufficiently graphic that the nature of the material to which they refer is clear—and, often, provocative.

TIP While coding, it is inevitable that you will notice important patterns in the data. Your evolving ideas and observations should be faithfully maintained in analytic memos.

Coding Qualitative Data

When a coding scheme has been developed, it should be reviewed and pilot-tested with a sample of texts. It is sometimes recommended that a single person apply the codes to the entire dataset, to ensure the highest possible coding consistency across interviews or observations, but team coding is recommended by others. It is often prudent to have at least a portion of the texts coded by two or more people early in the coding process, to evaluate and enhance reliability.

Researchers often create two products at this point. One is a master list of codes or *index*, usually in alphabetical order or in some hierarchical arrangement. The second is a *codebook*, which is a compilation of the codes with good descriptions and one or more excerpt that typifies content for that code. The Toolkit includes an example of a codebook from Beck's work. ✪

Once a coding scheme has been developed, the data are read in their entirety and coded for correspondence to the codes. Researchers may have difficulty deciding the most appropriate code or may not fully comprehend the underlying meaning of some data segments. It may take several readings of the data to grasp its nuances.

Researchers often discover during coding that the initial codes were incomplete. Concepts frequently emerge during coding that were not initially identified. When this happens, it is risky to assume that the concept was absent in materials that have already been coded. A concept might not be identified as salient until it has emerged several times. In such a case, it would be necessary to reread all previously coded material to ensure that the code is applied in a comprehensive fashion.

Another issue is that narrative materials seldom are linear. For example, paragraphs from transcribed interviews may contain elements relating to three or four different codes, embedded in a complex fashion. Table 25.1 provides an example of a paragraph with multiple codes.

Qualitative Data Management

Coding is an important early step in analyzing data in most qualitative studies, and it also plays an important role in data organization. Researchers must be able to gain access to parts of the data, without having repeatedly to reread the dataset in its entirety. Coding converts the data into smaller, more manageable units that can be retrieved and reviewed. Coding the data can be done manually using paper-and-pencil methods, followed by manual methods of data organization. Increasingly, however, special software is being used to code and manage the data.

Manual Methods of Managing Qualitative Data

Before the advent of computer software for managing qualitative data, a typical procedure was to develop **conceptual files.** In this approach, researchers begin with printed copies of the data with the codes in the margins. They create a physical file folder for each code and insert material relating to that code into the file by cutting up excerpts from the data. All of the content for a particular code can be retrieved by going to the applicable file folder.

Creating such files is cumbersome, especially when segments of the narratives have multiple codes. For example, for the data in Table 25.1, five copies of the paragraph, corresponding to the five codes, would be needed. Researchers must also provide enough context that the cut-up material can be understood, including material preceding or following the directly relevant materials. Finally, researchers must usually include pertinent administrative information. For example, for interview data, each excerpt would need to include the participant's ID number so that researchers could, if necessary, obtain additional information from the master copy of the transcript.

TIP Other methods of manual organization include the use of file cards that can be sorted into piles, or post-it notes that can be arrayed on a large surface. For small datasets with few codes, researchers sometimes use different colored fonts for excerpts with different codes.

Computer Software for Managing Qualitative Data

Computer-assisted qualitative data analysis software (**CAQDAS**) removes the work of cutting up pages of narrative material. These programs allow researchers to enter and store the entire data file on a computer, code each portion of the narrative, and then retrieve and display text tagged with specified codes for analytic reflection. Most software allows researchers to write analytic memos, and some offer transcription services. The software can also be used to examine relationships between codes. Software cannot, however, *do* the coding, and it cannot tell researchers how to analyze the data. Researchers must continue to be analysts and critical thinkers.

Dozens of CAQDAS have been developed. The main types of available packages include software for text retrieval, coding and retrieval, theory building, concept mapping, and data conversion/collection (Silver & Lewins, 2014). Tutorials on the mechanics of using various software packages are widely available on YouTube. Links to several CAQDAS programs are provided in the Toolkit. ⊗

A popular option is sophisticated *theory-building software,* which permits researchers to examine relationships between concepts, develop hierarchies of codes, construct diagrams, and generate hyperlinks to create nonhierarchical networks. Examples of theory-building packages include NVivo, ATLAS.ti, HyperRESEARCH, MAXQDA, Quirkos, and QDA Miner, most of which are available in Mac and PC versions.

> **TIP** Transana is an example of specialty software that enables the coding of large digital audio and video files. Dedoose is a cloud-based software known for its ability to work well in mixed methods studies with both qualitative and quantitative data.

Software for concept mapping permits researchers to construct more sophisticated diagrams than theory-building software. Concept maps are a means for organizing and representing knowledge (Novak & Cañas, 2006). CmapTools,

an example of concept mapping software, is available at no cost.

Data conversion and collection software, such as voice recognition software, converts audio into text. Such software may be attractive because of the time and expense needed to transcribe audio-recorded interviews—although a study by Johnson (2011) suggests that the time savings may not be great. Voice recognition software is designed for a single user. The software must be "trained" to recognize the voice of the user, typically an *oral transcriptionist.*

The performance of voice recognition software is variable and depends on such factors as computer capabilities, the quality of the microphone, and the amount of background noise. One disadvantage is the inability of voice recognition software to automatically punctuate. The oral transcriptionist must specifically state the punctuation, such as "period" and "comma." Oral transcriptionists also need to edit the text to correct errors. For instance, voice recognition programs often misinterpret common homonyms like "to," "too," and "two." Thus, the time-saving advantages in using voice recognition software may be modest.

Computer programs offer many advantages for managing qualitative data, but some people prefer manual methods as a means of getting closer to the data. Others have raised objections to having a process that is basically cognitive turned into an activity that is mechanical. Another disadvantage is that a considerable amount of time is typically needed to learn the software—but, once learned, the skills can be used for future projects. Despite concerns, many researchers have switched to computerized data management. Proponents insist that it frees up their time and permits them to pay greater attention to important conceptual issues.

Example of Using Computers to Manage Qualitative Data

Castro and Andrews (2018) explored the work-life narratives of nurses in accounts they posted in publicly accessible blogs. Four blogs written by nurses from different specialty areas (a total of 520 entries) were copied into NVivo10 for coding and analysis.

OVERVIEW OF ANALYTIC PROCEDURES

Data coding and *management* in qualitative research are reductionist in nature: They involve converting masses of data into smaller, manageable segments. By contrast, qualitative data *analysis* is constructionist: segments are put together into meaningful conceptual patterns. Qualitative analysis involves discovering pervasive ideas and searching for general concepts (*analytic generalization*) through an inductive process. Although there are various approaches to qualitative data analysis, some features are common to several of them.

The analysis of qualitative materials often begins with the identification of broad **categories**, which are clusters of codes that are connected conceptually. In Table 25.1, which shows a coded excerpt from Beck and Gable's (2012) study of nurses' secondary traumatic stress, two of the codes ("Feel like I failed my patient" and "I let my patient down") were clustered with other codes to form the category "Failing to Protect the Patient." Ideas for categories usually begin to emerge during coding or precoding and would likely be documented in analytic memos.

In many qualitative studies, the next phase involves the identification of themes. In their thorough review of how the term *theme* is used among qualitative researchers, DeSantis and Ugarriza (2000) offered this often-cited definition: "A **theme** is an abstract entity that brings meaning and identity to a current experience and its variant manifestations. As such, a theme captures and unifies the nature or basis of the experience into a meaningful whole" (p. 362).

Thematic analysis often relies on what Spradley (1979) called the similarity principle and the contrast principle. The *similarity principle* involves looking for units of information with similar content, symbols, or meanings. The *contrast principle* guides efforts to find out how content or symbols differ from other content or symbols—that is, to identify what is distinctive about themes or categories that are being identified.

During analysis, qualitative researchers distinguish between ideas that apply to all (or many) people, and aspects of the experience that are unique to particular participants because codes and categories are seldom found in every data source. Ayres, Kavanagh, and Knafl (2003) argued cogently for the importance of doing both across-case analysis and within-case analysis. The analysis of individual cases "enables the researcher to understand those aspects of experience that occur not as individual 'units of meaning' but as part of the pattern formed by the confluence of meanings within individual accounts" (p. 873). Themes that have explanatory or conceptual power both in individual cases and across the sample have the best potential for analytic generalization. Ayres and colleagues illustrated how within-case and across-case analyses were integrated in three nursing studies.

The analysis of themes involves not only discovering commonalities across participants, but also seeking natural variation. Themes are never universal. Researchers must attend not only to what themes arise but also to how they are patterned. Does the theme apply only to certain types of people? In certain contexts? At certain periods? What are the conditions that precede the observed phenomenon, and what are the apparent consequences of it? In other words, the qualitative analyst must be sensitive to *relationships* in the data.

Themes may be developed within categories, but thematic development often involves combining categories. For example, in Beck and Gable's (2012) study on secondary traumatic stress experienced by nurses, codes were clustered to create categories ("Helpless/Powerless," "Questioning One's Actions," and "Failing to Protect the Patient"), and these categories were the basis for the theme, "Agonizing over What Should Have Been" (Figure 25.2).

Researchers' search for themes and patterns sometimes can be facilitated by charting devices that enable them to summarize the evolution of behaviors, events, and processes. For example, for qualitative studies that focus on dynamic experiences—such as decision-making—it is sometimes useful to develop flowcharts or timelines that highlight time sequences, major decision points and events, and factors affecting the decisions (see examples in the Toolkit). ✹ Another device that

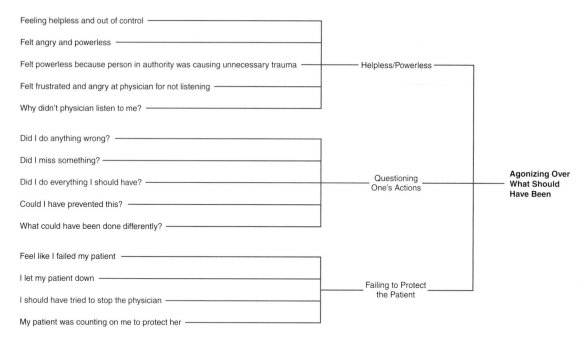

FIGURE 25.2 Codes and categories shown in a dendrogram for theme 3: *Agonizing Over What Should Have Been Done*. (Reprinted with permission from Beck, C. T., & Gable, R. [2012]. A mixed methods study of secondary traumatic stress in labor and delivery nurses. *Journal of Obstetric, Gynecologic, & Neonatal Nursing, 41*, 747–760.)

depicts the clustering of codes and categories is called a **dendrogram**, which is a tree diagram that illustrates the arrangement of clusters in a hierarchically ordered system. Figure 25.2 is a dendrogram from Beck and Gable's (2012) study of secondary traumatic stress.

Two-dimensional matrices are another method of displaying thematic material (Miles et al., 2014). Traditionally, each row of a matrix represents individual participants, and columns are used for codes or themes. The entries at the intersection are the raw data or summaries. Matrices can be constructed by hand, but computer spreadsheets enhance opportunities for sorting the data.

Some qualitative researchers—especially phenomenologists—use metaphors as an analytic strategy. A metaphor is a symbolic comparison, using figurative language to evoke a visual analogy. Metaphors can be a powerfully expressive tool for qualitative analysts. As a literary device, metaphors can permit greater insight and understanding in qualitative analysis and can help link together parts to the whole. Thorne and Darbyshire (2005), however, expressed concern about overusing metaphors. In their view, metaphoric allusions can be a compelling approach to depicting human experience but can run the risk of "supplanting creative insight with hackneyed cliché masquerading as profundity" (p. 1111). Carpenter (2008) also warned that when researchers mix metaphors, fail to follow through with metaphors, or use metaphors that do not fit, they can misrepresent their data. Hunter, on the other hand, in her study of resilience in adolescents, described how "the use of metaphors to capture the tenor of the voices of these adolescents brought life to my findings" (Hunter et al., 2002, p. 392).

Example of a Metaphor

Cuthbert and colleagues (2017) explored the experiences of cancer family caregivers who were participating in a physical activity program. The metaphor of a "downward spiral" characterized their experiences in the caregiving role, while the metaphor of an "upward spiral" represented their experiences in the special program.

TIP It is also possible to do an analysis of the metaphors that study participants themselves use. For example, Beck (2017) conducted a metaphorical analysis of mothers' descriptions of their experiences caring for children with obstetric brachial plexus injuries. Some of the metaphors used by the mothers to describe their experiences included a juggling act, a maze, a simmering pot, a dagger to the heart, and a roller coaster.

Identifying key categories and themes is seldom a tidy, linear process. Researchers derive themes from the narrative materials, go back to the materials with the themes in mind to see if the materials really do fit, and then refine the themes as necessary. Sometimes apparent insights early in the analysis need to be abandoned.

Some level of interpretation is essential in analyzing narrative materials, with interpretation and analysis occurring virtually simultaneously and iteratively. Interpretation is a challenging activity in qualitative analysis—and the most difficult to explain in a manner that makes clear how to achieve it. Although it is hard to provide guidance on interpretation, there is considerable agreement that the ability to "make meaning" from qualitative texts depends on researchers' immersion in and closeness to the data. **Incubation** is the process of *living* the data, a process in which researchers must try to understand the data's meanings, find their essential patterns, and draw legitimate, insightful conclusions. Another key ingredient in interpretation and meaning-making is researchers' self-awareness and the ability to reflect on their own world view and perspectives—that is, reflexivity.

Creativity also plays an important role in uncovering meaning in the data. Hunter and colleagues (2002) have written about the role of creativity in qualitative analysis and offer insights designed to "shed light on the magic of understanding the mysteries within data" (p. 388). Chandler, in writing about the transition from *saturation* to *illumination*, wrote that "Strategies for creativity take time and require incubation for new ideas to percolate" (Chandler in Hunter et al., p. 396). Researchers need to give themselves sufficient time to achieve the *aha* that comes with making meaning beyond the facts.

Researchers strive to weave thematic pieces together into an integrated whole. The various themes or categories need to be interrelated to provide an overall structure (such as an integrated description, model, or theory) to the data. The integration task is difficult because it demands ingenuity and intellectual rigor. In drawing conclusions, qualitative researchers are increasingly considering the transferability of the findings and the potential uses to which the qualitative evidence can be put. Like quantitative researchers, qualitative researchers need to give thought to the implications of their study findings for future research and for nursing practice.

QUALITATIVE ANALYSIS WITHIN RESEARCH TRADITIONS

In this section, we provide an overview of analytic approaches that have been advocated by researchers within the three main research traditions described in this book—ethnography, phenomenology, and grounded theory. These overviews are not sufficiently detailed to provide guidance on how to actually do an analysis; references are provided for further assistance.

Ethnographic Analysis

Analysis begins from the moment ethnographers set foot in the field. Ethnographers are continually looking for *patterns* in the behavior of participants, comparing one pattern against another, and analyzing many patterns simultaneously (Fetterman, 2010). As they become immersed in the everyday lives of participants, ethnographers acquire a deeper understanding of the culture being studied. Maps, flowcharts, and organizational charts are useful tools that help to crystallize and illustrate the data. Matrices (two-dimensional displays) can also help to highlight a comparison graphically, to cross-reference categories, and to discover emerging patterns.

Spradley's (1979) research sequence is sometimes used to analyze ethnographic data. His method is based on the premise that language is the primary means that relates cultural meaning in a culture. His sequence of 12 steps, which includes data collection and data analysis, is as follows:

1. Locating an informant
2. Interviewing an informant
3. Making an ethnographic record
4. Asking descriptive questions
5. Analyzing ethnographic interviews
6. Making a domain analysis
7. Asking structural questions
8. Making a taxonomic analysis
9. Asking contrast questions
10. Making a componential analysis
11. Discovering cultural themes
12. Writing the ethnography

Spradley's method involves four levels of data analysis, the first of which is **domain analysis**. Domains, which are units of cultural knowledge, are broad categories that encompass smaller ones. During this first level of data analysis, ethnographers identify relational patterns among terms in the domains that are used by members of the culture. The ethnographer focuses on the cultural meaning of terms and symbols (objects and events) used in a culture and their interrelationships.

In **taxonomic analysis**, the second level of data analysis, ethnographers decide how many domains the analysis will encompass. Will only one or two domains be analyzed in depth, or will several domains be studied less intensively? After making this decision, a **taxonomy**—a system of classifying and organizing terms—is developed to illustrate the internal organization of a domain and the relationship among the subcategories of the domain. In **componential analysis**, the ethnographer analyzes data for similarities and differences among cultural terms in a domain. Finally, in **theme analysis**, cultural themes are uncovered. Domains are connected in cultural themes, which help to provide a holistic view of the culture being studied. The discovery of cultural meaning is the outcome.

Example Using Spradley's Method

Kim and colleagues (2018) followed Spradley's analytic sequence in an ethnography of the experience of the hospital waiting area as perceived by hemodialysis patients and family carers; the goal was to develop an optimal social environment for providing nursing care. In the final analytic step, three cultural themes were derived: Sharing information and consoling, Inhabiting a separate area of ease and discomfort, and Experiencing vigilance and unsure stillness.

Other approaches to ethnographic analysis have been developed. For example, in Leininger's ethnonursing research method, as described in McFarland and Wehbe-Alamah (2015), ethnographers follow a four-phase ethnonursing data analysis guide. In the first phase, ethnographers collect, describe, and record data. The second phase involves identifying and categorizing descriptors. In phase 3, data are analyzed to discover repetitive patterns in their context. The fourth and final phase involves abstracting major themes and presenting findings.

Example Using Leininger's method

Salman and colleagues (2018) conducted a focused ethnography to understand Jordanian women's beliefs and values about breast cancer and how these beliefs influenced decisions for breast cancer screening. Using Leininger's four phases of data analysis, they identified three themes: Fear, denial, and lack of knowledge regarding breast cancer screening; Health care professionals were not quick to offer information and education; and Willingness to learn about breast cancer and prevention.

Phenomenologic Analysis

Many qualitative analysts use what might be called "fracturing" strategies that break down the data and rearrange them into categories. Phenomenologists tend to prefer holistic, "contextualizing" strategies that involve interpreting the narrative data within the context of a "whole text." We look briefly at three broad approaches to phenomenologic analysis.

Descriptive Phenomenology

Three frequently used methods for descriptive phenomenology are the methods of Colaizzi (1978),

Giorgi (1985), and van Kaam (1966). All three are from the Duquesne School of phenomenology, based on Husserl's philosophy.

Phenomenologic analysis using these methods involves a search for common patterns, but there are differences among these approaches, as summarized in Table 25.2. The basic outcome of all three methods is the description of the meaning of an experience, often through the identification of essential themes. Colaizzi's method, however, is the only one that calls for a validation of results by returning to study participants. Giorgi's analysis relies solely on researchers. His view was that it is inappropriate to return to participants to validate findings or to use external judges to review the analysis. Van Kaam's method requires that intersubjective agreement be reached with other expert judges.

Example of a Study Using Colaizzi's Method
Imani and co-researchers (2018) studied hospital nurses' lived experiences of intelligent resilience. The researchers conducted in-depth interviews with 10 nurses in Iranian hospitals. Colaizzi's seven-step analytic process was followed. Significant resilience-related statements were extracted from the interviews and 354 formulated meanings were generated. The nurses' experience of intelligent resilience was reflected in four main themes: Patience and wisdom; Reverence; Situational self-control; and Appealing to religiosity.

TIP Cheryl Beck, one of the authors of this book, has undertaken many studies using Colaizzi's method. Materials from some of her phenomenologic studies are included in the Toolkit.

The Utrecht School of Phenomenology

Another approach to phenomenology is the Utrecht School, which combines characteristics of descriptive and interpretive phenomenology. Van Manen's (1990) method is an example of this approach, in which researchers try to grasp the essential meaning of the experience being studied. According to van Manen, thematic aspects of experience can be uncovered from participants' descriptions of the experience by three methods: (1) the holistic approach, (2) the selective (highlighting) approach,

and (3) the detailed (line-by-line) approach. In the **holistic approach**, researchers view the text as a whole and try to capture its meanings. In the **selective approach,** researchers highlight or pull out statements or phrases that seem essential to the experience under study. In the **detailed approach**, researchers analyze every sentence. Once themes have been identified, they become the objects of reflection and interpretation through follow-up interviews with participants. Through this process, essential themes are discovered.

Van Manen (2006) emphasized that this phenomenologic method cannot be separated from the practice of writing. Writing up the results of qualitative analysis is an active struggle to understand and recognize the lived meanings of the phenomena studied. The text written by a phenomenologic researcher must lead readers to a "questioning wonder." Van Manen (2017) has recently asserted that "the outcomes of phenomenologic research are full-fledged reflective texts that induce the reader into a wondering engagement with certain questions that may be explored through the identification, critical examination, and eloquent elaboration of themes that help the reader recognize the meaningfulness of certain human experiences and events" (p. 777).

Example of a Study Using Van Manen's Method
Saxon and colleagues (2018) studied high-risk respiratory patients' experience of bronchoscopy with conscious sedation. Data from unstructured interviews with 13 patients were analyzed using van Manen's three-phase approach. Five themes emerged from the analysis: Frustration and fear; Comfort and safety; Choking and coughing; Being aware; and Consequences.

In addition to identifying themes from participants' words, van Manen also called for gleaning thematic descriptions from artistic sources. Van Manen urged qualitative researchers to keep in mind that literature, music, painting, and other art forms can provide experiential information that can increase insights as the phenomenologist tries to grasp the essential meaning of the experience being studied. Experiential descriptions in literature and art help challenge and stretch phenomenologists' interpretive sensibilities.

TABLE 25.2 • Comparison of Three Phenomenologic Analytic Methods

COLAIZZI (1978)	GIORGI (1985)	VAN KAAM (1966)
1. Read all protocols to acquire a feeling for them.	1. Read the entire set of protocols to get a sense of the whole.	1. List and group preliminarily the descriptive expressions that must be agreed upon by expert judges. Final listing presents percentages of these categories in that particular sample.
2. Review each protocol and extract significant statements.	2. Discriminate units from participants' description of phenomenon being studied.	2. Reduce the concrete, vague, and overlapping expressions of the participants to more descriptive terms. (Intersubjective agreement among judges needed.)
3. Spell out the meaning of each significant statement (i.e., formulate meanings).	3. Articulate the psychological insight in each of the meaning units.	3. Eliminate elements not inherent in the phenomenon being studied or that represent blending of two related phenomena.
4. Organize the formulated meanings into clusters of themes. a. Refer these clusters back to the original protocols to validate them. b. Note discrepancies among or between the various clusters, avoiding the temptation of ignoring data or themes that do not fit.	4. Synthesize all of the transformed meaning units into a consistent statement regarding participants' experiences (referred to as the "structure of the experience"); can be expressed on a specific or general level.	4. Write a hypothetical identification and description of the phenomenon being studied.
5. Integrate results into an exhaustive description of the phenomenon under study.		5. Apply hypothetical description to randomly selected cases from the sample. If necessary, revise the hypothesized description, which must then be tested again on a new random sample.
6. Formulate an exhaustive description of the phenomenon under study in as unequivocal a statement of identification as possible.		6. Consider the hypothesized identification as a valid identification and description once preceding operations have been carried out successfully.
7. Ask participants about the findings thus far as a final validating step.		

Interpretive Phenomenology and Hermeneutics

A third broad category of phenomenology is interpretive phenomenology (hermeneutics). As noted in Chapter 22, a key concept in a hermeneutic study is the *hermeneutic circle*. The circle signifies a methodologic process in which, to reach understanding, there is continual movement between the parts and the whole of the text being analyzed. Gadamer (1975) stressed that, to interpret a text, researchers cannot separate themselves from the meanings of the text and must strive to understand possibilities that the text can reveal. Ricoeur (1981) broadened this notion of text to include not just the written text but any human action or situation.

Example of Gadamerian Hermeneutics

Dalteg and colleagues (2017) explored the illness beliefs of couples in which one spouse had atrial fibrillation. The data from in-depth dyadic interviews with nine couples were analyzed and interpreted using an approach based on Gadamerian hermeneutics. The final stage of analysis involved identifying passages that seemed representative of the shared understanding between the researchers and the participant—a "fusion of horizons" (p. 3702).

Diekelmann, Allen, and Tanner (1989) proposed a seven-stage process of data analysis in hermeneutics that involves collaboration by a team of researchers:

1. All the interviews or texts are read for an overall understanding.
2. Interpretive summaries of each interview are written.
3. A team of researchers analyzes selected transcribed interviews or texts.
4. Any disagreements on interpretation are resolved by going back to the text.
5. Common meanings are identified by comparing and contrasting the text.
6. Relationships among themes emerge.
7. A draft of the themes with exemplars from texts is presented to the team. Responses or suggestions are incorporated into the final draft.

According to Diekelmann and colleagues, the discovery in step 6 of a **constitutive pattern**—a pattern that expresses the relationships among relational themes and is present in all the interviews or texts—is the highest level of hermeneutic analysis. A situation is constitutive when it gives actual content to a person's self-understanding or to a person's way of being in the world.

Example of a Diekelmann's Hermeneutic Analysis

Mirlashari and colleagues (2019) explored the lived experience of nurses implementing family-centered care in the neonatal intensive care unit (NICU) through in-depth interviews with 11 nurses. Using Diekelmann's approach, the research team identified four main themes: Strain to achieve stability; Bewildered by taking multiple roles; Accepting the family; and Reaching a bright horizon.

Benner (1994) offered another analytic approach for hermeneutics. Her interpretive analysis consists of three interrelated processes: the search for paradigm cases, thematic analysis, and the analysis of exemplars. **Paradigm cases** are "strong instances of concerns or ways of being in the world" (p. 113). Paradigm cases are used early in the analytic process as a strategy for gaining understanding. Thematic analysis is done to compare and contrast similarities across cases. Paradigm cases and thematic analysis can be enhanced by identifying **exemplars** that illuminate aspects of a paradigm case or theme. The presentation of paradigm cases and exemplars in reports allows readers to play a role in consensual validation of the results by deciding whether the cases support the researchers' conclusions. Crist and Tanner (2003) provide guidance for a hermeneutic interpretive process that includes features of both Benner's and Diekelmann's approaches.

Example Using Benner's Hermeneutic Analysis

Izumi and colleagues (2018) studied care coordination using Benner's approach. Fifteen care coordinators from 10 programs were interviewed over a 6-month period. The researchers found that the central theme of care coordination practice was "bridging the patient and the healthcare systems" (p. 49). Strong examples of care coordination practice were designated as paradigm cases, two of which were described in detail in their report.

Parse's (2016) Parsesciencing is another hermeneutic approach. Parse's second phase of inquiry, distilling-fusing, involves the researcher dwelling with transcribed interviews and audio recordings. A story is constructed that captures the central ideas about the phenomenon from each "historian's" (participant's) dialogue. These central ideas are labeled *essences*. Essences, written in the historian's language, are brought to a higher abstraction using the researcher's language. Next, the essences are fused and lead to a language art for each historian. A discerning extant moment of the universal humanuniverse living experience is created. In the final phase, heuristic interpreting entails transmogrifying, transsubstantiating, metaphorical emergings, and artistic expressions. In *transmogrifying*, language is shifted to a new level of abstraction. Then in *transsubstantiating*, the language is shaped into the core language of humanbecoming. The statements shared by the historians that are described in symbolic language are the *metaphorical emergings*. Lastly, the researcher's own personal choice for the art form to present the results of their Parsesciencing is the focus of artistic expression.

TIP Another approach mentioned in Chapter 22 is *reflective lifeworld research* (RLR). Dahlberg and colleagues (2008) presented steps for the analysis of data in both descriptive phenomenologic RLR studies and hermeneutic RLR studies. Sidenius and co-researchers (2017) used the RLR approach in their descriptive study of the lived experience of nature-based therapy in a therapy garden for those suffering from stress-related illness. Their paper presented a model showing their analytic process, and the model is included in the Toolkit.

TABLE 25.3 • Comparison of Alternative Grounded Theory Approaches

	GLASER	CORBIN AND STRAUSS	CHARMAZ
Initial data analysis	Breaking down and conceptualizing data, with comparisons so that patterns emerge	Breaking down and conceptualizing data, which include taking apart a single sentence, observation, or incident	Creating link between collecting data and developing emergent theory; defining what is occurring in data and beginning to analyze what it means
Types of coding	Open, selective, theoretical	Open, axial	Initial, focused
Connections between categories: strategies	18 coding families plus theoretical codes from different disciplines	Paradigm (conditions, actions-interactions, and consequences or outcomes) and the conditional/consequential matrix	Analytic strategies are emergent rather than procedural application; categories, subcategories, and links
Outcome	Emergent theory (discovery)	Conceptual description (verification)	An interpretive theory constructed through researcher's past and present involvement with persons, perspectives, and research practices

Grounded Theory Analysis

Grounded theory methods emerged in the 1960s in connection with Glaser and Strauss's (1967) research program on dying in hospitals. The two co-originators eventually split and developed divergent schools of thought, which have been called the "Glaserian" and "Straussian" versions of grounded theory (Walker & Myrick, 2006). A third grounded theory approach—constructivist grounded theory—has emerged more recently. The differences among these approaches mainly concern the analysis of the data (See Table 25.3).

Glaser and Strauss' Grounded Theory Method

Constant comparison is a core feature in all grounded theory analyses and in many other qualitative analyses. This method involves a comparison of elements present in one data source (e.g., in one interview) with those in another to determine if they are similar. The process continues until the content of each source has been compared to the content in all sources. In this fashion, commonalities are identified.

The concept of fit is a key element in Glaserian grounded theory analysis. By **fit,** Glaser meant that the developing categories of the substantive theory must fit the data. Fit enables the researcher to determine if data can be placed in the same category or if they can be related to one another. However, Glaser (1992) warned qualitative researchers not to force an analytic fit, noting that "if you torture data enough it will give up!" (p. 123). Forcing a fit hinders the development of a viable theory. *Fit* is also an important issue when a grounded theory is applied in new contexts: the theory must closely "fit" the substantive area where it will be used (Glaser & Strauss, 1967).

In the classic Glaserian approach, the substance of the data is conceptualized through *substantive codes*, while *theoretical codes* provide insights into how substantive codes relate to each other.

See entry B2 in the Toolkit. ⚙ Substantive coding includes both open coding and selective coding. **Open coding,** used in the first stage of the constant comparative analysis, captures what is going on in the data. Through open coding, data are broken down into incidents and their similarities and differences are examined.

There are three levels of open coding, with increasing degrees of abstraction. **Level I codes** (or *in vivo codes*) are derived directly from the participants' words and have vivid imagery. Table 25.4 presents five level I codes from Beck's (2002) grounded theory study on mothering twins and interview excerpts associated with those codes. Researchers constantly compare new level I codes to previously identified ones and then condense them into broader **level II codes** (categories). For example, in Table 25.4, Beck's five level I codes were collapsed into the level II category, "Reaping the Blessings." **Level III codes** (or theoretical constructs) are the most abstract. These constructs "add scope beyond local meanings" (Glaser, 1978, p. 70) to the generated theory. Collapsing level II codes aids in identifying constructs. In Beck's study, the level II code of "Reaping the Blessings" was collapsed with another level II code ("Becoming manageable") into the level III code "Resuming Own Life." (A figure with Beck's hierarchy of open codes is in the Toolkit. ⚙)

Open coding ends when the core category is discovered and then selective coding begins. The **core category** is a pattern of behavior that is relevant for participants. The primary function of a core category is to integrate the theory and make it dense and saturated. The core category in Glaserian grounded theory earns its prominence by accounting for most of the variation in processing the participants' main concern that has emerged as the study focus and by explaining the latent pattern of behavior that accounts for its resolution (Holton, 2010). In **selective coding,** researchers code only those data that relate to the core variable. One kind of core variable is a **basic social process (BSP)** that evolves over time in two or more phases. All BSPs

TABLE 25.4 • Collapsing Level I Codes Into the Level II Code *"Reaping the Blessings"* (Beck, 2002)

QUOTE	LEVEL I CODE
I enjoy just watching the twins interact so much. Especially now that they are mobile. They are not walking yet but they are crawling. I will tell you they are already playing. Like one will go around the corner and kind of peek around and they play hide and seek. They crawl after each other.	Enjoying Twins
With twins it's amazing. She was sick and she had a fever. He was the one acting sick. She didn't seem like she was sick at all. He was. We watched him for like 6–8 hours. We gave her the medicine and he started calming down. Like WOW! That is so weird. Cause you read about it but it's like, Oh come on! You know that doesn't really happen and it does. It's really neat to see.	Amazing
These days it's really neat cause you go to the store or you go out and people are like "Oh, they are twins, how nice." And I say, "Yeah they are. Look, look at my kids."	Getting Attention
I just feel blessed to have two. I just feel like I am twice as lucky as a mom who has one baby. I mean that's the best part. It's just that instead of having one baby to watch grow and change and develop and become a toddler and school-age child you have two.	Feeling Blessed
It's very exciting. It's interesting and it's fun to see them and how the twin bond really is. There really is a twin bond. You read about it and you hear about it but until you experience it, you just don't understand. One time they were both crying and they were fed. They were changed and burped. There was nothing wrong. I couldn't figure out what was wrong. So I said to myself, "I am just going to put them together and close the door." I put them in my bed together and they patty-caked their hands and put their noses together and just looked at each other and went right to sleep.	Twin Bonding

From data for the study reported in the following paper: Beck, C. T. (2002). Releasing the pause button: Mothering twins during the first year of life. *Qualitative Health Research, 12,* 593–608.

are core variables, but not all core variables have to be BSPs. In Beck's (2002) study, the core category—a BSP—was "Releasing the Pause Button."

Glaser (1978) provided nine criteria to help researchers decide on a core category:

1. It must be central, meaning that it is related to many categories.
2. It must reoccur frequently in the data.
3. It takes more time to saturate than other categories.
4. It relates meaningfully and easily to other categories.
5. It has clear and grabbing implications for formal theory.
6. It has considerable carry-through.
7. It is completely variable.
8. It is a dimension of the problem.
9. It can be any kind of a theoretical code.

Theoretical coding, which typically begins while selective coding is still in progress, helps grounded theorists to weave the broken pieces of data back together. Theoretical codes connect the categories and constructs that relate to the core category. Theoretical codes have the power "to grab," which Glaser (2005) called "theoretical code capture" (p. 74). Theoretical codes provide a grounded theory with greater explanatory power because they enhance the abstract meaning of the relationships among categories. Glaser (1978)

BOX 25.1 Families of Theoretical Codes for Grounded Theory Analysis

1. The six Cs: causes, contexts, contingencies, consequences, covariances, and conditions
2. Process: stages, phases, passages, transitions
3. Degree: intensity, range, grades, continuum
4. Dimension: elements, parts, sections
5. Type: kinds, styles, forms
6. Strategy: tactics, techniques, maneuverings
7. Interaction: mutual effects, interdependence, reciprocity
8. Identity–self: self-image, self-worth, self-concept
9. Cutting point: boundaries, critical junctures, turning points
10. Means–goal: purpose, end products
11. Cultural: social values, beliefs
12. Consensus: agreements, uniformities, conformity
13. Mainline: socialization, recruiting, social order
14. Theoretical: density, integration, clarity, fit, relevance
15. Ordering/elaboration: structural ordering, temporal ordering, conceptual ordering
16. Unit: group, organization, collective
17. Reading: hypotheses, concepts, problems
18. Models: pictorial models of a theory

Adapted from Glaser, B. G. (1978). *Theoretical sensitivity*. Mill Valley, CA: Sociological Press.

first proposed 18 "families" of theoretical codes that researchers can use to conceptualize how substantive codes relate to each other (Box 25.1). Glaser (2005) later identified many new possibilities for theoretical codes, offering examples from biochemistry (bias random walk), economics (amplifying causal looping), and political science (conjectural causation). Glaser believed that the large array of theoretical codes available reduces a researcher's tendency to force a pet or favorite theoretical code on the developing theory.

Throughout coding and analysis, grounded theory analysts document their ideas about the data, categories, and emerging conceptual scheme in *memos*. Memos preserve ideas that may initially not seem productive but may later prove valuable once further developed. Memos also encourage researchers to reflect on and describe patterns in the data, relationships between categories, and emergent conceptualizations.

TIP Glaser (1978) offered guidelines for preparing effective memos to generate substantive theory, including the following:

- Keep memos separate from data.
- Stop coding when an idea for a memo occurs, so as not to lose the thought.
- A memo can be brought on by forcing it, by beginning to write about a code.
- Memos can be modified as growth and realizations occur.
- In writing memos, do not focus on persons; talk conceptually about substantive codes.
- When you have two ideas, write each idea up as a separate memo to prevent confusion.
- Always remain flexible with memoing approaches.

The Toolkit includes examples of memos from Beck's work.

Glaser's grounded theory method is concerned with the *generation* of categories and hypotheses rather than testing them. The product of the typical grounded theory analysis is a model that endeavors to generate "a theory of continually resolving the main concern, which explains most of the behavior in an area of interest" (Glaser, 2001, p. 103). Once a problem or central concern emerges, the grounded theorist goes on to discover the process these participants experience in coping with or resolving the problem.

Example of Glaser and Strauss Grounded Theory Analysis

Figure 25.3 presents Beck's (2002) model from a grounded theory study. "Releasing the Pause Button," the core category, was conceptualized as the process through which mothers of twins progressed as they attempted to resume their lives after giving birth. According to this model, the process involves four phases: Draining Power, Pausing Own Life, Striving to Reset, and Resuming Own Life. Beck used 10 coding families in her theoretical coding for the Releasing the Pause Button process. The bottom of Figure 25.3 shows the theoretical codes for the phases of her grounded theory: Conditions, Consequences, Strategies, and Consequences. Another theoretical code was the family *cutting point*. Three months seemed to be the turning point for mothers, when life started to become more manageable. Here is an excerpt that Beck coded as a cutting point: "Three months came around and the twins sort of slept through the night and it made a huge, huge difference."

Although Glaser cautioned against consulting the literature before a theory is stabilized, he also viewed grounded theory as an "ever-modifying process" (Glaser, 1978, p. 5) that could benefit from scrutiny of other work. Glaser discussed the evolution of grounded theories through the process of **emergent fit**, to prevent individual substantive theories from being "respected little islands of knowledge" (p. 148). Glaser pointed out that generating grounded theory does not necessarily require discovering all new categories or ignoring ones previously identified in the literature. Through constant comparison, researchers can compare concepts emerging from the data with similar concepts from existing theory or prior studies to assess which parts have emergent fit with the theory being generated.

In Glaser's (2001) view, grounded theory modification is an ongoing process. As data from new studies become available, the grounded theory can be modified to accommodate varying conditions, in an effort to increase the theory's power and completeness. Constantly comparing data from new research to the existing theory can illuminate new properties of the categories. When a grounded theory is continually modified, it is brought to a higher level of theoretical completeness.

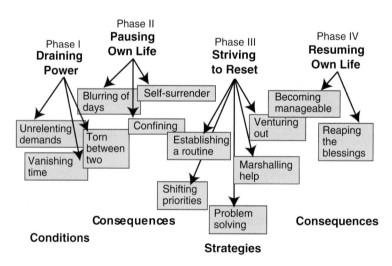

FIGURE 25.3 Beck's (2002) model of mothering twins. (Reprinted with permission from Beck, C. T. (2002). Releasing the pause button: Mothering twins during the first year of life. *Qualitative Health Research*, 12, 593–608.)

Corbin and Strauss Approach

The Corbin and Strauss (2015) approach to grounded theory analysis (the "Straussian" approach), differs from the original Glaser and Strauss method with regard to method, process, and outcomes, as summarized in Table 25.3.

Glaser believed that to generate a grounded theory, the basic problem must emerge from the data—it must be discovered. The theory is grounded in the data, rather than starting with a preconceived problem. Corbin and Strauss, however, argued that the research itself is only one possible source of a problem. Research problems can, for example, come from the literature, a researcher's personal and professional experience, an advisor or mentor, or a pilot project.

The Corbin and Strauss method involves two types of coding: open and axial coding. In **open coding**, data are broken down into parts and concepts identified for interpreted meaning of the raw data. In **axial coding**, the analyst groups the open codes according to conceptual categories that reflect commonalities among the codes. The term *axial coding* reflects the idea of clustering the open codes around "axes" or points of intersection. In axial coding, the analyst is "locating and linking action-interaction within a framework of subconcepts that give it meaning and enable it to explain what interactions are occurring, and why and what consequences real or anticipated are happening" (Corbin & Strauss, 2015, p. 156).

In the Corbin and Strauss approach, the *paradigm* is used as an analytic strategy to help integrate structure and process. The basic components of the paradigm include conditions, actions-interactions, and consequences or outcomes. Corbin and Strauss suggested the conditional/consequential matrix as an analytic strategy for considering the range of possible conditions and consequences that can enter into the context.

The first step in integrating the findings is to decide on the **central category** (also called the *core category*), which is the main theme of the research. Recommended techniques to facilitate identification of the central category are writing the storyline, using diagrams, and reviewing and organizing memos. The outcome of the Corbin and Strauss approach is, as Glaser (1992) termed it, a full conceptual description. The original Glaserian grounded theory method, by contrast, generates a theory that explains how a basic social problem that emerged from the data is processed in a social setting.

> **Example of Corbin and Strauss Grounded Theory Analysis**
> Huang and colleagues (2017) undertook a grounded theory study to understand the decision-making process of reproductive-age women with cancer in Taiwan. They conducted in-depth interviews with 18 women being treated for cancer; the data were analyzed using the Corbin and Strauss approach. After open coding, the researchers undertook axial coding in which "all coded elements were compared to explore for variations, similarities, and differences. We assigned codes to subcategories and categories by way of a coding scheme illustrating the context of the decision-making process regarding fertility" (p. 396). The model that these researchers developed and some coded excerpts are included in the Toolkit.

Constructivist Grounded Theory Approach

The constructivist approach to grounded theory is not dissimilar to a Glaserian approach. Charmaz's approach, however, puts more emphasis on interpretation and on the researcher's influence in data analysis. According to Charmaz (2014), in constructivist grounded theory, the "coding generates the bones of your analysis. Theoretical centrality and integration will assemble these bones into a working skeleton" (p. 113).

Charmaz distinguishes initial coding and focused coding. In **initial coding**, the pieces of data (e.g., words, lines, segments, incidents) are coded as the researcher begins to learn what participants view as problematic. Charmaz advises grounded analysts to "keep your initial codes short, simple, spontaneous—and analytic. The rest will fall in place" (p. 161).

In **focused coding** the analysis is directed toward using the most significant and frequent codes from the initial coding to help sort, integrate, and organize large chunks of data. The researcher decides which codes are most important for further analysis, which are then theoretically coded. Focused codes are more conceptual than initial codes and advance the direction of the developing theory. Charmaz encourages the use of theoretical sensitivity to aid in analyzing the data. *Theoretical sensitivity* is "the ability to understand and define phenomena in abstract terms and to demonstrate abstract relationships between studied phenomena" (p. 161).

Charmaz's method also involves a crucial step of memo writing where researchers stop, weigh, and analyze categories and their relationship to each other. Charmaz views *writing* as a strategy for developing a grounded theory. Use of prewriting exercises such as *clustering* helps to foster creativity and to organize analytic findings. Clustering produces a tentative map or chart: analysts make a circle for their main category and then use spokes from the circle to smaller circles to help illustrate properties and relationships. Charmaz advocates a writing style that is both literary and scientific—that is, analytic but also evocative of the participants' experiences. Her work provides guidance on making meaning from the data and rendering participants' words into accessible theoretical interpretations. She advocates for maintaining the participants' presence throughout the analysis and write-up.

TIP Hoare and colleagues (2012) provide a detailed description of how Charmaz's approach was used to code and analyze data relating to use of information by practice nurses.

Example of a Constructivist Grounded Theory Analysis

Brauer and colleagues (2018) explored the transition to self-care ("coming of age") among emerging adult survivors of cancer after hematopoietic cell transplantation. Their analysis was guided by Charmaz's constructivism. Beginning with initial coding, each transcript was studied in depth, followed by focused coding that allowed the researchers to group significant codes and form tentative categories. Using such devices as diagrams and memos, the authors explored and tested relationships among major categories. The researchers found that health-related setbacks disrupted the youth's journey toward self-care and their developmental trajectory toward adulthood.

QUALITATIVE ANALYSIS NOT LINKED TO A RESEARCH TRADITION

Broad guidelines for analyzing data from "generic" qualitative inquiries have been emerging to facilitate the analytic process and to make it less opaque and intimidating. Examples of analytic guidelines that have been used by nurse researchers include guides for qualitative content analysis (Zhang & Wildemuth, 2005), thematic analysis (Braun & Clarke, 2006), the Qualitative Analysis Guide of Leuven (QUAGOL) (Dierckx de Casterlé et al., 2012), and framework analysis (Gale et al., 2013) (examples of the first three can be found in the Toolkit) ⊗. In this section, we describe content analysis, a widely used approach in nursing studies, and framework analysis. Framework analysis is included because it is considered a useful method for beginning qualitative researchers, because it is often used by multidisciplinary teams, and because the literature is unusually rich with worked-out examples of its application. We also describe some special considerations in analyzing focus group data.

Qualitative Content Analysis

Content analysis is a family of analytic approaches ranging from intuitive and impressionistic analyses to strict systematic textual analyses. Indeed, quantitative researchers sometimes perform a content analysis—for example by counting words or phrases and formally testing hypotheses.

Qualitative content analysis is the analysis of the content of narrative data to identify prominent themes and patterns among the themes and is often used in descriptive qualitative studies. Patton (2015) defined qualitative content analysis as "any qualitative data reduction and sense-making effort that takes a volume of qualitative material and attempts to identify core consistencies and meaning" (p. 541).

Qualitative content analysis involves breaking down data into smaller units. The literature on content analysis often includes references to **meaning units**. In their widely cited paper on content analysis, Graneheim and Lundman

(2004) defined a meaning unit as "words, sentences or paragraphs containing aspects related to each other through their content and context" (p. 106). A meaning unit, essentially, is the smallest segment of a text that contains a recognizable piece of information.

The labels attached to meaning units are the codes (sometimes called *tags*). Codes are heuristic devices; "labelling a condensed meaning unit with a code allows the data to be thought about in new and different ways" (Graneheim & Lundman, 2004, p. 107). The success of a content analysis depends on the integrity of the coding process. Codes are, in turn, the basis for developing categories. In what is sometimes referred to as "secondary coding," the creation of categories involves gathering meaning units together that capture the substance of a topic—i.e., that fit into a cluster (Krippendorff, 2013).

In descriptive studies, qualitative researchers may decide to focus mainly on summarizing the data's manifest content (what the text actually says). Many content analysts also analyze what the text talks *about,* which involves interpretation of the meaning of its latent content. Interpretations vary in depth and level of abstraction and are usually the basis for themes.

Hsieh and Shannon (2005) discussed three different approaches to content analysis, based on the degree of involvement of inductive reasoning. In "conventional" content analysis (*inductive content analysis*), the codes are identified within the data and are defined during data analysis. In "directed" content analysis, researchers begin with a theory or earlier relevant findings, and codes are defined before data analysis and then expanded during the analysis. This approach is often used to validate or extend a theory or conceptual model. In "summative" content analysis, keywords are the starting point; keywords are identified before data analysis (e.g., from a literature review) as well as during data analysis (manifest content). This third approach has aspects that seem quantitative in nature at the outset (e.g., counting manifest content), but it seeks to explore words and indicators in an inductive manner as the process unfolds.

> **TIP** Elo and Kyngäs (2007) presented a good figure illustrating and distinguishing processes in inductive and deductive approaches to content analysis.

Example of a Content Analysis

Hilding and colleagues (2018) studied nurses' strategies for facilitating the transition from life-prolonging care to palliative care. Data from in-depth interviews with 14 nurses were content analyzed. Transcribed interviews were read thoroughly several times to identify meaning units, which were then condensed; out of the condensed units, codes were extracted. For example, here is one meaning unit: "I strive to be as honest as possible all the time, you strive towards being honest and telling what you maybe think they need." The two codes were "Nurses strive to be as honest as possible" and "Nurse tells what she thinks patients need" (p. 3). The final theme was "Striving for a balance between leading and following the patient and family" (p. 4).

Framework Analysis

Framework analysis was developed by social policy researchers in the United Kingdom but has emerged as a popular approach in healthcare research. It is an approach that is systematic but is also flexible and grounded in the data. Transparency at every phase of analysis is considered paramount. A step-by-step guide for the framework method for use by health researchers is available in an open-access article by Gale and colleagues (2013). They argued that the framework method can be used in multidisciplinary teams involving researchers and clinicians from different disciplines, and their paper illustrates how their team collaborated throughout the project.

Framework analysis is most often described as involving five main steps, with iteration often being necessary. Here are the five steps as described in papers by Hackett and Strickland (2019), Heath et al. (2012), Parkinson et al. (2016), Smith and Firth (2011), and Ward et al. (2013)—all of which provide rich worked-out examples of applying framework analysis in health studies:

Step 1. *Familiarization* through immersion in the data, to gain a sense of whole texts (such as interviews) before dividing the text into sections for coding. Familiarization involves listening to the data, reading and rereading transcripts, and noting key ideas in the margins of the transcripts.

Step 2. *Identification of an initial thematic framework* and developing a mechanism for labeling data in manageable units. Drawing upon recurrent concepts in the views or experiences of participants, an initial coding framework is developed and then pilot tested on a few narratives. An iterative process of refinement continues until a final thematic framework is agreed to by team members.

Step 3. *Coding and indexing* of the data by systematically applying the framework to data segments—usually using CAQDAS. The codes are then organized into categories reflecting prominent concepts in the dataset.

Step 4. *Charting,* which involves organizing the data for each theme into a two-dimensional matrix. Participants are arrayed in the rows of the matrix, and codes for the specified theme are represented in the columns. The data are then abstracted and allocated to the relevant cell for the participant and the code.

Step 5. *Mapping and interpretation* occur in the final step of a framework analysis. The analysts review the matrices and make connections within and between the cases and the codes. In this step, the analysts search for patterns and relationships and seek explanations for patterns within the data.

Charting the data into matrixes can be done in some CAQDAS programs such as NVivo or in spreadsheet software such as Excel. Gale and colleagues (2013) have noted an advantage of charting when working in teams: "Summarizing the data during charting…means that all members of a multi-disciplinary team, including lay, clinical and…academic members can engage with the data and offer their perspectives during the analysis process without necessarily needing to read all the transcripts or be involved in the more technical parts of the analysis" (p. 5). They also pointed out that the matrix format facilitates the recognition of not only patterns but

also inconsistencies and deviant cases. Another advantage of framework analysis is that the process leaves a clear *audit trail,* an issue we discuss in Chapter 26. However, one drawback of framework analysis is that it is time-consuming and resource-intensive.

Example of a Framework Analysis

Parsons and five colleagues (2018) explored the experience of gestational diabetes mellitus in a diverse sample of women attending a diabetes pregnancy unit in London. Framework analysis was used on data from 6 focus groups and 15 in-depth interviews. The research team, which included nurses and physicians, collaborated in the analysis. For example, in step 2 (identifying a thematic framework), three researchers independently coded a selection of transcripts and then met to achieve consensus on the framework. Two researchers coded all transcripts and met frequently throughout the process to address discrepancies. Their article included a dendrogram that portrays the relationship between women's experiences and care outcomes.

Analysis of Focus Group Data

Focus group interviews yield rich and complex data that pose special analytic challenges. Indeed, there is little consensus about analyzing data from focus groups, despite their widespread use.

A controversial issue in the analysis of focus group data is whether the unit of analysis is the group or individual participants. Some writers (e.g., Morrison-Beedy et al., 2001) maintain that the group is the proper unit of analysis. Analysis of group-level data involves a scrutiny of themes, interactions, and sequences within and between groups. Others, however (e.g., Carey & Smith, 1994; Kidd & Parshall, 2000), have argued that analysis should occur at both the group and individual level. Those who insist on only group-level analysis argue that what individuals say in focus groups cannot be treated as personal disclosures because they are inevitably influenced by the dynamics of the group. However, even in personal interviews, individual responses are shaped by social processes, and analysis of individual-level data (independent of group) is thought by some analysts to add important insights. Carey and Smith advocated a third level of analysis—namely, the analysis of individual responses *in relation* to group context (e.g., whether a participant's view is in accord with or in contrast to majority opinion.

For those who wish to analyze data from individual participants, it is essential to maintain information about what each person said—a task that is not possible if researchers rely solely on audio recordings. Video recordings, as supplements to audio recordings, are sometimes used to identify who said what in focus group sessions. More frequently, however, researchers have members of the research team in attendance at the sessions, and their job is to take detailed field notes about the order of speakers and about significant nonverbal behavior, such as pounding or clenching of fists, crying, aggressive body language, and so on.

Example of Integrating Focus Group Interview and Observational Data

Morrison-Beedy and colleagues (2001) provided several examples of integrating data across sources from their focus group research. For example, one verbatim quote was "It was no big deal." This was supplemented with data from the field notes that the woman's eyes were cast downward as she said this, and that the words were delivered sarcastically. The complete transcript for this entry, which included researcher interpretation in brackets, was as follows: "'It was no big deal.' (said sarcastically, with eyes looking downward). [It really was a very big deal to her, but others had not acknowledged that.]" (p. 52).

Because of group dynamics, focus group analysts must be sensitive to both the thematic content of these interviews and to how, when, and why themes are developed. Some issues that could be central to focus group analysis include the following:

- Does an issue raised in a focus group constitute a *theme* or merely a strongly held viewpoint of one or two members?
- Do the same issues or themes arise in more than one group?
- If there are group differences, why might this be the case—were participants different in characteristics and experiences, or did group processes affect the discussions?

- Are some issues sufficiently salient that not only are they discussed in response to specific questions posed by the moderator but also emerge spontaneously at multiple points in the session?

Some focus group analysts, such as Kidd and Parshall (2000), use quantitative methods as adjuncts to their qualitative analysis. Using CAQDAS, they conduct such analyses as assessing similarities and differences between groups, determining coding frequencies to aid pattern detection, examining codes in relation to participant characteristics, and examining how much dialogue individual members contributed. They use such methods not so that interpretation can be based on frequencies, but so that they can better understand context and identify issues that require further critical scrutiny and interpretation.

CRITICAL APPRAISAL OF QUALITATIVE ANALYSIS

It is not easy to evaluate a qualitative analysis as described in a report. Readers do not have access to the information they need to confirm that researchers exercised good judgment and insight in coding the narrative materials, developing a thoughtful analysis, and integrating materials into a meaningful whole. Researchers are seldom able to include more than a handful of examples of actual data in a journal article. Moreover, the process they used to abstract meaning from the data is difficult to describe and illustrate.

The report should provide information about the approach used to analyze the data. For example, a report for a grounded theory study should indicate whether the researchers used the Glaser, Corbin and Strauss, or constructivist method. It would, however, be inappropriate to criticize a grounded theory analysis for following Charmaz's approach rather than Glaser's approach. Both are respected methods of conducting a grounded theory study—although researchers themselves may have cogent reasons for preferring one approach over the other.

BOX 25.2 Guidelines for Critically Appraising Qualitative Analyses and Interpretations

1. Was the data analysis approach appropriate for the research design, the qualitative tradition, and nature of the data?
2. Were major analytic decisions communicated in the report (e.g., who did the analysis and transcription)? Were the decisions reasonable ones?
3. Were the coding process and coding scheme described? If so, does the process seem reasonable? Does the scheme appear logical and complete? Does there seem to be unnecessary overlap or redundancy in the codes?
4. Were manual methods used to index and organize the data, or was computer software used?
5. Does the report adequately describe the process by which the actual analysis was performed? If codes were collapsed into categories, does the resulting set of categories make sense?
6. Does the report indicate whose approach to data analysis was used (e.g., in grounded theory studies, Glaserian, Straussian, or constructivist)? Was this method consistently and appropriately applied?
7. What major themes or processes were gleaned from the data? If excerpts from the data were provided, do the themes appear to capture the meaning of the narratives—that is, does it appear that the researcher adequately interpreted the data and conceptualized the themes or categories? Is the analysis parsimonious—could two or more themes be collapsed into a broader conceptualization?
8. What evidence does the report provide that the analysis is accurate and appropriate? Were data shared in a manner that allows you to verify the researcher's conclusions?
9. Was a conceptual map, model, or diagram presented? Did it illuminate important processes, patterns, or relationships?
10. Was a metaphor used to communicate key elements of the analysis? Did the metaphor offer an insightful view of the findings, or did it seem contrived?
11. Was the context of the phenomenon adequately described? Does the report give you a clear picture of the social or emotional world of study participants?
12. Did the analysis yield a meaningful and insightful picture of the phenomenon under study—or is the resulting theory or description trivial and obvious?

One aspect of a qualitative analysis that *can* be appraised, however, is whether the researchers documented that they have used one approach consistently and have been faithful to the integrity of its procedures. Thus, for example, if researchers say they are using the Glaserian approach to grounded theory analysis, they should not mention axial coding from the Corbin and Strauss method. An even more serious problem occurs when, as sometimes happens, the researchers "muddle" traditions. For example, researchers who describe their study as a grounded theory study should not present *themes*, because grounded theory analysis does not yield themes.

Some guidelines that may be helpful in evaluating qualitative analyses are presented in Box 25.2.

RESEARCH EXAMPLES

We have illustrated different analytic approaches through examples of studies throughout this chapter. Here we present more detailed descriptions of two qualitative nursing studies.

Example of a Phenomenologic Analysis

Study: Posttraumatic growth after birth trauma: "I was broken, now I'm unbreakable" (Beck & Watson, 2016).

Statement of purpose: The purpose of this study was to explore women's experience of posttraumatic growth following a traumatic childbirth. Posttraumatic growth is a positive psychological change resulting from a struggle with challenging life circumstances.

Method: In this descriptive phenomenologic study, the researchers conducted Internet interviews with 15 women from four countries. The women were invited to participate through a recruitment notice posted on the website of the organization Trauma and Birth Stress (TABS), a charitable trust in New Zealand. The length of time since the traumatic births ranged from 5 months to 19 years. The women were asked to describe, in as much detail as they could remember, their experiences of positive changes in their lives that resulted from their traumatic birth. The descriptions, submitted through emails, ranged from one to seven single-spaced pages of text. Data collection continued over an 18-month period until data saturation was achieved.

Analysis: Colaizzi's method was used to analyze (manually) the data from the mothers' written descriptions. In a preliminary reading of the narratives, keywords and phrases were underlined. Then, all the significant statements from the interview that pertained to posttraumatic growth were extracted and their meanings were formulated. Here is an example:

Significant statement: "I am sharper, stronger, more balanced, more focused, more powerful than before because of what I have endured. I was broken. Now I am unbreakable."

Formulated meaning: "This mother felt sharper, stronger, more balanced, focused, and powerful than she had been before struggling with her traumatic birth. At first she felt broken but now she feels unbreakable."

In the next phase, the formulated meanings were categorized into themes. Finally, the themes were integrated into an exhaustive description of posttraumatic growth. No modifications to their analysis were necessary based on feedback from some participants.

Key findings: The analysis of the mothers' accounts of their posttraumatic growth yielded four themes: (1) Opening oneself up to a new present; (2) Achieving a new level of relationship nakedness; (3) Fortifying spiritual-mindedness; and (4) Forging new paths. The researchers used the metaphor of an earthquake to illustrate the "seismic power of a traumatic childbirth that can lead to posttraumatic growth" (p. 267). Some excerpts from theme 1 and the graphic used to illustrate their earthquake model are included in the Toolkit.

Example of a Grounded Theory Analysis

Study: Protecting: A grounded theory study of younger children's experiences of coping with maternal cancer (Furlong, 2017).

Statement of purpose: The purpose of this study was to develop a theory of children's day-to-day struggles living with their mothers who had been diagnosed for early-stage breast cancer and were receiving cancer treatment.

Method: This study used classic (Glaserian) grounded theory methods. The researcher collected data through in-depth interviews with twenty-eight 7- to 11-year-old children (14 boys and 14 girls) whose mothers had been diagnosed with breast cancer in the previous 4 months. The interviews, which lasted between 25 and 55 minutes, were conducted in the children's homes. The children were asked to describe their experience of having a mother with breast cancer. An interview guide was used but was continually revised as the ongoing analysis identified additional threads of inquiry. Sampling and data collection continued until theoretical saturation was achieved.

Analysis: The data for the study included interview transcripts, field notes, and memos that documented the researcher's analytic insights. Data were analyzed using constant comparison: "data, codes, and categories were compared with each other on an ongoing basis throughout data collection and analysis" (p. 15). NVivo was used for the storage and organization of the data. The analysis began with line-by-line open coding, then the open codes were used to generate categories that were collapsed and refined. Relationships among the categories were also identified. Theoretical coding was performed based on memos that had been written throughout the analysis.

Key findings: The children's main concern was navigating through the uncertainties in their lives and navigating complex changes. "*Protecting*" accounted for how these children problematized their experiences living with mothers with early-stage breast cancer. The children used the strategy of Protecting (the core category) which mediated three cyclical and iterative processes, which were labeled *Shifting normality, Shielding,* and *Transitioning.* The researcher stated that *Protecting* met the criteria for a core category "in that it constantly recurred in the data" and had "the most explanatory power to integrate all other categories" (p. 15). A diagram of Furlong's model depicting the grounded theory *Protecting* is provided in the Toolkit. ✪

SUMMARY POINTS

- Qualitative analysis is a challenging, labor-intensive activity, with few standardized rules—although guidelines have begun to appear to make the process less mystifying.
- Researchers make many decisions in analyzing qualitative data, including who will do the analysis and transcription; whether coding (if any) will be inductive or deductive; whether the focus will be on description or interpretation; whether both *manifest content* and *latent content* will be analyzed; whether computer software will be used to manage and organize the data; and whether the analysis will follow a formal guideline—and, if so, which one.
- Although there are no universal qualitative analytic methods, several broad and iterative processes are typical, including immersing oneself in the data; segmenting and coding the data; collapsing codes into broader and (usually) more interpretive categories; and then integrating and developing themes, models, or theories.
- Qualitative analysis usually begins with efforts to understand and manage the mass of narrative data by developing a *coding scheme*. Analysts use **codes** to identify (in a data segment, such as a sentence or paragraph) an interesting, salient, or essential feature of the data in relation to the phenomenon of interest. Data segments can be coded in different ways, depending on the goals of the research.
- Once a coding scheme is devised, researchers apply the codes to data segments, a process that allows analysts to retrieve data segments easily.
- Traditionally, researchers organized their data by developing **conceptual files**—physical files

in which excerpts of data relevant to specific codes are placed. Computer-assisted qualitative data analysis software (**CAQDAS**) is now widely used to index the data and to facilitate analysis.

- The analysis of qualitative materials often involves a search for broad **categories**, which are clusters of codes that are connected conceptually. In many qualitative studies, the next phase involves the identification of themes. A **theme**, which often cuts across several categories, is a recurring regularity that captures meaningful patterns in the data. Identifying themes involves the discovery not only of commonalities across participants but also of natural variation and patterns in the data.
- Some qualitative analysts use **metaphors** or figurative comparisons to evoke a visual and symbolic analogy. Analysts also use various graphic or charting devices, such as timelines and **dendrograms** (tree diagrams illustrating hierarchically ordered codes and categories).
- Interpreting qualitative data in efforts to make meaning from the data typically requires total immersion in the data and a period of **incubation** and creative reflection.
- In ethnographies, analysis begins as the researcher enters the field. Ethnographers continually search for *patterns* in the behavior and expressions of study participants.
- One approach to analyzing ethnographic data is Spradley's method, which involves four levels of data analysis: **domain analysis** (identifying *domains* or units of cultural knowledge), **taxonomic analysis** (selecting key domains and constructing **taxonomies** or systems of classification), **componential analysis** (comparing and contrasting cultural terms in a domain), and a **theme analysis** (uncovering cultural themes).
- Leininger's ethnonursing method involves four phases: collecting and recording data; categorizing descriptors; searching for repetitive patterns; and abstracting major themes.
- There are numerous approaches to phenomenologic analysis, including the descriptive methods of the Duquesne School. Colaizzi, Giorgi,

and Van Kaam recommend somewhat different procedures, but a common goal is to find recurrent patterns of experiences relating to a phenomenon of interest.

- In van Manen's approach, which involves efforts to grasp the essential meaning of the experience being studied, researchers search for themes, using either a **holistic approach** (viewing text as a whole); **selective approach** (pulling out key statements and phrases); or **detailed approach** (analyzing every sentence). Van Manen's approach is within the Utrecht school of phenomenology.

- Central to analyzing data in an interpretive phenomenologic (hermeneutic) study is the notion of the **hermeneutic circle**, which signifies a methodologic process in which there is continual movement between the parts and the whole of the text under analysis.

- There are several choices for hermeneutic data analysis, including the methods of Parse, Diekelmann, and Benner. Diekelmann's team approach calls for the discovery of a **constitutive pattern** that expresses the relationships among themes. Benner's approach consists of three processes: searching for **paradigm cases**, thematic analysis, and analysis of **exemplars**.

- Grounded theory researchers (as well as others) use the **constant comparative** method of analysis, which involves identifying characteristics in one piece of data and comparing them with those of others to assess similarity.

- One approach to grounded theory is the Glaser and Strauss (Glaserian) method, in which there are two broad types of codes: *substantive codes* (in which the empirical substance of the topic is conceptualized) and *theoretical codes* (in which higher-order relationships are conceptualized).

- Substantive coding involves **open coding** to capture what is going on in the data. Open codes begin with **level I (in vivo) codes**, which are collapsed into a higher level of abstraction in **level II codes** (categories). Level II codes are then used to formulate **level III codes**, which are theoretical constructs. **Selective coding** can then proceed, in which only data relating to a core category are coded. The **core category** is

a behavior pattern that has relevance for participants and can be used to integrate the theory; a **basic social process (BSP)** is one example of a core category. **Theoretical coding** helps weave the coded pieces of data back together.

- In Corbin and Strauss approach, an alternative grounded theory method, the outcome is a full conceptual description. Their method involves two types of coding: **open** (in which categories are generated) and **axial coding** (where categories are linked with subcategories and integrated).

- In Charmaz's constructivist grounded theory approach, coding can be word-by-word, line-by-line, or incident-by-incident. Such **initial coding** leads to **focused coding**. Her approach puts special emphasis on interpretation and on the researcher's influence in data analysis.

- Several systems have been developed to guide qualitative researchers who are not conducting a study within a disciplinary tradition. For example, researchers whose focus is qualitative description may use content analysis as their analytic method. **Qualitative content analysis** is an analysis of the content of narrative data to identify prominent themes or patterns. Content analysts using an inductive approach strive to identify **meaning units** that are then coded (tagged); the codes are the basis for developing categories.

- Another approach, used increasingly by multidisciplinary healthcare teams, is **framework analysis**. The five main steps in framework analysis are familiarization, identification of an initial thematic framework, coding and indexing, charting, and mapping and interpretation. The charting step involves the use of two-dimensional matrices that typically have participants in the rows and codes in the columns; raw data or data summaries are then entered in appropriate cells.

STUDY ACTIVITIES

Study activities are available to instructors on thePoint.

REFERENCES CITED IN CHAPTER 25

Ayres, L., Kavanagh, K., & Knafl, K. (2003). Within-case and across-case approaches to qualitative data analysis. *Qualitative Health Research, 13*, 871–883.

Beck, C. T. (2002). Releasing the pause button: Mothering twins during the first year of life. *Qualitative Health Research, 12*, 593–608.

Beck, C. T. (2017). Caring for a child with an obstetric brachial plexus injury: A metaphor analysis. *Journal of Pediatric Nursing, 36*, 57–63.

Beck, C. T., & Gable, R. (2012). A mixed methods study of secondary traumatic stress in labor and delivery nurses. *Journal of Obstetric, Gynecologic, & Neonatal Nursing, 41*, 747–760.

Beck, C. T., & Watson, S. (2016). Posttraumatic growth after birth trauma: "I was broken, now I'm unbreakable". *MCN: The American Journal of Maternal-Child Nursing, 41*, 264–271.

Benner, P. (1994). The tradition and skill of interpretive phenomenology in studying health, illness, and caring practices. In Benner, P. (Ed.), *Interpretive phenomenology* (pp. 99–127). Thousand Oaks, CA: Sage Publications.

Brauer, E., Pieters, H., Ganz, P., Landier, W., Pavlish, C., & Heilemann, M. (2018). Coming of age with cancer: Physical, social, and financial barriers to independence among emerging adult survivors. *Oncology Nursing Forum, 45*, 146–158.

*Braun, V., & Clarke, V. (2006). Using thematic analysis in psychology. *Qualitative Research in Psychology, 3*, 77–101.

Carey, M. A., & Smith, M. W. (1994). Capturing the group effect in focus groups: A special concern in analysis. *Qualitative Health Research, 4*, 123–127.

Carpenter, J. (2008). Metaphors in qualitative research: Shedding light or casting shadows? *Research in Nursing & Health, 31*, 274–282.

Castro, A., & Andrews, G. (2018). Nursing lives in the blogosphere: A thematic analysis of anonymous online nursing narratives. *Journal of Advanced Nursing, 74*, 329–338.

Charmaz, K. (2014). *Constructing grounded theory* (2nd ed.). Thousand Oaks, CA: Sage Publications.

Colaizzi, P. F. (1978). Psychological research as the phenomenologist views it. In Valle, R., & King, M. (Eds.), *Existential phenomenological alternatives for psychology*. New York: Oxford University Press.

Corbin, J., & Strauss, A. (2015). *Basics of qualitative research: Techniques and procedures for developing grounded theory*. Thousand Oaks, CA: Sage Publications.

Creswell, J. W. (2013). *Qualitative inquiry and research design: Choosing among five approaches* (3rd ed.). Thousand Oaks, CA: Sage Publications.

Crist, J. D., & Tanner, C. A. (2003). Interpretation/analysis methods in hermeneutic interpretive phenomenology. *Nursing Research, 52*, 202–205.

Cuthbert, C., Culos-Reed, S., King-Shier, K., Ruether, J., Bischoff, M., & Tapp, D. (2017). Creating an upward spiral: A qualitative study of caregivers' experience of participating in a structured physical activity programme. *European Journal of Cancer Care, 26*(6), e12684.

Dahlberg, K., Dahlberg, H., & Nyström, M. (2008). *Reflective lifeworld research*. Sweden: Studentlitteratur.

Dalteg, T., Sandberg, J., Malm, D., Sandgren, A., & Benzein, E. (2017). The heart is a representation of life: An exploration of illness beliefs in couples living with atrial fibrillation. *Journal of Clinical Nursing, 26*, 3699–3709.

DeSantis, L., & Ugarriza, D. (2000). The concept of theme as used in qualitative nursing research. *Western Journal of Nursing Research, 22*, 351–372.

Diekelmann, N. L., Allen, D., & Tanner, C. (1989). *The NLN criteria for appraisal of baccalaureate programs: A critical hermeneutic analysis*. New York: NLN Press.

Dierckx de Casterlé, B. D. Gastmans, C., Bryon, E., & Denier, Y. (2012). QUAGOL: A guide for qualitative data analysis. *International Journal of Nursing Studies, 49*, 360–371.

*Dykeman, C., Markle-Reid, M., Bortto, L., Bowes, C., Gagné, H., McGugan, J., & Orr-Shaw, S. (2018). Community service provider perceptions of implementing older adult fall prevention in Ontario, Canada: A qualitative study. *BMC Geriatrics, 18*, 34.

Elo, S., & Kyngäs, H. (2007). The qualitative content analysis process. *Journal of Advanced Nursing, 62*, 107–115.

Fetterman, D. M. (2010). *Ethnography: Step by step* (3rd ed.). Thousand Oaks, CA: Sage Publications.

**Furlong, E. P. (2017). Protecting: A grounded theory study of younger children's experiences of coping with maternal cancer. *Cancer Nursing, 40*, 13–21.

Gadamer, H. G. (1975). *Truth and method. G. Borden & J. Cumming (trans)*. London: Sheed and Ward.

*Gale, N., Heath, G., Cameron, E., Rashid, S., & Redwood, S. (2013). Using the Framework Method for the analysis of qualitative data in multi-disciplinary health research. *BMC Medical Research Methodology, 13*, 117.

Giorgi, A. (1985). *Phenomenology and psychological research*. Pittsburgh: Duquesne University Press.

Glaser, B. (1978). *Theoretical sensitivity*. Mill Valley, CA: The Sociology Press.

Glaser, B. (1992). *Emergence versus forcing: Basics of grounded theory analysis*. Mill Valley, CA: Sociology Press.

Glaser, B. (2001). *The grounded theory perspective: Conceptualization contrasted with description*. Mill Valley, CA: Sociology Press.

Glaser, B. (2005). *The grounded theory perspective III: Theoretical coding*. Mill Valley, CA: Sociology Press.

Glaser, B. G., & Strauss, A. (1967). *The discovery of grounded theory: Strategies for qualitative research*. New York: Aldine de Gruyter.

Graneheim, U., Lindgren, B., & Lundman, B. (2017). Methodological challenges in qualitative content analysis. *Nurse Education Today, 56*, 29–34.

*Graneheim, U., & Lundman, B. (2004). Qualitative content analysis in nursing research: Concepts, procedures and measures to achieve trustworthiness. *Nurse Education Today, 24,* 105–112.

Grigsby, S. (2018). Giving our daughters what we never received: African American mothers discussing sexual health with their preadolescent daughters. *Journal of School Nursing, 34,* 128–138.

Hackett, A., & Strickland, K. (2019). Using the framework approach to analyse qualitative data: A worked example. *Nurse Researcher, 26,* 8–13.

Heath, G., Cameron, E., Cummins, C., Greenfield, S., Pattison, H., Kelly, D., & Redwood, . (2012). Paediatric "care closer to home": Stake-holder views and barriers to implementation. *Health & Place, 18,* 1068–1073.

Hilding, U., Allvin, R., & Blomberg, K. (2018). Striving for a balance between leading and following the patient and family—nurses' strategies to facilitate the transition from life-prolonging care to palliative care. *BMC Palliative Care, 17,* 55.

Hoare, K., Mills, J., & Francis, K. (2012). Sifting, sorting and saturating data in a grounded theory study of information use by practice nurses: A worked example. *International Journal of Nursing Practice, 18,* 582–588.

*Holton, J. A. (2010). The coding process and its challenges. *Grounded Theory Review: An International Journal, 9,* 1.

*Hsieh, H., & Shannon, S. (2005). Three approaches to qualitative content analysis. *Qualitative Health Research, 15,* 1277–1288.

Huang, S., Hsieh, P., Hsiung, Y., Tseng, L., Chen, P., Hung, C. (2017). Decision-making process regarding fertility among reproductive-age women with cancer in Taiwan. *Cancer Nursing, 40,* 394–402.

Hunter, A., Lusardi, P., Zucker, D., Jacelon, C., & Chandler, G. (2002). Making meaning: The creative component in qualitative research. *Qualitative Health Research, 12,* 388–398.

Imani, B., Kermanshahi, S., Vanaki, Z., & Kazemnejad Lili, A. (2018). Hospital nurses' lived experiences of intelligent resilience: A phenomenological study. *Journal of Clinical Nursing, 27,* 2031–2040.

Izumi, S., Barfield, P., Basin, B., Mood, L., Neunzert, C., Tadesse, R., … Tanner, C. (2018). Care coordination: Identifying and connecting the most appropriate care to the patients. *Research in Nursing & Health, 41,* 49–56.

Johnson, B. E. (2011). The speed and accuracy of voice recognition software-assisted transcription versus the listen-and-type method: A research note. *Qualitative Research, 11,* 91–97.

Kidd, P. S., & Parshall, M. B. (2000). Getting the focus and the group: Enhancing analytic rigor in focus group research. *Qualitative Health Research, 10,* 293–308.

Kim, Y., Kim, M., Bhandari, P., & Choi, S. (2018). Experience of the waiting area as perceived by haemodialysis patients and family carers. *Journal of Advanced Nursing, 74,* 364–372.

Krippendorff, K. (2013). *Content analysis: An introduction to its methodology* (3rd ed.). Thousand Oaks, CA: Sage Publications.

McFarland, M. R., & Wehbe-Alamah, H. B. (2015). *Leininger's culture care diversity and universality: A worldwide nursing theory.* Burlington, MA: Jones & Bartlett Learning.

Miles, M., Huberman, M., & Saldaña, J. (2014). *Qualitative data analysis: A methods sourcebook* (3rd ed.). Thousand Oaks, CA: Sage Publications.

Mirlashari, J., Valizadhe, S., Navab, E., Craig, J., & Ghorbani, F. (2019). Dark and bright-two sides of family-centered care in the NICU: A qualitative study. *Clinical Nursing Research, 28,* 869–885.

Morgan, D. L. (2018). Themes, theories, and models. *Qualitative Health Research, 28,* 339–345.

Morrison-Beedy, D., Côté-Arsenault, D., & Feinstein, N. (2001). Maximizing results with focus groups: Moderator and analysis issues. *Applied Nursing Research, 14,* 48–53.

Morse, J. M., & Field, P. A. (1995). *Qualitative research methods for health professionals* (2nd ed.). Thousand Oaks, CA: Sage Publications.

*Novak, J., & Cañas, A. (2006). *The theory underlying concept maps and how to construct them.* (IHMC CmapTools Technical Report 2006-01). Pensacola, FL: Institute for Human and Machine Cognition.

Parkinson, S., Eatough, V., Holmes, J., & Stapley, E., & Midgley, N. (2016). Framework analysis: A worked example of a study exploring young people's experiences of depression. *Qualitative Research in Psychology, 13,* 109–129.

Parse, R. R. (2016). Parsesciencing: A basic science mode of inquiry. *Nursing Science Quarterly, 29,* 271–274.

*Parsons, J., Sparrow, K., Ismail, K., Hunt, K., Rogers, H., & Forbes, A. (2018). Experiences of gestational diabetes and gestational diabetes care: A focus group and interview study. *BMC Pregnancy & Childbirth, 18,* 25.

Patton, M. Q. (2015). *Qualitative research and evaluation methods* (4th ed.). Thousand Oaks, CA: Sage Publications.

Polit, D. F., London, A., & Martinez, J. (2000). *Food insecurity and hunger in poor, mother-headed families in four U.S. cities.* New York: MDRC.

Ricoeur, P. (1981). *Hermeneutics and the social sciences.* (J. Thompson, trans. & ed). New York: Cambridge University Press.

Saldaña, J. (2016). *The coding manual for qualitative researchers* (3rd ed.). Thousand Oaks, CA: Sage Publications.

Salman, K., Zoucha, R., & Nawafleh, H. (2018). Understanding Jordanian women's values and beliefs related to breast cancer: A focused ethnography. *Journal of Transcultural Nursing, 29,* 139–145.

Sandelowski, M. (2001). Real qualitative researchers do not count: The use of numbers in qualitative research. *Research in Nursing & Health, 24,* 230–240.

Saxon, C., Fulbrook, P., Fong, K., & Ski, C. (2018). High-risk respiratory patients' experiences of bronchoscopy with conscious sedation and analgesia. *Journal of Clinical Nursing, 27,* 2740–2751.

*Sidenius, U., Stigsdotter, U., Poulsen, D., & Bondas, T. (2017). "I look at my own forest and fields in a different way": The lived experience of nature-based therapy in a therapy garden when suffering from stress-related illness. *International Journal of Qualitative Studies in Health and Well-Being, 12,* 1324700.

Silver, C., & Lewins, A. (2014). *Using software in qualitative research: A step-by-step guide* (2nd ed.). Thousand Oaks, CA: Sage Publications.

Smith, J., & Firth, J. (2011). Qualitative analysis: The framework approach. *Nurse Researcher, 18,* 52–62.

Spradley, J. (1979). *The ethnographic interview.* New York: Holt Rinehart & Winston.

St. Pierre, E., & Jackson, A. (2014). Qualitative data analysis after coding. *Qualitative Inquiry, 20,* 715–719.

Thorne, S. & Darbyshire, P. (2005). Land mines in the field: A modest proposal for improving the craft of qualitative health research. *Qualitative Health Research, 15,* 1105–1113.

Van Kaam, A. (1966). *Existential foundations of psychology.* Pittsburgh, PA: Duquesne University Press.

Van Manen, M. (1990). *Researching lived experience: Human science for an action sensitive pedagogy.* London, Ontario: Althouse Press.

Van Manen, M. (2006). Writing qualitatively or the demands of writing. *Qualitative Health Research, 16,* 713–722.

Van Manen, M. (2017). But is it phenomenology? *Qualitative Health Research, 27,* 775–779.

Walker, D., & Myrick, F. (2006). Grounded theory: An exploration of process and procedure. *Qualitative Health Research, 16,* 547–559.

Ward, D., Furber, C., Tierney, S., & Swallow, V. (2013). Using Framework Analysis in nursing research: A worked example. *Journal of Advanced Nursing, 69,* 2423–2431.

*Zhang, Y., & Wildemuth, B. (2005). Qualitative analysis of content. *Analysis, 1*(2), 1–12.

A link to this open-access article is provided in the Toolkit for Chapter 25 in the **Resource Manual.** ⊗

**This journal article is available on* thePoint *for this chapter.*

26 | Trustworthiness and Rigor in Qualitative Research

Integrity in qualitative research is an all-encompassing concern that begins as questions are formulated and continues through writing the report. This is an important chapter for those learning to do qualitative research.

> **TIP** In thinking about quality enhancement in qualitative inquiry, attention needs to be paid to both "art" and "science." Creativity and insightfulness need to be encouraged and sustained but not at the expense of functional excellence—and the quest for rigor cannot sacrifice inspiration and elegant abstractions, or else the results are likely to be "perfectly healthy but dead" (Morse, 2006, p. 6). Good qualitative work is both descriptively sound and interpretively rich and innovative.

PERSPECTIVES ON QUALITY IN QUALITATIVE RESEARCH

Qualitative researchers agree on the importance of doing high-quality research, yet few issues in qualitative inquiry have generated more controversy than efforts to define what is meant by "high-quality." We provide an overview of some aspects of this debate to help you identify a position that is compatible with your philosophical and methodologic views.

Debates About Rigor and Validity

One contentious issue in the debate about quality concerns the use of terms such as *rigor* and *validity*. These terms are opposed by some critics because of their association with positivism—rigor and validity are not seen as suitable goals for the constructivist or critical paradigms. These critics argue that the philosophical underpinnings are fundamentally different from the positivist paradigm and require distinctive terminology. In their view, the concept of rigor does not fit into an interpretive approach that values insight and creativity (e.g., Denzin & Lincoln, 2000). As Sandelowski (1993a) put it, "We can preserve or kill the spirit of qualitative work; we can soften our notion of rigor to include the… soulfulness (and) imagination…we associate with more artistic endeavors, or we can further harden it by the uncritical application of rules. The choice is ours: rigor or rigor mortis" (p. 8).

Some qualitative researchers, however, argue for using the term rigor (e.g., Cypress, 2017; Morse, 2015). Others defend using the term *validity*. Whittemore and colleagues (2001), for example, argued that validity is an appropriate term in all paradigms, noting that the dictionary definition of validity (the quality of being sound, just, and well-founded) lends itself equally to qualitative and quantitative research. Morse and colleagues (2002) posited that the "concepts of reliability and validity can be applied to all research because the goal of finding plausible and credible outcome explanations is central to all research" (p. 3). A pragmatic argument favoring the use of "mainstream" terms like validity and rigor is precisely that they *are* mainstream. In the scientific community, whose criteria are used to make funding decisions, it may be useful to use recognizable terms and criteria.

Sparkes (2001) contended that there are four possible perspectives on the issue of validity. The first, which he called the *replication perspective*, is that validity is an appropriate criterion for assessing quality in both qualitative and quantitative studies, although qualitative researchers use different procedures to achieve it (e.g., Morse, 2015). Those who adopt a *parallel perspective* maintain that a separate set of evaluative criteria are needed for qualitative inquiry. This perspective resulted in the development of standards for the **trustworthiness** of qualitative research that parallel the standards of reliability and validity in quantitative research (Lincoln & Guba, 1985). The third perspective in Sparke's typology is the *diversification of meanings perspective*, which is characterized by efforts to establish new forms of validity that do not have reference points in quantitative research. As an example, Lather (1986) discussed *catalytic validity* in critical and feminist research as the degree to which the research process energizes study participants and alters their consciousness. The final perspective in Sparke's typology was what he called the *letting-go-of-validity perspective*, which involves a total abandonment of the concept of validity. Wolcott (1994), an ethnographer, represented this perspective in his discussion of the absurdity of validity. Yet, as Wolcott (1995) himself noted, validity can be dismissed, but the issue itself will not go away: "Qualitative researchers need to understand what the debate is about and *have* a position; they do not have to resolve the issue itself" (p. 170).

Generic Versus Specific Standards

Another controversial issue concerns whether there should be a generic set of standards or specific standards for different types of study—for example, for ethnographers or grounded theory researchers. Many writers have endorsed the notion that research conducted within different traditions must attend to different concerns, and that techniques for enhancing and demonstrating research integrity vary. Watson and Girard (2004), for example, proposed that quality standards must be "congruent with the philosophical underpinnings supporting the research tradition endorsed" (p. 875). Many writers have offered standards for specific forms of qualitative inquiry, such as grounded theory (Chiovitti & Piran, 2003; Cooney, 2011); phenomenology and hermeneutics (de Witt & Ploeg, 2006); ethnography (LeCompte & Goetz, 1982); descriptive qualitative research (Milne & Oberle, 2005); and critical research (Lather, 1986).

Some writers believe, however, that certain quality criteria are universal within the constructivist paradigm. For example, in their synthesis of criteria for developing evidence of validity in qualitative studies, Whittemore and associates (2001) proposed four primary criteria that they viewed as essential to all qualitative inquiry. For more information, see the Supplement to this chapter on thePoint. **Ⓢ**

Standards for Conduct Versus Appraisal of Qualitative Research

Yet another issue concerns whose point of view is being considered in the quality standards. Morse and colleagues (2002) contended that many of the established standards are relevant for *assessment* by readers rather than as guides to conducting high-quality qualitative research. They believe that Lincoln and Guba's criteria—often considered the gold standard—are best described as *post hoc* tools that reviewers can use to evaluate trustworthiness of a completed study: "While strategies of trustworthiness may be useful in attempting to *evaluate* rigor, they do not in themselves *ensure* rigor" (p. 9).

As an example of favoring the viewpoint of evaluators, one suggested indicator of integrity is **researcher credibility**—that is, the faith that can be put in the researcher (Patton, 1999, 2015). Such a criterion might affect readers' confidence in the integrity of the inquiry, but it clearly is not a *strategy* that researchers can adopt to make their study more rigorous.

Morse and colleagues (2002) emphasized the importance of verification strategies that researchers can use throughout the inquiry "so that reliability and validity are actively attained, rather than proclaimed by external reviewers on the completion of the project" (p. 9). In their view, responsibility for ensuring rigor should rest with researchers, not with external judges. They advocated a proactive stance involving self-scrutiny and verification. Morse (2006) noted that "good qualitative inquiry must be verified reflexively in each step of the analysis. This means that it is self-correcting" (p. 6).

From the point of view of qualitative researchers, the ongoing question must be: How can I be confident that my account is an accurate and insightful representation? From the point of view of a critical reader, the question is: How can I trust that the researcher has offered an accurate and insightful representation?

Terminology Proliferation and Confusion

The result of all these controversies is that there is no common vocabulary for quality criteria in qualitative research—nor, for that matter, for quality goals. Terms such as *goodness, integrity, truth value, rigor,* and *trustworthiness* abound, and for each proposed descriptor, several critics assert that the term is inappropriate.

Establishing a consensus on what the quality criteria for qualitative inquiry should be, and what they should be named, remains elusive. Some feel that the ongoing debate is healthy, but others feel that "the situation is confusing and has resulted in a deteriorating ability to actually discern rigor" (Morse et al., 2002, p. 5).

Given the lack of consensus and the heated arguments supporting and contesting various frameworks, it is difficult to offer definitive guidance. We present information about *criteria* from a widely used framework in the section that follows and then describe *strategies* for minimizing threats to integrity in qualitative research. We recommend that these strategies be viewed as points

of departure for explorations on how to make a qualitative study as rigorous/trustworthy/insightful/valid as possible.

THE LINCOLN–GUBA FRAMEWORK

Although not without critics, the quality criteria most often cited by qualitative researchers are those proposed by Lincoln and Guba, who in their original work (1985) proposed four criteria for enhancing the **trustworthiness** of a qualitative inquiry: credibility, dependability, confirmability, and transferability. These four criteria represent parallels to the positivists' criteria of internal validity, reliability, objectivity, and external validity, respectively. This framework provided the platform on which much of the current controversy on rigor emerged. Responding to numerous criticisms and to their own evolving conceptualizations, a fifth criterion that is more distinctively within the constructivist paradigm was added: authenticity (Guba and Lincoln, 1994).

Credibility

Credibility is viewed by Lincoln and Guba as an overriding goal of qualitative research, and is a criterion identified in several qualitative frameworks. **Credibility** refers to confidence in the truth of the data and interpretations of them. Qualitative researchers must strive to establish confidence in the truth of the findings for the particular participants and contexts in the research. Lincoln and Guba pointed out that credibility involves two aspects: first, carrying out the study in a way that enhances the believability of the findings and second, taking steps to *demonstrate* credibility in research reports.

Dependability

Dependability, the second criterion in the Lincoln–Guba framework, refers to the stability or reliability of data over time and conditions. The dependability question is: Would the findings of an inquiry be repeated if it were replicated with the same (or similar) participants in the same (or similar) context? Credibility cannot be attained in the absence of dependability.

Confirmability

Confirmability refers to objectivity, that is, the potential for congruence between two or more independent people about the data's accuracy, relevance, or meaning. Confirmability is enhanced by efforts to establish that the data represent participants' viewpoints, and that the interpretations of those data are not invented by the inquirer. For this criterion to be achieved, findings must reflect the participants' voice and the conditions of the inquiry and not the researcher's biases or perspectives.

Transferability

Transferability refers to the potential for extrapolation, i.e., the extent to which findings can be transferred to or have applicability in other settings or groups. Lincoln and Guba noted that investigators have a responsibility to provide sufficient descriptive data so that consumers can evaluate the relevance of the data to other contexts: "Thus the naturalist cannot specify the external validity of an inquiry; he or she can provide only the thick description necessary to enable someone interested in making a transfer to reach a conclusion about whether transfer can be contemplated as a possibility" (p. 316).

> **TIP** You may run across the term *fittingness,* a term Guba and Lincoln used earlier to refer to the degree to which research findings have meaning to others in similar situations. In later work, however, they used the term *transferability*. Similarly, they used the term *auditability*, a concept that was later refined and called *dependability*.

Authenticity

Authenticity refers to the extent to which researchers fairly and faithfully show a range of realities. Authenticity emerges in a report when it conveys the feeling tone of participants' lives as they are lived. A text has authenticity if it invites readers into a vicarious experience of the lives being described and enables readers to develop a heightened sensitivity to the issues being depicted. When a text achieves authenticity, readers are better able to understand the lives being portrayed "in the round," with some sense of the mood, feeling, experience, language, and context of those lives.

> **TIP** Whittemore, Chase, and Mandle (2001), who are nurse researchers, synthesized quality criteria from 10 prominent frameworks. In their view, four primary criteria are essential to all qualitative inquiry (credibility, authenticity, integrity, and criticality) and six secondary criteria provide supplementary benchmarks that are not relevant to every study. Researchers decide, based on the goals of their research, the optimal weight to give each criterion. The Whittemore et al. framework is described in the Supplement to this chapter on thePoint. 🅢

STRATEGIES TO ENHANCE QUALITY IN QUALITATIVE INQUIRY

The criteria for establishing integrity in a qualitative study pose challenges. Various strategies have been proposed to address these challenges, and this section describes many of them.

Quality-enhancing strategies often address multiple criteria simultaneously. For this reason, we have not organized strategies according to quality criteria. Instead, we have organized strategies according to different phases of an inquiry, namely data collection, coding and analysis, and report preparation. This organization is imperfect, due to the nonlinear and iterative nature of tasks in qualitative studies, and so we acknowledge that some activities described under one aspect of a study are likely to have relevance under another.

> **TIP** A table in the Toolkit of the accompanying *Resource Manual* suggests how various quality-enhancement strategies map onto the criteria in the Lincoln and Guba framework. ❽ A similar table is presented in the chapter Supplement for the criteria in the Whittemore framework. Most strategies discussed here contribute to credibility. 🅢

Quality-Enhancement Strategies in Collecting Data

Several strategies that qualitative researchers use to enrich and strengthen their studies have been mentioned in previous chapters and will not be elaborated here. For example, sampling an adequate number of information-rich and theoretically relevant data sources, intensive listening during an interview, careful probing to obtain rich and comprehensive data, audio-recording interviews for transcription, and monitoring transcription accuracy are all strategies to enhance data quality, as are methods to gain people's trust during fieldwork (Chapter 24). In this section we focus on additional strategies used during the collection of qualitative data.

Prolonged Engagement and Persistent Observation

An important step in establishing credibility is **prolonged engagement** (Lincoln & Guba, 1985)— the investment of sufficient time collecting data to have an in-depth understanding of the people under study, to test for misinformation and distortions, and to ensure saturation of key categories. Prolonged engagement is also essential for building trust and rapport with informants, which in turn makes it more likely that rich, detailed information will be obtained. In planning a qualitative study, researchers must ensure that they have adequate time and resources to stay engaged in fieldwork for a sufficiently long period.

> **TIP** *Premature closure* can undermine data quality (Thorne & Darbyshire, 2005). Without a commitment to prolonged engagement, researchers may make a claim of saturation simply because they have reached a convenient stopping point.

Example of Prolonged Engagement

Wright and colleagues (2018) studied relational engagement between nurses and their patients in the context of end-of-life delirium. The ethnographic fieldwork for this study, conducted in a residential hospice in Canada, spanned 15 months. Participant observations and interviews were undertaken during 80 visits to the hospice across day, evening, and night shifts.

High-quality data collection in qualitative inquiries also involves **persistent observation**, which concerns the salience of the data being gathered and recorded. Persistent observation refers to the researchers' focus on the characteristics or aspects of a situation or a conversation that are relevant to the phenomena being studied. As Lincoln and Guba (1985) noted, "If prolonged engagement provides scope, persistent observation provides depth" (p. 304).

Example of Persistent Observation

DeForge and an interprofessional team (2017) conducted a critical ethnography to understand how dementia home care practices are enacted and evaluated, especially at the interface of familial and formal caregiving. A total of 52 in-depth interviews were conducted with clients, family caregivers, and personal support workers. Participants were interviewed two or three times over a 19-month period. After each interview, "researchers dictated full field notes about their observations, perceptions, insights, nuances of communication, nonverbal expressions, caregiving behaviors and interactions between and among all participants" (p. 25).

Reflexivity Strategies

As noted in Chapter 8, reflexivity involves attending systematically and continually to the context of knowledge construction—and, in particular, to the researcher's effect on the collection, analysis, and interpretation of data. Reflexivity involves awareness that the researcher brings to the inquiry a unique personal background and set of values that can affect the research process.

The most widely used strategy for maintaining reflexivity and delimiting subjectivity is to maintain a reflexive journal or diary. Reflexive notes can be used to record, from the outset of the study and in an ongoing fashion, thoughts about the impact of previous life experiences and previous readings about the phenomenon on the inquiry. Through self-interrogation and reflection, researchers seek to be well-positioned to probe deeply and to grasp the experience, process, or culture under study through the lens of participants. Some argue that systematic efforts like maintaining a journal are not merely a means of constraining subjectivity—recognition of one's own perspectives can be exploited as an interpretive advantage because ultimately findings are cocreated by participants and respondents (Jootun et al., 2009).

Other reflexive strategies can be used. For example, researchers sometimes begin a study by being interviewed themselves regarding the phenomenon under study—an approach that only makes sense if the researcher has experienced that phenomenon. Other researchers ask a colleague to conduct a "bracketing interview." In such an interview, a person who is knowledgeable about reflexivity and about the study phenomenon queries the researcher about his or her a priori assumptions and perspectives.

Example of a Reflexive Interview

Lear and colleagues (2018) studied unfavorable experiences of nursing students studying abroad. A reflexive interview, conducted by a senior researcher unconnected to the study, was conducted to identify potential bias and to pilot test the interview questions. Answering these questions required introspection on the part of the researcher and revealed implicit biases. The article explained in detail the procedures used for reflexive interviewing.

Researchers often state in their reports that reflexivity was used or that bracketing was undertaken. Some researchers, however, provide a stronger description of addressing their initial perspectives or biases.

Example of Communicating "Preunderstandings"

Crowther and Smythe (2016) conducted a phenomenologic study of how relationships between care providers and mothers underpin safety in rural maternity care. The researchers included a section labeled "preunderstandings" in which they shared their experiences and judgments "as they shape the questions brought to the study and interpretation that followed" (p. 3).

Bradbury-Jones (2007) and Finlay and Gough (2003) provide further guidance on reflexivity. Also, Park and Zafran (2018) have written about reflexivity in teams of researchers.

Data and Method Triangulation

Triangulation refers to the use of multiple referents to draw conclusions about what constitutes

truth; it has been compared to convergent validation. The aim of triangulation is to "overcome the intrinsic bias that comes from single-method, single-observer, and single-theory studies" (Denzin, 1989, p. 313). Patton (1999) also encouraged triangulation, arguing that "no single method ever adequately solves the problem of rival explanation" (p. 1192). Triangulation can also help to capture a more complete and contextualized portrait of key phenomena. Denzin identified four types of triangulation (data triangulation, method triangulation, investigator triangulation, and theory triangulation), the first two of which we describe here because they relate to data collection.

Data triangulation involves the use of multiple data sources for the purpose of validating conclusions and can take several forms: triangulation over time, space, and persons. **Time triangulation** involves collecting data on the same phenomenon multiple times. Time triangulation can involve gathering data at different times of the day or at different times in the year. This concept is similar to test–retest reliability assessment—the point is not to study a phenomenon longitudinally to evaluate change but to assess congruence of the phenomenon over time. **Space triangulation** involves collecting data on the same phenomenon in multiple sites, to test for cross-site consistency. Finally, **person triangulation** involves collecting data from different types or levels of people (e.g., individuals, their family members, clinical staff), with the aim of validating data through multiple perspectives on the phenomenon.

Example of Person and Space Triangulation

Carduff and colleagues (2018) conducted a study to understand how healthcare professionals in the United Kingdom understand and address complex needs in palliative care. They gathered data from doctors, nurses, and allied health professionals in primary care, hospital, and hospice settings.

Method triangulation involves using multiple methods of data collection about the same phenomenon. In qualitative studies, researchers often use a rich blend of unstructured data collection methods (e.g., interviews, observations, documents) to develop a comprehensive understanding of a phenomenon. Multiple data collection methods provide an opportunity to evaluate the extent to which a consistent and coherent picture of a phenomenon or process emerges.

Example of Method Triangulation

Vasey and colleagues (2019) explored parental involvement in their children's acute pain care. Nurses, parents, grandparents, and children were involved in the study. The researchers collected data through nonparticipant observation of nurse-parent-child interactions in an acute children's ward, followed by semistructured interviews with participants.

Comprehensive and Vivid Recording of Information

In addition to taking steps to record interview data accurately, researchers need to prepare thoughtful field notes that are rich with descriptions of what transpired in the field. Even if interviews are the primary data source, researchers should maintain notes about the participants' demeanor and behaviors during the interactions and should thoroughly describe the interview context. Other record-keeping activities are also important. A log of decisions needs to be kept, reflexive journals should be maintained regularly with rich detail, and analytic memos are needed to facilitate a thoughtful analysis.

Researchers sometimes specifically develop an **audit trail**, that is, a systematic collection of materials and documentation that would allow an independent auditor (or other team members) to come to conclusions about the data. Types of records that are useful in creating an adequate audit trail include the following: (1) the raw data (e.g., interview transcripts); (2) data reduction and analysis products (e.g., annotated transcripts, codebooks, analytic memos); (3) materials relating to researchers' disposition (e.g., reflexive notes); and (4) data reconstruction products (e.g., charting matrixes, drafts of the final report). Many proponents of framework analysis, described in Chapter 25, have noted that one of the strengths of the approach is that the creation of a rich audit trail is built into its procedures (e.g., Gale et al., 2013; Ward et al., 2013).

TIP Diligent documentation does not in and of itself ensure the validity of the inquiry. Morse and colleagues (2002) pointed out that "audit trails may be kept as proof of the decisions made throughout the project, but they do not identify the quality of those decisions, the rationale behind those decisions, or the responsiveness and sensitivity of the investigator to data" (pp. 6-7).

Example of an Audit Trail

Chen and colleagues (2018) conducted a qualitative study to describe women's salient thoughts about their experiences of dysmenorrhea. One team member maintained an audit trail to document all methodologic and analytic decisions and draft products, and the audit trail was routinely reviewed by other team members.

Member Checking

Lincoln and Guba considered member checking a particularly important technique for establishing the credibility of qualitative data. In a **member check**, researchers provide feedback to participants about the study—including emerging interpretations—and elicit participants' reactions. The argument is that if researchers' understandings and interpretations are good representations of participants' realities, participants should be able to confirm their legitimacy.

Member checking can be carried out in an ongoing way as data are being collected (for example, through deliberate probing to ensure that participants' meanings were understood) and more formally after data have been processed or analyzed. Birt and colleagues (2016) identified five approaches to member checking:

- having participants review transcribed verbatim transcripts, to confirm accuracy;
- conducting a member checking interview with individual participants, using their transcribed interview as an opportunity to coconstruct the participants' meaning;
- conducting a member checking interview with individual participants, based on a preliminary interpretation of the original interview, to verify researcher's interpretation;

- conducting a member check focus group interview to review preliminary analyses of the data set; and
- conducting member checks (in writing or in person) with individual participants, using a synthesis of the analyzed data to confirm the interpretation.

TIP Hagens and colleagues (2009) assessed the approach of having participants review their transcribed interviews in a study that involved interviews with 51 key informants. They found that the review added little to the accuracy of the transcripts and in some cases resulted in biases when some participants wanted to remove valuable material.

Member checks are sometimes done in writing. For example, researchers can ask participants to review and comment on interpretive notes or thematic summaries. Member checks are often done in face-to-face discussions with individual participants.

Birt and colleagues (2016) developed a systematic approach to member checking, which they called *Synthesized Member Checking* (SMC). Their approach involves the preparation of a preliminary synthesis based on themes identified in the analysis, with interview excerpts included to illustrate the themes. The summary is sent to participants, with explicit questions, such as "Does this match your experience?" and "Do you want to change anything or add anything?" Their approach also includes careful documentation and analysis of participants who responded, so that readers can make judgments about the thoroughness of the validation. Participants' responses to the member check are considered a new data source and are coded and integrated with other data in the final interpretation.

TIP If member checking is used as a validation strategy, participants should be encouraged to provide critical feedback about errors or interpretive deficiencies. In writing about the study, it is important to be explicit about how member checking was done and what role it played as a validation strategy. Readers cannot develop much confidence in the study simply by learning that "member checking was done."

Despite the potential contribution that member checking can make to a study's credibility, several issues need to be kept in mind. First, not all participants are willing to engage in this process. Some—especially if the topic is emotionally charged—may feel they have attained closure once they have shared their experiences. Birt and colleagues (2016) have described several possible ethical concerns in member checking, especially in situations when member checking does not occur in face-to-face situations.

Another issue is that member checks can lead to misleading conclusions of trustworthiness if participants "share some common myth or front or conspire to mislead or cover up" (Lincoln & Guba, 1985, p. 315). Also, some participants might agree with researchers' interpretations either out of politeness or in the belief that researchers are "smarter" or more knowledgeable than they themselves are. Thorne and Darbyshire (2005), in fact, caution against what they irreverently called *Adulatory Validity*, which they described as "the epistemological pat on the back for a job well done, or just possibly it might be part of a mutual stroking ritual that satisfies the agendas of both researcher and researched" (p. 1110). They noted that member checking tends to privilege interpretations that place study participants in the most favorable light.

Thorne and Darbyshire are not alone in their concerns about member checking as a validation strategy. Indeed, few strategies for enhancing data quality are as controversial as member checking. Morse (1999, 2015), for example, disputed the idea that participants have more analytic and interpretive authority than the researcher. Morse and colleagues (2002), as well as Sandelowski (1993b), have worried that because study results have been synthesized, decontextualized, and abstracted across various participants, individual participants may not recognize their own experiences or perspectives in a member check. Even more scathingly, some critics view member checking as antithetical to the epistemology of qualitative inquiry. Smith (1993) criticized the philosophical contradictions inherent in this strategy, arguing that it is inconsistent with inquiry that purports to reveal multiple realities and multiple ways of knowing.

Example of Member Checking
Kurz (2018) conducted a grounded theory study of the reproductive decision-making process of women who were organ transplant recipients. Interviews were conducted with 10 women who were solid organ recipients. A two-page summary of the draft results were sent to participants, inviting them to comment on its accuracy. Seven women verified that the summary was accurate and that they had nothing new to add.

TIP For focus group studies, member checking often occurs in situ. That is, moderators develop a summary of major themes or viewpoints in real time and present that summary to focus group participants at the end of the session for their feedback. Rich data often emerge from participants' reactions to those summaries.

Quality-Enhancement Strategies Relating to Coding and Analysis

Excellent qualitative inquiry is likely to involve the concurrent collection and analysis of data, and so several strategies described in the preceding section are also relevant to promoting analytic integrity. Also, we discussed in Chapter 25 some strategies for analytic rigor (e.g., intensive and multiple readings of texts, preparing analytic memos). In this section, we introduce a few other strategies that relate to the coding, analysis, and interpretation of qualitative data.

Investigator and Theory Triangulation

The overall purpose of triangulation is to converge on the truth. Triangulation offers opportunities to discover the "truth" in the data through the use of multiple perspectives. Several types of triangulation are pertinent during analysis. **Investigator triangulation** refers to the use of two or more researchers to make coding, analysis, and interpretation decisions. The premise is that investigators can reduce the risk of biased judgments and idiosyncratic interpretations through collaboration.

Investigator triangulation, conceptually similar to interrater reliability in quantitative studies, is often used in coding qualitative data. Coding consistency depends on having clear codes and decision rules that are documented in a codebook. Researchers

sometimes formally compare two or more independent coding schemes or a subset of independent coding decisions. Some advice on developing a codebook and assessing coding reliability is offered by Fonteyn et al. (2008) and Burla et al. (2008).

Example of Independent Coding
Luck and Doucet (2018) studied the perceptions, experiences, and behaviors of healthcare providers after the implementation of a smoke-free hospital policy. Data were gathered in semistructured interviews with 28 providers. The two researchers independently coded randomly selected transcripts for comparison.

Collaboration is also often used at the analysis stage. If investigators bring to the analysis task a complementary blend of methodologic, disciplinary, and clinical expertise, the analysis and interpretation can potentially benefit from divergent perspectives. As noted in Chapter 25, some approaches to qualitative data analysis are explicitly designed for work in teams (e.g., framework analysis, Diekelmann's approach to hermeneutics).

TIP In focus group studies, immediate postsession debriefings are recommended. In such debriefings—which should be audio-recorded—team members who were present during the session meet to discuss issues and themes. They also should share their views about group dynamics, such as coercive group members, censoring of controversial opinions, individual conformity to group viewpoints, and discrepancies between verbal and nonverbal behavior.

With **theory triangulation**, researchers use competing theories or hypotheses in analyzing and interpreting the data. Qualitative researchers who develop alternative hypotheses while still in the field can test the validity of each because the flexible design of qualitative studies provides ongoing opportunities to direct the inquiry. Theory triangulation can help researchers to rule out rival hypotheses and to prevent premature conceptualizations.

Although Denzin's (1989) seminal work discussed four types of triangulation, other types have been suggested. For example, Kimchi and colleagues (1991) described **analysis triangulation** (i.e., using two or more analytic techniques to analyze the same set of data). This approach offers another opportunity to validate the meanings inherent in a qualitative data set. Analysis triangulation can also involve using multiple units of analysis (e.g., individuals, dyads, families). Renz and colleagues (2018), for example, described an intramethod analytic approach to triangulation in a study in which two different strategies of qualitative content analysis were used.

> **TIP** Farmer and colleagues (2006) provided a useful description of the triangulation protocol they used in the Canadian Heart Health Dissemination Project that illustrates how triangulation was operationalized.

Search for Confirming Evidence

Member checking with participants, as already noted, is one approach to validating the findings. Another verification strategy is to seek external evidence from other studies or from sources such as literary representations of the phenomenon. This is analogous to a strategy of seeking corroborating evidence to enhance credibility in quantitative studies (Chapter 21). Another possibility, and one that has implications for transferability, is to have people from other sites, or other disciplines, review preliminary findings.

> **Example of Confirming Evidence**
> Lavallée and colleagues (2018) studied barriers to and facilitators of pressure ulcer prevention in nursing homes. They identified four "barrier" domains and six "facilitator" domains. They noted that a strength of their study was that the findings were consistent with those of previous studies in pressure ulcer prevention.

Search for Disconfirming Evidence and Competing Explanations

A powerful verification procedure that occurs at the intersection of data collection and data analysis involves a systematic search for data that will challenge an emerging categorization or explanation. The search for disconfirming cases can occur through purposive or theoretical sampling methods, as described in Chapter 23. Clearly, this strategy depends on concurrent data collection and data analysis: researchers cannot look for disconfirming data unless they have a sense of what they need to know.

Member checking can also provide opportunities for soliciting disconfirming evidence. If participants are encouraged to give totally honest feedback, disconfirming voices can enrich the final analysis and interpretation.

> **Example of Disconfirming Evidence**
> Crispin and colleagues (2017) did an in-depth exploration of the exchange of information between patients and nurses in a teaching hospital in the United Kingdom. Patient–nurse interactions were observed, and in-depth interviews were conducted with 22 nurses and 19 patients. The researchers found some conflicting data between the interview and observational data, but they felt the discrepancies strengthened the analysis and "provided conflicting perceptions that needed further exploration" (p. 121).

Lincoln and Guba (1985) discussed the related activity of **negative case analysis.** This strategy is a process by which researchers search for cases (or data segments) that appear to disconfirm earlier hypotheses and then revise their interpretations as necessary. The goal of this procedure is to continuously refine a hypothesis or theory. Morse (2015) pointed out that negative cases may provide the key to understanding "the norm"—i.e., the most commonly occurring cases. She argued that data from negative cases should also be saturated.

> **Example of a Negative Case Analysis**
> Ong and colleagues (2018) studied the trajectory of critical care nurses' experience in providing end-of-life care. Ten nurses in a medical intensive care unit in Singapore were interviewed. Two researchers analyzed the data independently and then came to a consensus. Negative case analysis was "carried out by inspecting the themes in detail for issues that were internally conflicting with the themes, and themes were reframed to suit the data better" (p. 259).

Patton (1999) similarly encouraged a systematic exploration for rival themes and explanations during the analysis: "Failure to find strong supporting evidence for alternative ways of presenting the data or contrary explanations helps increase confidence in the original, principal explanation generated by the analyst" (p. 1191). This strategy can be addressed both inductively and logically. Inductively, the strategy involves seeking other ways of organizing the data that might lead to different conclusions and interpretations. Logically, it means conceptualizing other logical possibilities and then searching for evidence that could support those competing explanations.

Peer Review and Debriefing

External review is another quality-enhancement strategy. **Peer debriefing** involves sessions with peers to review and explore various aspects of the inquiry. Peer debriefing exposes researchers to the searching questions of others who are experienced in either the methods of qualitative inquiry, the phenomenon being studied, or both.

In a peer debriefing session, researchers might present written or oral summaries of the data, emergent categories and themes, and interpretations of the data. In some cases, recorded interviews might be played or transcripts might be shared with reviewers. Peer reviewers might be asked to address questions such as the following:

- Is there evidence of researcher bias? Have the researchers been sufficiently reflexive?
- Do the data adequately portray the phenomenon?
- Are there any apparent errors of fact?
- Are there possible errors of interpretation? Are there competing interpretations? More comprehensive or parsimonious interpretations?
- Have all important themes or patterns been identified?
- Are the themes and interpretations knit together into a cogent and creative conceptualization of the phenomenon?

TIP Morse (2015) expressed some concern about the use of peer review as a validation strategy. She recommended that researchers listen to alternative points of view, but that they need to take "final responsibility for the results, and its implications and applications" (p. 1215).

Example of Peer Review
Sarre and colleagues (2018) studied experiences in three English hospitals regarding the challenges of training and assessing healthcare support workers. The team's interpretations of the data were "tested" through consultation with two members of a project advisory group.

Inquiry Audits

A similar, but more formal, approach is to undertake an **inquiry audit**, which involves scrutiny of the data and supporting documents by an external reviewer. Such an audit requires careful documentation of all aspects of the inquiry, as previously discussed. Once the audit trail materials are assembled, the inquiry auditor proceeds to audit, in a fashion analogous to a financial audit, the trustworthiness of the data and the meanings attached to them. Although such auditing is complex, it can serve as a tool for persuading others that qualitative findings are worthy of confidence. Relatively few comprehensive inquiry audits have been reported in the literature, but some studies report partial audits. Rodgers and Cowles (1993) and Erwin and colleagues (2005) provide useful information about inquiry audits.

Example of an External Audit
Estebsari and an interprofessional team (2017) studied perspectives on "healthy death"—dealing with death positively—among patients and care providers in two Iranian hospitals. The team used both peer review and review by an external observer, who reviewed materials and also undertook independent coding. The reviewer's coding was 85% consistent with coding by the research team.

TIP In validating and refining themes, some researchers introduce **quasi-statistics**—a tabulation of the frequency with which certain themes or insights are supported by the data. The frequencies cannot be interpreted like frequencies in quantitative studies, but, as Becker (1970) pointed out, "Quasi-statistics may allow the investigator to dispose of certain troublesome null hypotheses. A simple frequency count of the number of times a given phenomenon appears may make untenable the null hypothesis that the phenomenon is infrequent" (p. 81).

Quality-Enhancement Strategies Relating to Presentation

The strategies discussed thus far are steps that researchers can undertake to convince *themselves* that their study has integrity and credibility. This section describes some issues relating to convincing *others* of the high quality of the inquiry.

Disclosure of Quality-Enhancement Strategies

A large part of demonstrating integrity to others involves providing a description of the quality-enhancement activities that were undertaken. Many research reports fail to include information that would give readers confidence in the integrity of the research. Some qualitative reports do not address the subject of validity or trustworthiness at all, while others pay lip service to such concerns, simply noting that, for example, member checking was undertaken. Just as clinicians seek *evidence* supporting healthcare decisions, readers of reports need *evidence* that the findings are credible. Readers can draw sensible conclusions about study quality only if they are provided with meaningful information about quality-enhancement strategies.

> **TIP** Avoid stating—as many researchers do—that your quality-enhancement strategies *assured* or *ensured* rigor or trustworthiness. Strategies are used to *enhance* or *promote* rigor, but nothing ensures it.

Thick and Contextualized Description

Thick description, as noted in previous chapters, refers to a rich, thorough, and vivid description of the research context, the people who participated in the study, and the experiences and processes observed during the inquiry. Transferability cannot occur unless investigators provide detailed information to permit judgments about contextual similarity. Lucid and textured descriptions, with the judicious inclusion of verbatim quotes from study participants, also contribute to the authenticity and vividness of a qualitative study.

> **TIP** Sandelowski (2004) cautioned that "…the phrase *thick description* likely ought not to appear in write-ups of qualitative research at all, as it is among those qualitative research words that should be seen but not written" (p. 215).

In high-quality studies, descriptions typically need to go beyond a faithful and thorough rendering of information. Powerful description often has an evocative quality and the capacity for emotional impact. Qualitative researchers must be careful, however, not to misrepresent their findings by sharing only the most dramatic or poignant stories. Thorne and Darbyshire (2005) cautioned against "lachrymal validity," a criterion for evaluating research based on the extent to which the report can wring tears from its readers. At the same time, they noted that the opposite problem with some reports is that they are "bloodless." Bloodless findings are characterized by a tendency of some researchers to "play it safe in writing up the research, reporting the obvious…, failing to apply any inductive analytic spin to the sequence, structure, or form of the findings" (p. 1109).

Researcher Credibility

In qualitative studies, researchers *are* the data collecting instruments—as well as creators of the analytic process. Therefore, researcher qualifications, experience, and reflexivity are relevant in establishing confidence in the findings. Patton (2015) argued that trustworthiness is enhanced if the report contains information about the researchers and their credentials. In addition, the report may need to make clear the personal connections researchers had to the people, topic, or community under study. For example, it is relevant for a reader of a report on AIDS patients' coping to know that the researcher is HIV positive. Patton recommended that researchers report "any personal and professional information that may have affected data collection, analysis and interpretation—either negatively or positively…" (p. 700).

> **Example of Researcher Credibility**
> DeMunnick and an interprofessional team (2017) explored the experiences of HIV nurses when discussing sexually risky behaviors with HIV-positive men. The report noted that "the lead researcher…is an experienced HIV nurse practitioner, who sees patients regularly and who has learned to critically assess current nursing care of HIV patients" (p. 60).

TIP Janice Morse (2015), an influential qualitative nurse researcher, disagrees with some aspects of the Lincoln and Guba framework. For example, she believes that member checking should never be done and that certain strategies described in this chapter are sometimes inappropriate. For instance, she believes that assessments of coder consistency are not suitable when the data are from unstructured interviews, and that prolonged engagement is a useful strategy only with observational research.

DEVELOPING A QUALITY-MINDED OUTLOOK

Conducting high-quality qualitative research is not just about what researchers *do*. It is also about who the researchers *are*—their outlook, self-demands, and ingenuity. As Morse and colleagues (2002) succinctly put it, "Research is only as good as the investigator" (p. 10). Attributes that good qualitative researchers must possess are difficult to teach, but it is important to know what those attributes are so they can be cultivated. We express several important attributes as *commitments* to which researchers should aspire.

1. **Commitment to Transparency.** Good qualitative inquiry cannot be a secretive enterprise that masks decisions, biases, and limitations from outside scrutiny. Conscientious qualitative researchers maintain the records needed to document and justify decisions. A commitment to transparency also means making efforts to have decisions reviewed by others. To the extent possible, researchers should seek opportunities to demonstrate transparency in their writing, including showing how themes and categories were formulated from the initial data.

2. **Commitment to Thoroughness and Diligence.** Meticulousness is essential to high-quality research. Researchers who are not thorough run the risk of having thin, unsaturated data that thwart rich description of phenomena. The concept of *replication* within the study is crucial: there must be sufficient, and redundant, data to account for all aspects of the phenomenon (Morse et al., 2002). In good qualitative research, investigators must commit to reading and rereading their data, returning repeatedly to check whether their interpretations are true to their data. Thoroughness also implies that researchers will seek opportunities to challenge early conceptualizations and to find sources of corroborating evidence both internally (i.e., within the study data) and externally (e.g., in the literature).

3. **Commitment to Verification.** Confidence in the data, and in the analysis and interpretation of those data, is possible only when researchers are committed to instituting verification and self-correcting procedures throughout the study. Morse and colleagues (2002) wrote at length about the importance of verification, noting that verification is "the process of checking, confirming, making sure, and being certain" (p. 9). A commitment to verification strengthens methodologic coherence and helps to promote the likelihood that errors and missteps are corrected before they undermine the enterprise.

4. **Commitment to Reflexivity.** While there is not always agreement about the forms that self-reflection will assume, there is widespread agreement that qualitative researchers need to devote time and energy to analyzing and documenting their presuppositions, biases, and ongoing emotions. Reflexivity involves a continuous self-scrutiny and asking: How might my previous experiences, values, background, and prejudices be shaping my methods, my analysis, and my interpretations?

5. **Commitment to Participant-Driven Inquiry.** In good qualitative research, the inquiry is driven forward by the participants, not the researcher. Researchers must continuously remain responsive to the flow and content of interactions with, and observations of, their informants. Participants shape the scope and breadth of questioning, and they help to guide sampling decisions. The analysis and interpretation must give voice to those who participated in the inquiry.

6. **Commitment to Insightful Interpretation.** Morse (2006) has written that *insight* is a major process in qualitative inquiry but has been neglected and overlooked in the literature—perhaps because it is not easily acquired. Morse argued that researchers must be *ready* for insight—they must have considerable knowledge about their data and be able to link them meaningfully to relevant literature. Immersion in one's own data and having good-quality data are essential. Morse also noted, however, that qualitative researchers need to give themselves "*permission* to use insight and the confidence to do it well" (p. 3). Relatedly, Morse and colleagues (2002) urged researchers to *think theoretically,* which "requires macro-micro perspectives, inching forward without making cognitive leaps, constantly checking and rechecking, and building a solid foundation" (p. 13).

CRITICAL APPRAISAL OF QUALITY IN QUALITATIVE STUDIES

For qualitative research to be judged trustworthy, investigators must *earn* their readers' trust. Many qualitative reports do not provide much information about the researchers' efforts to enhance trustworthiness. In a world that is very conscious about the quality of research evidence, qualitative researchers need to be proactive in doing high-quality research and sharing their quality-enhancement efforts with readers.

Part of the difficulty that qualitative researchers face in demonstrating trustworthiness and authenticity is that page constraints in journals impose conflicting demands. It takes a precious amount of space to report quality-enhancement strategies adequately and convincingly. Using space for such documentation means that there is less space for the thick description of context and the rich verbatim accounts that are also necessary in high-quality qualitative research. As Pyett (2003) has noted, qualitative research is often characterized by the need for critical compromises, which should be kept in mind when reading qualitative research reports.

Some guidelines that may be helpful in appraising qualitative studies are presented in Box 26.1, which can also be found in the Toolkit. ❂ Some additional questions that could be useful in evaluating the quality of qualitative reports are presented in the Supplement to this chapter. ❖

BOX 26.1   Guidelines for Critically Appraising Quality and Integrity in Qualitative Studies

1. Did the report discuss efforts to enhance or monitor the quality of the data and the overall inquiry? If so, was the description sufficiently detailed and clear? If not, was there other information that allowed you to draw inferences about the quality of the data, the analysis, and the interpretations?
2. Which specific techniques (if any) did the researcher use to enhance the trustworthiness and integrity of the inquiry? What quality-enhancement strategies were *not* used? Would additional strategies have strengthened your confidence in the study and its evidence?
3. Did the researcher adequately represent the multiple realities of those being studied? Do the findings seem *authentic*?
4. Were results interpreted in light of findings from other studies?
5. Did the report discuss any study limitations and their possible effects on the credibility of the results or on interpretations of the data?
6. Given the efforts to enhance data quality, what can you conclude about the study's validity/rigor/ trustworthiness?
7. Did the researchers discuss the study's implications for clinical practice or future research? Were the implications well-grounded in the study evidence?

RESEARCH EXAMPLE

Examples of various quality-enhancement strategies used by qualitative nurse researchers have been noted throughout this chapter. In this section, we describe more fully the strategies used by one team of researchers.

Study: "I do the best I can:" Personal care preferences of patients of size (Dial et al., 2018).

Statement of purpose: The purpose of this study was to identify successful self-care strategies that patients of size used to care for themselves, with the goal of helping nurses replicate these strategies in the hospital.

Method: In this qualitative descriptive study, the researchers recruited men and women whose body mass index was equal to or greater than 50 and who were admitted to a 500-bed Magnet hospital for a 2+ day hospitalization. Patients who were willing to participate were interviewed using a semistructured interview. For example, one question was: "We know that some people have concerns about keeping particular areas of their body clean and fresh while they are in the hospital. What concerns do you have about this?" A total of eight men (mean BMI = 60) and six women (mean BMI = 64) participated in the interviews. The analysis of the data resulted in 217 codes, which were categorized into nine themes.

Quality-enhancement strategies: The report included a subsection labeled "Trustworthiness," which provided good detail about efforts to enhance trustworthiness. A single PhD-prepared nurse scientist not caring for the patients completed all interviews "for consistency" (p. 260). The interviews, which were digitally recorded, took place in private rooms with the door closed. The nurse scientist "became immersed in listening deeply to what the participants were saying with their bodies as well as their words" (p. 261). Field notes were maintained to capture "any 'a-HA' thoughts" (p. 260) during the interview. Field notes were reflected on after the interview and were used as another data source during the analysis. Data saturation occurred after completing 14 interviews. The interviews and field notes were professionally transcribed. To promote consensus and standardized coding, all team members coded one record together. All interviews and field notes were read and coded by at least two researchers. Team members used bracketing to guard against biases. The research team maintained a comprehensive audit trail. In terms of researcher credibility, the research team members were the staff nurses and nurse manager who recruited the participants. The nurse scientist who conducted the interviews was experienced and trained in qualitative research methods. In terms of thick description, the researchers provided many vivid excerpts from the interviews and presented a demographic profile of the participants.

Key findings: The researchers identified nine categories that illuminated "the many structures and processes that people of size create to provide, as best as possible, their own hygienic self-care" (p. 262). The themes were collapsed within three broader categories: Caring, Self-care deficit, and Self-care, which were presented in a schematic model. The overarching theme was "I do the best I can."

SUMMARY POINTS

- Several controversies surround the issue of *quality* in qualitative studies, one of which involves terminology. Some have argued that terms such as *rigor* and *validity* are quantitative terms that are unsuitable goals in qualitative inquiry, but others think these terms are appropriate.

- Other controversies involve what criteria to use as indicators of integrity, whether there should be generic or tradition-specific criteria, and what strategies to use to address the quality criteria.

- The most-often used framework of quality criteria is that of Lincoln and Guba, who identified five criteria for evaluating the **trustworthiness** of the inquiry: credibility, dependability, confirmability, transferability, and authenticity.

- **Credibility,** which refers to confidence in the truth value of the findings, is sometimes said to be the qualitative equivalent of internal validity. **Dependability** refers to the stability of data over time and conditions and is somewhat analogous to reliability in quantitative studies. **Confirmability** refers to the objectivity or neutrality of the data. **Transferability**, the analog of external validity, is the extent to which findings from the data can be transferred to other settings or groups. **Authenticity** refers to the extent to which researchers fairly and faithfully show a range of different realities and convey the feeling tone of lives as they are lived.

- Strategies for enhancing the quality of qualitative data as they are being collected include **prolonged engagement**, which strives for adequate scope of data coverage; **persistent observation**, which is aimed at achieving adequate depth; reflexivity; comprehensive and vivid recording of information (including maintenance of an **audit trail** of key decisions and products); triangulation, and member checking.

- **Triangulation** is the process of using multiple referents to draw conclusions about what constitutes the truth. During data collection, key forms of triangulation include **data triangulation** (using multiple data sources to validate conclusions) and **method triangulation** (using multiple methods, such as interviews and observations, to collect data about the same phenomenon).

- **Member checks** involve asking participants to review and react to study data and emerging themes and conceptualizations. A procedure called *Synthesized Member Checking* (SMC) is an effort to make member checking more systematic. Member checking is among the most controversial methods of addressing quality issues in qualitative inquiry.

- Strategies for enhancing quality during the coding and analysis of qualitative data include **investigator triangulation** (independent coding and analysis of at least a portion of the data by two or more researchers); **theory triangulation** (use of competing theories or hypotheses in the analysis and interpretation of data); searching for confirming and disconfirming evidence; searching for rival explanations and undertaking a **negative case analysis** (revising interpretations to account for cases that appear to disconfirm early conclusions); external validation through **peer debriefings** (exposing the inquiry to the searching questions of peers); and launching a formal

inquiry audit (a formal scrutiny of audit trail documents by an independent external auditor).

- Strategies to convince qualitative report readers of high quality include disclosure of key quality-enhancement strategies; using **thick description** to vividly portray contextualized information about participants and the central phenomenon; and making efforts to be transparent about researcher credentials and reflexivity so that **researcher credibility** can be assessed.

- Doing high-quality qualitative research is not just about *method* and what the researchers *do*—it is also about who they *are*. To become an outstanding qualitative researcher, there must be a commitment to transparency, thoroughness, verification, reflexivity, participant-driven inquiry, and insightful and artful interpretation.

STUDY ACTIVITIES

Study activities are available to instructors on thePoint.

REFERENCES CITED IN CHAPTER 26

Becker, H. S. (1970). *Sociological work*. Chicago: Aldine.

Birt, L., Scott, S., Cavers, D., Campbell, C., & Walter, F. (2016). Member checking: A tool to enhance trustworthiness or merely a nod to validation? *Qualitative Health Research, 26*, 1802–1811.

Bradbury-Jones, C. (2007). Enhancing rigour in qualitative health research: Exploring subjectivity through Peshkin's I's. *Journal of Advanced Nursing, 59*, 290–298.

Burla, L., Knierim, B., Barth, J., Liewald, K., Duetz, M., & Abel, T. (2008). From text to codings: Intercoder reliability assessment in qualitative content analysis. *Nursing Research, 57*, 113–117.

*Carduff, E., Johnston, S., Winstanley, C., Morrish, J., Murray, S., Spiller, J., & Finucane, A. (2018). What does "complex" mean in palliative care? Triangulating qualitative findings from 3 settings. *BMC Palliative Care, 17*, 12.

*Chen, C., Draucker, C., & Carpenter, J. (2018). What women say about their dysmenorrhea: A qualitative thematic analysis. *BMC Women's Health, 18*, 47.

Chiovitti, R., & Piran, N. (2003). Rigour and grounded theory research. *Journal of Advanced Nursing, 44*, 427–435.

Cooney, A. (2011). Rigour and grounded theory. *Nurse Researcher, 18,* 17–22.

Crispin, V., Bugge, C., & Stoddart, K. (2017). Sufficiency and relevance of information for inpatients in general ward settings: A qualitative exploration of information exchange between patients and nurses. *International Journal of Nursing Studies, 75,* 112–122.

*Crowther, S., & Smythe, E. (2016). Open, trusting relationships underpin safety in rural maternity: A hermeneutic phenomenology study. *BMC Pregnancy and Childbirth, 16,* 370.

Cypress, B. S. (2017). Rigor or reliability and validity in qualitative research: Perspectives, strategies, reconceptualization, and recommendations. *Dimensions in Critical Care Nursing, 36,* 253–263.

DeForge, R., Ward-Griffin, C., St-Amant, O., Hall, J., McWilliam, C., Forbes, D., … Oudshoorn, A. (2017). Evaluating dementia home care practices: The reification of care norms. *Journal of Aging Studies, 43,* 23–31.

DeMunnick, A., den Daas, C., Ammerlaan, H., Kok, G., Raethke, M., & Vervoort, S. (2017). Let's talk about sex: A qualitative study exploring the experiences of HIV nurses when discussing sexual risk behaviours with HIV-positive men who have sex with men. *International Journal of Nursing Studies, 76,* 55–61.

Denzin, N. K. (1989). *The research act* (3rd ed.). New York: McGraw-Hill.

Denzin, N. K., & Lincoln, Y. S,. (Eds.). (2000). *Handbook of qualitative research* (2nd ed.). Thousand Oaks, CA: Sage Publications.

DeWitt, L., & Ploeg, J. (2006). Critical appraisal of rigour in interpretive phenomenological nursing research. *Journal of Advanced Nursing, 55,* 215–229.

Dial, M., Holmes, J., McGownd, R., & Wendler, M. (2018). "I do the best I can:" Personal care preferences of patients of size. *Applied Nursing Research, 39,* 259–264.

Erwin, E., Meyer, A., & McClain, N. (2005). Use of an audit in violence prevention research. *Qualitative Health Research, 15,* 707–718.

*Estebsari, F., Taghdisi, M., Mostafaei, D., & Rahimi, Z. (2017). Elements of healthy death: A thematic analysis. *Medical Journal of the Islamic Republic of Iran, 31,* 24.

Farmer, T., Robinson, K., Elliott, S., & Eyles, J. (2006). Developing and implementing a triangulation protocol for qualitative health research. *Qualitative Health Research, 16,* 377–394.

Finlay, L., & Gough, B,. (Eds.). (2003). *Reflexivity: A practical guide for researchers in health and social sciences.* Oxford: Blackwell Science.

Fonteyn, M., Vettese, M., Lancaster, D., & Bauer-Wu, S. (2008). Developing a codebook to guide content analysis of expressive writing transcripts. *Applied Nursing Research, 21,* 165–168.

*Gale, N., Heath, G., Cameron, E., Rashid, S., & Redwood, S. (2013). Using the Framework Method for the analysis of qualitative data in multi-disciplinary health research. *BMC Medical Research Methodology, 13,* 117.

Guba, E., & Lincoln, Y. (1994). Competing paradigms in qualitative research. In Denzin, N., & Lincoln, Y. (Eds.), *Handbook of Qualitative Research* (pp. 105–117). Thousand Oaks, CA: Sage Publications.

*Hagens, C., Dobrow, M., & Chafe, R. (2009). Interviewee transcript review: Assessing the impact on qualitative research. *BMC Medical Research Methodology, 9,* 47.

Jootun, D., McGhee, G., & Marland, G. (2009). Reflexivity: Promoting rigour in qualitative research. *Nursing Standard, 23,* 42–46.

Kimchi, J., Polivka, B., & Stevenson, J. S. (1991). Triangulation: Operational definitions. *Nursing Research, 40,* 364–366.

**Kurz, J. M. (2018). Pregnancy after solid organ transplantation. *MCN: The American Journal of Maternal-Child Nursing, 43,* 89–96.

Lather, P. (1986). Issues of validity in openly ideological research: Between a rock and a hard place. *Interchange, 17,* 63–84.

Lavallée, J., Gray, T., Dumville, J., & Cullum, N. (2018). Barriers and facilitators to preventing pressure ulcers in nursing home residents: A qualitative analysis informed by the Theoretical Domains Framework. *International Journal of Nursing Studies, 82,* 79–89.

Lear, H., Eboh, W., & Diack, L. (2018). A nurse researcher's guide to reflexive interviewing. *Nurse Researcher, 25,* 35–42.

LeCompte, M., & Goetz, J. (1982). Problems of reliability and validity in ethnographic research. *Review of Educational Research, 52,* 31–60.

Lincoln, Y. S., & Guba, E. G. (1985). *Naturalistic inquiry.* Newbury Park, CA: Sage Publications.

*Luck, K., & Doucet, S. (2018). What are the perceptions, experiences, and behaviors of health care providers after implementation of a comprehensive smoke-free hospital policy? *Global Qualitative Nursing Research, 5,* 29568792.

Milne, J., & Oberle, K. (2005). Enhancing rigor in qualitative description. *Journal of Wound, Ostomy, & Continence Nursing, 32,* 413–420.

Morse, J. M. (1999). Myth # 93: Reliability and validity are not relevant to qualitative inquiry. *Qualitative Health Research, 9,* 717–718.

*Morse, J. M. (2006). Insight, inference, evidence, and verification: Creating a legitimate discipline. *International Journal of Qualitative Methods, 5*(1), Article 8.

Morse, J. M. (2015). Critical analysis of strategies for determining rigor in qualitative inquiry. *Qualitative Health Research, 25,* 1212–1222.

*Morse, J. M., Barrett, M., Mayan, M., Olson, K., & Spiers, J. (2002). Verification strategies for establishing reliability and validity in qualitative research. *International Journal of Qualitative Methods, 1*(2), Article 2.

Ong, K., Ting, K., & Chow, Y. (2018). The trajectory of experience of critical care nurses in providing end-of-life care: A qualitative descriptive study. *Journal of Clinical Nursing, 27,* 257–268.

Park, M., & Zafran, H. (2018). View from the penthouse: Epistemological bumps and emergent metaphors as method for team reflexivity. *Qualitative Health Research, 28,* 408–417.

*Patton, M. (1999). Enhancing the quality and credibility of qualitative analysis. *Health Services Research, 34,* 1189–1208.

Patton, M. Q. (2015). *Qualitative research and evaluation methods* (4th ed.). Thousand Oaks, CA: Sage Publications.

Pyett, P. M. (2003). Validation of qualitative research "in the real world". *Qualitative Health Research, 13,* 1170–1179.

Renz, S., Carrington, J., & Badger, T. (2018). Two strategies for qualitative content analysis: An intramethod approach to triangulation. *Qualitative Health Research, 28,* 824–831.

Rodgers, B. L., & Cowles, K. V. (1993). The qualitative research audit trail: A complex collection of documentation. *Research in Nursing and Health, 16,* 219–226.

Sandelowski, M. (1993a). Rigor or rigor mortis: The problem of rigor in qualitative research revisited. *Advances in Nursing Science, 16,* 1–8.

Sandelowski, M. (1993b). Theory unmasked: The uses and guises of theory in qualitative research. *Research in Nursing & Health, 16,* 213–218.

Sandelowski, M. (2004). Counting cats in Zanzibar. *Research in Nursing & Health, 27,* 215–216.

Sarre, S., Maben, J., Aldus, C., Schneider, J., Wharrad, H., Nicholson, C., & Arthur, A. (2018). The challenge of training, support, and assessment of healthcare support workers: A qualitative study of experiences in three English acute hospitals. *International Journal of Nursing Studies, 79,* 145–153.

Smith, J. (1993). *After the demise of empiricism: The problem of judging social and educational inquiry.* Norwood, NJ: Ablex.

Sparkes, A. (2001). Myth 94: Qualitative health researchers will agree about validity. *Qualitative Health Research, 11,* 538–552.

Thorne, S., & Darbyshire, P. (2005). Land mines in the field: A modest proposal for improving the craft of qualitative health research. *Qualitative Health Research, 15,* 1105–1113.

Vasey, J., Smith, J., Kirshbaum, M., & Chimera, K. (2019). Tokenism or true partnership: Parental involvement in a child's acute pain care. *Journal of Clinical Nursing, 28,* 1491–1505.

Ward, D., Furber, C., Tierney, S., & Swallow, V. (2013). Using Framework Analysis in nursing research: A worked example. *Journal of Advanced Nursing, 69,* 2423–2431.

Watson, L., & Girard, F. (2004). Establishing integrity and avoiding methodological misunderstanding. *Qualitative Health Research, 14,* 875–881.

Whittemore, R., Chase, S. K., & Mandle, C. L. (2001). Validity in qualitative research. *Qualitative Health Research, 11,* 522–537.

Wolcott, H. (1994). *Transforming qualitative data.* London: Sage Publications.

Wolcott, H. (1995). *The art of fieldwork.* London: Sage Publications.

Wright, D., Brajtman, S., & Macdonald, M. (2018). Relational ethics of delirium care: Findings from a hospice ethnography. *Nursing Inquiry, 25,* e12234.

*A link to this open-access article is provided in the Toolkit for Chapter 26 in the **Resource Manual.** ✖

**This journal article is available on the Point for this chapter.*

Part 5

DESIGNING AND CONDUCTING MIXED METHODS STUDIES TO GENERATE EVIDENCE FOR NURSING

27 | Basics of Mixed Methods Research

OVERVIEW OF MIXED METHODS RESEARCH

A methodologic trend that has been gaining momentum in health research is the planned integration of qualitative and quantitative data within single studies or a coordinated series of studies. **Mixed methods research** in the health sciences has been called "a quiet revolution" (O'Cathain, 2009). Two decades ago, there was little guidance on conducting mixed methods research. Now there are abundant resources in the form of handbooks and textbooks (e.g., Creamer, 2018; Creswell et al., 2011; Creswell & Plano Clark, 2018; Morse, 2017; Plano Clark & Ivankova, 2016; Tashakkori & Teddlie, 2010) and many examples of mixed methods studies in the nursing and health care literature. New resources are becoming available continuously in this rapidly evolving field.

This chapter presents basic information about mixed methods research in nursing, and the next discusses the use of mixed methods in developing and testing nursing interventions. To streamline these chapters, we use the acronym MM to refer to mixed methods research.

Definition of Mixed Methods Research

The concept of combining qualitative and quantitative data in a study is straightforward, but definitions of MM research are not. This is partly because, in some

sense, most studies could be considered MM if the definition is too broad. For example, if a grounded theory researcher asks structured demographic questions about age and education at the end of an in-depth interview, does that count as mixed methods? Or, if a survey asks a broad open-ended question at the end of a questionnaire (e.g., "Is there anything else you would like to add?"), is that MM research? We do not consider such inquiries as MM research.

We use the definition offered in the first issue of *Journal of Mixed Methods Research*, which is that MM research is "research in which the investigator collects and analyzes data, *integrates* the findings, and *draws inferences* using both qualitative and quantitative approaches or methods in a single study or program of inquiry" (Tashakkori & Creswell, 2007, p. 4, emphasis added). MM research involves not just collecting qualitative and quantitative data, but also *integrating* the two at multiple points in the research process, giving rise to meta-inferences. A **meta-inference** is a conclusion generated by integrating inferences from the results of the qualitative and quantitative strands of an MM study.

Rationale for Mixed Methods Studies

The dichotomy between quantitative and qualitative data represents a key methodologic distinction in the behavioral and health sciences. Some have argued that the paradigms that underpin qualitative and quantitative research are fundamentally incompatible. Many people now believe, however, that health research can be enriched through the judicious integration of qualitative and quantitative data. The advantages and "added value" of mixed methods include the following:

- *Complementarity.* Qualitative and quantitative approaches are complementary—words and numbers are the two fundamental languages of human communication. By using mixed methods, researchers can allow each to do what it does best.
- *Practicality.* Given the complexity of phenomena, it is practical to not have one's hands tied by rigid adherence to one methodology. MM researchers often ask questions that cannot be answered with a single approach.
- *Enhanced validity.* When a hypothesis, model, or description is supported by complementary types of data, researchers can be more confident about the validity of their results. The integration of methods can provide opportunities for testing alternative interpretations, for obtaining corroboration, and for assessing whether context helped to shape the results.

Paradigm Issues and Mixed Method Studies

Although MM research has been around for decades, broad acceptance is recent. Mixed methods research emerged from the ashes of the so-called *paradigm wars* involving debates between the positivist and constructivist camps that erupted during the 1970s and 1980s. MM research gained momentum at the turn of the 21st century.

Discussions about an appropriate paradigmatic stance for MM research abound. Viewpoints range from those claiming the irrelevance of paradigms, to those advocating multiple paradigms. The paradigm called **pragmatism** is often associated with MM research—a paradigm that some consider offers an "umbrella worldview" for a study (Creswell & Plano Clark, 2018, p. 69). Pragmatist researchers consider that it is the *research question* that should drive the inquiry and the methods used. They reject a forced choice between the traditional positivists' and constructivists' modes of inquiry. In the pragmatist paradigm, both induction and deduction are important,

theory generation and theory verification can be accomplished, and a pluralistic view is encouraged. Pragmatism is practical: whatever works best to arrive at good evidence is appropriate.

> **TIP** The qualitative component of most MM studies is often "generic qualitative," i.e., not allied with a research tradition. However, some have discussed incorporating phenomenologic (Mayoh & Onwuegbuzie, 2015) and grounded theory (Guetterman et al., 2019) components into MM research.

Applications of Mixed Methods Research

Creswell and Plano Clark (2018) identified seven broad types of research situations that are especially well-suited to MM research:

1. Neither a qualitative nor a quantitative approach, by itself, is adequate in addressing the complexity of the research problem;
2. The findings from one approach can be greatly enhanced with a second source of data that has explanatory power;
3. The phenomenon needs to be explored in-depth before formal instruments can be developed and administered;
4. Quantitative results from an intervention study require qualitative data to help to explain and interpret the results;
5. Different types of cases need to be described and compared;
6. An effort is being made to involve study participants in the study; and
7. A program needs to be developed, implemented, and evaluated.

As this list suggests, mixed methods research can be used in various situations. Some specific applications are noteworthy because MM research has made important contributions in these areas in health disciplines.

Confirmation and Explication

Mixed methods studies are sometimes undertaken as a confirmatory strategy—that is, to converge on the truth. Additionally, some researchers deliberately collect qualitative data to explicate the *meaning* of quantitative findings. Quantitative methods can demonstrate that variables are systematically related but may fail to provide insights about *why* they are related. Such explications can corroborate statistical findings and guide the interpretation of results. Qualitative data can provide more global, dynamic, and contextualized views of the phenomena under study.

Example of Confirming and Explicating With Mixed Methods

Roberts and colleagues (2017) undertook an MM study of resilience in families of children with autism spectrum disorder (ASD) and sleep problems. They first surveyed a sample of parents of children with ASD and compared those who had or did not have sleep problems. Parents whose children had sleep problems had lower scores on a measure of resilience/family hardiness. The researchers then conducted in-depth interviews with a sample of the sleep-problem parents. The qualitative findings supported quantitative findings regarding the impact of sleep problems, but the qualitative data expanded the researchers' understanding by illustrating how sleep issues contributed to family strains and by describing their progression to greater resilience.

Instrumentation

Researchers sometimes collect qualitative data as a basis for developing structured instruments for research or clinical applications. Questions for a formal instrument are sometimes derived from clinical experience or prior research. When a construct is new, however, these mechanisms may be inadequate to capture its nuances. Thus, researchers sometimes gather qualitative data as the basis for generating items for quantitative instruments that are then rigorously tested, as described in Chapter 16.

Example of MM in Instrumentation

Hall and colleagues (2018) conducted a two-phase MM study focused on nurses' attitudes and behavior toward patients' use of complementary therapy. In-depth interviews with 19 Australian nurses led to four key themes (including Promoting safe care and Supporting holistic health care). The themes informed the development of a survey instrument that was administered to over 600 nurses online.

Intervention Development

Qualitative research is playing an increasingly important role in the development of promising nursing interventions. There is growing recognition that the development of effective interventions must take clients' perspective into account. Intervention research is increasingly likely to be MM research, a topic we address in the next chapter.

Example of MM in Intervention Development Research

Redeker and an interdisciplinary team (2018) published a protocol for an MM study of sleep in children from disadvantaged urban areas. They are launching a community-engaged study to understand the perspectives of key stakeholders (e.g., parents, pediatric health care providers) about children's sleep habits and difficulties. The team is collecting in-depth data through interviews with stakeholders and 9 days of objective sleep data (wrist actigraphy) from 30 infants and toddlers. Data from the study will be used to develop a contextually relevant program to promote sleep health.

Intervention and Program Evaluation

Program evaluations have a long history of using MM approaches (see Patton, 2015). As described in Chapter 11, impact analyses that evaluate the effectiveness of a program typically rely on quantitative data, but process evaluations that examine how a program *works* involve the integration of qualitative and quantitative information. *Realist evaluations* almost always used mixed methods approaches to program evaluation.

Example of Mixed Methods in Program Evaluation

Baron Nelson and colleagues (2018) evaluated a peer support program for parents of children with brain tumors. Their quasi-experimental study involved collecting quantitative data on parental resilience from parents in the intervention and comparison groups. Qualitative data were gathered in focus group sessions with program stakeholders to understand experiences with the program.

TIP In this book we have identified various types of studies, some qualitative and some quantitative (e.g., clinical trials, surveys, outcomes research). We provide a table in the Toolkit that illustrates how basic questions for these types of studies can be supplemented with questions that would require a mixed method approach.

The Issue of Integration in Mixed Method Studies

Integration is often considered a central feature of MM research—a centerpiece that sets it apart from other methodologies. Meaningful integration in MM research allows researchers to "produce a whole…that is greater than the sum of the individual qualitative and quantitative parts" (Fetters & Freshwater, 2015, p. 115). Mixed methods research can only achieve its full potential for providing enhanced insights when integration occurs.

Integration is a topic that has been given considerable recent attention. Leading thinkers have encouraged "divesting" from the term *triangulation* in MM research, using the newer language of *integration* of qualitative and quantitative methods (Fetters & Molino-Azorin, 2017a).

Some MM experts have provided guidance about the *when* and the *how* of integration. In all three editions of their widely used textbook on MM research, Creswell and Plano Clark (2018) have described options for integration at the analysis and interpretation stage, using broad analytic strategies such as mixing, merging, and connecting. For example, the data types can be *mixed* during the interpretation of the qualitative and quantitative findings. *Merging* can occur during data analysis, through a combined analysis. Integration also can occur during data collection by using a strategy of *connecting* in which the results from one strand influence data collection in a subsequent strand.

Creamer (2018), however, has advocated for fully integrated MM research in which there is an intention to mix or integrate throughout the planning and conduct of the study. She advocates for deliberative integration during these five stages:

planning and design, data collection, sampling, analysis, and inference development.

Similarly, the editors of the *Journal of Mixed Methods Research* recently wrote a lengthy editorial in which they suggest integration across 15 dimensions that encompass the entire range of activities in an MM study (Fetters & Molina-Azorin, 2017b). They defined integration as "the linking of qualitative and quantitative approaches and dimensions together to create a new whole or a more holistic understanding than achieved by either alone" (p. 293). They sought to identify integration approaches "at the philosophical, methodologic, and methods levels to inform an all-encompassing mixed methods research approach" (p. 293). Thus, MM researchers are urged to consider the issue of integration for every decision they make throughout the research process, including putting together a team, undertaking a literature review, and framing research questions. The Toolkit in the accompanying *Resource Manual* includes a table with some of the integration strategies suggested in the editorial.

Practical Issues: Skills and Resources for Mixed Methods

Mixed methods studies have become attractive to both new and seasoned researchers, but the decision to pursue such a study should not be made lightly. The researcher's skills should be critically evaluated in deciding whether to undertake an MM study because the researcher must have some level of competence in both qualitative and quantitative methods. Many courses are now available to teach mixed methods skills, and NIH offers mixed methods training programs. Also, a computer application (app) has been developed to help novice researchers plan an MM project (Luo & Creswell, 2016).

A team approach to MM research is often advocated. A research team provides opportunity for collaboration between qualitative and quantitative researchers working on similar problems. Although a team approach is a useful way to proceed because experts in both approaches can make contributions, all team members should be methodologically bilingual and have basic understanding of varied approaches. Increasingly, mixed methods collaboration involves teams of professionals in diverse disciplines (Hesse-Biber, 2016). Fetters and Molina-Azorin (2017c) noted that when working in teams MM researchers "need to understand the culture associated with disciplines that have been traditionally mono-method" (p. 428).

> **TIP** In dissertation MM research, the judicious selection of advisers with a mix of methodologic skills is imperative. Keep in mind, however, that advisers from different backgrounds may have conflicting views about the merit of your strategies and the emphasis given to different aspects of your study. Frels and colleagues (2015) have written about the important role of mentoring in MM research.

Mixed methods research can be expensive. Although funding agencies increasingly are looking favorably on MM studies, it is obviously costly to collect, analyze, and integrate two or more types of data. Relatedly, mixed methods studies are often time consuming. It is wise to develop a realistic timeline before embarking on an MM inquiry.

GETTING STARTED ON A MIXED METHODS STUDY

In this chapter, we discuss many aspects of mixed methods research, with emphasis on research design and the analysis of MM data. We begin, however, by considering the intent of an MM study and the kinds of questions that lend themselves to MM research.

The Purpose/Intent of a Mixed Methods Study

In an article in which several key scholars discussed current challenges of mixed methods research, one expert (Tashkkori) advised new researchers to use mixed methods only if MM is *required* (Fetters & Molina-Azorin, 2017c, p. 427). This implies that researchers need to develop and state a justifiable mixed methods purpose, as expressed in a purpose statement.

In writing mixed methods purpose statements, researchers should communicate the purpose of both the quantitative and qualitative components. They should also articulate a mixed methods purpose that states the overall **intent** of integrating the two approaches. The study's MM intent is what drives the study design, and so it is important to clarify what that intent is (e.g., To explore? To explicate or explain? To confirm? To compare?). Creswell and Plano Clark's (2018) book offers useful "scripts" for writing MM purpose statements.

> **Example of a Mixed Methods Purpose Statement**
> Bhandari and Kim (2016) studied the self-care behaviors of Nepalese adults with type 2 diabetes. Their quantitatively dominant study involved developing a path analytic model to predict diabetes self-care with data from a survey of 230 adults. The qualitative component involved in-depth interviews with 13 participants. The MM purpose was to "enhance model interpretation through qualitative input" (p. 204).

Research Questions for Mixed Methods Research

In mixed methods studies, the research questions are the driving force behind the scope of the inquiry. Investigators in MM studies typically pose questions that can *only* be addressed (or that can *best* be addressed) with more than one type of data.

In mixed methods research, there are inevitably at least two research questions, each of which requires a different approach. For example, MM researchers may simultaneously ask exploratory (qualitative) questions and confirmatory (quantitative) questions. MM researchers can examine causal *effects* in a quantitative component but can also shed light on causal *mechanisms* in a qualitative component.

In addition to mono-method questions, MM studies should ask a specific MM question relating to the integration of qualitative and quantitative data, and that makes explicit what will be answered through such integration. Examples include such questions as, "To what extent do the two types of data confirm each other?" and "How does one type of data help to explain the results from the other type?"

TIP Creswell and Plano Clark's (2018) book includes a table with a series of mixed methods questions (p. 169–170). An adapted version of a portion of this table is included in the Toolkit of the accompanying *Resource Manual*.

Example of a Mixed Methods Research Question
Beck and colleagues (2016) conducted an MM study to investigate vicarious posttraumatic growth in labor and delivery nurses who cared for women during traumatic births. The researchers asked five research questions, including two quantitative questions, two qualitative questions, and the following mixed methods question: "How do the quantitative and qualitative results develop a more complete picture of vicarious posttraumatic growth in labor and delivery nurses who cared for women during traumatic birth?" (p. 805).

MIXED METHODS DESIGNS

Mixed methods designs are continuing to evolve as greater thought is given to fruitful approaches—and as greater experience in conducting MM research occurs. Over a dozen design typologies have been developed by mixed methods scholars, so it is challenging to discuss this important topic. We begin by noting some key design issues, then present methods of portraying designs through a notation system and diagrams, and finally describe the design typology offered by Creswell and Plano Clark (2018).

Key Decisions in Mixed Methods Designs

In designing an MM study, researchers make several important decisions, which we briefly review in this section.

Fixed Versus Emergent Designs

One issue concerns whether to establish a design at the outset. In some cases, the research intent will lead to a certain type of MM research design. Novice researchers are especially likely to benefit by having a "roadmap" to follow. Experienced researchers may, however, prefer the flexibility of allowing answers from an initial **strand** (e.g., the qualitative component) guide them in subsequent strands (e.g., the quantitative component). Emergent MM designs may result from issues that develop during a mono-method study—for example, an inadequacy in fully understanding the construct or phenomenon of interest.

As noted by Creswell and Plano Clark (2018), "fixed" and "emergent" designs are probably best understood as endpoints on a continuum rather than as a dichotomy. No typology of designs encompasses every possible MM design, because a hallmark of the MM approach is that it permits creativity and paths to deeper understanding. Typologies and nomenclatures for designs are useful primarily because of their role in communicating an approach to others in proposals, IRB applications, and research articles. The designs we describe in this chapter are ones that have been adopted in many studies, but other possibilities exist for structuring an MM study, and the possibilities may emerge during a study that initially had a fixed design.

Sequencing in Mixed Methods Designs

There are three options for sequencing the strands of a mixed methods study: qualitative data are collected first, quantitative data are collected first, or both types are collected simultaneously (or at approximately the same time). When the two types of data are not collected at the same time, the approach is called **sequential**. When the data are collected at the same time, the approach is called **concurrent** (or *simultaneous*). Concurrent designs occur in a single phase, whereas sequential designs unfold in two or more phases. In well-conceived sequential designs, the analysis and interpretation in one phase informs the collection and analysis of data in the second. Another possibility is *multiphase timing*, which occurs when researchers launch a multiphase project that includes several sequential and/or concurrent substudies over a program of study. In an analysis of 294 MM studies in nursing, Beck and Harrison (2016) found that slightly more than half (53%) used a concurrent design.

Prioritization in Mixed Methods Designs

Researchers may decide whether one strand will be given greater weight or emphasis. One option is that the two components are given equal, or roughly equal, weight. Often, however, one strand is given **priority**. The distinction is sometimes referred to as *equal status* versus *dominant status*.

The overall intent of the study usually affects the priority decision, as we discuss later in this section. The researcher's worldview is another influence. Researchers' philosophical orientation (positivist or constructivist) leads them to tackle research problems for which one approach is dominant, and the other is viewed as a useful supplementary data source. Practical considerations also may influence the weighting decision. If resources are limited, or if the researcher's skills are stronger in qualitative or quantitative methods, these issues will probably result in an MM study in which one approach has dominant status.

The issue of priority, however, has become somewhat controversial. Some experts worry about designating a priority based on relatively superficial criteria such as the amount of data rather than the information value of different strands (Fetters & Molina-Azorin, 2017c). Nevertheless, design notation continues to be used to represent prioritization decisions—although in Beck and Harrison's (2016) review of MM nursing studies, only a minority of researchers specified priority.

Notation and Diagramming in Mixed Methods Designs

Morse (1991), a prominent nurse researcher, made a crucial contribution to the MM literature by proposing a notation system that has been adopted across disciplines. Her notation system concerns the sequencing and prioritization decisions and is thus useful in quickly summarizing major features of an MM design.

In Morse's system, priority is designated by upper case and lower case letters: QUAL/quan designate a mixed methods study in which the dominant approach is qualitative, while QUAN/qual designates the reverse. If neither approach is dominant (i.e., both are equal), the notation stipulates QUAL/QUAN. Sequencing is indicated by the symbols + or →. The arrow designates a sequential approach. For example, QUAN → qual is the notation for a primarily quantitative MM study in which qualitative data collection occurs in Phase II. When both approaches occur concurrently, a plus sign is used (e.g., QUAL + quan).

> **TIP** Other notations symbols have been suggested (e.g., parentheses, brackets, double-sided arrows), but the notations for sequence and priority are the ones most frequently used.

In addition to the notation system, MM designs can be visually diagrammed. Such diagrams can be useful in illustrating processes to reviewers and can also provide guidance to researchers themselves. Figure 27.1 illustrates a basic diagram for a QUAN + QUAL study. Additional information can be added under the boxes in the diagram to provide richer detail. For example, under the first box (Quantitative data collection and analysis), there might be a notation such as: "Administered survey to 281 patients," and under the second box for the qualitative strand, there might be another notation (e.g., "Conducted focus group interviews with 24 patients").

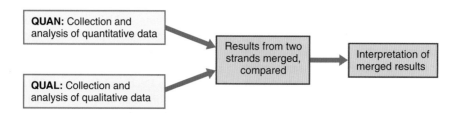

FIGURE 27.1 Diagram of a mixed methods convergent design.

TIP Creswell and Plano Clark (2018) offer ten guidelines for drawing visual diagrams of MM studies (Figure 3.2, p. 64). Their book also includes dozens of such visual diagrams that can serve as models.

Core Mixed Methods Designs

Although numerous design typologies have been developed by different MM methodologists, we focus on the one proposed by Creswell and Plano Clark (2018), two leading experts on MM research. They identified three designs that they call *core MM designs*, which we briefly describe in this section. Notations for these three designs are shown in Table 27.1. It should be noted that many published MM nursing studies do not fall exactly into the current Creswell-Plano Clark typology.

Convergent Design

The purpose of the **convergent design** is to obtain different, but complementary, data about the central phenomenon under study. In this design, qualitative and quantitative data are collected simultaneously and, most often, with equal priority. The notation for a typical convergent design is QUAN + QUAL. The diagram in Figure 27.1 illustrates this design.

The convergent design is appropriate if the researcher wants to (1) compare the QUAL and QUAN results with the goal of obtaining a more complete understanding of a problem, (2) validate findings from one strand with those from another, (3) illustrate quantitative results with qualitative findings or vice versa, or (4) contrast people's answers to structured and unstructured questions. The overall goal of this design is to converge on "the truth" about a problem or phenomenon.

With the convergent design, researchers analyze the two datasets separately. They then use various strategies to merge and compare the datasets. For example, they may seek to identify the similarities and differences within one set of results based on dimensions that are prominent in the other set.

The convergent design has several variants. The most conventional is the *parallel databases variant* (Creswell & Plano Clark, 2018). In this variant, QUAN data are collected and analyzed in parallel with the collection and analysis of QUAL data. The results of the two separate analyses are brought together for an overall interpretation of results. The goal is to develop internally confirmed conclusions about a single phenomenon.

Another variant is called the *data transformation variant*. This design also involves the separate but concurrent collection of QUAL and QUAN data, followed by QUAL and QUAN analysis. A novel step in this variant involves transforming the QUAL data into quan data (or the QUAN data into qual data) and then comparing and interrelating the datasets. Data transformations are described later in this chapter.

A third variant is the *questionnaire variant* in which both closed-ended questions and probing open-ended questions are included on a questionnaire. The open-ended questions are analyzed thematically and used to confirm or validate the quantitative results. Such a variant might in some cases be notated as QUAN + qual if the main use of the qualitative data is to illustrate the quantitative findings with interesting quotes.

TABLE 27.1 • Core Mixed Methods Designs

DESIGN NAME[a]	NOTATION AND PROCESS
Convergent	QUAN + QUAL → Results merged → Interpretation
Explanatory Sequential	QUAN → qual (QUAN results explained by qual) → Interpretation **OR** quan → QUAL (quan results explained by QUAL) → Interpretation
Exploratory Sequential	QUAL → Development (e.g., qual + quan) → QUAN (Testing) → Interpretation

[a]Design names are based on Creswell and Plano Clark (2018).

A major advantage of convergent designs is that they are efficient: both types of data are collected concurrently. A major drawback, however, is that these designs, which usually give equal weight to QUAL and QUAN strands, may be difficult for a single researcher working alone to do. Another potential problem can arise if the data from the two strands are not congruent.

> **Example of a Convergent Design**
> Fletcher and an interprofessional team (2019) used a convergent MM design to better understand functional communication in head and neck cancer survivors. Survivors completed structured questionnaires that included measures of quality of life and symptoms of anxiety and depression. Survivors also participated, concurrently, in in-depth interviews that probed their experiences of communication. The two types of data were analyzed separately, and the results were then integrated.

Explanatory Sequential Designs

Explanatory designs are sequential designs with quantitative data collected in the first phase, followed by qualitative data collected in the second phase. Either the qualitative or the quantitative data can be given a stronger priority in explanatory designs. That is, the design can be either QUAN → qual or quan → QUAL; the former sequence is more typical.

In explanatory designs, data from the second phase are used to build on or explain data from the initial phase. A QUAN → qual design is especially suitable when the quantitative results are surprising (for example, significant serendipitous results), when results are complicated and tricky to interpret, or when the sample has numerous outliers that are difficult to explain. Thus, this design is used to inform data collection for the second stage after the first-stage data have been analyzed. In reporting the use of this design, specific QUAN/quan results that were followed up should be identified.

Creswell and Plano Clark (2018) described two variants of the explanatory design. In the *follow-up explanations variant*, the researcher collects qual data that can best help to explain the initial QUAN findings. The primary emphasis is on the quantitative aspects of the study, and the analysis involves connecting data between the two phases. This model is one that is often attractive to researchers who are primarily quantitative, but who recognize that their study can be enriched by adding a follow-up qualitative component.

The second variant is the *case selection variant* in which first-stage quan data are in service of the second-phase QUAL component. In this model, information about the characteristics of a large group, as identified in the first phase, is used to purposefully select cases in the second dominant phase—for example, using extreme case sampling or stratified purposive sampling (Chapter 22).

> **TIP** In describing a design in a proposal or a report, it is probably best to combine words and notation. A citation should be provided for specifically named designs. For example, a design might be summarized as follows: "A sequential, qualitative-dominant (quan → QUAL) explanatory design (Creswell & Plano Clark, 2018), will be adopted in the proposed research." A visual diagram is a good supplement if space allows.

Advantages of explanatory designs are that they are straightforward, are easy to describe, and can be done by a single researcher. Another attractive feature, given page constraints in journals, is that the results can often be summarized in two separate papers. On the other hand, explanatory designs can be time consuming—the second phase cannot begin until data from the first phase are analyzed. Also, it may be difficult to secure upfront approval from funders or ethical review boards because details of the Phase II design are seldom known in advance.

> **Example of an Explanatory Sequential Design**
> Alabdulaziz and colleagues (2017) used an explanatory sequential (QUAN → qual) design to study pediatric nurses' perceptions and practice of family-centered care in Saudi hospitals. In the first phase, 234 nurses from six hospitals completed the Family-Centered Care Questionnaire. The survey results indicated that the nurses perceived family-centered care as necessary but were not likely to incorporate elements into their practice. The qualitative phase involved observations of pediatric nurses' practice in one hospital, which supported the survey findings. In-depth interviews with 14 nurses provided explanations, revealing that the nurses had limited and superficial understanding of what family-centered care means as a model of care.

TIP Creswell and Plano Clark's explanatory sequential design requires analysis of the QUAN data, with results serving as the springboard for making decisions for the qual strand. Many studies, however, have a sequential approach that does not involve a preliminary analysis of the QUAN data—the qual component is completed in a second phase, but the intent is to compare and contrast results (rather than to explain the QUAN findings), and is thus more like a convergent design.

Exploratory Sequential Designs

The **exploratory sequential design** is a three-phase MM design in which qualitative data are collected first. The design has as its central premise the need for initial in-depth exploration of a phenomenon, often to better understand contextual or cultural issues relevant to a phenomenon. Its intent is to use rich contextualized information to inform the development of a quantitative feature, such as a new measure, survey, intervention, or digital tool such as a website or app.

Findings from the initial qualitative phase are used to develop (phase II) and test (phase III) an innovation. The development phase can involve gathering additional quan or qual data (e.g., qual in a "think aloud" cognitive interview, quan in a pilot test). The final phase is a QUAN evaluation of the new product. For example, in instrument development studies, the researchers would undertake a psychometric assessment of the measure in phase III. The notation for this design might be QUAL → quan + qual → QUAN, but alternative decisions about prioritization might make sense. Creswell and Plano Clark (2018) described several variants of an exploratory design, such as the *new variable development variant,* the *survey (instrument) development variant,* and the *intervention-development variant.*

Example of an Exploratory Sequential Design
Yang and colleagues (2016) developed a checklist for assessing thirst in patients with advanced dementia. The items on the checklist were developed through in-depth interviews with nurses caring for patients with advanced dementia. The checklist was then tested quantitatively (e.g., for reliability) with caregivers from 8 facilities.

The advantages and disadvantages of an explanatory MM design also apply to exploratory MM designs. Separate phases make the inquiry easy to explain, implement, and report. A major challenge is that this design is time consuming and almost inevitably requires two or more rounds of sampling.

TIP In an earlier edition of their MM textbook, Creswell and Plano Clark described a design called the *embedded design.* An embedded design is one in which a second type of data is totally subservient to the other type of data. Creswell and Plano Clark (2018) now see embedding as an analytic strategy rather than as a design type.

Other Mixed Methods Designs

In some projects, core designs do not adequately characterize the complex series and sequences of mixing qualitative and quantitative data. Many advanced MM design options exist, including ones that are multiphase (progressing in multiple phases with various quan/qual combinations in each phase) and ones that are multilevels (gathering different combinations of qual/quan data from multiple tiers of an organizational system). Thus, although the core categories are a useful way to begin thinking about an MM study—especially for novice MM researchers—the typologies should not be used to force what should be a fluid and creative process into oversimplified boxes.

Creswell and Plano Clark (2018) described several *complex MM designs* that involve intersecting the core designs with other research approaches or frameworks. One is the *mixed methods experimental/intervention design,* using multiple methods and intricately related components that unfold over time. This type of MM research is described in the next chapter. *Participatory-social justice designs* are MM designs within a critical framework. A third complex design is the *mixed methods case study design,* which involves the use of one of the core designs within the framework of case study research. The fourth complex design is the *mixed methods evaluation design,* some features of which we described in Chapter 11.

TIP Mixed methods research is considered one category of *multimethod research* (Fetters & Molino-Azorin, 2017a). Other categories include quantitative studies with two or more approaches and qualitative studies with two or more approaches. Morse (2012), for example, has argued that a qualitative-qualitative study is a legitimate form of inquiry, using either a concurrent or sequential design. One of the qualitative methods is a "complete" method (e.g., grounded theory, phenomenology), and the other is supplemental (e.g., QUAL + qual or qual → QUAL). The supplementary strategy is not sufficiently complete to stand on its own.

TIP MM designs are often portrayed as cross-sectional, even when they are sequential—i.e., the goal in sequential designs usually is not to understand how a phenomenon unfolds over time. Plano Clark and colleagues (2015) have presented a conceptualization of longitudinal mixed methods designs.

Selecting a Mixed Methods Design

The most critical issue in selecting a design is its appropriateness for the research questions. The *design* should correspond to the study *intent*. Having a name for a design is less important than having a strong rationale for structuring a study in a certain way.

Practical issues are also relevant in designing a study. For example, few researchers are equally skillful in qualitative and quantitative methods. This suggests three options: (1) selecting a design in which your methodologic strengths are dominant; (2) working as a team with researchers whose strengths are complementary; or (3) strengthening your skills in your nondominant area. The first option is likely to be most realistic for many students. Practical concerns such as resource availability and time constraints also play a role in choosing a design. Concurrent designs often require shorter time commitments, and dominant designs can often be less resource-intensive.

It is advisable to learn the details of a particular MM design before making a selection. In addition to reading methodologic writings of MM scholars, it is useful to examine the methods section of reports that have used a design you are considering. Teddlie and Tashakkori (2009) also advised that "you should look for the most appropriate or single best available research design, rather than the 'perfect fit.' You may have to combine existing designs, or create new designs, for your study" (p. 163).

SAMPLING AND DATA COLLECTION IN MIXED METHODS STUDIES

When a study design has been selected, an MM researcher can then plan how best to collect the needed data. Sampling and data collection in MM studies are often a blend of approaches that we described in earlier chapters. A few special sampling and data collection issues for an MM study merit brief discussion.

Sampling in a Mixed Methods Study

Mixed methods researchers can combine sampling designs in various creative ways. The quantitative component is likely to rely on a sampling strategy that enhances the researcher's ability to generalize to a broader population. As noted in Chapter 13, probability samples are well-suited to selecting a representative sample of participants, but nurse researchers often must compromise, using such designs as consecutive samples or quota samples to enhance representativeness. For the qualitative strand of the study, MM researchers usually adopt purposive sampling methods (Chapter 23) to select information-rich cases.

Sample sizes are often different in the qualitative and quantitative components, in predictable ways—i.e., larger samples for the quantitative strand. Ideally, MM researchers should use power analyses to guide sample size decisions for the quantitative component, to diminish the risk of Type II errors in statistical analyses. In the qualitative sample, saturation is the principle often used to decide when to stop sampling.

A unique sampling issue in MM studies concerns whether the same people will be in both the qualitative and quantitative strands. The best strategy depends on the study purpose and the research design, but using overlapping samples can be advantageous. Having the same people in both parts of an MM study offers opportunities for convergence and for comparison between the two datasets.

Onwuegbuzie and Collins (2007) categorized mixed methods sampling designs according to the *relationship* between the qualitative and quantitative components. The four relationships are identical, parallel, nested, or multilevel. An **identical** relationship occurs when the same people are in both strands of the study—a situation that is especially likely in convergent designs. This approach might occur if everyone in a survey or intervention study was asked a series of probing, open-ended questions—or if everyone in a primarily QUAL study was administered a formal instrument, such as a self-efficacy scale.

Example of Identical Sampling
Moreland and Santacroce (2018) studied illness uncertainty and posttraumatic stress disorder (PTSD) in young adults with congenital heart disease, using a convergent design. The 25 study participants completed a questionnaire that included a measure of posttraumatic stress. They were also asked to tell their stories in unstructured interviews. The narrative analysis revealed a relationship between the severity of PTSD and the appraisal and management of uncertainty.

In a **parallel** relationship, the samples in the two strands are completely different, although they are usually drawn from the same population. Like identical sampling, parallel sampling can occur in either concurrent or sequential designs, and with any prioritization scheme. Parallel sampling is especially common in exploratory sequential designs: a phenomenon is explored with a relatively small sample of participants, and different samples are used to develop and test a new QUAN feature.

Example of Parallel Sampling
In a sequential qual → QUAN study, VanDevanter and colleagues (2014) explored challenges of nurses' deployment to New York City hospitals in the aftermath of a disaster, Hurricane Sandy. Initially, in-depth data were collected from a maximum variation sample of 20 nurses. Subsequently, an Internet-based survey was sent to all RNs employed at a New York Medical Center ($N = 1,668$).

In a **nested** relationship, participants in the qualitative strand are a subset of the participants in the quantitative strand. Nested sampling is especially common in studies with an explanatory design. Indeed, as discussed in the previous section, a variant of an explanatory design is geared to participant selection from the QUAN phase for in-depth scrutiny in the qual phase, to help explain the QUAN results. Examples of the kinds of nested sampling strategies include the sampling of participants who are "typical," who are "outliers," or who differ in their scores on significant predictors in the QUAN analysis. If the intent of a qualitative component is to offer detail and elaboration about phenomena and relationships captured quantitatively, then a nested sample is likely to enrich the researcher's understanding.

Example of Nested Sampling
Schneerson and Gale (2015) used framework analysis in their explanatory sequential study of cancer survivorship and self-management. Quantitative data were first collected in a survey of 445 adult cancer survivors with 10 different types of cancer. The researchers used purposive (nested) sampling to obtain a diverse sample for in-depth interviews. They sampled on three dimensions of diversity, using survey responses to guide the selection of 40 participants: cancer type, sociodemographic characteristics (age, gender, ethnicity), and patterns of cancer self-management.

Finally, a **multilevel** relationship involves selecting samples from different levels of a hierarchy. Usually this means sampling from different but related populations (e.g., hospital administrators, clinical staff, and patients).

Example of Multilevel Sampling
Horne and co-researchers (2015) studied practices and experiences of mouth hygiene in stroke care units in the UK. Questionnaires about policies and practices were completed by senior nurses in 11 stroke units. Qualitative data were collected in two focus groups with 10 healthcare professionals and by in-depth interviews with 5 stroke survivors.

The overall mixed method sampling plan should generate thorough datasets about the phenomenon under study and should be consistent with the intent of the mixed methods design.

Data Collection in a Mixed Methods Study

All data collection methods discussed in Chapters 14 (structured methods) and 24 (unstructured methods) can be creatively combined in a mixed method study. Thus, possible sources of data for MM studies include group and individual interviews, psychosocial scales, observations, biomarkers, records, diaries, performance tests, Internet postings, photographs, and physical artifacts. Mixed methods studies can involve both *intramethod mixing* (for example, structured and unstructured self-reports), and *intermethod mixing* (for example, biomarkers and in-depth interviews). Moreover, researchers can add a second strand to a study in which a secondary analysis of an existing dataset was undertaken.

Example of Mixed Methods With a Secondary Analysis

Kagawa and colleagues (2017) sought to understand the challenges in attaining the maternal role among women who began childbearing as adolescents in rural Mexico. They did a secondary analysis of baseline data from 1,381 mothers who had participated in a cluster-randomized trial in 2008, which yielded measures of mothers' well-being and parenting practices. In-depth data were obtained 5 years later in interviews with 30 mothers from towns that had been included in the trial (a parallel sample), and these data provided insight into the women's challenges in attaining the maternal role.

In selecting data sources for each strand of an MM study, a goal should be to use each method to address the research questions in a manner that enhances overall understanding of the problem. An important consideration concerns the methods' complementarity—that is, having the limitations of one method be offset by the strengths of the other.

Another consideration concerns the focus of the data being collected. For example, if the intent of the study is to compare or contrast results in the two strands, then common constructs/phenomena should be included in both datasets.

TIP Self-reports are the most common data source in both qualitative and quantitative nursing studies, and blending unstructured and structured self-report data is the most common approach in MM research as well (Beck & Harrison, 2016).

In concurrent designs, data collection decisions are made upfront. In sequential designs, however, MM researchers may have an emergent approach, with the types of data to be collected in the second phase shaped to some extent by findings in the first phase. Sequential designs thus have rich potential for incremental findings that build on one another.

In planning a data collection strategy, MM researchers may need to consider whether one method could introduce bias in the other method. For example, do closed-ended questions about a phenomenon affect how participants think about the phenomenon when asked in an unstructured fashion (or vice versa)? In other words, researchers should give some thought to whether one of the methods is an "intervention" that could influence people's behavior or responses.

One final issue concerns the possible need for additional data at the analysis and interpretation stage. If findings from the qualitative and quantitative strands conflict, it is sometimes useful to collect supplementary data to shed light on and possibly resolve contradictions or inconsistencies.

ANALYSIS OF MIXED METHODS DATA

Mixed methods data analysis involves analytic techniques applied to both the quantitative and qualitative datasets—and the integration of the two strands—to answer mixed methods questions. MM data analysis is one of the greatest challenges in doing mixed methods research. It is not uncommon, unfortunately, for the two strands of data to be analyzed and reported separately, without any integration of the findings. Beck and Harrison (2016), for example, found that nearly half of the 294 MM nursing studies they reviewed had no analytic or interpretive integration.

Integration is the central feature of a high-quality MM data analysis. The real benefits of MM research cannot be realized if there is no attempt to merge or connect results from the two strands, and to develop interpretations based on integrated understandings. As eloquently observed by Sandelowski (2003), a high-quality MM analysis merges measurement with meaning, graphs with graphical accounts, and tables with tableaux. Some MM researchers acknowledge that analytic integration "was the key to unfolding the complex relationships in the topic of the study" (Bazely, 2009b, p. 205).

Students often want specific guidance about how to analyze their data, but there are no rules for MM data analysis and integration. Decisions about how to blend the datasets hinge on several factors. Research design, especially sequencing of strands, strongly affects analytic choices. Sampling is another important factor. Several analytic techniques are appropriate only for identical and nested samples, i.e., for sampling plans with both qualitative and quantitative data obtained from the same people.

This section describes a few analytics considerations in MM studies, but our presentation is far from comprehensive. Additional resources should be consulted, such as the work of Bazely (2009a, 2009b, 2012) and Creswell and Plano Clark (2018).

Decisions in Analyzing Mixed Methods Data

Before pursuing a specific analytic strategy, MM researchers often make several preliminary decisions that will affect how they proceed. Our list is not exhaustive but is meant to encourage preanalytic thinking about several issues.

1. *What will be the unit of analysis?* The unit usually is individual participants, but other options include events (Happ et al., 2006) or subgroups of people. If the MM design is multilevel, the levels are usually the unit of primary interest.
2. *Will either type of data be converted or transformed?* Sometimes researchers convert their qualitative data into quantitative data, and vice versa. We discuss such strategies later in this section and in the Supplement to this chapter on thePoint. **S**
3. *Will direct comparisons be made between the qualitative and quantitative data—and, if so, at what level will the comparisons be made?* In nested and identical sampling designs, comparisons can be made at the individual level—for example, comparing each participant's score

on a health promotion scale with how he or she described lifestyle and activities in in-depth interviews. Comparisons can also be made between subgroups—for example, how high scorers on the health promotion scale differ from low scorers in terms of themes that emerge in the qualitative analysis. Finally, overall comparisons are possible—for example, is the picture of the salience of health promotion consistent in the qualitative and quantitative datasets? Comparisons are a major feature of convergent designs but are sometimes used in other MM designs.

4. *Will integration involve the use of specialized software?* Tremendous advances have been made regarding software for analytic integration in MM studies. Leading software include Dedoose, QDA Miner, and MAXQDA. Statistical packages such as SPSS now have text analyses software than can categorize text responses and combine them with other quantitative variables. Even if specialized software for combining qualitative and quantitative data is not used, MM researchers can use basic spreadsheets to good advantage.

Integration Intent in Mixed Methods Data Analysis

The intent of analytic integration in MM studies reflects the researcher's analytic goal. As discussed earlier, intent is a key issue in selecting an MM design, and the design affects the analytic procedures that are feasible and productive. In QUAL + QUAL convergent designs, the integration intent is to *merge* the results, and to develop integrated mixed methods results and interpretations that are comprehensive and confirmatory and that expand understanding.

In explanatory sequential designs, the intent is to *connect* the results in a sequential integration. The connected results are used to provide a strong explanation (from the qual strand) of specific results from the QUAN strand. The analytic goal is to shed light on particular quantitative findings with rich, insightful, and nuanced information—not to compare or contrast findings from the two strands. The integrated interpretation should reveal the added value of the qualitative component.

Sequential integration is also a feature in exploratory designs, in which the intent is to *build* (generate) a contextually appropriate quantitative feature (e.g., an intervention or measure) based on an in-depth exploration in the initial phase. Integrated interpretations are designed to reveal how the quantitative results support the integrity and contextual specificity of the newly developed feature.

In developing an analytic plan, it is also important to consider intent in terms of evidence-based practice goals: how can the data best be analyzed and integrated to yield high-quality evidence for practicing nurses?

> **TIP** Uprichard and Dawney (2019) have observed that while data integration is a sensible *goal*, it is not always successfully achieved. They challenge "the presupposition that it is necessarily the optimal *outcome* of mixed methods research" (p. 19). They offered suggestions for how to use a strategy they call *diffraction* as an approach that supports instances where the data strands do not integrate or "cohere."

Data Analysis Procedures in Mixed Methods Research

This section describes some specific MM analytic procedures, many of which are especially common in convergent designs. In such designs, quantitative data are analyzed using statistical techniques and qualitative data are analyzed using qualitative analysis methods (often via content or framework analysis), both according to standards of excellence for each method. Findings from the two separate analyses are then drawn together to answer the mixed methods question.

In convergent designs, the focus of the MM analysis is on *comparing* and *contrasting* the two sets of findings. The two sets of results for a given construct are compared to explore ways in which they confirm, disconfirm, qualify, or expand each other. One approach to facilitate the comparison is to create

matrices, and another strategy is to transform the data. Both methods are described later in this section.

Some researchers formally "audit" the extent to which there is congruence. For example, Tonkin-Crine and colleagues (2016) used a "triangulation protocol" to compare four sets of data in a multinational trial of the effectiveness of physician training in communication skills. The protocol was used to classify pairwise findings from two strands (QUAL and QUAN) and two perspectives (physicians and patients) into one of four categories: agreement, partial agreement, dissonance, or "silence" (i.e., an instance in which only one dataset of the two being compared contained data on a particular finding).

> **Example of Analytic Integration in a Convergent Design**
>
> Goldsmith and colleagues (2018) studied the pain management experiences of recently discharged adult trauma patients and the discharge practices of the treating hospital, based on data from hospital records and patients' responses to a structured questionnaire. Twelve patients were purposively recruited to participate in in-depth interviews. Data relating to pain management from both datasets were merged and compared to produce a greater understanding of the reasons for patients' pain management practices.

Analytic integration can also occur in sequential designs—although such integration is often what Bazely (2009a) called "integration 'on the way'" (p. 92) rather than formal integration at the end of the study. That is, the analysis of one data strand is interpreted and used to inform the design and analysis of the second strand. An overall integration of the two strands should also occur to address the MM question, but sometimes such integration does not occur.

Bazely (2009a) has described what she called *iterative analysis*, which involves ongoing interpretive feedback loops. Iterative analysis involves "taking what is learned in one stage of a project into a further stage to inform that data collection or analysis, and then on again for refinement or development through one or more subsequent iterations" (p. 109). She offered as an example a study in which a researcher developed a formal instrument based on themes from in-depth phenomenologic interviews.

The factor analytic results from psychometric testing of the scale were then taken back to the phenomenologic data for further thematic exploration. Similarly, Mendlinger and Cwikel (2008) provided a useful illustration of how "spiraling" between qualitative and quantitative data contributed to an integration of their data strands—a strategy that has been used by nurse researchers trying to resolve problems with the Japanese translation of a widely used measure of depression (St. Arnaud et al., 2016).

Constructing Meta-Matrices

One approach to analytic integration in MM studies involves the use of matrices, a method that can be used to identify patterns and make comparisons across data sources if identical or nested sampling was used. Matrices are a method that has been advocated for qualitative data analysis (Miles et al., 2014) and are an explicit feature of framework analysis, which we described in Chapter 25 (Gale et al., 2013). The concept has gained popularity among MM researchers.

In a meta-matrix, researchers array information from qualitative and quantitative data sources. In a typical case-by-variable meta-matrix, the rows correspond to cases—to individual participants. Then, for each participant, data from multiple data sources are entered in the columns, so that the analyst can see at a glance such information as demographic information, scores on psychosocial measures, responses to probing open-ended questions (e.g., verbatim narratives), hospital record data (e.g., biomarker data), and observational field notes. A third dimension can be added if, for example, there are multiple sources of data relating to multiple constructs (e.g., depression, pain). A third dimension can also be used if the qualitative and quantitative data have been collected longitudinally.

Patterns of regularities, as well as anomalies, often come to light through detailed inspection of meta-matrices. Their key advantage is that they allow for fuller exploration of all data sources simultaneously. The construction of a meta-matrix also allows researchers to explore whether statistical conclusions are supported by the qualitative data for individual study participants, and vice versa.

A simplified example of a meta-matrix for a study of sleep problems is presented in Figure 27.2. This example shows only five cases and a handful of variables/constructs, but it illustrates how diverse information can be displayed to facilitate inferences about patterns and relationships. It also suggests, however, that such meta-matrices may be unwieldy with large samples—although one strategy is to have separate matrices for distinct subgroups within a large sample (e.g., in our example, those with high vs. low levels of fatigue). Meta-matrix data such as those portrayed in Figure 27.2 can easily be entered in spreadsheet software and several analytic software packages. Software has important advantages over manual methods—in particular, the ability to sort and re-sort the data to identify patterns.

> **Example of a Study Using a Meta-Matrix**
> Valenta and colleagues (2018) are undertaking a mixed method study to test the side effects of a pain self-management intervention for cancer outpatients. Their protocol describes the collection of quantitative data on side effects and patient knowledge and qualitative data on family caregivers' involvement. They described how "quantitative and qualitative results will be combined within a mixed method matrix" (p. 1).

Transforming Quantitative and Qualitative Data

A technique that can be used in analytic and interpretive integration in mixed methods research involves converting data of one type into data of another type. Qualitative data are sometimes converted into numeric codes that can be analyzed quantitatively (**quantitizing**). It is also possible to transform quantitative data into qualitative information (**qualitizing**). Such transformed data can be included in meta-matrices.

Although some qualitative researchers believe that quantitizing is inappropriate, Sandelowski (2001) argued that some amount of quantitizing occurs regularly. She noted that every time qualitative researchers use terms such as *a few, many,* or *most*, they are implicitly conveying quantitative information about the frequency of occurrence of a theme or pattern. Quantification of qualitative

Case	Pseudonym	Age	Sex	Average Hours of Sleep Daily	Current Fatigue Level Rating[a]	Use of Sleep Medi-cation[b]	Fatigue Narrative
1	Anna	57	F	6.0	9	1	I *never* sleep through the night. I usually don't have much trouble falling asleep, but I just can't *stay* asleep. There is never a day when I don't wake up exhausted.
2	Jonathan	45	M	5.5	5	1	I've never really needed all that much sleep. Ever since I was in college, I get by with just a few hours and I feel just fine.
3	Claire	49	F	8.0	2	1	I'm a good sleeper, I can fall asleep anywhere, anytime. So, I get what I need.
4	Rosalind	51	F	7.0	7	2	I sleep just fine, but my husband is an insomniac, and a pain in my neck. When he's awake, he wants me awake, too!
5	Michael	54	M	7.5	6	3	I like my shut-eye. I can't concentrate if I don't get enough. I do what I have to, which usually means going to bed before anyone else and taking sleeping pills.

[a]Rating scale anchors: 0 = extremely energetic, 10 = totally exhausted
[b]Use of medication codes: 1 = Never, 2 = Occasionally, 3 = Regularly

FIGURE 27.2 Fictitious example of a meta-matrix with raw qualitative data.

data can sometimes offer benefits. Sandelowski described how this strategy can be used to achieve two important goals:

- *Generating meaning from qualitative data.* If qualitative data are displayed in a quantitative fashion (e.g., by displaying frequencies of certain phenomena), *patterns* sometimes emerge with greater clarity than they might have had the researchers simply relied on their impressions.
- *Documenting and confirming conclusions.* The use of numbers can assure people that researchers' conclusions are valid. Researchers can be more confident that the data are fully accounted for if they document the extent to which emerging patterns were observed—or *not* observed. Sandelowski noted that quantitizing can address some pitfalls of qualitative analysis, which include giving too much weight to dramatic or vivid accounts, giving too little weight to disconfirming cases, and smoothing out variation to clean up some of the "messiness" of human experience.

In a more recent article, Sandelowski and her colleagues (2009) noted that quantitizing can also serve the critical function of encouraging researchers to think about and interact with their data. They noted that quantitizing, "when used creatively, critically, and reflexively, can show the complexity of qualitative data and, thereby the 'multivariate nature' of the experiential worlds researchers seek to understand" (p. 219). Such higher-level understanding of a phenomenon is an overarching goal of many MM studies.

Procedures for qualitizing quantitative data and quantitizing qualitative data are described in the Supplement to this chapter on thePoint. 🔊

Presenting Integrated Mixed Methods Results: Joint Displays

Integrated mixed methods results are often reported in a narrative fashion. In convergent designs, narrative presentations often take the form of direct comparisons of the QUAN and QUAL findings, or QUAL data are used to illustrate the statistical findings using direct quotes. Narrative presentations are often supplemented with tables or figures that highlight features of the integrated results. A **joint display** has been defined as a way "to integrate the data by bringing the data together through a visual means to draw out new insights beyond the information

Use of Sleep Medication	Themes from In-Depth Interviews		
	The Role of Others	**Health Issues**	**Patterns of Sleep**
Never (*n* = 18, 45%)	• No one in household with sleeping problems • No pets in household	• No special health problems • Avoids *all* medication	• Never a problem falling asleep • Lifelong history of being good sleeper • Despite problems, averse to sleeping aids
Occasionally (*n* = 16, 40%)	• Spouse sleeping problems • Teens coming home late • Pet disturbances	• Stressful job • On a diet causing jitters • Anxiety about upcoming medical procedures/tests	• Problem staying asleep, not falling asleep • Sleeping only a problem if under stress • Frequent napping
Regularly (*n* = 6, 15%)	• Spouse works late or irregular shift • Infant in household • Severely ill family member	• Recent hospitalization • Diagnosed with life-threatening illness • Severely depressed	• Problems arise if medications not taken • Daily battles with insomnia

FIGURE 27.3 Ficitious example of a summary meta-matrix.

gained from the separate quantitative and qualitative results" (Fetters et al., 2013, p. 2143).

Guetterman and colleagues (2015) have written about the importance of joint displays in helping readers understand how mixed methods contribute new insights and enriched understanding. Their paper provides example of joint displays for all three Creswell and Plano Clark's (2018) core designs from the health literature.

Although there are no "rules" or standard formats for joint MM displays, certain types are especially common. One is a two-dimensional *statistics-by-theme* display, a kind of crosstabulation table that can be used when some (or all) participants are in both strands of a convergent or explanatory MM study. For example, for our fictitious sleep problem study (Figure 27.2), we could create a joint display that summarizes key themes from the QUAL data for subgroups defined by responses to a structured question on the use of sleep medication, as shown in Figure 27.3. Another statistics-by-theme possibility, again for our fictitious sleep study, would be to divide the sample into subgroups based on a QUAN measure (e.g., high scorers vs. low scorers on the fatigue measure), and then include actual quotes from the QUAL strand in the display.

Another type of joint display is what Guetterman and colleagues (2015) refer to as a *side-by-side*

joint display. Such displays typically put statistical results in one column and relevant qualitative results or data in another column. Side-by-side displays can be presented in tables or in figures.

Happ and colleagues' (2006) article is another useful resource for thinking about joint MM displays. Their paper included examples of using bar charts to show frequencies of quantitized qualitative data. Another type of joint display is a *modified stem leaf plot*. In their example from a study of health locus of control in lung transplant recipients, behaviors that were considered "internality behaviors" from unstructured data sources were listed on one side, and the identification numbers of the lung transplant recipients who exhibited those behaviors were listed on the right. The result was a re-presentation of the qualitative data in a quantitative manner that "provided a visual sense of the proportion of recipients who exhibited the internality behaviors" (p. S46). The display prompted further analyses about commonalities and differences among recipients' behaviors.

Another clever use of visualization in the Happ et al. (2006) paper involved the construction of a scatterplot. The values along the vertical axis were internality scores, those along the horizontal axis were externality scores. The scatterplot space was divided into quadrants (e.g., high internality, high externality) that corresponded to four profiles of health locus of control beliefs. The identification numbers of participants were then plotted in the two-dimensional space. This visual display allowed the researchers to more clearly identify clusterings and "outliers" that were difficult to identify from quantitative analysis alone. This and other joint displays from the Happ paper are included in the Toolkit of the accompanying *Resource Manual.* ⊗

Although most joint displays are for studies in which the QUAN and QUAL samples are identical or nested, joint displays from studies using parallel samples can sometimes be created. For example, Guetterman and colleagues (2015) showed a joint display for an instrument development MM study (exploratory), in which information from the QUAL strand was shown in one column and corresponding items from the QUAN strand in another.

Innovative ideas for joint displays appear regularly in mixed methods papers. For example, Johnson and colleagues (2019) described a technique they called the "Pillar Integration Process," which is an approach for building a "pillar" to integrate QUAN data and QUAL codes. Clearly, data analysis in mixed methods research is ripe with opportunities for creative blending and juxtaposition of data visually. Further advice regarding joint displays of information from mixed methods analyses is provided by Onwuegbuzie and Dickinson (2008) and Creswell and Plano Clark (2018).

Example of an MM Study With Joint Displays

Pedersen and colleagues (2017) undertook an MM study of women being treated for breast cancer to better understand the association between changes in their body weight and their perceptions of their bodies and their selves. Joint displays of the women's physiological data and their responses to probing questions about their changing bodies suggested that even small weight gains and weight losses were associated with feared recurrence of breast cancer. Two of their joint displays are shown in the Toolkit. ⊗

Meta-Inferences in Mixed Methods Research

It has been argued that the most important step in mixed methods studies is when the integrated findings from the qualitative and quantitative components are incorporated into an overall conceptualization that effectively answers the overarching mixed methods question. To achieve this, *active* interpretation and exploration of the results are required.

In convergent designs, interpretations focus on making sense of the degree to which the findings converge. Most researchers consider that an ideal situation occurs when findings from each strand are consistent and shed complementary perspectives on the phenomenon of interest. Yet, many MM scholars have noted the critical role that divergent results can play in advancing knowledge because they may yield opportunities for further generative work.

Moffatt and colleagues (2006) suggested possible steps to take when MM findings conflict. Their study involved quantitative data from 126 participants in a clinical trial and in-depth data from a purposive nested sample of 25 of them. The quantitative results suggested that the intervention (which was designed to improve health and social outcomes for older people) was not successful, yet the qualitative data suggested wide-ranging improvements. The researchers suggested six ways of further exploring the discrepancy: (1) treating the methods as fundamentally different; (2) examining rigor in the respective strands; (3) exploring dataset comparability; (4) collecting additional data; (5) exploring intervention processes; and (6) exploring whether the outcomes of the two components were really matched. Creswell and Plano Clark (2018) suggest that perhaps the easiest way to address discordant results is to return to the databases to look for clues and ways to resolve the discrepancy.

Although many MM scholars discuss convergence-divergence of results as a dichotomy, in fact, it is often the case that interpretive integration leads to a nuanced portrayal of the phenomenon because results are neither precisely convergent nor divergent. Thus, although the MM research question being addressed may be, "To what extent do the quantitative and qualitative data converge?", another important question might be, "How do the findings from one strand qualify, delimit, or temper findings from the other?".

An example comes from an MM study of one of this book's authors, whose convergent design involved a survey of nearly 4,000 low-income women and in-depth interviews with 67 women from a parallel sample (Polit et al., 2000). The analyses focused on hunger and food insecurity, and in both samples, about half the women were food insecure—results that appeared convergent. Yet, the in-depth interviews revealed that the term "food secure" in low-income urban families may be misleading: Mothers in the qualitative sample had to *struggle* enormously to be food secure, piecing together with great effort numerous strategies to provide an adequate amount of food for themselves and their children. This led the authors to hypothesize that *food security* is experienced differently in poor versus middle-class families— and is perhaps a totally different phenomenon.

In explanatory designs, interpretations are typically geared to understanding how the qualitative results provide a deeper understanding of the statistical results. In some cases, the interpretation could suggest possible new quantitative analyses based on the qualitative-informed explanations. Interpretations in exploratory sequential designs hinge on an analysis of how the new quantitative feature (e.g., a new instrument) was enriched through the insights provided in the initial qualitative strand.

In arriving at meta-inferences in an MM study, researchers must actively engage in meaning making. Interpretation can be enhanced by allowing the two strands of a study to "talk to each other" in a meaningful, reflexive, and thought-provoking way. Teddlie and Tashakkori (2009) offered several guidelines for making appropriate inferences at the interpretive stage of an MM study. Their "golden rule" is especially noteworthy: "*Know thy participants*" (p. 289). Mixed methods research offers great potential for getting a rounded picture of the complex lives of human beings.

QUALITY CRITERIA IN MIXED METHODS RESEARCH

The issue of quality criteria for mixed methods research has received considerable recent attention, in part because several controversies have emerged. One issue is similar to the one discussed in Chapter 26—what to *call* the quality goal. Terms like *quality, rigor,* and *validity* have been recommended by some, but rejected by others. Some experts have proposed terms that are deliberately different from those used in QUAN or QUAL studies. One prominent team of scholars, for example, have proposed *inference quality* as the MM substitute for validity (Teddlie & Tashakkori, 2009), while another team suggested the term *legitimation* (Onwuegbuzie & Johnson, 2006). Creswell and Plano Clark (2018) and other experts are urging greater consistency in quality terminology, but it is too early in the development of MM methodology to know what terms will be adopted.

> **TIP** In Teddlie and Tashakkori's (2009) classic framework, *inference quality* incorporates notions of both internal validity and statistical conclusion validity within a quantitative framework, and credibility within a qualitative framework. Inference quality essentially refers to the believability and accuracy of the inductively and deductively derived conclusions from an MM study. They also proposed *inference transferability* as a criterion that encompasses external validity (QUAN) and transferability (QUAL). Inference transferability is the degree to which the mixed methods conclusions can be applied to other similar people, contexts, settings, and time periods.

In terms of criteria to guide efforts to attain high quality, dozens of quality criteria frameworks for MM studies have been proposed. Fàbregues and Molina-Azorin (2017) undertook a systematic review of the MM literature and offered a metasummary of the most prevalent quality criteria that have been proposed. Some criteria concern excellence in reporting MM research and are helpful to those wishing to critically appraise a mixed methods study. Several criteria for *doing* high-quality mixed methods research, as proposed in many frameworks in Fàbregues and Molina-Azorin's (2017) review, are as follows:

1. A strong rationale exists for collecting and analyzing both QUAN and QUAL data.
2. The QUAN and QUAL strands are well implemented and adhere to the quality criteria of each tradition.

3. The QUAN and QUAL components of the study are well integrated.
4. The sampling, data collection, and data analysis procedures for both strands are linked to the study intent and the research questions.
5. Inferences are consistent with the study findings and with the study intent.

In a subsequent study, Fàbregues and colleagues (2018) compared how researchers in different disciplines conceptualized and operationalized quality in MM research. An international sample of 44 MM researchers, including 11 in nursing, were interviewed about their perspectives on quality. All five quality criteria noted earlier were highly rated by these experts, and the most frequently mentioned quality criteria were equally prevalent in the four disciplinary groups. However, nurses were especially likely to believe that the MM research community should reach a consensus on a set of quality criteria for conducting and appraising MM studies.

CRITICAL APPRAISAL OF MIXED METHODS RESEARCH

Individual components of mixed methods studies can be critically appraised using guidelines we have offered throughout this book. Key appraisal questions for quantitative studies (Box 5.2) and qualitative studies (Box 5.3) were presented in Chapter 5.

Box 27.1, which is also found in the Toolkit, offers supplementary questions that are specific to the mixed methods aspects of a study. ✪ Many of these questions were derived from the systematic review of Fàbregues and Molina-Azorin (2017) and therefore reflect a synthesis of widely promoted criteria for critical appraisals of mixed methods study. Formal tools for appraising mixed methods studies, such as the Mixed Methods Appraisal Tool (MMAT) have also been developed (Hong et al., 2018).

BOX 27.1   Guidelines for Critically Appraising Mixed Methods Studies

1. Did the researcher provide an explicit and persuasive rationale for conducting a mixed methods (MM) study?
2. Did the researcher state an overarching MM intent and an explicit MM question?
3. Did the researcher identify the research design? Was the design clearly described in terms of purpose, sequencing, and priority? Is the design appropriate for the research questions and study intent? Was the design concurrent or sequential? Which strand (if either) was given priority? Was mixed methods design notation (or a visual diagram) used to communicate key aspects of the design?
4. What sampling strategy was used (identical, parallel, nested, multilevel), and was this strategy appropriate for the study intent? Was the sampling strategy described in sufficient detail?
5. How were study data gathered? Were the methods appropriate for the study intent? In sequential designs, did the second-phase data collection (and sampling) flow from the analysis of data gathered in the initial phase?
6. Were the qualitative and quantitative components carefully implemented? Were procedures used to enhance rigor/trustworthiness of the components?
7. Were data analysis procedures sufficiently described? What specific analytic techniques were used to promote analytic integration (e.g., was data transformation or a meta-matrix used)? Do the findings answer the mixed methods question? Were joint displays effectively used to communicate mixed methods findings?
8. Was the process of integrating the strands described? How did integration occur? Were the components integrated in an effective manner?
9. Do the integrated findings yield richly textured information and added-value insights? If there were inconsistencies between the strands, were they sufficiently described? If the findings from each strand are conflicting or qualifying, are well-conceived explanations for the discrepancies offered?
10. Are the researcher's meta-inferences consistent with the individual findings? Are the inferences consistent with the study intent? Do the meta-inferences adequately encompass and integrate inferences from each strand?

The overarching consideration in MM studies is whether true integration of the strands occurred and contributed to strong meta-inferences about the phenomenon under scrutiny. Integration is the cornerstone for the added value of MM research—it is a foundational principle. Researchers who report their QUAL and QUAN findings in separate papers should, ideally, write a third integrative paper. The separate single-method (QUAL or QUAN) papers should communicate, in the Discussion section, the kinds of integrative work that has been or will be undertaken.

> **TIP** In critically appraising single-method qualitative or quantitative studies, it is worth considering whether a mixed methods approach would have enhanced the insights and value of the research.

RESEARCH EXAMPLE OF A MIXED METHODS STUDY

Study: Secondary traumatic stress in NICU nurses: A mixed methods study (Beck, Cusson, & Gable, 2017).

Statement of Purpose: The purposes of this study were to assess the pervasiveness of secondary traumatic stress (STS) in NICU nurses and to explore nurses' traumatic experiences caring for critically ill infants. The researchers asked three research questions: (1) What are the prevalence and severity of STS in nurses who care for critically ill infants in the NICU? (2) What are the traumatic experiences of nurses who care for critically ill infants in the NICU? And (3) How do the quantitative and qualitative sets of results develop a more complete picture of secondary traumatic stress in NICU nurses?

Methods: A convergent design (QUAL + QUAN) was used, i.e., independent strands of equal-priority data were collected in a single phase. (A diagram showing their MM design is presented in the Toolkit. ✪) Members of the National Association of Neonatal Nurses were sent an email invitation that included a link to an online survey. A total of 175 nurses completed the survey, which included the 17-item Secondary Traumatic Stress Scale (STSS) to measure the existence and severity of STS. Respondents were also asked to respond to the following probing question: "Please describe in as much detail as you can remember your traumatic experiences caring for critically ill infants in the NICU. Specific examples of points that you are making are extremely valuable" (p. 480). A nested sample of 109 nurses provided in-depth answers to the QUAL question.

Data Analysis and Integration: Statistical methods were used to answer research question 1. For example, descriptive statistics were used to characterize the prevalence and severity of STS, and correlation procedures were used to assess the relationship between NICU nurses' background characteristics and their STSS scores. Question 2 was addressed using a content analysis of the qualitative data on the nurses' actual experiences. Some qualitative data were also quantitized. For example, the researchers coded qualitative segments according to their correspondence to the three subscales of the STSS—Arousal, Intrusion, and Avoidance. These codes were then counted for presence/absence in the in-depth responses to the open-ended question. The mixed methods question was addressed by integrating quotes and statistics, and by creating joint displays.

Key Findings: In this sample, 29% of the NICU nurses reported high to severe STS; 35% screened positive for PTSD due to attending traumatic births. The total STSS scores were unrelated to any demographic characteristics, such as gender, age, or years practicing in the NICU. The subscale with the highest mean score was Arousal (e.g., "I had trouble sleeping"). The next highest score was for Intrusion (e.g., "I thought about my work with patients when I didn't want to"). Intrusion-related comments from the nurses' narrative descriptions were especially frequent. Figure 27.4 shows a side-by-side joint display with quantitative subscale results on the left and illustrative qualitative results on the right. In the content analysis of the qualitative data, five themes emerged: What intensified NICU nurses' traumatic experiences: Multiple scenarios; Parents insisting on aggressive treatment: So distressing; Baby torture: Performing painful procedures; Questioning their skills: Did I do enough?; and The grief of the family: It is contagious. (A dendrogram for the first theme is included in the Toolkit. ✪) The integrated QUAL and QUAN results provided a richer and more complete picture of both the prevalence of STS in NICU nurses and their complex experiences with it.

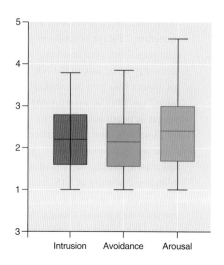

A highly traumatic experience that continues to haunt me in my dreams. These situations pop into my head randomly, even when I'm not at work, and continue to upset me enough to bring tears.

I have anxiety every time I enter that room and try to avoid caring for infants there. I go home wanting to hide and not talk to anyone about the event.

I can't sleep before going to work. I'm impulsive and irritable around others. I feel mentally drained and have difficulty concentrating. It takes me longer to finish a task.

FIGURE 27.4 Joint display from Beck et al.'s (2017) study of secondary traumatic stress in NICU nurses. The vertical axis shows values of scale item responses, from 1 (*never*) to 5 (*very often*). Each boxplot represents the middle 50% of cases, between the 25th and 75th percentiles. The right side includes illustrative quotes from the NICU nurses' qualitative data. Color coding of the boxplot and the quotes helps to match the quantitative and qualitative responses. (Adapted with permission from Beck, C. T., Cusson, R., & Gable, R. (2017). Secondary traumatic stress in NICU nurses: A mixed methods study. *Advances in Neonatal Care, 17*, 478–488.)

SUMMARY POINTS

- **Mixed methods** (MM) research involves the collection, analysis, and integration of both qualitative and quantitative data within a study or coordinated set of studies, often with an overarching goal of achieving enhanced insights.
- Mixed methods research has numerous advantages, including the complementarity of qualitative and quantitative data and the practicality of using methods that best address a question. MM research has many applications, including the development and testing of instruments, interventions, and programs.
- The paradigm often associated with MM research is **pragmatism**, which is considered to offer an umbrella worldview and has as a major tenet "the dictatorship of the research question."
- Mixed methods studies involve asking at least two questions that require different types of data, but high-quality MM research also asks integrative questions that focus on linking the two strands.

- **Integration** is a central feature of MM research—a centerpiece that distinguishes it from other methodologies. Integration ideally occurs throughout a project.
- Key decisions in designing an MM study involve how to sequence the components, which **strand** (if either) will be given priority, and how to integrate the two strands. Researchers also decide whether to use a "fixed" MM design or an emergent one that is devised as the study unfolds.
- In terms of **sequencing**, MM designs are either **concurrent designs** (both strands occurring in one simultaneous phase) or **sequential designs** (one strand occurring prior to and informing the second strand).
- Notation for MM research often designates both **priority**—all capital letters for the *dominant strand* and all lower-case letters for the *nondominant strand*—and sequence. An arrow is used for sequential designs, and a "+" is used for concurrent designs. QUAL → quan, for example, is a sequential, qualitative-dominant design.
- *Core designs* for MM research in the Creswell and Plano Clark taxonomy include the

convergent design (QUAL + QUAN); **explanatory sequential design** (QUAN → qual or quan → QUAL); and **exploratory sequential design** (e.g., QUAL → quan + qual → QUAN). More complex MM designs are sometimes adopted, involving intersecting core designs with other components or approaches.

- Sampling strategies can be described as **identical** (the same participants are in both strands); **nested** (some participants from one strand are in the other strand); **parallel** (participants are either in one strand or the other, drawn from the same population); or **multilevel** (participants are not the same and are drawn from different populations at different levels in a hierarchy).
- Data collection in MM research can involve all methods of structured and unstructured data. In sequential designs, decisions about data collection for the second phase often are based on findings from the first phase.
- Data analysis in MM research should involve integration of the strands, to arrive at **meta-inferences** about the phenomenon under study. The integrative focus in many concurrent designs is to assess congruence and to explore complementarity.
- Methods of integration of qualitative and quantitative data during analysis include **data transformations**, such as qualitizing quantitative data or quantitizing qualitative data, and the use of a **meta-matrix** in which both qualitative and quantitative data are arrayed in a spreadsheet-type matrix.
- **Joint displays** are visual displays, either in tables or figures, that present integrated findings from both the qualitative and quantitative strands.
- Goals and criteria for the integrity of MM studies are still evolving. One framework proposes the goals of *inference quality* (the believability and accuracy of inductively and deductively derived conclusions) and *inference transferability* (the degree to which conclusions can be applied to other similar people or contexts).
- A key criterion for the conduct of an MM study is the rigorous implementation of both strands, each according to the quality criteria of each. Another criterion is thoughtful and thorough integration of the two strands.

STUDY ACTIVITIES

Study activities are available to instructors on thePoint.

REFERENCES CITED IN CHAPTER 27

Alabdulaziz, H., Moss, C., & Copnell, B. (2017). Paediatric nurses' perceptions and practices of family-centred care in Saudi hospitals: A mixed methods study. *International Journal of Nursing Studies, 69*, 66–77.

Baron Nelson, M., Riley, K., & Arellano, K. (2018). Adding a parent to the brain tumor team: Evaluating a peer support intervention for parents of children with brain tumors. *Journal of Pediatric Oncology Nursing, 35*, 218–228.

Bazely, P. (2009a). Analysing mixed methods data. In Andrew, S., & Halcomb, E. (Eds.), *Mixed methods research for nursing and the health sciences* (pp. 84–117). Oxford: Blackwell-Wiley.

Bazely, P. (2009b). Integrating data analyses in mixed methods research. *Journal of Mixed Methods Research, 3*, 203–207.

Bazely, P. (2012). Integrative strategies for mixed data sources. *American Behavioral Scientist, 56*, 814–828.

Beck, C. T., Cusson, R., & Gable, R. (2017). Secondary traumatic stress in NICU nurses: A mixed methods study. *Advances in Neonatal Care, 17*, 478–488.

Beck, C. T., Eaton, C., & Gable, R. (2016). Vicarious post-traumatic growth in labor and delivery nurses. *Journal of Obstetric, Gynecologic, & Neonatal Nurses, 45*, 801–812.

**Beck, C. T., & Harrison, L. (2016). Mixed methods research in the discipline of nursing. *Advances in Nursing Science, 39*, 224–234.

Bhandari, P., & Kim, M. (2016). Self-care behaviors of Nepalese adults with Type 2 diabetes. *Nursing Research, 65*, 202–214.

Creamer, E. (2018). *An introduction to fully integrated mixed methods research*. Thousand Oaks, CA: Sage Publications.

*Creswell, J., Klassen, A., Plano Clark, V., & Smith, K. (2011). *Best practices for mixed methods research in the health sciences*. Washington, DC: NIH.

Creswell, J. W., & Plano Clark, V. L. (2018). *Designing and conducting mixed methods research* (3rd ed.). Thousand Oaks, CA: Sage Publications.

Fàbregues, S., & Molina-Azorin, J. (2017). Addressing quality in mixed methods research: A review and recommendations for a future agenda. *Quality & Quantity, 51*, 2847–2863.

Fàbregues, S., Pare, M., & Meneses, J. (2018). Operationalizing and conceptualizing quality in mixed methods research: A multiple case study of the disciplines of education, nursing, psychology, and sociology. *Journal of Mixed Methods Research*. doi:10.1177/1558689817751774.

*Fetters, M., Curry, L., & Creswell, J. (2013). Achieving integration in mixed methods designs: Principles and practices. *Health Services Research, 48*, 2134–2156.

Fetters, M., & Freshwater, D. (2015). The 1 + 1 = 3 integration challenge. *Journal of Mixed Methods Research, 9*, 115–117.

Fetters, M., & Molina-Azorin, J. (2017a). Principles for bringing new and divesting of old language of the field. *Journal of Mixed Methods Research, 11*, 3–10.

Fetters, M., & Molina-Azorin, J. (2017b). The mixed methods research integration trilogy and its dimensions. *Journal of Mixed Methods Research, 11*, 291–307.

Fetters, M., & Molina-Azorin, J. (2017c). Perspectives of past editors on the current state of the field and future directions. *Journal of Mixed Methods Research, 11*, 423–432.

Fletcher, B., Schumacher, K., Cohen, M., Kupzyk, K., & Lydiatt, W. (2019). Understanding functional communication in head and neck cancer survivors using a mixed methods design. *Cancer Nursing, 42*, 119–128.

Frels, R., Newman, I., & Newman, C. (2015). Mentoring the next generation in mixed methods research. In Hesse-Biber, S., & Johnson, R., (Eds.), *The Oxford handbook of multimethod and mixed methods research inquiry* (pp. 333–353). New York, NY: Oxford University Press.

*Gale, N., Heath, G., Cameron, E., Rashid, S., & Redwood, S. (2013). Using the Framework Method for the analysis of qualitative data in multi-disciplinary health research. *BMC Medical Research Methodology, 13*, 117.

Goldsmith, H., McCloughen, A., & Curtis, K. (2018). Using the trauma patient experience and evaluation of hospital discharge practices to inform practice change: A mixed methods study. *Journal of Clinical Nursing, 27*, 1589–1598.

Guetterman, T., Babchuk, W., Smith, M., & Stevens, J. (2019). Contemporary approaches to mixed methods-grounded theory research. *Journal of Mixed Methods Research, 93*, S154–S163.

*Guetterman, T., Fetters, M., & Creswell, J. (2015). Integrating quantitative and qualitative results in health science mixed methods research through joint displays. *Annals of Family Medicine, 13*, 554–561.

Hall, H., Brosnan, C., Cant, R., Collins, M., & Leach, M. (2018). Nurses' attitudes and behavior towards patients' use of complementary therapies: A mixed methods study. *Journal of Advanced Nursing, 74*, 1649–1658.

Happ, M., Dabbs, A., Tate, J., Hricik, A., & Erlen, J. (2006). Exemplars of mixed methods data combination and analysis. *Nursing Research, 55*, S43–S49.

Hesse-Biber, S. (2016). Doing interdisciplinary mixed methods health care research. *Qualitative Health Research, 26*, 649–658.

Hong, Q., Gonzalez-Reyes, A., & Pluye, P. (2018). Improving the usefulness of a tool for appraising the quality of qualitative, quantitative and mixed methods studies, the Mixed Methods Appraisal Tool (MMAT). *Journal of Evaluation in Clinical Practice, 24*, 459–467.

Horne, M., McCracken, G., Walls, A., Tyrrell, P., & Smith, C. (2015). Organisation, practice and experiences of mouth hygiene in stroke unit care: A mixed methods study. *Journal of Clinical Nursing, 24*, 728–738.

Johnson, R., Grove, A., & Clarke, A. (2019). Pillar Integration Process: A joint display technique to integrate data in mixed methods research. *Journal of Mixed Methods Research, 13*, 301–320.

Kagawa, R., Deardorff, J., Esponda, R., Craig, D., & Fernald, L. (2017). The experience of adolescent motherhood. *Journal of Advanced Nursing, 73*, 2566–2576.

Luo, S., & Creswell, J. (2016). Designing and developing an app for a mixed methods research design approach. *International Journal of Designs for Learning, 7*, 62–71.

Mayoh, J., & Onwuegbuzie, A. (2015). Toward a conceptualization of mixed methods phenomenological research. *Journal of Mixed Methods Research, 9*, 91–107.

Mendlinger, S., & Cwikel, J. (2008). Spiraling between qualitative and quantitative data on women's health behaviors: A double helix model for mixed methods. *Quantitative Health Research, 18*, 280–293.

Miles, M., Huberman, M., & Saldaña, J. (2014). *Qualitative data analysis: A methods source book* (3rd ed.). Thousand Oaks, CA: Sage Publications.

*Moffatt, S., White, M., Mackintosh, J. & Howel, D. (2006). Using quantitative and qualitative data in health services research—what happens when mixed method findings conflict? *BMC Health Services Research, 6*, 28.

Moreland, P., & Santacroce, S. (2018). Illness uncertainty and posttraumatic stress in young adults with congenital heart disease. *Journal of Cardiovascular Nursing, 33*, 356–362.

Morse, J. M. (1991). Approaches to qualitative-quantitative methodological triangulation. *Nursing Research, 40*, 120–123.

Morse, J. M. (2012). Simultaneous and sequential qualitative mixed method designs. In Munhall, P. L. (Ed.), *Nursing research: A qualitative perspective* (pp. 553–569). Sudbury, MA: Jones & Bartlett Learning.

Morse, J. M. (2017). *Essentials of qualitatively-driven mixed-method designs*. New York, NY: Routledge.

*Onwuegbuzie, A., & Collins, K. (2007). A typology of mixed methods sampling designs in social science research. *The Qualitative Report, 12*, 281–316.

*Onwuegbuzie, A., & Dickinson, W. (2008). Mixed methods analysis and information visualization: Graphical display for effective communication of research results. *The Qualitative Report, 13*, 204–225.

*Onwuegbuzie, A., & Johnson, R. (2006) The validity issue in mixed methods research. *Research in the Schools, 13*, 48–63.

O'Cathain, A. (2009). Mixed methods research in the health sciences: A quiet revolution. *Journal of Mixed Methods Research, 3*, 3–6.

Patton, M. Q. (2015). *Qualitative research & evaluation methods* (4th ed.). Thousand Oaks, CA: Sage Publications.

Pedersen, B., Groenkjaer, M., Flkmer, U., & Delmar, C. (2017). Understanding the essential meaning of measured changes in weight and body composition among women during and after adjuvant treatment for breast cancer. *Cancer Nursing, 40*, 433–444.

Plano Clark, V. L., Anderson, N., Wertz, J., Zhou, Y., Schumacher, K., & Miaskowski, C. (2015). Conceptualizing longitudinal mixed methods designs: A methodological review of health sciences research. *Journal of Mixed Methods Research, 9,* 297–319.

Plano Clark, V., & Ivankova, N. (2016). *Mixed methods research: A guide to the field.* Thousand Oaks, CA: Sage Publications.

Polit, D. F., London, A., & Martinez, J. (2000). *Food security and hunger in poor, mother-headed families in four U.S. cities.* New York: MDRC.

Redeker, N., Ordway, M. Banasiak, N., Caldwell, B., Canapari, C., Crowley, A., … Sadler, L. (2018). Community partnership for healthy sleep: Research protocol. *Research in Nursing & Health, 41,* 19–29.

Roberts, C., Hunter, J., & Cheng, A. (2017). Resilience in families of children with autism and sleep problems using mixed methods. *Journal of Pediatric Nursing, 37,* e2–e9.

Sandelowski, M. (2001). Real qualitative researchers do not count: The use of numbers in qualitative research. *Research in Nursing & Health, 24,* 230–240.

Sandelowski, M. (2003). Tables or tableaux? The challenges of writing and reading mixed methods studies. In Tashakkori, A., & Teddlie, C. (Eds.), *Handbook of mixed methods in social and behavioral research* (pp. 321–350). Thousand Oaks, CA: Sage Publications.

*Sandelowski, M., Voils, C., & Knafl, G. (2009). On quantitizing. *Journal of Mixed Methods Research, 3,* 208–222.

Schneerson, C., & Gale, N. (2015). Using mixed methods to identify and answer clinically relevant research questions. *Qualitative Health Research, 25,* 845–856.

*St. Arnaud, D., Hatashita, H., & Suzuki, H. (2016). Semantic examination of a Japanese Center for Epidemiologic Studies Depression: A cautionary analysis using mixed methods. *Canadian Journal of Nursing Research, 48,* 80–92.

Tashakkori, A., & Teddlie, C,., (Eds.). (2010). *Handbook of mixed methods in social and behavioral research* (2nd ed.). Thousand Oaks, CA: Sage Publications.

Tashakkorri, A., & Creswell, J. (2007). The new era of mixed methods. *Journal of Mixed Methods Research, 1,* 3–7.

Teddlie, C., & Tashakkori, A. (2009). *Foundations of mixed methods research.* Thousand Oaks, CA: Sage Publications.

*Tonkin-Crine, S., Anthierens, S., Hood, K., Yardley, L., Cals, J., Francis, N., … Little, P. (2016). Discrepancies between qualitative and quantitative evaluation of randomised controlled trial results: Achieving clarity through mixed methods triangulation. *Implementation Science, 11,* 66.

*Uprichard, E., & Dawney, L. (2019). Data diffraction: Challenging data integration in mixed methods research. *Journal of Mixed Methods Research, 13,* 19–32.

*Valenta, S., Spirig, R., Miaskowski, C., Zaugg, K., & Spichiger, E. (2018). Testing a pain self-management intervention by exploring reduction of analgesics' side effects in cancer outpatients and the involvement of family caregivers. *BMC Nursing, 17,* 54.

VanDevanter, N., Kovner, C., Raveis, V., McCollum, M., & Keller, R. (2014). Challenges of nurses' deployment to other New York City hospitals in the aftermath of Hurricane Sandy. *Journal of Urban Health, 91,* 603–614.

Yang, Y. P., Wang, C., & Wang, J. (2016). The initial development of a checklist for assessing thirst in patients with advanced dementia. *Journal of Nursing Research, 24,* 224–230.

A link to this open-access article or document is provided in the Toolkit for Chapter 27 in the Resource Manual. ✪

****This journal article is available on** thePoint *for this chapter.*

28 | Developing Complex Nursing Interventions Using Mixed Methods Research

This chapter discusses research-based efforts to develop innovative nursing interventions. Historically, there has been much more guidance on how to test interventions than on how to develop them, but that situation is changing. There is a growing recognition that new interventions should be designed based on research evidence and strong conceptualizations of the problem. Such endeavors benefit from mixed methods designs.

NURSING INTERVENTION RESEARCH

The term *intervention research* is used by nurse researchers to describe a research approach characterized not only by its research methods but by a distinctive *process* of developing, implementing, testing, and disseminating interventions (e.g., Richards & Rahm Hallberg, 2015; Sidani, 2015; Sidani & Braden, 2011). Naylor (2003) defined **nursing intervention research** as "studies either questioning existing care practices or testing innovations in care that are shaped by nursing's values and goals, guided by a strong theoretical basis, informed by recent advances in science, and designed to improve the quality of care and health of individuals, families, communities, and society" (p. 382).

Some nursing interventions are simple and do not require extensive development. For example, Lee and colleagues (2018) undertook a randomized

controlled trial (RCT) to test the effect of music on anxiety, heart rate, and blood pressure in patients undergoing mechanical ventilation in the intensive care unit. The intervention was relatively simple—one 30-minute session of music therapy—and the researchers did not "develop" the intervention; rather, they developed a protocol for its implementation. Many nursing interventions that are currently being tested, however, are complex and created by nurses by themselves or in interprofessional teams, usually within a focused program of research involving an integrated series of studies.

Complex Interventions

The term **complex intervention** has become a buzzword in research circles and has been the topic of dozens of discussion articles, including several in the nursing literature (e.g., Bleijenberg et al., 2018; Corry et al., 2013). We begin by discussing what the term means.

The Medical Research Council (MRC) in the United Kingdom proposed an influential framework for developing and testing complex interventions (Craig et al., 2008a, 2008b). According to the MRC report, complexity in an intervention can arise along several dimensions, including the following:

- The number of different components within the intervention ("bundling") and interactions between the components;

- The number of different behaviors required by those delivering or receiving the intervention, and the difficulty level of those behaviors;
- The number of different groups or organizational levels targeted by the intervention;
- The number and diversity of intervention outcomes targeted; and
- The degree to which the intervention can be tailored to individual patients.

Intervention complexity exists along a continuum, not as a dichotomy. There is no single point at which a simple intervention becomes complex. Lewin and colleagues (2017) have developed a complexity assessment tool in which interventions can be evaluated for complexity along 10 dimensions. (The 10 dimensions are shown in the Toolkit of the accompanying *Resource Manual.* ⊗) Nursing interventions often are complex along multiple dimensions.

Complex interventions are likely to be needed when complex problems are being treated, when a conceptual framework suggests multiple mediating forces, or when prior research suggests that simple interventions are ineffective. The more complex the intervention, the stronger the need for an intervention framework.

> **TIP** The issue of complexity has received considerable recent attention. Some writers have, for example, criticized the MRC framework for its absence of engagement with complexity theories (e.g., De Silva et al., 2014). One concern is that the interaction between interventions and *context* has not been conceptualized as a key complexity issue (Fletcher et al., 2016).

Frameworks for Developing and Testing Complex Interventions

Proponents of using a framework to guide the intervention development and testing process have rejected the simplistic and atheoretical approach that has often been used with healthcare interventions. The widely recommended process for intervention research involves an in-depth understanding of the problem and the target population, careful integration of diverse evidence, and the use of a guiding intervention theory. The recommendations call for a systematic, progressive sequence that places evidence-based developmental work at a premium.

Several frameworks for health interventions have been proposed. Table 28.1 lists a few of these frameworks, including two that have long served in the development of health promotion interventions (the Intervention Mapping and PRECEDE–PROCEED models) and one for nursing interventions. The Toolkit offers more detail about several of these frameworks. ⊗

The most prominent framework to date for complex health interventions is the **Medical Research Council framework**, which was first described in the literature in 2000 (Campbell et al., 2000). The original MRC framework was conceptualized as a five-phase process and is similar in some regards to the four-phase sequence delineated by the National Institutes of Health for clinical trials, as described in Chapter 11.

In 2008, the Medical Research Council published a revised framework, which reflects suggestions made by critics who thought the process outlined in the original was too linear. (Note that the MRC is updating their framework in 2019, but it was not available when this book was in press.) Figure 28.1 shows that the MRC framework consists of a set of four interconnected "elements" of the intervention process: (1) development, (2) feasibility and piloting, (3) evaluation, and (4) implementation. Although these elements are not connected in a linear, nor even in a cyclical fashion, Craig and colleagues (2008a) noted that it is often "useful to think in terms of stages" (p. 8), and so we have organized much of this chapter in terms of four broad "phases" corresponding to the MRC elements. The central focus of this chapter is on the initial development phase.

Key Features of Complex Intervention Research

In the past decade, considerable effort has been put into fleshing out—and using—the MRC guidance. It has become clear that certain features of intervention research are critical to success. Here we identify a few key features.

TABLE 28.1 • Frameworks for Health-Related Intervention Development

FRAMEWORK	COMMENTS
Intervention Mapping framework (Bartholomew et al., 2016)[a]	Six-phase model geared to the development of health promotion interventions
PRECEDE–PROCEED model (Green & Kreuter, 2005)[a]	A model with two major components: PRECEDE (a series of planned assessments in five phases) and PROCEED (strategic implementation in four phases); used in health promotion programs
6SQuID (Wight et al., 2016)[a]	Framework with six "essential" steps for quality intervention Development (6SQuID), aimed primarily at public health interventions
Behavior Change Wheel (Michie et al., 2011)	A model that identifies intervention functions and policy categories for interventions in which behavioral change is sought
Evidence-based Nursing Interventions (van Meijel et al., 2004)	A model to guide the development of nursing interventions, involving strong development of interventions with a theoretical rationale
Medical Research Council Framework (Craig et al., 2008)[a]	An iterative framework with four broad stages for developing and testing complex health interventions

[a]These frameworks are described in the Toolkit for this chapter in the accompanying *Resource Manual.*

FIGURE 28.1 Medical Research Council's Revised Framework for Developing and Testing Complex Healthcare Interventions. (Adapted with permission from Craig, P., Dieppe, P., Macintyre, S., Michie, S., Nazareth, I., & Petticrew, M. (2008a). *Developing and evaluating complex interventions: New guidance.* London: MRC and Craig, P., Dieppe, P., Macintyre, S., Michie, S., Nazareth, I., & Petticrew, M. (2008b). Developing and evaluating complex interventions: The new Medical Research Council guidance. *BMJ, 337,* 979–983.)

First, there is strong support for *mixed methods approaches*. In moving from a problem to be solved to the rigorous testing of a new intervention, a wide variety of questions that require diverse methods need to be answered. Borglin (2015) has described the value of mixed methods in complex intervention research.

Second, intervention research is undertaken in the context of coordinated *teamwork*, and efforts to develop high-quality complex interventions are often multidisciplinary. Nurses are increasingly collaborating with other health professionals (e.g., physicians, physical therapists, psychologists, nutritionists) on thorny problems requiring a multifaceted solution.

Another feature of intervention research is that it requires many years of work. The MRC framework calls for a sequence of activities that involve a long investment of time to "get it right." Commentators have begun to note that there is a lot of *research waste*—research that gets little or no *return on investment* (ROI) because some researchers do not ask the right questions, do not take into account what is already known, use weak research methods, or fail to disseminate their work promptly and effectively (e.g., Chalmers et al., 2014; Ioannidis, 2016). Research on complex interventions benefits from being embedded in an ongoing, dedicated program of research (Rahm Hallberg, 2015). Coordinated efforts to understand a problem, integrate relevant evidence, develop and test an intervention, and promote its wider adoption are strategies for reducing research waste.

Finally, there is growing realization that *patient and public involvement* (PPI) is imperative throughout the process of developing and testing complex interventions (Richards, 2015a). The literature on complex interventions is filled with cautions about potential challenges and pitfalls. Many pitfalls concern resistance on the part of patients, family members/caretakers, and healthcare staff in the settings where interventions get tested (Tables in the Supplement to this chapter on thePoint identify some major pitfalls. 🅢) In embarking on the pathway of complex intervention research, it is important to understand that a lot of things *can* go wrong, and so strategies should be designed to prevent them from happening to the extent possible. That is why skillful foundational work during the development phase is so crucial, including attempts to understand the perspectives of patients and other stakeholders.

> **TIP** One common pitfall is that intervention developers tend to be overly optimistic and fail to develop or identify evidence to support the links in the chain between the problem, the intervention components, and the outcomes of interest (Wight et al., 2016).

Desirable Features of Nursing Interventions

Nursing interventions are developed to improve health outcomes. Before embarking on an intervention development project, nurse researchers should carefully consider the relative importance of achieving certain goals.

Box 28.1 identifies features that may be considered "ideal" for nursing interventions—although in any situation, some features would be more vital than others. In some cases, the desirable features compete with one another—for example, cost and efficacy often involve trade-offs. Indeed, most of the ideals could plausibly be achieved if cost were not an issue.

Yet, practical issues *are* important considerations. Especially in this time of heightened consciousness about healthcare costs, an intervention should be one that has potential to be cost-effective. In designing new ways to address health needs, nurse researchers should give upfront thought to whether the intervention is feasible from a resource perspective in real-world settings. As noted by Richards (2015b), "We should consider the 'implementability' of our complex interventions from the moment we begin the process of design, testing, and evaluation" (p. 333). Some of the ideals in Box 28.1 may need to be relaxed in the face of cost constraints, but this should be a conscious decision and not left to serendipity. One ideal feature that should never be relaxed is the first one on the list—having an intervention that addresses a pressing problem.

BOX 28.1 Features of an "Ideal" Nursing Intervention

An ideal clinical intervention would be:
- **Salient**—addresses a pressing problem
- **Efficacious**—leads to improved client outcomes
- **Safe**—avoids any adverse outcomes, burdens, or stress
- **Conceptually sound**—has a theoretical underpinning
- **Cost-effective**—is affordable and has economic benefits to clients or society
- **Feasible**—can be implemented in real-world settings and integrated into current models of care
- **Developmentally appropriate**—is suitable for the age group for whom it is intended
- **Culturally sensitive**—demonstrates sensitivity to various groups
- **Accessible**—can be easily accessed by the people for whom it is intended
- **Acceptable**—is viewed positively by clients and other stakeholders, including family members, nurses, physicians, administrators, policy makers
- **Adaptable**—can be tailored to local contexts
- **Readily disseminated**—can be sufficiently described and packaged for adoption in other locales

PHASE 1: INTERVENTION DEVELOPMENT

The best current practice is to develop interventions in a systematic fashion, drawing on good evidence and an appropriate theory of how the intervention would achieve desired effects. In other words, interventions should be evidence-based from the start, and this can require extensive and diverse types of foundational work.

Each phase in the intervention development and testing process can be thought of as having three aspects: (1) key *issues* that must be addressed during this stage, (2) *actions* and strategies that can be brought to bear on those issues, and (3) *products* that pave the way for moving on to the next phase. Table 28.2 summarizes issues, actions, and products during Phase I development.

Key Issues in Intervention Development

Conceptualization and in-depth understanding of the problem are key issues during Phase 1. The starting point of an intervention project is the problem itself, which must be thoroughly understood. In Chapter 5, we discussed how those doing a literature review must "own" the literature. When it comes to intervention development, researchers must "own" the problem.

A thorough understanding of the target group—their needs, fears, preferences, and circumstances—is part of that ownership. It is only through such understanding that researchers can know whether key intervention pitfalls might be relevant in their situation. Ownership of the problem also requires a thorough grasp of existing evidence on similar interventions—and an understanding of current practices and why they are deficient.

Another development issue involves identifying key *stakeholders*—people who have a stake in fixing the problem—and getting them "on board." Interventions sometimes fail because researchers have not developed the relationships needed to ensure that the intervention will be given a fair test. In addition to the target group, stakeholders might include family members, advocates, community leaders, service providers in multiple disciplines, intervention agents, healthcare administrators, support staff in intervention settings, and content experts. The intervention team should think broadly about whose support could affect their ability to undertake the project.

Relationship building can contribute to the content of the intervention itself, because stakeholders can offer insight into the scope and depth of the problem. Relationships with stakeholders are also important because researchers must figure out not only *what* to deliver but also *how* to deliver it. The

TABLE 28.2 • Key Issues, Activities, and Products of Phase I Developmental Work for Nursing Interventions

KEY ISSUES	MAJOR ACTIVITIES	PRODUCTS AND OUTCOMES
<ul><li>Conceptualization of the problem</li><li>Understanding of current practices and why they are deficient</li><li>Articulation of an evidence base for the intervention</li><li>Conceptualization of the context</li><li>Conceptualization of solutions, strategies, and outcomes</li><li>Construct validation of the intervention</li><li>Identification of potential pitfalls within the implementation context</li><li>Cultivation of relationships</li></ul>	<ul><li>Critical synthesis of relevant literature</li><li>Concept and theory development</li><li>Exploratory and descriptive research</li><li>Consultation with experts; content validation</li><li>Brainstorming with colleagues, team building, partnerships with stakeholders</li><li>Modeling and designing the intervention</li></ul>	<ul><li>An intervention theory</li><li>Preliminary specification of the content, intensity, dose, timing, setting, and delivery method of the intervention</li><li>Preliminary identification of key outcomes</li><li>Strategies to overcome pitfalls in implementing and testing the intervention</li><li>An implementation plan</li><li>A design for a pilot study</li><li>A plan for sponsorship of the pilot study</li></ul>

intervention must be delivered in a manner that will gain the support of administrators and healthcare staff, appeal to the target group, enhance recruitment and retention of participants, and strengthen intervention fidelity in later phases.

Relatedly, the project team should develop a firm understanding of the context in which the intervention will be implemented. As noted by Hawe and colleagues (2009), contextual factors will almost surely shape how an intervention is delivered, how it will work, and who is likely to benefit. Fletcher and colleagues (2016) have emphasized the value of conceptualizing the contextual conditions necessary for the intervention mechanisms to function as planned.

Activities and Strategies in Intervention Development

Developmental issues can be addressed through a variety of activities. The importance of adequate development cannot be overemphasized.

Synthesizing Existing Evidence

As shown in the MDC framework in Figure 28.1, development work includes "identifying the evidence base," and thus development work often begins with close scrutiny of the literature. The research team needs to thoroughly understand the nature and scope of the problem, and how it is manifested in different groups or settings. The literature also needs to be searched for guidance about the content and mechanisms of possible interventions—the active ingredients. Systematic reviews may be available for evidence about specific strategies but preparing a new or updated one might be necessary (Chapter 30).

Researchers' efforts to understand the problem and possible solutions are an important, but not exhaustive, part of a literature review effort. Table 28.3 provides examples of other questions that should be addressed through a scrutiny of existing evidence during the development phase. When relevant literature is thin or nonexistent, other sources to address remaining uncertainties need to be pursued.

Example of Using Systematic Reviews in Intervention Research

Holloway and colleagues (2017) described their procedures for developing a complex intervention to address alcohol problems in male remand prisoners. Their development work included a scrutiny of several relevant systematic reviews. They acknowledged the need for further exploratory research on alcohol problems and treatments in their population.

TABLE 28.3 • Examples of Literature Review Questions for Designing an Evidence-Based Intervention

ISSUE	QUESTIONS FOR WHICH EVIDENCE CAN BE SOUGHT IN A LITERATURE REVIEW
Conceptualizing the problem	What is known about the nature and causes of this problem and possible solutions? What theories help to explain the problem? What are key mediators in the pathway between the causes or contributing factors and the outcomes?
Focusing the target group	Who or what have been the targets of efforts to address the problem—individuals? families? healthcare providers? healthcare systems? What populations appear to be most amenable to the intervention?
Developing intervention content and components	What is the content of other similar interventions? Is the presence of certain types of components linked to better outcomes? Are interventions generic or individualized?
Selecting outcomes and assessment strategies	What behaviors or outcomes have been targeted by similar interventions? Have the interventions had significant effects on these outcomes? Have they had an effect on key mediators? What assessment approaches and measures have been used with other similar interventions?
Making decisions about dose	How intense have other similar interventions been? Has dose been found to be related to outcomes?
Making decisions about timing of intervention	When are interventions of this type typically delivered? Is timing related to outcomes?
Making decision about mode of delivery	How have similar interventions been delivered? In face-to-face situations (group or individual delivery)? by telephone? Internet? video? Is there evidence that some delivery modes are especially effective?
Making decisions about timing of outcome measurement	When have data for this type of intervention typically been collected? Does the literature suggest that effects deteriorate?
Making decisions about settings and agents	Where (in what types of settings) have interventions of this type been delivered? Do impacts vary by type of setting? Who usually delivers them? Do outcomes vary by type of agent?
Assessing acceptability of the intervention	Is there evidence of strong (or weak) rates of participation in interventions of this type? Have recruitment or retention problems been reported?
Assessing cultural appropriateness	Is there evidence that cultural issues affect implementation of similar interventions? Is there cultural variation in outcomes?

Exploratory and Descriptive Research

Most researchers find that evidence from the literature is insufficient to satisfactorily address the questions suggested in Table 28.3. Almost inevitably, the developmental phase involves undertaking mixed methods exploratory and descriptive research. Insights from qualitative inquiries are virtually essential to the success of intervention development efforts. Morden and colleagues (2015) offer a compelling argument about the importance of qualitative research in developing and implementing complex interventions.

As previously noted, efforts to design acceptable and efficacious interventions require understanding clients' perspectives. Examples of questions that could be pursued in exploratory research with clients include: What is it like to have this problem? What strategies to address it have been tried and why have they not worked? What are clients' goals—what do *they* want as an intervention outcome? (Additional exploratory research questions are noted in the Supplement to this chapter on thePoint. 🅢) Answers to questions such as these could help to shape the intervention and make it more effective, tolerable, and appropriate for the group for whom the intervention is designed.

Exploratory research with other stakeholders can also be valuable. Many of the pitfalls of intervention research involve lack of cooperation, support, or trust among key stakeholders, including those who deliver the intervention. Stakeholders should be engaged in the development process to the extent possible.

Exploratory work can also be undertaken to understand the context within which an intervention would unfold (Bleijenberg et al., 2018; McGuire et al., 2000). It may also be important to understand institutional issues such as staff turnover, staff morale, nurse workload, and nurse autonomy. Van Meijel and colleagues (2004) recommended undertaking a "current practice analysis" to understand the status quo of how the problem under scrutiny is being addressed.

The nursing literature has hundreds of examples of descriptive or exploratory studies done as part of intervention development. Research strategies can include a wide range of approaches, such as focus group interviews, needs assessment surveys, in-depth or critical-incident interviews, records reviews, and observations in clinical settings. It is not unusual for researchers to conduct three or four small descriptive studies during the development phase of an intervention project.

Example of Qualitative Research for Developing a Nursing Intervention
Duggleby and Williams (2016) discussed methodologic and epistemologic considerations in using qualitative research to develop interventions. They illustrated the discussion with insights from their own developmental research for a psychosocial hope intervention for patients with advanced cancer. They undertook a qualitative study of the hope experience and a grounded theory study of hope in older palliative care patients to better understand processes of change.

Consultation With Experts

Experts in the content area of the problem can play a crucial role during the development of an intervention. Expert consultants are especially useful if the evidence base is thin and resources for exploratory research are limited. Many of the questions in Table 28.3 that are not answered by evidence in the research literature or from new descriptive studies are good candidates for discussion with experts. As an example, Duggleby and Williams (2016), in their intervention development project just described, used a Delphi survey to ask a five-member expert panel to identify themes emerging from their qualitative study that were most important to fostering hope, which led to the development of hope exercises.

TIP In selecting expert consultants, think in an interdisciplinary fashion. For example, the use of a cultural consultant may be valuable to assess the cultural sensitivity and appropriateness of some interventions. A developmental psychologist could help assess developmental suitability.

Often, experts are asked to review preliminary intervention protocols, to corroborate their utility, and to make suggestions for strengthening them. Curiously, this process is less often formalized than the process for reviewing new measurement scales. Procedures used to assess the *content validity* of new instruments using an expert panel (Chapter 16) can also be used to review draft intervention protocols. If the intervention is intended for use in diverse settings or contexts, content validation is likely to be a valuable approach.

> **Example of Content Validation of a Nursing Intervention**
> Lu and Haase (2011) used an interdisciplinary panel of six scientists and clinicians to assess the content validity of the Daily Enhancement of Meaningful Activity (DEMA) program, an intervention for mild cognitive impairment patient–spouse dyads.

Brainstorming and Team Building

Development work is usually interpersonal and involves cultivating relationships. At the team level, this entails putting together an enthusiastic and committed project team with diverse clinical and research skills. (If development work is undertaken for a dissertation, the "team" includes the dissertation committee, so members of this committee should be chosen carefully.)

Ideally, brainstorming sessions occur frequently during the development period to discuss evidence summaries, descriptive findings, expert feedback, and preliminary protocols. Technological advances such as videoconferencing make it possible to include team members from different locations. The team may include key stakeholders as participating partners.

> **TIP** It is wise to develop mechanisms for ongoing communication and collaboration with stakeholders. For example, it can be useful to form an advisory group of stakeholders and to have a project-specific website or Facebook page.

Intervention Theory Development

A critical activity in the development phase is to delineate the conceptual basis for the intervention (Craig et al., 2008a, 2008b). An **intervention theory** offers an explanation for the problem and guides what must be done to achieve desired outcomes. The theory provides a theoretical rationale for why an intervention should "work." In conceptualizing what is causing a problem, the research

team needs to identify which factors are modifiable and which would have the greatest impact on improving outcomes of interest.

The intervention theory can be an existing one that has been well-validated. Examples of theories that have been used in nursing intervention studies include the Health Promotion Model, the Transtheoretical Model, Social Cognitive Theory, the Health Belief Model, and the Theory of Planned Behavior (see Chapter 6). These theories provide guidance on how to fashion an intervention because they propose mechanisms to explain human behavior and behavior change. Abraham and colleagues (2015) offer perspectives on the theoretical basis of behavior change interventions.

Intervention theories can also be developed from qualitatively derived theory, a point made most eloquently by Morse (2006). Morse and colleagues (2000) developed a strategy called *qualitative outcome analysis* (QOA), which is a process for extending the findings of a qualitative study by identifying intervention strategies related to the phenomenon of concern.

> **Example of a Qualitatively Derived Intervention Theory**
> Harvey Chochinov and other researchers (including nurse researchers) developed a theory of dignity based on in-depth interviews with hospice patients. The theory formed the basis for an intervention (Dignity Therapy) to promote dignity and reduce stress at the end of life. Hall and colleagues (2009, 2013) evaluated a Dignity Therapy intervention for older people in care homes and undertook further qualitative research as part of the trial. Dignity Therapy has also been used in a nursing intervention for people living with dementia (Johnston et al., 2016).

Modeling and Designing the Intervention

The MRC framework (Figure 28.1) includes "modeling processes and outcomes" as a component of intervention development. Modeling involves synthesizing the information gleaned during the development phase (Figure 28.2), constructing components of the intervention and visualizing the pathways that patients will take in going through

FIGURE 28.2 Synthesis of evidence sources for intervention development.

the intervention. As described by Sermeus (2015), the aim of modeling is to unravel the "black box" between intervention components and desired outcomes.

An evidence-based intervention theory lays the groundwork for proceeding with the modeling task and developing intervention content. A visual *logic model* for the intervention should identify the active components and show how they are expected to work on the outcomes of interest. It should also describe how the active components relate to each other.

> **TIP** The Kellogg Foundation has prepared a guide for developing logic models. A link to the report is provided in the Toolkit.

Example of a Logic Model in a Complex Intervention Study

Saal and colleagues (2018) described the development of a complex intervention to improve the social participation of nursing home residents with joint contractures. The logic model for their intervention—Participation Enabling CAre in Nursing or PECAN—provides information about the "What" and the "How" of the intervention, mechanisms of impact (including elements from the Theory of Planned Behavior), process-influencing factors, and health outcomes.

Intervention content can sometimes be adapted from other similar interventions. In addition to content, however, the research team needs to make many decisions about the intervention's ingredients, including decisions about the following:

1. **Dose and intensity.** The treatment must be sufficiently powerful to achieve a desired, measurable effect on outcomes of interest, but cannot be so powerful that it is cost-prohibitive or burdensome to clients. Among the dose-related issues that need to be decided are the *potency* or *intensity* of the treatment (how much content is appropriate, and will it be given individually or in groups?); the *amount* of dose per session; the *frequency* of administering doses (number of sessions); and the *duration* of the intervention over time.

2. **Timing.** In some cases, it is important to decide when, relative to other events, the intervention will be delivered. The question is, When is the optimal point (in terms of an illness or recovery trajectory, individual development, or severity of a problem) to administer the intervention? Ideally, the intervention theory would suggest the most advantageous timing.

3. **Outcomes.** Two major decisions concern which outcomes will be targeted and when they will be measured. Thought should be given to selecting outcomes that are nursing sensitive and important to clients. One issue is whether the focus will be on proximal outcomes or more distal ones. *Proximal outcomes* are immediate and directly connected to the intervention—and thus usually most sensitive to intervention effects. For example, knowledge gains from a teaching component of an intervention are proximal. *Distal outcomes* are potentially more important, but more difficult to affect (e.g., eating behavior). Consideration should also be given to the information needs of people making decisions about using the intervention—what outcomes would affect uptake by administrators or policy makers? Another crucial outcome is cost: interventions are hard to "sell" without information about monetary costs and benefits.

4. **Setting.** Another design decision involves the setting for the intervention. Settings can vary in terms of ease of implementation, costs, and access. In deciding about settings (and sites),

researchers need to think about the type of setting that will be acceptable and accessible to clients, offer good potential for impacts, provide needed resources or supports, and serve clients whose needs and characteristics are compatible with the intervention.

5. **Agents.** Researchers must decide who will deliver the intervention, and how intervention agents will be trained. In many cases, the agents will be nurses, but nurses are not necessarily the best choice. For example, some clients might feel more comfortable if the interventionists were community members or patients who have experienced a similar illness or problem (i.e., peers).

6. **Delivery mode.** With technological innovations occurring regularly, options for delivering interventions—or components of interventions—have broadened tremendously. Among the possibilities are face-to-face delivery, video or audio recordings, print materials, telephone communication, texts, emails, Internet discussion boards, and social networking sites. Care should be taken to match any technological delivery methods to the needs of the clients and to the requirements of the content. The latest technology is not always optimal.

7. **Individualization.** Another decision concerns the extent to which the intervention will be tailored to the needs and circumstances of a particular group (e.g., older adults) or individualized to particular clients. When individual information is used to guide content, the intervention is inherently more complex than a one-size-fits-all treatment but may be more effective and attractive to participants (Lauver et al., 2002).

These various decisions should be evidence-based to the extent possible, using synthesized evidence from various sources. The development work should provide the basis for the intervention to be piloted in the next phase. As noted by the authors of the MRC framework, "the intervention must be developed to the point where it can reasonably be expected to have a worthwhile effect" (Craig et al., 2008b, p. 980).

Products of Phase 1 Development

Phase I typically results in several products (Table 28.2). These include an intervention theory and a conceptual map or logic model, preliminary intervention components and protocols, and an implementation plan that includes strategies for addressing potential implementation pitfalls. Hopefully, the research team will have documented the development work and major decisions in an ongoing fashion. Detailed written information about the theory, the intervention components and strategies, and expected outcomes will be valuable for writing reports about the intervention and for making funding requests.

> **TIP** A matrix can often be useful in summarizing *key decisions* in one column and *supporting evidence* for those decisions in another. Such a matrix is a good communication tool for discussing decisions with others. A worksheet for such a matrix is included in the Toolkit for this chapter in the *Resource Manual.*

If the development work provides support for moving forward with a pilot test of the intervention, another product of Phase 1 work will be a design for a pilot study, usually in the form of a research proposal (Chapter 33).

OTHER PHASES OF INTERVENTION RESEARCH

Other phases of intervention research include feasibility and pilot testing; a rigorous evaluation to assess efficacy; and implementation of the intervention (should it prove to be effective) into real-world settings with ongoing monitoring and longer-term follow-up. These other phases are briefly described next.

Phase 2: Pilot Testing an Intervention

The second phase of intervention research is a pilot test of the newly developed intervention. Key issues in this phase are *feasibility* (Can the intervention be implemented as conceptualized?), *acceptability* (Do recipients and other key stakeholders find the intervention relevant and appropriate?), and *promise* (Is it plausible that the intervention will result in desired effects on key outcomes?). The central *activities* of Phase 2 are undertaking a **pilot study** and analyzing pilot data. An important *product* of a pilot study is documentation of the results and the "lessons learned."

Although each pilot test yields its own context-specific and intervention-specific lessons, some "lessons" are recurrent. In particular, you should expect the reality of piloting the intervention to be different from the intervention that was developed on paper, and these differences—and reasons for them—should be documented. If the intervention proves feasible and promising, Phase 2 products include a formal intervention protocol for testing in a full Phase 3 trial. Another product is a formal plan for a Phase 3 evaluation, often in the form of a grant application. Chapter 29 discusses pilot tests of interventions in greater detail.

Example of a Mixed Methods Pilot Intervention Study

Barley and colleagues (2012, 2014) developed a personalized care intervention (UPBEAT) for coronary heart disease patients, after doing extensive developmental work. The 6-month nurse-led intervention was pilot tested with 81 patients. The researchers concluded that the intervention was feasible and acceptable. The team's program of research on UPBEAT is described in Tylee et al. (2016).

Phase 3: Evaluation of the Intervention

The third phase of a complex intervention project is a full test of the intervention, almost always using a randomized design. Many important issues of a Phase 3 evaluation were discussed in Chapter 10, which outlined various threats to the validity of quantitative studies and presented some strategies to address those threats. Whereas construct validity is particularly salient in the development phase of an intervention project, internal validity and statistical conclusion validity are key issues during the evaluation.

Although a major goal of Phase 3 is to assess the *efficacy* of the intervention, it is better to think of the trial as ongoing development rather than as simply "confirmatory." Even with a strong pilot study, problems and issues almost always emerge in the full test. As part of a process analysis (Chapter 11), problems should be identified, and researchers should make recommendations for how the intervention could be improved, how its implementation could be made smoother, or how context helped to shape the delivery or efficacy of the intervention.

The MRC has provided useful guidance about planning and implementing a process evaluation of complex evaluations (Moore et al., 2015), and a mixed methods approach is strongly advocated. Some of the goals of collecting qualitative data during Phase 3 might include the following:

1. **Assessing Intervention Fidelity.** Mixed methods research is needed to inform judgments about whether the intervention was faithfully implemented, and how it was delivered in real-world settings. If intervention effects are modest, one possibility is that it was not implemented according to the plan. The protocols or training materials, for example, might need revamping.

2. **Clarifying the Intervention.** A qualitative component in a randomized trial can help to clarify the nature and course of the intervention in its natural context. It is useful to understand how intervention recipients and other stakeholders experience the intervention in real life—and to identify possible barriers to widespread implementation.

3. **Understanding the Context.** Factors external to the intervention can facilitate or impede its implementation. Some of these factors can be measured (e.g., population characteristics, staff–patient ratios), but a full understanding of context usually requires deeper exploration. Pfadenhauer and colleagues (2017) have developed a framework to facilitate the conceptualization of context and implementation of complex interventions.

4. **Probing for Clinical Significance.** Quantitative results from a randomized trial indicate whether the results are statistically significant, and methods have been developed to quantitatively assess clinical significance (Chapter 21). Qualitative information could shed additional

light—clinically relevant effects sometimes can be discerned qualitatively even when treatment effects are not statistically significant.

5. **Interpreting Results.** Quantitative results indicate *whether* an intervention had beneficial effects—but do not explain *why* effects occurred. A strong conceptual framework offers a theoretical rationale for explaining the results but may not tell the whole story if the effects were weaker than expected or if they were observed for some outcomes but not for others. Moreover, even if there are specific theory-driven intervention effects, it is inevitable that people will pose "black box" questions about what is *driving* the results. Such questions often stem from practical concerns, reflecting a desire to streamline successful interventions when resources are tight.

Example of Using Qualitative Data to Interpret Evaluation Results

Berg and co-researchers (2015) conducted a trial to test the effectiveness of a complex cardiac rehabilitation intervention for patients with implantable cardioverter defibrillators. Nearly 200 patients were randomized in the Phase III trial, and intervention effects were found for several outcomes (peak oxygen uptake, general health, and mental health). The researchers embedded a qualitative component involving in-depth interviews with 10 patients, and the qualitative findings helped them explain the mechanisms of the effects.

TIP Quantitative results do not have much "sex appeal." As astutely pointed out by Sandelowski (1996), qualitative research embedded in intervention studies can enhance the power of the study findings: "...Storied accounts of scientific work are often the more compelling and culturally resonant way to communicate research results to diverse audiences, including patient groups and policy-makers" (p. 361).

A Phase 3 evaluation, then, includes both an analysis of intervention effectiveness and an in-depth process evaluation that provides rich information about the roll-out of the intervention and the processes of change that occurred. One final evaluation component is crucial to the intervention's

potential for widespread adoption: a cost-benefit analysis. Interventions are unlikely to be integrated into healthcare systems if their cost outweighs any benefits, and so the evaluation team should strive to understand economic implications. Payne and Thompson (2015) provide an overview of economic evaluations of complex interventions.

The primary product of Phase 3 is a report summarizing the evaluation results. Often, single papers are insufficient for providing the full range of information about the project, particularly if a mixed methods approach was used. Ideally, one report would integrate findings from the qualitative and quantitative components and offer recommendations for further adoption of (or revisions to) the intervention.

TIP Several groups have called for researchers to undertake *realist evaluations* (Chapter 11) in coming to conclusions about complex interventions (e.g., Fletcher et al., 2016; Hansen & Jones, 2017). Their position is that realist evaluations do a better job than traditional evaluations of answering questions about what works, for whom, and under what circumstances. The realist approach involves developing and testing theories about **context-mechanism-outcome (CMO)** configurations. Realist evaluations almost inevitably used mixed methods designs.

Phase 4: Implementation

In the MRC framework, the final phase of intervention research is the *implementation* of a complex intervention that has been found to have beneficial effects and favorable economic results. Implementation involves embedding a new and promising intervention into routine health and nursing services. The process of implementation is sometimes called *normalization*.

Increasingly, researchers have come to recognize that their work does not end with the publication of a research report on the findings from a Phase 3 trial. A whole new field of *implementation science* has burgeoned in efforts to help researchers plan for implementation challenges. (See the Supplement to Chapter 11 on the Point. 🅢)

Several conceptual models and frameworks have been devised to guide the implementation process.

One widely used framework is called **normalization process theory (NPT)** (May, 2013; May et al., 2016). NPT is an action theory that focuses on how new interventions or programs become embedded within social contexts. NPT involves four core constructs that represent the kinds of work and activity that people do when implementing a new practice: Coherence, Cognitive Participation, Collective Action, and Reflexive Monitoring. A measure called NoMAD (Normalization MeAsure Development) is available to assess these four constructs in practice settings (Finch et al., 2013). A table in the Toolkit provides brief description of the four NPT constructs. Several chapters in Richards and Rahm Hallberg (2015) are devoted to issues of relevance during the implementation of complex interventions.

Example of Using Normalization Process Theory
Gillespie and colleagues (2018) used NPT in their evaluation of the implementation of a complex intervention involving the introduction of a surgical safety checklist. Their mixed methods study involved having surgical teams complete the NoMAD instrument and participate in in-depth interviews about their experiences with the checklist. Their evaluation helped to explain what facets of the checklist use led to integration in practice.

MIXED METHODS DESIGNS FOR INTERVENTION RESEARCH

The full cycle of research activity for developing and testing complex interventions addresses myriad questions that can only be answered using a rich blend of methods. Creswell and Plano Clark (2018) identified as a possible advanced mixed methods design what they called the *mixed methods intervention design,* which involves incorporating qualitative data into a trial before, during, and (or) after the experimental treatment has been implemented. They also identified another complex design, the *mixed methods program evaluation design,* which is consistent with the Medical Research Council's intervention framework.

Visual diagrams for two possible two-stage mixed methods intervention designs are presented in Figure 28.3. Models such as these can work reasonably well for interventions that are closer to the "simple" end of the simple → complex continuum. They might also be appropriate for a small-scale study (such as a dissertation project) in which the main QUAN component is essentially a pilot study.

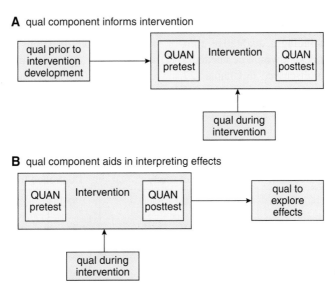

FIGURE 28.3 Mixed Methods Designs for a Two-Phase Intervention Project. (Adapted from Creswell, J. W., & Plano Clark, V. L. [2018]. *Designing and conducting mixed methods research* [3rd ed.]. Thousand Oaks, CA: Sage.)

For complex interventions such as those described in the MRC framework, it is better to think of a separate design structure for each phase, because each has its own purpose, research questions, design, sampling plan, and data collection strategy. For the project overall, QUAN typically has priority. Yet, foundational work in the development phase often involves QUAL-dominant research.

Figure 28.4 shows some design possibilities for a three-phase intervention project, and many others are possible. The overall project design is inherently sequential, but within each phase, the design could be either sequential or concurrent. Both qualitative and quantitative approaches are often used in each phase.

It is difficult to offer guidance on which of design to adopt because many factors influence which is most appropriate. Fewer design components may be required for simpler interventions, for "mainstream" target populations, for studies in a familiar site, and for studies of adaptations of well-tested interventions. Also, resources may force researchers to forego components they would have liked to include. The design for the Phase 3 trial is also likely to be affected by which of the five goals for qualitative inquiry (as described in the previous section) is most salient. For example, if the desire to monitor intervention fidelity is the primary objective of including a qualitative component, a QUAN + qual design would be needed.

Sampling designs, as discussed in Chapter 27, also differ in the three phases. During Phase 1, a multilevel sampling approach is often used to gather in-depth QUAL data from different populations—for example, from patients, family members, and healthcare staff. In Phases 2 and 3, by contrast, sampling is likely to be either identical or nested—although multilevel sampling may also be useful for understanding intervention fidelity. Samples for qualitative questions are typically purposively selected along dimensions likely to influence the implementation and effectiveness of the intervention.

In summary, researchers can be creative in developing an overall design that matches their needs, circumstances, and budgets. Inevitably, however, strong research for developing and testing complex interventions will rely on a mixed methods design.

CRITICAL APPRAISAL OF INTERVENTION RESEARCH

Many chapters of this book offer guidelines for evaluating methodologic aspects of studies that would be included in an intervention project. For example, guidelines in Chapters 9 and 10 would be useful for critically appraising the Phase 3 design. Qualitative components can be evaluated using guidelines in Chapters 22 through 26, and the previous chapter included suggestions for appraising mixed methods research.

Box 28.2, also found in the Toolkit, offers a few additional questions on intervention issues, with many of them focusing on intervention development. ✪ Of course, your ability to answer the questions in Box 28.2 will depend on the care researchers took in documenting the full effort.

Nursing Intervention Diagram

Phase 1 Development	Phase 2 Pilot Study	Phase 3 Controlled Trial
QUAL + quan or QUAL + QUAN or QUAL → quan or QUAL → qual	QUAN + qual or QUAN + QUAL or QUAN → qual or QUAN → QUAN	QUAN + qual or QUAN + qual → qual or QUAN → qual

FIGURE 28.4 Possible Mixed Methods Designs for a Three-Phase Nursing Intervention Project.

BOX 28.2 Guidelines for Critically Appraising Aspects of Intervention Projects

1. On a simple-to-complex continuum, where would you locate the intervention? If the intervention is complex, along which dimensions is complexity found (e.g., number of components, complexity of behaviors required, number of intervention sessions, time required, and so on)?
2. Is there an intervention theory, and is it adequate? Is there an explanation of how the theory was selected, adapted, or developed? Was a logic model presented?
3. What strategies were used to identify and create evidence in support of intervention development? Was a systematic review performed? Were expert consultants involved? Were descriptive or exploratory studies undertaken? Overall, was developmental work adequate?
4. What *was* the intervention? Was it described in sufficient detail in terms of content, target population, dose, outcomes, timing, individualization, intervention agents, and so on?
5. Was there a pilot study? Was pilot work sufficient for a decision to move forward with a full clinical trial?
6. For the overall project and for individual phases, was a mixed methods approach used? Which design was adopted, and is the design appropriate for the goals of different phases of the project?
7. Does the final report integrate key findings from the various strands of research?
   Does the report offer recommendations for replication, extension, or adaptation of the intervention or for use in different settings or with different populations?

Most often, the development and testing of an intervention are reported in separate articles, but the team should strive to prepare a summary report that integrates qualitative and quantitative findings from all phases and that offers evidence-based recommendations for how to proceed with implementing the intervention in everyday practice settings.

EXAMPLE OF MIXED METHODS INTERVENTION RESEARCH

Study: The development and testing of a proactive nurse-led care program (U-CARE) to maintain physical functioning of frail older people in primary care in the Netherlands.

Statement of purpose: The overall purpose of this research was to develop and test the efficacy of a theory-based complex intervention to preserve physical functioning and enhance the quality of life of frail older people. The development process and details of the intervention were described "to allow its replication" (Bleijenberg et al., 2013a, p. 230). The researchers followed the MRC framework for complex interventions.

Phase 1: Developmental work for this project unfolded over several years. The study team, which included nurses and physicians with clinical experience in primary care, did a thorough literature review. After studying the existing evidence, the researchers concluded that the most promising elements for an intervention would be ones based on the Chronic Care Model, which provided a theoretical framework. The emerging U-CARE program was developed to comprise three steps: a frailty assessment to identify frail patients, a comprehensive geriatric assessment of frail patients at home, and then an individualized care plan with evidence-based interventions. The researchers also explored measures to use in the intervention, such as an assessment tool for measuring frailty (e.g., Drubbel et al., 2014). The "face validity" of the intervention and the assessment procedures were discussed with a panel of experienced nurses in 10 meetings. The research team also sought input from other geriatric experts, and a few adaptations to care plans were made based on their recommendations. The content of U-CARE was also "assessed and approved by a panel of five independent older people" (p. 233), who met twice.

Phase 2: Small pilot and feasibility studies of the U-CARE program were undertaken, involving the collection of both quantitative and qualitative data.

In terms of feasibility, a mixed methods approach (QUAN → qual) was used to gather information from a sample of 32 general practitioners and 21 practice nurses. The study explored the participants' expectations and experiences with regard to a proactive and structured care program for frail elders (Bleijenberg et al., 2013b). This revealed several potential barriers, but participants affirmed the feasibility of such an approach in primary practices. The researchers also undertook a small-scale 6-week pilot test of the intervention with 30 patients. Patient outcomes were not formally assessed, but the nurses who delivered the pilot intervention reported gains in their own knowledge and their understanding of patients' needs.

Phase 3: A full-scale mixed methods evaluation (called U-PROFIT) of two related interventions was undertaken in 39 clusters of general practices in the Netherlands (Bleijenberg et al., 2012, 2016a). Using a cluster randomized design, a total of 3,092 community-dwelling elders were randomized to one of three arms: (1) the use of an electronic frailty screening instrument using routine medical records data to identify patients at risk for frailty, followed by GP care in which the reports were used proactively (U-PRIM); (2) use of the screening tool, followed by the nurse-led U-CARE program; or (3) usual care. Prior to undertaking the full trial, 21 nurses with experience working with older people were recruited and trained, and careful attention was paid to matters of intervention fidelity (Bleijenberg et al., 2016b). The primary outcome of the trial was level of activities of daily living (ADL). Secondary outcomes included quality of life, mortality, nursing home admission, emergency department visits, and caregiver burden. Outcome data were collected at baseline, and at 6-month and 12-month follow-ups. The researchers found that participants in both intervention arms experienced less decline in activity of daily living at the 12-month follow-up than those in the usual care arm. The groups did not differ significantly on other outcomes. An in-depth study of a sample of patients in the second arm revealed that the nurse-led care was well-received, and that the nurses' role as monitors (assessing potential risk) was perceived as especially important (Bleijenberg et al., 2015). In the team's cost-effectiveness analysis, it was found that total costs per patient were lower in both intervention groups compared to usual care, although the combined intervention showed less value for money (Bleijenberg et al., 2017).

SUMMARY POINTS

- **Nursing intervention research** involves a distinctive *process* of developing, implementing, testing, and disseminating nursing interventions—particularly complex interventions.
- *Complexity* in **complex interventions** can arise along several dimensions, including number of components, number of outcomes targeted, number and complexity of behaviors required, and the time needed for the full intervention to be delivered.
- Several frameworks for developing and testing complex interventions have been proposed. The most widely cited one is the **Medical Research Council (MRC) framework** (United Kingdom), which was published in 2000 and then revised in 2008.
- Most frameworks emphasize the critical importance of strong development efforts at the outset, followed by pilot tests of the intervention, and then a rigorous controlled trial to assess efficacy and evaluate the implementation process. The frameworks are idealized models; the process is rarely linear. Virtually all frameworks for intervention development and testing call for mixed methods (MM) research.
- Conceptualization and in-depth understanding of the problem and the target population are key issues during Phase 1 development work. An important product during Phase 1 is a carefully conceived **intervention theory** from which the design of the intervention flows. The theory indicates what inputs are needed to effect improvements on specific outcomes and is often incorporated into a *logic model*.
- In addition to theory, resources for creating an evidence-based intervention and intervention strategies during Phase 1 development include systematic reviews, descriptive research with

the target population or key stakeholders, consultation with experts, and brainstorming with a dedicated and diverse team.

- In developing an intervention, researchers must make decisions about not only the *content* of the intervention but also about dose and intensity, timing of the intervention, outcomes to target and when to measure them, intervention setting, intervention agents, mode of delivery, and individualization.

- In a Phase 2 **pilot study**, the preliminary intervention is tested for feasibility and preliminary effectiveness. Pilots often include supplementary qualitative components to understand the experience of being in the intervention and any problems with recruitment, retention, and acceptability.

- A mixed methods approach can strengthen the test of the intervention during the Phase 3 controlled trial. The inclusion of qualitative components can shed light on intervention fidelity, clinical significance, and interpretive ambiguities.

- Mixed methods designs are appropriate in all phases of an intervention project. Broadly speaking, the design is sequential, but each phase can involve the use of various mixed methods designs. In Phase 1, QUAL often has priority, while in Phases 2 and 3, QUAN is usually dominant.

STUDY ACTIVITIES

Study activities are available to instructors on thePoint.

REFERENCES CITED IN CHAPTER 28

Abraham, C., Denford, S., Smith, J., Dean, S., Greaves, C., Lloyd, J., … Wyatt, K. (2015). Designing interventions to change health-related behaviour. In Richards, D., & Rahm Hallberg, I. (Eds.), *Complex interventions in health: An overview of research methods* (pp. 103–110). Oxford, UK: Routledge.

*Barley, E., Haddad, M., Simmonds, R., Fortune, Z., Walters, P., Murray, J., … Tylee, A. (2012). The UPBEAT depression and coronary heart disease programme: Using the UK Medical Research Council framework to design a nurse-led complex intervention for use in primary care. *BMC Family Practice, 13*, 119.

*Barley, E., Walters, P., Haddad, M., Phillips, R., Achilla, E., McCrone, P., … Tylee, A. (2014). The UPBEAT nurse-delivered personalized care intervention for people with coronary heart disease who report current chest pain and depression: A randomised controlled pilot study. *PLOS One, 9*, e98704.

Bartholomew Eldredge, L., Markham, C., Ruiter, R., Fernandez, M., Kox, G., & Parcel, G. (2016). *Planning health promotion programs: An intervention mapping approach* (4th ed.). San Francisco: Jossey-Bass.

**Berg, S. K., Moons, P., Christensen, A., Zwisler, A., Pedersen, P., & Pedersen, P. (2015). Clinical effects and implications of cardiac rehabilitation for implantable cardioverter defibrillator patients. *Journal of Cardiovascular Nursing, 30*, 420–427.

Bleijenberg, N., Boeije, H., Onderwater, A., & Schuurmans, M. (2015). Frail older adults' experiences with a proactive, nurse-led primary care program: A qualitative study. *Journal of Gerontological Nursing, 41*, 20–29.

*Bleijenberg, M., de Man-van Ginekl, J., Trappenburg, J., Ettema, R., Sino, C., Heim, N., … Schuurmans, M. (2018). Increasing value and reducing waste by optimizing the development of complex interventions: Enriching the development phase of the Medical Research Council (MRC) framework. *International Journal of Nursing Studies, 79*, 86–93.

*Bleijenberg, N., Drubbel, I., Neslo, R., Schuurmans, M., Ten Dam, V., Numans, M., … de Wit, N. (2017). Cost-effectiveness of a proactive primary care program for frail older people: A cluster randomized controlled trial. *Journal of the American Medical Directors Association, 18*, 1029–1036.

Bleijenberg, N., Drubbel, I., Schuurmans, M., Dam, H., Zuithoff, N., Numans, M., & de Wit, N. (2016a). Effectiveness of a proactive primary care program on preserving daily functioning of older people: A cluster randomized controlled trial. *Journal of the American Geriatrics Society, 64*, 1779–1788.

*Bleijenberg, N., Drubbel, I., ten Dam, V., Numans, M., Schuurmans, M., & de Wit, N. (2012). Proactive and integrated primary care for frail older people: Design and methodological challenges of the Utrecht primary care PROactive frailty intervention trial (U-PROFIT). *BMC Geriatrics, 12*, 16.

Bleijenberg, N., ten Dam, V., Drubbel, I., Numans, M., de Wit, N., & Schuurmans, M. (2013a). Development of a proactive care program (U-CARE) to preserve physical functioning of frail older people in primary care. *Journal of Nursing Scholarship, 45*, 230–237.

Bleijenberg, N., ten Dam, V., Drubbel, I., Numans, M., de Wit, N., & Schuurmans, M. (2016b). Treatment fidelity of an evidence-based nurse-led intervention in a proactive primary care program for older people. *Worldviews on Evidence-Based Nursing, 13*, 75–84.

Bleijenberg, N., ten Dam, V., Steunenberg, B., Drubbel, I., Numans, M., deWit, N., & Schuurmans, M. (2013b). Exploring the expectations, needs and experiences of general practitioners and nurses toward a proactive and structured care programme for frail older patients: A mixed methods study. *Journal of Advanced Nursing, 69*, 2262–2273.

Borglin, G. (2015). The value of mixed methods for researching complex interventions. In Richards, D., & Rahm Hallberg, I. (Eds.), *Complex interventions in health: An overview of research methods* (pp. 29–45). Oxford, UK: Routledge.

*Campbell, M., Fitzpatrick, R., Haines, A., Kinmouth, A., Sandercrock, P., Spiegelhalter, D., & Tryer, P. (2000). Framework for design and evaluation of complex interventions to improve health. *BMJ, 321*, 694–696.

Chalmers, I., Bracken, M., Djulbegovic, B., Garattini, S., Grant, J., Gulmezoglu, A, ... Oliver, S. (2014). How to increase value and reduce waste when research priorities are set. *The Lancet, 383*, 156–165.

Corry, M., Clarke, M., While, A., & Lalor, J. (2013). Developing complex interventions for nursing: A critical review of key guidelines. *Journal of Clinical Nursing, 22*, 2366–2386.

*Craig, P., Dieppe, P., Macintyre, S., Michie, S., Nazareth, I., & Petticrew, M. (2008a). *Developing and evaluating complex interventions: New guidance*. London: MRC.

*Craig, P., Dieppe, P., Macintyre, S., Michie, S., Nazareth, I., & Petticrew, M. (2008b). Developing and evaluating complex interventions: The new Medical Research Council guidance. *BMJ, 337*, 979–983.

Creswell, J. W., & Plano Clark, V. L. (2018). *Designing and conducting mixed methods research* (3rd ed.). Thousand Oaks, CA: Sage.

*De Silva, M., Breuer, E., Lee, L., Asher, L., Chowdhary, N., Lund, C., & Patel, V. (2014). Theory of Change: A theory-driven approach to enhance the Medical Research Council's framework for complex interventions. *Trials, 15*, 267.

*Drubbel, I., Numans, M., Kranenburg, G., Bleijenberg, N., deWit, N., & Schuurmans, M. (2014). Screening for frailty in primary care: A systematic review of the psychometric properties of the Frailty Index in community-dwelling older people. *BMC Geriatrics, 14*, 27.

Duggleby, W., & Williams, A. (2016). Methodological and epistemological consideration in utilizing qualitative inquiry to develop interventions. *Qualitative Health Research, 26*, 147–153.

*Finch, T., Rapley, T., Girling, M., Mair, F., Murray, E., Treweek, S., ... May, C. (2013). Improving the normalization of complex interventions: Measure development based on Normalization Process Theory (NoMAD). *Implementation Science, 8*, 43.

*Fletcher, A., Jamal, F., Moore, G., Evans, R., Murphy, S., & Bonnell, C. (2016). Realist complex intervention science: Applying realist principles across all phases of the Medical Research Council framework for developing and evaluating complex interventions. *Evaluation, 22*, 286–303.

*Gillespie, B., Harbeck, E., Lavin, J., Gardiner, T., Withers, T., & Marshall, A. P. 2018). Using Normalization Process Theory to evaluate the implementation of a complex intervention to embed the surgical safety checklist. *BMC Health Services Research, 18*, 170.

Green, L., & Kreuter, M. (2005). *Health program planning: An educational and ecological approach* (4th ed.). New York: McGraw Hill.

*Hall, S., Chochinov, H., Harding, R., Murray, S., Richardson, A., & Higginson, I. (2009). A phase II randomised controlled trial assessing the feasibility, acceptability and potential effectiveness of Dignity Therapy for older people in care homes. *BMC Geriatrics, 9*, 9.

Hall, S., Goddard, C., Speck, P., & Higginson, I. (2013). "It makes me feel that I'm still relevant": A qualitative study of the views of nursing home residents on Dignity Therapy and taking part in a phase II randomised controlled trial of palliative care psychotherapy. *Palliative Medicine, 27*, 358–366.

*Hansen, A., & Jones, A. (2017). Advancing "real world" trials that take account of social context and human volition. *Trials, 18*, 531.

Hawe, P., Shiell, A., & Riley, T. (2009). Theorising interventions as events in systems. *American Journal of Community Psychology, 43*, 267–276.

*Holloway, A., Landale, S., Ferguson, J., Newbury-Birch, D., Parker, R., Smith, P., & Sheikh, A. (2017). Alcohol Brief Interventions (ABIs) for male remand prisoners: Protocol for development of a complex intervention and feasibility study. *BMJ Open, 7*, e014561.

*Ioannidis, J. (2016). Why most clinical research is not useful. *PLoS Medicine, 13*, e1002049.

Johnston, B., Lawton, S., McCaw, C., Law, E., Murray, J., Gibb, J, ... Rodriguez, C. (2016). Living well with dementia: Enhancing dignity and quality of life, using a novel intervention, Dignity Therapy. *International Journal of Older People Nursing, 11*, 107–120.

Lauver, D. R., Ward, S. E., Heidrich, S. M., Keller, M. L., Bowers, B.J., Brennan, P.F, ... Wells, T. J. (2002). Patient-centered interventions. *Research in Nursing & Health, 25*, 246–255.

Lee, C., Lee, C., Hsu, M., Lai, C., Sung, Y., Lin, C., & Lin, L. (2018). Effects of music intervention on state anxiety and physiological indices in patients undergoing mechanical ventilation in the intensive care unit. *Biological Research for Nursing, 19*, 137–144.

*Lewin, S., Hendry, M., Chandler, J., Oxman, A., Michie, S., Shepperd, S., ... Noyes, J. (2017). Assessing the complexity of interventions within systematic reviews: Development, content and use of a new tool (iCAT_SR). *BMC Medical Research Methodology, 17*, 76.

*Lu, Y. Y., & Haase, J. (2011). Content validity and acceptability of the Daily Enhancement of Meaningful Activity program intervention for mild cognitive impairment patient-spouse dyads. *Journal of Neuroscience Nursing, 43*, 317–328.

*May, C. (2013). Towards a general theory of implementation. *Implementation Science, 8*, 8–18.

*May, C., Johnson, M., & Finch, T. (2016). Implementation, context and complexity. *Implementation Science, 11*, 141.

McGuire, D., DeLoney, V., Yeager, K., Owen, D., Peterson, D., Lin, L., & Webster, J. (2000). Maintaining study validity in a changing clinical environment. *Nursing Research, 49*, 231–235.

*Michie, S., van Stralen, M., & West, R. (2011). The Behaviour Change Wheel: A new method for characterizing and designing behavior change interventions. *Implementation Science, 6*, 42.

*Moore, G., Audrey, S., Barker, M., Bond, L., Bonell, C., Hardeman, W., … Baird, J. (2015). Process evaluation of complex interventions: Medical Research Guidance. *BMJ, 350*, h1258.

Morden, A., Ong, B., Brooks, L., Jinks, C., Porcheret, M., Edwards, J., & Dziedzic, K. (2015). Introducing evidence through research "push": Using theory and qualitative methods. *Qualitative Health Research, 25*, 1560–1575.

Morse, J. M. (2006). The scope of qualitative derived clinical interventions. *Qualitative Health Research, 16*, 591–593.

Morse, J., Penrod, J., & Hupcey, J. (2000). Qualitative outcome analysis: Evaluating nursing interventions for complex clinical phenomena. *Journal of Nursing Scholarship, 32*, 125–130.

Naylor, M. D. (2003). Nursing intervention research and quality of care. *Nursing Research, 52*, 380–385.

Payne, K., & Thompson, A. J. (2015). Economic evaluations of complex interventions. In Richards, D., & Rahm Hallberg, I. (Eds.), *Complex interventions in health: An overview of research methods* (pp. 326–333). Oxford, UK: Routledge.

*Pfadenhauer, L., Gerhardus, A., Mozygemba, K., Lydashi, K., Booth, A., Hofmann, B., … Rehfuess, E. (2017). Making sense of complexity in context and implementation: The Context and Implementation of Complex Interventions (CICI) framework. *Implementation Science, 12*, 21.

Rahm Hallberg, I. (2015). Knowledge for health care practice. In Richards, D., & Rahm Hallberg, I. (Eds.), *Complex interventions in health: An overview of research methods* (pp. 16–28). Oxford, UK: Routledge.

Richards, D. A. (2015a). The critical importance of patient and public involvement for research into complex interventions. In Richards, D., & Rahm Hallberg, I. (Eds.), *Complex interventions in health: An overview of research methods* (pp. 46–50). Oxford, UK: Routledge.

Richards, D. A. (2015b). A few final thoughts. In Richards, D., & Rahm Hallberg, I. (Eds.), *Complex interventions in health: An overview of research methods* (pp. 326–333). Oxford, UK: Routledge.

Richards, D. A., & Rahm Hallberg, I., (Eds.). (2015). *Complex interventions in health: An overview of research methods.* Oxford, UK: Routledge.

*Saal, S., Meyer, G., Beutner, K., Klingshirn, H., Strobl, R., Grill, E., … Muller, M. (2018). Development of a complex intervention to improve participation of nursing home residents with joint contractures: A mixed method study. *BMC Geriatrics, 18*, 61.

Sandelowski, M. (1996). Using qualitative methods in intervention studies. *Research in Nursing & Health, 19*, 359–365.

Sermeus, W. (2015). Modelling process and outcomes in complex interventions. In Richards, D., & Rahm Hallberg, I. (Eds.), *Complex interventions in health: An overview of research methods* (pp. 111–126). Oxford, UK: Routledge.

Sidani, S. (2015). *Health intervention research: Understanding research design & methods.* Thousand Oaks, CA: Sage.

Sidani, S., & Braden, C. J. (2011). *Design, evaluation, and translation of nursing interventions.* New York: Wiley-Blackwell.

*Tylee, A., Barley, E., Walters, P., Achilla, E., Borschmann, R., Leese, M., … Mann, A. (2016). UPBEAT-UK: A programme of research into the relationship between coronary heart disease and depression in primary care patients. *Programme Grants for Applied Research, 4*(8).

Van Meijel, B., Gamel, C., van Swieten-Duijfjes, B., & Grypdonck, M. (2004). The development of evidence-based nursing interventions. *Journal of Advanced Nursing, 48*, 84–92.

*Wight, D., Wimbush, E., Jepson, R., & Doi, R. (2016). Six steps in quality intervention development. *Journal of Epidemiology and Community Health, 70*, 520–525.

A link to this open-access article or document is provided in the Toolkit for Chapter 28 in the Resource Manual. ⊗

**This journal article is available on the Point for this chapter.*

29 | Feasibility and Pilot Studies of Interventions Using Mixed Methods

In the Medical Research Council's (MRC) framework for complex interventions, as described in Chapter 28, mixed methods are used to develop a preliminary intervention (Craig et al., 2008). In the next phase, researchers assess whether the intervention, and ideas about rigorously testing it, make sense—that is, whether it is feasible, acceptable, and shows promise of positive effects.

There is considerable agreement in the health care literature that pilot studies are often poorly designed and reported. Until recently, there was little guidance on planning and conducting pilot work. Indeed, in their often cited "tutorial" on pilot studies, Thabane and colleagues (2010) stated with regard to coverage of pilot work in research methods textbooks, "We are not aware of any textbook that dedicates a chapter on this issue" (p. 2). We have remedied this situation by devoting this chapter to a discussion of feasibility assessments and pilot tests of interventions. Many other resources that offer excellent and cutting-edge advice for conducting pilot work have become available (e.g., Arain et al., 2010; Moore et al., 2011; Richards & Rahm Hallberg, 2015), and an open-access journal devoted to this topic (*Pilot and Feasibility Studies*) was inaugurated in 2015.

> **TIP** Wisdom regarding the value of advance planning can be seen in many cultures. For example, a 10th century bowl with a Kufic inscription on display in the Metropolitan Museum of Art in New York bears a relevant Iranian proverb: "Planning before work protects you from regret." Another proverb comes from Africa: "Only a fool tests the depth of a river with both feet."

BASIC ISSUES IN PILOTING INTERVENTIONS

This section lays the groundwork for conducting successful pilot work, the focus of which is to address *uncertainties* about the intervention or the planned evaluation.

Definition of Pilot and Feasibility Studies

The term *pilot study* has been defined in dozens of ways in the research literature and the terms pilot study and feasibility study are often used interchangeably. An international panel of experts recently came to a consensus about definitions and interrelationships, as delineated in a recent conceptual framework (Eldridge et al., 2016).

According to the expert panel, pilot studies are a subset of feasibility studies. *Feasibility* is an overarching concept—all pilot studies are feasibility studies, but not all feasibility studies are pilots. A **feasibility study** addresses whether something can be done: Should the team proceed with a project and, if so, how? The broad category of feasibility study includes three types of studies: randomized pilot studies, nonrandomized pilot studies, and other feasibility studies that are not pilots.

A **pilot study** is designed to assess the feasibility of mounting an intervention, but also has a specific goal of testing, on a smaller scale, features of a larger, more definitive future study. Pilot studies are designed to support refinements of the protocols, methods, and procedures to be used in a larger scale trial of an intervention. The emphasis in pilot studies is on assessing the feasibility of an entire set of procedures for a full-scale evaluation, including recruitment, protocol implementation, data collection procedures, outcome measurement, blinding, and the capacity to avoid contamination across treatment groups. Some pilot studies involve a randomized design—for example, to test whether people are willing to be randomized to treatment groups. Other pilot studies adopt quasi-experimental designs. Taylor and colleagues (2015) offer suggestions for when a pilot study requires randomization.

The third type of feasibility study is what the expert panel called "other" feasibility studies—which in this chapter we will call *feasibility assessments*. Such studies are often undertaken to test specific and discrete aspects of a new intervention or potential trial. For example, a feasibility assessment might evaluate whether a 10-week intervention is feasible and acceptable. Or, a feasibility assessment might explore whether a sufficient number of sites can be enlisted to participate in a multisite trial. Feasibility studies do not focus on intervention outcomes, but rather examine parameters that are integral to the conduct of a full intervention trial. Feasibility assessments typically do not use a randomized design.

For some interventions, it might be necessary for researchers to undertake both a feasibility assessment and a pilot trial. Lessons learned in an early feasibility assessment might, for example, lead to further development work, as suggested in the MRC framework (Figure 28.1). In other cases, especially if there is a strong evidence base and a well-conceived intervention theory, a single pilot study might suffice.

The distinction between a feasibility assessment and a pilot study is important for researchers doing them—for example, a study should be properly labeled in seeking funding or in publishing findings. However, to streamline our presentation in this chapter, we will for the most part describe activities under a general rubric of *pilot work*. Pilot work is sometimes undertaken for nonintervention studies (e.g., for a large-scale survey), but in this chapter we focus on intervention research.

> **TIP** Some writers distinguish between an internal and external pilot. An *external pilot* is a stand-alone study, the findings from which inform the design and implementation of a full RCT. An *internal pilot* is an early phase of a large trial and the findings are typically used to adjust sample size projections. In this chapter, we primarily discuss stand-alone (external) pilot work.

Overall Purpose of Pilot Work

The overall purpose of pilot work is to avoid a costly fiasco. Fully powered RCTs are extremely expensive. Without piloting, a full-scale trial can result in wasted resources and erroneous conclusions. A strong pilot can enhance the likelihood that a full test will be methodologically and conceptually sound, ethical, and informative. As mentioned in Chapter 28, there is growing concern about waste and inefficiency in health care research (e.g., Ioannidis, 2016), and pilots represent an important tool in combatting these problems in a responsible manner (Treweek & Born, 2014). Large-scale trials often cannot get funded without adequate pilot work.

> **TIP** Thousands of studies in the healthcare literature are described as "pilots," but many are inappropriately labeled—they are often simply small studies. The term should not be used unless there is an explicit goal of learning how best to design and implement a larger and more definitive study.

Recent guidance on pilot work has emphasized an important point that is often not appreciated by those conducting pilots: *the purpose of a pilot is not to test hypotheses about the efficacy of the intervention.* That is, a goal should *not* be to test the effectiveness of an intervention on key outcomes—and if statistical hypothesis tests are used in pilot work, they should be interpreted cautiously (Arain et al., 2010; Thabane et al., 2010). Given the small sample size of pilots, hypothesis tests are typically underpowered and result in effect size estimates that are unreliable. We discuss this issue again later in the chapter.

TIP Moore and colleagues (2011) bemoaned the cycle of nonproductive work than can ensue when young researchers undertake a pilot, find nonsignificant results, abandon their ideas, and then pursue another topic. When hypothesis testing is a major objective of a pilot, disappointment is typically high, and results are often unreported.

Lessons From Pilot Work

An important product of pilot work is a description of the "lessons learned." Almost inevitably, the pilot will reveal that the intervention did not play out in "real life" the way it was designed "on paper." A review of published reports on lessons learned in pilot studies reveals some recurrent themes. The following are among the most frequently mentioned lessons from pilot intervention studies:

- Fewer people meet the eligibility criteria than anticipated
- Recruitment of participants is more difficult and takes longer than expected
- Materials intended for direct use by participants (e.g., pamphlets, educational materials) need to be simplified
- Participant burden, especially regarding data collection, needs to be reduced
- Effect sizes tend to be larger in the pilot than in the main trial
- Key ingredients of the intervention should be front-loaded—i.e., delivered early—because greater attention and higher attendance occurs early

- When there is a control condition, diffusion and contamination are recurrent problems
- Even expert interventionists need to be trained (including researchers themselves)
- Relationships with others need to be continuously nurtured

Researchers who undertake pilot work should keep these lessons in mind and try to design their study in such a way that frequently occurring problems are avoided or minimized.

Example of an Important Lesson Learned in Pilot Work

Beebe (2007) provided a good example of how her pilot study of an exercise intervention for outpatients with schizophrenia revealed an unexpected need. She and her coresearchers found that some of their participants lacked appropriate footwear for the intervention. They learned the need to plan for "the provision of footwear in the budgets for future projects" (p. 216).

OBJECTIVES AND CRITERIA IN PILOT WORK

Writers who offer advice about the conduct of feasibility and pilot studies almost invariably encourage researchers to carefully articulate explicit objectives. For any given pilot study, the specific objectives can be wide-ranging. Thabane and colleagues (2010) organized pilot objectives into four broad categories: process, resources, management, and scientific. We use this organization to describe some objectives that are good targets for pilot work. Our examples are not exhaustive, but hopefully they will suggest ideas for how pilot work can inform decisions about a full trial of an intervention.

Process-Related Objectives

Process-related objectives focus on the feasibility of planned procedures for launching and maintaining the study. These include such issues as eligibility criteria, recruitment, retention, comprehension, adherence, acceptability, and ethics. Each objective can be addressed by gathering data to answer various questions, examples of which are shown in Table 29.1. As the table indicates, process-related

TABLE 29.1 • Examples of Process-Related Objectives and Questions for Pilot Work

OBJECTIVE	QUESTIONS (QUANTITATIVE)	QUESTIONS (QUALITATIVE)
Recruitment: To assess the feasibility of recruiting an adequate number of study participants	• How many people were screened for eligibility each week/month? • What percentage of eligible people agreed to participate (and what percentage actually did participate)? • How many eligibles are enrolled each week/month? • What are the characteristics of those who do versus those who did not agree to participate? • How long did it take to recruit the needed sample?	• Why did eligibles decline to participate? What would make the intervention (or study participation) more appealing? Was randomization a factor in their decision? • What barriers exist in the research sites regarding successful recruitment? • Did certain recruitment strategies work well? Work poorly?
Eligibility Criteria: To assess the adequacy of the eligibility criteria	• How many eligible people are there in each site? What proportion of all clients/patients are eligible? • Which eligibility criterion was associated with the biggest loss of potential participants? • Was attrition from the pilot associated with a particular eligibility criterion?	• Were procedures for identifying eligibles clear and manageable? • Would loosening or tightening the eligibility criteria be acceptable to some stakeholders (e.g., family members)? Would it affect ease of recruitment?
Retention: To assess the ability to retain an adequate proportion of participants	• What percentage of initial study participants remained in the study as they moved through the trial? • Were there differences in attrition by study group (intervention vs. control)? • What were the characteristics of those who remained and those who did not? • At what point did attrition occur?	• Why did participants decide to withdraw from the study? • What factors in the research sites contributed to poor retention?
Protocol Adherence: To assess the degree to which participants adhere to protocols	• What percentage of participants got the full "dose" of the intervention? What "dose" of the intervention did the typical participant get? • What are the characteristics of those who adhered and those who did not? • Were there particular components for which adherence was especially poor?	• Why did participants not adhere to the intervention protocol (or not adhere to particular components)? • What factors in the research sites contributed to successful adherence?

(table continues on page 636)

TABLE 29.1 • **Examples of Process-Related Objectives and Questions for Pilot Work** (Continued)

OBJECTIVE	QUESTIONS (QUANTITATIVE)	QUESTIONS (QUALITATIVE)
Acceptability: To assess the extent to which the intervention/research is acceptable to recipients and key stakeholders	• How satisfied were recipients (or other stakeholders) with the intervention, or with specific components of the intervention? • What percentage of recipients were allocated to their preferred treatment condition? • To what extent did recipients feel overburdened by the data collection demands?	• What did recipients/ stakeholders like and dislike about the intervention? What changes to the intervention protocol would make it more acceptable? • What did recipients most dislike about research aspects (e.g., the amount of time needed, the frequency of data collection?)
Ethics: To assess the adequacy of human protections	Were there any breeches of human protections (e.g., privacy, confidentiality)?	Did participants feel that they their rights and privacy were adequately protected?

objectives are often best addressed by collecting both quantitative and quantitative data. Pilot studies and feasibility assessments are a good way of investigating potential problems in mounting an intervention—and exploring ways to remedy those problems.

Although preliminary answers to some of the questions in Table 29.1 are sometimes obtained during intervention development, those answers often need to be confirmed. For example, there may be a big difference between patients saying they *would be* interested in an intervention and actually *agreeing* to participate. Moreover, a person might be willing to participate in an intervention but may *not* be willing to be randomized to a control group. Or, even if a person is willing and interested, motivation may wane over the course of a multisession intervention. Thus, development work alone cannot answer important questions about feasibility of an intervention implemented in real-world settings.

Pilot work can reveal the adequacy of the initial eligibility criteria and suggest how eligibility criteria affect recruitment, retention, and protocol adherence. Decisions about eligibility criteria must address numerous concerns, including substantive

ones (Should some people be excluded because they might not benefit?), ethical ones (Might certain people be harmed?), methodologic ones (How will eligibility criteria be measured? Will the criteria yield an adequate pool for the full-scale trial?), and scientific ones (Will eligibility criteria constrain the generalizability of the findings?). Pilot data can be used to fine-tune decisions about eligibility and about the time needed to recruit a sufficiently large sample.

TIP Unfounded optimism about the size of the pool of eligibles is common—indeed, it is so common that it has been given a name: *Lasagna's law* (van der Wouden et al., 2007). Carlisle and colleagues (2015) found, in analyzing nearly 500 trials that had either terminated because of failed sample accrual or completed with a much smaller sample than intended, that unsuccessful accrual was strongly associated with having a high number of eligibility criteria.

A particularly important process issue concerns recruitment—not only of study participants, but also of sites and research staff. If a multisite trial is envisioned for the full RCT, the feasibility of enlisting cooperative sites should be explored early. It is not just an issue of getting enough sites to achieve an adequate sample size, but also of making sure that there are sites that represent the diversity of the target population of participants. Also, if exploration of sites suggests a high rate of refusals, researchers might want to explore what factors led to refusals by administrators—especially if those factors are relevant for the eventual uptake of the intervention, should the RCT reveal promising results. For example, if concerns about staff time are a key consideration, the intervention may have little hope of being translated on a large scale.

Recruitment of participants is a perennial problem in clinical trials and is becoming more challenging. For example, a study found that in publicly funded trials in the United Kingdom, 45% failed to reach the targeted sample size (Sully et al., 2013), and similar findings were reported by Walters et al. (2017). Quantitative data from pilot work can answer questions about the feasibility of recruiting a sufficient number for a full trial, but qualitative data may suggest how key barriers could be eliminated or how additional recruitment techniques could be pursued. Treweek (2015) offers useful advice about participant recruitment.

Poor retention of participants in the study and low protocol adherence (on the part of participants or intervention agents) are two other problems that are strong candidates for scrutiny in pilot work. Attrition can reduce the final sample size for analyses and can also lead to biases in estimating the intervention's potential benefits. High attrition, low adherence to protocols, and low levels of satisfaction suggest that an intervention is not yet ready for a full RCT.

Ethical issues also can be explored during the pilot phase. In particular, researchers need to be vigilant during a pilot regarding any unanticipated ethical transgressions that would need to be remedied before a main trial could be undertaken. Pilots are also a good place to get feedback about the consent process. Several commentators have pointed out the absence of any special guidelines for the ethical conduct of pilot studies. There is some agreement, however, that researchers have an obligation to disclose the feasibility nature of pilot studies during informed consent procedures (Arain et al., 2010; Thabane et al., 2010).

Example of Pilot Work Addressing Process Objectives

Himes and colleagues (2017) described the pilot testing of a web-based intervention, Healthy Beyond Pregnancy, which is designed to improve adherence to postpartum care. The feasibility objectives included determining the proportion of eligible women willing to participate in a randomized trial of the intervention and the proportion of women willing to complete the web-based program.

Resource-Related Objectives

Pilot work is often a useful way to get a handle on the resources that would be needed in a full-scale trial. Resource objectives typically concern the following aspects of a study:

- Monetary costs
- Time demands
- Institutional capacity
- Personnel requirements and availability
- Other resource needs such as equipment, technology, and lab facilities

Tickle-Degnen (2013) provided some good examples of resource-related questions asked in a pilot study of a self-management intervention for patients with Parkinson disease. Here are a few of them: (1) Do we have the capacity to handle the desired number of participants? (2) Do we have phone and communication technology capacity to stay in touch with and coordinate participants? and (3) Do we have institutional willingness and capacity to carry through with project-related tasks and to support investigator time and effort? Some additional questions relating to resource objectives are suggested in a table (analogous to Table 29.1 for process-type objectives) in the Supplement to this chapter on thePoint. Ⓢ

A full scale RCT of a complex intervention costs many thousands of dollars. A pilot study can help researchers develop a realistic budget for such a trial. It can also shed light on whether the costs of the intervention are likely to be commensurate with the benefits. Even at an early stage, researchers should consider whether it is realistic to pursue a costly trial for an intervention that is unlikely to be translated into real-world applications because of prohibitive costs or modest benefits.

Example of Pilot Work and Resource Objectives
Signorelli and colleagues (2018) described a pilot test of a nurse-led eHealth intervention to re-engage, educate, and empower childhood cancer survivors. The researchers plan to gather data about the cost consequences of the intervention, including the costs of delivering it and costs of referrals and medical care received.

Management-Related Objectives

Another category of objectives for pilot work concerns the ability for the research team to manage the effort and work productively as a team. Pilot work can help to identify management "glitches" that should be addressed before moving on to a full-scale trial. The management-related objectives in pilot work include assessing feasibility in terms of the following:

- Viability of the site or sites
- Motivation and competence of project staff
- Adequacy of reporting, monitoring, technological, and other systems
- Ability to manage or nurture interpersonal relationships

In articles that have described "lessons learned" from pilot work, a recurrent theme is that interpersonal relationships can create problems. These can be the result of tensions among staff, between staff and management, and between staff and study participants or their family members. Researchers have found that it is often useful to give various stakeholders a sense of ownership, and an opportunity to make suggestions or air complaints.

In the previously mentioned paper on pilot work for a self-management intervention for patients with Parkinson disease, Tickle-Degnen (2013) addressed various feasibility questions relating to management objectives. For example, what are the challenges and strengths of the investigators'

administrative capacity to: (1) Manage the planned RCT? (2) Design systems to document participant progress through the trial? (3) Enter data and perform quality checks? and (4) Manage the ethical aspects of the trial? Additional examples of questions relating to management objectives are presented in Table 2 of the Supplement on thePoint. 🅢

Scientific-Related Objectives: Substantive Issues

Scientific objectives are the fourth category in Thabane and colleagues' (2010) classification system. For this crucial class of objectives, we discuss two subcategories. The first set of scientific objectives is substantive, concerning the intervention itself. The second set of scientific objectives is methodologic, concerning the feasibility of rigorously testing the intervention. In this section, we discuss substantive scientific objectives for pilot work.

Intervention Attributes

A pilot test provides an opportunity to evaluate whether the decisions made during the development phase regarding intervention content, dose, timing, setting, sequencing, and so on were sensible ones (Feeley & Cossette, 2015). A pilot study is an ideal time to revise the intervention protocols, based on feedback from participants and intervention staff and on such indicators as attendance and attrition. Table 3 in the Supplement provides examples of questions relating to the attributes of the intervention than can be addressed in a pilot study. 🅢

Safety and Tolerability

Assessing the safety of patients in trials of a new intervention and the tolerability of the intervention are crucial objectives of many pilot studies. Unfortunately, it is widely acknowledged that pilots do a poor job of providing reliable safety and tolerability data because of small sample sizes. For example, in a pilot with 30 patients, observing no adverse events does not necessarily mean that there are no safety risks.

Leon and colleagues (2011) advised that group-specific adverse events rates in pilots should be reported, with 95% confidence intervals. They further recommended that when no adverse event is observed, the *rule of three* should be used to estimate the upper bound of the 95% CI. This "rule" uses as the upper bound the value of $3/n$. Thus, if there are 30 participants per group, and zero adverse events are observed in the intervention group, the 95% CI for the adverse event rate for that group would be estimated as 0% to 10% (3/30 = 10). Such a calculation, which suggests the possibility that one out of 10 participants could experience an adverse event, illustrates the tenuous nature of pilot data relating to safety and tolerability.

It is nevertheless important to monitor safety and tolerability if the intervention has potential for even minor adverse events such as fatigue or dizziness. Moreover, as noted by Leon et al. (2011), pilots are useful for testing the adequacy of safety monitoring systems. Pilots may also suggest the desirability of requiring permission to participate in the trial from participants' physicians. Feedback from participants about perceptions of safety and tolerability are also very useful for evaluating potential safety problems. Some specific questions about safety and tolerability are included in the chapter Supplement. **S**

Example of Pilot Work and Safety Assessment

Chan and colleagues (2017) undertook a pilot test of a central venous access device and dressing for peripherally inserted central catheters (PICC) in adult acute hospital patients. The feasibility outcomes included the safety of the intervention. In their pilot with 124 patients, the researchers monitored such outcomes as dressing failure, skin complications, PICC removal for local infection, and catheter-associated bloodstream infection.

Intervention Efficacy

Most pilot studies are undertaken with the objective of gaining preliminary evidence of the intervention's potential to be beneficial. As previously noted, hypothesis testing is not considered appropriate in pilot tests because of the high risk of making a Type II error—i.e., falsely concluding that the intervention is not effective, even when it was.

Effect size (ES) estimates provide information about the potential of an intervention to achieve beneficial effects on key outcomes, but extreme caution is needed in interpreting pilot ES results. We illustrate the problem by presenting 95% confidence intervals around effect size estimates (d) of different magnitude for various sample sizes that are common in pilot studies (Table 29.2). As a reminder, the effect size d is computed by dividing the difference between two group means (i.e., intervention and control group postintervention means on an outcome) by the pooled standard deviation. For example, suppose that in a pilot study with 40 participants (20 per group) we calculated d for the primary outcome to be .50, which is a moderately strong ES. As Table 29.2 indicates, in this scenario there is a 95% probability that the *true* effect size lies somewhere between -0.13 (i.e., the intervention is mildly detrimental) and $+1.13$ (i.e., the intervention is extremely beneficial). Increasing the sample size decreases the width of the estimated range and thus offers stronger evidence of the intervention's potential effectiveness. For example, with a sample size of 100 pilot participants (50 per group), the 95% CI for a d of .50 ranges from .10 (mildly favorable) to .90 (strongly favorable). (As we discuss later, a 95% CI is considered by some experts to be too stringent for pilot work, although it is the conventional standard.) The pilot effect size should at least be encouraging. For example, an obtained d of 0.02 is unlikely to instill confidence about the intervention's benefits.

Because the objective in a pilot is to obtain preliminary (and not definitive) evidence of the intervention's potential benefits, researchers should use additional methods to draw conclusions about an intervention's effects. In-depth interviews with program participants and intervention agents concerning their perceptions of benefits or disappointments are an especially important means of augmenting statistical results. For example, the plausibility of weak beneficial effects (based on the lower limit of the confidence limit) can sometimes be challenged

TABLE 29.2 • 95% Confidence Intervals[a] Around d, for Various N's and d's

d	N = 20 10 PER GROUP	N = 30 15 PER GROUP	N = 40 20 PER GROUP	N = 50 25 PER GROUP	N = 60 30 PER GROUP	N = 100 50 PER GROUP
0.20	−0.69 to 1.09	− 0.53 to 0.93	−0.43 to 0.83	−0.37 to 0.77	−0.32 to 0.72	−0.20 to 0.60
0.30	−0.59 to 1.19	−0.43 to 1.03	−0.33 to 0.93	−0.27 to 0.87	−0.22 to 0.82	−0.10 to 0.70
0.40	−0.49 to 1.29	−0.33 to 1.13	−0.23 to 1.03	−0.17 to 0.97	−0.12 to 0.92	0.00 to 0.80
0.50	−0.39 to 1.39	−0.23 to 1.23	−0.13 to 1.13	−0.07 to 1.07	−0.02 to 1.02	0.10 to 0.90
0.60	−0.29 to 1.49	−0.13 to 1.33	−0.03 to 1.23	0.03 to 1.17	0.08 to 1.12	0.20 to 1.00
0.70	−0.19 to 1.59	−0.03 to 1.43	0.07 to 1.33	0.13 to 1.27	0.18 to 1.22	0.30 to 1.10

[a]Approximation of 95% CI using formula provided in Leon et al., 2011: $d + (4 \div \sqrt{N})$; assumes two groups of equal size.

through participants' feedback about the intervention's value to them. If there is a consistent pattern of positive ES estimates for several key outcomes, and if there is corroborating qualitative data, researchers may be well poised to conclude that intervention efficacy is promising.

Example of Pilot Work and Effect Size Estimates
Wang and colleagues (2018) conducted a pilot trial to test a behavioral lifestyle intervention for overweight or obese adults with type 2 diabetes. They found a moderately large effect size for weight loss (0.40) and an effect size of 0.28 for glycemic control.

TIP Major changes to the intervention based on pilot work (e.g., to the intervention content or dose) may put into question the accuracy of the pilot effect size as an estimate of what would be obtained in a full trial.

Clinical Significance

Another possible objective for pilot work is an early assessment of the intervention's clinical significance. At the group level, effect size estimates are often used to draw conclusions about clinical significance, as discussed in Chapter 21. This means that the researchers should establish in advance the size of the effect that would be

regarded as clinically significant. The criterion could be based on a consensus reached by an advisory panel. Arnold and colleagues (2009) advised that an intervention can be declared to have potential efficacy if the 95% CI around the estimated effect size includes a predesignated minimal for clinical significance. However, given the width of 95% CIs when the sample is small, this may be too liberal a standard. For example, with a sample of 50 pilot participants (25 per group), and a criterion of 0.50 for a clinically significant d, even an obtained d of 0.00 would meet this criterion (95% CI = −0.57 to + 0.57). Thus, it might be more prudent for the advisory group to establish not only the criterion for clinical significance, but also the acceptable range. For example, if the criterion were 0.50, experts might set the lower bound for clinical significance at an ES of 0.20.

As described in Chapter 21, there is another approach to evaluating clinical significance. If the primary outcome is one with an established MIC (minimal important change) benchmark, the percentage of participants who achieved a clinically significant change can be computed. Even in the absence of statistical significance, if a sizeable percentage of intervention recipients had clinically meaningful improvement, this could support the conclusion that the intervention showed promise.

Scientific-Related Objectives: Methodologic Issues

Scientific objectives encompass not only substantive concerns about the intervention, but also methodologic concerns about the feasibility of undertaking a rigorous controlled trial. This section focuses on pilot objectives relating to the methods of testing a new intervention.

Research Design

Preliminary evidence about feasibility can be obtained in feasibility assessments using fairly simple designs, such as a one-group pretest–posttest design. However, for a pilot study, the design ideally should be a trial run of the full-scale test. Many experts recommend that a pilot study use a randomized design rather than a quasi-experimental one to gain confidence that an RCT of the full trial is feasible (e.g., Conn et al., 2010; Thabane et al., 2010). As noted by Leon and colleagues (2011), the inclusion of a randomized control group in a pilot study "allows for a more realistic examination of recruitment, randomization, implementation of intervention, blinded assessment procedures, and retention" (p. 627).

A crucial issue in randomized trials is whether there is any contamination between the treatment groups. Pilot trials provide a good opportunity to assess whether any cointerventions could inflate intervention benefits (if those in the intervention receive them) or dilute benefits (if control group members receive them). Some questions about the viability of various design features, as well as other methodologic objectives, are provided in Table 4 of the chapter Supplement on thePoint. 🅢

Intervention Fidelity

Pilot studies offer researchers the opportunity to examine whether intervention agents can successfully implement the intervention as planned. Researchers also can assess the adequacy of intervention fidelity procedures for the full trial. Both quantitative and qualitative data play an important role in helping researchers understand how successful the implementation of the intervention

was, and identify barriers to full enactment of the intervention protocols. Quantitative data can be used to calculate actual rates of achieving fidelity, and qualitative data can help researchers understand factors that made fidelity difficult to accomplish.

Example of Pilot Work and Intervention Fidelity
Coppell and colleagues (2017) pilot tested a primary-care nurse-led dietary intervention for prediabetes in New Zealand. The intervention involved the use of a structured dietary tool in visits at baseline, 2 weeks, 3 months, and 6 months. Fidelity was monitored by observing nurse training sessions, reviewing documents, and interviewing key informants and patients. The researchers concluded that implementation fidelity was high during the pilot.

Data Collection Protocols and Instruments

Researchers make many decisions about data collection instruments and procedures for intervention studies, and a pilot trial offers researchers an opportunity to assess those decisions. Data quality and participant burden are two key areas of inquiry. A pilot provides an opportunity to examine patterns of missing data, to evaluate internal consistency of any scales, to assess participant comprehension, to explore variability in responses, and to estimate how much time is required to administer the research instruments. Given the evidence that people often drop out of studies because of a burdensome schedule of data collection, it is important to understand the practicality of proposed methods. Lengthy data collection instruments are not only risky in terms of attrition, but also have cost implications for data collection staff, data entry, and analysis. The pilot study might lead researchers to eliminate one or more outcomes, to select shorter instruments, or to alter the schedule for measuring outcomes. Van Teijlingen and Hundley (2001) offer explicit advice about pilot testing instruments for use in a full-scale study.

Sample Size

Many pilot studies are conducted to inform sample size decisions for the main trial, but using a pilot effect size in a power analysis is risky. A large pilot effect size (e.g., $d = .80$) could reflect an inflated positive result. If this d were used as the estimated effect size in a power analysis, it likely would result in an underpowered full-scale trial—i.e., the sample size projection would be too small. On the other hand, small pilot ES estimates could reflect a Type II error and could lead to a decision to abandon a potentially promising intervention.

> **TIP** Vickers (2003) found that many trials published in four major medical journals were considerably underpowered when sample size needs were estimated based on a pilot trial. He found, for example, that about one out of four of the full-scale trials needed five times as many participants as had been estimated.

Several approaches to this problem have been proposed. One is to calculate confidence intervals around the pilot ES and then use the lower limit of the CI in the power calculations. However, because the 95% CI results in a range that is unreasonably large with small pilot samples (Table 29.2), less conservative CIs have been suggested, such as an 80% CI (Cocks & Torgerson, 2013; Lancaster et al., 2004), a 75% CI (Lee et al., 2014), or a 68% CI (Hertzog, 2008).

As an example, suppose that in a pilot study with 30 participants (15 per group), we estimated the pilot ES as $d = 0.50$. As shown in Table 29.2, the 95% CI around 0.50 for this sample size ranges from -0.23 to $+1.23$. However, the 80% CI around a d of 0.50 ranges from -0.03 to 0.97, and the 68% CI ranges from 0.12 to $+ 0.88$. Using the lower limit for d of 0.12, the needed sample size for the final trial would still be prohibitive—over 1,000 subjects per group for power = .80 and alpha = .05 for a two-tailed test.

In many cases, researchers can draw on additional evidence to support their sample size projections. For example, if there were consistent evidence from trials of similar interventions that group differences on the primary outcome would favor the intervention group, we might be willing to

use a one-tailed test. This would result in a needed sample size of about 850 per group for the main trial for an estimated d of $+ 0.12$.

Additional avenues for deriving sample size estimates can be pursued when there is evidence from trials of similar interventions. To continue with our example of an observed $d = 0.50$ from our pilot, suppose there were three prior RCTs of a similar intervention. In these trials, the values of d were 0.26, 0.34, and 0.42 for the same primary outcome (e.g., pain)—values that all fall within the 95% CI of our pilot d of 0.50. We could argue that triangulating the evidence provides the best basis for estimating sample size requirements for a full-scale RCT. We might choose to use $d = 0.26$ (because it is the most conservative of the four estimates); or we might elect to use $d = 0.34$ (if the study with that ES was the most rigorous); or we might use $d = 0.38$ (the average of the four trials, including our own pilot. (Essentially, this is analogous to conducting a crude mini meta-analysis.) For a two-tailed test, these decisions would result in projected sample size needs of 233, 136, and 109, respectively, per group. If we had simply used our $d = 0.50$ in a power analysis, our projected sample size needs would have been 63 per group, which very well could have resulted in an underpowered full trial and a Type II error with nonsignificant results. On the other hand, if we had used $d = 0.12$ (the lower bound of the 68% CI around 0.50), we likely would not have pursued a full trial because it would have required a total sample size of over 2,000 participants.

A supplementary strategy is to factor in clinical significance in the power calculations (Kraemer et al., 2006). The rationale is that if the intervention cannot achieve benefits that are significant clinically, it may not matter that the trial is underpowered. Thus, in our example, suppose the judgment of the research team or an advisory group is that the effect size would need to be at least 0.40 to be clinically significant. In other words, there is a consensus that an ES of 0.40 is the threshold below which clinicians are unlikely to be interested in the intervention. If we used $d = 0.40$, the estimated sample size for the full trial would be about 100 per group for a two-group design. Based on our pilot results, an ES of 0.40 is plausibly attainable because it falls well within a 95% CI for a *d* of 0.50. And its attainability is supported by the results from another trial of a similar intervention in which *d* = 0.42 was obtained.

In short, the most defensible strategy for sample size calculation is to consider a totality of evidence to estimate the size of the effect that is plausibly attainable and clinically meaningful in a main test. More detailed and sophisticated guidance is provided by Ukoumunne et al. (2015) and Bell et al. (2018).

Criteria and Pilot Objectives

We have presented a wide range of objectives as potentially relevant in pilot work for interventions. Clearly, no pilot or feasibility study can address all the objectives we described. It is crucial to identify the objectives of the pilot work in advance, however, because important design and data collection decisions for the pilot depend on what the objectives are.

We recommend that researchers select pilot objectives based on several considerations. First, choose objectives for which information is genuinely lacking—that is, objectives that address key *uncertainties*. You may already have a good estimate of how much attrition to expect, for example, based on your own previous work with the target population or based on attrition rates in other similar trials. Second, select objectives that impinge most significantly on the feasibility of a full-scale trial. For example, if you cannot recruit a sufficient number of participants for the pilot, a large trial may be impossible. Thus, assessing and enhancing recruitment would be important objectives. And third, focus on objectives about which funders will be particularly vigilant. These might include recruitment and efficacy, for example, and might also include resource requirements.

The importance of articulating key pilot objectives stems from the fact that pilot work should lead to a decision about "next steps." Essentially,

there are three options. One decision would be to proceed to a full clinical trial. A second decision would be to revise the intervention protocols, methodologic protocols, or procedural processes. The decision to make changes might lead to further Phase I (developmental) work, and perhaps to a second pilot if the revisions are major. A third decision would be to abandon the entire effort because of poor prospects of feasibility or lack of adequate evidence that the intervention could be effective.

How do researchers make the critical decision about what course to take next? One widely advocated approach is to articulate not only objectives but also the criteria for making decisions (e.g., Arain et al., 2010; Arnold et al., 2009; Thabane et al., 2010). Prior to launching the pilot, the research team should formulate threshold criteria for claiming the feasibility of a full-scale RCT.

> **TIP** An alternative (or supplementary) approach to decision-making after a pilot study has been suggested by Bugge and colleagues (2013). Their framework involves a systematic analysis of pilot problems and assessments of possible solutions.

Table 29.3 (available in the Toolkit as a worksheet ✪) provides examples of pilot objectives and criteria for drawing conclusions about the feasibility of a full trial. As these examples suggest, the quantitative criteria can be expressed either as raw numbers or as rates. For example, the second and third entries in this table focus on the objective of assessing recruitment in the pilot. In objective #2, the benchmark for success involves having a certain percentage of all eligible people agreeing to participate in the pilot (in this example, 60%). In objective #3, by contrast, recruitment success is defined as getting a specific number of eligible people each week to agree to participate in the pilot.

The criteria would be based on judgments of the research team, but the judgments ideally would be informed by evidence gathered during the development phase (e.g., based on recruitment rates from other similar trials). The

TABLE 29.3 • **Examples of Pilot Objectives and Criteria for Success**

OBJECTIVE	CRITERION	MEASUREMENT
1. To assess the willingness of the site to screen prospective participants for eligibility	At least 50 patients per month will be screened for eligibility	Number of patients screened per month (and, possibly, number of patients not screened)
2. To assess the feasibility of recruiting study participants	60% of eligible people will agree to participate	Number agreeing to participate, divided by all eligibles
3. To assess the feasibility of recruiting study participants	At least three participants per week will be successfully recruited at each study site	Number of people agreeing to participate, per site
4. To assess the willingness of people to sign consent forms and be randomized	95% of people who agree to participate will be randomized to a treatment group	Number randomized, divided by number originally agreeing to participate
5. To assess the initiation of the intervention in a timely manner	90% of the people randomized to the intervention group will begin within 7 days of randomization	Number beginning the intervention within 7 days of randomization, divided by total number randomized
6. To assess adherence to the intervention	80% of those in the intervention group will complete at least 8 of the 10 intervention sessions	Number completing 8+ sessions, divided by the number randomized to the intervention
7. To assess the efficiency of the data collection protocols	90% of participants will complete the data collection package in < 30 minutes	Number completing package within 30 minutes, divided by all completing the package
8. To assess trial retention rates	80% of participants in both study groups will complete 3-month follow-up instruments	Number of people in each group completing 3-month follow-ups, divided by number randomized to each group
9. To assess the intervention's acceptability	75% of participants will say they are "satisfied" or "completely satisfied" with the intervention	Number of patients who are satisfied, divided by number of intervention participants
10. To assess the preliminary efficacy of the intervention	Lower limit of the 68% confidence interval (CI) around the value of d will be at least 0.20	Lower limit of d for 68% CI around obtained d
11. To assess the clinical significance of the intervention	40% of those in the intervention group will have a reduction of 8+ cm on a visual analog scale (VAS) for pain (the minimal important change [MIC]) at 3 months post-baseline	Number in the intervention group whose follow-up VAS pain score is > 8 cm lower than that at baseline, divided by the number randomized to the intervention group

criteria should achieve a balance between what is ideal (e.g., 100% recruitment success) and what is realistic. Proposed criteria often can best be developed with the aid of an advisory group of experts and stakeholders. We emphasize that the criteria included in Table 29.3 are only *examples*—they should not be adopted literally without considering the actual context of pilot work, including the nature of the intervention, the site, and the target population.

Articulating criteria for the pilot's success makes decision-making about "next steps" easier. In the recruitment example, if only 30% of eligible patients in the pilot agreed to participate, the next step probably should not be to move forward to a full trial. Exploratory (qualitative) inquiry might help to reveal why the recruitment effort went awry. Perhaps different recruitment techniques are needed, perhaps the intervention or the research is too burdensome, or perhaps the eligibility criteria need to be adjusted. Without criteria for a pilot's success, researchers may be tempted to overinterpret their pilot data in the desired direction—i.e., to move forward to a full trial before it is wise to do so.

The decision about "next steps" is likely to depend on how many criteria are not met, and the degree of deficiency in meeting them. For example, a 30% recruitment rate when 60% or higher was the benchmark might lead to major rethinking of the project, but a 50% recruitment rate might lead to adjustments to enhance recruitment. If identified problems cannot readily be rectified, then researchers might be forced to "go back to the drawing board" in efforts to address a clinical problem.

The decision to move forward to a full trial should be a carefully considered one. In preparing a proposal to fund a rigorous RCT, the research team should be persuaded that: (1) the intervention and the research methods are feasible; (2) any pitfalls for a rigorous test have been identified and solutions to potential problems have been identified; (3) there is preliminary evidence that the intervention will be effective; and (4) important stakeholders are "on board."

Example of Stakeholder Issues

Bird and her colleagues (2011) described experiences from an evaluation of a complex rehabilitation intervention for patients undergoing stem cell transplantation. The intervention had not been rigorously piloted, and several problems were identified during the actual trial. One problem was resistance to the trial by staff, one of whom commented that "the trial killed the intervention" (p. 5).

THE DESIGN AND METHODS OF PILOT STUDIES

In this section we offer recommendations relating to the design and conduct of pilot work.

Research Design in Pilot Work

We encourage using a randomized design for a pilot trial, especially if the plan is to use the pilot as the basis for requesting funding for a full-scale trial. To the extent possible, all design features for the full trial should be tested, including the control group strategy, procedures for blinding, outcome measures, and the schedule of data collection. Arnold and colleagues (2009) have suggested that it might be constructive to conduct a pilot trial in multiple sites. A multisite pilot gives project managers experience in multisite supervision.

In a feasibility assessment, simpler designs are usually adequate. Simple descriptive designs may suffice—for example, if a major goal is to assess the number of eligible people or to estimate how many sites could be recruited. One-group designs are often used to assess aspects of the intervention itself, such as whether participants find the intervention acceptable.

It is advantageous to use mixed methods (MM) designs in pilot work, because feasibility questions concern not only whether key objectives can be met, but also why they might have fallen short. Thus, in many cases, the appropriate design for a pilot trial will be either concurrent MM designs (e.g., QUAN + qual or QUAN + QUAL) or sequential ones (e.g., QUAN → qual or QUAN → QUAL).

Example of a Research Design for a Pilot Study

Sin and colleagues (2013) provided a detailed description of their design for a pilot trial to test an online, multicomponent intervention for siblings of patients with an episode of psychosis. The intervention was designed using the MRC framework. Their plan was to recruit and randomize 120 eligible siblings and assign them to one of 4 groups (3 treatment groups, 1 control group). The mixed methods QUAN → qual design included follow-up interviews with a subsample of participants in all treatment groups to better understand their experiences. The researchers successfully recruited and randomized 144 siblings, but they did experience recruitment challenges that were explored in the in-depth interviews (Sin et al., 2017).

Sampling in Pilot Work

The sample used in pilot work should be drawn from the same population as that for the main trial. This means that the eligibility criteria should be the same—although these criteria might be adjusted during the pilot if researchers run into unanticipated problems.

The sample size for pilot studies is typically small. Hertzog (2008) examined pilot studies that had been funded by the National Institute of Nursing Research between 2002 and 2004 and found that for studies with two-group designs, the median number of participants per group was about 25. Billingham and colleagues (2013) did an audit of 79 pilot clinical studies in the United Kingdom and found that the median sample size per group in publicly funded trials was 33.

Several experts have suggested using confidence intervals around feasibility outcomes to estimate the sample size needed in the pilot (Arnold et al., 2009; Hertzog, 2008; Thabane et al., 2010). For example, suppose we decided that a full-scale trial would be feasible if the rate of attrition from the study was no more than 20% at a 3-month follow-up. Based on evidence from other similar trials or Phase I development work, we predict that the *actual* rate of attrition will be 12%. If we used a confidence interval of 95% around the expected rate of 12%, we would need a total sample size of 64 for the upper bound of the confidence interval

not to exceed the criterion of 20% attrition (95% CI around 12% = 4% to 20% for $N = 64$). If we relaxed our standard to a less stringent 90% CI for the same scenario, the needed total sample size for the pilot would be 46 (90% CI around 12% = 4% to 20% for $N = 46$). A table in the Toolkit provides examples of 95%, 90%, and 68% CIs around selected percentages and sample sizes. ⊗

The ideal sample size for a pilot will vary from study to study because of differences in objectives and populations. Bell and colleagues (2018) provide "rules of thumb" for pilot size as a function of the targeted effect size. For example, if the target effect size is a *d* between 0.10 and 0.30 for an 80% powered main trial, they recommend a sample of 20 per arm in the pilot, but if the target *d* is greater than 0.70, a sample of 10 per arm would suffice. Hertzog (2008), however, has recommended a pilot size of at least 30 to 40 per group if funding for the pilot is being sought.

Data Collection in Pilot Work

The data collection plan for pilots is typically complex, because the pilot data serve two purposes: to test the viability of the instruments that would be used in the main trial and to address the various objectives of the pilot itself.

In terms of the second purpose, the type of data to be collected depends on the objectives. For example, if a key objective is to assess the acceptability of the intervention (Table 29.3), then a quantitative measure of participant satisfaction would be needed.

Detailed documentation about the trial and its progress should be maintained to help illuminate what went right and what went wrong. It is useful to keep a diary or journal to record impressions and observations about the pilot experience. Diary entries are probably best organized thematically rather than chronologically. For example, journal sections could be devoted to each pilot objective. Entries for each objective should be made at least weekly.

Thought needs to be given to how best to "get inside" the workings of the pilot through the collection of in-depth data. This is likely to include unstructured observations of various intervention activities (e.g., recruitment, consent procedures, intervention sessions). Participants in both the intervention and control groups could be asked to complete **exit interviews.** Focus group interviews could also be conducted with various stakeholders, including participants, family members, and pilot study staff.

Example of Data Collection in a Pilot Trial

Plow and Golding (2017) assessed several feasibility objectives in their randomized pilot test of using mHealth technology in a self-management intervention to promote physical activity in adults with chronic disabling conditions. They collected quantitative data for various process objectives (e.g., attrition, fidelity) and patient outcomes (physical activity, self-efficacy, self-regulation). The researchers also collected qualitative data on participants' subjective experience in the interventions.

Data Analysis in Pilot Work

The analysis of quantitative data from a pilot study focuses mainly on the pilot objectives and, therefore, tends to involve mainly descriptive statistics. For example, the analysis might indicate what percentage of eligible people agreed to participate or consented to be randomized. Means and SDs are likely to be calculated (e.g., mean number of sessions completed, mean length of time to complete the data collection forms). Effect size estimates may also be computed. In most of these cases, it is a good idea to compute confidence intervals around estimates. An upfront decision should be made about the desired level of precision (e.g., 68%, 80%, etc.).

It has been argued that researchers should pay more attention to individual results in pilot studies than to group averages. Shih and colleagues (2004), for example, suggest that the emphasis should be on testing whether *any* individual experienced a beneficial effect, and provided statistical guidance for such an approach. One method is to assess whether, for each person, a reliable improvement has occurred (Chapter 15), or whether clinically significant change has occurred in a *responder analysis* (Chapter 21). If the main outcomes are ones for which minimal important change (MIC)

benchmarks have not been established, the research team can decide how large an improvement is needed to be deemed meaningful.

The results of the quantitative data analysis from pilots can be used to guide decisions about how to proceed, based on a comparison of the results to the preestablished criteria. Analysis of the qualitative can confirm the wisdom of that decision and can also help researchers make modifications to improve the likelihood that a full trial will be successful in giving the intervention a fair test.

PRODUCTS OF PILOT WORK

Pilot work should result in several products. As previously noted, one product should be a description of "lessons learned," which ideally would be drafted and reviewed by the research team, advisory panel, and key stakeholders for accuracy and completeness. Other products may include the following:

- Revised protocols for the intervention, its implementation, and the research plan (or, if major revisions are needed, a plan for further descriptive and exploratory research)
- A finalized list of outcomes
- A formal proposal for a full Phase III trial (or for another pilot) and a plan for seeking funding
- A written manuscript for publication in a professional journal

There has been considerable discussion about the desirability—and the obligation—of publishing results from pilots (e.g., Conn et al., 2010; Thabane et al., 2010). Moore and colleagues (2011) lamented that some researchers fail to publish pilot results because they "didn't find anything" (p. 3). This may well be the conclusion of researchers who focus on hypothesis tests of the intervention's efficacy, which are often nonsignificant. However, as we have discussed in this chapter, the main purpose of pilot work is *not* to test the statistical significance of intervention effects, but to assess the feasibility of a full-scale rigorous trial.

Even if a pilot trial suggests that the intervention has little hope of being effective, that knowledge should be shared. Others working on the same or a similar problem can benefit from learning about failures as well as successes. A related issue is the importance of including findings from pilots in meta-analyses and systematic reviews, especially if the pilot does not translate into a full trial. As we discuss in Chapter 30, meta-analysts struggle with the issue of *publication bias*—that is, the tendency of researchers to publish studies only when there are statistically significant results. Such a tendency does a disservice to evidence-based practitioners who are then using a biased subset of the evidence.

Several commentators have also noted that there is an ethical obligation to communicate the results from a pilot (e.g., Thabane et al., 2010; van Teijlingen et al., 2001). The argument is that participants have agreed to volunteer their time for an endeavor they believed would be helpful scientifically, and researchers fail to fulfill their end of the bargain if the findings are not shared. Moreover, precious research funds spent on pilots are wasted if the results are not published so that others can learn from what was done.

The quality of reporting of pilot studies has been criticized by many recent writers. Reports should clearly state the objectives of the pilot, as well the criteria used to make decisions about next steps. Given that the emerging advice on pilot testing is relatively new, researchers may have to "educate" reviewers and journal editors about the focus on feasibility objectives and not on hypothesis testing, citing the leading experts' advice about the risks of interpreting *p* values in pilots. We offer further suggestions about reporting pilot work in the Supplement to Chapter 32. 🛈

> **TIP** Researchers sometimes wonder if the data from an external pilot can be pooled with the data from a main study—in other words, treating the pilot participants as the early participants in the larger trial. This practice is considered acceptable only if there have been no changes in the intervention or study protocols, and if the population is the same. This is not likely to be the case in most circumstances. Lancaster et al. (2004) discuss the biases that can result from the practice of pooling data from the pilot into a main trial.

CRITICAL APPRAISAL OF FEASIBILITY AND PILOT STUDIES

Reports of pilot studies should provide descriptions of the study methods (e.g., the design, sampling and data collection plans, and so on). The intervention theory and development of the intervention should be explained, or a reference should be provided to any previously published papers on intervention development work. Readers should be able to draw their own conclusions about the potential feasibility and efficacy of the intervention, and so information about the key features of the intervention itself needs to be included.

A critical appraisal of pilot work should focus on the researchers' description of the pilot objectives, the criteria used to make decisions about feasibility, and the methods associated with the assessments. Readers should question the omission of explicitly stated objectives. If objectives and criteria were reported, readers can assess their reasonableness and judge whether the methods used to test them were adequate.

We have stressed that the small sample sizes of pilot trials make hypothesis testing for intervention efficacy a risky business. However, we do not recommend that pilot studies be criticized for including such information. Many journals expect such analyses, and editors may reject manuscripts that do not report them. Confidence intervals around the point estimates for outcomes or around effect size estimates would ideally be provided. However, if a pilot study does report the results of hypothesis testing, the researchers should be cautious in their interpretation of the results. Whether the results are statistically significant or not, the researchers should warn readers that the results are preliminary and that the sample size precludes definitive conclusions.

Box 29.1, which is also found in the Toolkit, ✖ offers some questions that can be used to appraise a report of a pilot study. The overarching question is whether the researchers were successful in securing the data needed to make a decision about what the next steps should be.

BOX 29.1 Guidelines for Critically Appraising Aspects of Pilot Work

1. Did the title and abstract of the paper describe the study as a pilot or feasibility study? Which term was used? Was the term "pilot" used appropriately—or was the study simply a small-scale or exploratory study with no mention of its role as part of a larger-scale effort?
2. Did the report state the explicit objectives of the study? Were specific feasibility outcomes identified, and was a description of how they were measured provided?
3. If objectives were stated, were they ones that would provide important knowledge about the design and conduct of a full-scale trial? Were potentially important objectives overlooked? Were too many objectives tested?
4. Did the researchers state the criteria that would be used as a basis for decision-making about "next steps"? If no, was there any discussion of how decisions might be made?
5. If there were explicit criteria for the pilot objectives, were the criteria reasonable ones? Were they too liberal or too strict?
6. To what extent did the design mirror the likely design for a full-scale trial? If randomization was not used, was that decision adequately justified?
7. How large was the pilot sample? Was the sample size adequate for addressing the study objectives?
8. Was the data collection plan adequate for measuring feasibility outcomes and for testing data collection protocols for a larger trial? Were both quantitative and qualitative data judiciously collected and integrated to provide a strong portrayal of feasibility?
9. Were confidence intervals around key variables reported? Was intervention effectiveness tested for key outcomes using statistical hypothesis testing procedures? If so, was sufficient caution used in interpreting the results?
10. Did the report describe important lessons learned? Did the discussion section describe how the intervention or the trial methods might be altered on the basis of the pilot?
11. Overall, was pilot work sufficient for a decision to move forward with a full clinical trial?

EXAMPLE OF A PILOT TRIAL

Study: Web-based symptom management for women with recurrent ovarian cancer: A pilot randomized controlled trial of the WRITE Symptoms intervention (Donovan et al., 2014).

Statement of Purpose: The overall purpose of this research was to pilot test the Written Representational Intervention To Ease Symptoms (WRITE Symptoms), an intervention designed for women with recurrent ovarian cancer.

Intervention: WRITE-Symptoms is an educational intervention delivered through asynchronous web-based message boards between a participant and a nurse. It was based on the Representational Approach (RA) to patient education and was the first RA intervention using a web-based delivery mode. The

approach included 7 elements to be covered over the course of the intervention (e.g., identifying gaps and confusions, goal setting and planning).

Objectives: A major objective of the pilot trial was to assess the "feasibility of conducting the study via message boards" (p. 218). Feasibility was assessed by examining participant retention and the time and number of postings from the date of the first message to the date of the last one. The researchers also addressed another process-type objective, the acceptability of the intervention. A third objective was a management-related one: to assess the usability of the web-based system. Finally, the researchers sought preliminary information about the intervention's efficacy in terms of such outcomes as symptom severity, distress, consequences, and controllability.

Design and Sample: A total of 271 women responded to various recruitment solicitations; 84 of the women met eligibility criteria, and of these, 68 eligible women (81%) completed consent forms. The actual pilot study participants were 65 eligible women recruited from 25 states, who were randomized with equal allocation to either the intervention group or to a wait-list control group. Random assignments were generated using minimization techniques that used race/ethnicity as a stratifying factor. Quantitative data relating to intervention outcomes were collected online at baseline and 2 and 6 weeks after the intervention. Open-ended comments and suggestions were also solicited.

Results: A total of 56 of the 65 study participants (88%) were retained in the study. Most participants assigned to the intervention (76%) completed all elements of the intervention, and only two women never posted to the message board. The mean length of participants' posts were 260 words, and the mean length of nurses' posts were 300 words. It took the nurse-participant dyads an average of 79 days to complete all elements of the intervention. Responses to questions on a satisfaction survey indicated that patients were very satisfied with the program. For example, the mean response to the item "I enjoyed participating in the symptom management program" was 6.35 on a 7-point satisfaction scale. On a scale that measured usability of the message boards, there was strong agreement that the website was easy to learn to use. Individual complaints concerned being timed out of the message board and needing to check and re-check the message board to see if a nurse had posted a message. The researchers also reported evidence of "preliminary efficacy." Women in the intervention group reported significantly lower distress than those in the control group. Group differences were also encouraging (although not at conventional levels of statistical significance) for symptom severity.

Conclusions: The researchers concluded that the study "supports the feasibility, acceptability, and efficacy of web-based educational interventions" (p. 228). The pilot served as the foundation for a larger RCT, with funding from the National Institute of Nursing Research. Although final results on the intervention's effectiveness were not yet reported, some papers based on the trial have been published (e.g., Hagan et al., 2017; Hay et al., 2016).

SUMMARY POINTS

- Although the terms *feasibility study* and *pilot study* are sometimes used interchangeably in intervention research, an emerging trend is for greater definitional precision. A **feasibility study** is undertaken to assess whether something can be done (is feasible). *Feasibility* is an umbrella term.

- A **pilot study** is a small-scale version of a full trial, designed to assess feasibility and an entire set of procedures for implementing and evaluating an intervention, often using a randomized design. Pilot studies are feasibility studies but not all feasibility studies are pilots. Nonpilot *feasibility assessments* can be undertaken to test specific, discrete aspects of an emerging intervention, often using a simple design.

- Full-scale evaluations of new interventions are costly. The overall purpose of pilot work is to avoid a costly failure.

- There is a growing consensus among experts in pilot study methods that the purpose of pilot work should *not* be to test hypotheses about the effectiveness of the intervention, because sample sizes in pilots are too small to yield reliable results.

- Pilot work can address a variety of objectives, and researchers should articulate their objectives at the outset. The objectives can focus on processes (e.g., recruitment, retention, acceptability); resources (e.g., monetary costs, time demands); management issues (e.g., system adequacy, interpersonal relationships); and scientific issues.

- Scientific objectives can concern the substantive aspects of the intervention, such as intervention content and dose, safety, preliminary evidence of efficacy, and clinical significance.

- Preliminary effect size estimates for key outcomes are often computed from pilot data, together with confidence intervals (CIs). Because only preliminary evidence of efficacy is sought in pilots, CIs that are not stringent (e.g., 68% CI) may be sufficient.

- Scientific objectives also concern questions about methodologic aspects of a trial, such as whether randomization is feasible. A major issue in many pilots is the estimation of the sample size that would be needed to adequately power a full trial. Using the effect size estimate from a pilot to estimate sample size needs directly is unwise, because such an estimate often leads to Type II errors—i.e., underpowered full-scale trials.

- Pilot studies are meant to inform the decision about whether to (1) move forward with a full trial, (2) make revisions that require an additional pilot, or (3) abandon the project altogether. To make this decision, researchers should articulate criteria for each objective in advance and then assess the degree to which the criteria were met.
- Mixed methods designs are especially well suited for pilot work. Quantitative data can be used to assess whether feasibility criteria were met, and qualitative data can elucidate *why* they were not met, or how the intervention or study protocols could be improved.
- Sample sizes for pilots are typically small. Some experts recommend at least 30 to 40 subjects per group, especially if funding for the pilot is sought.
- A major product from pilot work is a description of "lessons learned." Another product, if the intervention has been found to be feasible, acceptable, and promising, is a proposal for a full-scale trial.
- Ideally, regardless of the outcome, the findings from pilot work will be published so that others can benefit from learning about both successes and failures.

STUDY ACTIVITIES

Study activities are available to instructors on the**Point**.

REFERENCES CITED IN CHAPTER 29

*Arain, M., Campbell, M., Cooper, C., & Lancaster, G. (2010). What is a pilot or feasibility study? A review of current practice and editorial policy. *BMC: Medical Research Methodology, 10*, 67.

**Arnold, D., Burns, K., Adhikari, N., Kho, M., Meade, M., & Cook, D. (2009). The design and interpretation of pilot trials in clinical research in critical care. *Critical Care Medicine, 37*, S69–S74.

Beebe, L. (2007). What can we learn from pilot studies? *Perspectives in Psychiatric Care, 43*, 213–218.

*Bell, M., Whitehead, A., & Julious, S. (2018). Guidance for using pilot studies to inform the design of intervention trials with continuous outcomes. *Clinical Epidemiology, 10*, 153–157.

*Billingham, S., Whitehead, A., & Julious, S. (2013). An audit of sample sizes for pilot and feasibility trials being undertaken in the United Kingdom registered in the United Kingdom Clinical Research Network database. *BMC Medical Research Methodology, 13*, 104.

*Bird, L., Arthur, A., & Cox, K. (2011). "Did the trial kill the intervention?" Experiences from the development, implementation and evaluation of a complex intervention. *BMC Medical Research Methodology, 11*, 24.

*Bugge, C., Williams, B., Hagen, S., Logan, J., Glazener, C., Pringle, S., & Sinclair, L. (2013). A process for Decision-making after Pilot and feasibility Trials (ADePT): Development following a feasibility study of a complex intervention for pelvic organ prolapse. *Trials, 14*, 353.

*Carlisle, B., Kimmelman, J., Ramsay, T., & LacKinnon, N. (2015). Unsuccessful trial accrual and human subjects protections: An empirical analysis of recently closed trials. *Clinical Trials, 12*, 77–83.

*Chan, R., Northfield, S., Larsen, E., Mihala, G., Ullman, A., Hancock, P., … Rickard, C. (2017). Central venous Access device SeCurement And Dressing Effectiveness for peripherally inserted central catheters in adult acute hospital patients (CASCADE): A pilot randomised controlled trial. *Trials, 18*, 458.

Cocks, K., & Torgerson, D. (2013). Sample size calculations for pilot randomized trials: A confidence interval approach. *Journal of Clinical Epidemiology, 66*, 197–201.

Conn, V. S., Algase, D., Rawl, S., Zerwic, J., & Wyman, J. (2010). Publishing pilot intervention work. *Western Journal of Nursing Research, 32*, 994–1010.

*Coppell, K., Abel, S., Freer, T., Gray, A., Sharp, K., Norton, J., … Whitehead, L. (2017). The effectiveness of a primary care nursing-led dietary intervention for prediabetes: A mixed methods pilot study. *BMC Family Practice, 18*, 106.

*Craig, P., Dieppe, P., Macintyre, S., Michie, S., Nazareth, I., & Petticrew, M. (2008). *Developing and evaluating complex interventions: New guidance*. London: MRC.

*Donovan, H. S., Ward, S., Serieka, S., Knapp, J., Sherwood, P., Bender, C., … Ingel, R. (2014). Web-based symptom management for women with recurrent ovarian cancer: A pilot randomized controlled trial of the WRITE symptoms intervention. *Journal of Pain & Symptom Management, 47*, 218–230.

*Eldridge, S., Lancaster, G., Campbell, M., Thabane, L., Hopewell, S., Coleman, C., & Bond, C. (2016). Defining feasibility and pilot studies in preparation for randomised controlled trials: Development of a conceptual framework. *PLoS One, 11*, e0150205.

Feeley, N., & Cossette, S. (2015). Testing the waters: Piloting a complex intervention. In D. Richards, & I. Rahm Hallberg (Eds.), *Complex interventions in health: An overview of research methods* (pp. 166–174). Oxford, UK: Routledge.

*Hagan, T., Arida, J., Hughes, S., & Donovan, H. (2017). Creating individualized symptoms management goals and strategies for cancer-related fatigue for patients with recurrent ovarian cancer. *Cancer Nursing, 40*, 305–313.

*Hay, C., Courtney-Brooks, M., Lefkowits, C., Hagan, T., Edwards, R., & Donavan, H. (2016). Symptom management in women with recurrent ovarian cancer: Do patients and clinicians agree on what symptoms are most important? *Gynecological Oncology, 143*, 367–370.

Hertzog, M. A. (2008). Consideration in determining sample size for pilot studies. *Research in Nursing & Health, 31*, 180–191.

*Himes, K., Donovan, H., Wang, S., Weaver, C., Grove, J., & Facco, F. (2017). Health Beyond Pregnancy, a web-based intervention to improve adherence to postpartum care: Randomized controlled feasibility trial. *JMIR Human Factors, 4*, e26.

*Ioannidis, J. P. (2016). Why most clinical research is not useful. *PLoS Medicine, 13*, e1002049.

Kraemer, H. C., Mintz, J., Noda, A., Tinklenberg, J., & Yesavage, J. (2006). Caution regarding the use of pilot studies to guide power calculations for study proposals. *Archives of General Psychiatry, 63*, 484–489.

Lancaster, G., Dodd, S., & Williamson, P. (2004). Design and analysis of pilot studies: Recommendations for good practice. *Journal of Evaluation in Clinical Practice, 10*, 307–312.

*Lee, E., Whitehead, A., Jacques, R., & Julious, S. (2014). The statistical interpretation of pilot trials: Should significance thresholds be reconsidered? *BMC Medical Research Methodology, 14*, 41.

Leon, A., Davis, L., & Kraemer, H. (2011). The role and interpretation of pilot studies in clinical research. *Journal of Psychiatric Research, 45*, 626–629.

*Moore, C., Carter, R., Nietert, P., & Stewart, P. (2011). Recommendations for planning pilot studies in clinical and translational research. *Clinical & Translational Science, 4*, 332–337.

*Plow, M., & Golding, M. (2017). Using mHealth Technology in a self-management intervention to promote physical activity among adults with chronic disabling conditions. *JMIR mHealth and uHealth, 5*, e185.

Richards, D. A., & Rahm Hallberg, I. (Eds.). (2015). *Complex interventions in health: An overview of research methods.* Oxford, UK: Routledge.

Shih, W. J., Ohman-Strickland, P., & Lin, Y. (2004). Analysis of data and early phase studies with small sample sizes. *Statistics in Medicine, 23*, 1827–1842.

*Signorelli, C., Wakefield, C., Johnston, K., Fardell, J., Brierley, M., Thornton-Benko, E., … Cohn, R. (2018). "Re-engage" pilot study protocol: A nurse- led eHealth intervention to re-engage, educate and empower childhood cancer survivors. *BMJ Open, 8*, e022269.

*Sin, J., Henderson, C., Pinfold, V., & Norman, I. (2013). The E-Sibling Project—Exploratory randomised controlled trial of an online multi-component psychoeducational intervention for siblings of individuals with first episode psychosis. *BMC Psychiatry, 13*, 123.

*Sin, J., Henderson, C., Spain, D., Gamble, C., & Norman, I. (2017). What factors influence successful recruitment of siblings of individuals with first episode psychosis to e-health interventions? A qualitative study. *Health Expectations, 20*, 696–704.

*Sully, B., Julious, S., & Nicholl, J. (2013). A reinvestigation of recruitment to randomised controlled, multicenter trials: A review of trials funded by two UK funding agencies. *Trials, 14*, 166.

Taylor, R., Ukoumunne, O., & Warren, F. (2015). How to use feasibility and pilot trials to test alternative methodologies and methodological procedures prior to a full-scale trial. In D. Richards, & I. Rahm Hallberg (Eds.), *Complex interventions in health: An overview of research methods* (pp. 136–144). Oxford, UK: Routledge.

*Thabane, L., Ma, J., Chu, R., Cheng, J., Ismaila, A., Rios, L., & Robson, R. (2010). A tutorial on pilot studies: The what, why and how. *BMC Medical Research Methodology, 10*, 1.

*Tickle-Degnen, L. (2013). Nuts and bolts of conducting feasibility studies. *American Journal of Occupational Therapy, 67*, 171–176.

Treweek, S. (2015). Addressing issues in recruitment and retention using feasibility and pilot trials. In D. Richards, & I. Rahm Hallberg (Eds.), *Complex interventions in health: An overview of research methods* (pp. 155–165). Oxford, UK: Routledge.

*Treweek, S., & Born, A. (2014). Clinical trial design: Increasing efficiency in evaluating new healthcare interventions. *Journal of Comparative Effectiveness Research, 3*, 233–236.

Ukoumunne, O., Warren, F., Taylor, R., & Ewings, P. (2015). How to use feasibility studies to derive parameter estimated in order to power a full trial. In D. Richards, & I. Rahm Hallberg (Eds.), *Complex interventions in health: An overview of research methods* (pp. 145–154). Oxford, UK: Routledge.

*Van Teijlingen, E. R., & Hundley, V. (2001). The importance of pilot studies. *Social Research Update, 35*.

Van Teijlingen, E. R., Rennie, A., Hundley, V., & Graham, W. (2001). The importance of conducting and reporting pilot studies: The example of the Scottish Births Survey. *Journal of Advanced Nursing, 34*, 289–295.

Van der Wouden, J., Blankenstein, A., Huibers, M., van der Windt, D., Stalman, W., & Verhagen, A. (2007). Survey among 78 studies showed that Lasagna's law holds in Dutch primary care research. *Journal of Clinical Epidemiology, 60*, 819–824.

Vickers, A. J. (2003). Underpowering in randomized trials reporting a sample size calculation. *Journal of Clinical Epidemiology, 56*, 717–720.

*Walters, S., Henriques-Cadby, B., Bortolani, O., Flight, L., Hind, D., Jacques, R., … Julious, S. (2017). Recruitment and retention of participants in randomised controlled trials: A review of trials funded and published the United Kingdom Health Technology Assessment Programme, *BMJ Open, 7*, e015276.

*Wang, J., Cai, C., Padhye, N., Orlander, P., & Zare, M. (2018). A behavioral lifestyle intervention enhanced with multiple-behavior self-monitoring using mobile and connected tools for underserved individuals with type 2 diabetes and comorbid overweight or obesity. *JMIR mHealth and uHealth, 6,* 4.

*A link to this open-access article or document is provided in the Toolkit for Chapter 29 in the **Resource Manual.** ✪*

**This journal article is available on the Point *for this chapter.*

Part 6

BUILDING AN EVIDENCE BASE FOR NURSING PRACTICE

30 | Systematic Reviews of Research Evidence

This chapter discusses systematic reviews, which are considered a cornerstone of evidence-based practice (EBP). As noted in Chapter 2, systematic reviews are at the pinnacle of most evidence hierarchies and level-of-evidence scales.

RESEARCH INTEGRATION AND SYNTHESIS

A **systematic review (SR)** carefully and transparently integrates research evidence about a specific research question using methodical procedures that are spelled out in advance. Systematic reviewers use methods that are disciplined, reproducible, and verifiable. Compared to a simple literature review, systematic reviews involve the rigorous development of, and adherence to, a protocol with explicit rules for gathering data from **primary studies**, i.e., original research inquiries that addressed a specific question.

The field of research integration is expanding rapidly, in terms of both the number of reviews being conducted and techniques used to perform them. Page and colleagues (2016), in an analysis of systematic reviews published in 2014, estimated that 25 new systematic reviews were indexed *every day* in MEDLINE—and that number has certainly grown since 2014.

Methods for conducting systematic reviews are also evolving, making it challenging to offer guidance. We provide only a brief introduction to this complex topic. Our advice for those embarking on a review project is to keep abreast of developments in this field and to seek more detailed information in websites devoted to the topic—or to participate in training that has become available through organizations focused on evidence integration, such as the Cochrane Collaboration and the Joanna Briggs Institute (JBI).

TIP The Cochrane Collaboration's reviewer's manual is a major resource for the conduct of systematic reviews. The 5.1 version of the manual, published in 2011 (Higgins & Green, 2011), is referenced extensively in this chapter and is available online (http://handbook-5-1.cochrane.org/). A new reviewer's manual, version 6.0, was published in late 2019, but its release occurred after this book went to press. The Cochrane Collaboration training team explained major changes to the manual in an online webinar in early 2019, and so we have pointed out several important revisions. Five introductory chapters of the revised manual are available online, but the main content is in a published book (Higgins & Thomas, 2020). The Toolkit of the accompanying *Resource Manual* includes further information about version 6, including its table of contents.

TYPES OF SYSTEMATIC REVIEWS

Systematic reviews can take various forms and result in different products. No simple taxonomy for classifying systematic reviews has emerged; we look at review types along several dimensions.

Systematic Reviews of Quantitative, Qualitative, and Mixed Methods Research

Systematic reviews in health care fields have largely been syntheses of quantitative evidence from randomized controlled trials (RCTs)—syntheses that focus on the question: Does *this* work? In other words, systematic reviews have most often integrated evidence from primary studies that addressed Therapy/intervention questions. In Page et al.'s (2016) analysis of systematic reviews indexed in MEDLINE in 2014, 55% were classified as therapeutic reviews. Researchers have also conducted systematic reviews of other types of quantitative research, such as reviews of studies addressing etiology, prognosis, or diagnosis questions (Munn et al., 2018).

Qualitative researchers have also created techniques to integrate evidence from multiple studies, and nurse researchers have played an important role in this area. Their products are often called **metasyntheses**. Metasyntheses typically involve integrations of studies focused on abstract phenomena and experiences (e.g., grief following the death of a child). However, there is an emerging interest among health care researchers in synthesizing information on qualitative aspects of interventions, such as patient acceptance, implementation processes, and barriers to implementation (e.g., Shaw et al., 2014). Such reviews are often called **qualitative evidence syntheses (QES)**.

A recent development involves systematic reviews that integrate findings from qualitative *and* quantitative studies and from mixed methods studies. **Mixed studies reviews** (or *mixed research syntheses*) are currently a "hot topic." Methodologic developments in the years ahead will likely lead to greater clarity on how best to undertake such reviews.

Narrative Versus Statistical Integration (Meta-Analysis)

In systematic reviews, the "data" are findings from studies that addressed a question of interest. Data from the included studies can be integrated in a narrative fashion or statistically. Qualitative systematic reviews, and some quantitative reviews, involve a narrative synthesis.

Many systematic reviews of quantitative studies—especially those that focus on intervention effects—use statistical integration, in what are called **meta-analyses**. The essence of a meta-analysis is that information from each study in the review is used to develop a common metric, an *effect size*. Effect sizes are averaged across studies, yielding aggregated information about not only the *existence* of a relationship between variables, but also an estimate of its *magnitude*. Most systematic reviews in the Cochrane Collaboration involve a meta-analysis. In Page et al.'s (2016) review of systematic reviews indexed in MEDLINE in 2014, 63% involved a meta-analysis.

For integrating quantitative evidence, meta-analysis offers these advantages:

- *Objectivity.* In narrative reviews, reviewers use unidentified or subconscious criteria to integrate disparate results. In a meta-analysis, decisions are explicit, and the integration itself is objective. Two meta-analysts using the same dataset would reach the same conclusions.
- *Power.* Power is the probability of detecting a true relationship between variables (Chapter 18). By combining results from multiple studies, power is increased. In a meta-analysis it is possible to conclude, with a given probability, that a relationship is real (e.g., that an intervention is effective), even when several small studies yielded nonsignificant findings. In a narrative review, multiple nonsignificant findings would likely be interpreted as lack of evidence of a relationship, which could be erroneous.
- *Precision.* Meta-analysts draw conclusions about the size of an intervention's effect, with a specified probability that the results are accurate. Estimates of effect size across multiple studies yield smaller confidence intervals than individual studies, and thus precision is enhanced.

Special Types of Review

Most of this chapter is devoted to "basic" systematic reviews. However, in the evolving field of evidence synthesis, special types of review have emerged, and references to them are appearing regularly in the literature. In this section, we briefly describe a few special review types.

Scoping Reviews

A strategy that is gaining momentum is to undertake a **scoping review** (or *scoping study*) as a means of refining the specific question for a systematic review. Although scoping studies have been defined in many ways (Davis et al., 2009), we refer here to scoping as a preliminary investigation that clarifies the range and nature of the evidence base. Unlike a systematic review, a scoping review addresses broad questions and uses flexible procedures and typically does not formally evaluate evidence quality. Scoping reviews can suggest strategies for a full systematic review and can indicate whether statistical integration (meta-analysis) is feasible. Scoping reviews are also used to identify areas in need of further research. Arksey and O'Malley (2005) have written a classic paper on the conduct of scoping reviews, and Daudt et al. (2013) and Khalil et al. (2016) have elaborated on their framework. JBI (2015) has developed a manual for scoping reviews.

Example of a Scoping Review
Pedersen and colleagues (2019) conducted a scoping review on changes in weight and body composition among women in adjuvant therapy for breast cancer. After reviewing 19 studies, they concluded that the large differences in study designs, measuring points, and cutoff values for weight change "make it difficult to synthesize findings and provide strong evidence for use in clinical practice" (p. 91).

Rapid Reviews

A type of evidence synthesis called a **rapid review** has emerged as "a streamlined approach to synthesizing evidence" (Khangura et al., 2012). Systematic reviews are considered the "gold standard" in knowledge synthesis, but they typically require up to 2 years to complete. Rapid reviews of research evidence are done within a period of weeks, do not involve statistical integration, and involve a less rigorous search for available evidence—often a single database is searched. In other words, rapid reviews are evidence syntheses in which aspects of the systematic review process are simplified or omitted to produce the review in a timely manner (Tricco et al., 2015). Rapid reviews are often used to inform emergent decisions facing clinicians in health care settings (Munn et al., 2015). The Cochrane Collaboration has a special methods group devoted to rapid reviews (Garrity et al., 2016).

Example of a Rapid Review
Carroll and colleagues (2017) undertook a rapid review to assess the efficacy of nonpharmacologic interventions (e.g., relaxation techniques) on the psychological distress of patients as they undergo a cardiac catheterization. The researchers synthesized findings from 29 intervention studies and acknowledged that their search "may not have identified all relevant studies…" (p. 93). They did not integrate the evidence statistically.

Overview of Reviews (Umbrella Reviews)

With the dramatic rise in the number of systematic reviews being undertaken, reviews that integrate findings from multiple reviews now appear in the literature with some regularity. The Cochrane Collaboration calls these **overviews of reviews**, and a chapter in their handbook on systematic reviews is devoted to their conduct (Higgins & Green, 2011, Chapter 22). Others use the term **umbrella review** to refer to reviews in which the unit of analysis is another review (e.g., Aromataris et al., 2015). Hunt et al. (2018) noted that "overviews have evolved to address a growing need to filter the information overload" (p. 1).

Example of an Umbrella Review
Jadczak and an interdisciplinary team (2018) undertook an umbrella review of the effectiveness of exercise interventions on physical function in community-dwelling frail older people. Seven systematic reviews, which covered 58 relevant RCTs, were included in the umbrella review.

Living Systematic Reviews

Systematic reviews can quickly get out-of-date (Elliott et al., 2014). The time between starting and publishing a review is typically over a year, and (for one study) the median time from primary study publication to inclusion in a published systematic review ranged from 3 to 7 years. Elliott and his group have proposed the conduct of timely **living systematic reviews** that are updated as new research becomes available and are published as online-only evidence summaries. Their approach relies, in part, on new methods of automating the retrieval and extraction of relevant information. Guidelines for living systematic reviews were presented in a series of papers in the *Journal of Clinical Epidemiology* (e.g., Elliott et al., 2017; Thomas et al., 2017).

"Next-Generation" Systematic Reviews

Ioannidis (2017), in a medical journal editorial, mentioned several "next-generation" types of quantitative systematic reviews, including the following two:

- **Individual patient-level meta-analysis.** Reviewers sometimes obtain the raw data from multiple trialists and then use the individual-level data in the analysis. A primary benefit of this approach is the ability to make statistical adjustments for confounding variables and to perform analyses for distinct subgroups (Higgins & Green, 2011, Chapter 18; Higgins & Thomas, 2020, Chapter 26).
- **Network meta-analysis (NMA).** Systematic reviews of interventions typically make direct pairwise comparisons, such as differences in outcomes between an intervention group versus a control group—often a placebo or "usual care." Network reviews involve incorporating direct and indirect evidence to draw conclusions about the effects of alternative interventions for a health problem—even if they have not been directly compared in trials (Tonin et al., 2017). This approach is popular in comparative effectiveness research. The new Cochrane reviewer's manual devotes a chapter to NMA (Higgins & Thomas, 2020, Chapter 11).

> **Example of a Network Meta-Analysis**
> Norman and colleagues (2018) conducted a network meta-analysis to assess the effect of dressings and topical agents for treating venous leg ulcers. Their sample of studies included RCTs that compared the effects of any dressing or topical agent with any other intervention in the treatment of venous leg ulcers. The primary studies involved 25 different interventions.

PLANNING A SYSTEMATIC REVIEW

Systematic reviews follow many of the same steps as for primary studies. Like other research endeavors, the conduct of a systematic review requires advance preparation and planning. We briefly discuss a few things to consider when planning a review.

Broad Steps in a Systematic Review

Despite the evolution of methods for conducting systematic reviews, some steps are fairly standard in rigorous efforts to synthesize research evidence. In sections that follow, we describe aspects of systematic review procedures in greater detail, but here is a brief summary of steps that are typical, especially for quantitative reviews:

1. Formulate the question(s) for the review
2. Define eligibility criteria for the primary studies
3. Prepare a protocol for the review
4. Search for and retrieve primary studies
5. Select studies for inclusion in the review
6. Assess the quality of the selected primary studies
7. Extract data from the studies
8. Analyze and synthesize the data
9. Evaluate the degree of confidence in the results
10. Present the findings in a systematic review report

Progress in conducting the review is less linear than this list suggests—there are typically feedback loops in the process.

Preparing to Conduct a Systematic Review

Some activities need to be addressed even before the actual review process gets underway.

Preliminary Groundwork

Before initiating a systematic review project, reviewers need to make sure that a review is necessary. One of the Institute of Medicine's standards for the conduct of high-quality systematic reviews is this: Confirm the need for a new review (IOM, 2011, Standard 2.5.1). An early search of important databases (including ones dedicated to systematic reviews) is warranted. Such a search might not reveal reviews that are underway, so it is important to also search for reviews in **PROSPERO**, an international prospective registry of systematic reviews. As of 2017, some 30,000 systematic reviews had been registered, and nearly 1,000 were being added each month (Page et al., 2018).

The Review Team

Unlike literature reviews, systematic reviews require a team. Assembling the right team is an important planning activity. Several tasks in a systematic review (e.g., appraising study quality) require two reviewers and often a third who can serve as a tie-breaker. With multiple reviewers, the work load is shared and subjectivity is reduced. The team should involve content experts and a methodologic or statistical expert who is familiar with systematic review methods. The team should include a librarian or information specialist who has training in systematic reviews.

Review teams for systematic reviews increasingly include other stakeholders, such as patients and other members of the public. The Cochrane Collaboration explicitly encourages "the involvement of healthcare consumers, either as part of the review team or in the editorial process" (Higgins & Greene, 2011, Chapter 2). An advisory group can be established to solicit input from people with a range of experiences.

The Review Auspices

Review teams may decide to undertake a systematic review independently—for example, in response to a locally identified problem. Some teams prepare a systematic review under the auspices of a national or international organization, such as the Cochrane Collaboration, the Joanna Briggs Institute (JBI), the Agency for Healthcare Research and Quality, or the Centre for Reviews and Dissemination. The process differs depending on the organization, but typically a review idea is submitted for approval prior to its conduct. Major review organizations also offer guidance to review teams working independently, through training opportunities and handbooks such as those by the Cochrane Collaboration (Higgins & Green, 2011; Higgins & Thomas, 2020) and JBI (Aromataris & Munn, 2017). These handbooks focus primarily on quantitative reviews but have chapters on qualitative synthesis.

Computer Software

Systematic reviews involve massive amounts of data that need to be managed and analyzed. Computer software is usually used to facilitate the process. Dozens of software packages have been created, including text mining software (e.g., SWIFT-Review, TERMINE), citation management software (e.g., EndNote, Mendeley, RefWorks), deduplication software (e.g., DistillerSR), software to assist in screening (e.g., Covidence, DistillerSR, Rayyan), data extraction software (DistillerSR, Covidence), and software for meta-analysis (e.g., DistillerSR, Meta-Easy). Macros are also available for doing meta-analyses within major software packages such as SPSS and SAS. For qualitative systematic reviews, researchers often use NVivo or other software described in Chapter 25. The Cochrane Collaboration's popular software, called *RevMan*, includes tools that perform many of the functions for systematic reviews. Similarly, the Joanna Briggs Institute (JBI) offers a comprehensive package of review software called *SUMARI*. The SRToolbox is a resource for identifying relevant software (http://systematicreviewtools.com/index.php).

Schedule for a Systematic Review

Systematic reviews typically take 9 to 18 months to complete. Before embarking on the project, a timeline should be constructed to help the project stay on track. Typically, the most time-consuming activities in the systematic review process are searching for and retrieving relevant studies, following up to obtain information that is missing in the study reports, and undertaking quality assessments.

In developing a project schedule, the team should plan for pilot tests of important decisions. For example, early in the search process, it is a good idea to pilot test the eligibility criteria to ensure that relevant primary studies are not filtered out. Quality assessment strategies and data extraction methods should also be pilot tested to ensure optimal results.

SYSTEMATIC REVIEWS OF QUANTITATIVE RESEARCH

In this section, we describe major steps in the conduct of a systematic review of quantitative research. The guidance applies to systematic reviews of quantitative research in general, but most advice has been developed for studies that address Therapy questions. Supplementary advice is available in both the JBI and Cochrane reviewers' manuals for integrating findings from observational studies, public health initiatives, economic evaluations, and diagnostic test accuracy research. The Agency for Healthcare Research and Quality (AHRQ, 2015) has also issued guidelines for reviews of comparative effectiveness studies.

Formulating the Review Question

A focused systematic review begins with a carefully framed question. Good review questions often follow the PICO format described in Chapter 2, with specification of the Population, the Intervention or Influence, the Comparison against which the intervention/influence is contrasted, and Outcomes. Question templates such as those provided in Chapters 2 or 4 (and provided in the Toolkit) serve as a good starting place. ✪

> **TIP** Munn and colleagues (2018) suggest question formats for several types of systematic review. For example, for prevalence and incidence reviews, they use the acronym CoCoPop (Condition, Context, Population).

Systematic review questions vary in scope. For example, a review might address a broad question regarding whether exercise interventions (in general) are effective as a weight-loss therapy for obese adolescents. Alternatively, a review might address

whether a particular intervention (e.g., high-intensity interval training) is an effective weight-loss strategy. Table 5.6.a in the Cochrane manual (Higgins & Greene, 2011) summarizes advantages and disadvantages of broad versus narrow review questions. Broad reviews tend to be demanding of time and resources.

Finalizing the review question is likely to involve multiple iterations of refinement. Team members should all be "on board" with the question, and the process is likely to benefit from the opinions of a diverse group of stakeholders. Scoping reviews sometimes play a vital role in formulating the question for a systematic review.

The reviewers need to be careful about specifying outcomes for the review. The handbook for Cochrane reviews recommends developing a list of possible outcomes and then prioritizing them. The "main outcomes" are those that are essential for decision-making and usually include two to three primary outcomes and a small number of secondary outcomes. For intervention studies, outcomes should include possible adverse effects.

> **Example of a Question From a Quantitative Systematic Review**
> Sherifali and an interprofessional team (2018) conducted a systematic review and meta-analysis that addressed the question of whether Internet-based interventions (I), compared to the absence of an Internet-based intervention (C), have positive effects on the mental health (O) of caregivers caring for adults with a chronic health problem (P).

Defining Eligibility Criteria

In systematic reviews, inclusion and exclusion criteria must be specified before a search for primary studies gets underway. Sampling criteria for a systematic review typically cover substantive, methodologic, and practical elements, such as the following:

- **Study participants.** Inclusion criteria normally indicate the disease or condition of interest (e.g., patients with cancer, low-birth-weight babies) and any relevant demographic characteristics, such as age.

- **Intervention/influence.** Reviewers need to stipulate the essential characteristics of the intervention or influence of interest, including features such as mode or timing of delivery.
- **Study design.** Some reviews stipulate a study design for eligible primary studies—most often, a randomized design when the review focuses on a Therapy question.
- **Other criteria.** From a practical standpoint, the criteria might exclude reports written in a language other than English, or reports published before a certain date. The criteria might also stipulate whether both published and unpublished reports will be included in the review, a topic we discuss in a later section.

For some reviews, the inclusion criteria specify the outcomes of interest. However, for reviews focused on Therapy questions, the handbook for Cochrane reviews cautions against including or excluding studies with specific outcomes: "A Cochrane review would typically seek all rigorous studies... of a particular comparison of interventions in a particular population of participants, irrespective of the outcomes measured or reported" (Higgins & Green, 2011, 5.1.2).

TIP Criteria for eligibility are not always straightforward. A table in the Toolkit of the accompanying *Resource Manual* includes a list of questions to consider in establishing eligibility criteria for a systematic review.

Example of Eligibility Criteria for a Quantitative Review
Whitehouse and colleagues (2018) conducted a systematic review of the effectiveness of smoking cessation interventions for patients with tuberculosis (TB). The eligibility criteria were as follows: "Peer-reviewed journal articles were included if they evaluated any smoking cessation intervention among patients with suspected or confirmed TB. Any studies that did not report on smoking cessation outcomes were excluded. The search included publications written in English, French, Spanish, Portuguese, and Korean" (p. 38).

Preparing a Review Protocol

Review teams are increasingly expected to prepare—and often to publish—a **protocol** of the proposed systematic review. The protocol, which promotes transparency, serves as the road map for the review. Review protocols, which are typically 10 to 15 single-spaced pages, usually include the following information:

- The title of the review
- Members of the review team
- Proposed schedule, with beginning and end dates
- The research questions
- Background/argument for the review
- Eligibility criteria for studies in the review
- Search strategy (anticipated databases, keywords, supplementary search strategies)
- Review methods (assessment of methodologic quality, method of data extraction, analysis methods, assessment of bias)
- Assessment of confidence in the findings

TIP Some software for systematic reviews, such as the software for Cochrane and JBI reviews, provide fill-in-the-blank forms for creating protocols. The Toolkit in the accompanying *Resource Manual* includes an outline for a Cochrane protocol.

Once a protocol has been developed, it is advisable to register the protocol with PROSPERO and, if relevant, with the Cochrane Collaboration, Joanna Briggs Institute, or other review group.

Example of a Systematic Review Protocol
Hutchinson and an interdisciplinary team (2018) published a protocol in *BMJ Open* for a systematic review focused on organizational interventions to reduce rates of caesarean birth. The review was registered in PROSPERO, and the registration number was provided in the article.

Searching for and Screening Primary Studies

Systematic reviewers should aim for an exhaustive search of primary studies that meet the eligibility criteria. Exhaustive searching requires a greater emphasis on sensitivity (ensuring retrieval of all relevant studies) than on specificity (minimizing retrieval of nonrelevant results). Preliminary search plans are spelled out in the protocol, but reviewers need to continuously assess and refine their strategies.

Traditionally, the keywords are the main research variables; many researchers use the PICO elements as keywords for a literature search. There is some evidence, however, that the use of a full PICO query may fail to retrieve all relevant articles. Ho et al. (2016), for example, found that using two or three of the PICO terms retrieved more articles than using all four, findings similar to those of Agoritsas et al. (2012). The chapter on searching in the Cochrane Handbook explicitly recommends against including Outcome or Comparison as search terms for systematic reviews of interventions (Higgins & Green, 2011, Chapter 6). Pilot testing alternative search strategies is recommended.

TIP Aromataris and Riitano (2014) provide advice on searching. They suggest creating a *logic grid* that begins as a matrix with PICO elements in four columns. An early step in a search is to identify alternative terms or synonyms for the concepts in the grid, and to then add them into the grid. An illustration of a logic grid is included in the Toolkit.

Searching for primary studies should be undertaken in multiple bibliographic databases and should include repositories of existing systematic reviews such as the Cochrane and JBI databases. Searching in MEDLINE, EMBASE, and CINAHL is essential. The Cochrane handbook (Higgins & Greene, 2011) includes lists of numerous national and regional databases, subject-specific databases, and citation indexes to consider. Bramer and colleagues (2017) estimated that 60% of published reviews fail to retrieve 95% of all relevant references as a result of not searching important databases. Their

analysis suggested that Google Scholar should be included in the search strategy.

TIP It seems likely that technologic advances soon will result in new algorithms for automating several activities in producing systematic reviews, including search and screening activities (e.g., Beller et al., 2018; Tsafnat et al., 2018).

There is some disagreement about whether reviewers should limit their sample to published studies or should cast as wide a net as possible and include **grey literature**—that is, studies with a more limited distribution, such as dissertations, conference presentations, and so on. Some people restrict their sample to published reports in peer-reviewed journals, arguing that the peer review system is an important, tried-and-true screen for findings worthy of consideration as evidence.

The limitations of excluding nonpublished findings, however, have been widely noted. A primary issue is **publication bias**—the tendency for published studies to overrepresent statistically significant findings. (This bias is increasingly being referred to as one type of **dissemination bias**.) Publication bias is widespread: authors tend to refrain from submitting manuscripts with negative findings, reviewers and editors tend to reject such papers when they are submitted, and users of evidence tend to ignore the findings when they are published. The exclusion of grey literature in a systematic review can lead to the overestimation of effects (Conn et al., 2003; Dwan et al., 2013).

TIP In addition to the bias favoring publication of reports with statistically significant results, there is good evidence of another type of dissemination bias—selective reporting of only those outcomes with positive results, sometimes called *outcome reporting bias*. Dissemination bias and resources for searching the grey literature are described in Supplement A to this chapter on thePoint.

We recommend retrieving as many relevant studies as possible, because methodologic weaknesses in unpublished reports can be dealt with later. Aggressive search strategies are essential and may include the following:

- **Handsearching** journals known to publish relevant content—i.e., doing a manual search of the tables of contents of a few key journals
- *Snowballing* (the ancestry approach or footnote chasing, i.e., tracking down references in bibliographies of relevant studies) and *digital snowballing* (using "related citations" features in electronic databases)
- Identifying and contacting key researchers in the field to see if they have done studies that have not (yet) been published, and networking with researchers at conferences
- Doing an "author search" of key researchers in the field in databases and on the Internet
- Reviewing abstracts from trial registries and conference proceedings
- Searching for unpublished reports, such as dissertations and theses, government reports, and registries of studies in progress (e.g., in the United States, through the NIH RePORTER http://projectreporter.nih.gov/reporter.cfm)
- Contacting foundations, government agencies, or corporate sponsors of the type of research under study to get leads on work in progress or recently completed

Once potentially relevant studies are identified, the search results should be merged (often, using reference management software), and duplicates should be removed. The next step is to perform an initial screening of abstracts to remove obviously irrelevant articles. Next, full-texts of the articles that passed the screening need to be retrieved and reviewed to determine if they do, in fact, meet the eligibility criteria. All decisions relating to exclusions should be made by at least two reviewers, with conflicts resolved either by consensus or by a third reviewer.

Example of a Search Strategy From a Systematic Review

Capezuti and colleagues (2018) conducted a systematic review of nonpharmacologic interventions to improve nighttime sleep among long-term care residents. They conducted searches in five databases (MEDLINE, Embase, CINAHL, Scopus, Cochrane Library). Tables in their report listed search terms for each database. After removing duplicates, their search yielded 6,747 articles whose abstracts were independently assessed for eligibility by two authors, with discrepancies resolved by a third author. Initial screening resulted in 445 articles that were retrieved as full-texts. Two teams of two authors performed the final screening, resulting in the removal of another 311 articles.

TIP The reports of studies that meet the sampling criteria do not always contain complete information needed for a meta-analysis. Be prepared to devote time and resources to communicating with researchers to obtain supplementary information.

Evaluating Study Quality and Risk of Bias

In systematic reviews, the evidence from primary studies needs to be evaluated to determine how much confidence to place in the findings. Assessments of study quality sometimes involve quantitative ratings of study features. Dozens of quality assessment scales that yield summary scores of overall study quality have been developed (Zeng et al., 2015). A frequently used scale to appraise RCTs is the Jadad scale (Jadad et al., 1996). The Newcastle-Ottawa Scale (Stang, 2010) can be used to appraise nonrandomized studies. A carefully developed scale, called ROBINS-I, was developed to assess bias in nonrandomized studies but is also used for RCTs (Sterne et al., 2016). Scales, however, are sometimes criticized because of concerns about their validity and reliability. Quality criteria vary from instrument to instrument, and the result is that study quality can be rated differently with different assessment tools and by different assessors (Jüni et al., 2001).

Another strategy is to use a quality assessment checklist with several discrete items that are not summed. An important example is the Critical Appraisal Tools developed by the Joanna Briggs Institute for evaluating different types of primary studies (e.g., RCTs, prevalence studies, case–control studies). The JBI Critical Appraisal tool for RCTs includes 13 items, each of which is rated as yes, no, unclear, or not applicable. For example, one item is, "Were outcomes measured in a reliable way?" After completing the checklist, the appraiser makes an assessment about whether to include the study in the review, exclude it, or seek more information.

The Cochrane Collaboration takes an approach that emphasizes risk of bias rather than study quality, using a "component" approach (Higgins & Green, 2011, Chapter 8). **Risk of bias** in intervention studies refers to the likelihood of an inaccuracy in the estimate of a causal effect—i.e., a threat to internal validity. In Cochrane reviews, reviewers rate each study for seven bias risks (Table 30.1).

Each component is rated low risk, high risk, or unclear risk of bias. Cochrane's risk-of-bias tool is primarily relevant for studies addressing Therapy questions; a comparable domain-based tool for nonrandomized studies, called ACROBAT-NRSI, has been developed (Bilandzic et al., 2016).

Regardless of approach, quality appraisals should be undertaken by at least two qualified individuals. If there are disagreements between the reviewers, there should be a discussion until a consensus has been reached or, if necessary, a third person should resolve the difference. Interrater reliability can be calculated to demonstrate adequate agreement on study quality.

TIP In the revised Cochrane Collaboration's reviewer's manual (Higgins & Thomas, 2020), the risk of bias (RoB) tool has been modified and is referred to as RoB2. A table in the Toolkit compares RoB1 and RoB2.

TABLE 30.1 • The Cochrane Collaboration's Tool for Assessing Risk of Bias

COMPONENT	SPECIFIC RISK
Selection bias	**Random sequence generation:** Was random sequence generation likely to produce comparable groups?
	Allocation concealment: Was the allocation sequence adequately concealed?
Performance bias	**Blinding of participants and personnel:** Were steps taken to blind participants and study personnel regarding receipt of the intervention?
	Blinding of outcome assessment: Were outcome assessors blinded to which intervention a participant received?
Attrition bias	**Incomplete outcome data:** How complete are the data for each outcome, including attrition and exclusions from the analysis?
Reporting bias	**Selective reporting:** Were all outcomes reported or was there selective reporting of outcomes?
Other bias	**Other sources of bias:** Are there important concerns about other types of bias not previously covered?

Adapted from Higgins, J. P. T., & Green, S. (Eds.). (2011). *Cochrane handbook for systematic reviews of interventions (version 5.1.0).* The Cochrane Collaboration. Retrieved from http://training.cochrane.org/handbook, Table 8.5.a. Each primary study is rated as "low risk of bias," "high risk of bias," or "unclear risk of bias" for each risk factor. A new Risk of Bias tool has been developed, as outlined in the Toolkit to the accompanying *Resource Manual.*

There is some disagreement about what to do with quality appraisal information. JBI recommends using their checklists as the basis for excluding studies of low quality (Porritt et al., 2014). Jüni and colleagues (2001), however, who advocated Cochrane's component approach, noted that excluding low-quality studies might sometimes be justified "but could exclude studies that might contribute valid information" (p. 45). They recommended excluding only studies with "gross deficiencies," and then handling quality at the analysis phase. Further information about quality assessments in systematic reviews is provided by Cooper (2017) and Viswanathan et al. (2018).

Example of Quality Assessments in a Systematic Review

Aghajafari and an interdisciplinary team (2018) conducted a systematic review of evidence on the link between vitamin D deficiency and antenatal and postpartum depression. Two team members independently appraised each primary study using the 9-point Newcastle-Ottawa scale (NOS). Disagreements were resolved in meetings with the full team. The review included a table showing the quality assessment ratings for all 12 observational studies included in the review.

Extracting and Encoding Data for Analysis

The next step in a systematic review is to extract information about study characteristics and findings from each report. A data extraction form must be developed, along with a coding manual to guide those who will be extracting information. Reviewers often begin with paper-and-pencil forms, but then input the data into an electronic system. Options include spreadsheets (e.g., Excel), database software (e.g., Access), web-based surveys repurposed for data extraction (e.g., SurveyMonkey), and review software such as Cochrane's RevMan (Elamin et al., 2009).

TIP A basic data extraction form is included in the Toolkit as a Word document that can be adapted for use in systematic reviews. ✪ A paper-and-pencil form such as this one should be developed and pretested but moving to a computerized platform is advantageous.

Basic data source information should be recorded for all studies. This includes such features as year of publication, country of participants, and language in which the report was published. Supplementary information might include whether the study was funded (and by whom) and the year in which data were collected.

In terms of methodologic information, a critical element is sample size. Design information also needs to be coded (e.g., RCT, quasi-experiment, case–control). Measurement issues may be important. For example, codes can be used to designate specific instruments used to measure outcomes. For scales, information is needed about whether a high or low score is desirable. In longitudinal studies, rates of attrition and length of time between waves of data collection are essential. Quality appraisal information needs to be included in the record for each study.

In intervention studies, features of the intervention should be recorded, such as type of setting, dose or length of intervention, and modality of delivering the intervention. Attributes of the comparison condition also needed to be extracted and recorded.

Characteristics of the study participants must be encoded as well, including both clinical and demographic traits. Categorical characteristics that could be represented as percentages include sex, race/ethnicity, educational level, and illness/treatment information (e.g., percentages of participants with comorbidities). Age usually should be recorded as mean age of sample members.

Finally, the findings must be encoded. Either effect sizes (discussed in the next section) or statistical information for computing effect sizes is essential for a meta-analysis. Effect size information is often recorded for multiple outcomes and may also be recorded for different subgroups of study participants (e.g., effects for males versus females).

Extraction and coding of information should be completed by two or more people, for at least a portion of the studies, to allow for an assessment of interrater agreement. Reviewer training in data extraction and monitoring is essential: studies have found high rates of extraction errors in systematic reviews (Mathes et al., 2017). Further guidance on data extraction and the creation of data extraction forms is offered by Higgins and Green (2011, Chapter 7), and Pedder et al. (2016).

Example of Data Extraction in a Systematic Review
Son and colleagues (2018) conducted a systematic review of the effects of psychosocial interventions on the quality of life of patients with colorectal cancer. Data were extracted from eight primary studies meeting eligibility criteria using a "predesigned data extraction form" (p. 3). When information was missing, the reviewers contacted the authors. Data were independently extracted by three reviewers and any disagreements were resolved through discussion.

Analyzing and Synthesizing the Data

Once data extraction for the eligible studies has been completed, reviewers can proceed to analyze their data. In quantitative studies, a major analytic goal is to gain insight into *effects*—i.e., the effect of an intervention or other causative factor on outcomes. Whether the analysis is narrative or statistical, reviewers are typically interested in integrating the data to answer the following questions: (1) What is the direction of the effect? (e.g., are there positive effects for the intervention group?); (2) How big is the effect? and (3) How consistent is the effect across studies? Supplementary questions may include the following: (4) Are effects similar for different subgroups of participants? and (5) Are effects similar for studies that vary in quality?

Narrative syntheses involve the creation of evidence summary tables and then the use of judgment to answer these questions, but reviewers often prefer to answer them by performing a meta-analysis. Statistical integration is not always possible, however, so reviewers often begin by considering the feasibility of a meta-analysis.

TIP We focus mainly on meta-analytic procedures, but the Institute of Medicine (2011) recommends beginning with a narrative integration to gain insights, even if meta-analysis is ultimately performed. An older approach to quantitatively integrating results, called *vote counting*, involves adding up significant and nonsignificant findings to assess the preponderance of evidence. Yet another alternative is to construct graphic displays known as *harvest plots* to synthesize evidence when meta-analysis is not possible (Ogilvie et al., 2008; Higgins & Thomas, 2020, Chapter 12).

Criteria for Using Meta-Analysis in a Systematic Review

A basic criterion for a meta-analysis is that the research question across studies is the same. This means that the independent variable, outcomes, and study populations must be sufficiently similar to merit integration. Variables may be operationalized differently, to be sure. Interventions to promote physical activity among diabetics could take the form of a 4-week clinic-based program in one study and a five-session web-based intervention in another, for example. The outcome (physical activity levels) could be measured differently across studies. Yet, a study of the effects of a 1-hour lecture to improve *attitudes* toward physical activity among obese adults would be a poor candidate to include in such a meta-analysis. This is frequently called the "apples and oranges" or "fruit" problem. A meta-analysis should not be about *fruit*—i.e., a broad, encompassing category—but about a specific question addressed in multiple studies—i.e., "apples."

A second criterion concerns whether there is a sufficient knowledge base for statistical integration. If there are only a few studies, or if all studies are weakly designed and harbor extensive bias, it usually is not sensible to compute an "average" effect.

A final issue concerns consistency of the evidence. When the same hypothesis has been tested in multiple studies and results are highly conflicting, meta-analysis usually is not appropriate. As an extreme example, if half the studies testing an intervention found benefits for those in the intervention group, but the other half found benefits for the controls, it would be misleading to compute an average effect. A more appropriate strategy would be to do an in-depth narrative analysis of why the findings are at odds. As we shall see, the issue of *heterogeneity* of results is important even when a decision is made to move forward with a meta-analysis.

Example of Decision Not to Conduct a Meta-Analysis
Denk and colleagues (2018) did a systematic review of evidence on the association between hand grip strength and hip fracture incidence. They identified 11 relevant studies and used narrative integration: "…studies were not comparable with regard to design, analyses, populations, primary objectives and dynamometer brands. Pooling data for meta-analysis was therefore…not possible" (p. 3).

Calculating Effects in a Meta-Analysis

Meta-analyses involve the calculation of an index that encapsulates the relationship between the independent variable (the intervention or influence) and the outcome in each study. Because effects are captured differently depending on the variables' level of measurement, there is no single formula for calculating an effect size. In nursing, the most common situations for meta-analysis involve comparisons of two groups on a continuous outcome (e.g., the body mass index or BMI), comparisons of two groups on a dichotomous outcome (e.g., obese versus not obese), or correlations between two continuous variables (e.g., the correlation between BMI and depression scores).

For simplicity, much of our discussion focuses on the first situation, comparison of group means. When the outcomes across studies are on identical scales (e.g., weight in pounds), the effect can be captured by simply subtracting the mean for one group from the mean for the other in each study. For example, if the mean weight in an intervention group were 182.0 pounds and that for a control group were 190.0 pounds, the effect would be −8.0. Outcomes often are measured on different scales, however. For example, postpartum depression might be measured by Beck's Postpartum Depression Screening Scale in one study and by the Edinburgh Postnatal Depression Scale in another. In such situations, mean differences across studies cannot be averaged—we need an index that is neutral to the metric used in the primary study. Cohen's d, described in Chapter 18, is the effect size (ES) index often used. It may be recalled that the formula for d is the group difference in means, divided by the pooled standard deviation, or:

$$d = \frac{\overline{X}_1 - \overline{X}_2}{SD_P}$$

where $\overline{X}_1$ is the mean of group 1, $\overline{X}_2$ is the mean of group 2, and SD_P is the pooled standard deviation. This effect size index transforms all effects to standard deviation units. That is, if d were 0.50, it means that the mean for one group was one-half a standard deviation higher than that for the other group—regardless of the original measurement scale.

> **TIP** The term for the effect size d in Cochrane reviews is **standardized mean difference** or SMD. Cooper (2017) describes another similar index, called the g *index*, which adjusts d for possible bias in the SD estimate when study samples are small.

If meta-analysis software is used in the meta-analysis, effect size statistics do not need to be calculated manually—the program can calculate them based on means and SDs. But what if this information is absent from the report? Fortunately, there are alternative formulas for calculating d from information in primary study reports. For example, it is possible to derive the value of d when the report gives the value of t or F, an exact probability value, or a 95% confidence interval around the mean group difference. (The Toolkit in the *Resource Manual* ⊗ includes alternative formulas for computing d.) If the necessary statistical information is not available in a report, authors must be contacted for additional information.

When the outcomes in the primary studies are dichotomies, meta-analysts have a choice of effect size index, but the most usual are ones we discussed in earlier chapters—the relative risk (RR) index, the odds ratio (OR), and absolute risk reduction (ARR, also called the risk difference). Guidance on computing these indexes was provided in Table 16.6. The selection of a summary effect index depends on several criteria, such as mathematical properties, ease of interpretation, and consistency. The odds ratio is difficult for many users of systematic reviews to interpret but is often used as the effect size index for dichotomous outcomes in the nursing literature.

For nonexperimental studies, a common statistic used to express the relationship between an influence and an outcome is Pearson's r. If the primary studies in a meta-analysis provide statistical information in the form of a correlation coefficient, the r itself serves as the indicator of the magnitude and direction of effect.

Sometimes findings are not all reported using the same level of measurement. For example, if the variable *weight* (a continuous variable) was our key outcome, some studies might present findings for weight as a dichotomous outcome (e.g., *obese* versus *not obese*). One approach is to reexpress some of the effect indicators so that all effects can be pooled. For example, an odds ratio can be converted to *d*, as can a value of *r*—and vice versa. Formulas for converting effect size information are available online (http://cebcp.org/practical-meta-analysis-effect-size-calculator/).

> **TIP** Our discussion of calculating effects sizes glosses over several complexities. Alternative methods sometimes may be needed—e.g., when the unit of analysis was not individual people, if a crossover design was used, if data were severely skewed, etc. Those embarking on a complex meta-analysis project should seek guidance from statisticians.

Analyzing Data in a Meta-Analysis

Meta-analysis is a two-step analytic process. In the first step, a summary statistic that captures an effect is computed for each study, as just described. In the second step, a pooled effect estimate is computed as a **weighted average** of the effects for individual studies. A weighted average is defined as follows, with ES representing effect size estimates from each study:

$$\text{weighted average} = \frac{\text{sum of (ES} \times \text{weight for that ES)}}{\text{sum of the weights}}$$

Weights reflect the amount of information that each study provides. The bigger the weight given to a study, the more that study will contribute to the weighted average. One widely used approach is the **inverse variance method**, which uses the inverse of the variance of the effect size estimate (that is, one divided by the square of its standard error) as the weight. Larger studies, which have smaller standard errors, are given greater weight than smaller ones. The data needed for this type of analysis are the estimate of the effect size and its standard error, for each study.

Meta-analysts make many decisions during the analysis. In this brief overview, we present basic information about the following topics: identifying and testing heterogeneity; deciding whether to use a fixed effects or random effects model; incorporating clinical and methodologic diversity into the analysis; and handling study quality.

Testing for Heterogeneity. An important analytic issue concerns the consistency of results across primary studies, which is referred to as **statistical heterogeneity**. Just as there is variation within studies (participants do not have identical scores on outcomes), there is inevitably variation in effects across studies. If results are highly variable (e.g., conflicting results), a meta-analysis may be inappropriate. But heterogeneity is a concern for analysts even when statistical pooling is justified.

Visual inspection of heterogeneity can most readily be accomplished by constructing a forest plot, which can be generated using meta-analysis software. **Forest plots** graph the estimated effect size for each study and the 95% CI around each estimate. Figure 30.1 depicts two forest plots for situations in which there is low (A) and high (B) heterogeneity for five studies that used the odds ratio as the effect size index. In Panel A, all ES estimates favor the intervention group and are statistically significant for three of them (studies 2, 4, and 5). In Panel B, results are "all over the map": two studies favor controls at significant levels (studies 1 and 5) and two favor the treatment group (studies 2 and 4). A meta-analysis is not appropriate for the studies in B.

A procedure should be used to test the null hypothesis that heterogeneity across studies reflects random fluctuations. The test—traditionally the *Q test*—yields a *p* value indicating the probability of obtaining ES differences as large as those observed if the null hypothesis were true. An alpha of .05 is usually used as the significance criterion but, because the test is underpowered when the meta-analysis involves a small number of studies, an α of .10 is sometimes considered an acceptable criterion. Reviewers now often use the I^2 **test**, which adjusts for the number of studies in the analysis. This index yields values on a scale from 0% to 100%; a value greater than 50% usually is considered as moderate to high heterogeneity.

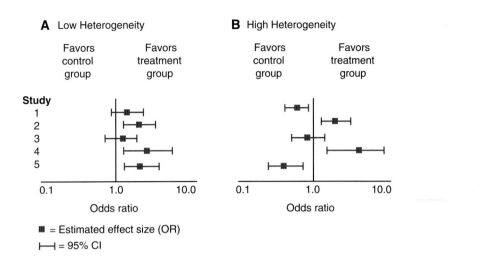

FIGURE 30.1 Two forest plots for five studies with low (A) and high (B) heterogeneity of effect size estimates.

Deciding on a Statistical Model. Two basic statistical models can be used in a meta-analysis, and the choice relates to heterogeneity. In a **fixed effects model**, it is assumed that a single true effect size underlies all study results and that observed estimates vary only as a function of chance. The error term in a fixed effects model represents only within-study variation; between-study variation is ignored. A **random effects model**, by contrast, assumes that each study estimates different, yet related, true effects, and that the estimates are normally distributed around a mean effect size. A random effects model takes both within- and between-study variation into account.

When there is little heterogeneity, both models yield nearly identical results. With extensive heterogeneity, however, the analyses yield different estimates of the average effect size. Moreover, when there is heterogeneity, the random effects model yields wider confidence intervals than the fixed effects model and so is more conservative. But it is precisely when there *is* extensive heterogeneity that a random effects model should be used.

Some argue that a random effects model is needed only when the test for heterogeneity is statistically significant (or when $I^2 > 50\%$). Others argue that a random effects model is almost always more tenable. A recommended approach is to perform a **sensitivity analysis**—a test of how sensitive the results of an analysis are to changes in the way the analysis was done. This would involve using both models to assess how the results are affected. If the results differ substantially, it is prudent to report estimates from the random effects model.

Examining Factors Affecting Heterogeneity. Many meta-analysts seek to understand determinants of effect size variation through formal analyses. Such analyses should always be considered exploratory because they are inherently nonexperimental (observational)—any causal interpretations are necessarily speculative. To be considered scientifically appropriate, explorations of heterogeneity should be specified before doing the review (i.e., in the protocol), to minimize the risk of finding spurious associations.

Heterogeneity across studies could reflect systematic differences regarding clinical or methodologic characteristics, and both can be explored. *Clinical heterogeneity* can result from participant differences (e.g., men versus women) or in the way that the independent variable was operationalized. For example, in intervention studies, variation in effects could reflect who the agents were (e.g., nurses versus others) or what the setting or delivery mode was.

Methodologic heterogeneity could reflect design features, such when the outcomes were measured (e.g., 3 versus 4 months after an intervention) or whether a randomized design was used. Explorations of methodologic diversity focus mainly on the possibility that results are affected by bias. Explorations of clinical diversity, on the other hand, are more substantively relevant: they examine the possibility that effects differ in relation to clinically relevant factors (e.g., are effects larger for certain types of people?).

Two strategies can be used to explore *moderating effects* on effect size: subgroup analysis and meta-regression. **Subgroup analysis** involves splitting effect size information from studies into distinct subgroups—for example, gender groups. Effects for studies with all-male (or predominantly male) samples could be compared to those for studies with all or predominantly female samples, using some threshold for predominance (e.g., 80% or more of participants). Of course, if it is possible to derive separate effect size estimates for males and females directly from study data, it is advantageous to do so, but this is seldom possible without contacting the researchers. Caution is important in undertaking subgroup analyses, as subgroup effects are often found to be spurious. (Subgroup analyses in primary studies are discussed at length in Chapter 31.)

When variables thought to influence study heterogeneity are continuous (e.g., "dose" of the intervention), or when there is a mix of continuous and categorical factors, then meta-regression might be appropriate. **Meta-regression** involves predicting the effect size based on possible explanatory factors. As in ordinary regression, the statistical significance of regression coefficients indicates a nonrandom linear relationship between effect sizes and the explanatory variable.

Example of Investigating Heterogeneity

Lim and colleagues (2018) studied the prevalence of depression in the community, using studies conducted in 30 countries between 1994 and 2014. The aggregate point prevalence of depression (using a random effect model) was 12.9%, with a high level of heterogeneity (I^2 = 99.8%). Subgroup analyses were performed to test hypotheses about clinical heterogeneity (e.g., gender, urban/rural setting) and methodologic heterogeneity (assessment by self-report versus clinical interview, year of publication). Point prevalence of depression was significantly higher in women, in studies published more recently, and in those using self-report instruments. In a meta-regression, the reviewers found that higher response rates were associated with higher rates of depression.

Addressing Study Quality. There are four basic strategies for dealing with study quality in a meta-analysis. One is to set a quality threshold for study inclusion. Exclusions could reflect requirements for certain features (e.g., only randomized studies) or for a sufficiently high score on a quality assessment scale. We prefer other alternatives that allow reviewers to summarize the full range of evidence in an area, but quality-based exclusions might in some cases be justified.

A second strategy is to perform sensitivity analyses to see whether the exclusion of lower-quality studies changes the results. Conn and colleagues (2003) described as one option beginning the meta-analysis with high-quality studies and then sequentially adding studies of progressively lower quality to evaluate how robust the effect size estimates are to variation in quality.

Example of a Sensitivity Analysis for Study Quality

Chaboyer and colleagues (2018) did a meta-analysis to assess the incidence and prevalence of pressure injuries in adult ICU patients. The reviewers used a validated risk-of-bias scale, and in a sensitivity analysis, they compared results for studies with low risk of bias to results for all studies and found the results were essentially the same.

A third approach is to test indicators of bias as factors influencing heterogeneity of effects. For example, do effects vary as a function of the study's score on a quality assessment scale? Individual study components ratings (as in Table 30.1) and overall study quality can be used in subgroup analyses and meta-regressions.

A fourth strategy is to weight studies according to quality criteria. Meta-analyses routinely give more weight to larger studies, but effect sizes can also be weighted by quality scores, thereby placing more weight on the estimates from rigorous studies. Jüni and colleagues (2001), however, warned that this approach is problematic for several reasons, such as the unknown validity of quality assessment scales and the unreliability of ratings.

A mix of strategies, with appropriate sensitivity analyses, is probably the most prudent approach to dealing with variation in study quality.

TIP Quality information, using a scale or component approach, is important descriptively and should be reported. For example, with a 25-point quality scale, reviewers should report the mean scale score across primary studies, or the percentage scoring above a threshold (e.g., 20 or higher).

Graphic Output from a Meta-Analysis. Dedicated meta-analysis software generates graphics to summarize aspects of the review. The most important graphic is the previously mentioned *forest plot*. A forest plot (Figure 30.2) visually communicates the effect in each primary study in the review (the point estimate for which is shown as a square with lines extending to show the 95% CI) and the overall meta-analysis results (shown as a diamond). The size of the squares corresponds to the weight assigned to each study, based on sample size. In this example, the overall effect for the risk ratio effect size, using a random effects model, was 1.49, a statistically significant effect favoring those in the experimental group (*p* = .02). Heterogeneity for the three studies in the analysis was not significant ($\chi^2 = 1.54$, $p = .46$, $I^2 = 0\%$).

Meta-analysis software often provides other graphics to facilitate interpretation. For example, Cochrane's RevMan software creates a figure that summarizes risk of bias ratings for the components

in Table 30.1 for every study in the review, as illustrated in Figure 30.3. Another useful risk-of-bias graph (available in the Toolkit) illustrates the proportion of studies with each of the three risk appraisal ratings (low, high, unclear) for the six bias components.

Example of Graphic Output

Palacios and colleagues (2017) did a meta-analysis of the effects of Internet-delivered self-management support for improving coronary heart disease and self-management outcomes. They applied the Cochrane tool for assessing risk of bias to the seven studies in their review. They produced a table, which is available in the Toolkit, summarizing bias risk for the studies.

Interpreting Results and Assessing Degree of Confidence: GRADE

Until a few years ago, reviewers typically moved from analyzing their data to writing a report of the findings. Increasingly, reviewers are taking one further step. Many systematic reviews now include a systematic effort to appraise the entire body of evidence—that is, to draw conclusions about how much *confidence* can be placed in the results of the review. Numerous organizations internationally, including the Cochrane Collaboration and JBI, have adopted the Grading of Recommendations, Assessment, Development and

FIGURE 30.2 Annotated illustration of a forest plot from meta-analysis software. (Reprinted with permission from Munn, Z., Tufanaru, C., & Aromataris, E. (2014). JBI's systematic reviews: Data extraction and synthesis. *American Journal of Nursing, 114*(7), 49–54.)

Study	A	B	C	D	E	F
Allen et al., 2017	+	−	+	+	+	−
Chisolm & Evans, 2016	+	+	+	+	+	?
Denny et al., 2018	+	?	−	−	?	−
Friesen et al., 2015	+	?	+	+	+	+
Koretzky & Forman, 2017	+	+	+	+	+	+
Strohl & O'Connor, 2018	+	+	−	−	?	−

KEY: **A** = Random sequence generation
B = Allocation concealment
C = Blinding participants/ personnel
D = Blinding of outcome assessment
E = Incomplete outcome data
F = Reporting bias

Green (+) = Low risk of bias
Red (−) = High risk of bias
Yellow (?) = Unclear risk of bias

FIGURE 30.3 Example of a risk of bias summary figure for studies in a review. (Adapted from Figure 8.6.c in Higgins, J. P. T., & Green, S. (Eds.). (2011). *Cochrane handbook for systematic reviews of interventions (version 5.1.0)*. The Cochrane Collaboration. Retrieved from http://training.cochrane.org/handbook.)

Evaluation (**GRADE**) approach to grading quality of evidence (Guyatt et al., 2008, 2011).

GRADE involves a two-part process designed to facilitate the development of clinical guidelines. In the first part of the process, the quality of the evidence about an intervention's effect is graded for each outcome. In the second part, a recommendation is made about using/not using the intervention, together with the strength of the recommendation (strong or weak). For those preparing a systematic review, only the first part is completed—that is, reviewers do not make clinical recommendations.

GRADE ratings are done on an outcome-by-outcome basis and usually are applied to only a subset of outcomes in a review—the patient-important outcomes judged to be critical to those making decisions about an intervention. Thus, an initial step is to decide which outcomes from the review will be graded.

> **TIP** GRADE was developed initially for evaluating the quality of a body of evidence for studies addressing Therapy questions, but guidelines have been developed for grading other types of studies, such as prognosis studies (Iorio et al., 2015), economic evaluations (Brunetti et al., 2013), and diagnostic test assessments (Schünemann et al., 2008).

Although evidence quality lies on a continuum, GRADE involves making a categorical determination of the *confidence* one can place in the systematic review results—that is, whether confidence in the evidence for a specified outcome (regardless of effect size) is High (++++), Moderate (+++), Low (++), or Very low (+). The second column of Table 30.2 shows GRADE's description of these classifications. A rating of High, for example, corresponds to high confidence that the *true* effect is close to the effect estimated in the review.

The review team begins by assigning an a priori "High" score (corresponding to 4 points) if the review integrated findings from randomized studies (column 1 of Table 30.2) or a "Low" score (2 points) if the primary studies were observational (nonexperimental). Evidence can be downgraded based on assessments of five criteria (column 3 of Table 30.2):

- **Risk of bias.** Important limitations in RCTs include lack of allocation concealment, lack of blinding, loss to follow up, and selective outcome reporting bias. Key limitations in observational studies include failure to control confounders, flawed measurement of exposure and outcome, and faulty eligibility criteria. Reviewers make a judgment about risk of bias (low, serious, very serious) *across all studies in the review* for the specified outcome.
- **Inconsistent results.** Results are inconsistent if point estimates vary widely across studies, the CIs for studies show minimal overlap, the test for heterogeneity has a low *p*-value, and/or the I^2 is large.
- **Indirectness of evidence.** Direct evidence comes from studies that directly compare interventions on outcomes of interest (e.g., not surrogate outcomes) in populations of direct interest (e.g., population of interest is people in long-term care but evidence is from hospital patients).

TABLE 30.2 • GRADE Scoring for the Quality of Evidence for the Effect of an Intervention on a Specific Outcome[a]

STUDY DESIGN	QUALITY OF EVIDENCE	SUBTRACT POINTS IF:	ADD POINTS IF:
Randomized controlled trials (RCTs) (Start at 4 points, High)	**High (++++):** We are very confident that the true effect lies close to that of the estimate of the effect.	**Risk of bias** −1 Serious risk −2 Very serious risk **Inconsistent results:** −1 Serious concern −2 Very serious concern	**Large magnitude of effect:** +1 Large +2 Very large **Dose-response gradient:** +1 Evidence of a gradient
Downgraded RCTs or Upgraded observational studies	**Moderate (+++):** We are moderately confident in the effect estimate: The true effect is likely to be close to the estimate of the effect, but there is a possibility that it is substantially different.	**Indirectness of evidence:** −1 Serious concern −2 Very serious concern **Imprecision (Wide CIs):** −1 Serious concern	**All plausible confounding:** would reduce a demonstrated effect or would suggest a spurious effect when results show no effect
Observational studies or double-downgraded RCTs	**Low (++):** Our confidence in the effect estimate is limited: The true effect may be substantially different from the estimate of the effect.	−2 Very serious concern **Publication bias:** −1 Likely −2 Very likely	+1
Downgraded studies of all types of design	**Very low (+):** We have very little confidence in the effect estimate: The true effect is likely to be substantially different from the estimate of effect		

[a]This table is a composite/adaptation of several tables created by the GRADE group.

- **Imprecision.** Wide CIs for the specified outcome for studies in the review (usually because of small sample size) may result in downgrading the rating.
- **Publication bias.** Publication bias can result in substantial overestimates of effects, so a body of evidence can be downgraded if the risk of publication bias is likely.

The rating for a specific outcome in non-RCTs can be upgraded under three circumstances (column 4 of Table 30.2):

- **Large effect.** Confidence in evidence from observational studies can be upgraded when an effect is so large that the biases common to such studies could not account for the magnitude of the effect.
- **Dose-response gradient.** Confidence is enhanced when the effect is proportional to the degree of exposure.
- **Implausible confounders.** The score can be upgraded when possible confounders would probably *diminish* the observed effect, and so the actual effect likely is larger than the calculated effect size suggests.

The use of GRADE inevitably involves subjective judgments. For example, would a review of

10 RCTs be downgraded from High to Moderate if only 2 studies did not use blinding? The developers of GRADE acknowledge the need to "take an overall or gestalt view of the body of evidence" in scoring (Guyatt et al., 2011, p. 154). Evaluating confidence in the evidence using GRADE is not completely objective, but what it offers is transparency, requiring reviewers to explicitly provide a rationale for grading decisions.

Systematic reviewers who apply the GRADE approach often use software called GRADEpro, which generates two types of tables. The first is an **evidence profile** that provides detailed information about the grading judgments for each outcome. The rows of evidence profiles indicate each outcome that has been graded. Columns correspond to features of the scoring—such as risk of bias, inconsistency, and so on. The entries in the cells explain why any downgrading occurred. An example of an evidence profile is included in the Toolkit.

GRADEpro can also produce **Summary of Findings** (SoF) tables. These tables show, for each outcome (shown in the rows), the results of the meta-analysis, number of participants and studies on which the effect size was based, and then the quality of evidence score.

Example of Using GRADE

Milazi and colleagues (2017) did a systematic review of the effectiveness of educational or behavioral interventions on adherence to phosphate control in adults receiving hemodialysis. The review integrated findings for several outcomes, one of which was rated using GRADE. A meta-analysis was performed for eight RCTs that compared intervention receipt to standard care with regard to serum phosphate levels. The Summary of Findings table (Table 30.3) shows a significant benefit for those in an intervention group; confidence in the effect size was Moderate. The footnote at the bottom indicates why evidence from the studies, all of which were RCTs, was downgraded.

Writing a Quantitative Systematic Review

The final step in a systematic review project is to prepare a report to disseminate the results. Such reports typically follow much the same format as reports for primary studies, with an introduction,

method section, results section, and discussion (see Chapter 32).

Particular care should be taken in preparing the method section. Readers of the review need to be able to assess the rigor of the review, and so methodologic decisions and their rationales should be described. Often, reports of systematic reviews include several appendixes that show details (e.g., the search strategy or quality appraisals of individual studies). If the reviewers decided that a meta-analysis was not justified, the reason for this decision must be made clear. The Cochrane *Handbook* (Higgins & Greene, 2011) offers excellent suggestions for preparing reports for a systematic review. There is also an explicit reporting guideline for meta-analyses of RCTs called **PRISMA** or Preferred Reporting Items for Systematic reviews and Meta-Analyses (Liberati et al., 2009) and another for meta-analyses of observational studies called **MOOSE** (Meta-analysis of Observational Studies in Epidemiology, Stroup et al., 2000). Our critical appraisal guidelines later in this chapter also suggest types of information to include.

A thorough discussion section is also important. The discussion should present an assessment of the overall quality of the body of evidence and the consistency of findings across studies—as well as an interpretation of why there might be inconsistencies. If GRADE was used to evaluate confidence in the results, that information is usually included in the discussion section. Implications of the review should also be described, including a discussion of further research needed to improve the evidence base and the clinical implications of the review.

Tables and figures typically play a key role in reports of systematic reviews. Forest plots are almost always presented, as well as Summary of Findings tables. A table usually summarizes characteristics of studies in the review. A template for such a table is included in the Toolkit. Also, the PRISMA guidelines call for the inclusion of a flow chart that documents the identification, screening, and inclusion of studies in a systematic review.

Finally, full citations for the entire sample of studies included in the review should be provided in the bibliography. Often these are identified separately from other references—for example, by noting them with asterisks.

TABLE 30.3 • Summary of Findings Table

Educational or behavioral interventions compared to standard care for adherence to phosphate control in adults receiving hemodialysis

Patient or population: Adults receiving hemodialysis

Intervention: Educational or behavioral interventions

Comparison: Standard care

Outcome	Number of Participants			Mean Difference[a]	Test for Overall Effect	Quality of the Evidence (GRADE)
	Education or Behavioral Intervention	Standard Care	Total			
Serum phosphate level	n = 408	n = 382	n = 790 (8 RCTs)	$d = -0.23$ mmol/L 95% CI (-0.37, -0.08)	$Z = 3.01$, $p = .003$	⊕⊕⊕◯ MODERATE[b]

[a]Mean difference in serum phosphate level is expressed as intervention group minus standard care group.

[b]No explanation was given on blinding of data collectors and allocation concealment in four studies.

CI, Confidence interval; d, Mean difference; Z, Z-score.

Reprinted with permission from Milazi, M., Bonner, A., & Douglas, C. (2017). Effectiveness of educational or behavioral interventions on adherence to phosphate control in adults receiving hemodialysis: A systematic review. *JBI Database of Systematic Reviews and Implementation Reports, 15*(4), 971–1010.

QUALITATIVE SYSTEMATIC REVIEWS

The systematic integration of qualitative findings is a rapidly evolving and sometimes perplexing field. Dozens of approaches have been proposed and hundreds of articles describing, explaining, or critiquing them have been published in the last 10 years alone. The field is also filled with controversies and debates. Some prominent qualitative scholars have challenged the prominence of *systematic* reviews as an approach to synthesizing healthcare knowledge (e.g., Greenhalgh et al., 2018). Others have embraced the expansion of systematic reviews to include qualitative evidence.

Terminology in this field can also be confusing. Indeed, there is not even a consensus on what to call the entire enterprise. The most frequently used "umbrella" terms are *qualitative metasynthesis, qualitative systematic review, qualitative evidence synthesis,* and *qualitative research synthesis* (Booth et al., 2016).

It is beyond the scope of this book to provide detailed descriptions of the various approaches to synthesizing qualitative evidence. Even summarizing the state of this field adequately is challenging. Several groups have put effort into developing comparison tables for various approaches along multiple dimensions as aids to helping reviewers select the "right" approach. We provide information about these comparative reviews in Supplement B on thePoint. Ⓢ Our goal in this chapter is to present a broad overview of a few approaches.

Aggregative and Interpretive Qualitative Reviews

Several scholars have characterized systematic reviews as being either *aggregative* or *interpretive/configurative* (e.g., Booth et al., 2018; Gough et al., 2012). We will use the aggregative/interpretive distinction to highlight several features of qualitative reviews, but we emphasize that most qualitative reviews have elements of both aggregation and interpretation and that the boundaries between these two broad categories are permeable.

The decision on which broad (and specific) qualitative synthesis approach to use depends on several factors, including the nature of the question and the philosophical leanings of the reviewers. Other important factors may include time and resource constraints, the expertise of the review team, and the intended audience for the review (Booth et al., 2018; Paterson, 2013). For students, the decision may also be affected by the preferences of their advisers.

Aggregative Qualitative Reviews

Qualitative reviews that are predominantly aggregative are similar in many respects to quantitative systematic reviews. Aggregative reviews involve the *pooling* of findings (that is, themes, categories, or processes) across the qualitative studies in the review. Other features that make aggregative qualitative reviews similar to quantitative systematic reviews include the following:

- The review process tends to be fairly structured, following a well-defined series of steps;
- The questions these reviews address are predetermined and, often, fairly focused;
- Exhaustive searching for primary studies is expected;
- Assessment of the quality of the primary studies is considered essential;
- Efforts are made to minimize subjectivity or bias; and
- A goal of the review is to provide direct and usable guidance for action.

Certain research questions are especially well-suited to an aggregative qualitative approach. Often these questions concern how best to address a healthcare problem—questions typically addressed in descriptive qualitative inquiries. Examples of such questions include the following: Why do people who know the risks of smoking continue to smoke? What strategies do people use in efforts to quit smoking? What are patients' barriers to participating in a smoking cessation intervention? What features of a smoking intervention lead to lapses in implementation fidelity?

Both the Joanna Briggs Institute (JBI) and the Cochrane Collaboration, who typically use the umbrella term **qualitative evidence synthesis (QES)**, provide guidance for reviews that would best be characterized as aggregative. At JBI, qualitative reviews use an approach to evidence synthesis called **meta-aggregation** (Aromataris & Munn, 2017; Hannes & Lockwood, 2011). The JBI approach is described in a later section.

Interpretive Qualitative Reviews

Qualitative reviews that are predominantly interpretive in nature emphasize the creation of integrated conceptualizations and theories by interpreting and reconfiguring findings from qualitative studies. Interpretive syntheses tend to have the following features:

- The approach tends not to be highly structured;
- The questions addressed by interpretive reviews often evolve during a process of discovery;
- Purposive sampling of studies is sometimes preferred to comprehensive searching;
- Assessment of the quality of the primary studies is not always considered essential;
- Interpreters' insights are valued; and
- The goal of the review is to provide enlightenment through new ways of understanding phenomena.

Interpretive syntheses most often focus on questions about meanings, feelings, experiences, and processes—questions typically addressed through phenomenologic, ethnographic, or grounded theory research. Examples of such questions include the following: What is it like for smokers to lose a loved one to lung cancer? Is smoking an important part of the culture among those in the military? What is the process by which previous smokers succeed in quitting?

In nursing, the term **metasynthesis** has predominated as the umbrella term for qualitative synthesis, usually referring to syntheses that are interpretive. In fact, nurse researchers have contributed more to the field of qualitative research synthesis than scholars in other health-related disciplines (Tricco et al., 2016). In the next section, we discuss metasynthesis but note that nurse researchers have used other interpretive synthesis approaches, including formal grounded theory (Eaves, 2001), critical interpretive synthesis or CIS (Dixon-Woods et al., 2006), and thematic synthesis (Thomas & Harden, 2008).

> **TIP** The book by Hannes and Lockwood (2012) has completely worked out examples of a meta-ethnography, a critical interpretive synthesis, and a meta-aggregation.

Metasynthesis

Over a decade ago, five leading thinkers on qualitative integration used the term metasynthesis as an umbrella term, with metasynthesis broadly representing "a family of methodologic approaches to developing new knowledge based on rigorous analysis of existing qualitative research findings" (Thorne, Jensen, Kearney, Noblit, and Sandelowski, 2004, p. 1343). There are diverse approaches to doing a metasynthesis.

There is more agreement on what a metasynthesis is not than on what it is. Metasynthesis is not a literature review—i.e., not a collation of research findings—nor is it a concept analysis. Many writers have followed the definition of metasynthesis offered by Schreiber and colleagues (1997): "...the bringing together and breaking down of findings, examining them, discovering the essential features and, in some way, combining phenomena into a transformed whole" (p. 314). Most metasyntheses involve a transformational process.

Two important approaches to interpretive metasynthesis are **meta-ethnography** (Noblit & Hare, 1988) and **metastudy** (Patterson et al., 2001). An approach called **metasummary** (Sandelowski & Barrosso, 2007) is more of an aggregative than interpretive approach; it is described in this section because of its link to metasynthesis. For the most part, differences in these approaches concern how the data from qualitative studies are analyzed and synthesized.

Preliminary Steps in a Metasynthesis
Many of the steps in qualitative syntheses are similar to ones we described for quantitative systematic reviews, and so details will not be repeated

here. However, we point out a few distinctive issues relating to qualitative integration.

Formulating the Question. In metasynthesis, researchers begin with a broad research question or an investigative focus. Booth et al. (2018) have described the research question in an aggregative review as an "anchor," but more like a "compass" in interpretive reviews. One issue concerns the scope of the inquiry. Finfgeld (2003) recommended that the scope be broad enough to fully capture the phenomenon of interest, but sufficiently focused to yield findings that are meaningful to clinicians or other researchers.

In metasyntheses, the research question may evolve over the course of the review. It may not be evident at first whether the initial question can be answered, or whether the scope of the review should be expanded or contracted. In their reports, metasynthesists sometimes state an overall study purpose rather than a research question.

> **Example of a Statement of Purpose in a Meta-Ethnography**
> Nybakkan and colleagues (2018) stated that their aim was "to explore how formal caregivers perceive and interpret aggressive behaviors in nursing home residents living with dementia, by synthesizing knowledge from published qualitative studies" (p. 2713).

Designing a Metasynthesis. Metasyntheses require advance planning. Having a team of at least two researchers to design and implement the study is often advantageous. Investigator triangulation is one strategy for enhancing the integrity of the metasynthesis.

> **TIP** Meta-analyses often are undertaken by researchers who did not do one of the primary studies in the review. Metasyntheses, by contrast, are often completed by researchers whose area of interest has led them to do both original studies and metasyntheses on the same topic. Prior work in an area offers advantages in terms of researchers' ability to grasp subtle nuances and to think abstractly about a topic, but a disadvantage may be a certain degree of partiality about one's own work.

Metasynthesists make several decisions about sampling. One issue is whether their sample of studies will be exhaustive (i.e., including all relevant studies) or purposive. Some approaches to metasynthesis, notably meta-ethnography, may involve purposive strategies in which studies are selected for conceptual purposes. For those opting for a purposive strategy, one guideline for sampling adequacy is whether categories in the metasynthesis are theoretically saturated (Finfgeld, 2003; Toye et al., 2014). Thus, the number of studies included in a metasynthesis is likely to be affected by the conceptual richness of the studies themselves. When purposive sampling is adopted, it is often difficult to articulate an up-front sampling strategy.

Another issue is whether to include findings only from peer-reviewed journals in the synthesis. One advantage of including nonpublished sources is that journal articles are constrained in what can be reported because of space limitations. Finfgeld (2003), in her metasynthesis on *courage*, used dissertations even when a peer-reviewed journal article was available from the same study because the dissertation offered richer data.

An aspect of sampling that has been controversial in metasynthesis concerns whether to integrate studies from different research traditions. Some researchers have argued against combining studies from different traditions. Others, however, advocate combining findings across traditions and methods. Which path to follow is likely to depend on the focus of the inquiry, its intent vis-à-vis theory development, and the nature of the available evidence.

Example of Sampling Decisions

Polita and colleagues (2018) conducted a metasynthesis of qualitative findings on the care provided by fathers to a child with cancer. The 16 primary studies in the review used phenomenology ($n = 6$), grounded theory ($n = 3$), qualitative description ($n = 5$), and mixed methods ($n = 2$).

Regardless of whether sampling for the review will be exhaustive or purposive, metasynthesists must develop inclusion and exclusion criteria.

These are likely to include language restrictions, and perhaps restrictions on settings (e.g., rural; long-term care settings), demographic characteristics (e.g., people older than 60 years), or research tradition.

Searching the Literature for Data. It is sometimes difficult to find relevant qualitative studies for a synthesis. Booth (2016) identified numerous challenges in searching for qualitative studies, including nonstandardized terminology, inadequate database indexing, interdatabase differences in indexing terminology, and the variety of qualitative methodologies. It is likely to be helpful to search using not only broad search terms (qualitative) but also specific names of traditions (e.g., grounded theory, phenomenolog*, ethnograph*). Booth's suggested search terms include *interview* and *experience*. Further search guidance is offered by DeJean et al. (2016).

> **TIP** Mnemonics other than PICO have been proposed for qualitative evidence searches (Booth, 2016). These include 3WH (What [topic], Who [population], When [temporal], and How [methodologic]); SPIDER (Sample, Phenomenon of Interest, Design, Evaluation, Research type), and PICo (Population, phenomenon of Interest, Context).

Appraising Study Quality. In general, there is less of an emphasis on assessing the methodologic quality of primary studies in interpretive syntheses than in aggregative ones. Nevertheless, critical appraisal is often used in metasyntheses, sometimes simply to describe the sample of studies in the review but in other cases to make sampling decisions.

There is no consensus about whether quality should be a criterion for eliminating studies for a metasynthesis. Sandelowski and Barroso (2003a) advocated inclusiveness: "Excluding reports of qualitative studies because of inadequacies in reporting…, or because of what some reviewers might perceive as methodologic mistakes, will result in the exclusion of reports with findings valuable to practice that are not necessarily invalidated by these errors" (p. 155). Finfgeld (2003) suggested that, at a minimum, studies included in the review must have used accepted qualitative methods and must have findings that are supported by raw data—i.e., quotes from participants.

Noblit and Hare (1988) advocated including all relevant studies, but also suggested giving more weight to higher-quality studies. A more systematic application of assessments in a metasynthesis is to use quality information in a sensitivity analysis that explores whether interpretations are altered when low-quality studies are removed (Thomas & Hardin, 2008).

Several instruments have been created to appraise qualitative studies for a metasynthesis. Many nurse researchers use the 10-question assessment tool from the Critical Appraisal Skills Programme (CASP) of the Centre for Evidence-Based Medicine in the United Kingdom (CASP, 2016). Others use the tool created for JBI qualitative evidence summaries, which we describe later in this chapter. Majid and Vanstone (2018) undertook a detailed analysis of appraisal instruments and recommended that those who are novices or looking for an easy-to-follow tool should use CASP.

Example of a Quality Appraisal in a Metasynthesis

Fogarty and colleagues (2018) did a meta-ethnography of studies on the experiences of women with an eating disorder perinatally. The 12 included studies were appraised using the CASP instrument, with two reviewers undertaking independent appraisals. The team used the ratings to describe the studies. No studies met all CASP criteria, but most studies were of good quality.

Extracting Data for Analysis. Information about various features of the study need to be abstracted and coded as part of the project. Metasynthesists usually record data source information (e.g., year of publication, country), characteristics of the sample (e.g., number of participants, mean age, gender distribution), and methodologic features (e.g., research tradition).

Most important, information about study findings must be extracted and recorded. Sandelowski and Barroso (2003b) have defined *findings* as the "data-based and integrated discoveries, conclusions, judgments, or pronouncements researchers offered regarding the events, experiences, or cases under investigation (i.e., their interpretations, no matter the extent of the data transformation involved)" (p. 228). Others characterize findings as the key themes, metaphors, categories, concepts, or phrases from each study.

As Sandelowski and Barroso (2002) have noted, however, *finding* the findings is not always easy. Qualitative researchers intermingle data with interpretation and findings from other studies with their own. Noblit and Hare (1988) advised that, just as primary study researchers must read and reread their data before they can proceed with a meaningful analysis, metasynthesists must read the primary studies multiple times to fully grasp the categories or metaphors being explicated. A metasynthesis becomes "another 'reading' of data, an opportunity to reflect on the data in new ways" (McCormick et al., 2003, p. 936).

Synthesizing and Interpreting the Data

Strategies for metasynthesis diverge most at the analysis stage. We briefly describe three approaches and advise you to consult other resources for more guidance. Regardless of approach, metasynthesis is a complex task that involves "carefully peeling away the surface layers of studies to find their hearts and souls in a way that does the least damage to them" (Sandelowski et al., 1997, p. 370).

Meta-Ethnography. Noblit and Hare's (1988) meta-ethnographic approach has been influential among nurse researchers. Noblit and Hare argued that the synthesis should focus on constructing interpretations rather than analyses (i.e., interpretation in lieu of aggregation). Their approach includes seven phases that overlap and repeat as the synthesis progresses, the first three of which are preanalytic: (1) deciding on the phenomenon, (2) deciding which studies are relevant for the synthesis, and (3) reading and rereading each study. Phase 7 involves writing up the synthesis. Phases 4 through 6 concern the analysis:

Phase 4: Deciding how the studies are related to each other. In this phase the researcher makes a list of the key metaphors in each study and their relation to each other. Noblit and Hare used the term "metaphor" to refer to themes, perspectives, and/or concepts that emerged from the primary studies. Studies can be related in three ways: *reciprocal* (directly comparable), *refutational* (in opposition to each other), and in *lines of argument* rather than either reciprocal or refutational.

Phase 5: Translating the qualitative studies into one another. Noblit and Hare noted that "translations are especially unique syntheses because they protect the particular, respect holism, and enable comparison. An adequate translation maintains the central metaphors and/or concepts of each account in their relation to other key metaphors or concepts in that account" (p. 28). *Reciprocal translation analysis* (RTA) involves exploring and explaining similarities and contradictions between studies and is similar to constant comparison.

Phase 6: Synthesizing translations. In this phase, the challenge is to make a whole into more than the individual parts imply. Syntheses involve building up a new picture of the whole (e.g., a whole culture or phenomenon) from a scrutiny of its parts.

Atkins and colleagues (2008), noting that some aspects of meta-ethnography were not well-defined by Noblit and Hare, offered further guidance. Campbell and colleagues (2011) prepared a useful open-access document that presents an evaluation of meta-ethnographic methods. More recently, Toye and colleagues (2014) identified challenges and offered suggestions for building on the meta-ethnographic approach.

Example of a Meta-Ethnography

Schmied and an interdisciplinary team (2017) used meta-ethnography to synthesize findings on migrant women's experiences with postpartum depression. Team members mainly used reciprocal translation "because the similarities across the studies dominated" (p. 5). Four key metaphors were identified, one of which was: "I am alone, worried and angry—this is not me!" (p. 2).

Metastudy. Paterson and colleagues' (2001) metastudy method of metasynthesis involves three components: metadata analysis, metamethod, and metatheory. These components often are conducted concurrently, and the metasynthesis results from the integration of findings from these three components. Paterson and colleagues define **metadata analysis** as the study of results of reported research in a specific substantive area of investigation by means of analyzing the "processed data." **Metamethod** is the study of the methodologic approaches and rigor of the studies included in the metasynthesis. Lastly, **metatheory** refers to the analysis of the theoretical underpinnings on which the studies are grounded. Metastudy uses metatheory to describe and deconstruct theories that shape a body of inquiry. The end product is a metasynthesis that results from bringing back together the findings of these three components.

Example of a Metastudy

Aagard and colleagues (2018) did a metastudy of parents' experiences of neonatal transfer. Metatheory analysis revealed that caring, transition, and family-centered care were main theoretical frames in primary studies. The metadata analysis showed that neonatal transfer was scary and threatening for the parents. "Wavering and wandering" was the metaphoric representation of the parents' experiences.

Sandelowski and Barroso's Metasummary and Metasynthesis. The strategies developed by Sandelowski and Barroso (2007) are the results of a multiyear methodologic project. They proposed a continuum relating to how much data transformation occurs in a primary study. Further, they dichotomized studies based on level of synthesis and interpretation. Reports are described as *summaries* if the findings are descriptive synopses of the qualitative data, usually with lists and frequencies of topics and themes, without conceptual reframing. *Syntheses* are findings that are more interpretive and explanatory and that involve conceptual or metaphorical reframing. Sandelowski and Barroso argued that only syntheses should be used in a metasynthesis.

Both summaries and syntheses can, however, be used in a **metasummary**, which can lay a foundation for a metasynthesis. Sandelowski and Barroso

(2003a) provided an example of a metasummary in which they used both summaries and syntheses of mothering within the context of HIV infection. The first step, extracting findings, resulted in almost 800 complete sentences from the 45 reports. The 800 sentences were then reduced to 93 thematic statements, or abstracted findings.

The next step in the metasummary was to calculate **manifest effect sizes,** i.e., effect sizes calculated from the manifest content pertaining to motherhood within the context of HIV as represented in the 93 abstracted findings. Qualitative effect sizes should not be confused with treatment effects: the "…calculation of effect sizes constitutes a quantitative transformation of qualitative data in the service of extracting more meaning from those data and verifying the presence of a pattern or theme" (Sandelowski & Barroso, 2003a, p. 231). They argued that by calculating effect sizes, integration can avoid the possibility of over- or under-weighting findings.

Two types of manifest effect size can be calculated. A **frequency effect size**, which indicates the magnitude of a finding, is the number of reports with unduplicated information that contain a given finding, divided by all unduplicated reports. For example, Sandelowski and Barroso (2003a) calculated an overall frequency effect size of 60% for the finding of mothers struggling with whether or not to disclose their HIV status to their children. In other words, 60% of the 45 reports had a finding of this nature. Such effect size information can be calculated for subgroups of reports—e.g., for published versus unpublished reports, for reports from different research traditions, and so on.

An **intensity effect size** indicates the concentration of findings *within* each report. It is calculated by dividing the number of different findings in a report, divided by the total number of findings in all reports. As an example, one primary study had 29 out of the 93 findings, for an intensity effect size of 31% for that study (Sandelowski & Barroso, 2003a).

Metasyntheses can build on metasummaries, but require findings that are interpretive, i.e., from reports characterized as syntheses. Metasyntheses require reviewers to piece the individual syntheses together and craft a new coherent explanation of a target event or experience. Several analytic methods can be used to achieve this goal, including, "… for example, constant comparison, taxonomic analysis, the reciprocal translation of in vivo concepts, and the use of imported concepts to frame data" (Sandelowski in Thorne et al., 2004, p. 1358).

Example of Sandelowski and Barroso's Approach

Ludvigsen and colleagues (2016) undertook a metasummary and metasynthesis of patients' experiences with transfers and transitions. They provided a step-by-step description of using Sandelowski and Barroso's approach. They noted that "calculating effect sizes increased our understanding of the power of the reports and the relationship between themes and individual reports; it also assisted us in generating theory through team discussions about the summaries" (p. 325).

Writing a Metasynthesis Report

Metasynthesis reports are similar to quantitative systematic review reports, except that the results section contains the new interpretations rather than quantitative findings. When a metasummary has been done, meta-findings would typically be presented in a table, a template for which is available in the Toolkit. ✪

The method section of a metasynthesis report should describe the sampling criteria, search procedures, study appraisal methods, and efforts to enhance the integrity of the integration. Key features of the sample of studies are usually summarized in a table. A PRISMA-type flowchart highlighting sampling decisions and outcomes is often included. Reporting guidelines for qualitative systematic reviews are called **ENTREQ** (Enhancing Transparency in Reporting the synthesis of Qualitative research) (Tong et al., 2012). France et al. (2019) offer reporting guidelines for meta-ethnographies.

Meta-Aggregation

The Joanna Briggs Institute uses an aggregative, structured approach to synthesizing qualitative evidence. JBI maintains that regardless of whether the evidence is quantitative or qualitative, the same review process should be used, with certain steps tailored to accommodate the special nature of the findings. Hannes and Lockwood (2011) have described the JBI approach as aligned with pragmatism, wherein the synthesis is connected to the idea of "practical usefulness." The JBI **meta-aggregation** method is aimed at delivering synthesized findings to inform clinical decision-making.

The JBI reviewer's manual (Aromataris & Munn, 2017) offers prescriptive guidance on preparing a *qualitative evidence synthesis* using meta-aggregation. Researchers at JBI have also published a series of articles describing their approach to systematic reviews in *The American Journal of Nursing* in 2014 (e.g., Munn et al., 2014a; Porritt et al., 2014). Additionally, the qualitative working group at the Cochrane Collaboration has published guidance on QES in six papers published in the *Journal of Clinical Epidemiology* (e.g., Noyes et al., 2018; Tugwell et al., 2018). Although less prescriptive than JBI, the Cochrane guidelines also favor aggregative approaches. In this section we briefly touch on a few issues relating to the JBI approach.

Preliminary Steps in a JBI Qualitative Evidence Synthesis

In a meta-aggregation synthesis, an explicit review question is formulated upfront. JBI recommends using the PICo format (**P**opulation, phenomenon of **I**nterest, **Co**ntext) for articulating the question (Stern et al., 2014). Reviewers are expected to do comprehensive and exhaustive searching for relevant evidence, including a search of the grey literature. For JBI reviews, a protocol describing plans for the QES—including the review question, search strategies, and inclusion criteria—must be prepared. Data are extracted by two independent reviewers using a JBI extraction form, and the information is input into the JBI software, SUMARI. In the extraction form, findings are listed, together with a supporting illustrative quote from the study's raw data.

Quality appraisals of the studies are undertaken using the 10-item JBI Critical Appraisal Checklist for Qualitative Research. In addition to appraising each study for its overall methodologic quality, the JBI approach calls for ratings of the *credibility* of each finding in a study. Reviewers assign a rating of *unequivocal* (a finding is beyond a reasonable doubt), *credible* (finding is open to challenge), and *unsupported* (findings not supported by the data).

Analysis Through Meta-Aggregation

Data synthesis using meta-aggregation is a three-step process that begins with the extraction of findings and illustrations from all included studies. In the second step, findings that are sufficiently similar or related conceptually are collapsed into categories. Each category must have two or more findings. In the final step, the reviewers develop one or more synthesized findings that encompass at least two categories. Reviewers are expected to explain what data they considered as a "finding," the process by which findings were identified, and how findings were grouped to create categories.

Munn et al. (2014a) presented a figure illustrating the analysis for a meta-aggregation of qualitative evidence on how patients experience high-technology medical imaging like MRIs. For example, three findings were: "An alien experience," "Being in another world," and "Swallowed and sinking," and these were grouped into the category "Out of this world, alien experience." One of the synthesized findings derived from this and other categories was this: "Scanning is a unique, out-of-this world experience that must be experienced by the person to be truly understood" (p. 53). The full meta-aggregation figure from the Munn et al. article is included in the Toolkit. ✪

Assessment of Confidence

Inspired by the GRADE rating system for quantitative reviews, a working group at JBI developed a system to rate confidence in the synthesized findings of a QES (Munn et al., 2014b). The **ConQual** approach, as it is called, requires a score—on a scale from 4 (high) to 1 (very low)—summarizing the reviewers' confidence in each finding. Essentially, a synthesized qualitative finding is given an initial score of "high" that can be downgraded because of low credibility (e.g., a mix of unequivocal and credible findings results in the loss of a point) or low dependability. The dependability score is based on answers to five specific questions from the critical appraisal tool.

The end product is a Summary of Findings table, similar to the one produced using GRADE. The table presents a synthesized finding for the meta-aggregation analysis in each row, together with the following information: type of research, dependability score, credibility score, the ConQual score, and comments explaining the scoring.

> **TIP** A separate effort was undertaken by a group working with GRADE to develop a means of rating confidence in the findings from a qualitative synthesis. A seven-paper series was published in the journal *Systematic Reviews* in 2018 to explain the **GRADE-CERQual** (Confidence in the Evidence from Reviews of Qualitative Research) (see Lewin et al., 2018). The GRADE-CERQual approach considers four aspects for each finding: methodologic limitations, coherence, data adequacy, and relevance. Dissemination bias also plays a role. The system yields a Summary of Qualitative Findings table and an evidence profile. Like GRADE, there are four levels of confidence: High, Moderate, Low, and Very Low confidence. Although ConQual and CERQual develop similar rankings, the criteria for scoring in the two systems differ.

Writing a Meta-Aggregation Report

JBI's reviewer's manual provides explicit direction on preparing a qualitative evidence report. Many JBI reviews include a table that lists the studies included in the review in the rows and then answers to the 10 critical appraisal questions in the columns (yes, no, unclear, or not applicable). A diagram showing the progression from findings to categories and then to synthesized findings is encouraged. A Summary of Findings table, with ConQual ratings, is essential. Discussing the relevance of the findings to key stakeholders (e.g., patients, clinicians) is recommended.

> **Example of the JBI Meta-Aggregation Approach**
>
> Parsons and colleagues (2018) undertook a JBI qualitative review of studies on older nurses' experiences of providing direct care in hospitals. Based on 12 studies, the team identified 75 findings, which were grouped into 12 categories and then into three synthesized findings. The review provided a Summary of Findings table for the three synthesized findings, with ConQual information. For example, one of the findings was: "It's a changing job; can I keep up?". This finding was elaborated on in the table ("Older nurses voice many concerns; some have memory problems, some are exhausted… many have concerns if they can move quickly enough in an emergency…" (p. 671). The ConQual score was downgraded one level for dependability but was not downgraded for credibility, resulting in an overall confidence score of Moderate.

SYSTEMATIC MIXED STUDIES REVIEWS

The growing recognition of the complexity of health care problems has given rise to interest in systematic reviews that integrate findings from a methodologic array of studies. Reviews that integrate qualitative and quantitative evidence have been called *mixed methods systematic reviews* (Pearson et al., 2014); *mixed methods reviews* (Harden & Thomas, 2005); *mixed research syntheses* (Sandelowski et al., 2013); *mixed-method syntheses* (Noyes et al., 2018); and *mixed-method research synthesis* (Heyvaert et al., 2017).

We use the term systematic **mixed studies review** (Pluye & Hong, 2014; Pluye et al., 2016) to refer to a systematic review that uses disciplined procedures to integrate and synthesize findings from qualitative, quantitative, and mixed methods studies. We prefer a term that does not include the phrase "mixed method," to clarify that such reviews are not syntheses of mixed-methods studies alone, but rather efforts to synthesize findings from diverse primary studies.

Rationale for Mixed Studies Reviews

Mixed studies reviews (MSRs) reflect the growing awareness that single-method reviews can seldom provide full information for making health care decisions in real-world settings. MSRs combine information about the human experience of illness and health with information on the prevalence of health problems, the effectiveness of interventions, or the prognosis of disease conditions. Syntheses of qualitative studies give voice to the concerns and experiences of clients and providers, and syntheses of quantitative studies provide information about outcomes and effects. Single-method reviews often present an incomplete picture that constrains their utility in evidence-based decisions. MSRs "have the capacity to present a very high level of evidence" (Pearson et al., 2014, p. 16).

In a review of MSRs, Hong and colleagues (2017) identified 459 published MSRs and found that the number had increased by 1000% (from 10 to 101) between 2007 and 2014. The reasons for performing an MSR fell into several categories, including: (1) to acknowledge the complexity of the problem itself; (2) to address related but different questions (what, how, and why); (3) to attain a thorough understanding or provide a complete picture; (4) to strengthen confidence in results through corroboration; and (5) to provide more meaningful evidence for practice.

TIP The advantages of MSRs need to be considered within the context of potential obstacles. MSRs are more time consuming and expensive than single-method reviews and require a team with diverse skills. Moreover, the evidence may be insufficient in one of the strands to provide meaningful integration.

Another impetus for MSRs is the growing interest in complex interventions. As noted by Petticrew and colleagues (2015), complex interventions present "unique challenges" for those conducting systematic reviews. A growing body of papers to guide MSRs for complex interventions has emerged, including a series of seven papers published in the *Journal of Clinical Epidemiology* in 2017 (e.g., Pigott et al., 2017). The revised Cochrane Manual includes a chapter on reviews relating to intervention complexities (Higgins & Thomas, 2020, Chapter 17).

Conducting Mixed Studies Reviews

In this section, we briefly review some issues relating to the conduct of MSRs but acknowledge that this is a field with new ideas and methods emerging weekly. We do not describe steps in the conduct of MSRs that are covered in earlier sections of this paper, such as searching for reports or extracting findings, but focus instead on issues unique to MSRs.

TIP An issue that has led to debate and controversy in all systematic reviews concerns quality appraisal of included studies; MSRs are no exception. Criteria for appraising the quality of quantitative, qualitative, and mixed-methods study for MSRs have been proposed and tested (e.g., Pace et al., 2012; Pluye et al., 2009).

Research Questions for MSRs

As in mixed methods research, the "dictatorship of the research question" is a driving force behind mixed studies reviews. Harden and Thomas (2005), whose work focused on health promotion interventions, noted that their reviews "were beginning to answer multiple questions" and that their reviews increasingly involved "more than one section in which the results of studies are brought together" (p. 261).

In an MSR, there must be at least two questions, one requiring quantitative data and the other needing qualitative data. In many cases, the quantitative question in a mixed studies review concerns the effects of an intervention, which is the case for all MSRs undertaken within the Cochrane Collaboration (Harden et al., 2018). In such reviews, there is a Therapy question and sometimes a question about intervention costs (economic evaluations). Qualitative questions can address diverse intervention-related issues, such as: What are patients' experiences with an intervention or with the health problem the intervention was designed to address? What are the experiences of patients unable to access the intervention? In what contexts was the intervention implemented and how did context shape the implementation and the outcomes? Which components or aspects of the intervention are perceived as most or least beneficial? MSRs can also address non-Therapy questions, including Prognosis, Etiology, and prevalence questions.

Although not always explicitly stated, MSR reviewers also address integrative questions. That is, the diverse evidence needs to be integrated to discern whether the qualitative findings corroborate, qualify, refute, or expand the quantitative ones.

Example of Questions in a Mixed Studies Review

Beck and Woynar (2017) conducted a mixed studies review on posttraumatic stress in mothers whose preterm infants stayed in a newborn intensive care unit (NICU). Using findings from 37 studies (25 quantitative, 12 qualitative), the review addressed 4 questions: (1) What is the prevalence of posttraumatic stress symptoms of mothers whose preterm infants are in the NICU? (2) What interventions have been tested to decrease those symptoms? (3) What are the NICU experiences of the mothers while their infants are hospitalized? And (4) How do the mixed results develop a more complete picture of mothers' posttraumatic stress while their infants are in the NICU?

Designs for Mixed Studies Reviews

Mixed studies reviews are a relatively new endeavor; both terminology and approaches are evolving at a rapid pace. Several typologies have been developed, some of which rely on category schemes associated with mixed-methods designs (e.g., Heyvaert et al., 2013; Pluye and Hong, 2014).

A basic design issue concerns the timing of the reviews—that is, whether the review of quantitative results and the review of qualitative results are conducted concurrently (*convergent* designs) or *sequentially* (Hong et al., 2017). MSRs for the Cochrane Collaboration are all sequential; often a "post hoc" qualitative review is undertaken following a standard Cochrane review on intervention effectiveness, to offer enriched guidance to clinicians (Harden et al., 2018).

Margarete Sandelowski has been in the forefront of MSR development. She and colleagues (Sandelowski et al., 2006) described three MSR designs that vary in approach and goals. In a *segregated design,* two separate syntheses are undertaken, one of qualitative and the other of quantitative

findings, and then the mixed synthesis integrates the two. This approach is appropriate when qualitative and quantitative findings are seen as complementing each other, as opposed to confirming or refuting each other. Complementarity occurs when the qualitative and quantitative research has addressed different but connected questions. The segregated design model characterizes many mixed studies reviews and has been found to be useful in integrating information about both effectiveness and context/processes in intervention research. The Joanna Briggs Institute has adopted segregated designs as its approach to mixed studies review (Pearson et al., 2014).

The second model is an *integrated design* (Sandelowski et al., 2006), which can be used when qualitative and quantitative findings in an area of inquiry are perceived as able to confirm, extend, or refute each other. In an integrated design, studies are grouped not by method but by findings viewed as answering the same research question. The analytic approach may involve transforming the findings (quantitizing qualitative findings or qualitizing quantitative findings) to enable them to be combined.

A third model is a *contingent design* (Sandelowski et al., 2006) that involves a coordinated and sequential series of syntheses. In such a design, the findings from the systematic synthesis to answer one research question are used to address a second research question—which may lead to yet another synthesis addressing a different question. For example, a qualitative synthesis can precede a quantitative review and may help to define key outcomes or key variables for an analysis of heterogeneity for the meta-analysis.

In Hong et al.'s (2017) review of 459 MSRs, fewer than 5% were contingent/sequential. Most MSRs used what they called "data-based convergent" designs, which they described as being most akin to Sandelowski et al.'s (2006) integrated design.

> **TIP** The chapter on mixed studies reviews in the JBI reviewer's manual (Chapter 8) has figures that diagram Sandelowski's three MSR designs (Pearson et al., 2014). Note that at the writing of this book, Chapter 8 of the JBI manual was under revision.

Approaches to Analysis and Integration

Many approaches to analysis and integration in MSRs have been described. Techniques such as textual narrative, content analysis, narrative summary, thematic synthesis, and critical interpretive synthesis (an adaptation of meta-ethnography) were identified in Hong et al.'s (2017) review of MSRs; the most common method was thematic synthesis.

Another approach is *Bayesian synthesis*, which is used in MSRs at the Joanna Briggs Institute. Bayesian synthesis involves transforming data into a compatible format—that is, either converting qualitative findings to quantitative ones or vice versa (e.g., Voils et al., 2009). The JBI method involves transforming quantitative data into qualitative themes that are then synthesized through meta-aggregation (Pearson et al., 2014).

> **TIP** Lucas and colleagues (2007) provide a worked-out example of two alternative approaches to MSRs (thematic synthesis and textual narrative) and Flemming (2010) offers a step-by-step guide to using critical interpretive synthesis in an MSR. A chapter in the book by Hannes and Lockwood (2012) includes a worked example of a Bayesian approach to MSRs.

The Cochrane working group identified five "tools" or methods for integrating qualitative evidence with intervention effectiveness reviews: (1) juxtaposing findings in a matrix; (2) using logic models or conceptual frameworks; (3) analyzing intervention theory; (4) testing hypotheses derived from qualitative evidence statistically via subgroup analysis; and (5) qualitative comparison analysis (Harden et al., 2018). All five tools can be used with MSRs whose design is sequential/contingent, but only the first three can be used with convergent designs.

The third tool, analyzing intervention or program theory, is a strategy often associated with realist reviews. The aim of **realist reviews** (or *realist syntheses*) is to understand theory-driven *Context-Mechanism-Outcome (CMO)* configurations in studies of interventions—especially complex interventions.

The overall goal of a realist review is to gain insights into what works, for whom, and under what circumstances (Emmel et al., 2019; Pawson, 2013).

According to a realist perspective, interventions work by altering the context for the people acting within it. Contexts are defined as the institutional or spatial locations in which interventions are situated. Context includes the norms, values, and interrelationships within the intervention setting, all of which establish boundaries on intervention mechanisms. The mechanisms, in turn, include the beliefs, feelings, choices, and motivations of people and groups of people, which affect behaviors that are considered outcomes. Realist reviews combine qualitative and quantitative findings to "unpack" how an intervention works in different contexts, through the development of theoretical explanations. Evidence from RCTs usually contributes to the outcome and mechanism components of a realist CMO analysis, and evidence from qualitative and implementation studies contributes to the context and mechanism components.

In Hong et al.'s (2017) review of 459 MSRs, only 6 were realist reviews, but interest in realist reviews is growing and several nurse researchers have been on teams that completed such reviews.

> **Example of a Realist Review**
> O'Halloran and colleagues (2018) undertook a systematic realist review relating to advance-care planning with patients who have end-stage kidney disease. The reviewers sought to identify factors that help or hinder implementation of advance-care planning and to develop a theory on how the intervention may work. A total of 62 papers were included in the review.

It is almost certain that guidance (and debate) on how best to conduct mixed studies reviews will continue in the years ahead.

CRITICAL APPRAISAL OF SYSTEMATIC REVIEWS

Systematic reviews should be appraised before the findings are deemed trustworthy and relevant. Box 30.1, available in the Toolkit, offers some guidelines for evaluating systematic reviews. Although these guidelines are broad, not all questions apply equally well to all types of systematic review, and the questions are not comprehensive. Supplementary questions are likely to be needed for some reviews— for example, for mixed studies reviews.

Several tools have been developed to assess systematic reviews. One rigorously developed tool is called Assessment of Multiple Systematic Reviews (AMSTAR) (Shea et al., 2007). Although AMSTAR has been revised (AMSTAR 2), there continue to be debates about some limitations, and further study into its reliability and usability is underway (Gates et al., 2018). The PRISMA guidelines are an additional resource for assessing whether a review included sufficient information.

BOX 30.1 Guidelines for Critically Appraising Systematic Reviews

The Problem
- Did the report clearly state the research problem and/or research questions? Is the scope of the project appropriate?
- Is the topic of the review important for nursing?
- Were concepts, variables, or phenomena adequately defined?

Search Strategy
- Did the report clearly describe criteria for selecting primary studies, and are those criteria reasonable?
- Were the databases used by the reviewers identified, and are they appropriate and comprehensive? Were search terms identified, and are they exhaustive?
- Did the reviewers use adequate supplementary efforts to identify relevant studies?
- Was a PRISMA-type flow chart included to summarize the search results?

The Sample
- Were inclusion and exclusion criteria clearly articulated, and were they defensible?
- Did the search strategy yield a strong and comprehensive sample of studies? Were strengths and limitations of the sample identified?
- If an original report was lacking key information, did reviewers attempt to contact the original researchers for additional information—or did the study have to be excluded?
- If studies were excluded for reasons other than insufficient information, did the reviewers provide a rationale for the decision?

Quality Appraisal
- Did the reviewers appraise the quality of the primary studies? Did they use a defensible and well-defined set of criteria or a respected quality appraisal scale?
- Did two or more people do the appraisals and was interrater agreement reported?
- Was the appraisal information used in a well-defined and defensible manner in the selection of studies or in the analysis of results?

Data Extraction
- Was adequate information extracted about methodologic and administrative aspects of the study, sample characteristics, and study findings?
- Were steps taken to enhance the integrity of the dataset (e.g., were two or more people used to extract and record information for analysis)?

(Continued)

BOX 30.1 Guidelines for Critically Appraising Systematic Reviews (Continued)

Data Analysis—General
- Did the reviewers explain their method of pooling, integrating, and synthesizing the data?
- Was the analysis of data thorough and credible?
- Were tables, figures, and text used effectively to summarize findings?
- Did the reviewers use GRADE or another approach to evaluate confidence in the review findings?

Data Analysis—Quantitative
- If a meta-analysis was not performed, was there adequate justification for using a narrative integration method? If a meta-analysis *was* performed, was this justifiable?
- •For meta-analyses, were appropriate procedures followed for computing effect size estimates for relevant outcomes?
- Was heterogeneity of effects adequately dealt with? Was the decision to use a random effects model or a fixed effects model sound?
- Were appropriate subgroup analyses undertaken—or was the absence of subgroup analyses justified?
- Was the issue of publication bias adequately addressed?

Data Analysis—Qualitative
- Was the analytic approach mainly aggregative or interpretive?
- In a metasynthesis, did the reviewers describe the techniques they used to compare the findings of each study, and did they explain their method of interpreting their data?
- If a metasummary was undertaken, did the abstracted findings seem appropriate and convincing? Were appropriate methods used to compute effect sizes? Was information presented effectively?
- In a metasynthesis, did the synthesis achieve a fuller understanding of the phenomenon to advance knowledge? Do the interpretations seem well-grounded? Was there a sufficient amount of data included to support the interpretations?
- In a meta-aggregation, does the integration of findings into categories and categories into synthesized findings appear insightful and justifiable?

Conclusions
- Did the reviewers draw reasonable conclusions about the quality, quantity, and consistency of evidence relating to the research question?
- Were limitations of the review/synthesis noted?
- Were implications for nursing practice and further research clearly stated?

	All systematic reviews/research syntheses
	Systematic reviews of quantitative studies
	Metasyntheses/qualitative evidence syntheses

In drawing conclusions about a research synthesis, a major issue concerns the nature of the decisions the reviewers made. Sampling decisions, approaches to handling quality of the primary studies, and analytic methods should be carefully evaluated. Another aspect, however, is envisioning how you might use the evidence in clinical practice.

RESEARCH EXAMPLES

We conclude this chapter with a description of two systematic reviews. Two reviews (a meta-analysis and a meta-ethnography) appear in their entirety in the accompanying *Resource Manual*.

Example 1: Systematic Review and Meta-Analysis

Study: The effects of care bundles on patient outcomes: A systematic review and meta-analysis (Lavallée et al., 2017).

Purpose: The purpose of the review was to examine the effects of care bundles on patient outcomes, as well as the healthcare workers' behavior vis-à-vis implementation. A protocol for the review was registered in PROSPERO.

Eligibility Criteria: A study was considered eligible for the meta-analysis if it met the following criteria: Design: the study was either an RCT or quasi-experiment; Participants: the sample included patients of any age, in any setting, and with any condition; Intervention: any type of care bundle; Outcomes: adverse patient outcomes (mortality, infections) and providers' adherence to a care bundle. The reports were limited to those written in English, published between 2001 and 2017.

Search Strategy: A search was undertaken in 9 databases, one of which was a database of the grey literature (OpenGrey). An appendix file listed all search terms for each database. Two reviewers independently screened titles and abstracts.

Quality Assessment: Two reviewers assessed the included studies for risk of bias using the Cochrane risk-of-bias tool. Interrater reliability for the ratings was adequate. The reviewers had planned to perform a sensitivity analysis comparing effects for studies with and without high risk of bias, but few studies were rated as being at low risk of bias.

Sample and Data Extraction: The search generated 5,796 records. After removing duplicates and performing an initial screening, 503 full-text articles were reviewed for eligibility. A total of 37 studies were included in a narrative analysis, but only 34 studies were included in the meta-analysis because of data insufficiencies. Three reviewers independently extracted data on study design, patient population, health care setting, intervention content, outcomes, and duration of follow-up.

Statistical Analysis and Findings: The relative risk index (RR) was used as the effect size index for negative patient outcomes. There was considerable variation in the effect of care bundles on patient outcomes across the studies, ranging from an RR of 0.08 (small benefit of the care bundle) to 1.88 (care bundle associated with increased risk). Because of strong heterogeneity ($I^2 = 86\%$), the data were not pooled into one analysis. Rather, subgroup analysis using a random effects model was used to explore whether certain intervention aspects or methodologic features influenced the effects. For example, a significant benefit was not observed for patients in studies with randomized designs (RR = 0.97, 95% CI = 0.71 to 1.34), but was observed for controlled before–after studies (RR = 0.66, 95% CI = 0.59 to 0.75). The reviewers generally found fidelity to the care bundles to be adequate.

GRADE assessment: Using GRADE, the reviewers rated the evidence as a whole to be of low quality, with downgrades arising for risk of bias, inconsistency, and indirectness. The low-quality evidence from before–after studies did suggest that care bundles may reduce the risk of negative patient outcomes compared with usual care, but better-quality evidence from 6 RCTs yielded less certainty about beneficial effects.

Example 2: A Meta-Ethnography

Study: "Trapped in an empty waiting room"—the existential human core of loneliness in old age: A meta-synthesis (Kitzmüller et al., 2018).

Purpose: The purpose of the meta-ethnography was to synthesize qualitative studies on older adults' subjective experiences of loneliness.

Eligibility Criteria: A study was included if it used a qualitative (or mixed methods) approach, was published in a scientific journal, and dealt with the phenomenon of loneliness from the perspective of older adults, defined as persons older than age 60. Studies were excluded if the participants suffered a mental illness or were in a palliative situation. Articles published in English, Finnish, or German between 2001 and 2016 were included.

Search Strategy: A systematic search strategy was developed during a preliminary pilot period. A search of seven electronic databases was undertaken (e.g., CINAHL, MEDLINE, EMBASE, PsycInfo). An ancestry search was conducted, using the reference lists of eligible studies. Manual searches in well-known journals with content relevant to the care of older adults were also undertaken.

Quality Appraisal: The researchers used a 32-item checklist to appraise the retrieved studies. Two studies that scored less than 25 on the checklist were excluded from the synthesis.

Sample: A total of 11 studies met the eligibility criteria. Study participants were 290 older adults ranging in age from 62 to 103. A majority were widowed. Five studies were phenomenologic, two were hermeneutic, and the others were descriptive.

Data Analysis: The synthesis was based on Noblit and Hare's approach. The researchers read the selected articles independently and in pairs, and then extracted metaphors and concepts from each. The relationships between the studies' concepts were found to be analogous, with the possibility of further analysis as reciprocal. The studies were then translated into one another by developing themes. The analysis was characterized as an iterative process in which the reviewers moved back and forth, comparing and contrasting findings in the studies.

Key Findings: The translation process illuminated four main themes, which were interpreted as the existential core of loneliness in old age, expressed by the metaphor "trapped in an empty waiting room." The four themes were: (1) A wall of sadness in an anxious space of being—negative emotions of loneliness; (2) "Give me back my past"—the loss of meaningful interpersonal relationships; (3) Feeling useless, unconnected, and unable to keep up—loneliness and the perception of self; and (4) Struggling to maintain the energy to endure—ways of dealing with loneliness.

Discussion: The reviewers concluded that the collaboration of health care providers, volunteers, and family members is needed to break the vicious circle of loneliness in older adults.

SUMMARY POINTS

- Evidence-based practice relies on rigorous integration of research evidence on a topic through systematic reviews. A **systematic review** methodically and transparently integrates findings from multiple **primary studies** about a specific research question using careful procedures that are spelled out in advance in a **protocol**.

- Systematic reviews are undertaken to synthesize quantitative findings, qualitative findings, or mixed findings. Reviews of quantitative studies often involve statistical integration of findings through **meta-analysis**, a procedure whose advantages include objectivity, enhanced power, and precision; meta-analysis is not appropriate, however, for broad questions or when there is substantial inconsistency of findings.

- In the rapidly evolving field of evidence synthesis, new types of review have emerged. **Scoping reviews** are preliminary efforts to map the literature on a topic and assess the possibility of a systematic review. **Rapid reviews** are less rigorous than systematic reviews but are intended to yield timely information. **Umbrella reviews** are systematic reviews of multiple systematic reviews. **Network meta-analyses** are reviews in which multiple interventions are compared using both direct and indirect comparisons.

- Major steps in a systematic review typically involve the following: formulating the question, defining eligibility criteria, preparing a protocol, searching for and selecting primary studies, evaluating study quality, extracting data, analyzing the data, interpreting the findings and evaluating confidence in them, and reporting the findings. To minimize the risk of duplication, a systematic review protocol can be registered in a database called **PROSPERO**.

- In most cases, reviewers undertake a comprehensive search, using a wide range of methods, including a search in multiple bibliographic databases, **handsearching** in key journals, *snowballing,* and searching in trial registries.

- Reviewers are increasingly likely to search for **grey literature**—i.e., unpublished reports—out of concern for **publication bias** (a form of **dissemination bias**) that results in the underrepresentation of nonsignificant findings in published literature.

- There are many approaches to appraising the quality of evidence of primary studies, including the use of various scales and checklists. In the Cochrane approach, each study is rated on separate **risk-of-bias** domains.

- In a meta-analysis, findings from primary studies are represented by an **effect size** index that quantifies the magnitude and direction of relationship between variables (e.g., an intervention and its outcomes). Common effect size indexes include d (the **standardized mean difference** or SMD), the odds ratio (OR), relative risk index (RR), and Pearson's r.
- Effects from individual studies are pooled to yield an estimate of the population effect size by calculating a **weighted average** of effects, often using the **inverse variance** as the weight—which gives greater weight to larger studies.
- **Statistical heterogeneity** (diversity in effects across studies) affects decisions about using a **fixed effects model** (which assumes a single true effect size) or a **random effects model** (which assumes a distribution of effects). Heterogeneity can be examined using a **forest plot** and tested statistically—most often using a chi square test or the I^2 **test**.
- Nonrandom heterogeneity (moderating effects) can be explored through **subgroup analyses** or **meta-regression**, in which the purpose is to identify clinical or methodologic features systematically related to variation in effects.
- Quality assessments are sometimes used to exclude weak studies from reviews, but they can also be used to differentially weight studies or in **sensitivity analyses** to test whether including or excluding weaker studies changes conclusions.
- Systematic reviewers are increasingly likely to use the **GRADE** (Grading of Recommendations, Assessment, Development, and Evaluation) approach to rate the degree of *confidence* that the review team has in the estimated effect, for outcomes in a review.
- Qualitative systematic reviews have been described as either **aggregative** (in which findings from multiple studies are pooled) or **interpretive** (in which the goal is to discover new ways of understanding phenomena). Aggregative reviews are often called **qualitative evidence syntheses**; the umbrella term most often used in nursing for interpretive reviews is **metasynthesis**. Most qualitative reviews in nursing have elements of both aggregation and interpretation.
- Metasynthesis methods often used by nurse researchers include meta-ethnography, meta-study, and metasummary.
- Metasynthesists do not necessarily start with a predetermined question—questions often emerge during the process of discovery. Metasynthesists may not undertake an exhaustive review—the sampling of studies may be purposive.
- One approach to qualitative integration, **meta-ethnography** as proposed by Noblit and Hare, involves listing key themes or metaphors across studies and then reciprocally translating them into each other. Key metaphors can be translated in one of three ways: *reciprocal, refutational,* or *lines-of-argument.*
- Paterson and colleagues' **metastudy** method integrates three components: (1) **metadata analysis,** the study of results in a specific substantive area through analysis of the "processed data"; (2) **metamethod,** the study of the studies' methodologic rigor; and (3) **metatheory,** the analysis of the theoretical underpinnings on which the studies are grounded.
- Sandelowski and Barroso distinguish qualitative findings in terms of whether they are *summaries* (descriptive synopses) or *syntheses* (interpretive explanations of the data). Both summaries and syntheses can be used in a **metasummary**, which can lay the foundation for a metasynthesis.
- A metasummary involves developing a list of abstracted findings from the primary studies and calculating **manifest effect sizes. A frequency effect size** is the percentage of studies in a sample of studies that contain a given finding. An **intensity effect size** indicates the percentage of all findings that are contained within any given report.
- In the Sandelowski and Barroso approach, only studies described as *syntheses* can be used in a metasynthesis, which can use a variety of approaches to analysis and interpretation (e.g., constant comparison).
- The approach to qualitative evidence synthesis used at the Joanna Briggs Institute (JBI) is **meta-aggregation**, which is more structured than a metasynthesis and relies on comprehensive searching and systematic quality appraisals. In a meta-aggregation, similar findings across

studies are grouped into *categories,* which in turn are grouped into *synthesized findings.* In JBI qualitative reviews, confidence in the findings is assessed using a rating system called **ConQual.** Another similar system, inspired by GRADE, is called **GRADE-CerQual.**

- **Systematic mixed studies reviews (MSRs)** are systematic reviews that use disciplined procedures to integrate and synthesize findings from qualitative, quantitative, and mixed methods studies.

- Designs for MSRs are either concurrent/convergent (qualitative and quantitative syntheses undertaken concurrently) or sequential. Sandelowski proposed three designs: *segregated* (two separate syntheses followed by integration); *integrated* (when qualitative and quantitative findings are viewed as answering the same question); or *contingent* (a coordinated, sequential series of syntheses). JBI MSRs use a segregated design, while Cochrane MSRs use a sequential design.

- Many approaches have been suggested for analyzing and synthesizing data in an MSR, including content analysis, narrative summary, critical interpretive synthesis, and *Bayesian synthesis.*

- A special type of MSR is called a **realist synthesis,** the goal of which is to understand theory-driven *Context-Mechanism-Outcome* (CMO) configurations. Realist syntheses are often used in reviews of complex interventions.

- **PRISMA** (Preferred Reporting Items for Systematic reviews and Meta-Analyses) is a useful reporting guideline for writing up a systematic review of RCTs; another called **MOOSE** (Meta-analysis of Observational Studies in Epidemiology) is for meta-analyses of observational studies. **ENTREQ** is a reporting guideline for qualitative systematic reviews.

- Most systematic reviews include a flow chart (showing search efforts and results), forest plots (for meta-analyses), and a **summary of findings** (SoF) table.

STUDY ACTIVITIES

Study activities are available to instructors on thePoint.

REFERENCES CITED IN CHAPTER 30

Aagard, H., Hall, E., Ludvigsen, M., Uhrenfeldt, L., & Fegran, L. (2018). Parents' experiences of neonatal transfer: A meta-study of qualitative research 2000-2017. *Nursing Inquiry, 25,* e12231.

*Agency for Healthcare Research and Quality. (2014). *Methods guide for effectiveness and comparative effectiveness reviews.* Washington, DC: AHRQ.

*Aghajafari, F., Letourneay, N., Mahinpey, N., Cosic, N., & Giesbrecht, G. (2018). Vitamin D deficiency and antenatal and postpartum depression: A systematic review. *Nutrients, 10,* 478.

*Agoritsas, T., Merglen, A., Courvoisier, D., Combescure, C., Garin, N., Perrier, A., & Perneger, T. (2012). Sensitivity and predictive value of 15 PubMed search strategies to answer clinical questions rated against full systematic reviews. *Journal of Medical Internet Research, 14,* e85.

Arksey, H., & O'Malley, L. (2005). Scoping studies: Toward a methodologic framework. *International Journal of Social Research Methodology, 8,* 19–32.

Aromataris, E., Fernandez, R., Godfrey, C., Holly, C., Khalil, H., & Tungpunkom, P. (2015). Summarizing systematic reviews: Methodological development, conduct, and reporting of an umbrella review approach. *International Journal of Evidence-Based Healthcare, 13,* 132–140.

Aromataris, E., & Munn, Z. (Eds.). (2017). *Joanna Briggs Institute Reviewer's Manual.* Adelaide, Australia: JBI. Retrieved from https://reviewersmanual.joannabriggs.org/.

Aromataris, E., & Riitano, D. (2014). Constructing a search strategy and searching for evidence: A guide to the literature search for a systematic review. *American Journal of Nursing, 114*(5), 49–56.

*Atkins, S., Lewin, S., Smith, H., Engel, M., Fretheim, A., & Volminck, J. (2008). Conducting a meta-ethnography of qualitative literature: Lessons learned. *BMC Medical Research Methodology, 8,* 21.

Beck, C. T., & Woynar, J. (2017). Posttraumatic stress in mothers while their preterm infants are in the newborn intensive care unit: A mixed research synthesis. *Advances in Nursing Science, 40,* 337–355.

*Beller, E., Clark, J., Tsafnat, G., Adams, C., Diehl, H., Lund, H., … Glasziou, P. (2018). Making progress with the automation of systematic reviews. *Systematic Reviews, 7,* 77.

*Bilandzic, A., Fitzpatrick, T., Rosella, L., & Henry, D. (2016). Risk of bias in systematic reviews of non-randomized studies of adverse cardiovascular effects of thiazolidinediones and Cyclooxygenase-2 inhibitors: Application of a new Cochrane risk of bias tool. *PLoS Medicine, 13,* e1001987.

*Booth, A. (2016). Searching for qualitative research for inclusion in systematic reviews: A structured methodological review. *Systematic Reviews, 5,* 74.

*Booth, A., Noyes, J., Flemming, K., Gerhardus, A., Wahlster, P., van der Wilt, G., … Rehfuss, E. (2016). *Guidance on choosing qualitative evidence synthesis methods for use in health technology assessments of complex interventions.* Retrieved from http://www.integrate-hta.eu/downloads/.

Booth, A., Noyes, J., Flemming, K., Gerhardus, A., Wahlster, P., van der Wilt, G., … Rehfuss, E. (2018). Structured methodology review identified seven (RETREAT) criteria for selecting qualitative evidence synthesis approaches. *Journal of Clinical Epidemiology, 99*, 41–52.

*Bramer, W., Rethlefsen, M., Kleijnen, J., & Franco, O. (2017). Optimal database combination for literature searches in systematic reviews: A prospective exploratory study. *Systematic Reviews, 6*, 245.

Brunetti, M., Shemilt, I., Pregno, S., Vale, L., Oxman, A., Lord, J., … Schünemann, H. (2013). GRADE guidelines: 10. Considering resource use and rating the quality of economic evidence. *Journal of Clinical Epidemiology, 66*, 140–150.

*Campbell, R., Pound, P., Morgan, M., Daker-White, G., Britten, M., Pill, R., … Donovan, J. (2011). Evaluating meta-ethnography: Systematic analysis and synthesis of qualitative research. *Health Technology Assessment, 15*, 1–164.

*Capezuti, E., Sagha-Zadeh, R, Pain, K., Basara, A., Jiang, N., & Krieger, A. (2018). A systematic review of non-pharmacological interventions to improve nighttime sleep among residents of long-term care settings. *BMC Geriatrics, 18*, 143.

Carroll, D., Malecki-Ketchell, A., & Astin, F. (2017). Non-pharmacological interventions to reduce psychological distress in patients undergoing diagnostic cardiac catheterization: A rapid review. *European Journal of Cardiovascular Research, 16*, 92–103.

Chaboyer, W., Thalib, L., Harbeck, E., Coyer, F., Blot, S., Bull, C., … Lin, F. (2018). Incidence and prevalence of pressure injuries in adult intensive care patients: A systematic review and meta-analysis. *Critical Care Medicine, 46*, e1074–e1081.

Conn, V., Valentine, J., Cooper, H., & Rantz, M. (2003). Grey literature in meta-analyses. *Nursing Research, 52*, 256–261.

Cooper, H. (2017). *Research synthesis and meta-analysis: A step-by-step approach.* (5th ed.). Thousand Oaks, CA: Sage Publications.

Critical Appraisal Skills Programme. (2016). *CASP qualitative research checklist.* Retrieved from http://www.cask-uk.net/casp-tools-checklists.

*Daudt, H., van Mossel, C., & Scott, S. (2013). Enhancing the scoping study methodology: A large, inter-professional team's experience with Arksey and O'Malley's framework. *BMC Medical Research Methodology, 13*, 48.

Davis, K., Drey, N., & Gould, D. (2009). What are scoping studies? A review of the nursing literature. *International Journal of Nursing Studies, 46*, 1386–1400.

DeJean, D., Giacomini, M., Simeonov, D., & Smith, A. (2016). Finding qualitative research evidence for health technology assessment. *Qualitative Health Research, 26*, 1307–1317.

Denk, K., Lennon, S., Gordon, S., & Jaarsma, R. (2018). The association between decreased grip strength and hip fracture in older people: A systematic review. *Experimental Gerontology, 111*, 1–9.

*Dixon-Woods, M., Cavers, D., Agarwal, S., Annandale, E., Arthur, A., Harvey, J., … Sutton, A. (2006). Conducting a critical interpretive synthesis of the literature on access to healthcare by vulnerable groups. *BMC Medical Research Methodology, 6*, 35.

*Dwan, K., Gamble, X., Williamson, P., & Kirkham, J. (2013). Systematic review of the empirical evidence of study publication bias and outcome reporting bias: An updated review. *PLoS One, 8*, e66844.

Eaves, Y. D. (2001). A synthesis technique for grounded theory data analysis. *Journal of Advanced Nursing, 35*, 654–663.

Elamin, M., Flynn, D., Bassler, D., Briel, M., Alonso-Coello, P., Karanicolas, P., … Montori, V. (2009). Choice of data extraction tools for systematic reviews depends on resources and review complexity. *Journal of Clinical Epidemiology, 62*, 506–510.

Elliott, J., Synnot, A., Turner, T., Simmonds, M., Akl, E., McDonald, S., … Thomas, J. (2017). Living systematic review: 1. Introduction—the why, what, when, and how. *Journal of Clinical Epidemiology, 91*, 23–30.

*Elliott, J., Turner, T., Clavisi, O., Thomas, J., Higgins, J., Mavergames, C., & Gruen, R. (2014). Living systematic reviews: An emerging opportunity to narrow the evidence-practice gap. *PLoS Medicine, 11*, e1001603.

Emmel, N., Greenhalgh, J., Manzano, A., Monaghan, M., & Dalkin, S. (Eds.). (2019). *Doing realist research.* Thousand Oaks, CA: Sage Publications.

Finfgeld, D. (2003). Metasynthesis: The state of the art—So far. *Qualitative Health Research, 13*, 893–904.

Flemming, K. (2010). Synthesis of quantitative and qualitative research: An example using Critical Interpretive Synthesis. *Journal of Advanced Nursing, 66*, 201–217.

*Fogarty, S., Elmir, R., Hay, P., & Schmied, V. (2018). The experience of women with an eating disorder in the perinatal period: A meta-ethnographic study. *BMC Pregnancy & Childbirth, 18*, 121.

*France, E., Cunningham, M., Ring, N., Uny, I., Duncan, E., Jepson, R., … Noyes, J. (2019). Improving reporting of meta-ethnography: The eMERGe reporting guidance. *Journal of Advanced Nursing, 75*, 1126–1139.

*Garritty, C., Stevens, A., Gartlehner, G., King, V., & Kamel, C. (2016). Cochrane Rapid Review Methods Group to play a leading role in guiding the production of informed high-quality, timely research evidence syntheses. *Systematic Reviews, 5*, 184.

*Gates, A., Gates, M., Duarte, G., Cary, M., Becker, M., Prediger, B., … Hartling, L. (2018). Evaluation of the reliability, usability, and applicability of AMSTAR, AMSTAR 2, and ROBIS: Protocol for a descriptive analytic study. *Systematic Reviews, 7*, 85.

*Gough, D., Thomas, J., & Oliver, S. (2012). Clarifying differences between review designs and methods. *Systematic Reviews, 1*, 28.

*Greenhalgh, T., Thorne, S., & Malterud, K. (2018). Time to challenge the spurious hierarchy of systematic over narrative reviews? *European Journal of Clinical Investigation, 48*, e12931.

*Guyatt, G. H., Oxman, A., Akl, E., Kunz, R., Vist, G., Brozek, J., … Schunemann, H. (2011). GRADE guidelines: 1. Introduction—GRADE evidence profiles and summary of findings tables. *Journal of Clinical Epidemiology, 64*, 383–394.

*Guyatt, G., Oxman, , Vist, G., Kunz, R., Falck-Ytter, Y., Alonso-Coello, P, & Schünemann, H. (2008). GRADE: An emerging consensus on rating quality of evidence and strength of recommendations. *BMJ, 336*, 924–926.

Hannes, K., & Lockwood, C. (2011). Pragmatism as the philosophical foundation for the Joanna Briggs meta-aggregative approach to qualitative evidence synthesis. *Journal of Advanced Nursing, 67*, 1632–1642.

Hannes, K., & Lockwood, C. (2012). *Synthesizing qualitative research: Choosing the right approach*. Chichester, UK: Wiley-Blackwell.

Harden, A., & Thomas, J. (2005). Methodologic issues in combining diverse study types in systematic reviews. *International Journal of Social Research Methodology, 8*, 257–271.

Harden, A., Thomas, J., Cargo, M., Harris, J., Pantoja, T., Flemming, K., … Noyes, J. (2018). Cochrane Qualitative and Implementation Methods Group guidance series—paper 5: Methods for integrating qualitative and implementation evidence within intervention effectiveness reviews. *Journal of Clinical Epidemiology, 97*, 70–78.

Heyvaert, M., Hannes, K., & Onghena, P. (2017). *Using mixed methods research synthesis for literature reviews*. Thousand Oaks, CA: Sage Publications.

Heyvaert, M., Maes, B., & Onghena, P. (2013). Mixed methods research synthesis: Definition, framework, and potential. *Quality and Quantity, 47*, 659–676.

*Higgins, J. P. T., & Green, S. (Eds.). (2011). *Cochrane handbook for systematic reviews of interventions (version 5.1.0)*. The Cochrane Collaboration. Retrieved from http://training. cochrane.org/handbook.

Higgins, J. P. T., & Thomas, J. (Eds.). (2020). *Cochrane handbook for systematic reviews of interventions (version 6)*. Hoboken, NJ: Wiley Blackwell.

*Ho, G., Liew, S., Ng, C., Shunmugam, R., Glasziou, P. (2016). Development of a search strategy for an evidence-based retrieval service. *PLoS One, 11*, e0167170.

*Hong, Q., Pluye, P., Bujold, M., & Wassef, M. (2017). Convergent and sequential synthesis designs: Implications for conducting and reporting systematic reviews of qualitative and quantitative evidence. *Systematic Reviews, 6*, 61.

*Hunt, H., Pollock, A., Campbell, P., Estcourt, L., & Brunton, G. (2018). An introduction to overviews of reviews: Planning a relevant research question and objective for an overview. *Systematic Reviews, 7*, 39.

*Hutchinson, A., Nagle, C., Kent, B., Bick, D., & Lindberg, R. (2018). Organisational interventions designed to reduce caesarean section rates: A systematic review protocol. *BMJ Open, 8*, e021120.

*Institute of Medicine. (2011). *Finding what works in health care: Standards for systematic reviews*. Washington, DC: The National Academies Press.

Ioannidis, J. (2017). Next-generation systematic reviews: Prospective meta-analysis, individual-level data, network and umbrella reviews. *British Journal of Sports Medicine, 51*, 1456–1458.

Iorio, A., Spencer, F., Falavigna, M., Alba, C., Lang, E., Burnard, B., … Guyatt, G. (2015). Use of GRADE for assessment of evidence about prognosis. *BMJ, 350*, h870.

Jadad, A. R., Moore, R., Carroll, D., Jenkinson, C., Reynolds, D., Gavaghan, D., & McQuay, H. (1996). Assessing the quality of reports of randomized controlled trials. *Controlled Clinical Trials, 17*, 1–12.

Jadczak, A., Makwana, N., Luscombe-Marsh, N., Visvanathan, R., & Schultz, T. (2018). Effectiveness of exercise interventions on physical function in community-dwelling frail older people: An umbrella review of systematic reviews. *JBI Database of Systematic Reviews and Implementation Reports, 16*, 752–775.

*Joanna Briggs Institute. (2015). *The Joanna Briggs Institute Reviewers' Manual 2015: Methodology for JBI scoping reviews*. Adelaide, Australia: JBI.

*Jüni, P., Altman, D., & Egger, M. (2001). Systematic reviews in health care: Assessing the quality of controlled clinical trials. *BMJ, 323*(7303), 42–46.

Khalil, H., Peters, M., Godfrey, C., McInerney, P., Soares, C., & Parker, P. (2016). An evidence-based approach to scoping reviews. *Worldviews on Evidence-Based Nursing, 13*, 118–123.

*Khangura, S., Konnyu, K., Cushman, R., Grimshaw, J., & Moher, D. (2012). Evidence summaries: The evolution of a rapid review approach. *Systematic Reviews, 1*, 10.

Kitzmüller, G., Clancy, A., Vaismoradi, M., Wegener, C., & Bondas, T. (2018). "Trapped in an empty waiting room"—the existential human core of loneliness in old age: A meta-synthesis. *Qualitative Health Research, 28*, 213–230.

*Lavallée, J., Gray, T., Dumville, J., Russell, W., & Cullum, N. (2017). The effects of care bundles on patient outcomes: A systematic review and meta-analysis. *Implementation Science, 12*, 142.

*Lewin, S., Booth, A., Glenton, C., Munthe-Kaas, H., Rashidian, A., Wainwright, M., … Noyes, J. (2018). Applying GRADE-CERQual to qualitative evidence synthesis findings: Introduction to the series. *Implementation Science, 13*(Suppl. 1).

*Liberati, A., Altman, D., Tetzlaff, J., Mulrow, C., Gotzsche, P., Ioannidis, J., … Moher, D. (2009). The PRISMA statement for reporting systematic reviews and meta-analyses of studies that evaluate health care interventions: Explanation and elaboration. *Journal of Clinical Epidemiology, 62*, e1–e34.

*Lim, G., Tam, W., Lu, XY., Ho, C., Zhang, M., & Ho, R. (2018). Prevalence of depression in the community from 30 countries between 1994 and 2014. *Scientific Reports, 8*, 2861.

*Lucas, P., Baird, J., Arai, L., Law, C., & Roberts, H. (2007). Worked examples of alternative methods for the synthesis of qualitative and quantitative research in systematic reviews. *BMC Medical Research Methodology, 7*, 4.

Ludvigsen, M., Hall, E., Meyer, G., Fegran, L., Aagard, H., & Uhrenfeldt, L. (2016). Using Sandelowski and Barroso's meta-synthesis method in advancing qualitative evidence. *Qualitative Health Research, 26*, 320–329.

Majid, U., & Vanstone, M. (2018). Appraising qualitative research for evidence syntheses: A compendium of quality appraisal tools. *Qualitative Health Research, 28*, 2115–2131.

*Mathes, T., Klassen, P., & Pieper, D. (2017). Frequency of data extraction errors and methods to increase data extraction quality. *BMC Medical Research Methodology, 17*, 152.

McCormick, J., Rodney, P., & Varcoe, C. (2003). Reinterpretations across studies: An approach to meta-analysis. *Qualitative Health Research, 13*, 933–944.

Milazi, M., Bonner, A., & Douglas, C. (2017). Effectiveness of educational or behavioral interventions on adherence to phosphate control in adults receiving hemodialysis: A systematic review. *JBI Database of Systematic Reviews and Implementation Reports, 15*(4), 971–1010.

Munn, Z., Lockwood, C., & Moola, S. (2015). The development and use of evidence summaries for point of care information systems: A streamlined rapid review approach. *Worldviews on Evidence-Based Nursing, 12*, 131–138.

*Munn, Z., Porritt, K., Aromataris, E., & Parson, A. (2014b). Establishing confidence in the output of qualitative research synthesis: The ConQual approach. *BMC Medical Research Methodology, 14*, 108.

*Munn, Z., Stern, C., Aromataris, E., Lockwood, C., & Jordan, Z. (2018). What kind of systematic review should I conduct? A proposed typology and guidance for systematic reviewers in the medical and health sciences. *BMC Medical Research Methodology, 18*, 5.

Munn, Z., Tufanaru, C., & Aromataris, E. (2014a). JBI's systematic reviews: Data extraction and synthesis. *American Journal of Nursing, 114*(7), 49–54.

Noblit, G., & Hare, R. D. (1988). *Meta-ethnography: Synthesizing qualitative studies*. Newbury Park, CA: Sage Publications.

Norman, G., Westby, M., Rithalia, A., Stubbs, N., Soares, M., & Dumville, J. (2018). Dressings and topical agents for treating venous leg ulcers. *Cochrane Database of Systematic Reviews, 6*, CD012583.

Noyes, J., Booth, A., Cargo, M., Flemming, K., Garside, R., Hannes, K., ... Thomas, J. (2018). Cochrane Qualitative and Implementation Methods Group guidance series—Paper 1: Introduction. *Journal of Clinical Epidemiology, 97*, 35–38.

Nybakken, S., Strandås, M., & Bondas, T. (2018). Caregivers' perceptions of aggressive behaviour in nursing home residents living with dementia: A meta-ethnography. *Journal of Advanced Nursing, 74*, 2713–2726.

*Ogilvie, D., Fayter, D., Petticrew, M., Sowden, A., Thomas, S., Whitehead, M., & Worthy, G. (2008). The harvest plot: A method for synthesizing evidence about differential effects of interventions. *BMC Medical Research Methodology, 8*, 8.

*O'Halloran, P., Noble, H., Norwood, K., Maxwell, P., Shields, J., Fogarty, D., ... Brazil, K. (2018). Advance care planning with patients who have end-stage kidney disease: A systematic realist review. *Journal of Pain and Symptom Management, 56*, 795–807.

Pace, R., Pluye, P., Bartlett, G., Macauley, A., Salsberg, J., Jagosh, J., & Seller, R. (2012). Testing the reliability and efficiency of the pilot Mixed Methods Appraisal Tool (MMAT) for systematic mixed studies review. *International Journal of Nursing Studies, 49*, 47–53.

*Page, M., Shamseer, L., Altman, D., Tetzlaff, J., Sampson, M., Tricco, A., ... Moher, D. (2016). Epidemiology and reporting characteristics of systematic reviews of biomedical research. *PLoS Medicine, 13*(5), e1002028.

*Page, M., Shamseer, L., & Tricco, A. (2018). Registration of systematic reviews in PROSPERO: 30,000 records and counting. *Systematic Reviews, 7*, 32.

*Palacios, J., Lee, G., Duaso, M., Clifton, A., Norman, I., Richards, D., & Barley, E. (2017). Internet-delivered self-management support for improving coronary heart disease and self-management-related outcomes: A systematic review. *Journal of Cardiovascular Nursing, 32*, E9–E23.

Parsons, K., Gaudine, A., & Swab, M. (2018). Older nurses' experiences of providing direct care in hospital nursing units: A qualitative systematic review. *JBI Database of Systematic Reviews and Implementation Reports, 16*, 669–700.

Paterson, B. (2013). Metasynthesis. In Beck, C. T. (Ed.). *Routledge international handbook of qualitative nursing research* (pp. 331–346). New York: Routledge.

Paterson, B. L., Thorne, S. E., Canam, C., & Jillings, C. (2001). *Meta-study of qualitative health research*. Thousand Oaks, CA: Sage Publications.

Pawson, R. (2013). *The science of evaluation: A realist manifesto*. Thousand Oaks, CA: Sage Publications.

Pearson, A., White, H., Bath-Hextall, F., Apostolo, J., Salmond, S., & Kirkpatrick, P. (2014). *Methodology for JBI mixed methods systematic reviews. The Joanna Briggs Institute Reviewers' Manual 2014, chapter 8*. Adelaide, Australia: JBI.

*Pedder, H., Sarri, G., Keeney, E., Nunes, V., & Dias, S. (2016). Data extraction for complex meta-analysis (DECiMAL) guide. *Systematic Reviews, 5*, 212.

**Pedersen, B., Delmar, C., Lörincz, T., Falkmer, U., & Grønkjaer, M. (2019). Investigating changes in weight and body composition among women in adjuvant treatment for breast cancer: A scoping review. *Cancer Nursing, 42*, 92–105.

Petticrew, M., Anderson, L., Elder, R., Grimshaw, J., Hopkins, D., Hahn, R., ... Welch, V. (2015). Complex interventions and their implications for systematic reviews: A pragmatic approach. *International Journal of Nursing Studies, 52*, 1211–1216.

*Pigott, T., Noyes, J., Umscheid, C., Myers, E., Morton, S., Fu, R., ... Beretvas, S. (2017). AHRQ series on complex intervention systematic reviews-Paper 5: Advanced analytic methods. *Journal of Clinical Epidemiology, 90*, 37–42.

Pluye, P., Gagnon, M., Griffiths, F., & Johnson-Lafleur, J. (2009). A scoring system for appraising mixed methods research, and concomitantly appraising qualitative, quantitative, and mixed methods primary studies in Mixed Studies Reviews. *International Journal of Nursing Studies, 46*, 529–546.

Pluye, P., & Hong, Q.N. (2014). Combining the power of stories and the power of numbers: Mixed methods research and mixed studies reviews. *Annual Review of Public Health, 35*, 29–45.

Pluye, P., Hong, Q.N., Bush, P., & Vedel, I. (2016). Opening up the definition of systematic literature review: The plurality of worldview, methodologies, and methods for reviews and syntheses. *Journal of Clinical Epidemiology, 73*, 2–5.

*Polita, N., Alvarenga, W., Leite, A., Araújo, J., Santos, L., Zago, M., … Nascimento, L. (2018). Care provided by the father to the child with cancer under the influence of masculinities: Qualitative meta-synthesis. *Revista Braseileira de Enfarmagem, 71*, 185–194.

Porritt, K., Gomersall, J., & Lockwood, C. (2014). JBI's systematic reviews: Study selection and critical appraisal. *American Journal of Nursing, 114*(6), 47–52.

Sandelowski, M., & Barroso, J. (2002). Finding the findings in qualitative studies. *Journal of Nursing Scholarship, 34*, 213–219.

Sandelowski, M., & Barroso, J. (2003a). Toward a metasynthesis of qualitative findings on motherhood in HIV-positive women. *Research in Nursing & Health, 26*, 153–170.

Sandelowski, M., & Barroso, J. (2003b). Creating metasummaries of qualitative findings. *Nursing Research, 52*, 226–233.

Sandelowski, M., & Barroso, J. (2007). *Handbook for synthesizing qualitative research*. New York: Springer Publishing Company.

Sandelowski, M., Docherty, S., & Emden, C. (1997). Qualitative metasynthesis: Issues and techniques. *Research in Nursing & Health, 20*, 365–377.

*Sandelowski, M., Voils, C., & Barroso, J. (2006). Defining and designing mixed research synthesis studies. *Research in the Schools, 13*, 29.

Sandelowski, M., Voils, C. I., Crandell, J. L., & Leeman, J. (2013). Synthesizing qualitative and quantitative research findings. In Beck, C. T. (Ed.), *Routledge international handbook of qualitative nursing research* (pp. 347–356). New York: Routledge.

*Schmeid, V., Black, E., Naidoo, N., Dahlen, H., & Liamputtong, P. (2017). Migrant women's experiences, meanings, and ways of dealing with postnatal depression: A meta-ethnographic study. *PLoS One, 12*, e0172385.

Schreiber, R., Crooks, D., & Stern, P. N. (1997). Qualitative meta-analysis. In Morse, J. M. (Ed.), *Completing a qualitative project* (pp. 311–326). Thousand Oaks, CA: Sage Publications.

*Schünemann, H., Oxman, A., Brozek, J., Glasziou, P., Jaeschke, R., Vist, G., … Guyatt, G. (2008). Grading quality of evidence and strength of recommendations for diagnostic tests and strategies. *BMJ, 336*, 1106–1110.

*Shaw, R., Larkin, M., & Flowers, P. (2014). Expanding the evidence within evidence-based healthcare: Thinking about the context, acceptability and feasibility of interventions. *Evidence-Based Medicine, 19*, 201–203.

*Shea, B., Grimshaw, J., Wells, G. Boers, M., Andersson, N., Hamel, C., … Bouter, L. (2007). Development of AMSTAR: A measurement tool to assess the methodological quality of systematic reviews. *BMC Medical Research Methodology, 7*, 10.

*Sherifali, D., Ali, M., Ploeg, J., Markle-Reid, M., Valaitis, R., Bartholomew, A., … McAiney, C. (2018). Impact of internet-based interventions on caregiver mental health: A systematic review and meta-analysis. *Journal of Medical Internet Research, 20*, e10668.

*Son, H., Son, Y., Kim, H., & Lee, Y. (2018). Effect of psychosocial interventions on the quality of life of patients with colorectal cancer: A systematic review and meta-analysis. *Health and Quality of Life Outcomes, 16*, 119.

Stang, A. (2010). Critical evaluation of the Newcastle-Ottawa scale for the assessment of the quality of nonrandomized studies in meta-analysis. *European Journal of Epidemiology, 25*, 603–605.

*Sterne, J., Herman, M., Reeves, B., Savovic, J., Berkman, N., Viswanathan, M., … Higgins, J. (2016). ROBINS-I: A tool for assessing risk of bias in non-randomised studies of interventions. *BMJ, 355*, i4919.

Stern, C., Jordan, Z., & McArthur, A. (2014). JBI's systematic reviews: Developing the review question and inclusion criteria. *The American Journal of Nursing, 114*,(4), 53–56.

Stroup, D., Berlin, J., Morton, S., Olkin, I., Williamson, G., Rennie, D., … Thacker, S. (2000). Meta-analysis of observational studies in epidemiology: A proposal for reporting. Meta-analysis Of Observational Studies in Epidemiology (MOOSE). *Journal of the American Medical Association, 283*, 208–212.

*Thomas, J., & Harden, A. (2008). Methods for the thematic synthesis of qualitative research in systematic reviews. *BMC Medical Research Methodology, 8*, 45.

*Thomas, J., Noel-Storr, A., Marshall, I., Wallace, M. McDonald, S., Mavergames, C., … Elliott, J. (2017). Living systematic reviews: 2. Combining human and machine effort. *Journal of Clinical Epidemiology, 91*, 31–37.

Thorne, S., Jensen, L., Kearney, M., Noblit, G., & Sandelowski, M. (2004). Qualitative metasynthesis: Reflections on methodologic orientation and ideological agenda. *Qualitative Health Research, 14*, 1342–1365.

*Tong, A., Flemming, K., McInnis, E., Oliver, S., & Craig, J. (2012). ENhancing Transparency in REporting the synthesis of Qualitative research. *BMC Medical Research Methodology, 12*, 181.

*Tonin, F., Rotta, I., Mendes, A., & Pontarolo, R. (2017). Network meta-analysis: A technique to gather evidence from direct and indirect comparisons. *Pharmacy Practice, 15*, 943.

*Toye, F., Seers, K., Allcock, N., Briggs, M., Carr, E., & Barker, K. (2014). Meta-ethnography 25 years on: Challenges and insights for synthesizing a large number of qualitative studies. *BMC Medical Research Methodology, 14*, 80.

*Tricco, A., Antony, J., Zarin, W., Strifler, L., Ghassemi, M., Icory, J., … Straus, S. (2015). A scoping review of rapid review methods. *BMC Medicine, 13*, 224.

Tricco, A., Soobiah, C., Antony, J., Cogo, E., MacDonald, H., Lillie, E., … Kastner, M. (2016). A scoping review identifies multiple emerging knowledge synthesis methods, but few studies operationalize the method. *Journal of Clinical Epidemiology, 73*, 19–28.

*Tsafnat, G., Glasziou, P., Karystianis, G., & Coiera, E. (2018). Automated screening of research studies for systematic reviews using study characteristics. *Systematic Reviews, 7*, 64.

Tugwell, P., Knottnerus, J., McGowan, J., & Tricco, A. (2018). Systematic Review Qualitative Methods Series reflect the increasing maturity in qualitative methods. *Journal of Clinical Epidemiology, 97*, vii-viii.

Viswanathan, M., Patnode, C., Berkman, N., Bass, E., Chang, S., Hartling, L., … Kane, R. (2018). Recommendations for assessing risk of bias in systematic reviews of healthcare interventions. *Journal of Clinical Epidemiology, 97*, 26–34.

*Voils, C., Hasselblad, V., Crandell, J., Chang, Y., Lee, E., & Sandelowski, M. (2009). A Bayesian method for the synthesis of evidence from qualitative and quantitative reports: The example of antiretroviral medication adherence. *Journal of Health Services Research & Policy, 14*, 226–233.

*Whitehouse, E., Lai, J., Golub, J., & Farley, J. (2018). A systematic review of the effectiveness of smoking cessation interventions among patients with tuberculosis. *Public Health Action, 8*, 37–49.

Zeng, X., Zhang, Y., Kwong, J., Zhang, C., Li, S., Sun, F., … Du, L. (2015). The methodological quality assessment tools for preclinical and clinical studies, systematic review and meta-analysis, and clinical practice guideline: A systematic review. *Journal of Evidence-Based Medicine, 8*, 2–10.

***A link to this open-access article is provided in the Toolkit for Chapter 30 in the* Resource Manual**. ⊗

****This journal article is available on* thePoint *for this chapter.*

31

Applicability, Generalizability, and Relevance: Toward Practice-Based Evidence

This chapter covers new ground in this edition. It differs from some of the other chapters in that it is not prescriptive—that is, it does not outline the steps that researchers should take to enhance the integrity of their inquiries. Rather, it presents a rationale for why greater attention should be paid to the *applicability* and *relevance* of research evidence in real-world settings and offers several suggestions for accomplishing these goals. This chapter reflects emerging trends in developing and testing targeted, personalized, and precision healthcare initiatives.

> **TIP** Because this chapter covers a lot of new ideas, we have included an extensive reference list with many open-access articles. The Toolkit offers links to other relevant papers that are not cited in this chapter.

EVIDENCE-BASED PRACTICE AND PRACTICE-BASED EVIDENCE

The evidence-based practice (EBP) movement has made significant and enduring contributions to the well-being of human beings. Clinicians no longer rely exclusively on a repository of knowledge acquired during their training—they are expected to be lifelong learners who seek and utilize evidence from rigorous studies about how best to address pressing health problems.

Yet, evidence-based practice has limitations that are not always acknowledged. In particular, concerns are increasingly expressed that EBP fails to provide "evidence to guide decisions in clinical care for individual patients" (Horwitz & Singer, 2017). Several commentators have noted that high-quality patient care requires **practice-based evidence**—evidence that is developed in real-world settings and is responsive to the needs and circumstances of specific patients and contexts (Concato, 2012; Horwitz et al., 2017; Sacristán & Dilla, 2018).

In this section, we briefly point out some limitations of evidence-based practice with respect to the applicability of research findings for clinical decision-making. Many concerns stem from EBP's reliance on randomized controlled trials (RCTs), which are considered the "gold standard" design for understanding intervention effects on health outcomes. An entire issue of the journal *Social Science & Medicine* was devoted to discussions about RCTs (e.g., Deaton & Cartwright, 2018; Horwitz & Singer, 2018), and although commentators acknowledged that RCTs are "clearly indispensable," they noted ways in which they are "often flawed" or "mostly useless" (Ioannidis, 2018, p. 53).

Evidence-Based Practice and Population Models

EBP is based on evidence about *populations* of people, such as a population of preterm infants or a population of obese adolescents. Systematic reviews of randomized controlled trials, at the pinnacle of evidence hierarchies, are the cornerstone of EBP. Yet, systematic reviews of RCTs cannot affirm that *all* patients receiving an effective intervention will benefit from it—only that the "average" patient in a specified population probably would. Clinicians, however, do not treat "average" patients—they care for people with varying and distinctive traits, preferences, and health risks.

Subramanian and colleagues (2018) were especially eloquent about this issue, noting that inferences about **average treatment effects** can be misleading or even harmful when responses to an intervention diverge—a situation that is called **heterogeneity of treatment effects (HTE).** They noted that the "average patient" is a construct, not a reality, and provided some evidence for their claim that "most people taking RCT-validated, effective treatments derive no benefit from them" (p. 78). For a few interventions, it is possible that beneficial effects from an intervention are nearly universal—but this is unlikely to be the case for nursing interventions aimed at affecting complex behaviors or emotions. Universal effects should seldom be assumed. Subramanian et al. provided one example regarding evidence that the widely used drug Nexium, although found to be effective based on RCT results, "works for only 1 in 25 people who take it for heartburn" (p. 78)—i.e., the number needed to treat (NNT) is 25. Yet, not unreasonably, clinicians recommend Nexium to treat heartburn because, *on average,* patients who used it in trials had a lower incidence of heartburn than those who did not. It is not that trial information about average effects is unimportant, but it is often insufficient. For an individual patient, the average effect is of little interest—an intervention either is or is not beneficial.

> **TIP** Randomized trials were initially used in agriculture: different strategies were experimentally tested with the goal of improving crop yield. However, those experimental strategies were never about the welfare of individual plants (Rolfe, 2009).

Average treatment effects, such as the ones estimated in systematic reviews, are problematic from another perspective: averages strip away *context.* Context shapes how interventions are implemented and influences their effectiveness. However, population models of EBP provide context-free conclusions about the delivery of effective care.

Evidence-Based Practice and External Validity

In Chapter 10, we pointed out the tensions between efforts to enhance a study's internal validity (inferences that an intervention *caused* an effect) and external validity (inferences that causal claims generalize across persons, settings, and time). Strategies to reduce threats to internal validity tend to negatively impact external validity and vice versa.

Researchers who seek to generate evidence for practice have traditionally resolved the tension between internal and external validity in favor of internal validity. Evidence hierarchies, for example, rank study designs based on their ability to eliminate threats to internal validity; external validity is ignored. In systematic reviews, evaluations of study quality almost invariably focus on internal rather than external validity. The GRADE system for evaluating reviewers' *confidence* in evidence from systematic reviews (Chapter 30), which emphasizes internal validity, gives a nod to external validity by including a criterion of consistency of results (Table 30.2), but the underlying concern is the *replicability* of a causal inference and not its generalizability (i.e., not whether the results are maintained across different settings or populations).

Traditional RCTs undermine the generalizability of the results in diverse ways. Table 31.1 lists features often used to enhance the internal validity of RCTs. These features indicate that RCTs have typically been conducted under ideal conditions rather than in normal, real-world situations. All aspects of the study are tightly controlled, including what the exact intervention is, who the interventionists are, where the study takes place, and who participates in the study.

Sampling issues are particularly troublesome for generalizing the results of RCTs. To reduce confounding, trialists often impose exclusion criteria

TABLE 31.1 • Constraints on Generalizability in Traditional (Explanatory) Randomized Controlled Trials (RCTs)[a]

TYPE OF ISSUE	NATURE OF THE PROBLEM
Research Design	Confounding influences on the outcomes are tightly controlled, unlike what typically occurs.
	Follow-up period in the trial is often shorter than what a usual course of treatment might be; long-term outcomes are seldom studied to see if benefits are sustained or if harms emerge.
	Participants are prohibited from receiving other treatments, unlike what happens in the normal course of life.
	Comparing the intervention to no treatment or to a placebo leaves questions about clinical decision-making unanswered.
Intervention	The trial is often undertaken in high-skill, resource-rich settings, not in "typical" settings.
	Intervention typically is administered by highly skilled and well-trained staff, unlike what occurs in normal settings.
	The intervention is adequately funded and carefully managed.
	Participants often undergo stringent tests/screenings to be eligible to participate, unlike what occurs in normal settings.
	The intervention in trials may be limited to a specified time interval rather than having treatment determined by need.
	Adherence and intervention fidelity are higher in trials than in normal practice settings.
Sampling	Exclusion criteria often eliminate people who might most benefit from (or who might most be harmed by) the intervention (e.g., older patients, ones with comorbidities).
	Low rates of participation in trials result in biases; RCT samples include only those willing to be randomized and might exclude people (or clinicians) who have strong treatment preferences.
Outcomes/Measurement	Studies are not always focused on outcomes of greatest interest to patients (e.g., quality of life).
	Studies seldom focus on outcomes of greatest interest to administrators (costs, resource requirements).
	Insufficient information on adverse events is gathered.
	Heavy response burden can contribute to attrition from the study.
Analysis	Focus is on "average" effects, not on the distribution of effects.
	Subgroup analyses, when undertaken, are not well conceived.

[a]Identified in such papers as those by Gross and Fogg (2001) and Rothwell (2005b; 2006).

that eliminate key groups of people—often, older people and those with comorbidities, who might especially benefit from, or be harmed by, the intervention under study. Other groups are often left out simply because they are not served in large healthcare centers where the trials are conducted (e.g., low income groups, rural residents). These limits on generalizability are compounded by low rates of participation in RCTs, with refusal rates sometimes approaching 90%. The bottom line is that, in general, patients are usually very different from those included in RCTs.

> **Example of an RCT With a High Rate of Refusal**
> Lin and an interprofessional team (2018) undertook an RCT to test a cell phone intervention to promote weight loss in young adults. Of the 1,743 who were screened and deemed eligible for the trial, 1,378 declined to participate (79%).

The combined effect of relying on a population model of average effects and using data from highly select study participants is that EBP is often based on evidence of whether an intervention works for a hypothetical "average" patient under ideal, context-neutral conditions. Although the RCT results may be unbiased from an internal validity standpoint, they may be less useful than one would hope in making decisions about individual patients who are neither "ideal" nor "average."

Applicability, Generalizability, and Relevance

The terms *generalizability* and *applicability* have often been used interchangeably, but there is a growing view that they are quite distinct (Sacristán & Dilla, 2018; Treweek & Zwarenstein, 2009). Generalizability is a term associated with populations—researchers identify characteristics of a population to which their findings might reasonably be generalized. As astutely noted by Lincoln and Guba (1985), however, "The trouble with generalizations is that they don't apply to particulars" (p. 110).

We define **applicability** as the degree to which research evidence can be applied to individuals, small groups of individuals, or local contexts. Applicability is relevant to clinical decision-making because of human heterogeneity—averages are not of much value as decision guides if there is wide diversity in whether an intervention works or how it is viewed, experienced, adhered to, or incorporated into normal life. Sacristán and Dilla (2018) noted that "As health care decisions are becoming more patient centric, the term 'applicability' should evoke 'individual patient' rather than 'average patient'" (p. 165).

Figure 31.1 shows a hypothetical continuum along which evidence can move from generalizable to applicable. The bottom of the figure shows examples of strategies that researchers can use along the continuum. We discuss several ideas for enhancing applicability and generalizability—as well as relevance—in this chapter. In the context of practice-based evidence, we define **relevance** as evidence that is important to key stakeholders and has the potential to be actionable. **Patient-centered research**, which focuses on developing evidence that is meaningful and valuable to patients, involves efforts to attain relevance.

Producing evidence that is applicable, relevant, and generalizable requires researchers to be vigilant, creative, and insightful in an ongoing way. The

FIGURE 31.1 Generalizability and applicability.

task of applying research evidence to solve health-care problems is a responsibility of practitioners, but researchers need to take steps to enrich the readiness of their evidence for "reasonable extrapolation" (Patton, 2015).

New Directions in Healthcare Research

Concern about the limitations of evidence-based practice for guiding decisions about individuals in real-world contexts has led to the emergence of new ideas and innovative methods for *optimizing* evidence. Efforts at optimization have taken various forms, such as *precision healthcare, individualized healthcare, stratified healthcare, personalized healthcare,* and *patient-centered healthcare*. Research in these domains has gone in broadly similar directions, but sometimes with different emphases. Such research typically strives for evidence that is practice-based.

Comparative effectiveness research (CER) is an important manifestation of emerging directions in healthcare research. CER emphasizes patient-centeredness and involves direct comparisons of clinical interventions to facilitate decision-making (Chapter 11). As noted by Greenfield and Kaplan (2012), "CER calls for substantial changes in the way clinical research is conducted, interpreted, and practically applied …the evolving CER paradigm requires …innovations that address three basic questions: what works? for whom? and in whose hands?" (p. 263).

The Institute of Medicine's (2009) report on priorities for comparative effectiveness research offered six defining characteristics of CER:

1. *CER's objective is to directly inform clinical decisions.* CER places a high value on the ability to generalize results to real-world decision-making. Because the goal is to contribute to important decisions, a broad range of relevant stakeholders and decision-makers (including patients) should be included in setting priorities, designing studies, and implementing results.
2. *CER involves comparisons of two or more alternative treatments, each of which has potential to be "best practice."* CER avoids the use of placebos, attention controls, or no intervention as comparators in testing an intervention. For this reason, CER trials are sometimes referred to as "head-to-head" trials.
3. *CER seeks evidence at both the population and the subgroup level.* A goal of CER is to help providers and patients in individualizing decisions—going beyond "average effects" to effects for people with similar characteristics.
4. *CER uses outcomes that are important to patients.* CER strives to include and give weight to patient-reported outcomes and to attend to benefits, harms, and unintended consequences of healthcare interventions. In turn, this means that CER is often focused on long-term outcomes. Costs are also considered important in CER because they can influence decisions.
5. *CER uses diverse research designs and methods.* Some comparative effectiveness studies involve experimental designs, but CER also uses other designs, including nonexperimental (observational) approaches. CER also draws on diverse data sources, such as data from electronic health records (EHRs), administrative claims, and clinical registries.
6. *CER is conducted in real-world settings.* CER studies the effectiveness of interventions in settings similar to those where an intervention would actually be used.

These characteristics of CER diverge in many important respects from the research model that has come to be established under EBP, which focuses on internal validity and adheres rather rigidly to evidence from RCTs. (A table in the Toolkit identifies major distinguishing features ✪.) Note that these characteristics of CER embody concerns about generalizability (defining characteristic 1), applicability (defining characteristic 3), and relevance (defining characteristic 4). In the remainder of this chapter, we offer some suggestions for optimizing evidence and generating practice-based evidence. Many of these suggestions rely on ideas emerging in the context of comparative effectiveness research, methods for which are still evolving.

STRATEGIES TO ENHANCE APPLICABILITY, GENERALIZABILITY, AND RELEVANCE

We organize this section on strategies to develop practice-based evidence according to major steps of a research project. We consider our suggestions merely a starting place and hope that we will inspire insights on how to make evidence more useful to practitioners in real-world settings.

Planning a Study for Practice-Based Evidence

A good place to begin with efforts to enhance applicability is to ask the right questions—questions that patients and clinicians want answered. There is a growing awareness of the importance of "co-designing" studies with a range of stakeholders and *end-users* of research evidence (Rycroft-Malone, 2012). Collaboration with patients, practitioners in varied disciplines, and administrators throughout the research process can result in better interprofessional "buy-in" and greater relevance of research results. Stakeholder involvement can also offer practical advantages, including greater ease of recruiting study participants and study sites. The Patient-Centered Outcomes Research Institute (PCORI) has played a lead role in spurring stakeholder involvement in health research and is a key funder of CER projects (Forsythe et al., 2018; Newhouse et al., 2015).

> **TIP** Several models of stakeholder and patient engagement have been proposed (e.g., Concannon et al., 2014; Sofolahan-Oladeinde et al., 2017). Research thus far suggests that stakeholder involvement can be challenging but results in research deemed to be highly relevant.

Site selection is important. A local focus, as in quality improvement projects or action research, greatly enhances applicability but may constrain generalizability. In planning a project, consideration needs to be given to which of these goals is more salient. Implementing the project in multiple sites is often a useful strategy, but then a decision must be made about whether the sites are essentially

replicates (in a manner that might enhance applicability to certain contexts) or are deliberately selected to allow conclusions to be generalized to different types of contexts or people. In the latter case, care must be taken to identify key dimensions of difference for the selected sites (e.g., rural/urban; public/private institutions, etc.).

As Figure 31.1 suggests, one approach to moving from generalizability to greater applicability is to study whether intervention effects differ for different subpopulations. We encourage researchers to give thought early in the planning process to studying *subgroup effects*, so that appropriate design and sampling strategies, described later, can be put in place. It is especially important to develop hypotheses about subgroup effects in advance and to develop a cogent rationale for such hypotheses.

During the planning stage, researchers should also consider using a framework to guide the design and implementation of a study aimed at enhancing relevance. One such framework is called **R**each, **E**ffectiveness, **A**doption, **I**mplementation, and **M**aintenance or **RE-AIM** (Battaglia & Glasgow, 2018). RE-AIM was explicitly developed with the goal of elevating awareness about external validity. The supplement to this chapter describes the RE-AIM framework. ⓢ

> **TIP** Numerous frameworks have been devised to facilitate translation and implementation projects. This chapter is not designed to assist researchers who are focused on translating evidence from efficacy trials into real-world settings. Rather, our goal is to illustrate how researchers can take steps to enhance relevance and applicability from the get-go. Although RE-AIM is most often used in implementation science, some of its strategies are useful to any researcher interested in developing practice-based evidence.

Designing a Study for Practice-Based Evidence

Table 31.1 identifies several features of a traditional RCT—all of which suggest opportunities for design modifications that could increase the relevance of intervention research. Here we mention a few design considerations, most of which are consistent with CER, but we acknowledge that this is an area in which innovations occur daily and which is ripe for further methodologic creativity.

Pragmatic Clinical Trials

As we have noted, features of the traditional RCT designs are so tightly controlled that the relevance of the findings to real-life situations can be questioned. Concern about this problem has led to interest in **pragmatic clinical trials (PCTs)**, which are designed to maximize external validity with minimal negative effect on internal validity (Ford & Norrie, 2016; Glasgow et al., 2005; Treweek & Zwarenstein, 2009). Tunis and colleagues (2003), in a seminal paper, defined pragmatic (practical) clinical trials as "trials for which the hypotheses and study design are formulated based on information needed to make a decision" (p. 1626). Thus, pragmatic trials are consistent with the goals of CER.

> **TIP** Pragmatic trials are more squarely focused on *effectiveness* rather than *efficacy* (Chapter 10). Pragmatic trials sometimes are part of a translational project—that is, they involve tests in usual care settings of an intervention previously found to be efficacious in a traditional RCT. But *pragmatism* as a construct can be applied in most studies. As noted by Sacristán and Dilla (2018), pragmatism is not so much a design type but a "mindset"—pragmatic attitudes can be used in all types of research. Indeed, pragmatism is the paradigm underlying mixed methods research.

Compared to more traditional **explanatory trials** conducted under optimal conditions with carefully selected participants, pragmatic clinical trials address practical questions about the benefits and risks of an intervention—as well as its costs—as they would unfold in routine clinical practice. Tunis and co-authors (2003) made these recommendations for PCTs: enrollment of diverse populations with fewer exclusions of high-risk patients; recruitment of participants from a variety of practice settings; follow-up over a longer period; inclusion of economic outcomes; and comparisons of clinically viable alternatives.

Trials cannot readily be categorized as *pragmatic* or *explanatory*, because they do not represent a dichotomy. As noted by Treweek and Zwarenstein (2009), "there is a continuum rather than a dichotomy... with the pragmatic attitude explicitly favouring design choices that maximise applicability of the trial results to usual care settings" (p. 2).

A tool called **PRECIS-2 (Preferred Explanatory Continuum Indicator Summary)** has been developed to help researchers evaluate how pragmatic their trial is and to help ensure that their designs are congruent with their intended aims (Loudon et al., 2015). The tool covers nine domains (e.g., patient eligibility, patient recruitment), each of which is rated from 1 (very explanatory) to 5 (very pragmatic). For example, the question for the eligibility domain is this: To what extent are the participants in the trial similar to those who would receive this intervention if it was part of usual care?

As shown in Figure 31.2, scoring for each PRECIS-2 domain is done on a "wheel." (Figure 31.2 is included in the Toolkit for this chapter for ease of reproduction ⊗). The more "filled in" the wheel is, the greater the degree of pragmatism. By scoring a planned trial, researchers can see how pragmatic the trial would be, and they can then decide whether to "tweak" design features to move in the direction of greater pragmatism. Ford and Norrie (2016) observed that many trials could be scored as pragmatic in one or two domains of the PRECIS-2 tool, but few trials are truly pragmatic on all of them. Nguyen and colleagues (2018) have described the application of the PRECIS-2 tool for the design and implementation of a PCT of physical activity coaching for patients with COPD.

> **TIP** Nurse researchers have demonstrated growing interest in PCTs. A methods conference at the 2017 meeting of the Council for the Advancement of Nursing Science (CANS) was devoted to pragmatic trials, and a special issue of *Nursing Outlook* included several papers based on presentations at the conference. In that issue, Battaglia and Glasgow (2018) asserted that pragmatic research "is an area of tremendous opportunity for the nursing science community" (p. 430). Littleton-Kearney (2018) described funding of PCTs at the National Institute of Nursing Research.

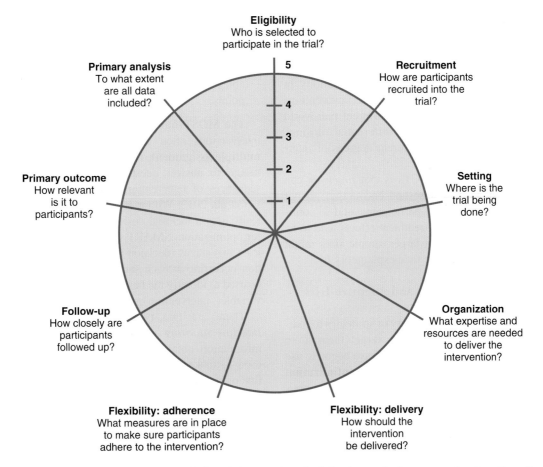

FIGURE 31.2 **The PRECIS-2 wheel.** Each domain is scored on the following scale: 1 = very explanatory; 2 = rather explanatory; 3 = equally pragmatic and explanatory; 4 = rather pragmatic; and 5 = very pragmatic. (Reprinted with permission from Loudon, K., Treweek, S., Sullivan, F., Donnan, P., Thorpe, K., & Zwarenstein, M. (2015). The PRECIS-2 tool: Designing trials that are fit for purpose. *British Medical Journal, 350*, h2147.)

Glasgow and colleagues (2005) proposed several research designs for pragmatic trials. The most promising (and widely used) include cluster randomization (randomization of groups rather than individuals) and delayed treatment designs (everyone gets the intervention eventually). When a delay-of-treatment strategy is combined with cluster randomization, the result is a **stepped wedge design**, which involves having clusters randomized to receive the intervention at different points (Battaglia & Glasgow, 2018).

Example of a PCT With Cluster Randomization

Chapman and colleagues (2018) undertook a multisite pragmatic cluster randomized trial in 41 community health stations (CHSs) in China. The CHSs were randomized to receive either usual care or a health coach intervention for managing individuals with type 2 diabetes mellitus. The researchers noted that the trial "was specifically tailored to be delivered in real world CHSs in urban China, hence maximizing external validity" (p. 12).

PCTs protect internal validity by using familiar bias-reducing strategies such as randomization, allocation concealment, and blinding. Moreover, cluster randomized pragmatic trials can promote internal validity by guarding against contamination of treatments. However, Eckardt and Erlanger (2018) have noted possible threats to validity in pragmatic trials. One issue is that the interventions are often less standardized in different real-world settings, perhaps resulting in differential "dosing" of the intervention and different degrees of intervention fidelity.

Another issue with PCTs is that *precision* can be affected: PCTs allow (and encourage) greater diversity in settings and participants, and so confidence intervals around treatment effects tend to be wider. This implies that larger sample sizes might be needed for pragmatic than explanatory trials.

Adaptive Interventions and Adaptive Trial Designs

Researchers are using a variety of strategies to individualize interventions and to target them more effectively. Recently, researchers have begun to use a framework called the **multiphase optimization strategy (MOST)**, which has been used for optimization in both fixed interventions and in dynamic multicomponent interventions that evolve over time (Collins et al., 2014).

Adaptive, dynamic treatments are common in clinical practice—clinicians begin with an intervention, assess whether it is working, and then make another decision (e.g., continuing with the treatment, strengthening it, trying something else). **Adaptive interventions** are ones in which there are multiple decision points over time, and decisions are based on individual responses. Adaptive interventions sometimes take the form of *stepped care interventions* in which care begins with a low-intensity strategy that is increased if goals are not reached, or with a high-intensity strategy that is stepped down if they are reached. Adaptive interventions involve four main components:

1. *Decision points.* Points in time when a treatment decision is made.
2. *Tailoring variables.* Information about individuals that is used to make treatment decisions.

3. *Intervention options.* Options regarding type, dose, intensity, duration, or delivery mechanism of the intervention.
4. *Decision rules.* Links between the tailoring variables and the treatment options at the decision points.

The MOST framework for optimizing adaptive interventions often involves using a **sequential, multiple assignment, randomized trial (SMART)** design to answer questions about individualized sequences of interventions (Almirall et al., 2014; Lei et al., 2012; Wilbur et al., 2016). SMART typically uses a factorial design to obtain information for optimization. SMART studies always involve at least two stages (decision points), with randomization occurring at each stage. SMART designs can be used to identify the best decision points, tailoring variables, intervention options, or decision rules.

There are two types of tailoring variables. *Baseline tailoring variables* are ones for which information obtained prior to the intervention is used to make tailored treatment decisions at the first or at a subsequent decision stage. For example, in a weight loss intervention, participants might be given longer or more intensive treatment in the first phase if they are classified as "obese" rather than "overweight." *Intermediate tailoring variables,* obtained after baseline, are often preliminary "outcomes," that is, indicators of whether the initial intervention has promise of effectiveness. Using a preestablished threshold, these tailoring variables are used to distinguish *responders* and *nonresponders* to the initial treatment, and this in turn is used to tailor the intervention in the second stage.

Figure 31.3 presents a hypothetical example in which an intermediate tailoring variable was used. At the outset, all study participants are randomized to Intervention A or Intervention B (in our example, individual [A] versus group [B] counseling for weight loss). Six weeks later, all study participants are evaluated for their response to the intervention—that is, whether they have reached the responder threshold based on a preestablished criterion (e.g., weight loss > 3.0% of baseline weight). Benchmarks might be established by a panel of stakeholders or by referencing established thresholds for clinical

PHASE I   **TREATMENT RESPONSE ASSESSMENT**   **PHASE II**

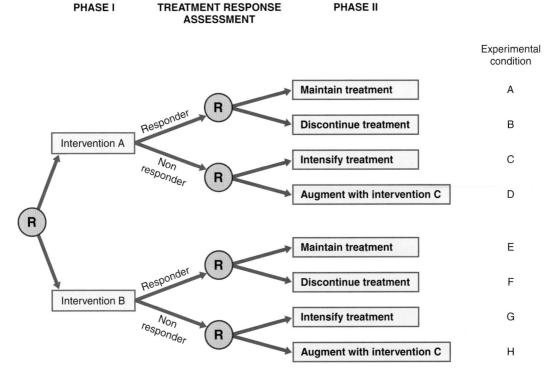

FIGURE 31.3 Example of a Sequential Multiple Assignment Randomized Trial (SMART).

Note: R = randomization to treatment condition.

significance on the primary outcome (Chapter 21). In both arms of the trial, responders and nonresponders are further randomized. Responders in both arms are randomized to either "maintenance" (e.g., continuation of the intervention) or discontinuation. Nonresponders are randomized to either an intensified version of the original treatment (e.g., longer or more frequent sessions) or to an augmented treatment (Intervention C) in which they receive a supplementary component (e.g., meal replacements).

In this example, the first *decision point* is at the outset (identifying overweight people who want to lose weight) and the second is 6 weeks later. The *tailoring variable* is whether the person showed adequate weight loss progress after getting an intervention. The *intervention options* included: (1) individualized weight loss counseling; (2) group weight loss counseling; (3) intensified counseling of both types; and (4) a supplementary intervention. The *decision rules*

were to offer an initial intervention and to then tailor it depending on the response.

The goal of a SMART study is to construct and optimize a tailored intervention before it is brought to a full traditional (or pragmatic) randomized trial. At each stage of a SMART, researchers use randomization to address a question about treatment options, and those options are tailored to individual circumstances or responses. Randomization in a SMART design permits unbiased comparisons between treatment components at each stage in the development of an adaptive intervention.

Several variants of SMART designs have been proposed. For example, Dai and Shete (2016) suggested a time-varying SMART design in which participants are re-randomized to the second stage interventions as soon as the predesignated intermediate response is observed—in our example, as soon as a participant achieves a weight loss greater than 3% of weight at baseline.

Example of SMART Design
Sikorskii and colleagues (2017) described a protocol for a trial in which a SMART design is being used to examine strategies to improve symptom management among patients with cancer. In the trial, dyads of solid tumor cancer patients and their caregivers are initially being randomized to 4 weeks of either reflexology or mindfulness practices, or to a control group. In the second phase, intervention group dyads in which the patients' fatigue levels have not improved (nonresponders) are re-randomized to receive either 4 more weeks with the initial therapy or the addition of the alternative therapy. This study is described more fully at the end of Chapter 10.

SMART studies are used to develop adaptive interventions, but they do not typically involve an **adaptive trial design** in which the trial design itself is altered during the course of the trial (Bhatt & Mehta, 2016). Adaptive designs are used to learn if a treatment is safe and effective and who will derive the most benefit (Heckman-Stoddard & Smith, 2014). In an adaptive trial design, the results of interim analyses are used to make adjustments to features of the study design. For example, the interim analyses may lead to stopping the trial early, adaptively assigning doses, dropping or adding study arms, focusing more attention on responder groups, or changing the proportion of participants randomized to each arm of the trial. Adaptive trial designs (and other innovative types of designs such as *basket* trials) are often used in tests of gene therapies in connection with precision healthcare (Biankin et al., 2015; Pallmann et al., 2018).

TIP The emergence of "just-in-time" adaptive interventions using mHealth (mobile health) technologies has given rise to other innovations in experimental design, including *microrandomization*, which involves randomly assigning intervention options at multiple decision points—i.e., at the points at which a particular component might be efficacious (Klasnja et al., 2015).

N-of-1 Trials

The ultimate approach to individualization is to test an intervention with individual study participants. **N-of-1 trials** (also called **single-subject experiments**) are studies in which different treatments are tested in an individual patient over time. N-of-1 trials typically are randomized crossover trials conducted on a single patient. These trials are characterized by alternating an active treatment phase and a placebo phase (or alternating two active treatments). The simplest N-of-1 trial design is exposure to one treatment condition (A) and then exposure to another condition (B). When the sequence is randomly determined, this results in an AB or BA allocations. However, preferred designs involve the repetition of treatment sequences to protect against various sources of biases—for example, designs such as ABAB or ABBAABBA. N-of-1 trials have been strongly advocated by proponents of patient-centered research: such designs are uniquely capable of leading to evidence-informed clinical decisions for individual patients. In some cases, N-of-1 studies can be profitably aggregated (Schork, 2018).

Example of a Single-Subject AB Design
Strahan and Elder (2015) used an AB single-subject design to assess video-game playing effects on obesity in an adolescent with autism spectrum disorder. The teenager played an inactive video game for 6 weeks, followed by an active video game for another 6 weeks. Physiological data and stress and anxiety were evaluated weekly.

The *Journal of Clinical Epidemiology* published a series of papers on N-of-1 trials in 2016, consistent with the growing research interest in the personalization of health care (e.g., Knottnerus et al., 2016; Vohra, 2016). Punja and colleagues (2016) identified numerous potential advantages of single-subject trials, including the following: (1) intervention approaches are individualized; (2) results are applicable and directly relevant to participants; (3) participants quickly learn the results; and (4) the cost is low compared to traditional RCTs. Methodologic safeguards are traditionally implemented in N-of-1 trials (e.g., randomization and blinding). Indeed, the Oxford Centre for Evidence-Based Medicine considers evidence from such trials as Level 1 evidence. Kravitz and Duan (2014) offer excellent guidance on single-subject trials.

TIP Some studies that are called "N-of-1" trials do not involve alternating treatments but rather are tests of interventions that are personalized for each participant.

Example of a Personalized (N-of-1) Study

Yoon and colleagues (2018) studied whether people randomized to receive a personalized (N-of-1) "activity fingerprint" message about personal predictors of exercise (based on behavioral analytics) increased their levels of physical activity relative to those who did not receive the personalized fingerprint.

Alternatives to Randomized Trials: Quasi-Experiments

Randomized designs are the gold standard for enhancing internal validity and coming to conclusions about causal relationships, but they are often removed from clinical realities. As pointed out by Gross and Fogg (2001), nurse researchers should consider "reasonable alternatives" to random assignment. Participation in an intervention study can be far more acceptable to prospective participants (and to research site administrators) if randomization of patients is not involved—which is precisely what makes cluster randomization attractive in pragmatic trials. Higher rates of participation, in turn, enhance generalizability.

Quasi-experimental designs are sometimes a useful alternative to an RCT, but researchers need to be strategic in designing quasi-experiments to minimize threats to internal validity. Supplement B to Chapter 10 offers guidance on designing powerful quasi-experimental tests of intervention effectiveness. Also, in 2017, the *Journal of Clinical Epidemiology* published a useful series of 13 papers on the utility of quasi-experimental designs (e.g., Bärnighausen et al., 2017; Rockers et al., 2017). Partially randomized patient preference designs (Chapter 9) can also be useful for enhancing applicability—such designs include both randomized and nonrandomized components and can provide valuable information about what patients prefer.

Alternatives to Randomized Trials: Nonexperimental Research

Observational (nonexperimental) studies are even lower than quasi-experiments on traditional evidence hierarchies. Yet, there is growing awareness that carefully conducted observational studies can yield evidence with high internal validity—and with far greater external validity than explanatory RCTs because they tend to involve broader and more representative samples (e.g., Booth & Tannock, 2013; Concato & Horwitz, 2018). Comparative effectiveness research embraces the contribution of observational studies in assessing the benefits and harms of alternative interventions (Marko & Weil, 2010).

Observational studies can be used to evaluate the effects of alternative interventions in situations in which patients have not been randomized to the treatment. Although there have been concerns about "overestimation bias" in observational studies of treatment effects when there is self-selection into treatments, new approaches to designing studies that mimic RCT protocols are emerging. Such methodologic strategies as aligning eligibility criteria to an RCT, establishing a "zero time" for treatment, and using sophisticated methods such as propensity score analysis and *instrumental variables* to address confounding variables are being pursued (Armstrong, 2012; Frieden, 2017).

Observational studies with large administrative or epidemiological databases can contribute to practice-based evidence in other ways. For example, large observational studies can help researchers to understand the representativeness of samples from traditional or pragmatic RCTs (Greenhouse et al., 2008). In that vein, some have suggested "nesting" RCTs within large population databases or electronic health record (EHR) databases to get a better handle on the generalizability of the RCT results (Angus, 2015; Dahabreh, 2018).

Other important uses of observational data from large databases include the following: learning the uptake and outcomes of new interventions in routine practice; identifying potential harms or adverse effects associated with new interventions; expanding tailored clinical decision support mechanisms (Angus, 2015); and developing prediction models about the types of people most likely to have a favorable response to an intervention (Iwashyna & Liu, 2014).

Booth and Tannock (2013) argued that RCTs and population-based observational research should be considered partners in the evolution of healthcare evidence. They recommend a two-prong approach in which rigorous RCTs powered to detect clinically meaningful improvements are followed by observational studies that "evaluate patterns of care, toxicity, and the effectiveness of treatment in routine practice" (p. 553).

Mixed Methods Designs

Developing practice-based evidence requires the thoughtful integration of qualitative and quantitative data, especially in studies of intervention effectiveness (Battaglia & Glasgow, 2018). Qualitative data offer insights into why, how, and with whom effects are observed.

There are several ways in which mixed methods designs are especially valuable with regard to the applicability of evidence. Qualitative information can provide a rich understanding of the *context* in which interventions are delivered. Contextualized understandings can lead to insights into the kinds of environments in which an intervention does or does not "work."

Qualitative data can also play a crucial role in untangling the enigma of "average treatment effects." For individual participants, the effects might be much greater than the average, while for others, the intervention might have no benefit. Sometimes quantitative subgroup analyses can be undertaken, but these are productive only if the dimension along which variation occurs is a measurable attribute about which hypotheses have been developed in advance. A qualitative study of participants who experienced the intervention differently could illuminate how to target the intervention more effectively in the future or how to improve it to reach a more diverse audience. A qualitative component also can lay the foundation for more formal subgroup analysis or for developing interventions tailored to individual needs and circumstances. Qualitative methods are well suited to exploring

the heterogeneity of treatment effects (Holtrop et al., 2018). Realist evaluations, described earlier in this book, usually use mixed methods to address a range of questions about an intervention, including applicability.

Sampling for Practice-Based Evidence

A major problem with the evidence from traditional RCTs—evidence that forms the basis for most clinical practice guidelines—is that the samples exclude many types of people to whom the evidence is supposed to be applied. Pragmatic trials, which typically have fewer exclusion criteria, tend to yield samples that are closer to real-world populations. Thus, one obvious suggestion for generating practice-based evidence is to make efforts to ensure that research samples reflect the full range of people who could benefit from an intervention.

Other advice concerning strategies to enhance applicability and generalizability includes the following:

- *Clearly identify the target population.* The starting point for selecting a heterogeneous "real-world" sample to which study results can be generalized is to clearly define the characteristics of the people (and settings) of interest. All too often, researchers seem to begin with a nonrepresentative sample from an ill-defined and restrictive population and then hope for the best. Stakeholder involvement in identifying the target population is likely to be productive.
- *Use purposive sampling strategies.* Convenience samples of "ideal" (e.g., no comorbidities) and cooperative people are all too common in quantitative research. Quota sampling is a step in the right direction—it is used to ensure a sufficient number of sample members within key population strata. In general, researchers would do far better at achieving representative samples if they had a more purposive approach to sampling (Polit & Beck, 2010). When researchers know in advance the characteristics of their target population, they can monitor sample characteristics in an ongoing fashion and then recruit types of participants who are not yet adequately

represented. Sampling totally by convenience is seldom justified if the goal is to produce practice-based evidence.

- *Sample from multiple sites.* It is often useful to recruit sample members from multiple sites, being strategic about site selection. For example, if people in a single site are homogeneous with regard to a characteristic that might affect intervention outcomes, then an important way to broaden understanding about intervention effects is to select sites that vary on important dimensions (e.g., low-income versus affluent communities).
- *Aim for a sample size that permits subgroup analyses.* The sample size should be large enough to support relevant subgroup analyses that are sufficiently powered. Sample size projections should also take into consideration requirements for studying clinical significance, which is more patient-centric than statistical significance.
- *Sample participants carefully for in-depth inquiry in mixed methods studies.* A nested sample (Chapter 27) of participants from the full sample may be especially useful for in-depth explorations of heterogeneity of effects, as well as other issues such as variation in adherence. Multilevel samples may provide rich insights into the research context.

Collecting Data for Practice-Based Evidence

Several steps can be taken to improve the data collection efforts of researchers striving for practice-based evidence. First and foremost, there is growing awareness that researchers do not always focus on the needs and interests of key stakeholders, including both patients and clinicians. Studies ideally would be co-created with people who can provide input regarding patient-important outcomes. For example, patients are much less likely to care about whether an intervention can bring about a 5-point improvement on a composite scale—or even a 5% decrease in blood pressure—than about functional outcomes (e.g., regaining the ability to walk up a flight of stairs). People are more likely to cooperate

in research if they perceive the research to be relevant to them, and selecting relevant outcomes is a path to patient-centered evidence.

In Chapter 15, we describe psychometric criteria for selecting high-quality measures for research purposes—notably reliability, validity, and responsiveness. Additional criteria should be considered for creating practice-based evidence. Glasgow and Riley (2013) offered four primary criteria for *"pragmatic measures"*:

- Important to stakeholders (outcomes are deemed important by diverse stakeholder groups);
- Low response burden (requires minimal time and effort to complete);
- Actionable (enhances application in busy, real-world settings; easy to interpret and useful in decision-making); and
- Sensitive to change (capable of tracking progress).

For certain outcomes, the use of measures from the Patient-Reported Outcome Measurement Information System (PROMIS®) offers many advantages (Kroenke et al., 2015). PROMIS® covers dozens of outcomes with high relevance to patients (e.g., pain, physical function, sleep disturbance), and, because of computer adaptive testing, the measures are extremely efficient yet precise. Another important feature of PROMIS® is that scoring is instantaneous and yields feedback about performance relative to normed samples (for many measures, separate norms by sex and age). Scoring is on a common metric (a T-score), where a score of 50 equals the mean of the U.S. general population—this, in turn, makes scores interpretable and actionable by patients and clinicians. Finally, PROMIS® includes measures that are sensitive to change and minimizes floor and ceiling effects. PROMIS® measures are available for use with the general population, as well as with adult and pediatric populations with chronic conditions. PROMIS® measures are available for free online, and most have been translated into several languages.

Patients and clinicians are likely to find the *clinical significance* of outcomes of greater relevance to them than statistical significance. This suggests the desirability of including outcome measures for which a minimal important change (MIC) benchmark has been estimated. (Alternatively, researchers can take steps to estimating it themselves, as we discuss in Chapter 21.) The best approach to estimating an MIC value involves getting input about meaningfulness directly from patients.

Qualitative data are also important for building practice-based evidence. Qualitative data can potentially shed light on *why* or *with whom* an intervention was effective—or why it was not. Qualitative data can also illuminate implementation processes and contextual features that are important to those interested in translating an intervention into other settings.

> **TIP** Information about study contexts are most often qualitative descriptions. However, in some cases, it might make sense to formally measure contextual elements—especially in multisite studies. Carole Estabrooks and her colleagues (2011), for example, have developed the Alberta Context Tool to measure organizational contextual factors.

In addition to traditional methods of measurement and data collection, thought should also be given to the use of Big Data in nursing studies, which can be used to address questions about broad groups and populations (with potential enhancements to generalizability) and about variations in treatment effects (with potential enhancements to applicability). **Big Data** refers to large, complex datasets that are often difficult to process using customary analytic methods. Big Data has been described as having three features: high volume of data, high velocity of data flow, and high variety of data types (Wang & Krishnan, 2014). Big Data can come from aggregated clinical datasets, administrative datasets (e.g., Medicare), electronic health record datasets, and from large dedicated surveys, such as data from the diverse 1 million-person research cohort "All of Us" in the United States (Lyles et al., 2018). As noted previously, observational data from large datasets can be exploited to improve both generalizability of results about treatment effects and to improve applicability with the development of predictive models to guide individualized decisions. Big Data has another important advantage over traditional clinical research methods—they are better

suited than data from RCTs for tracking people's health and symptoms trajectories over years or decades (Concato & Horwitz, 2018).

Finally, with the rapidly emerging interest in precision healthcare, researchers should consider gathering data on relevant biomarkers that might facilitate understanding of individual health. Corwin and Ferranti (2016) urge that nurse researchers integrate biomarkers into their studies to be "better able to precisely tailor and test nursing interventions to improve the health and well-being of patients and families across the lifespan" (p. 293). They argued that studying biomarkers and their contribution to disease and symptoms in observational studies can pave the way for precision nursing interventions.

Analyzing Data for Practice-Based Evidence

The analysis of research data is a major avenue for enhancing applicability. In particular, analytic strategies can be used to better understand heterogeneity of treatment effects. Strategies to enhance practice-based evidence range from simple approaches to complex, sophisticated ones.

Know Your Data

With the focus on *average effects* in many RCTs and systematic reviews, quantitative researchers may seldom feel the need to get close to their data. The sheer ease with which complex statistical analyses can be undertaken can result in a "disconnect" between researchers and their data—and this is especially true if statisticians are called in to do the analysis.

With respect to statistical analyses, it is always a good idea to begin with a thorough exploration of the dataset. Researchers should learn how the data on key outcomes are distributed—for example, whether heterogeneity is extensive, whether there are extreme outliers, whether the data are skewed, and so on. The Supplement to Chapter 20 offers some suggestions for early exploratory steps in data analysis. Focusing on heterogeneity is crucial—if there was no variation, the "average" would apply to everyone in the sample.

Qualitative researchers are expected to be immersed in their data; quantitative researchers could benefit from greater immersion as well. One strategy is for researchers to look at their data horizontally (within cases) and not simply vertically (across cases). By careful scrutiny of the complete records of selected cases—for example, people who improved greatly, deteriorated, remained unchanged, and so on—researchers often can illuminate "what is going on" in a dataset in a way that computing an average cannot (Polit & Back, 2010). (Approaches to qualitizing quantitative data were described in the Supplement to Chapter 27 on mixed methods.) Integrating quantitative information about extreme cases or typical cases with in-depth qualitative information about such cases can potentially lead to powerful insights into constraints on generalizability and approaches to enhancing applicability.

Exploring and Representing the Outcomes

It is inevitable that researchers will continue to calculate and report average treatment effects, but they should consider other ways to look at their data. For example, if the distribution for key outcomes is skewed, it would be wise to report both median and mean values (Green & Glasgow, 2006).

In analyzing data from clinical trials, researchers often test for group differences on mean postintervention outcomes for the intervention and control groups. Assuming that outcomes were measured at baseline, it is prudent to also examine the *change scores:* How diverse were the changes in the intervention group and what was typical? Both patients and clinicians are likely to find it more relevant to know what percentage of people receiving an intervention improved than what a mean value on an outcome is.

For insights into potential intervention effects on individuals, several experts have noted the importance of calculating the absolute risk reduction (ARR)—rather than relative risk—for key outcomes. Rothwell and colleagues (2005) noted that the "absolute risk reductions in large pragmatic RCTs are…the best guide to the probable effects of treatment of individuals in routine practice" (p. 257). The ARR, which indicates the probability that an individual will benefit from an intervention on a specified outcome, is the mathematic equivalent of

the number needed to treat (NNT). For example, an absolute risk reduction of 25% equals an NNT of 4: 1 patient out of 4 patients treated would benefit. As noted in Chapter 21, the NNT is considered an index of clinical significance at the group level.

ARRs and NNTs are calculated with dichotomous outcomes (e.g., did/did not fall), but continuous outcomes can be dichotomized. As described in Chapter 21, there are various approaches to estimating a benchmark for meaningful change (e.g., the minimal important change or MIC). Such benchmarks create an opportunity for dichotomizing outcomes (did/did not have meaningful change) and calculating the NNT. Even in the absence of an MIC benchmark, many measures have "cutpoints" for interpreting scores that can be used to dichotomize people—for example, a threshold for clinical depression on depression scales. Finally, some researchers use the median value of the outcome to divide a sample into responder and nonresponder groups.

It is particularly useful, from the point of view of patient-centeredness, to estimate the percentage of people who experienced clinically meaningful change. Researchers who are interested in developing relevant evidence should make efforts to analyze meaningful improvement (or deterioration), which is calculated at the level of individual participants. *Responder analyses* of those in intervention and control groups who have and have not had meaningful change is a vital tool in the analytic arsenal for improving applicability.

TIP Sometimes insights into differential effectiveness of an intervention can be gained by undertaking a *dose–response analysis*, i.e., whether getting different "doses" of an intervention or exposure results in different outcomes. Some researchers create treatment groups with different amounts of an intervention, but more often, in dose–response analyses, "dose" is not under the researchers' control. If the "dose" is not experimentally manipulated, then caution would be needed in coming to conclusions about whether different doses yielded different outcomes—or whether different people self-selected into different doses.

Heterogeneity of Treatment Effects and Subgroup Analyses

Many researchers try to develop evidence that is applicable to well-defined groups of people (rather than to entire populations) by conducting subgroup analyses. A **subgroup analysis** involves efforts to disentangle heterogeneity of treatment effects (HTE) for subpopulations of people. For example, a subgroup analysis might suggest that an intervention is effective for men but not for women, or more effective for people with comorbidities than for those without them.

Subgroup analyses, which are intuitively appealing to those interested in individualizing care, are often undertaken in the context of RCTs. Reviews of RCTs in medicine have consistently suggested that subgroup analyses of primary outcomes are undertaken and reported in 50% to 60% of published trials (Gabler et al., 2016, 2009; Sun et al., 2012). Evidence suggests that the rate of subgroup analysis is increasing, perhaps because of its prominence in CER. Subgroup analyses are also performed in many cohort studies that examine treatment effects (Dahan et al., 2018).

Subgroup analyses are, however, controversial, in part because they are frequently not undertaken properly (e.g., Burke et al., 2015; Sun et al., 2014). The struggle between wanting to go beyond population averages on the one hand and the statistical challenges of subgroup analysis on the other was described by renowned clinical epidemiologist Alvan Feinstein as a "clinicostatistical tragedy" (Feinstein, 1998, p. 297).

The statistical challenge in subgroup analyses involves addressing the strong risk of both Type I and Type II errors. False positives (Type I errors) are common because researchers often test multiple subgroups without making adjustments to probabilities. The probability of a false positive might be 5% for one test, but for three independent tests the risk is 14% (Chapter 18). This problem has resulted in many reported subgroup effects that could not be replicated. Potential subgroup effects are also at high risk of being missed because of a Type II error. If a study is adequately powered for the entire sample, it will likely be underpowered when the sample is divided into subgroups.

Because of increased interest in personalized healthcare, the number of scholarly papers devoted to subgroup analyses and HTE tripled between 2005 and 2014 (Tanniou et al., 2016). We describe a few of the recommended subgroup analyses strategies here, with particular emphasis on analyses within randomized trials, and urge readers to seek additional guidance in referenced papers.

● *Specify hypotheses in advance.* Subgroup analysis should be a hypothesis-testing effort, not a fishing expedition. Tables showing 5 to 10 subgroup test results, without a priori hypotheses, are common in reports of RCTs. Multiple subgroup tests are especially suspect when there is no overall significant effect—the researchers appear to be searching for a subgroup "rescue" for disappointing results. Hypotheses about differential effects should be based on sound theoretical reasoning, biological plausibility, or previous empirical evidence. This, in turn, means that hypotheses should be directional, specifying which group is expected to experience greater benefit. Plans for subgroup analyses should be specified in the trial protocol, and preferably the trial would be registered. When there is a strong basis for a subgroup hypothesis, researchers might consider using stratified randomization—although Kaiser (2016) found that stratification is not always needed for prespecified subgroup analyses.

TIP Burke et al. (2015) distinguished *primary* subgroup analyses (based on a priori hypotheses) and *secondary* subgroup analyses that are not stipulated in advance but can sometimes *generate* hypotheses. They reasoned that positive hypothesis-testing analyses can influence decisions about patient care, but that positive hypothesis-generating analyses require confirmatory research.

● *Restrict the number of subgroup analyses.* Burke and colleagues (2015) argued that only rarely should more than one or two primary subgroup analyses be performed. The problem with large numbers of tests is twofold. First, the risk of a Type I error increases as the number of tests goes up. Another problem is that the same people are in multiple subgroups. If we hypothesized, for example, that women would benefit more from an intervention than men (gender subgroup) and that younger people would benefit more than older people (age subgroup), what would be the expectation for older women or younger men? (This is an issue we discuss in the next section). It is probably safest to specify a single primary subgroup analysis and to consider subgroup tests beyond that one as exploratory and to adjust the probabilities using a Bonferroni-type procedure. For exploratory (hypothesis-generating) analyses, some have suggested relaxing the criterion for significance, for example to $p < .10$ (Gabler et al., 2009).

• *Restrict subgroup tests to the primary outcome.* Several experts have recommended that subgroup analyses should be undertaken only for the primary outcome in a trial, not for secondary ones (e.g., Assmann et al., 2000; Rothwell, 2005a).

• *Avoid severely underpowered subgroup analyses.* Many trials are powered to find an overall true treatment effect 80% of the time, but subgroup tests inevitably have lower statistical power. Power is probably closer to 20% to 30% for subgroup effect sizes that are similar in magnitude to the expected main treatment effect (Burke et al., 2015). This suggests the desirability of using a more stringent power standard for the overall sample (e.g., 90%-95% power) when a subgroup analysis is planned. Also, power is modestly enhanced if there are an equal proportion of participants in the subgroups (e.g., 50% male and female). Although the term "subgroup" suggests categorical groupings, the variable for which HTE is hypothesized can be continuous (e.g., age, body mass index [BMI]), and continuous variables can yield substantial improvements in statistical power (Hayward et al., 2006).

• *Base the analyses on variables defined at baseline.* As noted by Sun and colleagues (2014), subgroup analyses should be based on baseline characteristics, not on ones that emerge during the study (e.g., length of stay in the ICU). The

most frequently used variables for HTE analyses in medical RCTs include risk factors for the outcome (e.g., smoking status, disease severity, comorbidity), sex, and age (Gabler et al., 2009, 2016). In multisite studies, subgroup analyses are often undertaken to assess whether similar effects are observed across sites.

• *Analyze for subgroup differences using tests for interactions.* Most analyses for subgroup effects are done incorrectly (e.g., Gabler et al., 2009, 2016). The typical approach is to test for intervention effects *within* each subgroup—for example, testing intervention–control group differences separately for men and women—and then comparing the results. If, for example, there is a significant intervention effect for males but not for females, this is often considered evidence of a subgroup effect. However, such analyses could lead to totally erroneous conclusions—for example, the differences might simply be the result of differential subgroup sample sizes. The question that should be addressed in tests of HTE is this: *Are subgroup treatment effects significantly different from each other?* The null hypothesis is that the treatment effect is the same in the subgroups. To test this hypothesis, the analysis should test for an **interaction**, i.e., an interaction between the treatment variable and the subgroup variable. Such analyses of HTE are sometimes referred to as **moderator analyses** (Kraemer et al., 2006; Wang & Ware, 2013). When formal tests for interaction are undertaken, they should be reported as the estimated difference in the effect of the intervention in the subgroups, with a confidence interval.

• *Calculate ARRs/NNTs for subgroups if possible.* Rothwell and colleagues (2005) advise that both overall results and subgroup results should be expressed as absolute risk reductions.

Because the risk of statistical errors is high, it is wise to be cautious in interpreting subgroup results. The most convincing evidence for a subgroup effect comes from replicated results—especially if the effect is supported by a persuasive biologic or theoretic rationale. Corroboration can occur in the context of a systematic review (Chapter 30). As noted by Sun et al. (2014), it is appropriate to consider the likelihood of a true subgroup effect "on a continuum ranging from 'certainly true' to 'certainly false'" (p. 406).

> **TIP** Consistent *lack* of support for subgroup effects is also illuminating: it suggests that using the overall average may be appropriate in applying the evidence.

Example of a Subgroup Analysis

Bowen and an interdisciplinary team (2016) conducted a comparative effectiveness study that involved randomizing 150 adults with type 2 diabetes to either an attention control group or to one of two alternative diabetes self-management nutrition education approaches. The researchers prespecified a subgroup analysis: they hypothesized that patients with a baseline HbA$_{1C}$ between 7% and 10% would be most likely to benefit from educational interventions. They also had an exploratory subgroup analysis that involved assessing differential effects based on patients' numeracy skill level. Using appropriate tests of interaction, the researchers found that, 6 months after baseline, patients with moderately uncontrolled diabetes had improved HbA$_{1C}$ in both intervention groups, which "may allow improved targeting" (p. 1374) of the interventions. The subgroup analysis for numeracy skills was not statistically significant.

Multivariable Risk-Stratified Analyses

A growing number of experts have noted the limitations of subgroup analysis for understanding heterogeneity of treatment effects, even when analyses are rigorously conducted. The basic problem is that subgroup analysis is a "one-variable-at-a-time" approach—despite the fact that people may have many traits that could moderate the effects of an intervention and they belong to dozens of potential subgroups. Sometimes analysts create multifactorial subgroups by combining traits—for example, older men, older women, younger men, and younger women. However, this approach involves only two variables at a time and increases the risk of a Type II error.

An approach that is gaining momentum is **multivariable risk stratification** (MRS) in analyses

of intervention effects (e.g., Dahabreh et al., 2016; Hayward et al., 2006; Kent et al., 2010). To perform an MRS analysis, researchers use a tool that has been developed to predict the risk of the primary outcome. For example, if the intervention of interest was designed to reduce the risk of pressure ulcers (PUs), then a prediction tool such as the Braden Scale (Bergstrom et al., 1987) or other PU prediction tools (e.g., Deng et al., 2017) could be used. Scores on the risk index are then included in the MRS analysis instead of a subgroup variable in tests for interaction. The tool should be one that has been rigorously evaluated for discriminant validity—usually using receiver operating curves (ROCs)—and found to be adequate (e.g., area under the curve > .60). The components of risk prediction tools often are easily obtainable clinical variables that are available in electronic health records (e.g., age, sex, smoking status, BMI, etc.). Risk prediction tools have been developed for many outcomes of interest to nurse researchers. Some measures of disease severity (APACHE) have broad predictive scope and could be useful.

> **TIP** Experts typically recommend using an externally developed risk prediction tool in risk-stratified analyses. However, such tools are not always available. Kent and colleagues (2010) have discussed developing "internal" risk models using baseline data from the trial itself to predict the outcome, using blinded logistic regression analysis.

Table 31.2 presents an example of results from a risk-stratified analysis, using fictitious data from an RCT testing an intervention to prevent falls in hospitals. The table shows the absolute risk for those in the intervention and control groups, the relative risk reduction (RRR), and the number needed to treat (NNT) for study participants who were predicted to have low, moderate, or high risk of falling, based on their scores on a fall risk prediction scale. This table shows that those in the low-risk group did not benefit from the intervention, whereas those in the moderate- and (especially) high-risk groups did benefit. (An annotated version of Table 31.2 is provided in the Toolkit ⊗.) Typically, the actual risk-stratified analysis uses the full risk score rather

TABLE 31.2 • Risk-Stratified Analysis: Fictitious Example of Fall Outcomes in a Fall Prevention Intervention Trial, Stratified on Predicted Risk of Falling

PREDICTED RISK OF A FALL[a]	EXPERIENCED A FALL AT END OF TRIAL		RELATIVE RISK REDUCTION (RRR) (95% CI)	p	NUMBER NEEDED TO TREAT (NNT)
	INTERVENTION GROUP	CONTROL GROUP			
<3%	8/500 (1.6%)	6/500 (1.2%)	−33% (−28%, 50%)	.79	−250[b]
3%-10%	10/400 (2.5%)	24/400 (6.0%)	58% (14%, 80%)	.02	29
>10%	8/100 (8%)	20/100 (20%)	60% (14%, 82%)	.025	8
Overall	26/1,000 (2.6%)	50/1,000 (5.0%)	48% (17%, 67%)	.007	42

[a]The predicted risk of a fall is based on a score of a fall risk prediction tool. The results are shown in three risk categories to facilitate interpretation, but the risk-stratified analysis to test for heterogeneity of effects should be based on the full continuous scores on the risk prediction tool.

[b]The negative sign indicates the number needed to **harm**; this was not statistically significant.

than creating risk subgroups—unless there are reasons to suspect that the effect of the risk variable is nonlinear; however, results may be easier to communicate in a subgroup format.

When a risk-stratified analysis is possible, it offers many advantages over subgroup analysis for understanding heterogeneity of treatment effects. First, MRS analyses are consistent with the fact that outcomes are affected by multiple independent contributing factors. Second, this analytic approach uses the full sample size because it does not divide the sample into discrete subgroups. This means that MRS analyses almost invariably have superior statistical power to subgroup analyses (Hayward et al., 2006). The results of a risk-stratified MRS analysis provide insights into who best can benefit from an intervention—or who might not be helped very much. In turn, this can help to target interventions to the people for whom they are most likely to be effective.

Heterogeneity in treatment effects can arise for different reasons (Hayward et al., 2006). One is that people differ in their risk for a bad outcome (e.g., a fall) even before any intervention. Risk-stratified analysis is especially useful to help with targeting

decisions in such situations. If, however, HTE reflects differential benefits from the treatment itself, then a subgroup analysis based on a strong theoretical rationale may be advantageous. Thus, Hayward et al. suggest that a risk-stratified analysis should sometimes supplement rather than replace subgroup analyses.

Risk-stratified analyses of trial data are less common than subgroup analyses, but this approach is growing in popularity in medical RCTs. Gabler and colleagues, in their reviews of studies exploring HTE, found only three studies that used MRS in their 2009 review of 319 trials (0.9%), compared to 33 studies in their 2016 review of 416 trials (7.9%). Kent and colleagues (2016) illustrate how such analyses are done, using data from 32 large clinical trials.

TIP MRS analyses offer avenues of opportunity for innovative nursing research. For example, risk-stratified analyses of HTE sometimes can be undertaken as a reanalysis of trial data by researchers not involved in the trial. Another opportunity lies in developing and validating risk prediction tools for outcomes of importance to nursing.

Precision/Personalized Healthcare

A fundamental tenet of **precision healthcare** (a term sometimes used interchangeably with *personalized healthcare* or *stratified healthcare*) is that interventions can be individually tailored to people based on their unique genetic, physiologic, behavioral, lifestyle, and environmental profile. The goal is not necessarily to develop a unique treatment for every individual, but rather to tailor interventions for those with tightly grouped biologic and other features—moving beyond what is possible with risk-stratified analyses. Personalized healthcare is being driven by advances in molecular genomics and is heavily dependent on data linkages and integration, data analytics, and machine learning for the identification of patterns in large datasets (Big Data).

The term *precision healthcare* has been strongly connected with advances in genomics. However, genomics and other "omic" data (e.g., metabolomics, proteomics) are not the only sources of data in personalized healthcare. A wide range of biomarkers, data from EHRs, and data from wearable sensors are examples of data with relevance to precision healthcare, suggesting the inevitability of complex multivariate models that will be needed for mapping dynamic factors that affect individual health (Mutch et al., 2018). Multivariate stratification algorithms using machine learning systems are likely to play an important role.

At present, precision healthcare is only an emerging aspiration rather than a broad reality (Fröhlich et al., 2018) and many challenges remain. However, precision science is advancing rapidly, which bodes well for improving targeted and efficient health care with high levels of applicability. Hickey and colleagues (2019) provide a description of the Nursing Science Precision Health Model.

Example of Nursing Involvement in the National Precision Medicine Initiative

Oruche and colleagues (2016) conducted a study of adolescents with disruptive behavior. One of the goals of the study was to contribute to a statewide cohort assembly as part of the National Precision Medicine Initiative by providing biospecimens (saliva samples) of understudied families to the Indiana Biobank.

TIP Ralph Horwitz and his colleagues, proponents of practice-based evidence, have proposed the development of a large library of patient profiles that could be searched for tailored healthcare decisions for individual patients. The profiles would be derived from EHRs, clinical trials, and longitudinal observational studies. Their view is that the profiles would comprise an "*n* of many" comparison group of patients who have and have not been exposed to many different interventions (e.g., Horwitz & Singer, 2017, 2018).

Reporting Results for Practice-Based Evidence

Enhancing the applicability and relevance of research evidence requires that great care be taken in reporting study results and discussing their implications. We encourage researchers to provide sufficient information in their reports so that readers can make judgments about the utility of the information for individual patients or groups of patients. Here are a few specific suggestions:

- *Begin with an "applicability" attitude.* Committing to applicability as an important goal will likely sharpen efforts to have a strong dissemination plan. Researchers should ask themselves: What would I need to know if I were making a decision about using this evidence? Treweek and Zwarenstein (2009) noted that "trialists can and should report their trials in ways that make it easier for others to make judgements about their applicability" (p. 2).
- *Seek stakeholder input.* An important way to gain perspective on the applicability of the evidence is to involve key stakeholders in planning analyses, interpreting results, and reviewing drafts of reports. An explicit request for feedback on applicability should be made to diverse stakeholders.
- *Disseminate widely.* One way to enhance applicability is to share the evidence broadly. This means making deliberate efforts to disseminate results to various stakeholders (e.g., clinicians, patients, and their families, advocacy groups)—preferably in face-to-face meetings or at conferences. Especially when presenting results to lay audiences, be thoughtful about how results

are presented—for example, talking about the percentage of people who improved rather than mean improvement.

- *Seek opportunities to provide supplementary information.* Page constraints in journals may make it difficult to provide as much information to inform relevance/applicability judgments as desired. Open-access journals (Chapter 32) are often less restrictive in terms of article length than traditional journals, but many traditional journals offer the possibility of online supplements in which more extensive information can be included. Alternatively, researchers can publish a separate paper focused explicitly on study methods, with a focus on methods that enhance both rigor and applicability.
- *Clearly describe the sample.* Research reports almost always describe the research samples on key characteristics, but they may neglect to report important information, such as baseline risk on the primary outcome. If a risk prediction tool is available, it is useful to describe the distribution of risk, which can provide a richer understanding of the sample than one-variable-at-a-time descriptions (e.g., mean age, mean BMI).
- *Clearly describe the target population.* Research reports are not always clear about who the target population was. Users cannot envision the use of evidence in their own settings without understanding the intended population—which needs to be described beyond just stipulating the eligibility criteria. Readers should be able to discern whether the population is similar to the patients in their care.
- *Provide details about the research context.* Potential users of evidence judge the relevance of research evidence not only in terms of the target population but also in terms of the context in which the research was conducted. Rich qualitative descriptions about the study sites should be provided—together with information about how and why the research sites were selected. Make explicit efforts to evaluate whether contextual descriptions are sufficiently "thick," and involve others in this evaluation, if possible. Readers of the report should be able to draw conclusions about whether it would make sense to implement the findings of a study in their own practice setting.

- *Call readers' attention to aspects of the results that relate to applicability.* If possible, include information about the components identified in the PRECIS tool, whether the study is "pragmatic" or not. Also, an effort should be made to call readers' attention to the heterogeneity of the results, not just to "average" results.
- *Provide guidance in the discussion.* The discussion section of the report should emphasize constraints on applicability and generalizability. A discussion about what heterogeneity of effects might mean in terms of clinical decision-making—and future research—can help to shine a spotlight on applicability issues. If subgroup analyses were performed, readers should be cautioned about not overinterpreting their significance, but evidence supporting the consistency of subgroup results should be noted.

MOVING TOWARD PRACTICE-BASED EVIDENCE

The push for evidence-based practice has led to impressive improvements in health care in all health disciplines, and ongoing commitment to EBP is warranted. However, for maximum benefit, efforts to generate evidence based on population models will have to be integrated with evidence for individualized care.

Several forces in health research are converging to encourage greater demand for and interest in evidence that is patient-centered, practice-based, and personalized. These include frustration about the limitations of EBP on the part of many clinicians, the growth of interest in and funding for comparative effectiveness research, and the emerging excitement over opportunities that will become available through precision healthcare research and Big Data initiatives. The messages in this chapter are consistent with the priorities of the Patient-Centered Outcomes Research Institute in the United States—an institute in which nurse researchers have played a big role. For example, two of its research priorities are as follows: Identifying patient differences in response to therapy and Understanding differences in effectiveness across groups (Barksdale et al., 2014).

Conducting rigorous research has never been an easy process, but there have been well-accepted "blueprints" for minimizing bias and coming to conclusions about the quality of the resulting evidence. We are moving into an era that will be even more demanding because person-centered and practice-based evidence require greater creativity and scrupulous vigilance: researchers cannot make findings relevant to real-world settings and applicable to individuals by mechanically following standard "steps" of research. We have provided a few ideas about strategies for moving toward practice-based evidence, but we are confident that many nurse researchers will be inventive in their efforts to make their research relevant and applicable.

TIP We note that interprofessional collaboration is likely to prove vital to the advancement of person-centered research and practice-based evidence. Disciplinary "silos" are likely to be unproductive in efforts to personalize health care.

New challenges and new rewards are in store for those who wish to facilitate patient-centered care based on patient-centered evidence. Thus, the overall message of this chapter to those conducting research is this: Strive to consider in an ongoing way the needs of the users of evidence in planning and designing your studies, analyzing your data, interpreting your results, and reporting your findings.

CRITICAL APPRAISAL OF APPLICABILITY, GENERALIZABILITY, AND RELEVANCE

Box 31.1, included in the Toolkit , provides a few suggestions for those who wish to consider whether researchers have provided sufficient information for coming to conclusions about a study's applicability, generalizability, and relevance. In many cases, the

---

BOX 31.1 Guidelines for Critically Appraising a Study's Applicability, Generalizability, and Relevance*

1. Were patients or other stakeholders involved in co-designing the study? In what way were they involved (e.g., identifying the research question, designing the study, disseminating or using the results?) If there was no such involvement, what steps (if any) did the researcher take to enhance the relevance of the research?
2. Did the researchers mention that the study was comparative effectiveness research? If yes, did the study match the six characteristics of CER described in the text? If the study was a clinical trial, what was the comparator?
3. If the study was a clinical trial, where on the pragmatic-to-explanatory continuum did the trial lie? To what extent was the study conducted in "real-world" circumstances with a broad range of study participants? Did the researchers claim that the trial was pragmatic? Was the PRECIS-2 tool used?
4. To what extent could the measures used in the study be considered *pragmatic?*
5. If the study involved an intervention, did the researchers make any efforts to *tailor* the intervention to individual participants? Was there any effort to *target* the intervention to particular types of people—for example, was an adaptive intervention tested or was an adaptive trial design used?
6. What are some of the constraints on the generalizability of the results? For example, could the study context limit generalizability? Do the eligibility criteria for the sample constrain generalizability? Did a high percentage of people invited to participate in the study decline?
7. Were subgroup effects examined? If yes, were the subgroup analyses done properly (e.g., a priori hypotheses of a small number of subgroup effects; appropriate test for interaction)? Was a multivariable risk-stratified analysis undertaken?
8. Did the Discussion section of the report adequately address the issues of applicability, generalizability, and relevance?

---

*These questions are primarily relevant for quantitative or mixed methods studies, especially for trials of an intervention.

researchers' lack of attention to the issues discussed in this chapter may be disappointing. The absence of information on applicability may reflect page constraints in the journal. It may also reflect the fact that most researchers use conventional standards in preparing their articles—standards that have not taken applicability into account. Moreover, the peer review of most articles is undertaken by researchers who may not yet be attuned to changes taking place in healthcare research. We hope that in the future researchers will do more to help clinicians answer questions about applicability, generalizability, and relevance.

> **TIP** A carefully developed checklist for the appraisal of moderators and predictors (CHAMP) is available to appraise studies with subgroup analyses (van Hoorn et al., 2017). Another useful resource for appraisal is a guideline for reporting pragmatic clinical trials (Zwarenstein et al., 2008).

RESEARCH EXAMPLE

In this section, we present a description of a protocol for a project that incorporated several strategies described in this chapter.

Study: The ACHRU-CPP versus usual care for older adults with type-2 diabetes and multiple chronic conditions and their family caregivers: Study protocol for a randomized controlled trial (Markle-Reid et al., 2017).

Background: An interdisciplinary team in Canada has developed a program of research called the Aging, Community and Health Research Unit (ACHRU). The research program, which is devoted to research on the promotion of optimal aging at home for older adults with multimorbidities, is described by the team as patient-oriented and devoted to interagency and intersectoral partnerships with community-based agencies, policy makers, and health and social service agencies (Markle-Reid et al., 2018).

Program Objectives: The research program has numerous objectives, some of which include: (1) the codesign of integrated and person-centered interventions with older adults, family/friend caregivers, and

providers; (2) the assessment of newly designed interventions; (3) the examination of intervention context and implementation barriers and facilitators; and (4) the development of patient-oriented research strategies. Three pragmatic clinical trials are being undertaken, one of which is described here.

Trial Description: The research team is undertaking the implementation and testing of an intervention for older adults with type-2 diabetes and multiple comorbidities and their family caregivers. The intervention, a 6-month interprofessional, nurse-led program to promote self-management for older patients and to provide support to their caregivers, is being implemented through a community partnership program (CPP). The multicomponent intervention, involving in-home visits and group meetings, will be delivered by nurses and dietitians in coordination with partnering community organizations. Each client is considered "a key member of the care team and is fully engaged in the development of a care plan that is tailored to their individual needs and preferences" (p. 6). The intervention was pilot tested and then modified based on feedback from clients and interventionists.

Methods: The ACHRU-CPP intervention will be tested in two Canadian provinces. The plan is to enroll 160 participants, who will be randomly assigned to either the program or to usual care. The trial design is mixed methods and pragmatic: the program will be implemented under real-world conditions in community settings, including participants' homes. The inclusion criteria "were designed to be minimally stringent in order to facilitate the broad applicability of the results…" (p. 5). The sample size was calculated to detect a minimally important difference in the primary outcome. The primary outcome is the change in clients' physical functioning; secondary outcomes included self-efficacy and changes in mental functioning. Caregiver outcomes include quality of life and depressive symptoms. A wide range of implementation outcomes, many from the RE-AIM framework, will be monitored (e.g., Reach, Maintenance). Qualitative data will be collected to examine program implementation and team collaboration. Dose–response analyses are planned "to better understand the mechanisms underlying the outcome" (p. 9). The researchers will also undertake subgroup analyses to identify which clients benefit most from the treatment. Subgroup hypotheses were not stated, but several possible subgroup variables were identified (e.g., age, gender, number of comorbidities). The subgroup analyses will be conducted for the primary outcome using interaction terms.

SUMMARY POINTS

- The evidence-based practice (EBP) movement has made significant contributions to health care worldwide. However, a variety of forces are combining to demand greater attention to **practice-based evidence**—*patient-centered evidence* from real-world settings that is responsive to the needs and circumstances of specific patients and local contexts.

- EBP is based on evidence about populations of people; it relies heavily on results from randomized controlled trials (RCTs)—which (especially when integrated in systematic reviews) yield **average treatment effects** within the population of interest.

- **Applicability** is the degree to which research evidence can be applied to individuals, small groups of individuals, or local contexts.

- **Generalizability** concerns the ability to extrapolate evidence from samples to a specified population.

- **Relevance**, in the context of this chapter, is the degree to which research evidence is important to key stakeholders and has the potential to be actionable. A key strategy for developing practice-based evidence is to involve stakeholders as co-creators of the research process.

- RCTs are seldom designed with the goals of generalizability or applicability in mind. In traditional **explanatory trials**, researchers value internal validity at the expense of external validity and focus on average effects at the expense of understanding **heterogeneity of treatment effects (HTE)**—individual variation in response to interventions.

- Researchers have begun to address these issues with innovative methodologic strategies, some of which are described in this chapter. In

particular, there is growing interest in **comparative effectiveness research**, whose defining characteristics are in line with person-centered research and practice-based evidence.

- Concerns about explanatory RCTs (e.g., restrictive eligibility criteria, tight controls) have led to the development of **pragmatic clinical trials** that enroll diverse people from real-world settings and are designed to enhance external validity. The degree to which a trial is "pragmatic" can be evaluated using a tool called **PRECIS-2**.

- A strategy called the **multiphase optimization strategy (MOST)** is being used to develop targeted adaptive interventions. **Adaptive interventions** are ones that have multiple decision points, and decisions are based on individual responses. The MOST framework for adaptive interventions often uses a tool called **sequential, multiple assignment, randomized trial (SMART)**, which uses *targeting variables* (e.g., response to an initial intervention) to tailor an intervention in a second round of randomization.

- The ultimate design for individualization is an **N-of-1 trial** (**single-subject experiment**) in which different treatments are tested in an individual or a small number of patients over time. These trials usually are characterized by alternating an active treatment phase and a placebo phase (or alternating two active treatments), such as in an AB or ABAB arrangement.

- Randomized trials are considered the gold standard design for yielding rigorous evidence for EBP, but alternatives (e.g., quasi-experiments, observational designs) have attractive features in the movement toward personalized and precision healthcare. Mixed methods designs also are important for practice-based evidence because they can incorporate rich contextual information and in-depth insights into why "average effects" are misleading and provide clues into sources of variation of effects.

- Sampling strategies for practice-based evidence include clarifying the target population, using purposive sampling strategies, and recruiting a large enough sample for subgroup analyses.

- In terms of data collection, researchers should consider *pragmatic measures*—ones that are important to stakeholders, actionable, and sensitive to change and that minimize response burden (e.g., measures from the Patient-Reported Outcome Measurement Information System or PROMIS®).

- **Big Data** (large complex datasets) potentially can be exploited to improve generalizability of evidence about populations and to improve applicability through the development of predictive models to guide individualized decisions.

- **Subgroup analyses** are efforts to disentangle heterogeneity of treatment effects for subpopulations. Subgroup analyses have been controversial because of risks of both Type I and Type II errors, but guidance for rigorously conducting them has emerged (e.g., prespecification of hypotheses, limiting analyses to a small number of subgroups, testing for interactions).

- In lieu of "one-variable-at-a-time" subgroup analyses, it is sometimes possible to undertake **multivariable risk stratification** that uses a person's score on a multicomponent index of risk rather than a subgroup variable. The results of a risk-stratified analysis can provide insights into who can best benefit from an intervention.

- Advances in technology and research methods, coupled with increased interest in personalized and precision healthcare, will likely advance the promise of practice-based and patient-centered evidence and contribute to its applicability.

REFERENCES CITED IN CHAPTER 31

*Almirall, D., Nahum-Shani, I., Sherwood, N., & Murphy, S. (2014). Introduction to SMART designs for the development of adaptive interventions: With application to weight loss research. *Translational Behavioral Medicine, 4,* 260–274.

Angus, D. C. (2015). Fusing randomized trials with big data. *Journal of the American Medical Association, 314,* 767–768.

*Armstrong, K. (2012). Methods in comparative effectiveness research. *Journal of Clinical Oncology, 34,* 4208–4214.

Assmann, S., Pocock, S., Enos, L., & Kasten, L. (2000). Subgroup analysis and other (mis)uses of baseline data in clinical trials. *The Lancet, 355,* 1064–1069.

*Barksdale, D., Newhouse, R., & Miller, J. (2014). The Patient-Centered Outcomes Research Institute (PCORI): Information for academic nursing. *Nursing Outlook, 62,* 192–200.

Bärnighausen, T., Tugwell, P., Røttingen, J., Shemilt, I., Rockers, P., Geldsetzer, P., …Atun, R. (2017). Quasi-experimental study designs series—paper 4: Uses and value. *Journal of Clinical Epidemiology, 89,* 21–29.

Battaglia, C., & Glasgow, R. (2018). Pragmatic dissemination and implementation research models, methods and measures and their relevance for nursing research. *Nursing Outlook, 66,* 430–445.

Bergstrom, N., Braden, B., Laguzza, A., & Holman, V. (1987). The Braden Scale for predicting pressure sore risk. *Nursing Research, 36,* 205–210.

*Bhatt, D., & Mehta, C. (2016). Adaptive designs for clinical trials. *New England Journal of Medicine, 375,* 65–74.

Biankin, A., Piantadose, S., & Hollingsworth, S. (2015). Patient-centric trials for therapeutic development in precision oncology. *Nature, 526,* 361–370.

*Booth, C., & Tannock, F. (2013). Randomised controlled trials and population-based observational research: Partners in the evolution of medical evidence. *British Journal of Cancer, 110,* 551–555.

*Bowen, M., Cavanaugh, K., Wolff, K., Davis, D., Gregory, R., Shintani, A., … Rothman, R. (2016). The diabetes nutrition education study randomized controlled trial: A comparative effectiveness study of approaches to nutrition in diabetes self-management education. *Patient Education & Counseling, 99,* 1368–1376.

*Burke, J., Sussman, J., Kent, D., & Hayward, R. (2015). Three simple rules to ensure reasonably credible subgroup analyses. *British Medical Journal, 351,* h5651.

*Chapman, A., Browning, C., Enticott, J., Yang, H., Liu, S., Zhang, T., & Thomas, S. (2018). Effect of a health coach intervention for the management of individuals with type 2 diabetes mellitus in China: A pragmatic cluster randomized controlled trial. *Frontiers in Public Health, 6,* 252.

*Collins, L., Nahum-Shani, I., & Almirall, D. (2014). Optimization of behavioral dynamic treatment regimens based on the sequential, multiple assignment, randomized trial (SMART). *Clinical Trials, 11,* 426–434.

*Concannon, T., Fuster, M., Saunders, T., Patel, K., Wong, J., Leslie, L., & Lau, J. (2014). A systematic review of stakeholder engagement in comparative effectiveness and patient-centered outcomes research. *Journal of General Internal Medicine, 29,* 1692–1791.

Concato, J. (2012). Is it time for medicine-based evidence? *Journal of the American Medical Association, 307,* 1641–1643.

Concato, J., & Horwitz, R. (2018). Randomized trials and evidence in medicine. *Social Science & Medicine, 210,* 32–36.

Corwin, E., & Ferranti, E. (2016). Integration of biomarkers to advance precision nursing interventions for family research across the lifespan. *Nursing Outlook, 64,* 292–298.

Dahabreh, I. (2018). Randomization, randomized trials, and analyses using observational data. *Social Science & Medicine, 210,* 41–44.

*Dahabreh, A., Hayward, R., & Kent, D. (2016). Using group data to treat individuals: Understanding heterogeneous treatment effects in the age of precision medicine and patient-centred evidence. *International Journal of Epidemiology, 45*, 2184–2193.

*Dahan, M., Scemama, C., Porcher, R., & Biau, D. (2018). Reporting of heterogeneity of treatment effect in cohort studies: A review of the literature. *BMC Medical Research Methodology, 18*, 10.

*Dai, T., & Shete, S. (2016). Time-varying SMART design and data analysis methods for evaluating adaptive intervention effects. *BMC Medical Research Methodology, 16*, 112.

*Deaton, A., & Cartwright, N. (2018). Understanding and misunderstanding randomized controlled trials. *Social Science & Medicine, 210*, 2–21.

*Deng, X., Yu, T., Hu, A. (2017). Predicting the risk for hospital-acquired pressure ulcers in critical care patients. *Critical Care Nurse, 37*, e1–e11.

Eckardt, P., & Erlanger, A. (2018). Pragmatic study lessons learned: Methods and analyses. *Nursing Outlook, 66*, 446–454.

*Estabrooks, C., Squires, J., Hutchinson, A., Scott, S., Cummins, G., Kang, S., ... Stevens, B. (2011). Assessment of variation in the Alberta Context Tool: The contribution of unit level contextual factors and specialty in Canadian pediatric acute care settings. *BMC Health Services Research, 11*, 251.

Feinstein, A. R. (1998). The problem of cogent subgroups: A clinicostatistical tragedy. *Journal of Clinical Epidemiology, 51*, 297–299.

*Ford, I., & Norrie, J. (2016). The changing face of clinical trials: Pragmatic trials. *New England Journal of Medicine, 375*, 454–463.

*Forsythe, L., Heckert, A., Margolis, M., Schrandt, S., Frank, L. (2018). Methods and impact of engagement in research, from theory to practice and back again. *Quality of Life Research, 27*, 17–31.

*Frieden, T. R. (2017). Evidence for health decision-making: Beyond randomized, controlled trials. *New England Journal of Medicine, 377*, 465–475.

*Fröhlich, H., Balling, R., Beerenwinkel, N., Kohlbacher, O., Kumar, S., Lengauer, T., ... Zupan, B. (2018). From hype to reality: Data science enabling personalized medicine. *BMC Medicine, 16*, 150.

*Gabler, N., Duan, N., Liao, D., Elmore, J., Ganiats, T., & Kravitz, R. (2009). Dealing with heterogeneity of treatment effects: Is the literature up to the challenge? *Trials, 10*, 43.

*Gabler, N., Duan, N., Raneses, E., Suttner, L., Ciarametaro, M. Cooney, E., ... Kravitz, R. (2016). No improvement in the reporting of clinical trial subgroup effects in high-impact general medical journals. *Trials, 17*, 320.

Glasgow, R. E., Magid, D., Beck, A., Ritzwoller, D., & Estabrooks, P. (2005). Practical clinical trials for translating research to practice: Design and measurement recommendations. *Medical Care, 43* 551–557.

Glasgow, R., & Riley, W. (2013). Pragmatic measures: What they are and why we need them. *American Journal of Preventive Medicine, 45*, 237–243.

*Greenfield, S., & Kaplan, S. (2012). Building useful evidence: Changing the clinical research paradigm to account for comparative effectiveness research. *Journal of Comparative Effectiveness Research, 1*, 263–270.

Green, L., & Glasgow, R. (2006). Evaluating the relevance, generalization, and applicability of research. *Evaluation & the Health Professions, 29*, 126–153.

*Greenhouse, J., Kaizar, E., Kelleher, K., Seltman, H., & Gardner, W. (2008). Generalizing from clinical trial data: A case study. *Statistics & Medicine, 27*, 1801–1813.

Gross, D., & Fogg, L. (2001). Clinical trials in the 21st century: The case for participant-centered research. *Research in Nursing & Health, 24*, 530–539.

*Hayward, R., Kent, D., Vijan, S., & Hofer, T. (2006). Multivariable risk prediction can greatly enhance the statistical power of clinical trial subgroup analysis. *BMC Medical Research Methodology, 6*, 18.

*Heckman-Stoddard, B., & Smith, J. (2014). Precision medicine in clinical trials: Defining new treatment strategies. *Seminars in Oncology Nursing, 30*, 109–116.

Hickey, K., Bakken, S., Byrne, M., Bailey, D., Demiris, G., Docherty, S., & Grady, P. (2019). Precision health: Advancing symptom and self-management science. *Nursing Outlook, 67*, 462–475.

*Holtrop, J., Rabin, B., & Glasgow, R. (2018). Qualitative approaches to use of the RE-AIM framework: Rationale and methods. *BMC Health Services Research, 18*, 177.

*van Hoorn, R., Tummers, M., Booth, A., Gerhardus, A., Rehfuess, E., Hind, D., ... Kievet, W. (2017). The development of CHAMP: A checklist for the appraisal of moderators and predictors. *BMC Medical Research Methodology, 17*, 173.

Horwitz, R., Hayes-Conroy, A., Caricchio, R., & Singer, B. (2017). From evidence based medicine to medicine based evidence. *American Journal of Medicine, 130*, 1246–1250.

Horwitz, R., & Singer, B. (2017). Why evidence-based medicine failed in patient care and medicine-based evidence will succeed. *Journal of Clinical Epidemiology, 84*, 14–17.

Horwitz, R., & Singer, B. (2018). Introduction: What works? And for whom? *Social Science & Medicine, 210*, 22–25.

*Institute of Medicine of the National Academies. (2009). *Initial priorities for comparative effectiveness research.* Washington, DC: IOM.

Ioannidis, J. (2018). Randomized controlled trials: Often flawed, mostly useless, clearly indispensable. *Social Science & Medicine, 210*, 53–56.

*Iwashyna, T., & Liu, V. (2014). What's so different about Big Data? *Annals of the American Thoracic Society, 11*, 1130–1135.

Kaiser, L. D. (2016). Stratification of randomization is not required for a pre-specified subgroup analysis. *Pharmaceutical Statistics, 12*, 43–47.

*Kent, D., Nelson, J., Dahabreh, I., Rothwell, P., Altman, D., & Hayward, R. (2016). Risk and treatment effect heterogeneity: Re-analysis of individual participant data from 32 large clinical trials. *International Journal of Epidemiology, 45*, 2075–2088.

*Kent, D., Rothwell, P., Ioannidis, J., Altman, D., & Hayward, R. (2010). Assessing and reporting heterogeneity in treatment effects in clinical trials. *Trials, 11*, 85.

*Klasnja, P., Hekler, E., Shiffman, S., Boruvka, A., Almirall, S., Tewari, A., & Murphy, S. (2015). Micro-randomized trials: An experimental design for developing just-in-time adaptive interventions. *Health Psychology, 34*, 1220–1228.

Knottnerus, J., Tugwell, P., & Tricco, A. (2016). Individual patients are the primary source and the target of clinical research. *Journal of Clinical Epidemiology, 76*, 1–3.

Kraemer, H., Frank, E., & Kupfer, D. (2006). Moderators of treatment outcomes: Clinical, research, and policy importance. *Journal of the American Medical Association, 296*, 1286–1289.

*Kravitz, R. L., & Duan, N. (2014). *Design and implementation of N-of-1 trials: A user's guide*. Washington, DC: Agency for Healthcare Research and Quality.

*Kroenke, K., Monahan, P., & Kean, J. (2015). Pragmatic characteristics of patient-reported outcome measures are important for use in clinical practice. *Journal of Clinical Epidemiology, 68*, 1085–1092.

*Lei, H., Naum-Shani, I., Lynch, K., Oslin, D., & Murphy, S. (2012). A "SMART" design for building individualized treatment sequences. *Annual Review of Clinical Psychology, 8*, 21–48.

Lincoln, Y., & Guba, E. (1985). *Naturalistic inquiry*. Beverly Hills, CA: Sage.

*Lin, P., Grambow, S., Intille, S., Gallis, J., Lazenka, T., Bosworth, H., … Svetkey, L. (2018). The association between engagement and weight loss through personal coaching and cell phone interventions in young adults. *JMIR mHealth and uHealth, 6*, e10471.

Littleton-Kearney, M. (2018). Pragmatic clinical trials at the National Institute of Nursing Research. *Nursing Outlook, 66*, 470–472.

*Loudon, K., Treweek, S., Sullivan, F., Donnan, P., Thorpe, K., & Zwarenstein, M. (2015). The PRECIS-2 tool: Designing trials that are fit for purpose. *British Medical Journal, 350*, h2147.

*Lyles, C., Lunn, M., Obedin-Maliver, J., & Bibbins-Domingo, K. (2018). The new era of precision population health: Insights from the All of Us Research Program and beyond. *Journal of Translational Medicine, 16*, 211.

*Markle-Reid, M., Ploeg, J., Fraser, K., Fisher, K., Akhtar-Danesh, N., Bartholomew, A., … Upshur, R. (2017). The ACHRU-CPP versus usual care for older adults with type-2 diabetes and multiple chronic conditions and their family caregivers: Study protocol for a randomized controlled trial. *Trials, 18*, 55.

*Markle-Reid, M., Ploeg, J., Valaitis, R., Duggleby, W., Fisher, K., Fraser, K., … Williams, A. (2018). Protocol for a program of research from the Aging, Community and Health Research Unit: Promoting optimal aging at home for older adults with comorbidities. *Journal of Comorbidity, 8*, 1–16.

*Marko, N., & Weil, R. (2010). The role of observational investigations in comparative effectiveness research. *Value in Health, 13*, 989–997.

*Mutch, D., Zulyniak, M., Rudkowska, I., & Tejero, M. (2018). Lifestyle genomics: Addressing the multifactorial nature of personalized health. *Lifestyle Genomics, 1*, 1–8.

**Newhouse, R., Barksdale, & Miller, J. (2015). The Patient-Centered Outcomes Research Institute: Research done differently. *Nursing Research, 64*, 72–77.

Nguyen, H., Moy, M., Fan, V., Gould, M., Xiang, A., Bailey, A., … Coleman, K. (2018). Applying the pragmatic-explanatory continuum indicator summary to the implementation of a physical activity coaching trial in chronic obstructive pulmonary disease. *Nursing Outlook, 66*, 455–463.

Oruche, U., Carpenter, J., Renbarger, J., & Ross, S. (2016). Raising the level of nursing involvement in the National Precision Medicine Initiative. *Journal of Child and Adolescent Psychiatric Nursing, 29*, 85–88.

*Pallmann, P., Bedding, A., Choodari-Oskooei, B., Dimairo, M., Flight, L., Hampson, L., … Jaki, T. (2018). Adaptive designs in clinical trials: Why use them, and how to run and report them. *BMC Medicine, 16*, 29.

Patton, M. Q. (2015). *Qualitative research & evaluation methods* (4th ed.). Thousand Oaks, CA: Sage.

Polit, D. F., & Beck, C. T. (2010). Generalization in quantitative and qualitative research: Myths and strategies. *International Journal of Nursing Studies, 47*, 1451–1458.

Punja, S., Bukutu, C., Shamseer, L., Sampson, M., Hartling, L., Urichuk, L., & Vohra, S. (2016). N-of-1 trials are a tapestry of heterogeneity. *Journal of Clinical Epidemiology, 76*, 47–56.

Rockers, P., Tugwell, P., Røttingen, J., & Bärnighausen, T. (2017). Quasi-experimental study designs series—paper 13: Realizing the full potential of quasi-experiments for health research. *Journal of Clinical Epidemiology, 89*, 106–110.

Rolfe, G. (2009). Complexity and uniqueness in nursing practice. *International Journal of Nursing Studies, 46*, 1156–1158.

Rothwell, P. M. (2005a). Subgroup analysis in randomised controlled trials: Importance, indications, and interpretation. *The Lancet, 365*, 176–186.

Rothwell, P. M. (2005b). External validity of randomised controlled trials: "To whom do the results of this trial apply?" *The Lancet, 365*, 82–93.

*Rothwell, P. M. (2006). Factors that can affect the external validity of randomised controlled trials. *PLoS Clinical Trials, 1*, e9.

Rothwell, O. M., Mehta, Z., Howard, S., Gutnikov, S., & Warlow, C. (2005). From subgroups to individuals: General principles and the example of carotid endarterectomy. *The Lancet, 365*, 256–265.

Rycroft-Malone, J. (2012). Implementing evidence-based practice in the reality of clinical practice. *Worldviews on Evidence-Based Nursing, 9*, 1.

*Sacristán, J., & Dilla, T. (2018). Pragmatic trials revisited: Applicability is about individualization. *Journal of Clinical Epidemiology, 99*, 164–166.

Schork, N. J. (2018). Randomized clinical trials and personalized medicine. *Social Science & Medicine, 210*, 71–73.

Sikorskii, A., Wyatt, G., Lehto, R., Victorson, D., Badger, T., & Pace, T. (2017). Using SMART design to improve symptom management among cancer patients: A study protocol. *Research in Nursing & Health, 40*, 501–511.

Sofolahan-Oladeinde, Y., Newhouse, R., Lavallee, D. C., Huang, J. C., & Mullins, C. D. (2017). Early assessment of the 10-step patient engagement framework for patient-centred outcomes research studies. *Family Practice, 34*, 272–277.

*Strahan, B., & Elder, J. (2015). Video game playing effects on obesity in an adolescent with autism spectrum disorder. *Autism Research and Treatment, 2015*, 128365.

Subramanian, S., Kim, N., & Christakis, N. (2018). The "average" treatment effect: A construct ripe for retirement. *Social Science & Medicine, 210*, 77–82.

*Sun, X., Briel, M., Busse, J., Akl, E., Mejza, F., Bala, M., ... Guyatt, G. (2012). Credibility of claims of subgroup effects in randomised controlled trials: A systematic review. *British Medical Journal, 344*, e1553.

Sun, X., Ioannidis, J., Agoritsas, T., Alba, A., & Guyatt, G. (2014). How to use a subgroup analysis: Users' guide to the medical literature. *Journal of the American Medical Association, 311*, 405–411.

*Tanniou, J., van der Tweel, I., Teerenstra, S., & Roes, K. (2016). Subgroup analyses in confirmatory clinical trials: Time to be specific about their purposes. *BMC Medical Research Methodology, 16*, 20.

*Treweek, S., & Zwarenstein, M. (2009). Making trials matter: Pragmatic and explanatory trials and the problem of applicability. *Trials, 10*, 37.

Tunis, S. R., Stryer, D., & Clancy, C. (2003) Practical clinical trials: Increasing the value of clinical research for decision making in clinical and health policy. *Journal of the American Medical Association, 290*, 1624–1632.

Vohra, S. (2016). N-of-1 trials to enhance patient outcomes: Identifying effective therapies and reducing harms, one patient at a time. *Journal of Clinical Epidemiology, 76*, 6–8.

*Wang, W., & Krishnan, E. (2014). Big data and clinicians: A review of the state of the science. *Journal of Medical Informatics, 1*, e1.

*Wang, R., & Ware, J. (2013). Detecting moderator effects using subgroup analyses. *Prevention Science, 14*, 111–120.

Wilbur, J., Kolanowski, A., & Collins, L. (2016). Utilizing MOST frameworks and SMART designs for intervention research. *Nursing Outlook, 64*, 287–289.

Yoon, S., Schwartz, J., Burg, M., Kronish, I., Alcantara, C., Julian, J., ... Diaz, K. (2018). Using behavioral analytics to increase exercise: A randomized N-of-1 study. *American Journal of Preventive Medicine, 54*, 559–567.

*Zwarenstein, M., Treweek, S., Gagnier, J., Altman, D., Tunis, S., Haynes, B., ... Moher, D. (2008). Improving the reporting of pragmatic trials: An extension of the CONSORT statement. *British Medical Journal, 337*, a2390.

A link to this open-access article is provided in the Toolkit for Chapter 31 in the **Resource Manual.** ✪

**This journal article is available on thePoint *for this chapter.*

32 | Disseminating Evidence: Reporting Research Findings

No study is complete until the findings have been shared with others. This chapter offers guidance on disseminating research results. Several books on publishing research findings offer further assistance (e.g., Lang, 2010; Oermann & Hays, 2016; Wager, 2016). Also, the *American Journal of Nursing* published four articles that take nurses through the publication process (Roush, 2017a, 2017b, 2017c, 2017d).

GETTING STARTED ON DISSEMINATION

Researchers consider various issues in developing a dissemination plan, as we discuss in this section.

Selecting a Communication Medium and Outlet

Researchers can communicate their findings orally or in writing. Oral presentations (typically at professional conferences) can be a formal talk in front of an audience or integrated with written material in a *poster session*. Major advantages of conference presentations are that they can be done soon after study completion (or while it is in progress) and they offer opportunities for dialogue with people interested in the topic. Written reports can take the form of theses/dissertations or journal articles published in traditional or open-access journals. A major advantage of journal articles, especially ones that are open-access, is worldwide accessibility. Our advice is relevant for most types of dissemination, but publication in journals is featured.

Knowing the Audience

Good research communication requires researchers to think about the audience they hope to reach. Here are some questions to consider:

1. Will the audience be nurses only, or will it likely include professionals from other disciplines (e.g., physicians, psychologists, physical therapists)?
2. Will the audience be researchers, or will it include clinicians or other professionals (e.g., health care policy makers)?
3. Are patients or other lay people a potential audience?
4. Will the audience include people whose native language is not English?
5. Will reviewers, editors, and readers be experts in the field?

Researchers often write with multiple audiences in mind, which means writing clearly and avoiding technical jargon to the extent possible. It also means that researchers sometimes must develop a multiprong strategy—for example, publishing a report for researchers in a journal such *Nursing Research*, and then publishing a summary for clinicians in a specialty publication or an institutional newsletter.

> **TIP** Oermann and colleagues (2006) offer suggestions about presenting research results to clinical audiences. Their advice may also be useful if the audience includes patients.

Although writing for a broad audience may be a goal, it is also important to keep in mind the needs of the *main* intended audience. If the readers are mostly clinical nurses, it is essential to explain what the findings mean for practice. If the audience is administrators or policy makers, information should be included about implications for such outcomes as *cost* and *accessibility*. If researchers are the primary audience, information about methodologic strategies, study limitations, and implications for future research should be provided.

Developing a Plan

Before writing a report, researchers should have a plan, part of which involves how best to coordinate the actual tasks of preparing a **manuscript** (i.e., an unpublished paper).

Deciding on Authorship

When a study is undertaken by a team, division of labor and authorship must be addressed. The International Committee of Medical Journal Editors (ICMJE, 2017) advises that authorship credit should be based on (1) making a substantial contribution to the study's conception and design, or to data acquisition, data analysis, and interpretation; (2) drafting or revising the manuscript for intellectual content; (3) approving the final version of the manuscript to be published; and (4) agreeing to be accountable for all aspects of the work.

The **lead author**, usually the first-named author, has overall responsibility for the report. The lead author and co-authors should reach an agreement in advance about responsibilities for producing the manuscript. To avoid possible conflicts, they should also decide beforehand the order of authors' names. Ethically, it is most appropriate to list names in the order of authors' contribution to the work, not according to status. When contributions of co-authors are comparable, an alphabetical

listing is appropriate. The editorial board of the *Western Journal of Nursing Research* has prepared guidelines for co-authorship (Conn et al., 2015), as has the past editor of *Research in Nursing & Health* (Kearney, 2014).

> **TIP** A taxonomy called Contributor Roles Taxonomy (CRediT) has been created to help people identify specific author contributions to scholarly written work. A link to an article about CRediT is available in the Toolkit in the *Resource Manual* ⊗. A similar tool has been proposed by Clement (2014).

Deciding on Content

In many studies, more data are collected than can be presented in one report, and multiple publications are thus possible. And, if there are multiple research questions, more than one paper may be required to communicate results adequately. In such situations, an early decision involves which findings to present in a given paper. In mixed methods (MM) research, separate reports are sometimes needed to summarize qualitative and quantitative findings—although there should also be a report integrating findings from both strands.

It is, however, inappropriate and even unethical to write several papers when one would suffice—a practice that has been called "salami slicing" (Jackson et al., 2014). Each paper from a study should make an independent contribution. Editors, reviewers, and readers expect original work, so unnecessary overlap should be avoided. It is also unethical to submit essentially the same or similar paper to two journals simultaneously. Oermann and Hays (2016) offer guidelines regarding duplicate and redundant publications, and Happell (2016) provides practical tips for dealing with multiple papers from one dataset.

Assembling Materials

Planning also involves assembling the materials needed to begin a draft, including information about manuscript requirements. Traditional and online journals issue guidelines for authors, and these guidelines should be retrieved and understood.

Other materials also need to be gathered, including relevant literature; details about instruments used in the study; descriptions of the study sample; output of computer analyses; relevant analytic memos or reflexive notes; figures or photographs that illustrate some aspect of the study; and permissions to use copyrighted materials. Style manuals that provide information about both grammar and language use (e.g., Strunk & Campbell, 2018) are important tools, as are specific guides for writing professional and scientific papers (e.g., American Psychological Association, 2020; ICMJE, 2017).

> **TIP** For authors whose native language is not English but who plan to submit their work to an English-language journal, a review of the manuscript by someone proficient in English is advisable. For authors from developing countries, assistance may be available through AuthorAID (www.authoraid. info/en/).

Finally, a written outline and a timeline should be developed, especially if there are multiple co-authors who have responsibility for different sections of the paper. The overall outline and individual assignments, together with due dates, should be developed collaboratively.

Writing Effectively

Many people have a hard time putting their ideas down on paper. It is beyond the scope of this book to teach good writing skills, but we can offer a few suggestions. One suggestion, quite simply, is: *do it*. Get in the habit of writing, even if it is only 15 minutes a day. *Writer's block* is probably responsible for thousands of unfinished (or never-started) manuscripts each year. So, just begin somewhere, and keep at it regularly—writing gets easier with practice.

Writing *well* is, of course, important, and several resources offer suggestions on how to write compelling sentences, select good words, and organize your ideas effectively (e.g., Zinsser, 2006). It is usually better to write a draft in its entirety, and then go back later to rewrite awkward

sentences, correct errors, reorganize, and generally polish it up.

In a survey of 61 nursing journal editors, Northam and colleagues (2014) found that the two most common reasons for rejecting a manuscript were that (1) the article provided no new information and (2) it was poorly written. A frequently mentioned suggestion by these editors was to have others review the manuscript before submitting it. In another survey of 53 editors, Kennedy and colleagues (2017) reported common problems that editors found in student papers submitted to journals, such as failure to follow author guidelines, poor writing, and insufficient detail. Griffiths and Norman (2016) also noted that poor writing is a common concern of peer reviewers of papers submitted to the *International Journal of Nursing Studies*.

> **TIP** It should go without saying that plagiarism should be avoided. In some cases, this means avoiding "plagiarizing" yourself. Most journals now have powerful plagiarism detection software that will trigger an editorial response, and you may be asked to rewrite sentences that you "lifted" from your own prior publications.

CONTENT OF RESEARCH REPORTS

Research reports vary in terms of audience, purpose, and length. Theses or dissertations document students' ability to perform scholarly work and therefore tend to be long. Journal articles, by contrast, are short because they compete for limited journal space and are read by busy professionals. Nevertheless, the form and content of research reports are often similar. Chapter 3 summarized the major sections of research reports, and here we offer a few additional tips. Distinctions among various kinds of reports are described later in the chapter.

Quantitative Research Reports

Quantitative reports typically follow the **IMRAD format**, which involves organizing content into four sections—the **I**ntroduction, **M**ethod, **R**esults, **and**

Discussion. These sections, respectively, address the following questions:

- Why was the study done? (I)
- How was the study done? (M)
- What was learned? (R)
- What does it mean? (D)

The Introduction

The introduction acquaints readers with the research problem, its significance, and its context. The introduction sets the stage by describing existing literature, the study's conceptual framework, the problem, research questions, or hypotheses, and the study rationale. Although the introduction includes multiple components, it should be concise. A common critique of research manuscripts by reviewers is that the introduction is too long.

Introductions are often written in a funnel-shaped structure, beginning broadly to establish a framework for understanding the study and then narrowing to the specifics of what researchers sought to learn. The end point of the introduction should be a succinct delineation of the research questions or hypotheses, which provides a good transition to the method section.

> **TIP** An up-front, clearly stated problem statement is of immense value. The first paragraph should be written with special care, because the goal is to grab readers' attention.

The introduction typically includes a summary of related research to provide a pertinent context. Except for dissertations, the literature review should be a brief summary, not an exhaustive review. The summary should make clear what is known and what the deficiencies are, thus helping to clarify the contribution of the new study.

The introduction also should describe the study's theoretical or conceptual framework. The framework should be sufficiently explained so that readers who are unfamiliar with it can understand its main thrust.

The various background strands need to be convincingly and cogently interwoven to persuade readers that, in fact, the new study holds promise for adding evidence important to nursing. The introduction, in other words, lays out the *argument* for new research.

> **TIP** Many journals articles begin without an explicit heading labeled *Introduction*. In general, all the material before the method section is considered the introduction. Some introductions include subheadings such as *Literature Review* or *Hypotheses*.

The Method Section

To critically appraise the quality of a study's evidence, readers need to know exactly what methods were used to answer research questions. In traditional dissertations, the method section should provide sufficient detail that another researcher could replicate the study. In journal articles and conference presentations, the method section is condensed, but the degree of detail should permit readers to draw conclusions about the integrity of the findings. Faulty method sections are a leading cause of manuscript rejection by journals. Your job in writing the method section of a quantitative report is to persuade readers that evidence from your study is sufficiently robust to merit consideration.

> **TIP** The method section is often subdivided into several parts, which helps readers to locate vital information. As an example, the method section might contain the following subsections: Research Design; Sample; Data Collection Instruments; Procedures; and Data Analysis.

The method section usually begins with the description of the research design. The design is often given detailed coverage in clinical trials, with information about what specific design was adopted, how participants were assigned to groups, and whether and with whom blinding was used. Reports for studies with multiple points of data collection should indicate the number of times data were collected and the amount of time elapsed between those points. In all types of quantitative studies, it is important to identify the methods used to control confounding variables. The method section also addresses steps taken to safeguard participants' rights.

Readers also need to know about study participants. This subsection (which may be labeled *Research Sample*, *Subjects*, or *Study Participants*) normally specifies the eligibility criteria, to clarify the population to whom results can be generalized. The method of sample selection and its rationale, recruitment techniques, and sample size should be indicated. If a power analysis was undertaken to estimate sample size needs, this should be described. There should also be information about response rates and, if possible, about response bias (or attrition bias, if this is relevant). Basic characteristics of study participants (e.g., age, gender, health status) should also be described—although this is sometimes presented in the results section.

> **TIP** Readers who are interested in using study evidence in practice need to learn not only about characteristics of the sample, but also about key contextual features so they can judge whether study findings are relevant in their setting.

Data collection methods, another critical component of the method section, may be presented in a subsection called *Instruments*, *Measures*, or *Data Collection*. A description of study instruments, and a rationale for their use, should be provided. If instruments were constructed specifically for the project, the report should describe their development. Any special equipment that was used (e.g., to gather biomarker data) should be described, including information about the manufacturer. The report should also indicate who collected the data (e.g., the authors, research assistants, staff nurses) and how they were trained. The report must convince readers that data collection methods were sound. Information relating to data quality, and procedures used to evaluate reliability and validity, should be described.

In intervention research, there is usually a procedures subsection with information about the intervention. What exactly did the intervention entail? How and by whom was the treatment administered? What was the control group condition? How much time elapsed between the intervention and measurement of the outcome? How was intervention fidelity monitored?

Analytic procedures are also described in the method section. It is usually sufficient to identify the statistical tests used; formulas or references for commonly used statistics such as a multiple regression are not necessary. For unusual procedures, a technical reference justifying the approach should be noted. If confounding variables were controlled statistically, the variables controlled should be identified. The level of significance is typically set at .05 for two-tailed tests, which may not be stated; however, if a different significance level or one-tailed tests were used, this must be specified.

Explicit guidelines for reporting key information for various types of studies are now available (Table 32.1). The most well known is the Consolidated Standards of Reporting Trials or **CONSORT guideline**. This guideline focuses on reporting information about RCTs; extensions have been developed for specific designs, such as cluster randomized trials and pilot trials. The CONSORT guideline, included in the Toolkit, has been adopted by most major medical and nursing journals; it includes a checklist of 25 pieces of information to include in reports of RCTs (Moher et al., 2010) ⊗. The CONSORT website (www.consort-statement.org) offers an interactive checklist with detailed information about checklist components. A special reporting guideline has been prepared for pragmatic trials (Zwarenstein et al., 2008), which should be scrutinized by those interested in enhancing the applicability of their findings.

> **TIP** Reporting guidelines are also available for manuscripts using the style of the American Psychological Association (APA), a style used by many nursing journals. (A list of citation-related websites is included in the Toolkit. ⊗)

TABLE 32.1 • Reporting Guidelines for Various Types of Papers

TYPE OF STUDY	GUIDELINE
Parallel group randomized controlled trials (RCTs)	CONSORT[a]: CONsolidated Standards Of Reporting Trials (Moher et al., 2010)
Development and evaluation of complex interventions in health care	CReDECI 2: Criteria for Reporting the Development and Evaluation of Complex Interventions (Möhler et al., 2015)
Description of features of an intervention	TIDieR: Template for Intervention Description and Replication (Hoffman et al., 2014)
Protocols for clinical trials	SPIRIT: Standard Protocol Items: Recommendations for Interventional Trials (Chan et al., 2013)
Evaluations of interventions using quasi-experimental designs	TREND: Transparent Reporting of Evaluations with Nonrandomized Designs (Des Jarlais et al., 2004)
Nonexperimental (observational) studies	STROBE: Strengthening the Reporting of Observational Studies in Epidemiology (von Elm et al., 2014)
Implementation studies of complex interventions	StaRI: Standards for Reporting Implementation studies (Pinnock et al., 2017)
Observational studies using routinely collected health data	RECORD: Reporting of studies Conducted using Observational Routine-collected health Data (Benchimol et al., 2015)
Qualitative studies	SRQR: Standards for Reporting Qualitative Research (O'Brien et al., 2014)
Qualitative studies (focus groups and interview studies)	COREQ: COnsolidated criteria for REporting Qualitative research (Tong et al., 2007)
Studies of measurement reliability and agreement	GRRAS: Guidelines for Reporting Reliability and Agreement Studies (Kottner et al., 2011)
Diagnostic accuracy studies	STARD: Standards for Reporting of Diagnostic accuracy (Cohen et al., 2016)
Health care quality improvement studies	SQUIRE 2: Standards for QUality Improvement Reporting Excellence (Ogrinc et al., 2015)
Health economic evaluations	CHEERS: Consolidated Health Economic Evaluation Reporting Standards (Husereau et al., 2013)
Meta-analyses of RCTs	PRISMA[b]: Preferred Reporting Items for Systematic Reviews and Meta-Analyses (Moher et al., 2009)
Meta-analysis of observational studies	MOOSE: Meta-analysis Of Observational Studies in Epidemiology (Stroup et al., 2000)
Synthesis of qualitative research	ENTREQ: ENhancing Transparency in REporting the synthesis of Qualitative research (Tong et al., 2012)

[a]CONSORT extensions are available for several types of design-specific trials, such as the following: Pilot and feasibility trials (Eldridge et al., 2016); N-of-1 trials (Vohra et al., 2016); within-person (crossover) trials (Pandis et al., 2017); pragmatic trials (Zwarenstein et al., 2008); noninferiority and equivalence trials (Piaggio et al., 2012); cluster randomized trials (Campbell et al., 2012); trials of nonpharmacological interventions (Boutron et al., 2008); trials with patient reported outcomes (Calvert et al., 2013); and trials for psychological interventions (Montgomery et al., 2013).

[b]Numerous extensions of PRISMA have been developed. See http://www.equator-network.org/reporting-guidelines/prisma/.

Several guidelines recommend inclusion of a flow chart to track participants through a study, from eligibility screening through analysis of outcomes. Flow charts should be as detailed as possible, within space constraints, about reasons for losing participants during the study. Figure 32.1 provides an example of such a flow chart for a randomized controlled trial (RCT). This chart summarizes withdrawals from the intervention, as well as participant losses during follow-up. It also shows that data for all participants were analyzed in an intention-to-treat analysis, which is recommended in CONSORT (Polit & Gillespie, 2010).

In response to critiques about inadequate reporting of intervention features (e.g., Conn et al., 2008; Glasziou et al., 2008), several relevant guidelines have emerged. The **CReDECI** guidelines (Möhler et al., 2015) offer criteria for reporting the phases researchers have undertaken in developing, piloting, and evaluating complex interventions. CReDECI is useful for providing information about the *processes* of intervention research. The **TIDieR**

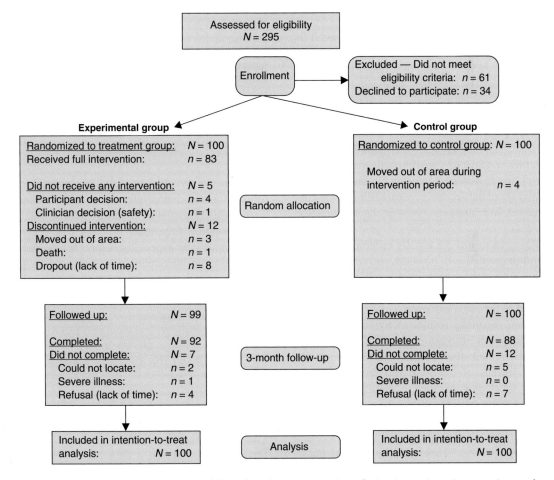

Figure 32.1 Example of CONSORT guidelines flowchart: progression of participants in an intervention study.

guidelines (Hoffmann et al., 2014) offer a template for a thorough description of interventions. Key intervention features should always be summarized in a report of a trial, but a separate article describing the intervention in greater detail might be needed.

> **TIP** Guidelines for various types of studies are regularly being updated or expanded. The EQUATOR Network (www.equator-network.org) is a useful resource for information on reporting guidelines and for tips on good reporting in health studies; it offers resources in Spanish and other languages. A list of resources for writing and disseminating research is included in the Toolkit ⊗.

The Results Section

Readers scrutinize the method section to learn if the study was done with rigor, but the results section is the heart of the report. In a quantitative study, the results of the statistical analyses are summarized in a factual manner. Descriptive statistics are ordinarily presented first, to provide an overview of study variables. If key research questions involve comparing groups with regard to dependent variables (e.g., in an experimental or case–control study), the results section often begins with information about the groups' comparability on baseline variables, so readers can evaluate the risk of selection bias.

Research results are usually ordered in terms of overall importance. If, however, research questions or hypotheses have been numbered in the introduction, the analyses addressing them should be ordered in the same sequence.

When reporting results of hypothesis-testing statistical tests, three pieces of information are typically stated: the value of the calculated statistic, degrees of freedom, and the exact probability level. For instance, a report might state, "Patients who received the intervention were significantly less likely to develop decubitus ulcers than patients in the control group (χ^2 = 8.23, df = 1, p = .008)." However, the current publication manual of the American Psychological Association (2020) urges authors to report confidence intervals: "Because confidence intervals

combine information on location and precision and can often be directly used to infer significance levels, they are, in general, the best reporting strategy" (p. 34). The manual also strongly encourages reporting effect sizes, which can facilitate meta-analyses.

When results from several statistical analyses are reported, they should be summarized in a **table**. Good tables, with precise titles, headings, and footnotes, are an important way to avoid dull, repetitive statements. When tables are used, the text should refer to the table by number (e.g., "As shown in Table 2, patients in the intervention group…"). Box 32.1 presents some suggestions regarding the construction of effective statistical tables. The table templates in the Toolkit (Chapters 17-19) can help you create clear and concise tables ⊗.

> **TIP** Do not simply repeat statistical information in text and tables. Tables should display information that would be monotonous to present in the text—and to display it in such a way that patterns are evident. The text can be used to highlight major findings.

Figures may also be used to communicate results. Figures that display the results in graphic form are used less as an economy than as a means of dramatizing important findings and relationships. Figures are especially helpful for displaying information on phenomenon over time or for portraying conceptual or empirical models.

> **TIP** Research evidence does not constitute *proof* of anything, and so the report should never claim that the data proved, verified, confirmed, or demonstrated that hypotheses were correct or incorrect. Hypotheses are supported or not supported, accepted or rejected.

The Discussion Section

The discussion section is devoted to a thoughtful (and, hopefully, insightful) analysis of the findings and their clinical and theoretical utility. A typical discussion section addresses the following

BOX 32.1 Guidelines for Preparing Statistical Tables

1. Number tables so they can be referenced in the text.
2. Give tables a brief but clear explanatory title.
3. Avoid both overly simple tables with information more efficiently presented in the text, and overly complex tables that intimidate or confuse readers.
4. Arrange data in such a way that patterns are obvious at a glance.
5. Give each column and row of data a heading that is succinct but clear. Table headings should establish the logic of the table structure.
6. Express data values to the number of decimal places justified by the precision of the measurement. In general, it is preferable to report numbers to one decimal place (or to two decimal places for correlation coefficients) because rounded values are easier to absorb than more precise ones. Report all values in a table to the same level of precision.
7. Make each table a "stand-alone" presentation, capable of being understood without referring to the text.
8. Indicate probability levels, either as actual p values or with confidence intervals. In correlation matrixes, use the system of asterisks with a probability level footnote. The usual convention is one asterisk when $p < .05$, two when $p < .01$, and three when $p < .001$.
9. Indicate units of measurement for numbers in the table whenever appropriate (e.g., pounds, milligrams).
10. Use footnotes to explain abbreviations or special symbols used in the table, except commonly understood abbreviations such as N.

questions: What were the main findings? What do the findings mean? What evidence is there that the results and the interpretations are valid? What limitations might threaten validity? How do the results compare with prior knowledge on the topic? What are the implications of the findings for future research? What are the implications for nursing practice?

TIP The discussion is often the most challenging section to write. It deserves your most intense intellectual effort—and careful review by peers. Peers should be asked to comment on how reasonable your inferences are, how well organized the section is, and whether it is too long—a common flaw. Griffiths and Norman (2016) noted that faulty conclusions are a common reason for rejecting manuscripts submitted to the *International Journal of Nursing Studies.*

Typically, the discussion section begins with a summary of key findings. The summary should be brief, however, because the focus of the discussion is on making sense of (and not merely repeating) the results.

Interpretation of results is a global process, encompassing the findings, methodologic strengths and limitations, sample characteristics, related research findings, clinical and contextual aspects, and theoretical issues. Researchers should justify their interpretations, stating why alternative explanations have been ruled out. If the findings conflict with those of earlier studies, tentative explanations should be offered. The generalizability of study findings should also be discussed.

Implications of study findings are speculative and so should be couched in tentative terms, as in the following example: "The results *suggest* that nurses' communication about advanced directives is inconsistent, and that nurses' years of experience affect the nature and amount of communication." The interpretation is, in essence, a hypothesis that can be tested in another study. The discussion should include recommendations for testing such hypotheses.

Finally, implications of the findings for nursing practice need to be discussed. Are aspects of the evidence clinically significant—and if so how might the evidence be used by nurses? The importance of addressing implications for nursing practice has been discussed by the editors of several nursing journals (e.g., Becker, 2009; Gennaro, 2010).

Other Aspects of the Report

The materials covered in the four IMRAD sections are found in some form in most quantitative research reports. Other aspects of the report deserve mention.

Title. Every research report needs a title articulating the nature of the study. Insofar as possible, the independent variables and outcomes (or central constructs under study) should be named in the title. It is also desirable to indicate the study population. Yet, the title should be brief (no more than about 15 words), so writers must balance clarity with brevity. The length of titles can often be reduced by omitting unnecessary terms such as "A Study of…" or "An Investigation to Examine the Effects of…" The title should communicate concisely what was studied and stimulate interest in the research. A few journals, however, such as the *International Journal of Nursing Studies* (IJNS), request that the basic method or design be stated in the title, often after a colon. For example, Markopoulos and colleagues (2019) published a paper in IJNS titled "Bladder training prior to urinary catheter removal in total joint arthroplasty: A randomized controlled trial."

Abstract. Research reports usually include abstracts—brief descriptions of the problem, methods, and findings of the study, written so that readers can decide whether to read the entire report. As noted in Chapter 3, journal abstracts are sometimes written as an unstructured paragraph of 100 to 200 words, or in a structured form with subheadings. Pearce and Ferguson (2017) offer tips on writing strong abstracts.

> **TIP** Take the time to write a compelling abstract, which is your first main point of contact with reviewers and readers. It should convey that your study is important clinically and that it was done with conceptual and methodologic rigor. The abstract should contain words that will help people find your paper if they search for articles on your topic.

Keywords. It is often necessary to include keywords that will be used in databases to help others locate your study. Sometimes authors are given a list of keywords from which to choose (often Medical Subject Headings or MeSH terms), but additional keywords sometimes can be added. Substantive, methodologic, and theoretical terms can be used as keywords.

References. Each report concludes with a list of references cited in the text, using a reference style specified by the journal or institution. References can be cumbersome to prepare, but software can facilitate the preparation of reference lists (e.g., EndNote, ProCite, Reference Manager, Format Ease). Penders (2018) offers some guidance on responsible referencing.

Acknowledgments. People who helped with the research but whose contribution does not qualify them for authorship can be acknowledged in the report. This might include statistical consultants, data collectors, or people who reviewed the manuscript. Acknowledgments should also give credit to organizations that made the project possible, such as funding agencies or organizations that helped with participant recruitment.

Checklist. A few journals, such as the *International Journal of Nursing Studies,* require the completion of an author checklist that obliges authors to state their compliance with various conditions, such as total word count, declaration of keywords, and so on.

> **TIP** Some specific advice on writing an article about pilot intervention studies is provided in Supplement A to this chapter on the**Point** Ⓢ.

Qualitative Research Reports

There is no single style for reporting qualitative findings, but qualitative research reports often follow the IMRAD format or something akin to it.

The Introduction

Qualitative reports usually begin with a problem statement, in a similar fashion to quantitative reports. The types of questions the researchers sought to answer are usually tied to the research tradition underlying the study (e.g., grounded theory, ethnography), which is usually stated in the introduction. Prior research on the phenomenon under study may be summarized in the introduction but is sometimes described in the discussion section.

In qualitative studies, it is essential to explain the study's cultural or social context. For studies with an ideologic orientation (e.g., critical theory), it is also important to describe the sociopolitical context. For studies using phenomenologic or grounded theory designs, the philosophy of phenomenology or symbolic interaction, respectively, may be described.

As another aspect of explaining the study's background, qualitative researchers sometimes provide information about relevant personal experiences or qualifications. If a researcher who is studying decisions about long-term care placements is caring for two elderly parents and participates in a caregiver support group, this is relevant for readers' understanding of the study. In descriptive phenomenologic studies, researchers may discuss their personal experiences in relation to the phenomenon being studied to communicate what they bracketed.

The concluding paragraph of the introduction usually offers a summary of the purpose of the study or the research questions.

The Method Section

Although the research tradition of the study usually is noted in the introduction, the method section elaborates on specific methods used in conjunction with that tradition. Design features such as whether the study was longitudinal should also be stated.

The method section should provide a good description of the research setting, so that readers can assess transferability of findings. Study participants and methods by which they were selected should also be described. Even when samples are small, it is often useful to provide a table summarizing participants' key characteristics. If researchers have a personal connection to participants, this connection should be noted. To disguise a group or institution, it may be necessary to omit or modify potentially identifying information.

Qualitative reports usually do not provide much specific information about data collection, but some researchers provide a sample of questions, especially if a topic guide was used. The description of data collection methods should include how data were collected (e.g., interview or observation), who collected the data, and how the data were recorded.

Information about quality and integrity is particularly important in qualitative studies. The more information included in the report about steps researchers took to ensure the trustworthiness of the data, the more confident readers can be that the findings are credible.

Quantitative reports typically have only brief descriptions of data analysis techniques because standard statistical procedures are widely understood. By contrast, analytic procedures are often described in some detail in qualitative reports because readers need to understand how researchers organized, synthesized, and made sense of their data.

The Results Section

In their results sections, qualitative researchers summarize their themes, categories, taxonomic structure, or theory. The results section can be organized in a number of ways. For example, if a process is being described, results may be presented chronologically, corresponding to the unfolding of the process. Key themes, metaphors, or domains are often used as subheadings, organized in order of salience to participants or to a theory.

Example of Organization of Qualitative Results

Lambert and colleagues (2018), in their descriptive phenomenologic study of the quality of care provided to South African women at the time of birth, interviewed 49 new mothers and 33 health care providers. The researchers identified eight themes that were used to organize their results section. Examples of themes include: Alone, exposed, and unsupported, and Mutual distrust.

Sandelowski (1998) emphasized the importance of developing a story line before beginning to write the findings. Because of the richness of qualitative data, researchers must decide which story, or how much of it, they want to tell. They must also decide how best to balance description and interpretation.

The results section in a qualitative paper, unlike that in a quantitative one, intertwines data and interpretations of those data. It is important, however, to give sufficient emphasis to the voices and experiences of participants themselves so that readers can appreciate their lives and worlds. Most often, this occurs through the inclusion of direct quotes to illustrate key points. Because of space constraints in journals, quotes cannot be extensive; great care must be exercised in selecting the best possible exemplars. Gilgun (2005) has offered guidance in writing up the results of qualitative research in a manner that has "grab."

> **TIP** Using quotes is a complex process. When inserting quotes in the results section, pay attention to how the quote is introduced and how it is put in context. Quotes should not be used haphazardly or listed one after the other in a string.

Figures, diagrams, and word tables that organize concepts are often useful in summarizing an overall conceptualization of the phenomena under study. Grounded theory studies are especially likely to benefit from a schematic presentation of the basic social process.

Discussion

In qualitative studies, findings and interpretation are typically interwoven in the results section because the task of integrating qualitative materials is essentially interpretive. The discussion section of a qualitative report, therefore, is not so much designed to give meaning to the results, but to summarize them, link them to other research, and suggest possible implications for theory, research, or nursing practice.

Other Aspects of a Qualitative Report

Qualitative reports, like quantitative ones, include abstracts, keywords, references, and acknowledgments. Abstracts for journals that feature qualitative reports (e.g., *Qualitative Health Research*) tend to be the traditional (single-paragraph) type, rather than structured abstracts.

The titles of qualitative reports usually state the central phenomenon under scrutiny. Phenomenologic studies often have titles that include such words as

"the lived experience of…" or "the meaning of…". Grounded theory studies often indicate something about the *findings* in the title—for example, mentioning the core category or basic social process. Ethnographic titles usually indicate the culture being studied. Two-part titles are not uncommon, with substance and method, research tradition and findings, or theme and meaning separated by a colon. For example, Wong and colleagues (2019) published a paper with this title: "The impact of social support networks on family resilience in an Australian intensive care unit: A constructivist grounded theory."

> **TIP** Preparing a report for a mixed methods (MM) study has challenges of its own—particularly regarding the integration of the qualitative and quantitative strands. Creswell and Plano Clark (2018) offer useful guidance for writing up integrated MM reports.

THE STYLE OF RESEARCH REPORTS

Research reports, especially for quantitative studies, are written in a distinctive style. Some style issues were discussed previously, but additional points are elaborated here.

A research report is not an essay. It is an account of how and why a problem was studied, and what was discovered as a result. The report should not include overtly subjective assertions or emotionally laden statements. This is not to say that the research story should be told in a dreary manner. Indeed, in qualitative reports there are ample opportunities to enliven the narration with rich description, direct quotes, and insightful interpretation. Authors of quantitative reports, although somewhat constrained by structure and the need to include numeric information, should strive to keep the presentation lively.

Quantitative researchers often avoid personal pronouns such as "I," "my," and "we" because impersonal pronouns, and use of the passive voice, may suggest greater impartiality. Qualitative reports, by contrast, are sometimes written in the first person and in an active voice. Even among quantitative researchers, however, there is a trend toward striking a greater balance between active and passive voice. If a direct presentation can be made without suggesting bias, a more readable product usually results.

It is not easy to write simply and clearly, but these are important goals of scientific writing. The use of technical jargon does little to enhance the communicative value of the report and should be avoided in conveying findings to practicing nurses. The style should be concise and straightforward. If writers can add elegance to their reports without interfering with clarity and accuracy, so much the better, but the product is not expected to be a literary achievement.

A common flaw in reports of novice researchers is inadequate organization. The overall structure is fairly standard, but organization within sections and subsections also needs attention. Sequences should be in an orderly progression with appropriate transitions. Continuity and logical thematic development are critical to good communication.

It may seem a trivial point, but methods and results should be described in the past tense. For example, it is inappropriate to say, "Nurses who receive special training perform triage functions significantly better than those without training." In this sentence, "receive" and "perform" should be changed to "received" and "performed" to reflect the fact that the statement pertains only to a particular sample whose behavior occurred in the past.

TYPES OF RESEARCH REPORTS

This section describes features of several major kinds of research reports: theses and dissertations, traditional or online journal articles, and presentations at professional meetings. Reports for class projects are excluded—not because they are unimportant but rather because they so closely resemble theses on a smaller scale.

Theses and Dissertations

Most doctoral degrees, and some master's degrees, are granted on the successful completion of a study. Most universities have a preferred format for their dissertations. Until recently, most schools used a traditional format with the following organization:

- Front Matter: Title Page; Abstract; Copyright Page; Approval Page; Acknowledgment Page; Table of Contents; List of Tables; List of Figures; List of Appendices
- Main Body: Chapter I. Introduction; Chapter II. Review of the Literature; Chapter III. Methods; Chapter IV. Results; Chapter V. Discussion and Summary
- Supplementary Pages: Bibliography; Appendices; Curriculum vita

The **front matter** (preliminary pages) for dissertations is similar to those for a scholarly book. The title page indicates such information as the title of the study, the author's name, the degree requirement being fulfilled, and the name of the university awarding the degree. The acknowledgment page gives writers the opportunity to thank those who contributed to the project. The table of contents outlines major sections and subsections of the report, indicating on which page readers will find material of interest. The lists of tables and figures identify by number, title, and page the tabular and graphic material in the text.

The main body of a traditionally formatted dissertation incorporates the IMRAD sections described earlier. The literature review often is so extensive that a separate chapter may be devoted to it. When a short review is sufficient, the first two chapters may be combined. In some cases, a separate chapter may also be required to elaborate the study's conceptual framework.

TIP In some traditional dissertations, the early chapters describe students' intellectual journey, including a description of the paths they took and decisions they made in selecting their final research question and methodology.

The supplementary pages include a bibliography or list of references and one or more appendixes. An appendix contains materials that are either too lengthy or too tangential to be incorporated into the body of the report. Data collection instruments, scoring instructions, codebooks, cover letters, permission letters, IRB approval, category schemes, and peripheral statistical tables are examples of appendix materials. Sometimes a *curriculum vita* of the author is required.

Some universities offer a new formatting option, what has been called the **paper format thesis** or **publication option** (Robinson & Dracup, 2008). In a typical paper format thesis, there is an introduction, two or more publishable papers, and a conclusion. This format permits students to move directly from dissertation to journal submission but can be more demanding than the traditional format on both students and their advisers. Formats for the paper format thesis vary and are typically decided by the dissertation committee. Some universities require that a certain number of the publishable papers (e.g., two out of three) be data-based—that is, reports of original research. Other papers within the dissertation, however, might be publishable systematic reviews, concept analyses, or methodologic papers (e.g., describing the development of an instrument). Some universities require that the papers be under review or *in press* (that is, accepted and awaiting publication), but others require that the papers be ready to submit.

If an academic institution does not accept paper format theses, students need to adapt their dissertations before submission to a journal. Ahern (2012) provides some guidance on converting a traditional dissertation into a manuscript. Roush (2016) has written a useful guide on writing theses and dissertations.

TIP Another innovation involves publishing theses and dissertations electronically. In some fields, online repositories of dissertations are widely used, but this has not been the case in nursing (Macduff et al., 2016). Electronic Theses and Dissertations (ETDs) have the advantage of making scholarly work widely accessible—and ETDs can incorporate such features as film and audio clips. A new initiative is underway to promote nursing's engagement with ETDs (www.inetdin.net).

Journal Articles

Traditional dissertations, which are too lengthy for widespread use and often difficult to access, are read only by a handful of people. Publication in a professional journal ensures broader circulation of research findings, and it is professionally advantageous to publish. This section discusses the publication of research reports in journals.

TIP The Nurse Author & Editor website at http://www.nurseauthoreditor.com/ is a valuable resource for nurse authors.

Traditional and Open-Access Journals

An important issue facing authors concerns whether to publish in a traditional journal or an open-access journal. Traditional journals are typically available both in print and online, but access to the online version is restricted to individuals and institutions paying a subscription fee. **Open-access journals** are available online free of charge to those with access to the Internet.

A major benefit is that open-access formats offer a worldwide audience of readers and hence can increase the visibility and impact of the authors' research. Also, unlike traditional journals in which the journal publishers maintain the copyright for all publications, open-access journals usually allow authors to retain copyright. The legal basis for open access is the consent of the copyright holder, i.e., the authors. In many cases, copyright holders demonstrate their consent to use open access by using something called the *Creative Commons licenses*. When authors consent to open access, they are usually consenting upfront to unrestricted access, reading, downloading, copying, printing, and sharing of the work.

An article accepted by an open-access journal typically gets published more quickly than is true for traditional print journals. Another advantage is that online journals are much less strict about page limits. Qualitative researchers may benefit from this feature because it allows them to include more extensive verbatim quotes. Quantitative researchers can include more figures and tables than is true in traditional journal articles (although some traditional journals publish online supplements that can be used to share additional material).

TIP In selecting examples of nursing studies in this edition, we deliberately sought studies published as open-access articles, so that readers around the world would be able to obtain them. We identify open-access articles in the chapter reference lists, and links to these articles are provided in the Toolkit ✪.

One drawback is that open-access journals usually charge a fee to cover the cost of producing the journal. For example, in 2019 the open-access journal *BMC Nursing* charged authors $2,170 (£1,480, €1,690) for an accepted article. However, many nurse authors are affiliated with institutions that are members of BioMed Central, in which case there is no fee. In other cases, institutions pay publication fees for faculty members. (The fee for open-access journal publication is often waived for authors from low-income countries and is sometimes reduced for students.) Another drawback for nurse researchers is that relatively few nursing journals are open access. The scarcity of open-access nursing journals has meant that nurse researchers who seek open-access publication often opt to send their manuscripts to nonnursing journals.

TIP The Directory of Open Access Journals (DOAJ) indexes and provides information for about 12,500 open-access journals, 90 of which were classified as having *Nursing* as a subject code in 2019 (www.doag.org). Examples include *Nursing Plus Open, SAGE Open Nursing, Global Qualitative Nursing Research,* and *BMC Nursing.* Many open-access nursing journals are subsidized by national governments (e.g., in Brazil and Iran). The Cochrane Collaboration has made a commitment to publishing their systematic reviews as open-access by 2020.

Many traditional journals have moved to a hybrid model, in which authors can elect to have individual articles published as open access, usually for an article-processing fee. However, many government agencies that fund health research (such as the National Institutes of Health [NIH] in the United States and Research Councils [United Kingdom]) now require that articles reporting government-funded studies be published as open access.

Some journals allow articles to be uploaded into *open-access repositories* in academic networks such as Research Gate or Academia.edu, or in institutional repositories. If open access is important but unaffordable, researchers should check a journal's policy about uploading to open-access repositories—including whether there is a period of *embargo*. When there is an embargo, an article cannot be uploaded to the repository for a period after it first appears in print (e.g., 12 months). As noted by Griffiths (2014), publishers and journals vary in their policies regarding costs and embargos (or permission to upload at all), so authors "need to be wary to avoid breaking copyright laws" (p. 690).

When the open-access movement got underway, many expressed concerns that low-quality articles would increasingly find their way into publication. And, in fact, there has been an alarming surge in **predatory journals** that charge fees, fail to provide adequate review and editorial services, and publish articles of poor quality (Oermann et al., 2018). In their study of predatory nursing journals in 2016, Oermann and colleagues identified 140 such journals, most of which solicit manuscripts through spam emails. Bradley-Springer (2015) offers advice on how to identify a predatory journal.

Nevertheless, many high-quality open-access journals are fully peer-reviewed, and many have attained high prestige. All major open-access initiatives insist on the importance of high-quality scientific review of submitted articles.

Selecting a Journal

Hundreds of nursing journals exist and are indexed in CINAHL and PubMed. Journals differ in focus, prestige, acceptance rates, word limits, and reference styles. Journals also vary in their goals, types of manuscript sought, review methods, and readership. These various factors need to be matched against personal ambitions and realistic assessments of the study. Writers should develop a clear idea of the journal to which a manuscript will be submitted before writing begins.

TIP Several "journal selection" websites have been created and are designed to help researchers identify appropriate journals (Cuschieri, 2018). Some services are free but others charge a fee. Links to a few services are provided in the Toolkit ⊗.

All journals release goal statements, as well as guidelines for preparing and submitting a manuscript. This information is published on journal websites.

Example of a of Journal Goal Statement From the Website

Qualitative Health Research is an international, interdisciplinary, refereed journal for the enhancement of health care and to further the development and understanding of qualitative research methods in health care settings. We welcome manuscripts in the following areas: the description and analysis of the illness experience, health and health-seeking behaviors, the experiences of caregivers, the sociocultural organization of health care, health care policy, and related topics. We also seek critical reviews and commentaries addressing conceptual, theoretical, methodologic, and ethical issues pertaining to qualitative enquiry.

Many authors would like to know a journal's acceptance rate, but this information is seldom available. Northam and colleagues (2014) conducted a survey of journal editors and reported on the acceptance rate for 61 nursing journals. Some journals were more competitive than others. For example, *Nursing Research* accepted only 20% of submitted manuscripts, whereas the acceptance rates for some specialty journals was greater than 50%. Competition for journal publication likely became keener in the years since the survey was conducted.

TIP Some nursing journals provide acceptance information on their websites. For example, the website for *Oncology Nursing Forum* stated in 2018 that the journal accepted 36% of manuscripts on first submission and 52% after revision. The website also noted that the peer review process took, on average, 6 to 8 weeks, and that the time to publication was 7 to 10 months. In a paper by editors of the prestigious *International Journal of Nursing Studies* (IJNS), Griffiths and Norman (2016) explained that about 70% of manuscripts submitted to IJNS are rejected even before being sent out for peer review.

Authors are often guided in their selection of a journal by the journal's *prestige*. Several metrics have been developed to capture a journal's impact, including indexes called *impact factor, Cite Score,* and *Source Normalized Impact per Paper (SNIP)*.

A journal's **impact factor (IF)** is the most widely used status index. The IF is a measure of citation frequency for an average article in a journal. Specifically, a journal's IF for, say, 2019 is the number of times in 2019 that articles published in the journal in the two prior years (2017 and 2018) were cited, divided by the number of the journal's articles in those 2 years that *could* have been cited (i.e., number of actual citations divided by the number of potentially citable articles) (Polit & Northam, 2011). As examples, the 2018 impact factor for *International Journal of Nursing Studies,* the highest ranked nursing journal in that year, was 3.57, while that for *Journal of Cardiovascular Nursing,* ranked sixth, was 2.51. Impact factor information can be found in *Journal Citation Reports* and on the websites of journals that have an IF. Many nursing journals are not evaluated for impact factor, but more than 100 are.

Open-access nursing journals are especially unlikely to have an impact factor. Only 4 of the 120 nursing journals with impact factors in 2018 were open-access journals, and only one of the four had an IF of 1.00 or greater. By contrast, many open-access medical journals have high impact factors. For example, *PLoS Medicine* had an impact factor of 11.05. Open-access journals have been found to have more citations overall than traditional journals (Cuschieri, 2018).

Because a journal's IF can be influenced by a single article that is cited numerous times, another potentially useful metric is the *percentage* of articles in a journal that are cited. For example, for the years 2016 to 2019, 53.5% of all articles in the *Western Journal of Nursing Research* were cited, compared to 7.2% of articles in *Oncology Nursing Forum* that were cited, even though these two journals had similar impact factors (1.46 and 1.44, respectively). This metric is available in InCites by Clarivate Analytics.

Impact factor information for 2018 for most nursing journals with a high concentration of research articles is shown in a table in Supplement B to this chapter ⑤. The table also shows information on acceptance rates for those journals participating in the Northam et al. (2014) survey, Cite Scores, and the InCites metric of percentage of articles cited.

> **TIP** Citation impact metrics are available not only for journals, but also for specific articles and for authors. The best-known measure of author-level citations is the *h-index*, which attempts to capture both the productivity and citation impact of a scholar's publications. An alternative approach (often referred to as *altmetrics*) is to measure impact based on usage data, such as the number of article downloads.

Query Letters

It is sometimes useful to send a **query letter** to a journal to ask the editor whether there is interest in a manuscript. The query letter should briefly describe the topic and methods, title, and a tentative submission date. Query letters are not essential if you have done a lot of homework about the journal's goals, but they might help to avoid impediments in some circumstances (e.g., if editors have recently accepted several papers on a similar topic and do not wish to consider another). Query letters can be submitted by e-mail using contact information provided on the journal's website.

Query letters can be sent to multiple journals simultaneously, but ultimately the manuscript can be submitted only to one—or rather, to one at a time. If several editors express interest in reviewing a manuscript, journals can be prioritized according to criteria previously described. The priority list should be preserved because the manuscript can be resubmitted to the next journal on the list if the journal of first choice rejects it.

> **TIP** A useful strategy in selecting a journal is to inspect your citation list. Journals that appear in your list have shown an interest in your topic and likely are good candidates for publishing new studies on that topic.

Preparing the Manuscript

Once a journal has been selected, the information in the journal's **Instructions to Authors** should be carefully reviewed. These instructions typically give authors such information as the maximum page length; permissible fonts and margins; the type of abstract desired; the reference style that should be used; and how to submit the manuscript online. It is important to adhere to the journal's guidelines to avoid rejection for nonsubstantive reasons. (The Toolkit section of the *Resource Manual* offers links to manuscript requirements for several nursing research journals.) ✖ In an informal survey of journal editors, Froman (2008) found that the most aggravating author behavior was "disregard for journal format or mission" (p. 399).

> **TIP** Before you begin to write, it can be helpful to examine a research article that can serve as a model. Select a journal article on a topic similar to your own in the journal you have selected as first choice. When you have written a draft, a review by colleagues or advisers can be invaluable in getting feedback about possible improvements.

Typically, a manuscript for journals should be no more than 15 to 20 pages, double-spaced, not counting references and tables. The greatest amount of space usually should be allocated to methods and results. A frequent complaint of journal editors is that submitted manuscripts are too long.

Care should be taken in using and preparing citations. Some nursing journals suggest that there be no more than 15 references in total or no more than three citations supporting a single point. In general, only published work can be cited (e.g., not papers presented at a conference). The reference style of the American Psychological Association (APA, 2020) is the style used by many nursing journals. Another popular style is that of the American Medical Association.

> **TIP** There is a wealth of resources to assist you ✖ with the APA style, including an APA "cribsheet" (http://www.docstyles.com) and tutorials at university libraries. Several websites are listed in the Toolkit for you to click on directly.

Submission of a Manuscript

When the manuscript is ready for journal submission, a *cover letter* should be drafted. The cover letter should state the title of the paper and the name and contact information of the **corresponding author** (the author who communicates with the journal, usually the lead author). The letter may include assurances that (1) the paper is original and has not been published or submitted elsewhere; (2) all authors have read and approved the manuscript; and (3) there are no conflicts of interest. Most traditional journals also require a signed *copyright transfer* form, which transfers all copyright ownership of the manuscript to the journal and warrants that all authors signing the form participated sufficiently in the research to justify authorship.

In submitting an article online, it is usually necessary to upload several files containing different parts of your manuscript. The title page, which has author-identifying information, should be in the first file. The next file usually contains the abstract, main text, and reference list. Tables and figures are submitted separately, one file at a time. In other words, if there are two tables and one figure, these would be submitted in three files. At the end of the process, a pdf file that contains all the elements is created for your review prior to submission. The entire process often requires a fair amount of time, but fortunately it is usually possible to begin the process and return later if you need to track down information, such as the addresses of co-authors.

> **TIP** Nurses publish articles in many health-related journals, not just in nursing journals. Nurse researchers, who increasingly work in interprofessional teams, are co-authors on papers published in diverse journals.

Manuscript Review

Most nursing journals with research content have a policy of independent **peer review** of manuscripts by two or more experts in the field. Reviewers are typically independent—they do not collaborate to achieve consensus. The ultimate decision rests in the hands of journal editors. Peer review usually is a *blind review,* the idea being that greater candor is possible if there is anonymity. In a double-blind review, reviewers do not know the identity of the authors, and authors do not learn the identity of reviewers. Journals with peer reviewers are **refereed journals** and are held in higher esteem than nonrefereed journals. When submitting a manuscript to a refereed journal, authors' names should not appear anywhere except on the title page.

> **TIP** It takes skill to be a good reviewer. In an ideal scenario, experienced reviewers would mentor their students in this important professional role. Montsivais (2016) offers suggestions on how to be responsive, focused, and compassionate as a reviewer. The website called Nurse Author & Editor provides guidance for reviewers (http://naepub.com/for-reviewers/).

Peer reviewers make recommendations to the editors about whether to accept the manuscript for publication, accept it contingent on revisions, or reject it. Relatively few manuscripts are accepted on first submission—substantive and editorial revisions are the norm.

> **Example of Reviewer Recommendation Categories**
> The journal *Research in Nursing & Health* asks reviewers to make one of five recommendations: (1) Accept; (2) Minor revision; (3) Major revision; (4) Reject and resubmit; and (5) Reject.

Authors are sent information about the editors' decision, together with reviewers' comments. In many cases, the initial review results in an invitation to resubmit the manuscript. As noted by Algase (2016), the revise-and-resubmit decision reflects the editor's view that the paper has appeal but has some flaws that make it unacceptable in its initial form. The editor typically gives a deadline for the revised submission. Authors can accept the invitation, but if the authors decline to resubmit, the paper should be withdrawn from consideration.

When resubmitting a revised manuscript to the same journal, each reviewer recommendation should be addressed, either by making the requested change, or by explaining in a cover letter the rationale for not revising (Bearinger et al., 2010). Defending some aspect of a paper against a reviewer's recommendation often requires a strong supporting argument and citations. Noble (2017) has offered advice about responding to reviewers. Typically, many months go by between submission of the original manuscript and the publication of a journal article, especially if there are revisions, as there usually are.

Example of Journal Timeline

Beck (2017) published a paper in the *Journal of Perinatal Education* titled, "The anniversary of birth trauma: A metaphor analysis." The timeline for acceptance and publication of this manuscript, which was relatively fast, is as follows:

October 27, 2016	Manuscript submitted to *Journal of Perinatal Education* for review
January 5, 2017	Letter from editor informing of a revise-and-resubmit decision
January 18, 2017	Revised manuscript resubmitted
January 21, 2017	Revised manuscript accepted for publication
Fall, 2017	Publication in *Journal of Perinatal Education*

Many manuscripts are rejected because of keen competition. If a manuscript is rejected, the reviewers' comments should be taken into consideration before submitting it to another journal.

TIP Author reviews of their experiences with journals are available in SciRev. The reviews for a specific discipline can be found at www.SciRev.sc by entering the discipline name in the search field; specific journals can also be searched.

Presentations at Professional Conferences

Many international, national, and regional organizations sponsor meetings at which nursing studies are presented, either in an oral report or as a visual display in a poster session. Professional conferences are good forums for presenting results to clinical audiences. Researchers can take advantage of meeting and talking with other conference attendees who are working on similar problems in different geographic regions. Becker's (2014) book on conference presentations is a useful resource, and Joshua (2017) has written about the learning opportunities of presenting at a conference.

TIP: Predatory conferences are set up to look like legitimate professional conferences but in reality are an exploitative method to make money from registration fees. Guidelines called "Think. Check. Attend." can be used to judge the legitimacy of a conference.

The mechanism for submitting a presentation to a conference is simpler than for journal submission. The association sponsoring the conference ordinarily publishes an announcement or **Call for Abstracts** on its website or sends an email to its members, 6 to 9 months before the meeting date. The notice indicates topics of interest, submission requirements, and deadlines for submitting a proposed paper or poster. Most universities and major health care agencies receive and post Call for Abstracts notices. In addition, Sigma Theta Tau posts a schedule of nursing conferences on its website (https://www.sigmanursing.org).

Oral Reports

Most conferences require prospective presenters to submit online abstracts of 250 to 1,000 words. Each conference has its own guidelines for abstract content and form. Abstracts are sometimes submitted to the organizer of a particular session; in other cases, conference sessions are organized after-the-fact, with related papers grouped together. Abstracts are evaluated based on the quality and originality of the research and the paper's appropriateness for the conference audience. If abstracts are accepted, researchers are committed to appear at the conference to make a presentation.

Oral reports at meetings usually follow the IMRAD format. The time allotted for presentation usually is about 10 to 15 minutes, with 5 minutes or so for audience questions. Thus, only the most important aspects of the study, with emphasis on the results, can be shared. It is especially challenging to condense qualitative findings to a brief oral summary without losing the rich, in-depth character of the data.

A handy rule of thumb is that a page of double-spaced text requires 2½ to 3 minutes to read aloud. Although presenters often prepare a written paper or a script, presentations are most effective if they are delivered informally or conversationally, rather than if they are read verbatim. The presentation should be rehearsed to gain comfort with the script and to ensure that time limits are not exceeded.

> **TIP** Most conferences presentations include visual materials—notably PowerPoint slides. Visual materials should be kept simple for biggest impact. Tables are difficult to read on a slide but sometimes can be distributed to the audience in hard copy form.

The question-and-answer period can be a good opportunity to expand on aspects of the research and to get early feedback. Audience comments can be helpful in turning the conference presentation into a manuscript for journal submission.

Poster Presentations

Researchers sometimes present their findings or study protocols in **poster sessions**. Abstracts, often similar to those required for oral presentations, must be submitted to conference organizers according to specific guidelines. In poster sessions, several researchers simultaneously present visual displays summarizing study features, and conference attendees circulate around the exhibit area perusing displays. Those interested in a poster topic can discuss the study with the researcher and bypass posters dealing with topics of less interest. Poster sessions are efficient and encourage one-on-one discussions. Poster sessions are typically 1 to 2 hours in length. Researchers are expected to stand near their posters throughout the session to allow discussion.

It is challenging to design an effective poster. The poster must convey essential information about the background, design, and results of a study, in a format that can be perused in minutes. Bullet points, graphs, and photos are useful for communicating information quickly. Large, bold fonts are essential, because posters are often read from a short distance. It is important to follow conference guidelines regarding such matters as poster size, format, and display materials. For those traveling long distances, lightweight fabric posters can be created.

Several authors have offered advice on preparing for poster sessions (e.g., Berg & Hicks, 2017; Kohtz et al., 2017; Siedlecki, 2017). Software for producing posters is available (e.g., www.postersw. com).

Electronic Dissemination

Computers and the Internet have changed forever how information is disseminated. Earlier we discussed publishing in open-access online-only journals, but there are other ways to disseminate research findings on the Internet. For example, some researchers or research teams develop their own web page with information about their studies. When there are hyperlinks embedded in the websites, consumers can navigate between files and websites to retrieve relevant information on a topic of interest. Links to unpublished papers can also be uploaded on to the websites of individual researchers, their institutions, special interest organizations, and online repositories.

Such online dissemination avenues ensure timely distribution of information. One drawback of such dissemination opportunities, however, is that the papers are not peer-reviewed. Researchers who want their evidence to have an impact on nursing practice should seek publication in outlets that subject manuscripts to expert external review.

> **TIP** McGrath and Brandon (2016) offer advice on how to "market" your research on social media, such as Facebook or Twitter.

CRITICAL APPRAISAL OF RESEARCH REPORTS

Although various aspects of study methodology can be evaluated using guidelines presented throughout this book, the manner in which study information is communicated in the research report can also be scrutinized in a comprehensive appraisal. Box 32.2, included in the Toolkit, summarizes major points to consider in evaluating the presentation of a research report ⊗.

BOX 32.2 Guidelines for Critically Appraising the Presentation of a Research Report

1. Does the report include a sufficient amount of detail to permit a thorough appraisal of the study's purpose, conceptual framework, design and methods, handling of ethical issues, analysis of data, and interpretation?
2. Is the report well written and grammatical? Are pretentious words or jargon used when simpler wording would have been possible?
3. Is the report well organized? Is there an orderly, logical presentation of ideas?
4. Does the report effectively combine text with tables or figures?
5. Are overt biases, exaggerations, and distortions avoided? Are conclusions logical?
6. Is the report written using appropriately tentative language?
7. Is sexist or insensitive language avoided?
8. Does the title of the report adequately capture the key concepts and the population under investigation? Does the abstract adequately summarize the research problem, study methods, and important findings?

An important issue is whether the report provided sufficient information for a thoughtful appraisal of other dimensions. When vital pieces of information are missing, researchers leave readers little choice but to assume the worst because this would lead to the most cautious interpretation of the results. For example, if there is no mention of blinding, then the safest conclusion is that blinding did not occur.

Styles of writing differ for qualitative and quantitative reports, and it is unreasonable to apply the standards considered appropriate for one paradigm to the other. Regardless of style, however, you should be alert to indications of overt biases or exaggerations.

In summary, a research report is meant to be an account of how and why a problem was studied and what results were obtained. The report should be clearly written, cogent, and concise, and written in a manner that piques readers' interest.

SUMMARY POINTS

- In developing a dissemination plan, researchers select a communication outlet (e.g., journal article, conference presentation), identify the audience whom they wish to reach, and decide on the content that can be effectively communicated.

- In the planning stage, researchers need to decide authorship credits (if there are multiple authors), who the **lead author** and **corresponding author** will be, and in what order authors' names will be listed.

- Quantitative reports (and many qualitative reports) follow the **IMRAD format**, with the following sections: Introduction, Method, Results, and Discussion.

- The *introduction* acquaints readers with the research problem. It includes the problem statement and study purpose, the research hypotheses or questions, a brief literature review, and description of a framework. In qualitative reports, the introduction indicates the research tradition and, if relevant, the researchers' connection to the problem.

- The *method section* explains what researchers did to address the research problem. It includes a description of the study design (or an elaboration of the research tradition); the sampling approach and a description of study participants; instruments and procedures used to collect and evaluate the data; and methods used to analyze the data.

- In the *results section*, findings from the analyses are summarized. Results sections in qualitative reports necessarily intertwine description and interpretation. Quotes from transcripts are essential for giving voice to study participants.

- Both qualitative and quantitative researchers include **figures** and **tables** that dramatize or succinctly summarize major findings or conceptual schema.
- The *discussion section* presents the interpretation of results, how the findings relate to earlier research, study limitations, and implications of the findings for nursing practice and future research.
- Standards for reporting methodologic elements now abound. Researchers reporting an RCT follow the **CONSORT guideline** (Consolidated Standards of Reporting Trials), which includes use of a flow chart to shows the flow of study participants. Guidelines for reporting aspects of an intervention include **CReDECI** and **TIDieR.**
- The major types of research reports are theses and dissertations, journal articles, and presentations at professional meetings.
- Theses and dissertations normally follow a standard IMRAD format, but some schools now accept **paper format theses**, which include an introduction, two or more publishable papers, and a conclusion.
- In selecting a journal for publication, researchers consider the journal's goals and audience, its prestige, and how often it publishes. Another major consideration is whether to publish in a traditional journal or in an online **open-access journal.** An advantage of open-access journals is speedy, worldwide dissemination.
- Researchers need to be wary of the many **predatory journals** that solicit manuscripts and collect article processing charges for a profit, but then fail to provide adequate editorial services and tend to publish articles of poor quality.
- One proxy for a journal's prestige is its **impact factor,** the ratio between citations to a journal and recent citable items published.
- Before beginning to prepare a **manuscript** for submission to a journal, researchers need to carefully to review the journal's **Instructions to Authors.**
- Most nursing journals that publish research reports are **refereed journals** with a policy of basing publication decisions on **peer reviews** that are usually **double-blind reviews** (identities of authors and reviewers are not divulged).

- Nurse researchers can also present their research at professional conferences, either through a 10- to 15-minute oral report to a seated audience, or in a **poster session** in which the "audience" moves around a room perusing research summaries attached to posters. Sponsoring organizations usually issue a **Call for Abstracts** for the conference 6 to 9 months before it is held.

STUDY ACTIVITIES

Study activities are available to instructors on thePoint.

REFERENCES CITED IN CHAPTER 32

Ahern, K. (2012). How to create a journal article from a thesis. *Nurse Researcher, 19*, 21–25.

Algase, D. L. (2016). Revise and resbumit: Now what? *Research and Theory for Nursing Practice, 28*, 195–198.

American Psychological Association. (2020). *Publication manual of the American Psychological Association* (7th ed.). Washington, DC: Author.

Bearinger, L., Taliaferro, L., & Given, B. (2010). When R & R is not rest and recovery but revise and resubmit. *Research in Nursing & Health, 33*, 381–385.

Beck, C. T. (2017). The anniversary of birth trauma: A metaphor analysis. *Journal of Perinatal Education, 26*, 219–228.

Becker, P. T. (2009). Thoughts on the end of the article: The implications for nursing practice. *Research in Nursing & Health, 32*, 241–242.

Becker, L. (2014). *Presenting your research: Conferences, symposiums, poster presentations and beyond.* Thousand Oaks, CA: Sage.

*Benchimol, E., Smeeth, L., Guttmann, A., Harron, K., Moher, D., Petersen, I., … Langan, S. (2015). The Reporting of studies Conducted using Observational Routinely-collected health Data (RECORD) statement. *PLoS Medicine, 12*, e1001885.

Berg, J., & Hicks, R. (2017). Successful design and delivery of a professional poster. *Journal of the American Association of Nurse Practitioners, 29*, 461–469.

Boutron, I., Moher, D., Altman, D., Schulz, K., Ravaud, P., for the CONSORT group, . (2008). Extending the CONSORT statement to randomized trials of nonpharmacologic treatment: Explanation and elaboration. *Annals of Internal Medicine, 148*, 295–309.

Bradley-Springer, L. (2015). Predatory publishing and you. *Journal of the Association of Nurses in AIDS Care, 26*, 219–221.

Calvert, M., Blazeby, J., Altman, D., Revicki, D., Moher, D., & Brundage, M. (2013). Reporting of patient-reported outcomes in randomized trials: The CONSORT PRO extension. *Journal of the American Medical Association, 309,* 814–822.

*Campbell, M., Elbourne, D., & Altman, D. (2012). CONSORT 2010 statement: Extension to cluster randomised trials. *British Medical Journal, 345,* e5661.

*Chan, A. W., Tetzlaff, J., Gotzsche, P., Altman, D., Mann, H., Berlin, J., … Moher, D. (2013). SPIRIT 2013 explanation and elaboration: Guidance for protocols of clinical trials. *British Medical Journal, 346,* e7586.

*Clement, T. (2014). Authorship matrix: A rational approach to quantify individual contributions and responsibilities in multi-author scientific articles. *Science and Engineering Ethics, 20,* 345–361.

*Cohen, J., Korevaar, D., Altman, D., Bruns, D., Gatsonis, C., Hooft, L., … Bossuyt, P. (2016). STARD 2015 guidelines for reporting diagnostic accuracy studies: Explanation and elaboration. *BMJ Open, 6,* e012799.

Conn, V. S., Cooper, P., Ruppar, T., & Russell, C. (2008). Searching for the intervention in intervention research reports. *Journal of Nursing Scholarship, 40,* 52–59.

Conn, V. S., Ward, S., Herrick, L., Topp, R., Alexander, G., Anderson, C., … Georgesen, S. (2015). Managing opportunities and challenges of co-authorship. *Western Journal of Nursing Research, 37,* 134–163.

Creswell, J. W., & Plano Clark, V. L. (2018). *Designing and conducting mixed methods research* (3rd ed.). Thousand Oaks, CA: Sage.

Cuschieri, S. (2018). Is open access publishing the way forward? A review of the different ways in which research papers can be published. *Early Human Development, 121,* 54–57.

*Des Jarlais, D., Lyles, C., Crepaz, N., & the TREND Group. (2004). Improving the reporting quality of nonrandomized evaluations of behavioral and public health interventions: The TREND statement. *American Journal of Public Health, 94,* 361–366.

*Eldridge, S., Chan, C., Campbell, M., Bond, C., Hopewell, S., Thabane, L., & Lancaster, G. (2016). CONSORT 2010 statement: Extension to randomised pilot and feasibility trials. *British Medical Journal, 355,* i5239.

Froman, R. (2008). Hitting the bull's eye rather than shooting yourself between the eyes. *Research in Nursing & Health, 31,* 399–401.

Gennaro, S. (2010). Closing the gap. *Journal of Nursing Scholarship, 42,* 357.

Gilgun, J. (2005). "Grab" and good science: Writing up the results of qualitative research. *Qualitative Health Research, 15,* 256–262.

*Glasziou, P., Meats, E., Heneghan, C. & Shepperd, S. (2008). What is missing from descriptions of treatment in trials and reviews? *British Medical Journal, 336,* 1472–1474.

*Griffiths, P. (2014). Open access publication and the International Journal of Nursing Studies: All that glitters is not gold. *International Journal of Nursing Studies, 51,* 689–690.

Griffiths, P., & Norman, I. (2016). Why was my paper rejected? Editors' reflections on common issues which influence decisions to reject papers submitted for publication in academic nursing journals. *International Journal of Nursing Studies, 57,* A1–A4.

Happell, B. (2016). Salami: By the slice or swallowed whole? *Applied Nursing Research, 30,* 29–31.

*Hoffmann, T. C., Glasziou, P. P., Boutron, I., Milne, R., Perara, R., Moher, D., … Michie, S. (2014). Better reporting of interventions: Template for intervention description and replication (TIDieR) checklist and guide. *British Medical Journal, 348,* g1687.

*Husereau, D., Drummond, M., Petrou, S., Carswell, C., Moher, D., Greenberg, , … Loder, E. (2013). Consolidated Health Economic Evaluation Reporting Standards (CHEERS) statement. *BMC Medicine, 11,* 80.

*International Committee of Medical Journal Editors, . (2017). *Recommendations for the conduct, reporting, editing, and publication of scholarly work in medical journals—updated 2017.* Retrieved from www.icmje.org.

Jackson, D., Walter, G., Daly, J., & Cleary, M. (2014). Multiple outputs from single studies: Acceptable division of findings vs. "salami" slicing. *Journal of Clinical Nursing, 23,* 1–2.

Joshua, B. (2017). Reflecting on the learning opportunities of presenting at a conference. *Nurse Researcher, 24,* 27–30.

Kearney, M. H. (2014). Be a responsible co-author. *Research in Nursing & Health, 37,* 1–2.

Kennedy, M., Newland, J., & Owens, J. (2017). Findings from the INANE survey on student papers submitted to nursing journals. *Journal of Professional Nursing, 33,* 175–183.

Kohtz, C., Hymer, C., & Humbles-Pegues, P. (2017). Poster creation: Guidelines and tips for success. *Nursing, 47,* 43–46.

Kottner, J., Audigé, L., Brorson, S., Donner, A., Gajeweski, B., Hróbjartsson, A., … Streiner, D. (2011). Guidelines for reporting reliability and agreement studies (GRRAS). *International Journal of Nursing Studies, 48,* 661–671.

*Lambert, J., Etsane, E., Bergh, A., Pattinson, R., & van den Broek, N. (2018). "I thought they were going to handle me like a queen but they didn't": A qualitative study exploring the quality of care provided to women at the time of birth. *Midwifery, 62,* 256–263.

Lang, T. A. (2010). *How to write, publish, and present in the health sciences.* Washington: American College of Physicians.

Macduff, C., Goodfellow, L., Leslie, G., Copeland, S., Nolfi, D., & Blackwood, D. (2016). Harnessing our rivers of knowledge: Time to improve nursing's engagement with Electronic Theses and Dissertations. *Journal of Advanced Nursing, 72,* 2255–2258.

Markopoulos, G., Kitridis, D., Tsikopoulos, K., Georgiannos, D., & Bisbinas, I. (2019). Bladder training prior to urinary catheter removal in total joint arthroplasty: A randomized controlled trial. *International Journal of Nursing Studies, 89,* 14–17.

*McGrath, J., & Brandon, D. (2016). Scholarly publication and social media: Do they have something in common? *Advances in Neonatal Care, 16*, 245–248.

*Moher, D., Hopewell, S., Schulz, K. F., Montori, V., Gotzsche, P., Devereaux, P., … Altman, D. (2010). CONSORT 2010 explanation and elaboration: Updated guidelines for reporting parallel-group randomised trials. *British Medical Journal, 340*, c869.

*Moher, D., Liberati, A., Tetzlaff, J., Altman, D., & The PRISMA Group, . (2009). Preferred reporting items for systematic reviews and meta-analyses: The PRISMA statement. *British Medical Journal, 339*, b2535.

*Möhler, R., Köpke, S., & Meyer, G. (2015). Criteria for Reporting the Development and Evaluation of Complex Interventions in healthcare: Revised guideline (CReDECI 2). *Trials, 16*, 204.

Monsivais, D. B. (2016). Taking a professional approach to peer reviewing. *Research and Theory for Nursing Practice, 30*, 195–197.

*Montgomery, P., Grant, S., Hopewell, S., MaDonald, G., Moher, D., Michie, S., & Mayo-Wilson, E. (2013). Protocol for CONSORT-SPI: An extension for social and psychological interventions. *Implementation Science, 8*, 99.

*Noble, W. S. (2017). Ten simple rules for writing a response to reviewers. *PloS Computational Biology, 13*, e1005730.

Northam, S., Greer, D., Rath, L., & Toone, A. (2014). Nursing journal editor survey results to help authors publish. *Nurse Educator, 39*, 290–297.

Oermann, M., Conklin, J., Nicoll, L., Chinn, P., Ashton, K., Edie, A., … Budinger, S. (2016). Study of predatory open access nursing journals. *Journal of Nursing Scholarship, 48*, 624–632.

Oermann, M., Galvin, E., Floyd, J., & Roop, J. (2006). Presenting research to clinicians: Strategies for writing about research findings. *Nurse Researcher, 13*, 66–74.

Oermann, M., & Hays, J. (2016). *Writing for publication* (3rd ed.). New York: Springer Publication.

Oermann, M., Nicoll, L., Chinn, P., Ashton, K., Conklin, J., Edie, A., … Willias, B. (2018). Quality of articles published in predatory nursing journals. *Nursing Outlook, 66*, 4–10.

*Ogrinc, G., Davies, L., Goodman, D., Batalden, P., Davidoff, F., & Stevens, D. (2015). SQUIRE 2.0 (Standards for QUality Improvement Reporting Excellence): Revised publication guidelines from a detailed consensus process. *Journal of Nursing Care Quality, 31*, 1–8.

O'Brien, B., Harris, I., Beckman, T., Reed, D., & Cook, D. (2014). Standards for Reporting Qualitative Research: A synthesis of recommendations. *Academic Medicine, 89*, 1245–1251.

*Pandis, N., Chung, B., Scherer, R., Elbourne, D., & Altman, D. (2017). CONSORT 2010 statement: Extension checklist for reporting within person randomised trials. *British Medical Journal, 357*, j2835.

Pearce, P., & Ferguson, L. (2017). How to write abstracts for manuscripts, presentations, and grants: Maximizing information in a 30-s sound bite world. *Journal of the American Association of Nurse Practitioners, 29*, 452–460.

*Penders, B. (2018). Ten simple rules for responsible referencing. *PLoS Computational Biology, 14* (4).

Piaggio, G., Elbourne, D., Pocock, S., Evans, S., & Altman, D. (2012). Reporting of noninferiority and equivalence randomized trials: Extension of the CONSORT 2010 statement. *Journal of the American Medical Association, 308*, 2594–2604.

*Pinnock, H., Barwick, M., Carpenter, C., Eldridge, S., Grandes, G., Griffiths, C., … Taylor, S. (2017). Standards for Reporting Implementation Studies (StaRI): Explanation and elaboration document. *BMJ Open, 7*, e013318.

Polit, D. F., & Gillespie, B. (2010). Intention-to-treat in randomized controlled trials: Recommendations for a total trial strategy. *Research in Nursing & Health, 58*, 391–399.

Polit, D. F., & Northam, S. (2011). Impact factors in nursing journals. *Nursing Outlook, 59*, 18–28.

Robinson, S., & Dracup, K. (2008). Innovative options for the doctoral dissertation in nursing. *Nursing Outlook, 56*, 174–178.

Roush, K. (2016). *A nurse's step-by-step guide to writing your dissertation or capstone*. Indianapolis: Sigma Theta Tau.

Roush, K. (2017a). Becoming a published writer. *American Journal of Nursing, 117*(3), 63–66.

Roush, K. (2017b). Writing your manuscript: Structure and style. *American Journal of Nursing, 117*(4), 56–61.

Roush, K. (2017c). What types of articles to write. *American Journal of Nursing, 117*(5), 68–71.

Roush, K. (2017d). Navigating the publishing process. *American Journal of Nursing, 117*(6), 62–67.

Sandelowski, M. (1998). Writing a good read: Strategies for representing qualitative data. *Research in Nursing & Health, 21*, 375–382.

**Siedlecki, S. L. (2017). Original research: How to create a poster that attracts an audience. *American Journal of Nursing, 117*, 48–54.

*Stroup, D., Berlin, J., Morton, S., Olkin, I., Williamson, G., Rennie, D., … Thacker, S. (2000). Meta-analysis of observational studies in epidemiology: A proposal for reporting. *Journal of the American Medical Association, 283*, 208–2012.

Strunk, W., & Campbell, V. (2018). *The elements of style: Simplified & illustrated for busy people*. Essex, UK: Campbell & Co. Literary.

*Tong, A., Flemming, K., McInnis, E., Oliver, S., & Craig, J. (2012). ENhancing Transparency in REporting the synthesis of Qualitative research. *BMC Medical Research Methodology, 12*, 181.

*Tong, A., Sainsbury, P., & Craig, J. (2007). Consolidated criteria for reporting qualitative research (COREQ): A 32-item checklist for interviews and focus groups. *International Journal for Quality in Health Care, 19*, 349–357.

*Vohra, S., Shamseer, L., Sampson, M. Bukutu, C., Schmid, C., Tate, R., … CENT group, . (2016). CONSORT extension for reporting N-of-1 trials (CENT) 2015 statement. *Journal of Clinical Epidemiology, 76*, 9–17.

*von Elm, E., Altman, D., Egger, M., Pocock, S., Gotzsche, P., & Vandenbroucke, J. (2014). The Strengthening the Reporting of Observational Studies in Epidemiology (STROBE) statement: Guidelines for reporting observational studies. *International Journal of Surgery, 12*, 1495–1499.

Wager, E. (2016). *Getting research published: An A-Z of publication strategy* (3rd ed.). London: Radcliffe Books.

Wong, P., Liamouttong, P., Koch, S., & Rawson, H. (2019). The impact of social support networks on family resilience in an Australian intensive care unit: A constructivist grounded theory. *Journal of Nursing Scholarship, 51*, 68–80.

Zinsser, W. (2006). *On writing well: The classic guide to writing nonfiction* (9th ed.). New York: Harper Collins.

*Zwarenstein, M., Treweek, S., Gagnier, J., Altman, D., Tunis, S., Haynes, B., … Moher, D. (2008). Improving the reporting of pragmatic trials: An extension of the CONSORT statement. *British Medical Journal, 337*, 1–8.

*A link to this open-access article is provided in the Toolkit for Chapter 32 in the **Resource Manual.**

**This journal article is available on thePoint for this chapter.

33 Writing Proposals to Generate Evidence

Research **proposals** communicate a research problem and proposed methods of solving it to an interested party. Research proposals are written both by students seeking faculty approval for studies and by researchers seeking financial support. In this chapter, we offer tips on how to improve the quality of research proposals and how to develop proficiency in **grantsmanship**—the set of skills needed to secure research funding.

OVERVIEW OF RESEARCH PROPOSALS

This section provides some general information about research proposals, most of which applies equally to dissertation proposals and grant applications.

Functions of a Proposal

Proposals are a means of opening communication between researchers and other parties. Those parties typically are either funding agencies or faculty advisers, whose job it is to accept or reject the proposed plan or to request modifications. An accepted proposal is a two-way contract: those accepting the proposal are effectively saying, "We are willing to offer our (professional or financial) support for a study that proceeds as proposed," and those writing the proposal are saying, "If you offer support, then the study will be conducted as proposed."

Proposals often serve as the basis for negotiating with other parties as well. For example, a proposal may be shared with administrators when seeking institutional approval to conduct a study (e.g., for gaining access to participants). Proposals may also be incorporated into submissions to research ethics committees or Institutional Review Boards.

Proposals help researchers to clarify their own thinking. By committing ideas to writing, ambiguities are eliminated at an early stage. When proposals are undertaken collaboratively, they help ensure that all parties are "on the same page" about how the study is to proceed. Reviewers also play an important role by suggesting conceptual and methodologic improvements.

Proposal Content

Proposal reviewers want a clear idea of what the researcher plans to study, why the study is needed, what methods will be used to achieve study goals, how and when tasks will be accomplished, and whether the researcher has the skills to complete the project successfully. Proposals are evaluated on a number of criteria, including the importance of the question, the adequacy of the methods, and, if money is requested, the reasonableness of the budget.

Proposal writers are usually given instructions about how to structure proposals. Funding agencies often supply an application kit that includes forms to be completed and specifies the format for organizing proposal content. Universities issue guidelines for dissertation proposals. The content and organization of most proposals are broadly similar to that for a research report, but proposals are written in the future tense (i.e., indicating what the researcher *will* do) and obviously do not include results and conclusions.

Proposals for Qualitative Studies

Preparing a proposal for qualitative research entails special challenges. Methodologic decisions typically evolve in the field, and therefore it is seldom possible to provide thorough information about such matters as sample size or data collection strategies. Sufficient detail needs to be provided, however, so that reviewers gain confidence that the researcher will assemble rich data from a good sample and will do justice to the data collected.

Qualitative researchers must persuade reviewers that the topic is important and worth studying, that they are sufficiently knowledgeable about the challenges of field work and adequately skillful in eliciting rich data, and, in short, that the project would be a good risk. Knafl and Deatrick (2005) offered 10 tips for successful qualitative proposals. The first tip is to make the case for the *idea*, not the method. They also advised qualitative researchers to avoid methodologic tutorials and to write for both experts and skeptics.

Resources are available to help qualitative researchers with proposal development. For example, an entire issue of the journal *Qualitative Health Research* was devoted to proposal writing (volume 13, issue 6). Useful advice is also available in Klopper (2008) and Padgett and Henwood (2009).

TIP DeCuir-Gunby and Schutz (2017) provide guidance on developing proposals for mixed methods studies.

Proposals for Theses and Dissertations

Dissertation proposals are sometimes a bigger hurdle than dissertations themselves. Many doctoral candidates founder at the proposal development stage rather than when writing or defending the dissertation. Much of our advice—especially in our "Tips" section later in the chapter—applies equally to proposals for theses and dissertations as for grant applications, but some additional advice might prove helpful.

The Dissertation Committee

Choosing the right dissertation adviser or chair (if a chair is chosen rather than appointed) is almost as important as choosing the right research topic. The ideal chair is a mentor, an expert with a strong reputation in the field, a good teacher, a patient and supportive coach and critic, and an advocate. Ideally, the chair also has sufficient time and interest to devote to your research and will stick with your project until its completion. This means that it might matter whether the prospective chair has plans for a sabbatical leave or is nearing retirement.

Dissertation committees often involve three or more members. If the chair lacks certain "ideal" characteristics, those characteristics can be balanced across committee members by seeking people with complementary talents. Putting together a group who will work well together can, however, be tricky. Advisers can usually offer suggestions about other committee members.

Once a committee has been formed, it is important to develop a good working relationship with members and to learn about their viewpoints before and during the proposal development stage. This means, at a minimum, becoming familiar with their research and the methodologic strategies they have favored. It also means meeting with them and sounding them out with ideas about topics and methods. If the suggestions from two or more members are at odds, it is prudent to seek your chair's counsel on how to resolve this.

TIP When meeting with your chair and committee members, take notes about their suggestions and write them out in more detail after the meeting while they are still fresh in your mind. The notes should be reviewed while developing the proposal.

Practices vary from one institution to another and from adviser to adviser, but some faculty require a *prospectus* before giving approval to prepare a full proposal. The prospectus is usually a three- to four-page paper outlining the research questions and proposed methods.

Content of Dissertation Proposals

Specific requirements regarding the length and format of dissertation proposals vary in different settings, and it is important to know at the outset what is expected. Typically, dissertation proposals are 20 to 40 pages in length. In some cases, however, committees prefer "mini-dissertations," that is, a document with fully developed sections that can be inserted with minor adaptation into the dissertation itself. For example, the review of the literature, theoretical framework, hypotheses, and the bibliography may be sufficiently refined at the proposal stage that they can be incorporated into the final product.

Literature reviews are often the most important section of a dissertation proposal, at least for quantitative studies. Committees may not desire lengthy literature reviews, but they want to be assured that students are in full command of knowledge in their field of inquiry.

Dissertation proposals sometimes include elements not normally found in proposals to funding agencies. One such element may be table shells (see Chapter 20), which can demonstrate that the student knows how to analyze data and present results effectively. Another element in proposals is the table of contents for the dissertation. The table of contents serves as an outline for the final product and demonstrates that the student knows how to organize material.

Several books provide additional advice on writing a dissertation proposal, including Locke et al. (2014), Roberts and Hyatt (2019), and Rudestam and Newton (2015). Bloomberg and Volpe (2016) have written specifically about qualitative dissertations.

FUNDING FOR RESEARCH PROPOSALS

Funding for research projects is becoming increasingly difficult to obtain because of keen competition. Successful proposal writers need to have good research and proposal-writing skills, and they must also know from whom funding is available. Wisdom and colleagues (2015), in their synthesis of grant-writing advice in 53 papers, emphasized the importance of doing appropriate background investigation to identify the goals and missions of potential funders.

TIP Because competition for research funding is fierce, Conn and colleagues (2015) suggested creative approaches to undertaking "science on a shoestring"—that is, research that is less costly to carry out. Examples include secondary analyses, research using data from electronic health records or social media, and collaborative efforts involving *practice-based research networks* (PRBNs).

Government Funding

Government Funding in the United States

The largest funder of research activities in the United States is the federal government. For healthcare researchers, the National Institutes of Health (NIH), the Agency for Healthcare Research and Quality (AHRQ), and the Patient-Centered Outcomes Research Institute (PCORI) are leading agencies. Two major types of federal disbursements are grants and contracts. **Grants** are awarded for studies conceived by researchers themselves, whereas **contracts** are for studies desired by the government.

There are several mechanisms for NIH grants, which can be awarded to researchers in both domestic and foreign institutions. Most grant applications are unsolicited and reflect the research interests of individual researchers. Unsolicited applications should be consistent with the broad objectives of an NIH institute, such as the National Institute of Nursing Research (NINR). Investigator-initiated applications are submitted in response to **Parent Announcements**, which are covered under omnibus *Funding Opportunity Announcements* (FOAs).

NIH also issues periodic **Program Announcements** (PAs) that describe new, continuing, or expanded program interests. For example, in November 2018, NINR issued a program announcement titled "Addressing caregiver symptoms through technological tools" (PA-19-023). The purpose of this PA, which expires in 2022, is to encourage applications for projects "to develop and test tools to address symptoms in caregivers."

Another grant mechanism allows federal agencies to identify a *specific* topic area in which they are interested in receiving proposals. **Requests for Applications** (**RFAs**) are one-time opportunities with a single submission date. As an example, NIH issued an RFA titled "Promoting research on music and health" in October 2018 (RFA-NS-19-008), with grant applications due in January 2019. The RFA states general guidelines and goals for the competition, but researchers can develop specific research questions within the broad area of interest. The *NIH Guide for Grants and Contracts* (available online at https://grants.nih.gov/funding/index.htm) contains announcements about RFAs, PAs, and Parent Announcements.

Some federal agencies—notably PCORI—award contracts to do specific studies. Contract offers are announced in a **Request for Proposals** (**RFPs**), which details the study that the government wants. Contracts, which are often awarded to only one competitor, constrain researchers' activities. Federal RFPs are announced in Federal Business Opportunities (https://www.fbo.gov/) or on the agencies' websites.

> **TIP** Kulage and colleagues (2015) have pointed out the very high costs associated with applying for NIH grants. An analysis in one school of nursing indicated that costs per grant application ranged from about $5,000 to $13,500.

Government Funding in Countries Other Than the United States

Government funding for nursing research is also available in many other countries. In Canada, for example, various types of health research are sponsored by the Canadian Institutes of Health Research (CIHR). In Australia, major government funding for health research comes from the National Health and Medical Research Council (NHMRC). In the United Kingdom, the major funder of health research is the Medical Research Council (MRC).

Private Funds

Healthcare research is supported by numerous philanthropic foundations, professional organizations, and corporations. Many researchers prefer private funding rather than government support because there is less "red tape."

Information about philanthropic foundations that support research in the United States is available through the Foundation Center (http://foundationcenter.org/). A comprehensive resource for identifying funding opportunities is the Center's *Foundation Directory*, available online for a fee. The directory lists the purposes and activities of foundations and information for contacting them. The Foundation Center also offers seminars and training on grant-writing and funding opportunities in many locations in the United States. Another resource for information on funding is the Community of Science's database on funding opportunities. Hassmiller (2017) noted that it may be easier to get initial funding from smaller regional foundations; the United Philanthropy Forum is a resource for such foundations.

> **TIP** The Robert Wood Johnson Foundation (RWJF) has been an especially strong supporter of nursing projects. It funds research to support a collaborative framework called a Culture of Health, which has as its goal that each person is able to live the healthiest life possible (Hassmiller, 2017).

Professional associations (e.g., the American Nurses' Foundation, Sigma Theta Tau, the American Association of Critical-Care Nurses) offer funds for conducting research. Health organizations, such as the American Heart Association and the American Cancer Society, also support research activities.

Finally, research funding is sometimes donated by private corporations, particularly those dealing with healthcare products. The Foundation Center publishes a directory of corporate grantmakers and provides links through its website to corporate philanthropic programs. Additional information about corporate requirements and interests should be obtained from the organization directly or from staff in the research administration offices of the institution with which you are affiliated. Conn and colleagues (2015) also noted that the local business community, which prefers supporting local causes, may be another resource worth exploring.

GRANT APPLICATIONS TO NIH

NIH funds many nursing studies through NINR and other institutes. Because of the importance of NINR as a funding source for nurse researchers, this section describes the process of proposal submission and review at NIH. AHRQ, which also funds nurse-initiated studies, uses the same application kit and similar procedures. Although the specifics of applying for funding vary across funders, many of the points made in this section are relevant for other funding sources.

> **TIP** NIH has 24 institutes and centers (ICs) that make grant awards, each of which has a website that explains its mission and priorities (e.g., for NINR: http://www.nih.gov/ninr). If you have an idea for a study and are not sure which type of grant program is suitable—or are unsure whether NINR or another NIH institute might be interested—you should contact NINR directly (Telephone number: 301-496-0207, email: info@ninr.nih.gov). NINR Program Officers can provide feedback about whether your proposed study matches NINR's program interests.

Types of NIH Grants and Awards

NIH awards different types of grants, and each has its own objectives and review criteria. The basic grant program—and the primary funding mechanism for independent research—is the traditional **Research Project Grant (R01)**. The objective of R01 grants is to support specific projects in areas reflecting the interests and competencies of a Principal Investigator (PI) and his or her team. It is NIH's most commonly used grant program. Note that there are two separate Parent Announcements for R01 grants—one for clinical trials and one for other types of projects.

Three other grant programs available through NIH are worth noting. A special program (R15) has been established for researchers working in institutions that have not been major participants in NIH programs. These **Academic Research Enhancement Awards (AREAs)** are designed to stimulate research in institutions that provide baccalaureate training for many individuals who go on to do health-related research. There is also a **Small Grant Program** (R03) that provides support for pilot or feasibility studies, methodology development, and secondary analyses. R03 grants provide a maximum of $50,000 of direct support for up to 2 years and are not renewable. Finally, the R21 grant mechanism—the **Exploratory/Developmental Research Grant Award**—is intended to encourage new, exploratory, and developmental projects by providing support for early stages of research.

NIH and other agencies also offer individual and institutional predoctoral and postdoctoral fellowships, as well as career development awards. Individual fellowship mechanisms available through the National Research Service Award (NRSA) program within NINR include the following:

- F31, Ruth Kirschstein Individual Predoctoral NRSA Fellowships, support nurses in a supervised training leading to a doctoral degree in areas related to the NINR mission.
- F32, Ruth Kirschstein Individual Postdoctoral NRSA Fellowships, support postdoctoral training to nurses to broaden their scientific background.

> **TIP** Advice on developing a proposal for an NRSA fellowship has been offered in papers by Parker and Steeves (2005) and Rawl (2014).

Three important Career Development Awards offered through NINR are as follows:

- K01, Mentored Research Scientist Development Award, available to doctorally prepared scientists who would benefit from a mentored experience with an expert sponsor

- K23, Mentored Patient-Oriented Research Career Development Award, supports the career development of investigators who are committed to focusing on patient-oriented research
- K99, Pathway to Independence Awards, provides for postdoctoral research activity leading to the submission of an independent research project application

TIP Botham and colleagues (2017) have described "10 simple rules" for preparing a career development award proposal. Also, Lor and colleagues (2019) have prepared a resource guide for postdoctoral opportunities for nurses.

NIH Forms and Processing Schedule

The SF424 application form, accessed through the online portal Grants.gov, is used for the types of grants and awards described in the previous section, although supplemental components are needed for some of them. Researchers use Adobe Reader to "fill in" and complete this application. There is abundant information online about the application process, and NIH offers training sessions on how to submit applications electronically. Several options can be used to submit an application, one of which is the use the NIH ASSIST system to prepare and submit the application and another is to use an institutional system-to-system process.

New grant applications are usually processed in three cycles annually. Different types of grants have different deadlines, as shown in Table 33.1. For most new applications, except fellowships in the F series and AIDS-related research, the deadline for receipt is in February, June, and October. The scientific merit review dates are about 4 to 5 months after each submission date. For example, applications submitted for the February cycle are reviewed in June or July; the earliest project start date for applications funded in that cycle would be in September or December (depending on when the applications are reviewed by the NIH Advisory Council). Individual applicants should begin a registration process through the Electronic Research Administration (eRA) Commons at least 6 weeks prior to the submission date. Once submitted, applications can be tracked through eRA Commons (https://commons.era.nih.gov/commons).

Preparing a Grant Application for NIH

Although many substantive aspects of the NIH grant application have remained stable, the forms and procedures for NIH grant applications have been changing. It is crucial to carefully review up-to-date instructions for grant application submission rather than relying on information in this chapter.

TABLE 33.1 • Schedule for Selected New Research Applications, National Institutes of Health

APPLICATION DUE DATE*	MECHANISM OF SUPPORT (TYPE OF AWARD)				
	R01 (NEW)	**R03, R21**	**R15**	**K SERIES**	**F SERIES**
Cycle I[a]	February 5	February 16	February 25	February 12	April 8
Cycle II[b]	June 5	June 16	June 25	June 12	August 8
Cycle III[c]	October 5	October 16	October 25	October 12	December 8

*Note: AIDS-related applications are on a different schedule: May 7, September 7, January 7 for new applications.

[a]Cycle I: Scientific Merit Review: June-July; Earliest start date: September or December.

[b]Cycle II: Scientific Merit Review: October-November; Earliest start date: April.

[c]Cycle III: Scientific Merit Review: February-March; Earliest start date: July.

Forms: Screens and Uploaded Attachments

The SF424 form set has numerous components. The "front matter" of SF424 consists of various forms that appear on a series of fillable screens. These forms help in processing the application. Some of the major forms include the following:

- *SF424 Form.* This form, used in all grant applications, collects information about the type of submission, type of applicant, proposed project dates, and other administrative data. Applicants must also state a brief descriptive title of the project.

> **TIP** The project title should be given careful thought. It is the first thing that reviewers see and should be crafted to create a good impression. The title, which is limited to 200 characters, should be concise, informative, and should also be compelling.

- *R&R Other Project Information Form.* This form is the mechanism for submitting key information for all grant applications. The form begins with questions about human subjects and vertebrate animals. The last few items require attachments to be uploaded, including a project summary, a project narrative, bibliography, and facilities and equipment information. Attachments, which must be in PDF format, have strict size limitations. The **Project Summary** serves as a succinct description of aims and methods of the proposed study and must be no longer than 30 lines. The **Project Narrative** is a brief (two to three sentences) description of the relevance of the research to public health. The *Bibliography* is a list of references cited in the research plan; any reference style is acceptable. The *Facilities* attachment is used to describe needed and available resources (e.g., laboratories). The *Equipment* attachment is used to list major items of equipment already available for the project.
- *Senior/Key Person Profile Form.* For each key person, the form requests basic identifying information and calls for an attachment, a Biographical Sketch. The sketch should list education and training, as well as the following:

(1) a Personal Statement describing the qualifications that make the person well-suited for his or her role; (2) Positions and Honors; (3) Contributions to Science in which up to five contributions are described, each of which can provide citations for up to four publications or interim research products relevant to that contribution; and (4) Research Support (ongoing and completed projects) and/or Scholastic Performance. A maximum of five pages is permitted for each person.

- *Budget Form.* For NIH applications, researchers must choose between two budget options—the R&R Budget Component or the PHS 398 Modular Budget Component. Detailed R&R budgets showing specific projected expenses are required if annual direct project costs exceed $250,000.

> **TIP** Cover letters are no longer recommended except under special circumstances (e.g., an application is late and a cover letter explains extraordinary circumstances that caused a delay). Requests to be assigned (or to *not* be assigned) to a particular review group should be submitted on a special form called the PHS Assignment Request Form. This form also allows applicants to identify individuals who should *not* review the application and the reason for such a request.

For grant applications to NIH and other public health service agencies, additional forms referred to as PHS 398 components are required and include the following:

- *PHS 398 Modular Budget Form.* **Modular budgets**, paid in modules of $25,000, are appropriate for R-series applications (e.g., R01s) from domestic organizations requesting $250,000 or less per year of direct costs. (**Direct costs** include specific project-related costs such as staff and supplies; **indirect costs** are institutional **overhead** costs.) This form provides budget fields for annual summaries of projected costs for up to 5 years of support. A *budget justification* attachment, detailing primarily personnel costs, must be uploaded.

TIP Even though modular budget forms ask only for summaries of the funds needed to complete a study, you should prepare a more detailed budget to arrive at a reasonable projection of needed funds. Beginning researchers are likely to require the assistance of a research administrator or an experienced, funded researcher in developing their first budget. Higdon and Topp (2004) and Bliss (2005) have offered advice on developing a budget.

- *PHS 398 Research Plan Form.* The PHS 398 Research Plan form requires information, in the form of attachments, about the proposed study and the research plan. Research plan requirements, the heart of the proposal, are described in the next section.
- *PHS Human Subjects and Clinical Trials Information.* Researchers who plan to collect data from human beings must submit a form relating to the protection of participants. Applicants must either address the involvement of humans and describe protections from research risks or provide a justification for exemption. The application must also include various types of information regarding the inclusion of women, minorities, and children. For example, applicants must complete an Inclusion Enrollment Report and Cumulative Inclusion Enrollment Report, which ask for expectations for enrollment of participants from various racial and ethnic categories, separately by gender. Additional attachments include a recruitment and retention plan and a study timeline. An attachment describing the data safety monitoring plan is required if the proposed study is a clinical trial.

TIP Examples of selected NIH forms are presented in the Toolkit of the *Resource Manual* in nonfillable form—i.e., they are included for information purposes only.

The Research Plan Component
The Research Plan component consists of 12 items, not all of which are relevant to every application—for example, item 1 is an Introduction but is required only for a resubmission or revision. Each item involves uploading a separate PDF attachment. In this section, we briefly describe guidelines for several items, with emphasis on items 2 and 3. We also present some advice based on a study (Inouye & Fiellin, 2005) in which the researchers content analyzed the criticisms in the review sheets of 66 applications (R01s) submitted to a clinical research review group (not NINR). Thus, the advice relating to specific pitfalls is "evidence-based," i.e., based on identified problems in actual applications. To our knowledge, this helpful analysis has not been updated.

TIP Based on their study, Inouye and Fiellin (2005) created a grant-writing checklist designed as a self-assessment tool for proposal developers. We have included an adapted and expanded checklist in the Toolkit of the accompanying *Resource Manual*.

Specific Aims. On this attachment, which is restricted to a single page, researchers must provide a succinct summary of the research problem and the specific objectives of the study, including any hypotheses to be tested. The aims statement should indicate the scope and importance of the problem. Care should be taken to be precise and to identify a problem of manageable proportions. Santen and colleagues (2017) describe the Specific Aims section as the "jewel in the crown" of a grant proposal—the most important component because reviewers read it first and form an immediate opinion.

Inouye and Fiellin (2005) found that the most frequent critique of the Specific Aims section was that the goals were overstated, overly ambitious, or unrealistic (18% of the reviews). Other complaints were that the project was poorly conceptualized (15%) or that hypotheses were not clearly articulated (12%).

TIP Some suggestions for describing the objectives of a pilot intervention study (see Chapter 29) are provided in the Supplement to this chapter on thePoint.

Research Strategy. Unless otherwise specified in a Funding Opportunity Announcement (FOA), the Research Strategy section is restricted to 12 pages for R01 and R15 applications and to 6 pages for R03, R21, and F-series applications. For other funding mechanisms, page restrictions are specified in the FOA.

> **TIP** Career Development Awards (K-series) involve completion of a special form, requiring attachments that include a description of the applicant's background, a statement of career goals and objectives, career development or training activities during the award period, and training in the responsible conduct of research. The applicant's institution and mentor must also submit a letter describing their commitment to the candidate and to his or her development.

The Research Strategy section is organized into three subsections: Significance, Innovation, and Approach. In the Significance section, researchers must convince reviewers that the proposed study idea has clinical or theoretical relevance and that the study will contribute to scientific knowledge or clinical practice. Applicants should describe how the concepts, treatments, services, or interventions that drive the field will be changed if the project aims are achieved. Researchers describe the study context in this section through a brief analysis of existing knowledge and gaps on the topic. Researchers should demonstrate command of current knowledge in a field, but this section must be very tightly written. Inouye and Fiellin (2005) found that a frequent critique expressed by reviewers about this section was that the need for the study was not adequately justified (29%).

In the Innovation section, researchers should describe how the proposed study challenges, refines, or improves current research or clinical practice paradigms. The application should describe novel theoretical concepts, instrumentation, or interventions to be developed or implemented, and explain their advantage over existing ones. An innovative grant application often proposes approaches to solve a persistent problem in new ways.

> **TIP** NINR launched an Innovative Questions (IQs) initiative that involved workshops with nursing researcher experts to develop creative questions for guiding future research directions. These innovative questions are organized into five topic areas: symptom science, wellness, self-management, end-of-life and palliative care, and innovation and technology (https://www.ninr.nih.gov/newsandinformation/iq).

The proposed design and methods for the study are described in the third subsection, Approach. This section, which is the heart of the application, should be written with extreme care and reviewed with a self-critical eye. The Approach section needs to be concise but with sufficient detail to persuade reviewers that methodologic decisions are sound and that the study will yield important and reliable evidence.

> **TIP** In 2018, NIH launched initiatives to enhance the accountability and transparency of clinical research—especially for clinical trials. A special website—Research Methods Resources—has been developed that offers help to investigators in satisfying new requirements (https://researchmethodsresources.nih.gov/).

The Approach section typically describes the following: (1) the research design, including comparison group strategies and methods of controlling confounding variables (for qualitative studies, the research tradition should be described); (2) the experimental intervention, if applicable, including a description of the treatment and control group conditions; (3) procedures, such as how participants will be assigned to groups and what type of blinding, if any, will be achieved; (4) the sampling plan, including eligibility criteria and sample size; (5) data collection methods and the measurement properties of measures that will be used; and (6) data analysis strategies. The Approach should identify potential methodologic problems and intended strategies for handling such problems. In proposals for qualitative studies, steps that will be taken to enhance the integrity and trustworthiness of the study should be described.

Inouye and Fiellin (2005) found that *all* of the reviews they analyzed had one or more criticism of this section, the most general of which was that the description of methods was underdeveloped (15%). A few of the most persistent criticisms were as follows:

- Inadequate blinding for outcome assessment (36%)
- Sample was flawed—biased or unrepresentative (36%)
- Important confounding variables inadequately controlled (32%)
- Inadequate sample size or inadequate power calculations (26%)
- Insufficient description of the approach to data analysis (24%)
- Outcome measures inadequately specified or described (23%)

Although some of these concerns relate to clinical trials (e.g., blinding), many have broad relevance. Small sample size, sample biases, and poorly described data collection and analysis plans can be problematic in any type of study.

The Approach section must also include information on Preliminary Studies. In new applications, researchers must describe the PI's preliminary or developmental studies and any experience pertinent to the application. This section must persuade reviewers that you have the skills and background needed to do the research. Any pilot work that has served as a foundation for the proposed project should be described. Inouye and Fiellin's (2005) analysis is especially illuminating with regard to Preliminary Studies. They found that the single biggest criticism across the 66 reviews was that more pilot work was needed, mentioned in 41% of the reviews.

Other Research Plan Sections. Most remaining items of the research plan (items 5-11) are not universally relevant. These include such items as a description and justification of the use of vertebrate animals (item 5) and a leadership plan if there are multiple principal investigators (item 7). One item (item 9), however, has relevance to many applications: Letters of support. This item requires you to attach letters from individuals agreeing to provide services to the project, such as consultants and collaborators. A letter of support should also be provided from proposed host organizations (preferably on their letterhead), indicating that the project is embraced by the organization and would be supported in moving forward as proposed.

Appendix Materials. In 2017, NIH initiated restrictions on appendix materials. Allowable materials include clinical trial protocols (for clinical trials), blank informed consent forms, and blank questionnaires or data collection instruments. Other items may be included only if the FOA requires it. The consequence of including disallowed items is nonreview of the application.

> **TIP** In terms of content, the research plan for NIH applications is similar to what is required in most research proposals—although emphases and page restrictions may vary and supplementary information may be required.

The Review Process

Grant applications submitted to NIH are reviewed for completeness, relevance, and adherence to instructions by the NIH Center for Scientific Review. Acceptable applications are assigned to an appropriate Institute or Center, and to a peer review group.

NIH uses a sequential, dual review system for informing decisions about its grant applications. The first level involves a panel of peer reviewers (not NIH employees), who evaluate applications for their scientific merit. These review panels are called **scientific review groups** (SRGs) or, more commonly, **study sections**. Each panel consists of about 10 to 20 researchers with backgrounds appropriate to the study section for which they have been selected and usually with a track record of NIH funding. Appointments to the review panels are for 4-year terms and are staggered so that about one-fourth of each panel is new each year.

TIP Applications by nurse researchers usually are assigned to the Nursing and Related Clinical Sciences Study Section (acronym NRCS). However, applications by nurse researchers can be reviewed in other study sections, such as Health Disparities and Equity Promotion (HDEP) or Health Services Organization and Delivery (HSOD).

The second level of review is by a National Advisory Council, which includes scientific and lay representatives. The Advisory Council considers not only the scientific merit of an application but the relevance of the proposed study to the programs and priorities of the Center or Institute to which the application has been submitted, as well as budgetary considerations.

During the first round of review in a study section, applications are assigned to primary and secondary (and sometimes a tertiary) reviewers for detailed analysis. Each assigned reviewer prepares comments and assigns scores according to five core review criteria.

1. *Significance.* Does this study address an important problem? If the aims of the application are achieved, how will scientific knowledge or clinical practice be advanced? What will be the effect of the study on the concepts or methods that drive this field?
2. *Investigator.* Is the PI appropriately trained and well-suited to carry out this work? Is the proposed work appropriate to the experience level of the PI and other researchers? Do Early-Stage Investigators have appropriate training and experience?
3. *Innovation.* Does the project employ novel concepts, approaches, or methods? Are the aims original and innovative? Does the project challenge existing paradigms or develop new methods or technologies?
4. *Approach.* Are the overall strategy, design, methods, and analyses adequately developed, and appropriate to the aims of the project? Does the applicant acknowledge potential problem areas and consider alternative tactics?

5. *Environment.* Does the scientific environment in which the work will be done contribute to the probability of success? Do the proposed experiments take advantage of unique features of the scientific environment or employ useful collaborative arrangements?

In addition to these five criteria, other factors are relevant in evaluating proposals, including the adequacy of protections for human or animal subjects and the appropriateness of the sampling plan in terms of including women, minorities, and children as participants. These factors are not, however, formally scored.

Scoring of applications changed in 2010. In the current system, each of the five core criteria is scored on a scale from 1 (exceptional) to 9 (poor). Assigned reviewers score applications and submit their scores before attending a study section meeting and submit a preliminary overall **impact score** (also called a **priority score**) on the same 1 to 9 scale. An impact score reflects a reviewer's assessment of the extent to which the study will exert a powerful influence in an area of research. Based on preliminary impact scores, applications with unfavorable scores (usually those in the lower half) are not discussed or scored by the entire study section in its meeting. This streamlined process was instituted so that study section members could focus their discussion on the most meritorious applications.

For applications that *are* discussed in the meeting, each study section member (not just those who were assigned as reviewers) designates an impact score, based on their own critique of the application and the committee's discussion. Individual impact scores from all committee members are averaged, and the mean is then multiplied by 10 to arrive at a final score. Thus, final impact scores for applications that are discussed can range from 10 (the best possible score) to 90 (the worst possible score). Final scores tend to cluster in the 10 to 50 range, however, because the least meritorious applications were previously screened out and not scored by the full study section. Among the scored applications, only those with the best priority scores actually obtain funding. Cutoff scores for funding vary from institute to institute and year to year, but a score of 20 or lower is usually needed to secure funding.

> **TIP** Some NIH institutes (but not NINR) calculate and publish a *payline*—a percentile-based funding cutoff point for impact scores, up to which nearly all R01 applications are funded.

Within a few days after a study section meeting, applicants can learn their priority score and percentile ranking online via the NIH eRA Commons, and within about 30 days they can access a summary of the evaluation. These **summary statements** include critiques written by the assigned reviewers, a summary of the study section's discussion, study section recommendations, and administrative notes of special consideration (e.g., human subjects issues). All applicants receive a summary sheet, even if their applications were unscored. Applicants of unscored applications also learn how the assigned reviewers scored the five core criteria.

Revisions and Resubmissions

Unless an unfunded proposal is criticized in some fundamental way (e.g., the problem area was not judged to be significant), applications often should be resubmitted, with revisions that reflect the concerns of the peer reviewers. Noble (2017) has offered "10 simple rules" for preparing a response to reviewers. Although his guidance was in relation to reviews of manuscripts submitted to a journal, the advice is also useful for addressing concerns of proposal reviewers. Examples of his tips include respond to every point raised by the reviewer; be polite and respectful of reviewers; and do what the reviewer asks, when possible.

When a proposal is resubmitted, the next review panel members are given a copy of the original application and the summary sheet so that they can evaluate the degree to which concerns have been addressed. Revised applications to NIH can be submitted only once.

TIPS ON PROPOSAL DEVELOPMENT

Although it is impossible to tell you exactly what steps to follow to produce a successful proposal, we conclude this chapter with some advice that might help to improve the process and the product. Many of these tips are especially relevant for those preparing proposals for funding. We draw heavily in this section on the many papers that have appeared in the healthcare literature on writing successful grant proposals and on a synthesis of advice by Wisdom and colleagues (2015). Further suggestions for writing effective grant applications may be found in Funk and Tornquist (2016), Gerin et al. (2018), and Karsh and Fox (2014).

Things to Do Before Writing Begins

Advance planning is essential to the development of a successful proposal. This section offers suggestions for things you can do to prepare for the actual writing.

Start Early

Writing a proposal and attending to the details of a formal submission process are time-consuming and almost always take longer than envisioned. Be sure to budget enough time that the product can be reviewed and rereviewed by members of the team (including any faculty mentors) and by willing colleagues. Build in adequate time for administrative issues such as securing permissions and getting budgets approved.

Having a proposal timeline is a good way to impose discipline on the proposal development process. Figure 33.1 presents one example, but the list of tasks is merely suggestive. Of course, it is advantageous to build pilot or preliminary work into your proposal development schedule, which may add many months to your timeline. As noted earlier, NIH reviewers frequently criticize the absence of adequate pilot work. Incremental knowledge building is attractive to reviewers. When you apply for funding, you are asking funders to make an *investment* in you; they will have the sense of being offered a better investment opportunity if some groundwork for a study has already been completed.

Task	Timeline (Months Before Submission)												
	12+	12	11	10	9	8	7	6	5	4	3	2	1
Identify/conceptualize the problem	X												
Undertake a literature review	X												
Identify and approach possible data collection sites	X												
Initiate descriptive or pilot work	X												
Analyze pilot data, assess feasibility	X	X	X	X	X								
Develop a "brief," outlining significance & preliminary thoughts about overall study design		X	X										
Identify methodologic and content experts; solicit input and possible collaboration		X	X	X									
Begin building a team of co-investigators and consultants		X	X	X	X								
Identify and contact funder/program officer (as needed)		X	X										
Obtain/download all application forms and instructions		X	X										
Review funding agencies' priorities; review recently funded grants		X	X	X									
Develop research plan, identify instruments, etc.; consult with statisticians, psychometricians, etc., as needed			X	X	X	X	X	X					
Collect site data for describing site, staff, clients				X	X	X							
Obtain written letters of agreement and/or support from data collection sites				X	X	X							
Prepare an outline of the proposal; develop writing assignments						X	X						
Write draft of proposal							X	X	X	X	X	X	X
Draft a budget								X	X				
Draft other ancillary components (bio sketches, etc.)								X	X				
Review application package internally (team members)									X	X	X		
Make revisions based on review										X	X	X	
Review application package externally by colleagues or mentors; convene mock review											X	X	X
Review all comments; make final revisions											X	X	X
Write abstract/summary												X	X
Finalize budget and other ancillary components													X
Prepare all final documents, get needed signatures													X

FIGURE 33.1 Example of a grant-writing timeline.

Select an Important Problem

A factor that is critical to the success of a proposal is selecting a problem that has clinical or theoretical significance. The proposal must articulate a persuasive argument that the research could make a contribution to evidence on a topic that is important and appealing to reviewers.

Researchers can sometimes profit by taking advantage of certain "hot topics" that have the special attention of the public and government officials. For example, *patient safety* emerged as a key topic in the early part of this century. Other recent "buzz words" in health care include *integrated care, patient-centered care,* and *precision medicine.* Sometimes there is an emerging hot topic that allows researchers to "catch and ride the wave" (Wiseman et al., 2013, p. 229). In the United States, one way of keeping abreast of emerging health topics is to visit the website for the "Healthy People" initiative that focuses on key health topics for the coming decade. For example, topics that were new for Healthy People 2020 included *sleep health; lesbian, gay, bisexual, and transgender health;* and *preparedness* (https://www.healthypeople.gov/2020/topics-objectives). Researchers should be sensitive to cultural and political realities.

Know Your Audience

Learn as much as possible about the audience for your proposal. For dissertations, this means getting to know your committee members and learning about their expectations, interests, and schedules. If you are writing a proposal for funding, you should obtain information about the funding organization's priorities. It is also a good idea to learn about recently funded projects. For NIH applications, you may be able to learn about the interests and preferred methods of reviewers by finding a roster of study section members for the likely review group.

Another aspect to "knowing your audience" concerns appreciating reviewers' perspective. Reviewers for funding agencies are busy professionals who are taking time away from their own work to consider the merits of proposed new studies. They are likely to be methodologically sophisticated and experts in *their* field—but they may have limited knowledge of your area of research. It is therefore imperative to help time-pressured reviewers to grasp the merits of your proposed study, without relying on jargon or specialized terminology.

Identify and Consult With a Mentor

An experienced grant-writer who is willing to provide guidance and support can play an invaluable role for novice researchers. A mentor may be willing to share their own experience in writing or reviewing proposals. Ideally, you would find a mentor who is willing to discuss early ideas, help you navigate the budgeting process, and review preliminary products. You should also ask your mentor to review your proposal timeline (and then commit to adhering to it). Mentors can often help young researchers through the "what-was-I-thinking" stage of proposal writing (Conn, 2013).

Review a Successful Proposal

Although there is no substitute for actually writing a proposal as a learning experience, novice proposal writers can profit by examining a successful proposal. It is likely that some of your colleagues or fellow students have written a proposal that has been accepted (either by a funding sponsor or by a dissertation committee), and some people are willing to share their successful efforts with others. Also, proposals funded by the government are usually in the public domain—that is, you can ask

for a copy of funded proposals. To obtain a funded NIH project, for example, you can contact the NIH Freedom of Information Coordinator for the appropriate institute. An important alternative is to communicate directly with the principal investigator of previously funded projects to inquire if they might be willing to share their proposal with you.

Several journals have published entire proposals, except for administrative/budgetary information. For example, the *Western Journal of Nursing Research* published a proposal for a qualitative study of adolescent fathers, together with reviewers' comments (Dallas et al., 2005a, 2005b). A chapter in the book by DeCuir-Gunby and Schutz (2017) includes a full mixed methods research proposal. Although the proposal is not in a health field and it is longer than proposals to NIH, it offers a useful perspective on good grant writing. Finally, one NIH institute (the National Institute of Allergy and Infectious Diseases [NIAID]) offers sample applications and summary statements for several types of funding mechanisms, such as R01, R03, R15, K01, and F31; a link is provided in the Toolkit. ✖

> **TIP** Appendix N of the accompanying *Resource Manual* includes the entire successful grant application to NINR by Deborah Dillon McDonald entitled "Older adults' response to health care practitioner pain communication," together with reviewers' comments and Dr. McDonald's response. Appendix O includes portions of a successful grant application for a NINR-funded project that is ongoing. Dr. Xiaomei Cong's application is entitled "Multi-omics analysis of pain/stress impact on neurodevelopment in preterm infants."

Create a Strong Research Team

For funded research, it is important to think strategically in putting together a team because reviewers often give considerable weight to researchers' qualifications. Having a team of competent people is insufficient—it is necessary to have the right *mix* of competence. Gaps and weaknesses can often be compensated for by the judicious use of consultants.

Another shortcoming of some project teams is that there are too many researchers with small-time commitments. It is unwise to propose a staff with five or more top-level professionals who can contribute only 5% to 10% of their time to the project. Such projects often run into management problems because no one is in control of the work flow. Although collaborative work is commendable, you should be able to justify the inclusion of every person.

Things to Do as You Write

If you have planned well and drafted a realistic schedule, the next step is to move forward with the development of the proposal. Some suggestions for the writing stage follow.

Adhere to Instructions

Funding agencies (and universities) provide instructions on what is required in a research proposal. It is crucial to read these instructions carefully and to follow them precisely. Proposals are sometimes rejected without review if they do not adhere to such guidelines as minimum font size or page limitations.

Build a Clear and Persuasive Case

In a proposal, whether or not funding is sought, you need to persuade reviewers that you are asking the right questions, that you are the right person to ask those questions, and that you will use rigorous methods to obtain valid and credible answers. You must also convince them that the answers will make a difference to nursing and its clients.

Beginning proposal writers sometimes forget that they are *selling* a product: themselves and their ideas. It is appropriate, therefore, to think of the proposal as a marketing opportunity. It is not enough to have a good idea and sound methods—you must have a persuasive presentation. When funding is at stake, the challenge is greater because *other applicants are trying to persuade reviewers that their proposal is more worthy of funding than yours.*

Reviewers know that most applications they review will *not* get funded. For example, in fiscal year 2018, the *success rate* for new and competing grant applications to NINR was approximately 11%. That means that nearly 9 out of 10 applications did

not receive funding. (For F-series training grants, the success rate tends to be higher, about 33%.) The reviewers' job is to identify the most scientifically worthy applications. In writing the proposal, you must consciously include features that will put your application in a positive light. That is, you should think of ways to gain a competitive edge. Be sure to give thought to issues persistently identified as problematic by reviewers (Inouye & Fiellin, 2005) and use a well-conceived checklist to ensure that you have not missed an opportunity to strengthen your proposal.

The proposal should be written in a positive, self-assured tone. If you do not sound convinced that the proposed study is important and will be rigorously done, then reviewers will not be persuaded either. It is unwise to promise what cannot be achieved, but you should think about ways to create enthusiasm.

Justify Methodologic Decisions

Many proposals fail because they do not instill confidence that key decisions have a good rationale. Methodologic decisions should be made carefully, keeping in mind the benefits and drawbacks of alternatives, and a compelling—if brief—justification should be provided. To the extent possible, make your decisions evidence-based and *defend* the proposed methods with citations demonstrating their utility. Insufficient detail and scanty explanation of methodologic choices can be perilous, although page constraints often make full elaboration impossible.

Address the Review Criteria

As you write, be conscious of the review criteria and emphasize the parts of the proposal that are relevant to those criteria. Every paragraph should be scrutinized to evaluate whether it addresses at least one of the criteria by which the proposal will be judged. If you ask others to review the proposal, be sure that they understand the review criteria.

Begin and End With a Flourish

The abstract or summary to the proposal should be crafted with extreme care. Because it is one of the first things that reviewers read, you need to be sure that it will create a favorable impression. (For NIH applications, nonassigned reviewers may read *only* the summary and not the entire application.) The ideal abstract is one that generates excitement and inspires confidence in the proposed study's rigor. Although abstracts appear at the beginning of a proposal, they are often written last.

Proposals typically conclude with material that is somewhat unexciting, such as a data analysis plan. A brief, upbeat concluding paragraph that summarizes the significance and innovativeness of the proposed project can help to remind reviewers of its potential to contribute to nursing practice and nursing science.

Pay Attention to Presentation

Reviewers are put in a better frame of mind if the proposals they read are well organized, grammatical, and easy to read. Glitzy figures are not needed, but the presentation should be professional and show respect for weary reviewers. In Inouye and Fiellin's (2005) study, 20% of the grant applications were criticized for such presentation issues as typographical or grammatical errors, poor layout, inconsistencies, and omitted tables.

Have the Proposal Critiqued

Before formal submission of a proposal, a draft should be reviewed by others. Reviewers should be selected for both substantive and methodologic expertise. If the proposal is being submitted for funding, one reviewer ideally would have first-hand knowledge of the funding source. If a consultant has been proposed because of specialized expertise that you believe will strengthen the study, he or she should be asked to participate by reviewing the draft and making recommendations for its improvement.

In universities, mock review panels are often convened prior to submission to a funding agency. Faculty and students are invited to these mock reviews and provide valuable feedback for enhancing a proposal. Kulage and Larson (2018) found, in one school of nursing, that applications that had undergone a mock review had a significantly higher rate of funding than those that had not. They describe protocols for mock reviews.

RESEARCH EXAMPLES

NIH makes available the abstracts of all funded projects through its Research Portfolio Online Reporting Tools (RePORTER). Abstracts can be searched by subject, researcher, institute, type of funding mechanism, year of support, and so on. Abstracts for two projects funded through NINR are presented here.

Example of a Funded Clinical Trial (R01) Project

Dr. Ji Yeon Choi, a postdoctoral fellow at the University of Pittsburgh School of Nursing, prepared the following abstract for a project entitled "Lung Transplant GO (LTGO): Improving self-management of exercise after lung transplantation." The application was reviewed by a Special Emphasis Panel and received NINR funding in May 2018. The project is scheduled for completion in March 2022. The total funding for this project is $569,238.

Project Summary: Lung transplantation is a costly procedure. Estimated costs, from 30 days prior to transplant to 6 months post surgery, exceed $1 million per patient and routine medical management costs $50,000 per year thereafter. Despite this extensive investment, major challenges remain. Prior to transplant, lung transplant recipients (LTRs) self-restrict activity due to severe ventilatory limitation, resulting in reduced muscle mass and qualitative changes in large exercising skeletal muscles. After transplant, despite improved lung function, prior studies consistently report LTR fail to reach predicted physical function or physical activity. Further, nearly 70% of LTR are at risk of developing hypertension within first 5 years due to their immunosuppressive regimen and an inactive lifestyle can worsen this risk. Consequently, full benefits of transplant may not be achieved. Few studies have tested ways to engage LTR to self-manage exercise and adopt an active lifestyle. Initiated by an Early-Stage New Investigator, we propose to test Lung Transplant Go (LTGO), a behavioral exercise intervention that provides individualized exercise training integrated with behavioral coaching for LTR in their home. Exercise training will focus on assisting LTR to learn and practice exercises to reverse muscle deconditioning. Behavioral coaching will engage LTR in developing skills to self-manage physical activity in their daily life and maintain this as a sustained habit using strategies that include incremental goal setting, self-monitoring, and feedback and problem solving. The LTGO intervention consists of two phases: Phase 1, intensive home-based exercise training and behavioral coaching via a telerehabilitation platform, VISYTER (Versatile and Integrated System for Telerehabilitation). Interactive intervention sessions will be delivered to the home via real-time video conferencing (10 sessions within 12 weeks); and Phase 2, transition to self-management. Four telephone sessions (one behavioral contract + three monthly counseling sessions) will be delivered over 12 weeks to provide behavioral coaching and exercise reinforcement. Our exciting pilot work successfully demonstrated the feasibility, safety, and ability of LTGO to improve physical function and physical activity and was enthusiastically received. We will conduct a two-group randomized controlled trial comparing LTGO against enhanced usual care (EUC). Participants will be 112 LTR randomized to LTGO or EUC (1:1). Outcomes will be measured at baseline, and 3 and 6 months post randomization. Primary outcomes are physical function (walking ability [6-Minute Walk Test], balance [Berg Balance Scale], lower body strength [30-second Chair Stand Test], and quadriceps muscle strength [Biodex System 3 Pro]) and physical activity (Actigraph GT3X). Secondary outcome is blood pressure control (preventing onset of hypertension or controlling existing hypertension). Potential mediators will be exercise self-efficacy and self-monitoring (Fitbit Charge HR). Potential moderators will be sex and clinical factors (symptoms, pre- and posttransplant clinical data). Findings will provide evidence regarding efficacy of the LTGO as a means to improve exercise self-management in LTR and, potentially, benefit in individuals living with other complex chronic conditions.

Example of a Funded Mixed Methods Training (F31) Project

Foster Baah, a doctoral student at the University of Pennsylvania, submitted a successful application for an NRSA predoctoral (F31) fellowship. The project was funded by NINR in September 2018 and is scheduled to end in June 2020. He prepared the following abstract for a study entitled "A mixed methods study to understand the relationship between social determinants of health and self-care in community dwelling patients with heart failure."

Project Summary: Prior research has focused on linking social determinants of health (SDH) to the distribution of chronic diseases such as heart failure (HF) within community groups. These studies reflect that racial, ethnic, and socioeconomic minority groups are the most burdened by HF. While adequate self-care in HF patients is known to significantly prevent exacerbations, reduce readmissions, improve quality of life and overall well-being, little is known about the relationship between SDH and HF self-care. Specifically, investigators are unsure of patients' fundamental situational needs that serve as operational mechanisms through which SDH limit the self-care choices of HF patients. These mechanisms may be the pathway through which SDH lead to the unequal distribution and inequity in HF burden among disparate population groups. Only by assessing the specific patient-identified needs that influence self-care behavior can interventions be targeted to improve health among vulnerable groups who suffer the negative effects of SDH. Therefore, this proposed research intensive application will prepare the applicant to conduct a mixed methods study to understand the relationship between SDH and HF self-care in hospitalized community-dwelling patients with HF. This goal will be achieved through three specific aims: (1) Quantitatively assess the relationship between SDH and HF self-care in 145 community-dwelling participants hospitalized for exacerbation of HF by testing seven SDH core domains (Race, Income, Education, Employment, Neighborhood, Housing status/stability, and Social integration/support), as predictors of HF self-care (maintenance, monitoring, management, and confidence) using backward elimination regression analyses, (2) Qualitatively explore the perceptions, beliefs, and experiences of extreme cases (poor and excellent self-care maintenance, N = 40) within the quantitative sample surrounding SDH and their self-care choices using the Gibb's reflective cycle in one-on-one interviews. This way, we will identify fundamental situational needs that are salient to participants and serve as operational mechanisms through which SDH limit the self-care choices of HF patients. In aim 3, we will describe differences in the self-reported SDH in relation to participants' self-care behavior by integrating the qualitative and quantitative data obtained from the extreme cases to identify patterns of differences or congruence in SDH and self-care behavior. The proposed study is first to use a mixed methods approach to explore the relationship between SDH and HF self-care and identify patient-specific fundamental needs as operational mechanisms through which SDH influence self-care. The proposed study aligns with the strategic plan of the National Institute of Nursing Research of promoting health, preventing illness, improving the health of individuals, and advancing health equity.

SUMMARY POINTS

- A **research proposal** is a written document specifying what a researcher intends to study; proposals are written by students seeking approval for dissertations and theses and by researchers seeking financial or institutional support. The set of skills associated with developing proposals for funding is called **grantsmanship**.

- Preparing proposals for qualitative studies is especially challenging because some methodologic decisions are made in the field; qualitative proposals need to persuade reviewers that the proposed study is important and a good risk.

- Students preparing a proposal for a dissertation or thesis need to work closely with a well-chosen committee and chair. Dissertation proposals are sometimes "mini-dissertations" that include sections that can be incorporated into the dissertation.

- The federal government is the largest source of research funds for health researchers in the United States. Regular grants programs are described through **Parent Announcements** (which are covered under *Funding Opportunity Announcements* or FOAs). Federal agencies such as the National Institutes of Health (NIH) also announce special opportunities in the form of **Program Announcements (PAs)** and **Requests for Applications (RFAs)** for **grants** and **Requests for Proposals (RFPs)** for **contracts**.

- Nurses can apply for a variety of grants from NIH, the most common being **Research Project Grants** (R01 grants), **AREA Grants** (R15), **Small Grants** (R03), or **Exploratory/Developmental Grants** (R21). NIH also awards training fellowships through the National Research Service Award (NRSA) program as F-series awards and Career Development Awards (K-series awards).

- Grant applications to NIH are submitted online using the SF424, which has a series of special forms (fillable screens) that require uploaded PDF attachments.

- The heart of an NIH grant application is the **research plan component**, which includes two major sections for new applications: *Specific Aims* and *Research Strategy*. The latter, which is restricted to 12 pages for R01 applications, includes subsections called Significance, Innovation, and Approach.

- NIH grant applications also require budgets, which can be abbreviated **modular budgets** if requested funds for R01 grants do not exceed $250,000 in direct costs per year.

- Grant applications to NIH are reviewed three times a year in a dual-review process. The first phase involves peer review by a **scientific review group** (SRG, usually called a **study section**) that evaluates each proposal's scientific merit; the second phase is a review by an Advisory Council.

- In NIH's review procedure, the study section assigns **priority (impact) scores** only to applications judged to be in the top half of proposals based on a preliminary appraisal by assigned reviewers. A final priority score of 10 by the study section is the best possible score and 90 is the poorest score.

- All applicants for NIH grants are sent a **summary statement**, which offers a critique of the proposal. Applicants of scored proposals also receive information on the impact/priority score and percentile ranking.

- Some suggestions for writing a strong proposal include several for the planning stage (e.g., starting early, selecting an important topic, learning about the audience, reviewing a successful proposal, creating a strong team) and several for the writing stage (adhering to proposal instructions, building a persuasive case, justifying methodologic decisions, ensuring that review criteria are addressed, beginning and ending with a flourish, and having the draft proposal critiqued by reviewers).

STUDY ACTIVITIES

Study activities are available to instructors on thePoint.

REFERENCES CITED IN CHAPTER 33

Bliss, D. Z. (2005). Writing a grant proposal, Part 6: The budget, budget justification, and resource environment. *Journal of Wound, Ostomy, & Continence Nursing, 32*, 365–367.

Bloomberg, L., & Volpe, M. (2016). *Completing your qualitative dissertation: A road map from beginning to end* (3rd ed.). Thousand Oaks: Sage.

*Botham, C., Arribere, J., Brubaker, S., & Beier, K. (2017). Ten simple rules for writing a career development award proposal. *PLoS Computational Biology, 13*, e1005863.

Conn, V. (2013). Welcome to the dark side of grant writing. *Western Journal of Nursing Research, 35*, 967–969.

Conn, V., Topp, R., Dunn, S., Hopp, L., Jadack, R., Jansen, , … Moch, D. (2015). Science on a shoestring: Building nursing knowledge with limited funding. *Western Journal of Nursing Research, 37*, 1256–1268.

Dallas, C., Norr, K., Dancy, B., Kavanagh, K., & Cassata, L. (2005a). An example of a successful research proposal: Part I. *Western Journal of Nursing Research, 27*, 50–72.

Dallas, C., Norr, K., Dancy, B., Kavanagh, K., & Cassata, L. (2005b). An example of a successful research proposal: Part II. *Western Journal of Nursing Research, 27*, 210–231.

DeCuir-Gunby, J., & Schutz, P. (2017). *Developing a mixed methods proposal: A practical guide for beginning researchers*. Thousand Oaks, CA: Sage.

Funk, S. G., & Tornquist, E. M. (2016). *Writing winning proposals for nurses and health care professionals*. New York: Springer Publishing Co.

Gerin, W., Kinkade, C., & Page, N. (2018). *Writing the NIH grant proposal: A step-by-step guide* (3rd ed.). Thousand Oaks, CA: Sage.

**Hassmiller, S. B. (2017). How to engage funders and get money: The 10Rs you need to know. *American Journal of Nursing, 117*, 63–65.

Higdon, J., & Topp, R. (2004). How to develop a budget for a research proposal. *Western Journal of Nursing Research, 26*, 922–929.

Inouye, S. K., & Fiellin, D. A. (2005). An evidence-based guide to writing grant proposals for clinical research. *Annals of Internal Medicine, 142*, 274–282.

Karsh, E., & Fox, A. (2014). *The only grant-writing book you'll ever need* (4th ed.). New York: Basic Books.

*Klopper, H. (2008). The qualitative research proposal. *Curationis, 31*, 62–72.

Knafl, K., & Deatrick, J. (2005). Top 10 tips for successful qualitative grantsmanship. *Research in Nursing & Health, 28*, 441–443.

Kulage, K., & Larson, E. (2018). Intramural pilot funding and internal grant reviews increase research capacity at a school of nursing. *Nursing Outlook, 66*, 11–17.

Kulage, K., Schnall, R., Hickey, K., Travers, J., Zezulinksi, K., Torres, F., … Larson, E. (2015). Time and costs of preparing and submitting an NIH grant application at a school of nursing. *Nursing Outlook, 63*, 639–649.

Locke, L., Spirduso, W., & Silverman, S. (2014). *Proposals that work: A guide for planning dissertations and grant proposals* (6th ed.). Thousand Oaks, CA: Sage.

Lor, M., Oyesanya, T., Chen, C., Cherwin, C., & Moon, C. (2019). Postdoctoral opportunities for nursing PhD graduates: A resource guide. *Western Journal of Nursing Research*. doi:10.1177/0193945918775691.

*Noble, W. S. (2017). Ten simple rules for writing a response to reviewers. *PLoS Computational Biology, 13*, e1005730.

Padgett, D., & Henwood, B. (2009). Obtaining large-scale funding for empowerment-oriented qualitative research: A report from personal experience. *Qualitative Health Research, 19*, 868–874.

Parker, B., & Steeves, R. (2005). The National Research Service Award: Strategies for developing a successful proposal. *Journal of Professional Nursing, 21*, 23–31.

Rawl, S. M. (2014). Writing a competitive individual National Service Award (F31) application. *Western Journal of Nursing Research, 36*, 31–46.

Roberts, C., & Hyatt, L. (2019). *The dissertation journey: A practical guide to planning, writing, and defending your dissertation* (3rd ed.). Thousand Oaks, CA: Sage.

Rudestam, K., & Newton, R. (2015). *Surviving your dissertation: A comprehensive guide to content and process* (4th ed.). Thousand Oaks, CA: Sage.

*Santen, R., Barrett, E., Siragy, H., Farhi, L., Fishbein, L., & Carey, R. (2017). The jewel in the crown: Specific aims section of investigator-initiated grant proposals. *Journal of the Endocrine Society, 1*, 1194–1202.

Wisdom, J., Riley, H., & Myers, N. (2015). Recommendations for writing successful grant proposals: An information synthesis. *Academic Medicine, 90*, 1720–1725.

*Wiseman, J., Alavi, K., & Milner, R. (2013). Grant writing 101. *Clinics in Colon and Rectal Surgery, 26*, 228–231.

*A link to this open-access article is provided in the Toolkit for Chapter 33 in the **Resource Manual.** ⊗

**This journal article is available on* thePoint *for this chapter.*

Appendix:
Statistical Tables of Theoretical Probability Distributions

TABLE A.1 • Critical Values for the *t* Distribution

df	α, 2-tailed test:	.10	.05	.02	.01	.001
	α, 1-tailed test:	.05	.025	.01	.005	.0005
1		6.314	12.706	31.821	63.657	636.619
2		2.920	4.303	6.965	9.925	31.598
3		2.353	3.182	4.541	5.841	12.941
4		2.132	2.776	3.747	4.604	8.610
5		2.015	2.571	3.376	4.032	6.859
6		1.953	2.447	3.143	3.707	5.959
7		1.895	2.365	2.998	3.449	5.405
8		1.860	2.306	2.896	3.355	5.041
9		1.833	2.262	2.821	3.250	4.781
10		1.812	2.228	2.765	3.169	4.587
11		1.796	2.201	2.718	3.106	4.437
12		1.782	2.179	2.681	3.055	4.318
13		1.771	2.160	2.650	3.012	4.221
14		1.761	2.145	2.624	2.977	4.140
15		1.753	2.131	2.602	2.947	4.073
16		1.746	2.120	2.583	2.921	4.015
17		1.740	2.110	2.567	2.898	3.965
18		1.734	2.101	2.552	2.878	3.922
19		1.729	2.093	2.539	2.861	3.883
20		1.725	2.086	2.528	2.845	3.850
21		1.721	2.080	2.518	2.831	3.819
22		1.717	2.074	2.508	2.819	3.792
23		1.714	2.069	2.500	2.807	3.767
24		1.711	2.064	2.492	2.797	3.745
25		1.708	2.060	2.485	2.787	3.725
26		1.706	2.056	2.479	2.779	3.707
27		1.703	2.052	2.473	2.771	3.690
28		1.701	2.048	2.467	2.763	3.674
29		1.699	2.045	2.462	2.756	3.659
30		1.697	2.042	2.457	2.750	3.646
40		1.684	2.021	2.423	2.704	3.551
60		1.671	2.000	2.390	2.660	3.460
120		1.658	1.980	2.358	2.617	3.373
∞		1.645	1.960	2.326	2.576	3.291

TABLE A.2 • **Critical Values for the F Distribution**

df_B df_W	α = .05 (Two-Tailed)									α = .025 (One-Tailed)
	1	**2**	**3**	**4**	**5**	**6**	**8**	**12**	**24**	**∞**
1	161.4	199.5	215.7	224.6	230.2	234.0	238.9	243.9	249.0	254.3
2	18.51	19.00	19.16	19.25	19.30	19.33	19.37	19.41	19.45	19.50
3	10.13	9.55	9.28	9.12	9.01	8.94	8.84	8.74	8.64	8.53
4	7.71	6.94	6.59	6.39	6.26	6.16	6.04	5.91	5.77	5.63
5	6.61	5.79	5.41	5.19	5.05	4.95	4.82	4.68	4.53	4.36
6	5.99	5.14	4.76	4.53	4.39	4.28	4.15	4.00	3.84	3.67
7	5.59	4.74	4.35	4.12	3.97	3.87	3.73	3.57	3.41	3.23
8	5.32	4.46	4.07	3.84	3.69	3.58	3.44	3.28	3.12	2.93
9	5.12	4.26	3.86	3.63	3.48	3.37	3.23	3.07	2.90	2.71
10	4.96	4.10	3.71	3.48	3.33	3.22	3.07	2.91	2.74	2.54
11	4.84	3.98	3.59	3.36	3.20	3.09	2.95	2.79	2.61	2.40
12	4.75	3.88	3.49	3.26	3.11	3.00	2.85	2.69	2.50	2.30
13	4.67	3.80	3.41	3.18	3.02	2.92	2.77	2.60	2.42	2.21
14	4.60	3.74	3.34	3.11	2.96	2.85	2.70	2.53	2.35	2.13
15	4.54	3.68	3.29	3.06	2.90	2.79	2.64	2.48	2.29	2.07
16	4.49	3.63	3.24	3.01	2.85	2.74	2.59	2.42	2.24	2.01
17	4.45	3.59	3.20	2.96	2.81	2.70	2.55	2.38	2.19	1.96
18	4.41	3.55	3.16	2.93	2.77	2.66	2.51	2.34	2.15	1.92
19	4.38	3.52	3.13	2.90	2.74	2.63	2.48	2.31	2.11	1.88
20	4.35	3.49	3.10	2.87	2.71	2.60	2.45	2.28	2.08	1.84
21	4.32	3.47	3.07	2.84	2.68	2.57	2.42	2.25	2.05	1.81
22	4.30	3.44	3.05	2.82	2.66	2.55	2.40	2.23	2.03	1.78
23	4.28	3.42	3.03	2.80	2.64	2.53	2.38	2.20	2.00	1.76
24	4.26	3.40	3.01	2.78	2.62	2.51	2.36	2.18	1.98	1.73
25	4.24	3.38	2.99	2.76	2.60	2.49	2.34	2.16	1.96	1.71
26	4.22	3.37	2.98	2.74	2.59	2.47	2.32	2.15	1.95	1.69
27	4.21	3.35	2.96	2.73	2.57	2.46	2.30	2.13	1.93	1.67
28	4.20	3.34	2.95	2.71	2.56	2.44	2.29	2.12	1.91	1.65
29	4.18	3.33	2.93	2.70	2.54	2.43	2.28	2.10	1.90	1.64
30	4.17	3.32	2.92	2.69	2.53	2.42	2.27	2.09	1.89	1.62
40	4.08	3.23	2.84	2.61	2.45	2.34	2.18	2.00	1.79	1.51
60	4.00	3.15	2.76	2.52	2.37	2.25	2.10	1.92	1.70	1.39
120	3.92	3.07	2.68	2.45	2.29	2.17	2.02	1.83	1.61	1.25
∞	3.84	2.99	2.60	2.37	2.21	2.09	1.94	1.75	1.52	1.00

TABLE A.2 • Critical Values for the *F* Distribution (Continued)

df_B / df_W	α = .01 (Two-Tailed)									α = .005 (One-Tailed)
	1	2	3	4	5	6	8	12	24	∞
1	4,052	4,999	5,403	5,625	5,764	5,859	5,981	6,106	6,234	6,366
2	98.49	99.00	99.17	99.25	99.30	99.33	99.36	99.42	99.46	99.50
3	34.12	30.81	29.46	28.71	28.24	27.91	27.49	27.05	26.60	26.12
4	21.20	18.00	16.69	15.98	15.52	15.21	14.80	14.37	13.93	13.46
5	16.26	13.27	12.06	11.39	10.97	10.67	10.29	9.89	9.47	9.02
6	13.74	10.92	9.78	9.15	8.75	8.47	8.10	7.72	7.31	6.88
7	12.25	9.55	8.45	7.85	7.46	7.19	6.84	6.47	6.07	5.65
8	11.26	8.65	7.59	7.01	6.63	6.37	6.03	5.67	5.28	4.86
9	10.56	8.02	6.99	6.42	6.06	5.80	5.47	5.11	4.73	4.31
10	10.04	7.56	6.55	5.99	5.64	5.39	5.06	4.71	4.33	3.91
11	9.65	7.20	6.22	5.67	5.32	5.07	4.74	4.40	4.02	3.60
12	9.33	6.93	5.95	5.41	5.06	4.82	4.50	4.16	3.78	3.36
13	9.07	6.70	5.74	5.20	4.86	4.62	4.30	3.96	3.59	3.16
14	8.86	6.51	5.56	5.03	4.69	4.46	4.14	3.80	3.43	3.00
15	8.68	6.36	5.42	4.89	4.56	4.32	4.00	3.67	3.29	2.87
16	8.53	6.23	5.29	4.77	4.44	4.20	3.89	3.55	3.18	2.75
17	8.40	6.11	5.18	4.67	4.34	4.10	3.78	3.45	3.08	2.65
18	8.28	6.01	5.09	4.58	4.29	4.01	3.71	3.37	3.00	2.57
19	8.18	5.93	5.01	4.50	4.17	3.94	3.63	3.30	2.92	2.49
20	8.10	5.85	4.94	4.43	4.10	3.87	3.56	3.23	2.86	2.42
21	8.02	5.78	4.87	4.37	4.04	3.81	3.51	3.17	2.80	2.36
22	7.94	5.72	4.82	4.31	3.99	3.76	3.45	3.12	2.75	2.31
23	7.88	5.66	4.76	4.26	3.94	3.71	3.41	3.07	2.70	2.26
24	7.82	5.61	4.72	4.22	3.90	3.67	3.36	3.03	2.66	2.21
25	7.77	5.57	4.68	4.18	3.86	3.63	3.32	2.99	2.62	2.17
26	7.72	5.53	4.64	4.14	3.82	3.59	3.29	2.96	2.58	2.13
27	7.68	5.49	4.60	4.11	3.78	3.56	3.26	2.93	2.55	2.10
28	7.64	5.45	4.57	4.07	3.75	3.53	3.23	2.90	2.52	2.06
29	7.60	5.42	4.54	4.04	3.73	3.50	3.20	2.87	2.49	2.03
30	7.56	5.39	4.51	4.02	3.70	3.47	3.17	2.84	2.47	2.01
40	7.31	5.18	4.31	3.83	3.51	3.29	2.99	2.66	2.29	1.80
60	7.08	4.98	4.13	3.65	3.34	3.12	2.82	2.50	2.12	1.60
120	6.85	4.79	3.95	3.48	3.17	2.96	2.66	2.34	1.95	1.38
∞	6.64	4.60	3.78	3.32	3.02	2.80	2.51	2.18	1.79	1.00

(Continued)

TABLE A.2 • **Critical Values for the *F* Distribution**   (Continued)

df_B	$\alpha = .001$ (Two-Tailed)									$\alpha = .0005$ (One-Tailed)
df_W	1	2	3	4	5	6	8	12	24	∞
1	405,284	500,000	540,379	562,500	576,405	585,937	598,144	610,667	623,497	636,619
2	998.5	999.0	999.2	999.2	999.3	999.3	999.4	999.4	999.5	999.5
3	167.5	148.5	141.1	137.1	134.6	132.8	130.6	128.3	125.9	123.5
4	74.14	61.25	56.18	53.44	51.71	50.53	49.00	47.41	45.77	44.05
5	47.04	36.61	33.20	31.09	29.75	28.84	27.64	26.42	25.14	23.78
6	35.51	27.00	23.70	21.90	20.81	20.03	19.03	17.99	16.89	15.75
7	29.22	21.69	18.77	17.19	16.21	15.52	14.63	13.71	12.73	11.69
8	25.42	18.49	15.83	14.39	13.49	12.86	17.04	11.19	10.30	9.34
9	22.86	16.39	13.90	12.56	11.71	11.13	10.37	9.57	8.72	7.81
10	21.04	14.91	12.55	11.28	10.48	9.92	9.20	8.45	7.64	6.76
11	19.69	13.81	11.56	10.35	9.58	9.05	8.35	7.63	6.85	6.00
12	18.64	12.97	10.80	9.63	8.89	8.38	7.71	7.00	6.25	5.42
13	17.81	12.31	10.21	9.07	8.35	7.86	7.21	6.52	5.78	4.97
14	17.14	11.78	9.73	8.62	7.92	7.43	6.80	6.13	5.41	4.60
15	16.59	11.34	9.34	8.25	7.57	7.09	6.47	5.81	5.10	4.31
16	16.12	10.97	9.00	7.94	7.27	6.81	6.19	5.55	4.85	4.06
17	15.72	10.66	8.73	7.68	7.02	6.56	5.96	5.32	4.63	3.85
18	15.38	10.39	8.49	7.46	6.81	6.35	5.76	5.13	4.45	3.67
19	15.08	10.16	8.28	7.26	6.61	6.18	5.59	4.97	4.29	3.52
20	14.82	9.95	8.10	7.10	6.46	6.02	5.44	4.82	4.15	3.38
21	14.59	9.77	7.94	6.95	6.32	5.88	5.31	4.70	4.03	3.26
22	14.38	9.61	7.80	6.81	6.19	5.76	5.19	4.58	3.92	3.15
23	14.19	9.47	7.67	6.69	6.08	5.65	5.09	4.48	3.82	3.05
24	14.03	9.34	7.55	6.59	5.98	5.55	4.99	4.39	3.74	2.97
25	13.88	9.22	7.45	6.49	5.88	5.46	4.91	4.31	3.66	2.89
26	13.74	9.12	7.36	6.41	5.80	5.38	4.83	4.24	3.59	2.82
27	13.61	9.02	7.27	6.33	5.73	5.31	4.76	4.17	3.52	2.75
28	13.50	8.93	7.19	6.25	5.66	5.24	4.69	4.11	3.46	2.70
29	13.39	8.85	7.12	6.19	5.59	5.18	4.64	4.05	3.41	2.64
30	13.29	8.77	7.05	6.12	5.53	5.12	4.58	4.00	3.36	2.59
40	12.61	8.25	6.60	5.70	5.13	4.73	4.21	3.64	3.01	2.23
60	11.97	7.76	6.17	5.31	4.76	4.37	3.87	3.31	2.69	1.90
120	11.38	7.31	5.79	4.95	4.42	4.04	3.55	3.02	2.40	1.56
∞	10.83	6.91	5.42	4.62	4.10	3.74	3.27	2.74	2.13	1.00

TABLE A.3 • Critical Values for the χ^2 Distribution

df	LEVEL OF SIGNIFICANCE				
	.10	.05	.02	.01	.001
1	2.71	3.84	5.41	6.63	10.83
2	4.61	5.99	7.82	9.21	13.82
3	6.25	7.82	9.84	11.34	16.27
4	7.78	9.49	11.67	13.28	18.46
5	9.24	11.07	13.39	15.09	20.52
6	10.64	12.59	15.03	16.81	22.46
7	12.02	14.07	16.62	18.48	24.32
8	13.36	15.51	18.17	20.09	26.12
9	14.68	16.92	19.68	21.67	27.88
10	15.99	18.31	21.16	23.21	29.59
11	17.28	19.68	22.62	24.72	31.26
12	18.55	21.03	24.05	26.22	32.91
13	19.81	22.36	25.47	27.69	34.53
14	21.06	23.68	26.87	29.14	36.12
15	22.31	25.00	28.26	30.58	37.70
16	23.54	26.30	29.63	32.00	39.25
17	24.77	27.59	31.00	33.41	40.79
18	25.99	28.87	32.35	34.81	42.31
19	27.20	30.14	33.69	36.19	43.82
20	28.41	31.41	35.02	37.57	45.32
21	29.62	32.67	36.34	38.93	46.80
22	30.81	33.92	37.66	40.29	48.27
23	32.01	35.17	38.97	41.64	49.73
24	33.20	36.42	40.27	42.98	51.18
25	34.38	37.65	41.57	44.31	52.62
26	35.56	38.89	42.86	45.64	54.05
27	36.74	40.11	44.14	46.96	55.48
28	37.92	41.34	45.42	48.28	56.89
29	39.09	42.56	46.69	49.59	58.30
30	40.26	43.77	47.96	50.89	59.70

TABLE A.4 • Critical Values of the *r* Distribution

	LEVEL OF SIGNIFICANCE FOR ONE-TAILED TEST				
	.05	.025	.01	.005	.0005
	LEVEL OF SIGNIFICANCE FOR TWO-TAILED TEST				
df	.10	.05	.02	.01	.001
1	.98769	.99692	.999507	.999877	.9999988
2	.90000	.95000	.98000	.990000	.99900
3	.8054	.8783	.93433	.95873	.99116
4	.7293	.8114	.8822	.91720	.97406
5	.6694	.7545	.8329	.8745	.95074
6	.6215	.7067	.7887	.8343	.92493
7	.5822	.6664	.7498	.7977	.8982
8	.5494	.6319	.7155	.7646	.8721
9	.5214	.6021	.6851	.7348	.8471
10	.4973	.5760	.6581	.7079	.8233
11	.4762	.5529	.6339	.6835	.8010
12	.4575	.5324	.6120	.6614	.7800
13	.4409	.5139	.5923	.5411	.7603
14	.4259	.4973	.5742	.6226	.7420
15	.4124	.4821	.5577	.6055	.7246
16	.4000	.4683	.5425	.5897	.7084
17	.3887	.4555	.5285	.5751	.6932
18	.3783	.4438	.5155	.5614	.5687
19	.3687	.4329	.5034	.5487	.6652
20	.3598	.4227	.4921	.5368	.6524
25	.3233	.3809	.4451	.5869	.5974
30	.2960	.3494	.4093	.4487	.5541
35	.2746	.3246	.3810	.4182	.5189
40	.2573	.3044	.3578	.3932	.4896
45	.2428	.2875	.3384	.3721	.4648
50	.2306	.2732	.3218	.3541	.4433
60	.2108	.2500	.2948	.3248	.4078
70	.1954	.2319	.2737	.3017	.3799
80	.1829	.2172	.2565	.2830	.3568
90	.1726	.2050	.2422	.2673	.3375
100	.1638	.1946	.2301	.2540	.3211

Glossary

5 Whys A process involving rounds of questioning that is used in some quality improvement projects to gain insight into the root cause of a problem.

6S hierarchy A 6-level hierarchy that ranks evidence sources (including preappraised evidence) in terms of ease of use in clinical settings.

absolute risk (AR) The proportion of people in a group who experienced an undesirable outcome.

absolute risk reduction (ARR) The difference between the absolute risk in one group (e.g., those exposed to an intervention) and the absolute risk in another group (e.g., those not exposed); sometimes called the *risk difference* or *RD*.

abstract A brief description of a completed or proposed study, usually located at the beginning of a report or proposal.

accessible population The population of people available for a particular study; often a nonrandom subset of the target population.

acquiescence response set A bias in self-report instruments, especially in psychosocial scales, created when participants characteristically agree with statements ("yea-say"), independent of content.

adaptive intervention An intervention in which there are multiple decision points over time and decisions are based on individual responses to the treatment.

adaptive trial design A strategy for testing an intervention that involves altering the design itself during the course of the trial (e.g., dropping or adding a study arm).

adherence to treatment The degree to which those in an intervention group adhere to protocols or continue getting the treatment.

after-only design An experimental design in which data are collected from participants only after an intervention has been introduced.

AGREE instrument A widely used instrument (Appraisal of Guidelines Research and Evaluation) for systematically assessing clinical practice guidelines.

allocation concealment The process used to ensure that the people enrolling participants into a clinical trial are unaware of upcoming assignments to treatment conditions.

alpha (α) (1) In tests of statistical significance, the significance criterion—the risk the researcher is willing to accept of making a Type I error; (2) in measurement, an index of internal consistency, i.e., Cronbach's alpha.

alternative hypothesis In hypothesis testing, a hypothesis different from the one actually being tested—usually, the alternative to the null hypothesis; sometimes called the *research hypothesis*.

analysis The organization and synthesis of data so as to answer research questions or test hypotheses.

analysis of covariance (ANCOVA) A statistical procedure used to test mean group differences on an outcome variable, while controlling for one or more covariate.

analysis of variance (ANOVA) A statistical procedure for testing mean differences among three or more groups by contrasting variability between groups to variability within groups, yielding an *F*-ratio statistic.

analytic generalization One of three models of generalization, concerning researchers' efforts to generalize from particulars to broader conceptualizations and theories.

ancestry approach In literature searches, using citations from relevant studies to track down earlier research on the same topic (the "ancestors"); also called *snowballing*, *footnote chasing*, and *pearl growing*.

anchor-based approach An approach to estimating a measure's responsiveness, and to developing a benchmark of importance for interpreting change scores, that relies on a "gold standard" criterion as the anchor.

anonymity Protection of participants' confidentiality such that even the researcher cannot link individuals with the data they provided.

applicability The degree to which research evidence can be applied to individuals, small groups of individuals, or local contexts (as opposed to broad populations).

applied research Research aimed at finding a solution to a practical problem.

area under the curve (AUC) In ROC analysis, an index of the performance of a diagnostic or screening measure vis-à-vis diagnostic accuracy, summarized in a single value that typically ranges from .50 (no better than random classification) to 1.0 (perfect classification).

argument An explanation of what a researcher wants to study, with supportive evidence and background material linked in a manner that provides a rationale.

arm A particular treatment condition to which participants are allocated (e.g., the intervention *arm* or control *arm* of a controlled trial).

ascertainment bias Systematic differences between groups being compared in how outcome variables are measured, verified, or recorded when data collectors have not been blinded; also called *detection bias.*

assent The affirmative agreement of an individual (e.g., a child) to take part in a study, typically to supplement formal consent by a parent or guardian.

associative relationship An association between two variables that cannot be described as causal.

assumption A principle that is accepted as being true based on logic or reason, without proof.

asymmetric distribution A distribution of data values that is skewed, with two halves that are not mirror images of each other.

attention control group A control group that gets a similar amount of attention as those in the intervention group, without receiving the "active ingredients" of the treatment.

attrition The loss of participants over the course of a study, which can create bias by changing the composition of the sample initially drawn.

AUC See *area under the curve.*

audio-CASI (computer-assisted self-interview) An approach to collecting self-report data in which respondents listen through headphones to questions being read and respond by entering information onto a computer.

audit trail The systematic documentation of material that would allow an independent auditor of a qualitative study to draw conclusions about trustworthiness.

authenticity The extent to which qualitative researchers fairly and faithfully show a range of different realities in the collection, analysis, and interpretation of data.

autoethnography An ethnographic study in which researchers study their own culture or group.

axial coding The second level of coding in a grounded theory study using the Strauss and Corbin approach, involving the process of categorizing, recategorizing, and condensing first level codes by connecting a category and its subcategories.

back translation The translation of a translated text back into the original language, so that original and back-translated versions can be compared to assess semantic equivalence.

baseline data Data collected at an initial measurement (e.g., prior to an intervention), to enable an assessment of changes.

basic research Research designed to extend the base of knowledge in a discipline for the sake of knowledge production or theory construction, rather than for solving a current problem.

basic social process (BSP) A central social process that is discovered through analysis of grounded theory data; a type of *core variable.*

before-after design A design in which data are collected from participants both before and after the introduction of an intervention.

benchmark In measurement, a threshold value on a measure that signifies an important value, such as a threshold for interpreting whether a change in scores is meaningful or clinically significant.

beneficence An ethical principle that seeks to maximize benefits for study participants, and prevent harm.

beta (β) In statistical testing, the probability of a Type II error.

beta (β) weight In multiple regression, the standardized coefficients indicating the relative weights of the predictor variables in the equation.

between-subjects design A research design in which different groups of people are compared (e.g., smokers and nonsmokers; intervention and control group members).

bias Any influence that distorts the results of a study and undermines validity.

bibliographic database Data files containing bibliographic (reference) information that can be accessed electronically in conducting a literature search.

Big Data Large, complex datasets that have high velocity of data flow, high volume of data, and high variety in data types; analyses involve a search for patterns, trends, and associations.

bimodal distribution A distribution of data values with two peaks (high frequencies).

binomial distribution A statistical distribution with known properties describing the number of occurrences of an event in a series of observations; forms the basis for analyzing dichotomous data.

biomarker An objective, measurable characteristic of a biological process or condition.

bivariate statistics Statistical analysis of two variables to assess the empirical relationship between them.

Bland–Altman plot A graphic depiction of the degree of agreement between two sets of scores, for people who have been measured twice on the same continuous measurement scale; the plot highlights random differences between the two measurements through the construction of a parameter called the *limits of agreement*.

Blind review The review of a manuscript or proposal such that neither the author nor the reviewer is identified to the other party.

blinding The prevention of those involved in a study (participants, intervention agents, data collectors, or healthcare providers) from having information that could lead to a bias, particularly information about which treatment group a participant is in; also called *masking*.

Bonferroni correction An adjustment made to establish a more conservative alpha level when multiple statistical tests are being run from the same data set; the correction is computed by dividing the desired α by the number of tests—e.g., .05/3 = .017.

bracketing In phenomenological inquiries, the process of identifying and holding in abeyance any preconceived beliefs and opinions about the phenomena under study; also called *epoché*.

bricolage The tendency in qualitative research to gather a complex array of data from a variety of sources, using a variety of methods.

calendar question A question used to obtain retrospective information about the chronology of events and activities in people's lives.

carryover effect The influence that one treatment (or measurement) can have on subsequent treatments (or measurements), notably in a crossover design or in test–retest reliability assessments.

Case study A study involving a thorough, in-depth analysis of an individual, group, or other social unit.

case–control design A nonexperimental design that compares "cases" (i.e., people with a specified condition, such as lung cancer) to matched controls (similar people without the condition), to examine differences that could have contributed to "caseness."

categorical variable A variable that involves discrete categories (e.g., blood type) rather than values along a continuum (e.g., weight).

category system In studies involving observation, the prespecified plan for recording the behaviors and events under observation; in qualitative studies, the system developed from the narrative data to organize the data.

causal modeling The development and statistical testing of an explanatory model of hypothesized causal relationships among phenomena.

causal (cause-and-effect) relationship A relationship between two variables wherein the presence or value of one variable (the "cause") affects the presence or value of the other (the "effect").

cause-probing research Research designed to illuminate the underlying causes of phenomena.

ceiling effect An effect resulting from restricted variation above a certain point on a measurement continuum, which limits discrimination at the upper end of the measure, constrains true variability, and reduces the amount of upward change that is detectable.

cell The intersection of a row and column in a table (matrix) with two or more dimensions; in a factorial design, the representation of an experimental condition in a schematic diagram.

census A survey covering an entire population.

central category The main category or pattern of behavior in grounded theory analysis; sometimes referred to as the *core category*.

central limit theorem A statistical principle stipulating that the larger the sample, the more closely the sampling distribution of the mean will approximate a normal distribution and that the mean of a sampling distribution will equal the population mean.

central tendency A statistical index of what is "typical" in a set of scores, derived from the center of the score distribution; indices of central tendency include the mode, median, and mean.

Certificate of Confidentiality A certificate issued by the National Institutes of Health in the United States to protect researchers against forced disclosure of confidential research information.

change score A person's score difference between two measurements on the same measure, calculated by subtracting the value at one point in time from the value at the other point.

chi-square test A statistical test used in various contexts, most often to assess differences in proportions; symbolized as χ^2.

classical test theory (CTT) A measurement theory that has traditionally been used in the development of multi-item scales; in CTT, any score on a measure is conceptualized as having a "true score" component and an error component, and the goal is to approximate the true score.

clinical practice guidelines Practice guidelines that typically combine a synthesis and appraisal of research evidence from systematic reviews with specific recommendations for clinical decisions.

clinical relevance The degree to which a study addresses a problem of significance to clinical practice.

clinical research Research designed to generate knowledge to guide practice in healthcare fields.

clinical significance The practical importance of research results in terms of whether they have genuine, palpable implications for patients' daily lives or for the healthcare decisions made on their behalf.

clinical trial A study designed to assess the safety, efficacy, and effectiveness of a new clinical intervention, sometimes involving several phases (e.g., Phase III typically is a *randomized controlled trial* using an experimental design).

clinimetrics An approach to the quantitative measurement of clinical phenomena such as symptoms and signs; an alternative approach to psychometrics for health measurement.

closed-ended question A question that offers respondents specific response options; also referred to as a *fixed alternative question.*

cluster randomization The random assignment of intact units or organizations (e.g., hospitals), rather than individuals, to treatment conditions.

cluster sampling A form of sampling in which large groupings ("clusters") are selected first (e.g., census tracts), typically with successive subsampling of smaller units (e.g., households) in a multistage approach.

Cochrane Collaboration An international organization that aims to facilitate well-informed healthcare decisions by sponsoring systematic reviews, primarily about the effects of healthcare interventions.

code of ethics The fundamental ethical principles established by a discipline or institution to guide researchers' conduct in research with human (or animal) participants.

codebook A record documenting categorization and coding decisions.

coding The process of transforming raw data into standardized form for data processing and analysis; in quantitative research, the process of attaching numbers to categories; in qualitative research, the process of identifying and indexing recurring salient words, themes, or concepts within the data.

coefficient alpha A widely used index of internal consistency, indicating the degree to which the items on a multi-item scale are measuring the same underlying construct; also referred to as *Cronbach's alpha.*

coercion In a research context, the explicit or implicit use of threats (or excessive rewards) to gain people's cooperation in a study.

cognitive questioning A method sometimes used in a pretest of an instrument in which respondents are asked to explain the process by which they answer questions; basic approaches include a *think-aloud* method and the use of targeted *probes*; also used in connection with content validity work.

cognitive test A performance test designed to assess cognitive skills or cognitive functioning (e.g., a test of cognitive impairment).

Cohen's *d* An effect size index for comparing two group means, computed by subtracting one mean from the other and dividing by the pooled standard deviation; also called *standardized mean difference* or *SMD.*

Cohen's kappa See *kappa.*

cohort design A nonexperimental design in which a defined group of people (a cohort) is followed over time to study outcomes for the cohorts or subgroups within it; also called a *prospective design.*

comparative effectiveness research (CER) A patient-centered research approach that focuses on comparisons of alternative approaches to bring about health improvements.

comparison group A group of study participants whose scores on an outcome are used to evaluate the outcome of the group of primary interest (e.g., nonsmokers as a comparison group for smokers); term often used in lieu of control group when the study design is not a randomized experiment.

complex intervention An intervention in which complexity exists along one or more dimensions, including number of components, number of targeted outcomes, and the time needed for the full intervention to be delivered.

composite scale A measure of an attribute, involving the aggregation of information from multiple items into a single numerical score that places people on a continuum with respect to the attribute.

computerized adaptive testing (CAT) An approach to measuring a latent trait in which computer algorithms are used to tailor a set of questions to individuals, usually using questions from an item bank created using item response theory; CAT offers precise measures of a trait with a small set of targeted items.

concealment A tactic involving the unobtrusive collection of research data without participants' knowledge or consent, used to obtain an accurate view of naturalistic behavior when the known presence of an observer would distort the behavior of interest.

concept An abstraction inferred from observation or self-reports of behaviors, situations, or characteristics (e.g., stress, pain).

concept analysis A systematic process of analyzing a concept or construct, with the aim of identifying its boundaries, definitions, and dimensionality.

conceptual definition The abstract or theoretical meaning of a concept of interest.

conceptual equivalence The extent to which a construct of interest is comparable in another culture; of relevance in the translation or cultural adaptation of an instrument.

conceptual files A manual method of organizing qualitative data, by creating file folders for each category in the coding scheme and inserting relevant excerpts from the data.

conceptual map A schematic representation of a theory or conceptual model that graphically represents key concepts and linkages among them; also called a *schematic model*

conceptual model Interrelated concepts assembled in a rational and often explanatory scheme to illuminate relationships, but less formally than a theory; sometimes called a *conceptual framework.*

concurrent design A mixed methods study design in which the qualitative and quantitative strands of data collection occur simultaneously; symbolically designated with a plus sign (e.g., QUAL + QUAN).

concurrent validity A type of criterion validity that concerns the degree to which scores on an instrument are correlated with an external criterion, measured at the same time.

confidence interval (CI) The range of values within which a population parameter is estimated to lie, at a specified probability (e.g., 95% CI).

confidence limit The upper (or lower) boundary of a confidence interval.

confidentiality Protection of study participants so that data provided are never publicly divulged.

confirmability A criterion for trustworthiness in a qualitative inquiry, referring to the objectivity or neutrality of the data and interpretations.

confirmatory factor analysis (CFA) A factor analysis designed to confirm a hypothesized measurement model, using maximum likelihood estimation; used in assessments of an instrument's structural validity.

confounding variable A variable that is extraneous to the research question and that confounds understanding of the relationship between the independent and dependent variables; confounding variables can be controlled in the research design or through statistical procedures.

consecutive sampling Involves sampling all the people from an accessible population who meet the eligibility criteria over a specific time interval or for a specified sample size.

consent form A written agreement signed by a study participant and a researcher concerning the terms and conditions of voluntary participation in a study.

CONSORT guidelines Widely adopted guidelines (Consolidated Standards of Reporting Trials) for reporting information for a randomized controlled trial, including a checklist and flow chart for tracking participants through the trial, from recruitment through data analysis.

constant comparison A procedure used in qualitative analysis (especially in grounded theory) wherein new data are compared in an ongoing fashion with data obtained earlier, to refine theoretically relevant categories.

constitutive pattern In hermeneutic analysis, a pattern that expresses the relationships among relational themes and is present in all the interviews or texts.

construct An abstraction or concept that is invented (constructed) by researchers, based on inferences from human behavior or human traits (e.g., health locus of control); sometimes referred to as a *latent trait.*

construct validity The degree to which evidence about study particulars supports inferences about the higher order constructs they are intended to represent; in measurement, the degree to which a measure truly captures the focal construct.

constructivist grounded theory An approach to grounded theory, developed by Charmaz, in which the grounded theory is constructed from shared experiences and relationships between the researcher and study participants and interpretive aspects are emphasized.

constructivist paradigm An alternative to the positivist paradigm that holds that there are multiple interpretations of reality and that the goal of research is to understand how individuals construct reality within their context; associated with qualitative research; also called *naturalistic paradigm.*

contamination The inadvertent, unwanted influence of one treatment condition on another treatment condition, as when members of the control group receive the intervention; sometimes called *treatment diffusion.*

content analysis An approach to extracting, organizing, and synthesizing material from documents, often narrative data from a qualitative study, according to key concepts and themes.

content validity The degree to which a multi-item instrument has an appropriate set of relevant items reflecting the full content of the construct domain being measured.

content validity index (CVI) An index summarizing the degree to which a panel of experts agrees on an instrument's content validity; both item content validity (I-CVI) and the overall scale content validity (S-CVI) can be assessed.

continuous quality improvement An approach to healthcare that involves creating an environment in which management and staff strive to constantly improve quality.

continuous variable A variable that can take on an infinite range of values along a specified continuum (e.g., height); less strictly, a variable measured on an interval or ratio scale.

Control group Participants in an experimental study who do not receive the intervention being tested and whose performance provides a counterfactual, against which the effects of the intervention can be compared (see also *comparison group*).

control, research The process of holding constant confounding influences on the outcome under study.

controlled trial A trial that has a control group, with or without randomization.

convenience sampling Selection of the most readily available persons as participants in a study.

convergent design A concurrent mixed methods design in which complementary qualitative and quantitative (usually equal priority) data are gathered about a phenomenon; often symbolized as QUAL + QUAN.

convergent validity A type of construct validity concerning the degree to which scores on a focal measure are correlated with scores on measures of constructs with which there is a hypothesized correlation (i.e., the degree of conceptual convergence).

core category (variable) In a grounded theory study, the central phenomenon that is used to integrate all categories of the data and that is central in explaining what is going on.

correlation An association or bond between variables, with variation in one variable systematically related to variation in another.

correlation coefficient An index summarizing the strength of relationship between variables, typically ranging from +1.00 (for a perfect positive relationship) through .00 (for no relationship) to −1.00 (for a perfect negative relationship).

correlation matrix A two-dimensional display showing the correlation coefficients between all pairs of variables in a set of several variables.

correlational design An observational research design that explores interrelationships among variables of interest without researcher intervention.

COSMIN The **Co**nsensus-based **S**tandards for the selection of health **M**easurement **In**struments, an initiative that developed an important measurement taxonomy and sought to standardize the definitions of measurement properties.

cost-benefit analysis An economic analysis in which both costs and outcomes of a program or intervention are expressed in monetary terms and compared.

cost-effectiveness analysis An economic analysis in which costs of an intervention are measured in monetary terms, but outcomes are expressed in natural units (e.g., costs per added year of life).

cost-utility analysis An economic analysis that expresses the effects of an intervention as overall health improvement and describes costs for some additional utility gain—usually in relation to gains in quality-adjusted life years (QALY).

counterbalancing The process of systematically varying the order of presentation of stimuli or treatments to control for ordering effects, especially in a cross-over design.

counterfactual The condition or group used as a basis of comparison in a trial, representing what would have happened *to the same people* exposed to a causal factor if they *simultaneously* were *not* exposed to the causal factor.

covariate A variable that is statistically controlled (held constant) in ANCOVA, typically a confounding influence on, or a preintervention measure of, the outcome variable.

covert data collection The collection of information in a study without participants' knowledge.

Cox regression A regression analysis in which independent variables are used to model the risk (or hazard) of experiencing an event at a given point in time, given that one has not experienced the event before that time.

Cramér's V An index describing the magnitude of relationship between nominal-level data, used when the contingency table to which it is applied is larger than 2×2.

credibility A criterion for evaluating trustworthiness in qualitative studies, referring to confidence in the truth of the data; analogous to internal validity in quantitative research.

Criterion sampling A purposive sampling approach used by qualitative researchers that involves selecting cases that meet a predetermined criterion of importance.

criterion validity The extent to which scores on a measure are an adequate reflection of (or predictor of) a criterion—i.e., a "gold standard" measure.

critical case sampling A qualitative sampling approach involving the purposeful selection of cases that are especially important or illustrative.

critical ethnography An ethnography that focuses on raising consciousness in the group or culture under study in the hope of effecting social change.

critical region The area in the sampling distribution representing values that are "improbable" if the null hypothesis is true.

critical theory An approach to studying phenomena that involves a critique of society, with the goal of envisioning new possibilities and effecting social change.

critique A critical appraisal that analyzes both weaknesses and strengths of a research report or proposal.

Cronbach's alpha A widely used index that estimates the internal consistency of a composite measure composed of several subparts (e.g., items); also called *coefficient alpha*.

cross-cultural validity The degree to which the items on a translated or culturally adapted scale perform adequately and equivalently, individually and in the aggregate, in relation to their performance on the original instrument; an aspect of construct validity.

crossover design An experimental design in which one group of participants is exposed to more than one condition or treatment, in random order.

cross-sectional design A study design in which data are collected at one point in time, in contrast to a longitudinal design; sometimes used to infer change over time when data are collected from different age or developmental groups.

crosstabulation A calculation of frequencies for two variables considered simultaneously—e.g., gender (male/female) crosstabulated with smoking status (smoker/nonsmoker).

cutoff point (cutpoint) The point in a distribution of scores used to classify or divide people into different groups, such as cases and noncases for a disease or health problem (e.g., the cutpoint for classifying newborns as low birthweight is 5.5 pounds [2500 g]).

d An effect size index for comparing two group means, computed by subtracting one mean from the other and dividing by the pooled standard deviation; also called *Cohen's d* or *standardized mean difference*.

data The pieces of information obtained in a study; the singular is *datum*.

data analysis The systematic organization and synthesis of research data and, in most quantitative studies, the testing of hypotheses using those data.

data cleaning The preparation of data for analysis by performing checks to ensure that the data are correct.

data collection plan The plan for the gathering of information needed to address a research problem.

data collection protocols The formal procedures researchers develop to guide the collection of data in a standardized fashion.

data saturation The collection of qualitative data to the point where a sense of closure is attained because new data yield redundant information.

data set The total collection of data on all variables for all participants in a study.

data transformation A step undertaken before quantitative data analysis, to put the data in a form that can be meaningfully analyzed (e.g., recoding of values); in mixed method studies, qualitizing quantitative data or quantitizing qualitative data.

data triangulation The use of multiple data sources for the purpose of validating conclusions.

debriefing Communication with study participants after participation is complete regarding aspects of the study.

deception The deliberate withholding of information, or the provision of false information, to study participants, usually to minimize potential biases.

deductive reasoning The process of developing specific predictions from general principles; see also *inductive reasoning*.

degrees of freedom (*df*) A statistical concept referring to the number of sample values free to vary (e.g., with a given sample mean, all but one value would be free to vary).

de-identified data Data or records from which identifying information is removed to protect the privacy of individuals.

delay of treatment design A design for an intervention study that involves putting control group members on a waiting list for the intervention until follow-up data are collected; also called a *wait-list design*.

Delphi survey A technique for obtaining judgments from an expert panel about an issue of concern; experts are questioned individually in several rounds, with a summary of the panel's views circulated between rounds, to achieve some consensus.

dendrogram A tree diagram sometimes used in qualitative studies to illustrate the arrangement of codes and categories in a hierarchically ordered system.

dependability A criterion for evaluating trustworthiness in qualitative studies, referring to the stability of data over time and over conditions; analogous to reliability in quantitative research.

dependent variable The variable hypothesized to depend on or be caused by the independent variable; the outcome variable of interest.

descendancy approach In literature searches, finding a pivotal early study and searching forward in citation indexes to find more recent studies ("descendants") that cited the key study.

Description question A question aimed at describing a health-related phenomenon.

descriptive research Research that has as a primary objective the accurate portrayal of people's characteristics or circumstances and/or the frequency with which certain phenomena occur.

descriptive statistics Statistics that describe and summarize data (e.g., means, percentages).

descriptive theory A broad characterization that thoroughly accounts for a phenomenon.

detection bias Systematic differences between groups being compared in how outcome variables are measured, verified, or recorded; a bias that can result when there is no blinding of data collectors.

determinism The belief that phenomena are not haphazard or random, but rather have antecedent causes; an assumption in the positivist paradigm.

deviation score A score computed by subtracting an individual score from the mean of all scores.

diagnostic accuracy The degree to which a measure is accurate in diagnosing or predicting "caseness" and "noncaseness" for a condition, as established by a gold standard criterion.

Diagnostic/assessment question A question about the accuracy and validity of instruments to screen, diagnose, or assess patients.

dichotomous variable A variable having only two values or categories (e.g., alive/dead).

differential item functioning (DIF) The extent to which an item functions differently for one group than for another, despite the groups' equivalence on the underlying latent trait.

direct costs Specific project-related costs incurred during a study (e.g., for salaries, supplies, etc.).

directional hypothesis A hypothesis that makes a specific prediction about the direction of the relationship between two variables.

disconfirming case In qualitative research, a case that challenges the researchers' conceptualizations; sometimes sought as part of a sampling strategy.

discourse analysis A qualitative tradition, from the discipline of sociolinguistics, that seeks to understand the rules, mechanisms, and structure of conversations.

discrete variable A variable with a finite number of values between two points, representing discrete quantities (e.g., number of children).

disproportionate sampling A sampling approach in which the researcher samples varying proportions of people from different population strata to ensure adequate representation from smaller strata.

dissemination bias A bias that occurs when the profile of a study's results depends on the direction or strength of its findings; one example is *publication bias.*

Distribution-based approach An approach to estimating a measure's responsiveness, and to developing a benchmark of importance for interpreting change scores, that relies on distributional properties of the data—often the distribution of change scores.

divergent validity An approach to construct validation that involves gathering evidence that the focal measure is not a measure of a different construct; also called *discriminant validity.*

domain analysis One of Spradley's levels of ethnographic analysis, focusing on the identification of domains, or units of cultural knowledge.

domain sampling model The model underpinning scale development in the classical test theory framework, which conceptually involves the random sampling of a homogeneous set of items from a hypothetical universe of items relating to the construct.

dose-response analysis An analysis to assess whether larger doses of an intervention are associated with greater benefits.

double-blind study A study (usually a clinical trial) in which two sets of people are blinded with respect to the group that a study participant is in; often a situation in which neither the participants nor those who administer the treatment know who is in the experimental or control group.

dummy variable Dichotomous variables created for use in many multivariate statistical analyses, typically using codes of 0 and 1 (e.g., smoker = 1, nonsmoker = 0).

ecological momentary assessment (EMA) Repeated assessments of people's feelings, experiences, or behaviors in real time, within their natural environment, using contemporary technologies such as smartphones.

ecological validity The extent to which study designs and findings have relevance and meaning in a variety of real-world contexts.

economic analysis An analysis of the costs and outcomes of alternative healthcare interventions.

effect A consequence of a causal factor (e.g., the effect of an intervention on an outcome).

effect size (ES) In quantitative research, an index summarizing the strength of relationship between variables; an example is *Cohen's d*; in metasynthesis, an index used to characterize the salience of a theme or category.

effectiveness study A clinical trial designed to test the effectiveness of an intervention under standard real-world conditions, often with an intervention already found to be efficacious in an efficacy study.

efficacy study A tightly controlled trial designed to establish the efficacy of an intervention under ideal conditions, using a design that maximizes internal validity; sometimes called an *explanatory trial.*

eigenvalue The value equal to the sum of the squared weights for a linear composite, such as a factor in a factor analysis, indicating how much variance is accounted for in the solution.

element The most basic unit of a population for sampling purposes, typically a human being.

eligibility criteria The criteria designating the specific attributes of the target population, by which people are selected for inclusion in a study or excluded from it.

emergent design A design that unfolds during the course of a qualitative study as the researcher makes ongoing design decisions reflecting what has already been learned.

emergent fit A concept in grounded theory that involves comparing new data and new categories with previous conceptualizations.

emic perspective An ethnographic term referring to the way members of a culture themselves view their world; the "insider's view."

empirical evidence Evidence rooted in objective reality and gathered using one's senses as the basis for generating knowledge.

endogenous variable In a causal model (path analysis), a variable whose variation is influenced by other variables within the model.

endpoint In a clinical trial, the target outcome of interest.

equivalence In the context of instrument translation, the degree to which the translated and original measures are comparable; types of equivalence include conceptual equivalence, content equivalence, semantic equivalence, technical equivalence, measurement equivalence, and factorial equivalence.

equivalence trial A trial designed to assess whether the outcomes of two treatments do *not* differ, by no more than a prespecified amount judged to be clinically unimportant.

error of measurement The difference between the hypothetical true scores and the obtained scores of a measured characteristic.

error term The mathematic expression (e.g., in a regression analysis) that represents all unknown or unmeasurable attributes that affect the outcome variable.

estimation procedures Statistical procedures that estimate population parameters based on sample statistics.

eta squared In ANOVA, a statistic calculated to indicate the proportion of variance in the dependent variable explained by the independent variables, analogous to R^2 in multiple regression.

ethics In research, a system of moral values that is concerned with the degree to which research procedures adhere to professional, legal, and social obligations to study participants.

ethnography A branch of human inquiry, associated with anthropology, that focuses on the culture of a group of people, with an effort to understand the world view and customs of those under study.

ethnonursing research The study of human cultures, with a focus on a group's beliefs and practices relating to nursing care and related health behaviors.

etic perspective In ethnography, the "outsider's" view of the experiences of a cultural group.

Etiology question A question about the underlying cause of a health problem, such as an environmental cause or personal behavior (e.g., smoking).

evaluation research Research that assesses how well a program, practice, or policy works.

event history calendar A data collection matrix that plots time on one dimension and events or activities of interest on the other.

event sampling A type of observational sampling that involves the selection of integral behaviors or events to be observed.

evidence-based practice (EBP) A practice that involves making clinical decisions based on clinical judgment, patient preferences, and on the best available evidence, which often is evidence from disciplined research.

evidence hierarchy A ranked arrangement of the strength of research evidence based on the rigor of the method that produced it; the traditional evidence hierarchy is appropriate primarily for cause-probing research.

exclusion criteria Criteria specifying characteristics that a target population does *not* have, stipulated for the purpose of sampling.

exogenous variable In a causal model (path analysis), a variable whose determinants lie outside the model.

expectation bias The bias that can arise when study participants (or research staff) have expectations about treatment effectiveness in intervention research; the expectations can result in altered behavior.

expectation maximization (EM) A sophisticated imputation process that generates an estimated value for missing data in two steps (an expectation or E-step and a maximization or M-step), using maximum likelihood estimation.

experimental group The study participants who receive the experimental treatment or intervention.

experimental research A study using a design in which the researcher controls (manipulates) the independent variable by randomly assigning participants to different treatment conditions; randomized controlled trials use experimental designs.

explanatory design A sequential mixed methods design in which quantitative data are collected in the first phase and qualitative data are collected in the second phase to build on or explain quantitative findings.

explanatory trial A traditional clinical trial, conducted under optimal conditions with carefully selected participants, in an effort to enhance internal validity.

exploratory design A sequential mixed methods design in which qualitative data are collected in the first phase and quantitative data are collected in the second phase based on the initial in-depth exploration.

exploratory factor analysis (EFA) A factor analysis undertaken to explore the underlying dimensionality of a set of variables.

exploratory research A study that explores the dimensions of a phenomenon or that develops or refines hypotheses about relationships between phenomena.

external validity The degree to which study results can be generalized to settings or samples other than the one studied.

extraneous variable A variable that confounds the relationship between the independent and dependent variables and that needs to be controlled either in the research design or through statistical procedures; often called *confounding variable*.

extreme response set A bias resulting from a respondent's consistent selection of extreme alternatives (e.g., *strongly agree* or *strongly disagree*) to scale items, regardless of item content.

***F*-ratio** The statistic obtained in several statistical tests (e.g., ANOVA) in which variation attributable to different sources (e.g., between-group variation and within-group variation) is contrasted.

face validity The extent to which a measuring instrument looks as though it is measuring what it purports to measure.

factor analysis A statistical procedure for disentangling complex interrelationships among items and identifying the items that "go together" as a unified dimension.

factor extraction The first phase of a factor analysis, which involves the extraction of as much variance as possible through the successive creation of linear combinations of the variables in the analysis.

factor loading In factor analysis, the weight associated with a variable or item on a given factor.

factor matrix In a factor analysis of scale items, a matrix with items on one dimension and factors on the other, with matrix entries being factor loadings of the items on the factors; factor matrices can be either *rotated* or *unrotated*.

factor rotation The second phase of factor analysis, during which the reference axes for the factors are pivoted to more clearly align items or variables with a single factor.

factorial design An experimental design in which two or more independent variables are simultaneously manipulated, permitting a separate analysis of the main effects of the independent variables and their interaction.

Failure Mode and Effect Analysis (FMEA) In quality improvement, a systematic approach to identifying and preventing problems before they occur.

feasibility study Research completed prior to a main intervention study to assess whether it is sensible to proceed with the project; as distinct from a *pilot study*, a *feasibility assessment* tests specific aspects of an intervention or the anticipated trial (e.g., the intervention's acceptability).

feminist research Research that seeks to understand how gender and a gendered social order shape women's lives and their consciousness.

field diary A daily record of events and conversations in the field; also called a log.

field notes The notes taken by researchers to record the unstructured observations made in the field, and the interpretation of those observations.

field research Research in which the data are collected "in the field" from people in their normal roles, with the aim of understanding the practices, behaviors, and beliefs of individuals or groups as they normally function in real life.

fieldwork The activities undertaken by qualitative researchers to collect data out in the field, i.e., in natural settings.

findings The results and interpretation of analyzed research data.

fishbone analysis A technique used in root cause analyses that is aimed at visualizing causal processes and identifying opportunities for quality improvement.

Fisher's exact test A statistical procedure used to test the significance of differences in proportions, used when the sample size is small or cells in the crosstabs table have no observations.

fit An element in Glaserian grounded theory analysis in which the researcher develops categories of a substantive theory that fit the data.

fixed effects model In meta-analysis, a model in which studies are assumed to be estimating a single true effect; a pooled effect estimate is calculated under the assumption that observed variation between studies is attributable to chance.

floor effect An effect resulting from restricted variation below a certain point on a measurement continuum, which limits discrimination at the lower end of the measure, constrains true variability, and reduces the amount of downward change that is detectable.

focus group interview An interview with a small group of individuals assembled to discuss a specific topic, usually guided by a moderator using a semistructured topic guide.

focused interview A loosely structured interview in which an interviewer guides the respondent through a set of questions using a topic guide.

follow-up study A study undertaken to ascertain the outcomes of individuals who have a specified condition or who received a specific treatment.

forest plot A graphic representation of effects across studies in a meta-analysis, permitting a visual assessment of heterogeneity.

formal grounded theory A theory of a substantive grounded theory's core category that is extended by sampling other studies in a range of substantive areas.

formative index A multi-item measure whose items are viewed as "causing" or defining the construct of interest, rather than being the effect of the construct; distinct from a *reflective scale.*

forward translation The translation of an item (or any text, such as scale instructions) from an original source language into a target language. See also *back translation.*

framework The conceptual underpinnings of a study—a *theoretical framework* in theory-based studies, or *conceptual framework* in studies based on a conceptual model.

framework analysis A method used to organize and manage qualitative analysis that yields a matrix that allows researchers, usually working in a team, to analyze data both by case and theme.

frequency distribution A systematic array of numeric values from the lowest to the highest, together with a count of the number of times each value was obtained.

frequency effect size In a qualitative metasummary, the percentage of reports that contain a given thematic finding.

frequency polygon A graphic display of frequency distribution information that shows the distribution's shape.

Friedman test A nonparametric analog of ANOVA, used with paired-groups or repeated measures situations.

full disclosure The communication of complete, accurate information to potential study participants.

functional relationship A relationship between two variables in which it cannot be assumed that one variable caused the other.

funnel plot A graphic display that plots a measure of study precision (e.g., sample size) against effect size, to explore the possibility of publication bias.

gaining entrée The process of gaining access to study participants through the cooperation of key gatekeepers in a selected community or site.

general linear model (GLM) A large class of statistical techniques (including regression analysis and ANOVA) that describe the relationship between a dependent variable and one or more independent variables using straight-line solutions.

generalizability The degree to which the research methods justify the inference that the findings are true for a broader group than study participants; usually, the inference that the findings can be generalized from the sample to the population.

global rating scale (GRS) A single item that provides a summary measurement of a person's status on a construct, or his/her perception of change on a construct over a specified interval; also referred to as a *health transition rating.*

"going native" A pitfall in ethnographic research wherein a researcher becomes emotionally involved with participants and loses the ability to observe objectively.

GRADE The Grades of Recommendation, Assessment, Development and Evaluation, an approach to grading the quality of an overall body of evidence.

grand theory A broad theory aimed at describing and explaining large segments of the physical, social, or behavioral world; also called a *macrotheory*.

grand tour question A broad question asked in an unstructured interview to gain a general overview of a phenomenon, on the basis of which more focused questions are subsequently asked.

grant A financial award made to a researcher to conduct a proposed study.

grantsmanship The set of skills and knowledge needed to secure financial support for a research idea.

graphic rating scale A scale in which respondents are asked to rate a concept along an ordered, numbered continuum, typically on a bipolar dimension (e.g., "very poor" to "excellent").

grey literature Unpublished, and thus less readily accessible, papers or research reports (e.g., a dissertation).

grounded theory An approach to collecting and analyzing qualitative data that aims to develop theories about social processes, grounded in data from real-world observations.

handsearching The searching of key journals on an article-by-article basis (i.e., by hand), to identify relevant reports that might be missed in electronic searches.

Hawthorne effect The effect on the outcome resulting from people's awareness that they are participants under study.

health transition rating scale A single item, often on a 7-point scale, that asks people to rate the extent to which they have improved/deteriorated (e.g., slightly, moderately, greatly), or stayed the same with regard to a focal attribute.

hermeneutic circle In hermeneutics, a methodologic and interpretive process in which, to reach understanding, there is continual movement between the parts and the whole of the text that are being analyzed.

hermeneutics A qualitative research tradition, drawing on interpretive phenomenology, that focuses on the lived experiences of humans and on how they interpret those experiences.

heterogeneity The degree to which objects are dissimilar (i.e., characterized by variability) on some attribute.

heterogeneity of treatment effects (HTE) Variation in the effectiveness of an intervention across a population—i.e., the intervention's benefits (or harms) are not universal.

hierarchical multiple regression A multiple regression analysis in which predictor variables are entered into the equation in a series of prespecified steps.

histogram A graphic display of frequency distribution information that shows the distribution's shape.

historical comparison group A comparison group chosen from a group observed at some time in the past or for whom existing data are available, often in records.

historical research Systematic studies designed to discover facts and relationships about past events.

history threat The occurrence of events external to an intervention, but concurrent with it, that can affect the outcome variable and threaten the study's internal validity.

homogeneity The degree to which objects are similar (i.e., characterized by low variability) on some attribute.

Hosmer–Lemeshow test A test used in logistic regression to evaluate the degree to which observed frequencies of predicted probabilities correspond to expected frequencies in an ideal model over the range of probability values; a good fit is indicated by lack of statistical significance.

hypothesis A statement of predicted outcomes, most often about predicted relationships between study variables.

hypothesis-testing validity The extent to which it is possible to corroborate hypotheses regarding how scores on a measure function in relation to scores on other variables; a key aspect of construct validity.

identical sampling An approach to sampling in mixed methods studies in which all participants are included in both the qualitative and quantitative strands.

impact analysis An evaluation of the effects of a program or intervention on outcomes of interest, net of other factors influencing those outcomes.

impact factor An annual measure of citation frequency for an average article in a given journal over a 2-year period, i.e., the ratio between citations and citable items published in the journal in that period.

implementation analysis In evaluations, a descriptive analysis of the process by which a program or intervention was implemented in practice.

implementation potential The extent to which an innovation is amenable to implementation in a new setting, an assessment of which is sometimes made in an evidence-based practice project.

implementation research Research that focuses on solving problems in the implementation of healthcare improvements (e.g., a new program).

implied consent Consent to participate in a study that a researcher assumes has been given based on participants' actions, such as returning a completed questionnaire.

improvement science An emerging field that focuses on explorations of how to accelerate quality improvement and to do it rigorously.

imputation A class of methods used to address missing values problems by estimating (imputing) the missing values.

IMRAD format The standard organization of a research report into four sections the **I**ntroduction, **M**ethod, **R**esults, **a**nd **D**iscussion sections.

incidence rate The rate of new cases with a specified condition, computed by dividing the number of new cases over a given period of time by the number at risk of becoming a new case (i.e. free of the condition at the outset of the time period).

independent variable The variable that is believed to cause or influence the dependent variable; in experimental research, the manipulated variable (the intervention).

index A multi-item measure, by convention differentiated from a *scale* in that the term *index* is used for a formative (rather than a reflective) measure.

indirect costs Administrative costs, over and above the specific (direct) costs of conducting the study; also called *overhead.*

inductive reasoning The process of reasoning from specific observations to more general rules (see also *deductive reasoning*).

inference In research, a conclusion drawn from study evidence, taking into account the methods used to generate that evidence.

inference quality An overarching criterion for the integrity of mixed methods studies, referring to the believability and accuracy of inductively and deductively derived conclusions.

inferential statistics Statistics that permit inferences about whether results observed in a sample are likely to be found in the population.

informant An individual who provides information to researchers about a phenomenon under study; term used mostly in qualitative studies.

informed consent An ethical principle that requires researchers to obtain people's voluntary participation, after informing them of possible risks and benefits.

inquiry audit An independent scrutiny of qualitative data and supporting documents by an external reviewer, to evaluate their dependability and confirmability.

insider research Research on a group or culture—usually in an ethnography—by a member of the group or culture; in ethnographic research, an *autoethnography.*

Institutional Review Board (IRB) A term used primarily in the United States to refer to the institutional group that convenes to review proposed and ongoing studies with respect to ethical considerations.

instrument The device used to collect data (e.g., a questionnaire or observation checklist).

instrumentation threat The threat to the internal validity of the study that can arise if the researcher changes the measuring instrument or measurement circumstances between two points of data collection.

intensity effect size In a qualitative metasummary, the percentage of all thematic findings that are contained in any given report.

intention-to-treat A strategy for analyzing data in a randomized controlled trial that includes all randomized participants in the group to which they were assigned, whether or not they received or completed the treatment associated with the group, and whether or not their outcome data were missing.

interaction effect The effect of two or more independent variables acting interactively on an outcome; subgroup analyses test for an interaction between a treatment variable and the subgroup variable.

intercoder reliability The degree to which two coders, working independently, agree on coding decisions.

internal consistency The degree to which the items on a composite scale are interrelated and are measuring the same attribute or dimension, usually as evaluated using coefficient alpha; a measurement property within the reliability domain.

internal validity The degree to which it can be inferred that an intervention (the independent variable), rather than confounding factors, caused the observed effect on the outcome.

Interpretability In measurement, the degree to which it is possible to assign qualitative meaning to an instrument's scores or change scores.

interpretation The process of making sense of the results of a study and examining their implications.

Interquartile range (*IQR*) A measure of variability, indicating the difference between Q_3 (the third quartile or 75th percentile) and Q_1 (the first quartile or 25th percentile).

interrater (interobserver) reliability The degree to which two raters or observers, operating independently, assign the same ratings or score values for an attribute being measured.

interval estimation A statistical estimation approach in which the researcher establishes a range of values that are likely, within a given level of confidence, to contain the true population parameter.

interval measurement A measurement level in which an attribute or a variable is rank ordered on a scale that has equal distances between points on that scale (e.g., Fahrenheit degrees).

intervention In experimental research (clinical trials), the treatment being tested.

intervention fidelity The extent to which the implementation of a treatment is faithful to its plan.

intervention protocol The specific details about what the intervention and alternative (or control) treatment conditions are, and how they should be administered.

intervention research Research involving the development, implementation, and testing of an intervention.

intervention theory The conceptual underpinning of a healthcare intervention, which articulates the theoretical basis for the achievement of desired outcomes.

interview A data collection method in which an interviewer asks questions of a respondent, either face-to-face or by telephone.

interview schedule The formal instrument that specifies the wording of questions to be asked orally of respondents in studies collecting structured self-report data.

intraclass correlation coefficient (ICC) The statistical index used to assess the reliability (e.g., test-retest reliability) of a measure.

intrarater reliability The extent to which a rater or observer assigns the same score values for an attribute being observed on two separate occasions, as an index of self-consistency.

intuiting The second step in descriptive phenomenology, which occurs when researchers remain open to the meaning attributed to the phenomenon by those who experienced it.

inverse relationship A relationship characterized by the tendency of high values on one variable to be associated with low values on the second variable; also called a *negative relationship*.

inverse variance method In meta-analysis, a method that uses the inverse of the variance of the effect estimate (one divided by the square of its standard error) as the weight in calculating a weighted average of effects.

investigator triangulation The use of two or more researchers to code, analyze, or interpret data, to enhance trustworthiness.

Iowa Model of Evidence-Based Practice A widely used framework that can be used to guide the development and implementation of a project to promote evidence-based practice.

item A single question on an instrument, such as on a scale.

item analysis A type of analysis used to assess whether items on a scale are tapping the same construct and are sufficiently discriminating.

item bank In item response theory, a large collection of previously tested items, usually with the aim of using the items in computerized adaptive testing (e.g., the PROMIS® item bank established by NIH).

item characteristic curve (ICC) In item response theory, a graphic representation of an item's performance that models the relationship between people's responses to the item and their level of the latent trait; typically an ICC is approximately S-shaped, and different parts of the curve yield information about different item parameters, such as difficulty and discrimination.

item discrimination A parameter in item response theory models that indicates the degree to which an item can differentiate between people with different levels of the latent trait.

item location A parameter in item response theory and Rasch models, indicating the amount of a latent trait a respondent must possess in order to "pass" (or endorse) an item; also referred to as *item difficulty*.

item pool A collection of items generated for possible inclusion in a multi-item scale.

item response theory (IRT) A "modern" measurement perspective, also called *latent trait theory*, that is gaining favor for developing precise multi-item measures of latent traits; in IRT, the focus is on understanding item characteristics, independent of the people who complete the items; an alternative to *classical test theory*.

joint display In mixed methods research, a visual display that presents integrated results from both the qualitative and quantitative strands.

jottings Short notes jotted down quickly while engaged in fieldwork so as to not distract researchers from their observations or their role as participating members of a group.

journal article A report (e.g., description of a study) appearing in a professional journal such as *Nursing Research* or *International Journal of Nursing Studies*.

journal club A group that meets in clinical settings (or online) to discuss and critically appraise research reports published in journals.

kappa A statistical index of chance-corrected agreement or consistency between two nominal or ordinal measurements, often used to assess interrater or intrarater reliability.

Kendall's tau A correlation coefficient used to indicate the magnitude of a relationship between ordinal-level variables.

key informant A person knowledgeable about a phenomenon or culture and who is willing to share information and insights with the researcher, most often in ethnographies.

keyword An important term used to search for references on a topic in a bibliographic database, provided by authors or indexers to enhance the likelihood that the report will be found.

knowledge translation (KT) The exchange, synthesis, and application of knowledge by relevant stakeholders within complex systems to accelerate the beneficial effects of research aimed at improving healthcare.

known-groups validity A type of construct validity that concerns the degree to which a measure is capable of discriminating between groups known or expected to differ with regard to the construct of interest; also called *discriminative validity.*

Kruskal–Wallis test A nonparametric test used to test the difference between three or more independent groups, based on ranked scores.

last observation carried forward (LOCF) A method of imputing a missing outcome using the previous measurement of that same outcome.

latent trait An abstract human trait that is not directly observable or measurable, but that can be inferred from people's behavior or their responses to a set of questions; term often used in the context of item response theory analyses, confirmatory factor analyses, and structural equations modeling. See also *construct.*

latent trait scale A scale developed within an *item response theory* framework, an alternative psychometric theory to *classical test theory.*

lean approach In quality improvement, a model whose aim is to improve quality and efficiency at lower costs; also called the Toyota Production System.

least-squares estimation A method of statistical estimation in which the solution minimizes the sums of squares of error terms; also called OLS (ordinary least squares).

level of evidence (LOE) scale A scale that rank orders evidence for cause-probing questions in terms of risk of bias, based on evidence hierarchies; level I evidence is typically a systematic review.

level of measurement A system of classifying measurements according to the nature of the measurement and the type of permissible mathematical operations; the levels are nominal, ordinal, interval, and ratio.

level of significance The risk of making a Type I error in a statistical analysis, with the criterion (alpha) established by the researcher beforehand (e.g., α = .05).

life history A narrative self-report about a person's life experiences vis-à-vis a topic of interest.

likelihood ratio (LR) For a screening or diagnostic instrument, the relative likelihood that a given result is expected in a person with (as opposed to one without) the target attribute; LR indexes summarize the relationship between specificity and sensitivity in a single number.

likelihood ratio test A test for evaluating the overall model in logistic regression, or to test improvement between models when predictors are added.

Likert scale A type of scale for measuring attitudes, involving the summation of scores on a set of items that respondents rate for their degree of agreement or disagreement; more loosely, the name used for many summated rating scales.

limits of agreement (LOA) An estimate of the range of differences in two sets of scores that could be considered random measurement error, typically with 95% confidence; graphically portrayed on Bland–Altman plots.

linear regression An analysis for predicting the value of a dependent variable from one or more predictors by determining a straight-line fit to the data that minimizes deviations from the line.

listwise deletion A method of dealing with missing values in a data set that involves the elimination of cases with missing data.

literature review A summary of research on a topic of interest, often prepared to put a research problem in context; typically less rigorously conducted than a systematic review.

log In participant observation studies, the observer's daily record of events and conversations; also called a *field diary.*

logical positivism The philosophy underlying the traditional scientific approach; see also *positivist paradigm.*

logistic regression A multivariate regression procedure that analyzes relationships between two or more independent variables and a categorical outcome.

logit The natural log of the odds, used as the outcome variable in logistic regression; short for logistic probability unit.

longitudinal design A study design that involves the collection of data at more than one point in time over an extended period, in contrast to a cross-sectional study.

macrotheory A broad theory aimed at describing and explaining large segments of the physical, social, or behavioral world; also called a *grand theory*.

main effect In a study with multiple independent variables, the effect of a single independent variable on the outcome.

manifest variable An observed, measured variable that serves as an indicator of an underlying construct/latent trait; term used often in a confirmatory factor analysis or structural equations modeling.

manipulation The deliberate introduction of an intervention or treatment in experimental or quasi-experimental studies to assess its effect on outcomes of interest.

Mann–Whitney *U* test A nonparametric statistic used to test the difference between two independent groups, based on ranked scores.

MANOVA See *multivariate analysis of variance*.

masking See *blinding*.

matching The pairing of participants in one group with those in another group based on their similarity on one or more dimension, to enhance the comparability of groups.

maturation threat A threat to the internal validity of a study that results when changes to the outcome variable result from the passage of time.

maximum likelihood estimation An estimation approach in which the estimators are ones that estimate the parameters most likely to have generated the observed measurements.

maximum variation sampling A sampling approach used by qualitative researchers involving the purposeful selection of cases with variation on dimensions of interest.

McNemar test A statistical test for comparing differences in proportions when values are derived from paired (nonindependent) groups.

mean A measure of central tendency, computed by summing all scores and dividing by the total number of cases.

mean substitution A relatively weak approach for addressing missing data problems that involves substituting missing values on a variable with the sample mean for that variable.

Meaning/process question A question about what health-related phenomena mean to people or about how a process unfolds.

measure A device designed to quantify an attribute or a construct, i.e. to yield quantitative scores.

measurement The process of assigning numbers to represent the amount of a construct or attribute that is present in a person (or object), according to specified rules.

measurement error The systematic and random error of a person's score on a measure, reflecting factors other than the construct being measured and resulting in an observed score that is different from a hypothetical true score; a measurement property within the reliability domain.

measurement model In structural equations modeling, the model that stipulates the hypothesized relationships among manifest and latent variables.

measurement parameter A statistical index that estimates a measurement property of a measure (e.g., Cronbach's alpha is a measurement parameter for the property of internal consistency).

measurement property A characteristic reflecting a distinct aspect of a measure's quality; properties include reliability, validity, reliability of change, and responsiveness.

median A measure of central tendency; the point in a score distribution above and below which 50% of the cases fall.

mediating variable A variable that mediates or acts like a "go-between" in a causal chain linking two other variables; also called a *mediator*.

Medical Research Council framework A framework developed in the United Kingdom for developing and testing complex interventions.

member check A method of validating the credibility of qualitative data through debriefings and discussions with study participants.

MeSH Medical Subject Headings, used to index articles in MEDLINE; recommended by several nursing journals to help authors identify keywords for their articles.

meta-aggregation An approach to the synthesis of qualitative evidence in which findings are categorized and summarized rather than transformed.

meta-analysis A technique for quantitatively integrating the results of multiple studies addressing the same research question.

meta-ethnography An approach to the integration of findings from qualitative studies by translating and interpreting concepts and metaphors across studies; developed by Noblit and Hare.

meta-inference A higher-order conclusion that can be gleaned in a mixed methods study when findings from the two strands (qualitative and quantitative) are integrated and interpreted.

meta-matrix A two-dimensional data array, sometimes used in a mixed methods study, that permits researchers to recognize important patterns and themes across data sources.

metaphor A figurative comparison used by some qualitative analysts to evoke a visual or symbolic analogy.

meta-regression In meta-analyses, a method for statistically examining clinical, demographic, and methodologic factors contributing to the heterogeneity of effects.

metasummary A type of qualitative research synthesis that uses quantitatively oriented methods to aggregate qualitative findings; it involves the development of a list of abstracted findings from primary studies and calculating manifest effect sizes (frequency and intensity effect size).

metasynthesis An interpretive translation produced by integrating findings from multiple qualitative studies.

method triangulation The use of multiple methods of data collection about the same phenomenon, to enhance coherence and validity.

methodologic study Research designed to develop or refine methods of obtaining, organizing, or analyzing data.

methods, research The steps, procedures, and strategies for designing a study and gathering and analyzing study data.

middle-range theory A theory that attempts to explain a piece of reality or human experience, focusing on a limited number of concepts (e.g., a theory of stress).

minimal important change (MIC) A benchmark for interpreting change scores that represents the smallest change that is meaningful to patients or clinicians, and thus establishes clinically significance.

minimal risk Anticipated risks from study participation that are no greater than those ordinarily encountered in daily life or during the performance of routine tests or procedures.

missing at random (MAR) Values that are missing from a data set in such a manner that missingness is unrelated to the value of the missing data, after controlling for another variable; missingness is unrelated to the value of the missing data but *is* related to values of other variables.

missing completely at random (MCAR) Values that are missing from a data set in such a manner that missingness is unrelated to either the value of the missing data, or the value of any other variable; the subsample with missing values is a totally random subset of the original sample.

missing not at random (MNAR) Values that are missing from a data set in such a manner that missingness *is* related to the value of the missing data and, usually, to values of other variables as well.

missing values Values missing in a dataset for some participants due to such factors as refusals, withdrawals from the study, failure to complete forms, or researcher error.

mixed design A design that lends itself to comparisons both within groups over time (within subjects) and between different groups of participants (between subjects).

mixed methods (MM) research Research in which both qualitative and quantitative data are collected and analyzed, to address different but related questions.

mixed studies review A systematic review that integrates and synthesizes findings from qualitative, quantitative, and mixed methods studies on a topic.

modality A characteristic of a frequency distribution concerning the number of peaks; i.e., values with high frequencies.

mode A measure of central tendency; the value that occurs most frequently in a distribution of scores.

model A symbolic representation of concepts or variables, and interrelationships among them.

moderator variable A variable that affects (moderates) the strength or direction of a relationship between the independent and dependent variables.

mortality threat A threat to the internal validity of a study, referring to differential loss of participants from different groups.

multicollinearity A problem that can occur in multiple regression when predictor variables are too highly intercorrelated, which can lead to unstable estimates of the regression coefficients.

multilevel sampling An approach to sampling in mixed methods studies in which participants in the two strands are not the same, and are drawn from different populations at different levels of a hierarchy (e.g., nurses, nurse administrators).

multimodal distribution A distribution of values with more than one peak (high frequency).

multiphase optimization strategy (MOST) A framework for optimizing behavioral and biobehavioral interventions and targeting them more effectively, often involving factorial designs.

multiple comparison procedures Statistical tests, normally applied after an ANOVA indicates statistically significant group differences, that compare all pairs of groups; also called *post hoc tests*.

multiple correlation coefficient An index that summarizes the strength of relationship between two or more independent (predictor) variables and a dependent variable; symbolized as *R*.

multiple imputation (MI) The gold standard approach for addressing missing values, involving the imputation of multiple (*m*) estimates of the missing value, which are later pooled and averaged.

multiple regression A statistical procedure for examining the effects of two or more independent (predictor) variables on a dependent variable.

multisite study A study in which data are collected in multiple sites, typically to enhance generalizability and to recruit a larger sample.

multistage sampling A sampling strategy that proceeds through stages from larger to smaller sampling units (e.g., from states, to census tracts, to households).

multitrait–multimethod matrix method A method of assessing an instrument's construct validity using multiple measures for a sample; the target instrument is valid to the extent that there is a strong relationship between it and other measures of the same attribute (convergent validity) and a weak relationship between it and measures presumed to measure a different attribute (divergent validity).

multivariable risk stratification An analytic approach designed to understand the link between patients' risks and their response to an intervention.

multivariate analysis of variance (MANOVA) A statistical procedure used to test the significance of differences between the means of two or more groups on two or more outcomes, considered simultaneously.

multivariate statistics Statistical procedures designed to analyze relationships among three or more variables (e.g., multiple regression, ANCOVA).

N The symbol designating the total number of participants (e.g., "the total *N* was 500").

n The symbol designating the number of participants in a subgroup or cell of a study (e.g., "each of the four groups had an *n* of 125, for a total *N* of 500").

N-**of-one trial** A trial that tests the effectiveness of an intervention with a single person, typically using a time series design; sometimes called a *single-subject experiment*.

Nagelkerke R^2 A pseudo R^2 statistic used as an overall effect size index in logistic regression, analogous to R^2 in least-squares multiple regression, but lacking the ability to capture the proportion of variance explained in the outcome variable.

narrative analysis A qualitative approach that focuses on the story as the object of the inquiry.

natural experiment A nonexperimental study that takes advantage of a naturally occurring event (e.g., an earthquake) that is explored for its effect on people's behavior or condition, typically by comparing people exposed to the event with those not exposed.

naturalistic setting A setting for the collection of research data that is natural to those being studied (e.g., homes, places of employment).

nay-sayers bias A bias in self-report scales created when respondents characteristically disagree with statements ("nay-say"), independent of content.

needs assessment A study designed to describe the needs of a group, community, or organization, usually as a guide to policy planning and resource allocation.

negative case analysis The refinement of a theory or description in a qualitative study through the search for and inclusion of cases that appear to disconfirm earlier hypotheses.

negative predictive value (NPV) A measure of the usefulness of a screening/diagnostic test that can be interpreted as the probability that a negative test result is correct; calculated by dividing the number with a negative test who do not have the target condition by the number with a negative test.

negative relationship A relationship between two variables in which there is a tendency for high values on one variable to be associated with low values on the other (e.g., as stress increases, emotional well-being decreases); also called an *inverse relationship*.

negative results Results that fail to support the researcher's hypotheses.

negative skew An asymmetric distribution of data values with a disproportionately high number of cases at the upper end; when displayed graphically, the tail points to the left.

nested sampling An approach to sampling in mixed methods studies in which some, but not all, of the participants from the quantitative strand are included in the sample for the qualitative strand.

net impact The effect of an intervention or program on an outcome, over and above standard care, and sometimes after controlling for the effect of covariates statistically (e.g., through ANCOVA).

network sampling The sampling of participants based on referrals from others already in the sample; also called *snowball sampling.*

nominal measurement The lowest level of measurement involving the assignment of numbers to categories (e.g., married = 1; not married = 2).

nondirectional hypothesis A research hypothesis that does not stipulate the expected direction of the relationship between variables.

nonequivalent control group design A quasi-experimental design involving a comparison group that was not created through random assignment.

nonexperimental research Studies in which the researcher collects data without introducing an intervention; also called *observational research.*

noninferiority trial A trial designed to assess whether the effect of a new treatment is not worse than a standard treatment, by no more than a prespecified amount judged to be clinically unimportant.

nonparametric statistical tests A class of statistical tests that do not involve stringent assumptions about the distribution of variables.

nonprobability sampling The selection of elements (e.g., participants) from a population using nonrandom procedures (e.g., convenience sampling).

nonrecursive model A causal model that predicts reciprocal effects (i.e., a variable can be both the cause of and an effect of another variable).

nonresponse bias A bias that can result when a nonrandom subset of people invited to be study participants decline to participate.

nonsignificant result The result of a statistical test indicating that group differences or observed relationships could have occurred by chance, at a given probability level; sometimes abbreviated as NS.

normal distribution A theoretical distribution that is unimodal, bell-shaped, and symmetrical; also called a *Gaussian distribution.*

norms Measurement standards, based on test or scale score information from a large, representative sample.

novelty effect A potential threat to design-related construct validity that can occur when participants or research agents alter their behavior because an intervention is new or different, not because of its inherent qualities.

null hypothesis A hypothesis stating no relationship between the variables under study; used primarily in statistical testing as the hypothesis to be rejected.

number needed to treat (NNT) An estimate of how many people would need to receive an intervention to prevent one undesirable outcome, computed by dividing 1 by the value of the absolute risk reduction.

nursing intervention research Studies either questioning existing care practices or testing innovations in care that are shaped by nursing's values and goals and are guided by an intervention theory.

nursing research Systematic inquiry designed to develop knowledge about issues of importance to the nursing profession.

nursing sensitive outcome A patient outcome that improves if there is greater quantity or quality of nursing care.

objectivity The extent to which two independent researchers would arrive at similar judgments or conclusions (i.e., judgments not biased by personal values or beliefs).

oblique rotation In factor analysis, a rotation of factors such that the reference axes are allowed to move to acute or oblique angles and hence the factors are allowed to be correlated.

observation A method of collecting information and measuring constructs by directly watching and recording behaviors and characteristics.

observational notes An observer's in-depth descriptions of events and conversations observed in naturalistic settings.

observational research A study that does not involve an experimental intervention—i.e., nonexperimental research in which phenomena are merely observed.

observed (obtained) score The actual score or numerical value assigned to a person on a measure.

Odds A way of expressing the chance of an event; the probability of an event occurring relative to the probability that it will not occur, calculated by dividing the number of people who experienced an event by the number who did not.

odds ratio (OR) The ratio of one odds to another odds, e.g., the ratio of the odds of an event in one group to the odds of an event in another group; an odds ratio of 1.0 indicates no difference between groups.

one-tailed test A statistical test in which only values in one tail of a distribution are considered in determining significance; sometimes used when the researcher states a directional hypothesis.

open-access journal A journal that allows free online access to articles, without user subscription costs (authors or their institutions typically pay publication costs); traditional journals may include some articles that are open-access.

open coding The first level of coding in a grounded theory study, referring to the basic descriptive coding of the content of narrative materials.

open-ended question A question in an interview or questionnaire that does not restrict respondents' answers to preestablished response options.

operational definition The definition of a concept or variable in terms of the procedures by which it is to be measured.

operationalization The process of translating research concepts into measurable phenomena.

ordinal measurement A measurement level that involves sorting people (or objects) based on their relative ranking on an attribute.

ordinary least squares (OLS) regression Regression analysis that uses a least-squares criterion for estimating the parameters in the regression equation.

orthogonal rotation In factor analysis, a rotation of factors such that the reference axes are kept at right angles, and hence the factors remain uncorrelated.

outcome analysis An evaluation of what happens to outcomes of interest after implementing a program or intervention, typically using a one group before-after design.

outcome variable A term often used, especially in intervention studies, to refer to the dependent variable, i.e., the outcome (endpoint) of an intervention.

outcomes research Research designed to document the effectiveness of healthcare services and the end results of patient care.

outlier A value that lies outside the normal range of values on a measure, especially in relation to other cases in a data set.

***p* value** In statistical testing, the probability that the obtained results are due to chance; the probability of a Type I error.

pairwise deletion A method of dealing with missing values in a data set that involves deleting cases with missing data selectively (i.e., on a variable by variable basis).

paradigm A way of looking at natural phenomena—a worldview—that encompasses a set of philosophical assumptions that guides one's approach to inquiry.

paradigm case In Benner's hermeneutic analysis, a strong exemplar of the phenomenon under study, often used early in the analysis to gain understanding of the phenomenon.

parallel sampling An approach to sampling in mixed methods studies in which the participants in one strand are completely different from those in the other strand, but sampling for both strands is from the same population.

parameter A characteristic of a population (e.g., the mean age of all practicing nurses).

parametric statistical tests A class of statistical tests that involves assumptions about the distribution of the variables and the estimation of a parameter.

pareto chart A chart used in quality improvement that graphically shows the distribution of factors contributing to a targeted problem and that can be useful in setting priorities.

partially randomized patient preference (PRPP) design A design that involves randomizing only patients without a strong preference for a treatment condition.

participant observation A method of collecting data through the participation in and in-depth observation of a group or culture, most often used in an ethnography.

participatory action research (PAR) A research approach with groups or communities that is based on the premise that the use and production of knowledge can be political and used to exert power.

path analysis A regression-based procedure for testing causal models, typically using correlational data.

path coefficient The weight representing the effect of one variable on another in a path analytic model.

path diagram A graphic representation of the hypothesized interrelationships and causal flow among variables.

patient-centered intervention (PCI) An intervention tailored to meet individual needs or characteristics.

patient-centered research Research that focuses on the development of evidence that is important and relevant to patients.

patient-reported outcome (PRO) A health outcome that is measured by directly asking the patient for information.

Pearson's *r* A correlation coefficient designating the magnitude of relationship between two variables measured on at least an interval scale; also called the *product-moment correlation coefficient.*

peer debriefing Sessions with peers to review and explore various aspects of a study, as an approach to enhancing trustworthiness in a qualitative study.

peer review A review and critique of a research report (or proposal) by one or more researcher, who makes a recommendation about publishing (or funding) the research.

pentadic dramatism An approach for analyzing narratives, developed by Burke, that focuses on five key elements of a story—act (what was done), scene (when and where it was done), agent (who did it), agency (how it was done), and purpose (why it was done).

per protocol analysis Analysis of data from a randomized controlled trial that excludes participants who did not obtain the protocol to which they were assigned (or who received an incomplete dose of the intervention); sometimes called an *on-protocol analysis.*

percentile A value indicating the percentage of people who score below a particular score on a measure; the 50th percentile is the median for the distribution of scores.

perfect relationship A correlation between two variables such that the values of one variable permit perfect prediction of the values of the other; designated as 1.00 or −1.00.

performance bias In clinical trials, systematic differences in the care provided to members of different groups of participants, apart from the intervention that is the focus of the inquiry, which can occur when there is no blinding.

performance ethnography A scripted, staged reenactment of ethnographically derived findings that reflect an interpretation of the culture.

performance test A measure designed to assess a person's physical or cognitive abilities or achievements.

permuted block randomization Randomization that occurs for blocks of participants (e.g., 6 or 8 at a time), to ensure a balanced allocation to groups within cohorts of participants; the size of the blocks is varied (permuted).

persistent observation A qualitative researcher's intense focus on the aspects of a situation that are relevant to the phenomena being studied.

person triangulation The collection of data from different levels or types of persons, with the aim of validating data through multiple perspectives on the phenomenon.

person-item map A graphic display of information from a Rasch analysis that shows the distribution of respondents on one side of a latent trait continuum or "ruler," and the distribution of items on the other side.

personal interview A face-to-face interview between an interviewer and a respondent.

phenomenography A qualitative approach in which researchers strive to understand the qualitatively different ways in which people experience a phenomenon.

phenomenology A qualitative research tradition, with roots in philosophy and psychology, that focuses on the lived experience of humans.

phenomenon The abstract concept under study; term often used by qualitative researchers in lieu of *variable.*

phi coefficient A statistical index describing the magnitude of relationship between two dichotomous variables.

photo elicitation An in-depth interview stimulated and guided by photographic images.

photovoice A method of collecting qualitative data that involves asking participants to take photographs of their culture or environment and then interpret the photos.

PICO framework A framework for asking well-worded questions, and for searching for evidence, where P = population, I = intervention or influence, C = comparison, and O = outcome.

pilot study A small scale version, or trial run, of a study done in preparation for a major study; designed to assess the feasibility of, and support refinements to, the protocols, methods, and procedures to be used in a larger scale study, such as a clinical trial.

placebo A sham or pseudo intervention, sometimes used as a control group condition.

placebo effect Changes in the outcome attributable to the placebo condition because of expectations.

Plan-Do-Study-Act (PDSA) A quality improvement model that involves systematic, rapid cycles of activities; sometimes called *Plan-Do-Check-Act (PDCA).*

plausibility analysis An analysis of the plausibility of alternative explanations (rival hypotheses) of study results; useful especially in designs without randomization.

point estimation A statistical procedure in which information from a sample (a statistic) is used to estimate the single value that best represents the population parameter.

point prevalence rate The number of people with a condition or disease divided by the total number at risk, multiplied by the total number for whom the rate is being established (e.g., per 1000 population).

population The entire set of individuals or objects having some common characteristics (e.g., all RNs in Canada); sometimes called *universe.*

positive predictive value (PPV) A measure of the usefulness of a screening/diagnostic test that can be interpreted as the probability that a positive test result is correct; calculated by dividing the number with a positive test who have the target condition by the number with a positive test.

positive relationship A relationship between two variables in which high values on one variable tend to be associated with high values on the other (e.g., as physical activity increases, heart rate increases).

positive results Research results that are consistent with the researcher's hypotheses.

positive skew An asymmetric distribution of values with a disproportionately high number of cases at the lower end; when displayed graphically, the tail points to the right.

positivist paradigm The paradigm underlying the traditional scientific approach, which assumes that there is an orderly reality that can be objectively studied; often associated with quantitative research.

post hoc test A test for comparing all possible pairs of groups following a significant test of overall group differences (e.g., in an ANOVA).

poster session A session at a professional conference in which several researchers simultaneously present visual displays summarizing their studies, while conference attendees circulate around the room perusing the displays.

posttest The collection of data after introducing an intervention.

posttest-only design An experimental design in which data are collected from participants only after the intervention has been introduced; also called an *after-only design.*

power The ability of a design or analysis to detect true relationships that exist among variables.

power analysis A procedure used to estimate sample size requirements prior to undertaking a study, or to estimate the likelihood of committing a Type II error.

practice-based evidence Research evidence that is developed in real-world settings and is responsive to the needs and circumstances of specific patients and contexts.

pragmatic (practical) clinical trial A trial that addresses practical questions about the benefits, risks, and costs of an intervention as it would unfold in routine clinical practice, to enhance clinical decision-making.

pragmatism The paradigm on which mixed methods research is often said to be based, in that it acknowledges the practical imperative of the "dictatorship of the research question."

PRECIS-2 instrument A widely used instrument (**P**referred **E**xplanatory **C**ontinuum **I**ndicator **S**ummary) for assessing where a trial design lies on a "pragmatic" to "explanatory" continuum.

precision The degree to which it can be inferred that repeated measurements (or parameter estimates) under unchanged conditions show the same results; usually expressed in terms of the width of the confidence interval.

precision healthcare A model that proposes the customization of healthcare, with decisions and treatments tailored to individual patients based on their unique genetic, physiologic, behavioral, lifestyle, and environmental profile.

prediction The use of empirical evidence to make forecasts about how variables will perform in a new setting and with a different sample.

predictive validity A type of criterion validity that concerns the degree to which a measure is correlated with a criterion measured at a future point in time.

predictor variable A variable (usually the independent variable) used to predict another variable (usually the outcome); term used primarily in the context of regression analysis.

pretest (1) The collection of data prior to an experimental intervention; sometimes called baseline data. (2) The trial administration of a newly developed measure to identify flaws or to gain better understanding of how the construct in question is conceptualized by respondents.

pretest-posttest design An experimental design in which data are collected from participants both before and after introducing an intervention; also called a *before-after design.*

prevalence The proportion of a population having a particular condition (e.g., ovarian cancer) at a given point in time.

primary source First-hand reports of facts or findings; in research, the original report prepared by the investigator who conducted the study.

primary study In a systematic review, an original study whose findings are the data in the review.

principal components analysis (PCA) An analysis that some consider a type of factor analysis; PCA analyzes all variance in the observed variables, not just common factor variance, with 1s on the diagonal of the correlation matrix.

principal investigator (PI) The person who is the lead researcher with primary responsibility for overseeing a study.

priority A feature of mixed methods designs, concerning which strand (qualitative or quantitative) will be given more emphasis; using symbols to represent a design, the dominant strand is in all capital letters, as QUAL or QUAN, and the nondominant strand is in lower case, as qual or quan.

PRISMA guidelines Guidelines for reporting meta-analyses of randomized controlled trials.

probability sampling The selection of elements (e.g., participants) from a population using random procedures (e.g., simple random sampling).

probe A method used in interviews to get detailed and reflective information from a respondent; in cognitive interviews, a method used to obtain information about how a question was processed and answered.

problem statement The articulation of a dilemma or disturbing situation that needs investigation.

process analysis In evaluations, a descriptive analysis of the process by which a program or intervention gets implemented and used in practice.

process consent In qualitative studies, an ongoing, transactional process of negotiating consent with study participants, allowing them to collaborate in decisions about their continued participation.

product moment correlation coefficient (*r*) A correlation coefficient designating the magnitude of relationship between two variables measured on at least an interval scale; also called *Pearson's r*.

Prognosis question A question about the consequences or long-term outcomes of a disease or health problem.

projective technique A data collection method designed to elicit information about a person's innermost feelings and emotions through the presentation of vague stimuli (e.g., the Rorschach inkblot test).

prolonged engagement In qualitative research, the investment of sufficient time during data collection to have an in-depth understanding of the group under study, thereby enhancing credibility.

propensity score A score that captures the conditional probability of exposure to a treatment, given various preintervention characteristics; can be used to match comparison groups or as a statistical control variable to enhance internal validity.

proportion of agreement In assessing agreement/consistency between two nominal or ordinal measurements, the proportion of cases for which there is total agreement.

proportional hazards model A model in which independent variables are used to predict the risk (hazard) of experiencing an event at a given point in time.

proportionate stratified sampling A sampling approach in which the researcher samples from different strata of the population in direct proportion to their representation in the population.

proposal A document for a proposed study that communicates a research problem, its significance, proposed methods for addressing the problem, and, when funding is sought, how much the study will cost.

prospective design A study design that begins with an examination of presumed causes (e.g., cigarette smoking) and then goes forward in time to observe presumed effects (e.g., lung cancer); also called a *cohort design.*

proximal similarity model A conceptualization relating to generalization that concerns the contexts that are more or less like the one in a study in terms of a *gradient of similarity* for people, settings, times, and contexts.

pseudo R^2 A type of statistic used to evaluate overall effect size in logistic regression, analogous to R^2 in least-squares multiple regression; the statistic does not, strictly speaking, indicate the proportion of variance explained in the outcome variable.

psychometric assessment An evaluation of the quality of an instrument, in which its measurement properties (i.e., its reliability, validity, and responsiveness) are estimated.

psychometrics A field of inquiry concerned with the theory of measurement of abstract psychological constructs, and the application of the theory in the development and testing of measures.

publication bias A bias resulting from the fact that published studies overrepresent statistically significant findings, reflecting the tendency to not publish nonsignificant results; a form of *dissemination bias*, also called a *bias against the null hypothesis.*

purposive (purposeful) sampling A nonprobability sampling method in which the researcher selects participants based on a judgment about which ones will be most informative.

Q sort A data collection method in which participants sort statements into piles (usually 9 or 11) according to some bipolar dimension (e.g., most helpful/least helpful).

qualitative analysis The organization and interpretation of narrative data for the purpose of discovering important underlying themes, categories, and patterns of relationships.

qualitative data Information in narrative (nonnumeric) form, such as the information provided in a conversational (open-ended) interview.

qualitative descriptive research Qualitative studies that yield rich descriptions of phenomena, but that are not embedded in a qualitative tradition such as phenomenology.

qualitative evidence synthesis (QES) A systematic review of qualitative evidence, typically using an aggregative approach to evidence synthesis and often focused on qualitative aspects of an intervention or program (e.g., barriers to participation).

qualitative research The investigation of phenomena, typically in an in-depth fashion, through the collection of rich narrative materials using a flexible research design.

qualitizing The process of reading and interpreting quantitative data in a qualitative manner.

quality improvement (QI) Systematic efforts to improve practices and processes, typically within a specific organization or patient group.

quantitative analysis The exploration of numeric data through statistical procedures for the purpose of describing phenomena or assessing the magnitude and reliability of relationships among them.

quantitative data Information collected in a numeric (quantified) form.

quantitative research The investigation of phenomena that lend themselves to precise measurement and quantification, often involving a rigorous and controlled design and statistical analysis of data.

quantitizing The process of coding and analyzing qualitative data quantitatively.

quasi-experiment A type of design for an intervention study in which participants are not randomly assigned to treatment conditions; also called a *nonrandomized trial.*

quasi-statistics An "accounting" system sometimes used to assess the validity of conclusions derived from qualitative analysis.

query letter A letter to a journal editor to ask if there is interest in a proposed manuscript, or to a funding source to ask if there is interest in a proposed study.

questionnaire A written or electronic instrument used to gather self-report data via self-administration of questions.

quota sampling A nonrandom sampling method in which "quotas" for certain subgroups (e.g., males, females) are established based on population proportions, to increase the representativeness of the sample.

r The symbol for a bivariate correlation coefficient (*Pearson's r*), summarizing the magnitude and direction of a relationship between two variables measured on an interval or ratio scale.

R The symbol for the multiple correlation coefficient, indicating the magnitude (but not direction) of the relationship between an outcome variable and multiple independent (predictor) variables, taken together.

R^2 The squared multiple correlation coefficient, indicating the proportion of variance in the dependent variable explained by a group of independent (predictor) variables.

random assignment The assignment of participants to treatment conditions in a random manner (i.e., in a manner determined by chance alone); also called *randomization.*

random effects model In meta-analysis, a model in which studies are not assumed to be measuring the same overall effect, but rather different, yet related effects; often preferred to a fixed effect model when there is extensive statistical heterogeneity.

random number table A table displaying hundreds of digits (from 0 to 9) in random order; each number is equally likely to follow any other.

random sampling The selection of a sample such that each member of a population has an equal probability of being included.

randomization The assignment of participants to treatment conditions in a random manner (i.e., in a manner determined by chance alone); also called *random assignment.*

randomized controlled trial (RCT) A full experimental test of an intervention, involving random assignment of participants to different treatment groups.

randomness An important concept in quantitative research, involving having certain features of the study established by chance rather than by design or personal preference.

range A measure of variability, computed by subtracting the lowest value from the highest value in a distribution of scores.

rapid review A streamlined and less rigorous approach to evidence synthesis than a systematic review, typically completed in a few weeks to meet information needs in a timely manner.

Rasch model A latent trait model, used to evaluate items for a scale or test, that estimates only item difficulty (location) parameters; mathematically similar to a one-parameter item response theory model.

rating scale A scale that requires ratings of an object or concept along a continuum.

ratio measurement A measurement level with equal distances between scores and a true meaningful zero point (e.g., body weight).

raw data Data in the form in which they were collected, without being transformed or analyzed.

reactivity A measurement distortion arising from the study participant's awareness of being observed, or, more generally, from the effect of the measurement procedure itself.

readability The ease with which materials (e.g., a questionnaire) can be read by people with varying reading skills, often empirically evaluated through readability formulas.

realist evaluation A theory-driven approach to evaluating complex programs, designed to examine "What works for whom and under what circumstances?"

realist review An approach to synthesizing qualitative and quantitative evidence on complex interventions that seeks to understand theory-driven Context-Mechanism-Outcome (CMO) configurations.

RE-AIM framework (*Reach, Efficacy, Adoption, Implementation,* and *Maintenance*) A model for designing and evaluating intervention research that addresses multiple forms of study validity, including external validity.

receiver operating characteristic curve (ROC curve) A statistical tool that involves plotting specificity against sensitivity for different scores on a measure to determine the best cutoff score for "caseness"; also used to generate an index (the *area under the curve*) that has relevance for assessing validity and responsiveness in some situations.

recursive model A path model in which the causal flow is unidirectional, without any feedback loops; distinct from a nonrecursive model.

reflective lifeworld research (RLR) Dahlberg's approach to phenomenologic research that enables researchers to reflect on taken-for-granted assumptions so that the phenomenon being studied can show itself more fully.

reflective notes Notes that document a qualitative researcher's personal experiences, reflections, and progress in the field.

reflective scale A multi-item scale whose items are conceptualized as having been "caused" by the underlying trait that is being measured; items are viewed as the "effects" of an underlying construct. See also *formative index.*

reflexivity In qualitative studies, critical self-reflection about one's own biases, preferences, and preconceptions.

regression analysis A statistical procedure for predicting values of a dependent variable based on one or more independent (predictor) variables.

relationship A bond or a connection between two or more variables.

relative risk (RR) An estimate of the risk of "caseness" in one group compared to another, computed by dividing the absolute risk for one group (e.g., a treated group) by the absolute risk for another (e.g., the untreated group); also called the *risk ratio.*

relative risk reduction (RRR) The estimated proportion of baseline (untreated) risk that is reduced through exposure to an intervention, computed by dividing the absolute risk reduction (ARR) by the absolute risk for the control group.

relevance In the context of patient-centered research, the degree to which evidence is meaningful and valuable to patients and other stakeholders and has the potential to be actionable.

reliability The accuracy and consistency of information in a study. In measurement, the extent to which a measurement is free from measurement error. In statistics, the degree to which the results support an inference about what is true in the population.

reliability coefficient A quantitative index, usually ranging in value from .00 to 1.00, that provides an estimate of how reliable an instrument is (e.g., the intraclass correlation coefficient).

reliable change index (RCI) An index used (used especially in psychotherapy) to estimate the threshold for a "real" change in scores—i.e., a change that, with 95% confidence, is beyond measurement error; similar in concept to the *smallest detectable change* but based on a different formula.

repeated-measures ANOVA An analysis of variance used when there are multiple measures of the outcome variable over time (e.g., in a crossover design).

repeated measures design A design that involves the collection of data multiple points in time, to track changes in an outcome.

replication The repetition of research procedures in a second investigation for the purpose of assessing whether earlier results can be confirmed.

representative sample A sample whose characteristics are comparable to those of the population from which it is drawn.

research Systematic inquiry that uses orderly, disciplined methods to answer questions or solve problems.

research control See *control, research.*

research design The overall plan for addressing a research question, including specifications for enhancing the study's integrity.

research hypothesis The actual hypothesis a researcher wishes to test (as opposed to the *null hypothesis*), stating the anticipated relationship between two or more variables.

research methods The techniques used to structure a study and to gather and analyze information relevant to a research question.

research misconduct Fabrication, falsification, plagiarism, or other practices that deviate from those that are commonly accepted within the scientific community for conducting or reporting research.

research problem An enigmatic or perplexing situation or condition that can be investigated through disciplined inquiry.

research proposal A document for a proposed study that communicates a research problem, its significance, proposed procedures for solving the problem, and, when funding is sought, how much the study will cost.

research question The specific query the researcher wants to answer to address a research problem.

research report A document (often a journal article) summarizing the main features of a study, including the research question, the methods used to address it, the findings, and the interpretation of the findings.

research utilization The use of some aspect of a study in an application unrelated to the original research.

researcher credibility The faith that can be put in a researcher, based on his or her training, qualifications, and experiences.

residuals In regression analyses, the error term, i.e., unexplained variance.

respondent In a self-report study, the person responding to questions posed by the researcher.

responder analysis An analysis that compares the percentage of people who are *responders*, i.e. who reach a benchmark on a change score, in different groups (e.g., a treatment group versus a control group).

response bias An influence that leads a person to select a response option that does not correspond to his or her hypothetical "true score" for an item.

response options The prespecified set of possible answers to a closed-ended question or item; also called *response alternatives*.

response rate The rate of participation in a study, calculated by dividing the number of people participating by the number of people invited to participate.

response set bias The systematic bias resulting from the tendency of some individuals to respond to items in characteristic ways (e.g., always agreeing), independently of item content.

responsiveness The ability of a measure to detect change over time in a construct that has changed, commensurate with the amount of change that has occurred.

results The answers to research questions, obtained through an analysis of collected data.

retrospective design A study design that begins with the manifestation of the outcome in the present (e.g., lung cancer), followed by a search for a presumed cause occurring in the past (e.g., cigarette smoking).

risk/benefit ratio The relative costs and benefits, to an individual person and to society at large, of participation in a study; also, the relative costs and benefits of implementing an innovation.

rival hypothesis An alternative explanation, competing with the researcher's hypothesis, for interpreting the results of a study.

root cause analysis (RCA) In quality improvement, systematic efforts to identify the underlying causes of a problem that needs to be addressed (e.g., using the "5 whys" process).

sample A subset of a population comprising those selected to participate in a study.

sample size The number of people who participate in a study; an important factor in the *power* of the analysis and in statistical conclusion validity.

sampling The process of selecting a portion of the population to represent the entire population.

sampling bias Distortions that arise when a sample is not representative of the population from which it was drawn.

sampling distribution A theoretical distribution of a statistic, using the values of a statistic (e.g., means) computed from an infinite number of samples as the data points in the distribution.

sampling error The fluctuation of the value of a statistic from one sample to another drawn from the same population.

sampling frame A list of all the elements in the population, from which the sample is selected.

sampling plan In quantitative research, a formal plan specifying a sampling method, desired sample size, and procedures for recruiting participants.

saturation The collection of qualitative data to the point where a sense of closure is attained because new data yield redundant information.

scale A composite measure of an attribute or trait, involving the aggregation of information from multiple items into a single numerical score that places people on a continuum with respect to the trait.

scatter plot A representation of the relationship between two continuous variables on a coordinate graph.

schematic model A representation of a theory or conceptual model that graphically represents key concepts and linkages among them; also called a *conceptual map*.

scientific merit The degree to which a study is methodologically and conceptually sound.

scientific method A set of orderly, systematic, controlled procedures for acquiring dependable, empirical—and typically quantitative—information; the methodologic approach associated with the positivist paradigm.

scoping review A preliminary review of research findings to clarify the range and nature of the evidence base, often to refine the questions and protocols for a systematic review.

score A numerical value derived from a measurement that communicates *how much* of an attribute is present in a person, or whether the attribute is present or absent.

screening instrument An instrument used to ascertain whether potential participants for a study meet eligibility criteria, or for determining whether a person tests positive for a specified condition.

secondary analysis A form of research in which the data collected in a study are reanalyzed by (usually by another investigator) to answer new questions.

secondary source Second-hand accounts of events or facts; in research, a description of a study prepared by someone other than the original researcher.

selection threat (self-selection) A threat to the internal validity of the study resulting from preexisting differences between groups under study; the differences affect the outcome variable in ways extraneous to the effect of the independent variable (e.g., an intervention).

selective coding A level of coding in a grounded theory study that begins once the core category has been discovered; involves limiting coding to only those categories related to the core category.

self-determination A person's right to voluntarily decide whether to participate in a study.

self-report A method of collecting data that involves a direct verbal report of information by the person who is being studied (e.g., by interview or questionnaire).

semantic differential A method used to measure attitudes in which respondents rate concepts of interest on a series of bipolar rating scales.

semantic equivalence In a translation or adaptation of an instrument, the extent to which the meaning of an item is the same in the target culture after the item is translated as it was in the original.

semistructured interview An interview in which the researcher has a list of topics to cover rather than specific questions to ask.

sensitivity The ability of a measure to correctly identify a "case" or true positive i.e., the correct diagnosis of a condition.

sensitivity analysis An effort to test how sensitive the results of a statistical analysis are to changes in assumptions or in the way the analysis was done (e.g., in a meta-analysis, assessing whether conclusions are sensitive to the quality of the studies included).

sequential clinical trial A trial in which data are continuously analyzed, and *stopping rules* are used to decide when the evidence about treatment efficacy is sufficiently strong that the trial can be stopped.

sequential design A mixed methods design in which one strand of data collection (qualitative or quantitative) occurs prior to the other, informing the second strand; symbolically shown with an arrow, as QUAL → QUAN.

sequential, multiple assignment, randomized trial (SMART) A trial design for optimizing adaptive interventions, involving multiple individualized sequences of interventions; used to identify the best decision points, decision rules, intervention options, and tailoring variables for patients with varying response to intervention components.

setting The physical location in which data collection takes place in a study.

simple random sampling Basic probability sampling, involving the random selection of sample members from a sampling frame.

simultaneous multiple regression A multiple regression analysis in which all predictor variables are entered into the equation simultaneously.

single-blind study A study in which only one group (e.g., data collectors) do not know participants' status, in terms of the group to which they have been assigned.

single-subject experiment An intervention study that tests the effectiveness of an intervention with a single person, typically using a time series design; often called an *N-of-1 experiment*.

site The overall location where a study is undertaken.

Six Sigma Model A quality improvement approach that focuses on improving outputs by minimizing variation in performance.

skewed distribution An asymmetric distribution of data values around a central point.

smallest detectable change (SDC) An index that estimates the threshold for a "real" change in scores—i.e., a change that, with 95% confidence, is beyond measurement error; the SDC is a change score that falls outside the limits of agreement on a Bland–Altman plot.

snowball sampling The selection of participants through referrals from earlier participants; also called *network sampling* and *chain sampling.*

social desirability response bias A bias in self-report instruments created when participants tend to misrepresent their opinions in the direction of views consistent with prevailing social norms.

space triangulation The collection of data on the same phenomenon in multiple sites, to assess cross-site consistency and enhance the validity of the findings.

Spearman's rank-order correlation (Spearman's rho) A correlation coefficient indicating the magnitude of a relationship between variables measured on an ordinal scale.

specificity The ability of a screening or diagnostic instrument to correctly identify noncases (true negatives).

stakeholder In the context of healthcare, a person or group that has a direct interest in a healthcare decision or action.

standard deviation A statistic that describes the "average" amount of variability in a set of scores.

standard error The standard deviation of a sampling distribution, such as the sampling distribution of the mean.

standard error of measurement (SEM) An index that quantifies the amount of "typical" error on a measure and indicates the precision of individual scores.

standard score A score expressed in terms of standard deviations from the mean, with raw scores typically transformed to have a mean of zero and a standard deviation of one; sometimes called a z score.

standardized mean difference (SMD) In meta-analysis, the effect size index for comparing two group means, computed by subtracting one mean from the other and dividing by the pooled standard deviation; also called Cohen's d.

statement of purpose A broad declarative statement of the overall goals of a study.

statistic An estimate of a parameter, calculated from sample data.

statistical analysis The organization and analysis of quantitative data using statistical procedures, including both descriptive and inferential statistics.

statistical conclusion validity The degree to which inferences about relationships from a statistical analysis of the data are correct.

statistical control The use of statistical procedures to control confounding influences on the outcome variable.

statistical heterogeneity Diversity of effects across primary studies included in a meta-analysis.

statistical inference An inference about the population based on information from a sample, using laws of probability.

statistical power The ability of a research design and analytic strategy to detect true relationships among variables.

statistical process control (SPC) A statistical method of monitoring a process unfolding over time; used originally to monitor quality in manufacturing processes, but SPC can be used to test hypotheses about changes over time (e.g., as the result of a quality improvement).

statistical significance A term indicating that the results from an analysis of sample data are unlikely to result from chance, at a specified level of probability.

statistical test An analytic tool used to estimate the probability that results from a sample reflect true population values.

stepped wedge design A design involving a delayed treatment strategy within a cluster randomized design (i.e., the clusters receive the intervention at different points in time).

stepwise multiple regression A multiple regression analysis in which predictor variables are entered into the equation in steps, in the order in which the increment to R is greatest.

stimulated recall interview An approach that involves video recording study participants in social situations and then discussing participants' behavior in follow-up interviews.

stipend A monetary payment to individuals participating in a study, as an incentive for participation and/or to compensate for time and expenses.

strata Subdivisions of the population based on a specified characteristic (e.g., gender); singular is *stratum.*

stratification The division of a sample of a population into smaller units (e.g., males and females), typically to enhance representativeness; used in both sampling and in allocation to treatment groups.

stratified random sampling The random selection of study participants from two or more strata of the population independently.

structural equations modeling (SEM) A statistical modeling procedures that involves equations representing the magnitude of hypothesized relations among sets of variables; typically used to test a model or theory in a path analysis using maximum likelihood estimation.

structural validity The extent to which an instrument captures the hypothesized dimensionality of a broad construct; an aspect of construct validity.

structured data collection An approach to collecting data from participants, either through self-report or observation, in which categories of information (e.g., response options) are specified in advance.

study participant An individual who participates and provides information in a study.

study section Within the National Institutes of Health, a group of peer reviewers who evaluate grant applications in the first phase of a dual-review process.

subgroup analysis Analytic efforts to understand whether intervention effects vary for well-defined groups of people (e.g., men versus women); undertaken to disentangle heterogeneity of treatment effects (HTE).

subject An individual who participates and provides data in a study; term used primarily in quantitative research.

subscale A subset of items that measures one aspect or dimension of a multidimensional construct.

summated rating scale A composite scale consisting of multiple items that are added together to yield an overall continuous measure of an attribute (e.g., a Likert scale).

superiority trial A trial in which the researchers hypothesize that the focal intervention is "superior to" (more effective than) the control condition; most clinical trials are superiority trials.

surrogate outcome An outcome used as a substitute or proxy for an actual outcome of interest (e.g., continued smoking as a proxy for eventual lung cancer).

survey research Nonexperimental research that involves gathering information about people's activities, beliefs, preferences, and attitudes via direct questioning.

survival analysis A statistical procedure used when the outcome variable represents a time interval between an initial event (e.g., onset of a disease) and an end event (e.g., death).

symmetric distribution A distribution of values with two halves that are mirror images of the each other.

systematic review A rigorous synthesis of research findings on a research question, using systematic sampling, data collection, and data analysis procedures and a formal protocol.

systematic sampling The selection of sample members such that every *kth* (e.g., every tenth) person or element in a sampling frame is chosen.

table shell A table without any numeric values, prepared in advance of data analysis to guide the analyses to be performed.

tacit knowledge Information about a culture that is so deeply embedded that members do not talk about it or may not even be consciously aware of it.

target population The entire population in which a researcher is interested and to which he or she would like to generalize study results.

taxonomy In an ethnographic analysis, a system of classifying and organizing terms and concepts, developed to illuminate the domain's internal organization and the relationship among the categories of the domain.

test statistic A statistic used to assess the reliability of relationships between variables (e.g., chi-squared, *t*); sampling distributions of test statistics are known for circumstances in which the null hypothesis is true.

test-retest reliability The type of reliability that concerns the extent to which scores for people who have not changed are the same when a measure is administered twice; an assessment of a measure's stability.

testing threat A threat to a study's internal validity that occurs when the administration of a pretest or baseline measure of an outcome variable results in changes on the variable, apart from the effect of the independent variable.

theme A recurring regularity emerging from an analysis of qualitative data.

theoretical notes In field studies, notes detailing the researcher's interpretations of observed behavior and events.

theoretical sampling In qualitative studies, especially in grounded theory studies, the selection of sample members based on emerging findings to ensure adequate saturation of important theoretical categories.

theory An abstract generalization that presents a systematic explanation about relationships among phenomena or that thoroughly describes a phenomenon.

Therapy/intervention question A question focused on the effects of an intervention on patient outcomes.

thick description A rich and thorough description of the research context, study participants, and the phenomenon of interest in a qualitative study narrative.

think aloud method A qualitative method used to collect data about cognitive processes (e.g., decision-making), in which people's reflections on decisions or problem-solving are captured as they are being made; sometimes used in cognitive questioning during a pretest of a new instrument.

threats to validity In research design, reasons that an inference (e.g., about the effect of an independent variable, such as an intervention, on an outcome) could be wrong.

time sampling In structured observations, the sampling of time periods during which observations will take place.

time series design A quasi-experimental design involving the collection of data over an extended time period, with multiple data collection points both before and after an intervention is introduced.

time triangulation The collection of data on the same phenomenon or about the same people at different points in time, to assess congruence and enhance trustworthiness.

topic guide A list of broad question areas to be covered in a semistructured interview or focus group interview.

tracing Procedures used to relocate participants to reduce attrition in a longitudinal study.

transferability The extent to which qualitative findings can be extrapolated to other settings or groups; an aspect of trustworthiness.

translational research Research that focuses on how study findings can best be translated into practice.

treatment An intervention; in experimental research (a clinical trial), the condition being manipulated.

treatment group The group receiving the intervention being tested; the experimental group.

trend study A form of longitudinal study in which different samples from a population are studied over time with respect to some phenomenon (e.g., annual polls on attitudes toward abortion).

triangulation The use of multiple methods to collect and interpret data about a phenomenon, so as to converge on an accurate representation of reality.

true score A hypothetical score that would be obtained if a measure were infallible.

trustworthiness The degree of confidence qualitative researchers have in their data and analyses, assessed using the criteria of credibility, transferability, dependability, confirmability, and authenticity.

***t*-test** A parametric statistical test for analyzing the difference between two group means.

two-tailed tests Statistical tests in which both ends of the sampling distribution are used to establish improbable values.

Type I error An error created by rejecting the null hypothesis when it is true (i.e., the researcher concludes that a relationship exists when in fact it does not—a false positive).

Type II error An error created by accepting the null hypothesis when it is false (i.e., the researcher concludes that *no* relationship exists when in fact it does—a false negative).

umbrella review A systematic review that integrates findings from multiple systematic reviews; also called an *overview of reviews.*

underpowered A characteristic of a study that lacks sufficient statistical power to minimize the risk of a Type II error (i.e., the risk of concluding that a relationship does not exist when, in fact, it does).

unidimensional scale A scale that measures only one construct or a unitary facet of a construct.

unimodal distribution A distribution of values with one peak (high frequency).

unit of analysis The basic unit or focus of a researcher's analysis—typically individual study participants.

univariate statistics Statistical analysis of a single variable for purposes of description (e.g., computing a mean).

unstructured interview An interview in which the researcher asks respondents questions without having a fixed plan regarding the content or flow of information to be gathered.

unstructured observation The collection of descriptive data through direct observation that is not guided by a formal, prespecified plan for observing, enumerating, or recording the information.

urn randomization A method of randomizing participants to groups, in which group balance is monitored and the allocation probability is adjusted when imbalances occur.

validity A quality criterion referring to the degree to which inferences made in a study are unbiased and well-founded; in measurement, the degree to which an instrument measures what it is intended to measure.

variability The degree to which values in a set of scores are dispersed.

variable An attribute that varies, that is, takes on different values (e.g., body temperature, heart rate).

variance A measure of variability or dispersion, equal to the standard deviation squared.

vignette A brief description of an event, person, or situation to which respondents are asked to express their reactions.

visual analog scale (VAS) A scaling procedure used to measure certain clinical symptoms (e.g., pain, fatigue) by having people indicate on a straight line the intensity of the symptom; usually measured on a 100 mm scale with values from 0 to 100.

vulnerable groups Special groups of people whose rights in studies need special protection because of their inability to provide meaningful informed consent or because their circumstances place them at higher-than-average risk of adverse effects (e.g., children, unconscious patients).

wait-list design A design for an intervention study that involves putting control group members on a waiting list for the intervention until follow-up data have been collected; also called a *delay of treatment design.*

Wald statistic A statistic used to evaluate the significance of individual predictors in a logistic regression equation.

web-based survey A questionnaire delivered over the Internet on a dedicated survey website for self-administration.

weighting A procedure used to adjust estimated population values when disproportionate sampling has been used.

Wilcoxon signed ranks test A nonparametric statistical test for comparing two paired groups, based on the relative ranking of values between the pairs.

wild code A coded value that is not legitimate within the coding scheme for that data set.

within-subjects design A research design in which a single group of participants is compared under different conditions or at different points in time (e.g., before and after surgery).

yea-sayers bias A bias in self-report scales created when respondents characteristically agree with statements ("yea-say"), independent of content.

***z* score** A standard score, expressed in terms of standard deviations from the mean; raw scores are transformed such that the mean equals zero and standard deviations are 1.

Index

Quick Guide to an Evidence Hierarchy of Designs for Therapy/Intervention Questions

I	**Level I:** Systematic review/meta-analysis of RCTs
II	**Level II:** Randomized controlled trial (RCT)
III	**Level III:** Nonrandomized trial (quasi-experiment)
IV	**Level IV:** Systematic review of nonexperimental (observational) studies
V	**Level V:** Nonexperimental/observational study
VI	**Level VI:** Systematic review/metasynthesis of qualitative studies
VII	**Level VII:** Qualitative study/descriptive study
VIII	**Level VIII:** Nonresearch source (e.g., internal evidence, expert opinion)

This list contains some commonly used symbols in statistics. The list is in approximate alphabetical order, with English and Greek letters intermixed. Nonletter symbols have been placed at the end.

a	Regression constant, the intercept
α	Greek alpha; significance level in hypothesis testing, probability of Type I error; also, a reliability coefficient
b	Regression coefficient, slope of the line
β	Greek beta, probability of a Type II error; also, a standardized regression coefficient (beta weight)
χ^2	Greek chi squared, a test statistic for several statistical tests
CI	Confidence interval around estimate of a population parameter
d	An effect size index, a standardized mean difference
df	Degrees of freedom
η^2	Greek eta squared, index of variance accounted for in ANOVA context
f	Frequency (count) for a score value
F	Test statistic used in ANOVA, ANCOVA, and other tests
H_0	Null hypothesis
H_A	Alternative hypothesis; research hypothesis
λ	Greek lambda, a test statistic used in several multivariate analyses (Wilks' lambda)
μ	Greek mu, the population mean
M	Sample mean (alternative symbol for $\overline{X}$)
MS	Mean square, variance estimate in ANOVA
n	Number of cases in a subgroup of the sample
N	Total number of cases or sample members
NNT	Number needed to treat
OR	Odds ratio
p	Probability that observed data are consistent with null hypothesis
r	Pearson's product-moment correlation coefficient for a sample
r_s	Spearman's rank-order correlation coefficient
R	Multiple correlation coefficient
R^2	Coefficient of determination, proportion of variance in *dependent variable* attributable to *independent variables*
RR	Relative risk
ρ	Greek rho, population correlation coefficient
SD	Sample standard deviation
SEM	Standard error of the mean
σ	Greek sigma (lowercase), population standard deviation
Σ	Greek sigma (uppercase), sum of
SS	Sum of squares
t	Test statistics used in *t*-tests (sometimes called Student's *t*)
U	Test statistic for the Mann-Whitney *U*-test
$\overline{X}$	Sample mean
x	Deviation score
Y'	Predicted value of Y, dependent variable in regression analysis
z	Standard score in a normal distribution
$\|\|$	Absolute value
$\leq$	Less than or equal to
$\geq$	Greater than or equal to
$\neq$	Not equal to